P9-CCI-464

CANINE *and* FELINE NEPHROLOGY *and* UROLOGY

Carl A. Osborne, DVM, PhD
Diplomate, American College of Veterinary Internal Medicine
Professor
Department of Small Animal Clinical Sciences
College of Veterinary Medicine
University of Minnesota

Delmar R. Finco, DVM, PhD
Diplomate, American College of Veterinary Internal Medicine
Professor
Department of Physiology and Pharmacology
College of Veterinary Medicine
University of Georgia

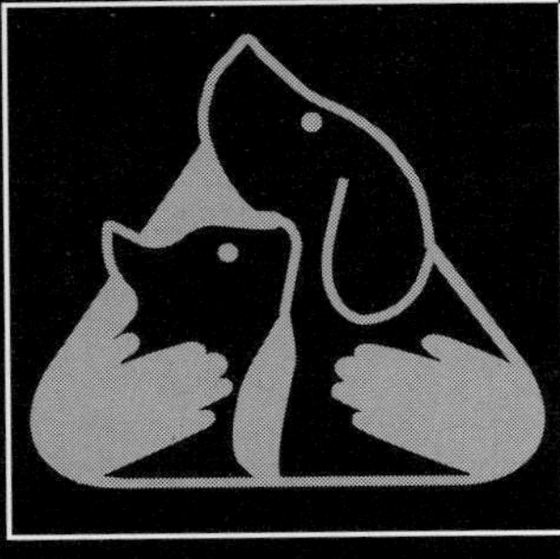

CANINE *and* FELINE NEPHROLOGY *and* UROLOGY

A Lea & Febiger Book

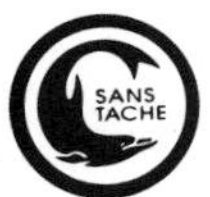

Williams & Wilkins

BALTIMORE • PHILADELPHIA • HONG KONG
LONDON • MUNICH • SYDNEY • TOKYO

A WAVERLY COMPANY
1995

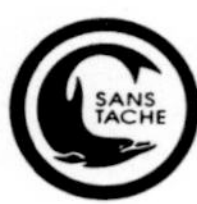

Executive Editor: Carroll C. Cann
Developmental Editor: Susan Hunsberger
Production Coordinator: Marette D. Magargle
Project Editor: Arlene C. Sheir-Allen

Rose Tree Corporate Center
1400 North Providence Road
Building II, Suite 5025
Media, PA 19063-2043 USA

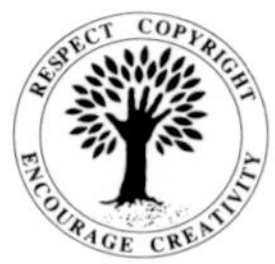

Accurate indications, adverse reactions, and dosage schedules for drugs are provided in this book, but it is possible they may change. The reader is urged to review the package information data of the manufacturers of the medications mentioned.

Printed in the United States of America

Library of Congress Cataloging in Publication Data
Canine and feline nephrology and urology/edited by Carl A. Osborne
and Delmar R. Finco.
p. cm.
"A Lea & Febiger book."
Includes bibliographical references and index.
ISBN 0-683-06666-8
1. Dogs—Diseases. 2. Cats—Diseases. 3. Veterinary nephrology.
4. Veterinary urology. I. Osborne, Carl A. II. Finco, Delmar R.
SF992.K53C35 1995
636.7′08966—dc 20 94-34694
CIP

The Publishers have made every effort to trace the copyright holders for borrowed material. If they have inadvertently overlooked any, they will be pleased to make the necessary arrangements at the first opportunity.

95 96 97 98 99
1 2 3 4 5 6 7 8 9 10

Reprints of chapters may be purchased from Williams & Wilkins in quantities of 100 or more. Call Isabella Wise, Special Sales Department, (800) 358-3583.

ISBN 0-683-06666-8

Dedication

We dedicate this book to our mentor and colleague, Donald G. Low. Our professional pursuits were initiated and nurtured by his competency, vision, and enthusiasm. In our eyes, he is a giant among contributors to the veterinary profession. It is with pleasure that we dedicate this book to Don.

Thank You, DGL . . .

for your patience, perseverance, and encouragement—so needed and appreciated during our years of training, as we struggled to master the concepts and assimilate the information that we found so essential during our subsequent professional endeavors.

Thank You, DGL . . .

for teaching us to question, and for training us to let facts form conclusions, rather than to draw conclusions and scurry for facts to justify them.

Thank You, DGL . . .

for showing us that as teachers, our obligation is not just to share and apply new knowledge: we also must create it.

Thank You, DGL . . .

for showing us that although "art is I, science is we."

And Most of all, Thank You, DGL . . .

for being our special friend.

Carl A. Osborne

Delmar R. Finco

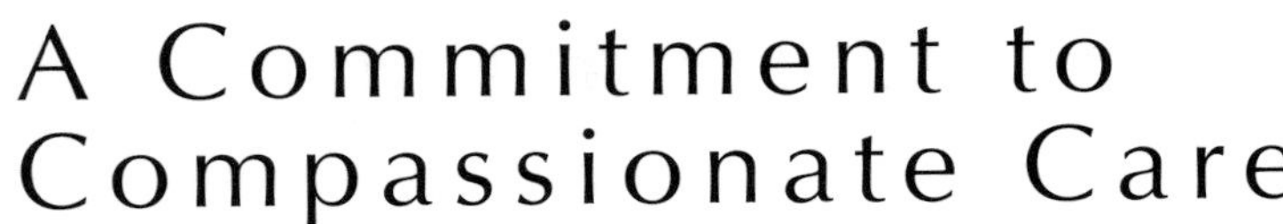

A Commitment to Compassionate Care

The logo on our cover and at the beginning of each chapter symbolizes our commitment to providing compassionate care to our patients. The design is similar to that used by the World Small Animal Veterinary Association.

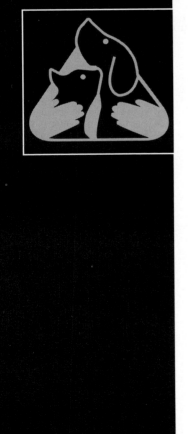

What is compassion? Compassion is derived from the Latin words *passio* and *cum*, which literally mean *to suffer with*. Thus, compassion encompasses feeling or emotion. By definition, to be compassionate, two complementary feelings must be combined. First, a person must have empathetic awareness of the suffering, distress, or troubles of another. Second, the person must have an empathetic desire to help correct the problems. Thus, compassion is not a form of pity that is satisfied by mere expression of sorrow. The feeling of sorrow does not transcend to a feeling of compassion until there is a strong desire to correct the cause, distress, or suffering of another. Meaning well is not enough. Compassion moves us to come to the aid of those needing help.

How might we, as participants in the profession of veterinary medicine, express our compassion? First, by striving to attain and maintain our professional competence, which is a major goal of this textbook. This is, in reality, an extension of the Golden Rule, which states: "Do unto others, as we would have them do unto us." Stated another way, we should strive to provide the quality of care that we would desire if we were the patients, rather than the doctors. We should always remember that there are some patients we cannot help, but there are none we cannot harm. No patient should be worse for having seen the doctor. We believe it necessary to avoid the pitfall of substituting stellar "bedside manner" for competency. Thoughtful, compassionate veterinarians recognize that dazzling the owner while mismanaging the case represents a total lack of compassion. Imposing questionable treatment, particularly technical skills ("a chance to cut is a chance to cure"), for ego gratification represents the antithesis of compassion.

But mastering the knowledge and technical skills of the science of veterinary medicine is not enough to make us compassionate. We must develop other qualities if we desire to be compassionate. Most of our clients won't care how much we know, until they know how much we care. To some, caring about the patient is more important than caring for the patient.

What are some of the qualities that will help us to become compassionate? One is the quality of generosity. The root in generosity is *gen*, meaning to create or produce. We must be generous, even when our efforts do not bring us remuneration or prestige. Our generosity should not be motivated by a sense of duty or obligation, or a desire to acquire prominence. Rather, it should come from our hearts. Likewise, giving is infinitely divisible. The person who has a little can always give a little. Hippocrates put it this way: "Sometimes give your services for nothing . . . and if there be an opportunity of serving one who is a stranger in financial straits, give full assistance to such."

Besides generosity, we must also be able to develop the quality of encouraging others, especially our clients, during difficult times. The root word in the term encourage is the Latin term *cor*, meaning heart. Therefore, to encourage means to give from the heart.

Another quality that we should develop is kindness. Kindness encompasses the desire to take interest in others, and to demonstrate our interest by helpful acts and considerate words. It is the attribute of kindness that attaches itself to a mission until its purpose in connection with that mission is realized. Kindness should not be motivated by self gain or profit.

Yet another important quality that will help us to become compassionate is humility. As a result of being humble, we will never feel that we are above or superior to those needing help. Despite our D.V.M., V.M.D., A.H.T., and Ph.D. degrees, we are all servants to all living beings. Our mission is to serve, not to be served. As we talk with others, we need to remember that our words, as our medical treatments, should first do no harm.

Ultimately, compassion can be measured only by the action it prompts.

Carl A. Osborne
Delmar R. Finco

Preface

"During our professional lifetimes, let us strive to practice 40 to 50 years of veterinary medicine, and not 1 year 40 to 50 times."

Donald G. Low

The purpose of *Canine and Feline Nephrology and Urology* is to bring together contemporary information about the causes, pathophysiology, diagnosis, prognosis, treatment, and prevention of diseases of the urinary system of companion animals. With the expertise of 41 contributing authors, this book has been prepared for students, interns, residents, veterinary technicians, and practitioners of veterinary medicine who have not specialized in urology and nephrology, but whose clinical practice (generalist or specialist) requires familiarity with available diagnostic and therapeutic techniques. The primary objective of the book is to provide information about urinary diseases in a simplified, systematic, and readily accessible outline form. To this end, the book has been divided into six major divisions:

I. Applied Anatomy and Physiology

II. Clinical Evaluation of the Urinary System

III. Diseases of the Kidney

IV. Diseases of the Ureters

V. Diseases of the Lower Urinary Tract

VI. Diseases of the Upper and Lower Urinary Tract

Throughout the book logic and common sense have been emphasized. Where possible, basic principles of physiology and pathology have been correlated with clinical manifestations, treatment, and prevention of disease in order to emphasize their interrelationships. It is our conviction that adequate patient care is best provided by individuals with knowledge of the pathophysiology of various disease processes, and the ability to apply this knowledge in a clinical setting. Putting knowledge into practice emphasizes the importance of practicality. But our commitment to practicality should not be misdirected. Practicality may be a virtue, provided that it is not used as an excuse for ignorance.

A 19th-century philosopher, Theodor Billroth, penned this thought: "It is a most gratifying sign of the rapid progress of our time that the best textbooks become antiquated so quickly." It is our hope that the information contained in this issue will become rapidly antiquated as a result of continued basic and applied research. This is the essence of Donald Low's admonition to us to practice 40 to 50 years of veterinary medicine during our professional lifetimes, rather than 1 year 40 or 50 times.

Time and experience have polished the thought that *a fact merely marks the point where we have agreed to let investigation cease.* It is undoubtedly a fact that, based on their investigations, not all of our colleagues will agree with the observations and interpretations advanced herein. To this end, we apologize for our shortcomings, and invite those who would help us to bring errors and different viewpoints to our attention. One way to advance truth is by vigorous and open interaction of opposing opinions.

Carl A. Osborne
Delmar R. Finco

Acknowledgments

We extend our appreciation to our co-authors who have so generously and capably contributed their knowledge and wisdom to this textbook. They were an essential catalyst in the completion of this work. Heartfelt thanks to Marcia Johnson and Lori Schultz for typing major portions of the text, and to Michelle Mero Riedel for help with illustrations.

Special thanks to Carroll C. Cann, Executive Editor, for his advice, encouragement, and patience for the past 20 years. He had confidence that this book would be completed when others said it would never happen. Carroll—you're special!

A wise philosopher once penned, "There is no limit to what a person can do if (s)he doesn't care who gets the credit." This thought reflects the qualities of other members of the Williams and Wilkins team who also were involved in the completion of this book. Thanks to Susan L. Hunsberger, Development Editor, for her positive "We can fix that—no problem" responses to our requests for help. Thanks to Arlene C. Sheir-Allen for her meticulous devotion to important details, and for her never-ending efforts to see situations from our viewpoint. We also thank Marette D. Magargle, Production Coordinator; Samuel Rondinelli, Director of Production; Michael DeNardo, Operations Manager; Susan Rockwell, Manuscript Editing Manager; Stephanie Carbo and Joanne Husovski, Editorial Assistants; and Karen Cuzzolino and Suzanne Boyd Enright, Freelance Editors, for their contributions to this work.

Carl A. Osborne
Delmar R. Finco

Contributors

Suzanne Barker, AHT
Nursing Supervisor, Critical Care Unit
Veterinary Teaching Hospital
Colorado State University
Fort Collins, CO

Jeanne A. Barsanti, DVM
Professor
Department of Small Animal Medicine
College of Veterinary Medicine
Internist, Veterinary Teaching Hospital
The University of Georgia
Athens, GA

Joseph W. Bartges, DVM, PhD
Assistant Professor
Department of Small Animal Medicine
College of Veterinary Medicine
University of Georgia
Athens, GA

Kathleen A. Bird, CVT
Senior Veterinary Technician
Department of Small Animal Clinical Sciences
College of Veterinary Medicine
University of Minnesota
St. Paul, MN

Cathy A. Brown, VMD, PhD
Diagnostic Pathologist
University of Georgia Diagnostic Laboratory
Athens, GA

Scott A. Brown, VMD, PhD
Associate Professor
Department of Physiology & Pharmacology
College of Veterinary Medicine
The University of Georgia
Athens, GA

Dennis D. Caywood, DVM, MS
Professor
Department of Small Animal Clinical Sciences
College of Veterinary Medicine
University of Minnesota
St. Paul, MN

Larry D. Cowgill, DVM, PhD
Professor
Department of Medicine and Epidemiology
School of Veterinary Medicine
University of California-Davis
Davis, CA

Wayne A. Crowell, DVM, PhD
Professor
Department of Pathology
College of Veterinary Medicine
The University of Georgia
Athens, GA

Stephen P. DiBartola, DVM
Professor of Medicine
Department of Veterinary Clinical Sciences
College of Veterinary Medicine
Ohio State University
Columbus, OH

Daniel A. Feeney, DVM, MS
Professor
Department of Small Animal Clinical Sciences
College of Veterinary Medicine
University of Minnesota
St. Paul, MN

Lawrence J. Felice, PhD
Associate Professor
Department of Diagnostic Investigation
College of Veterinary Medicine
University of Minnesota
St. Paul, MN

Delmar R. Finco, DVM, PhD
Professor
Department of Physiology and Pharmacology
College of Veterinary Medicine
The University of Georgia
Athens, GA

Thomas F. Fletcher, DVM, PhD
Professor of Anatomy
Department of Veterinary PathoBiology
University of Minnesota
St. Paul, MN

S. Dru Forrester, DVM, MS
Assistant Professor
Department of Small Animal Clinical Sciences
Virginia-Maryland Regional College of Veterinary Medicine
Virginia Polytechnic Institute and State University
Blacksburg, VA

Gregory F. Grauer, DVM, MS
Associate Professor
Department of Clinical Sciences
Staff Internist
Veterinary Teaching Hospital
College of Veterinary Medicine and Biomedical Sciences
Colorado State University
Fort Collins, CO

Clare R. Gregory, DVM
Associate Professor
Department of Surgical and Radiological Sciences
Chief, Small Animal Surgical Services
Veterinary Medical Teaching Hospital
School of Veterinary Medicine
University of California
Davis, CA

Gary R. Johnston, DVM, MS
Professor
Department of Small Animal Clinical Sciences
College of Veterinary Medicine
University of Minnesota
St. Paul, MN

Jeffrey S. Klausner, DVM, MS
Professor and Chairman
Department of Small Animal Clinical Sciences
College of Veterinary Medicine
University of Minnesota
St. Paul, MN

Lori A. Koehler, CVT
Senior Veterinary Technician
Department of Small Animal Clinical Sciences
College of Veterinary Medicine
University of Minnesota
St. Paul, MN

Donald R. Krawiec, DVM, MS, PhD
Associated Professor of Medicine
Department of Veterinary Clinical Medicine
College of Veterinary Medicine
University of Illinois
Urbana, IL

John M. Kruger, DVM, PhD
Associate Professor, Small Animal Clinical Sciences
College of Veterinary Medicine
Michigan State University
East Lansing, MI

India F. Lane, DVM, MS
Assistant Professor and Internist
Atlantic Veterinary College
University of Prince Edward Island
Charlottetown, Prince Edward Island, Canada

George E. Lees, DVM, MS
Professor
Department of Small Animal Medicine and Surgery
College of Veterinary Medicine
Texas A&M University
College Station, TX

Donald G. Low, DVM, PhD
Professor Emeritus, Department of Medicine
School of Veterinary Medicine
University of California, Davis
Davis, CA

Jody P. Lulich, DVM, PhD
Assistant Professor
Department of Small Animal Clinical Sciences
College of Veterinary Medicine
University of Minnesota
St. Paul, MN

Mary B. Mahaffey, DVM, MS
Associate Professor
Department of Anatomy and Radiology
College of Veterinary Medicine
University of Florida
Gainesville, FL

Lisa Neuwirth, DVM, MS
Assistant Professor of Radiology
Department of Small Animal Clinical Sciences
College of Veterinary Medicine
University of Florida
Gainesville, FL

Carl A. Osborne, DVM, PhD
Professor
Department of Small Animal Clinical Sciences
College of Veterinary Medicine
University of Minnesota
St. Paul, MN

David J. Polzin, DVM, PhD
Professor
Department of Small Animal Clinical Sciences
College of Veterinary Medicine
University of Minnesota
St. Paul, MN

J. E. Riviere, DVM, PhD
Burroughs Wellcome Distinguished Professor of Veterinary Pharmacology
Department of Anatomy, Physiological Sciences & Radiology
College of Veterinary Medicine
North Carolina State University
Raleigh, NC

Linda A. Ross, DVM, MS
Associate Dean for Clinical Programs and Hospital Director
Tufts University School of Veterinary Medicine
North Grafton, MA

David F. Senior, BVSc
Professor and Head
Department of Veterinary Clinical Sciences
College of Veterinary Medicine
Louisiana State University
Baton Rouge, LA

Jerry B. Stevens, DVM, PhD
Professor
College of Veterinary Medicine
North Carolina State University
Raleigh, NC

Laura L. Swanson, CVT
Senior Veterinary Technician
Department of Small Animal Clinical Sciences
College of Veterinary Medicine
University of Minnesota
St. Paul, MN

Rosama Thumchai, DVM
Research Assistant
Department of Small Animal Clinical Sciences
College of Veterinary Medicine
University of Minnesota
St. Paul, MN

Lisa K. Ulrich, CVT
Principle Veterinary Technician
Department of Small Animal Clinical Sciences
College of Veterinary Medicine
University of Minnesota
St. Paul, MN

Shelly L. Vaden, DVM, PhD
Assistant Professor of Internal Medicine
Department of Companion Animals and Special Species Medicine
College of Veterinary Medicine
North Carolina State University
Raleigh, NC

Deborah R. Van Pelt, MS, DVM
Assistant Professor, Critical Care & Emergency Medicine
Department of Clinical Sciences
College of Veterinary Medicine & Biomedical Sciences
Colorado State University
Fort Collins, CO

Patricia A. Walter, DVM, MS
Associate Professor
Department of Small Animal Clinical Sciences
College of Veterinary Medicine
University of Minnesota
St. Paul, MN

Wayne E. Wingfield, MS, DVM
Professor and Chief, Emergency and Critical Care Medicine
Veterinary Teaching Hospital
College of Veterinary Medicine
Colorado State University
Fort Collins, CO

Contents

PART IV
DISEASES OF THE URETERS

PART V
DISEASES OF THE LOWER URINARY TRACT

PART I

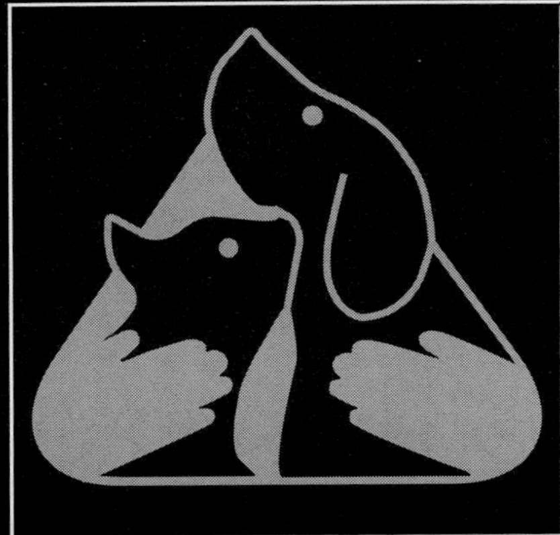

APPLIED ANATOMY AND PHYSIOLOGY

CHAPTER 1

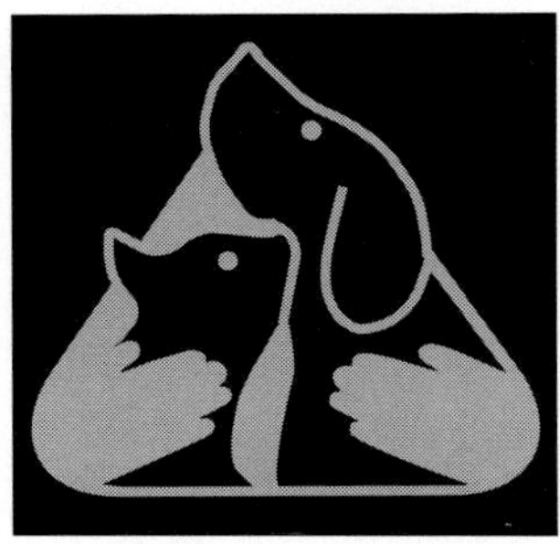

Applied Anatomy of the Urinary System with Clinicopathologic Correlation

CARL A. OSBORNE AND THOMAS F. FLETCHER

I. KIDNEYS

A. Appearance, size, and weight.

1. In dogs and cats, both kidneys are approximately equal in size and shape, and have a smooth surface contour. The surface of cat kidneys is grooved to accommodate prominent subcapsular vessels, which radiate toward the hilus to join the renal vein. The kidneys of dogs are bean shaped (or are beans kidney shaped?), whereas those of cats tend to be more spherical. In both species, a hilus is located on the concave surface through which pass vessels (artery, vein, and lymphatics), nerves, and the renal pelvis. Of these structures, the renal artery is most dorsal and the renal vein is most ventral.
2. Experimental and clinical studies have revealed that kidney length is the best radiographic parameter of kidney size.
   a. Results of studies utilizing ventrodorsal radiographic views indicate that 95% of normal dogs had a kidney length that ranged from 2.5 to 3.5 times the length of the 2nd lumbar vertebra.[30] For optimum evaluation of canine kidney length, radiographs should be obtained 5 minutes after injection of sodium iothalamate given at a dose of 400 mg of iodine per pound of body weight.[25,26]
   b. It has been reported that normal cat kidneys should range in size from 2.4 to 3.0 times the length of the 2nd lumbar vertebra.[35,50,53] Other investigators indicate that normal feline kidney length is equivalent to 1.5 to 2.0 vertebral bodies, including intervertebral disks.[56] Values outside these ranges suggest abnormal kidney size. Values within these ranges do not exclude the possibility of renal disease, however.
   c. Kidneys from male dogs have been reported to be proportionately larger than those from female dogs.[53]
   d. Kidneys from immature dogs have been reported to be proportionately larger than those from mature dogs.[53]
   e. Very young kittens and large male cats may have relatively large kidneys compared with those from other normal cats.[39]
3. Evaluation of the width of normal dog kidneys utilizing ventrodorsal radiographic views revealed that they were twice the length of the 2nd lumbar vertebral body (standard deviation = 0.2 times the width of L-2).[25] Measurements were made between a line tangent to the medial aspect of the cranial and caudal kidney poles and the furthermost point of the lateral aspect of the kidney. Evaluation of the width of normal feline kidneys on lateral radiographic views revealed that they were approximately 1.5 to 2.0 times the length of L-2.[53]
4. Varying degrees of prerenal fat surround the kidneys. Large quantities of prerenal fat enhance visualization of the kidneys by survey radiography.

5. The kidneys are surrounded by a relatively thick inelastic capsule, which is loosely attached to the underlying cortex.
   a. Numerous capillaries and lymphatics extend from the capsule into the renal parenchyma.
   b. The firmness of the renal capsule can often be detected when introducing a biopsy needle into the renal parenchyma.
   c. The renal capsule is often incriminated as one factor in the pathogenesis of obstructive uropathy and its sequela because its inelastic nature contributes to abnormal intrarenal pressure.
   d. In diseases characterized by generalized necrosis and repair by substitution with collagenous connective tissue, the renal capsule often becomes adherent to the underlying parenchyma.
6. Weight
   a. Normal right and left kidneys of the same individual are similar in weight.

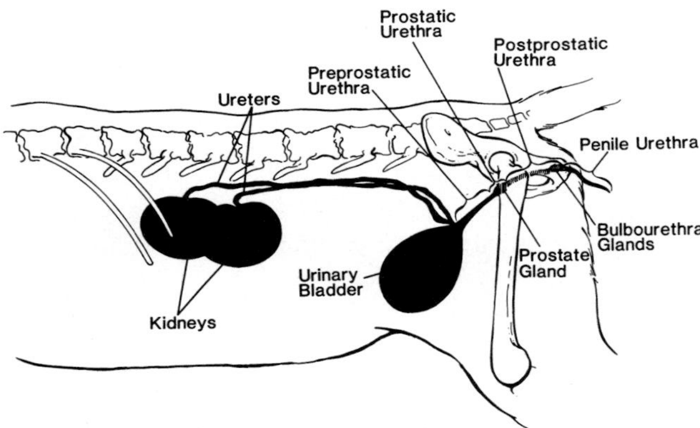

FIG. 1–1. Line drawing of a contrast radiograph illustrates the anatomic structures of the urinary system of a male cat.

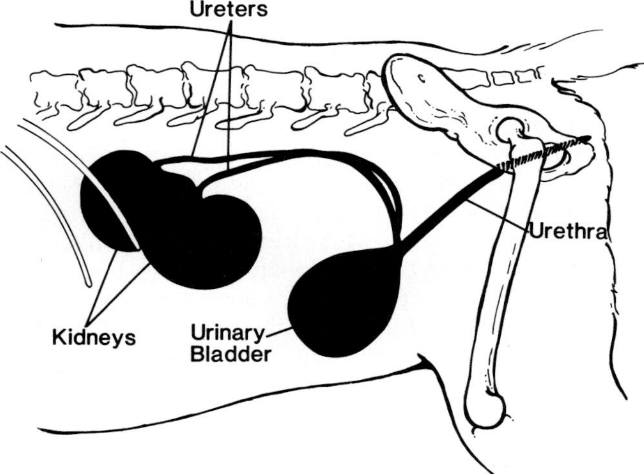

FIG. 1–2. Line drawing of a radiograph illustrates the anatomic structures of the urinary system of a female cat.

   b. In adult cats, kidney weight varies from 0.6 to 1.0% of body weight, with larger males having slightly heavier kidneys.[39]
   c. In adult dogs, kidney weight is approximately 0.5 to 1.0% of body weight.[1,45]
7. Other factors may also affect kidney size and weight.
   a. Factors leading to physiologic compensatory hypertrophy may increase renal size and weight.
   b. Renal hypertrophy may occur in dogs, especially when immature, if they consume diets containing large quantities of protein.
   c. Ammonium chloride causes renal hypertrophy in rats; the effect of ammonium chloride on the size and weight of canine and feline kidneys is as yet unknown.

B. Position.

1. In dogs and cats, the kidneys are completely enveloped by peritoneum and are loosely attached to the body wall. Therefore, they may move a short distance during respiration, or be slightly displaced by viscera or different body positions.[37]
   a. The right kidney of dogs is usually located between the 13th thoracic and 2nd lumbar vertebrae; the left kidney is usually located about one half of a kidney length caudal to the right kidney. The cranial pole of the right kidney lies in a deep fossa of the caudate lobe of the liver; for this reason, it is often difficult to visualize on survey radiographs. On ventrodorsal radiographs, the kidneys of normal dogs have been reported to be one-third the distance from the vertebrae to the outside body wall.[50]
   b. The right kidney of cats is usually cranial to the left kidney, although their position (approximately from L-2 to L-5) is variable because of loose attachment to the body wall (Figs. 1–1 and 1–2).
2. In dogs with generalized renal disease involving both kidneys, the right kidney is usually chosen for the "keyhole" technique of biopsy because its anatomic position is more constant than that of the left kidney.[71] This occurs because the right kidney is more firmly attached to the body wall than is the left.
3. Because the left kidney is more loosely attached to the body wall, it can often be evaluated by abdominal palpation.
4. In cats, both kidneys can readily be palpated per abdomen. The blind percutaneous technique may be used to obtain biopsy specimens from either the right or the left kidney because both kidneys can usually be localized and immobilized by digital palpation through the abdominal wall.[71]

C. Structural organization.

1. Overview.
   a. It is helpful to consider the kidneys in terms of glomerular, tubular, interstitial, or vascular

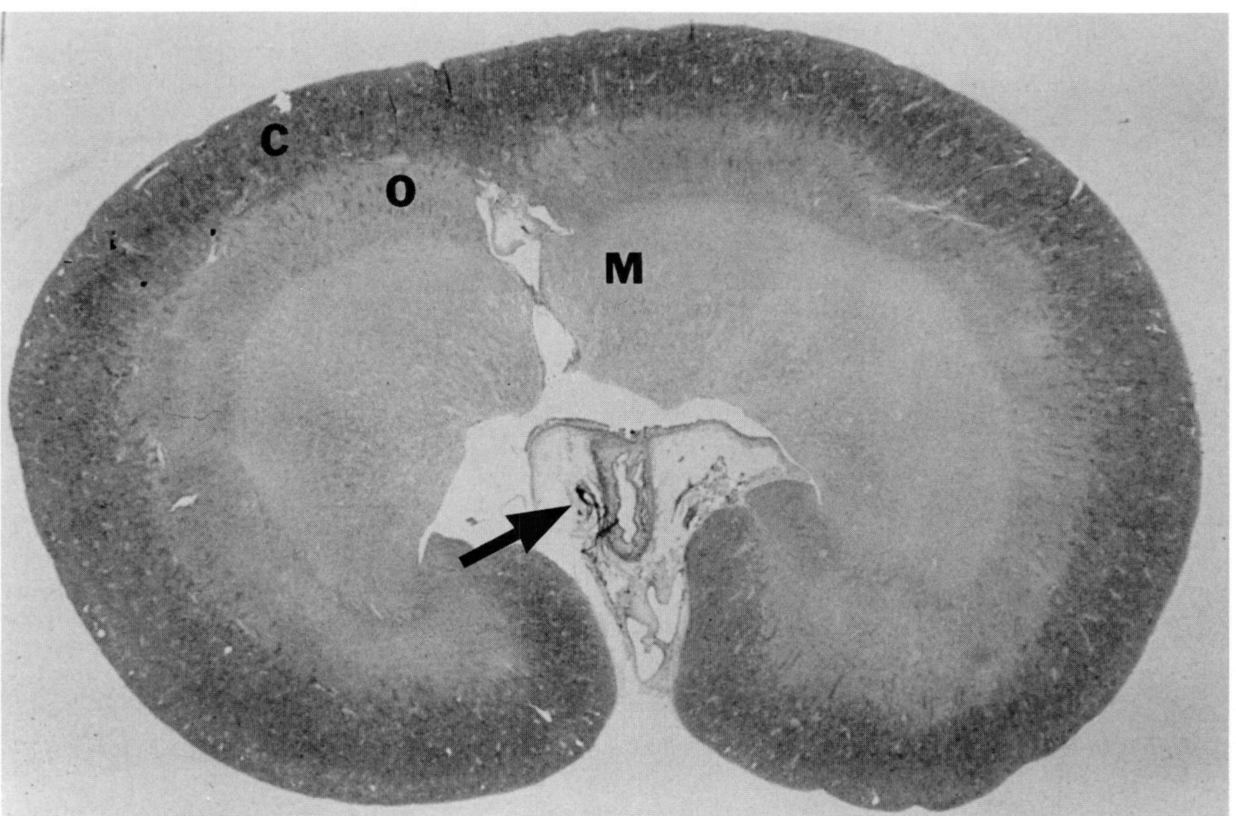

FIG. 1–3. Sagittal 1.5-mm section of kidney obtained from a normal adult mixed-breed dog illustrates renal cortex (C), outer medullar (O), inner medulla (M), and renal pelvis (arrow). Periodic acid–Schiff stain. (Courtesy of Dr. James W. Wilson.)

components when evaluating structure and function.

b. The cut surface of the bisected kidney may be grossly separated into a superficial dark-colored cortex, which completely surrounds an inner light-colored medulla. The medulla can be further divided into outer and inner zones (Fig. 1–3).
   (1). With the exception of a few ectopic pelvic glomeruli,[34] all glomeruli are located within the renal cortex. This anatomic fact is of considerable significance in proper procurement of renal biopsy samples. Unlike some species, dogs have no glomeruli in cortical tissue immediately adjacent to the renal capsule (Figs. 1–4 and 1–5).[11,79]
   (2). Both cortex and medulla contain renal tubules, vessels, and interstitial tissue.
   (3). The outer zone of the renal medulla contains portions of proximal tubules, distal tubules, loops of Henle, and collecting ducts; the inner zone of the medulla contains portions of loops of Henle and collecting ducts (see Fig. 1–3).
   (4). Kidneys of both dogs and cats are unipyramidal. Unlike in humans, cows, and some other species, the renal pelves of dogs and cats do not contain calyces.

2. The nephron.
   a. Numbers
      (1). Different species of animals have different numbers of nephrons (as estimated by number of glomeruli).
         (a). There are approximately 30,000 glomeruli per kidney in the rat, 190,000 per kidney in the cat, 400,000 in the dog, 1,000,000 in man, and 7,000,000 in elephants.[29,51,58,75,78]
         (b). In dogs, there is a correlation between glomerular diameter (an estimate of nephron size?) and body weight or surface area. There was no correlation between glomerular numbers and body weight or surface area.[29] Therefore, in dogs, anatomic and physiologic studies should be evaluated in context to body size.
      (2). The normal canine renal cortex contains sufficient glomeruli to expect an average of 25 glomeruli per punch biopsy sample

obtained with a Franklin-Silverman biopsy needle.[70]

b. Definitions
   (1). The anatomic and functional unit of the kidney is called the nephron.
   (2). Classically, nephrons have been divided into several components on the basis of certain histologic and functional characteristics. These segments are:
      (a). Renal (or malpighian) corpuscle, comprised of a tuft of highly branched capillaries (glomerulus) surrounded by a capsule (Bowman's capsule).
      (b). Proximal tubule.
      (c). Loop of Henle.
      (d). Distal convoluted tubule.
   (3). Each nephron in turn drains into a collecting duct. Collecting ducts drain multiple nephrons.
   (4). The space between the glomerulus and Bowman's capsule that collects glomerular filtrate is called the urinary space (or Bowman's space).

c. Heterogenicity of nephrons
   (1). Although all nephrons are similar in structure and function, they are not identical.[27,71]
      (a). In most mammals, nephrons with glomeruli located in outer portions of the renal cortex have relatively short loops of Henle, whereas nephrons with glomeruli located adjacent to the renal medulla (so-called juxtamedullary glomeruli) have relatively long loops of Henle that extend deep into the renal medulla.
      (b). Other differences between nephrons include those related to glomerular size, efferent arteriolar perfusion pattern, and intracellular enzyme composition, distribution, and quantity.[27]
      (c). Corticomedullary glomeruli are the most mature; subcapsular glomeruli are the least mature.
   (2). Knowledge of heterogenicity of nephrons within each kidney is of importance in evaluation of normal and abnormal structure and function.[66]

d. Glomeruli
   (1). Glomeruli produce large quantities of an ultrafiltrate of plasma, only a small portion of which ultimately is voided from the body as urine.
   (2). Glomeruli contain capillary endothelial cells, visceral epithelial cells, mesangial cells and mesangial matrix, and capillary basement membranes (Figs. 1–6 and 1–7).[67]
   (3). Glomerular capillary endothelial cells are similar to endothelial cells lining capillaries in other parts of the body, except that their cytoplasm contains numerous large pores (or fenestrae) (see Figs. 1–6 and 1–9 through 1–11). The functional significance of these pores is as yet unknown. They are too large to inhibit filtration of macromolecules with a molecular weight (MW) similar to that of plasma albumin (MW = 68,000 daltons). Although endothelial cells once were considered an insignificant barrier to all macromolecules at one time, the negative charge imparted by sialoproteins coating

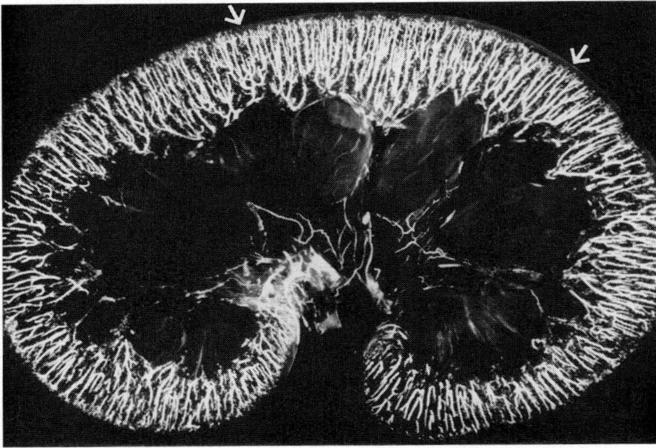

FIG. 1–4. Microangiogram of a 2-mm slice of kidney from a normal adult mixed-breed dog illustrates a thin aglomerular region immediately beneath the renal capsule (arrows). (Courtesy of Dr. James W. Wilson.)

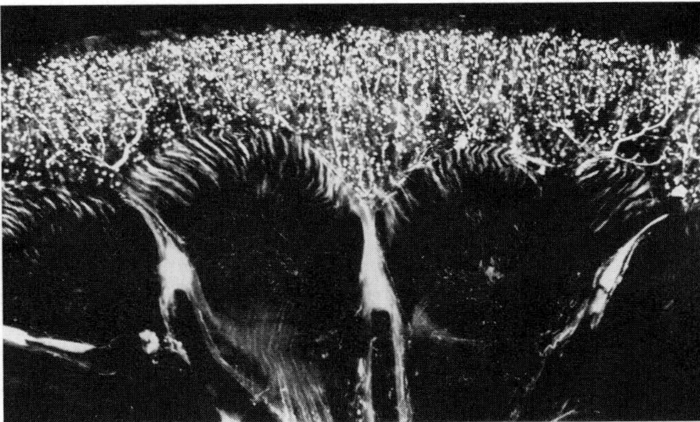

FIG. 1–5. Microangiogram of a 1.5-mm slice of kidney obtained from a normal adult mixed-breed dog illustrates afferent arterioles, glomeruli, and some peritubular vessels. There are no glomeruli immediately adjacent to the renal capsule. (Courtesy of Dr. James W. Wilson.)

endothelial cells has been shown to play a vital role in repelling the passage of negatively charged macromolecules including albumin.[7] Thus plasma proteins of a size that would readily pass through electrically neutral glomerular capillary endothelium are restricted from passage if they are negatively charged.

(4). The glomerular basement membrane (GBM) is located between endothelial cells and visceral epithelial cells in peripheral portions of capillaries, and between mesangial cells and visceral epithelial cells in other portions of the glomerular tuft (Figs. 1–6, 1–8, 1–9, and 1–11). The GBM does not surround the entire capillary lumen, as is the case with other capillaries in the body, but covers the glomerular tuft in a fashion somewhat analogous to the serosa of the abdominal cavity. It is not located between endothelial cells and mesangial cells. When viewed with the aid of an electron microscope, the GBM is characterized by three separate layers (lamina rara interna, lamina densa, and lamina rara externa). Like endothelial cells and visceral epithelial cells, the GBM contains fixed negatively charged sites that may influence the filtration of electrically charged macromolecules.[13] The GBM also appears to serve as a primary filtration barrier to noncharged, large, high-molecular-weight macromolecules present in plasma. It apparently does not prevent filtration of smaller noncharged molecules, however. Special structures (called slit-pore membranes) associated with the cytoplasm of visceral epithelial cells are thought to act as the filtration barrier for smaller substances.

(5). Glomerular capillaries are covered with visceral epithelial cells (commonly called podocytes) characterized by an elaborate layer of primary, secondary, and tertiary cytoplasmic processes (commonly called foot processes) that extend to the GBM (Figs. 1–6 and 1–8 through 1–12). Immediately adjacent foot processes originate from different visceral epithelial cells. The spaces between the epithelial foot processes are called filtration slits or slit pores (see Fig. 1–11). Ultrastructural studies have revealed the presence of thin mem-

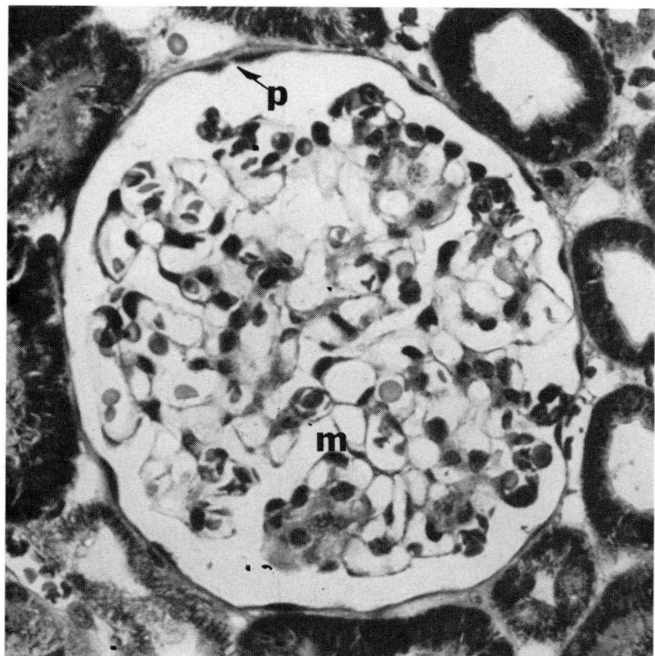

FIG. 1–7. Photomicrograph of a normal glomerulus obtained from an adult dog. Bowman's capsule is lined by flattened parietal epithelial cells (p). Visceral epithelial cells are adjacent to the glomerular basement membrane, which is of uniform thickness. Mesangial cells (m) are surrounded by glomerular capillary lumens. (PAS stain; 2-μm section; original magnification, 100×.)

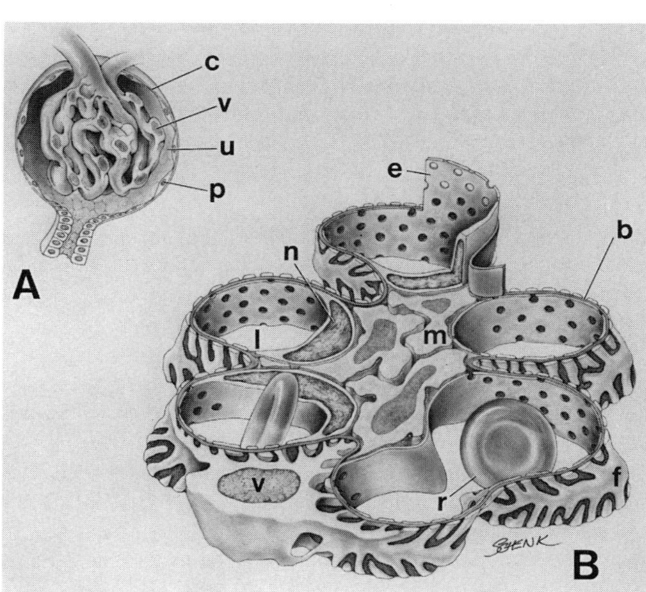

FIG. 1–6. A, Renal corpuscle with glomerular tuft, urinary space, and Bowman's capsule. c = Bowman's capsule; u = urinary space; p = parietal epithelial cell; v = nucleus of visceral epithelial cells. **B,** Cross section of a portion of a glomerulus. f = foot processes of visceral epithelial cell; b = basement membrane; n = nucleus of capillary endothelial cell; e = cytoplasm of capillary endothelial cell containing large pores; m = mesangial cells separated by space normally containing mesangial matrix; l = capillary lumen; r = red blood cell; v = nucleus of visceral epithelial cell.

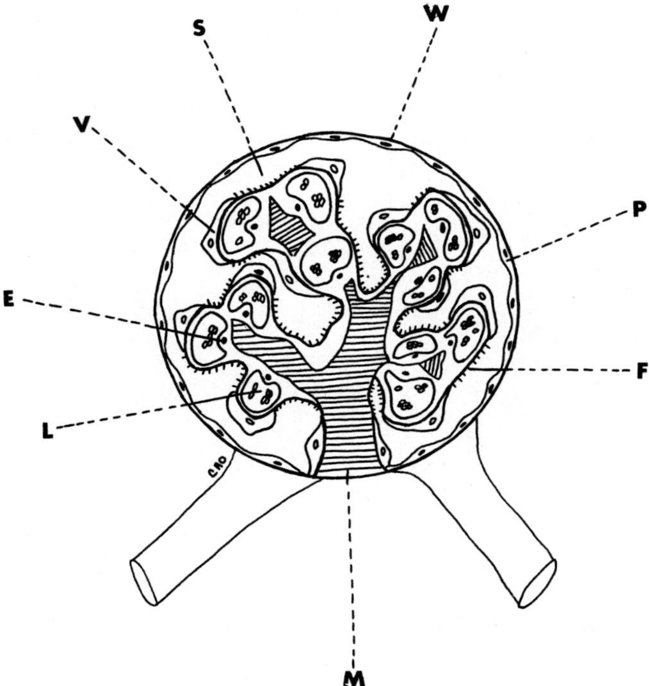

FIG. 1–8. Schematic drawing of a normal glomerulus. M = area occupied by mesangial cells and mesangial matrix; F = foot processes of visceral epithelial cells; P = parietal epithelium; W = Bowman's capsule; S = Bowman's space; V = visceral epithelial cells; E = endothelial cells; L = capillary lumen.

branes (slit-pore membranes) that close the spaces between the foot processes. Filtration presumably occurs at these sites. Visceral epithelium is also covered with negatively charged sialoprotein, which tends to inhibit passage of negatively charged macromolecules. The negative surface charge of visceral epithelial cell cytoplasm also plays an important role in maintaining the characteristic architecture of its cytoplasmic processes. In contrast, the negative charge of the glomerular capillary walls appears to enhance filtration of positively charged molecules. Visceral epithelium is thought to produce one or more components of the GBM.[67]

(6). Mesangial cells typically have an irregular shape caused by elongated cytoplasmic processes (see Figs. 1–6 through 1–9, 1–11). They occupy a space between capillaries and are separated from capillary lumina by endothelial cytoplasm and mesangial matrix rather than by GBM. Mesangial cell nuclei are larger and more dense than adjacent endothelial cell nuclei, thus aiding in their identification by light microscopy. Mesangial cells are separated from visceral epithelial cells by GBM (see Figs. 1–6, 1–8, 1–9, and 1–11). Mesangial cells are able to phagocytose material in a fashion similar to that of reticuloendothelial cells. The cells extend cytoplasmic processes between capillary endothelial cells and the GBM, where they remove filtration residues that might otherwise interfere with filtration or damage the GBM (see Figs. 1–6, 1–9, and 1–11). Mesangial cells also help to anchor (or support) the GBM, which does not completely surround glomerular capillary lumina. Mesangial cells are separated from each other by a variable quantity of dense basement membrane-like material called mesangial matrix. Some investigators have suggested that mesangial matrix is formed in part from deposition of "old" GBM following turnover and renewal of the GBM. Demonstration of contractile elements in the mesangium and of a contractile response of glomerular cells to several agents, including angiotensin II, has led to the hypothesis that the mesangium may also play a role in modulation of glomerular filtration by altering capillary surface area.[6] Changes in mesangial cells (hypercellularity) and mesangial matrix (increased accumulation) reflect much of the injury to glomeruli associated with inflammation, and these areas appear to

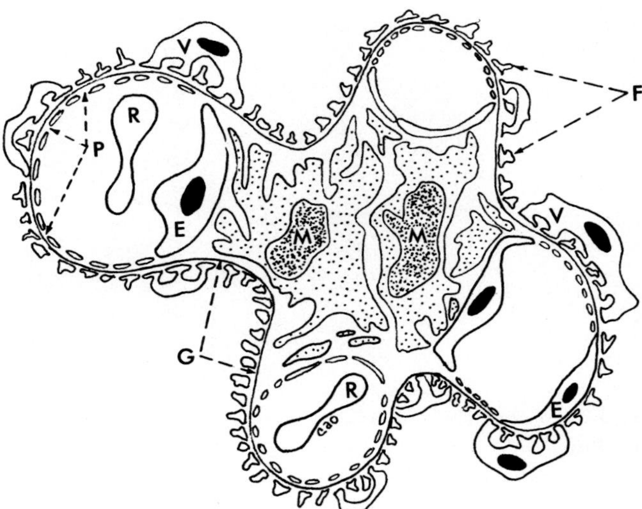

FIG. 1–9. Schematic illustration of the ultrastructure of a normal glomerulus. E = capillary endothelial cells; F = visceral epithelial cell foot processes; G = glomerular basement membrane; M = mesangial cell nuclei; P = pores (fenestrae) in capillary endothelial cells; R = red blood cells in capillary lumens; V = visceral epithelial cell cytoplasm.

be the sites where hyaline material accumulates in patients with diabetes mellitus and amyloidosis.

(7). The components of glomeruli function as a unit. Filtration of fluid through glomerular capillaries is influenced by several factors, including:
  (a). Perfusion of glomerular capillaries.
  (b). The size, shape, molecular configuration, and charge of molecules.
  (c). The architecture of glomerular capillary walls (Figs. 1–6 through 1–13).
  (d). Negatively charged sialoproteins that coat endothelial cells and visceral epithelial cells, facilitate passage of small

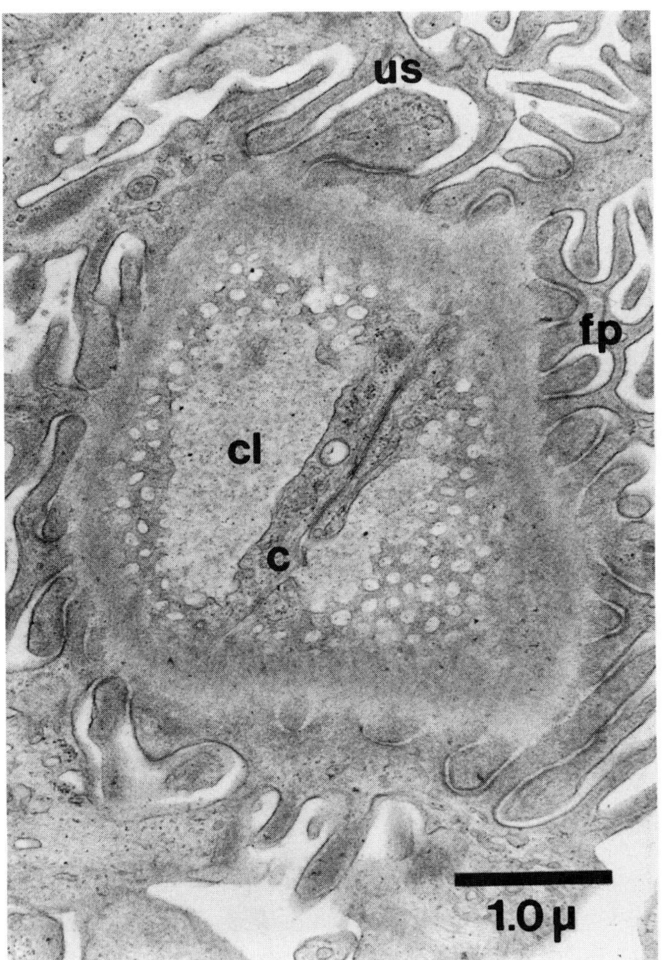

FIG. 1–10. Electron micrograph of a glomerular capillary obtained from an adult dog illustrates numerous fenestrations in endothelial cells. The cell junction between two endothelial cells is visible. c = cytoplasm of capillary endothelial cell; cl = capillary lumen; fp = foot processes of visceral epithelial cells; us = urinary space. (Courtesy of Dr. Robert F. Hammer, University of Minnesota.)

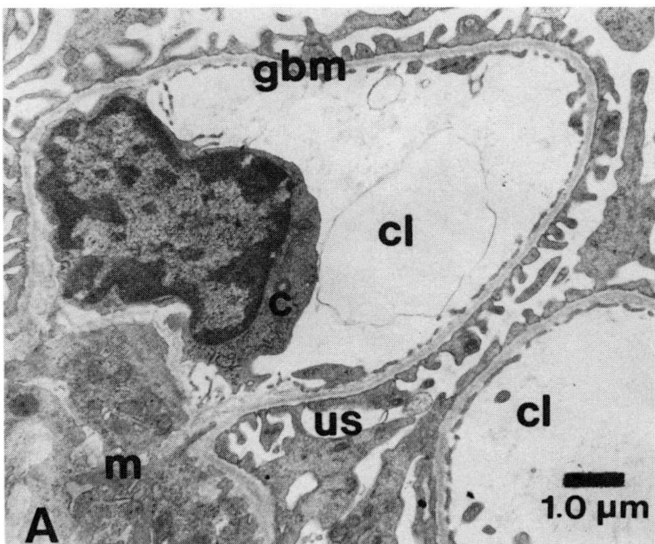

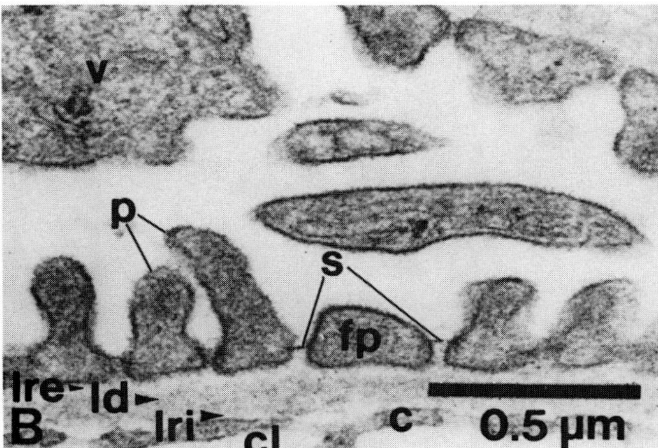

FIG. 1–11. Electron micrograph of a normal adult dog glomerulus. **A,** Low-power magnification illustrates patent capillary lumens (cl) surrounded by fenestrated endothelial cytoplasm (c), glomerular basement membrane (gbm), and foot processes of visceral epithelial cytoplasm. m = mesangium; us = urinary space. **B,** Higher magnification of glomerular capillary wall consists of fenestrated endothelial cytoplasm (c); glomerular basement membrane composed of three layers: lamina rara interna (lri), lamina densa (ld), and lamina rara externa (lre); and foot processes (fp) of visceral epithelial cytoplasm. Slit-pore membranes(s) are located between foot processes in the slit pores. Foot processes are covered with glomerular polyanion (p), v = cytoplasm of visceral epithelial cells; cl = patent capillary lumens. Reprinted with permission from Osborne, C.A., et al. The glomerulus in health and disease: A comparative review of domestic animals and man. Adv Vet Sci Comp Med. 1977; 21:207.

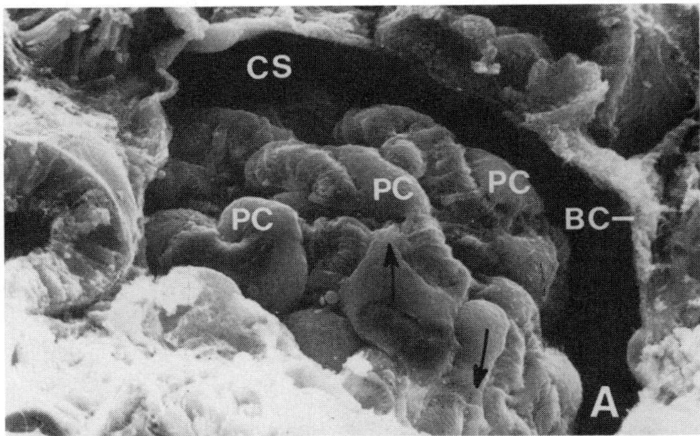

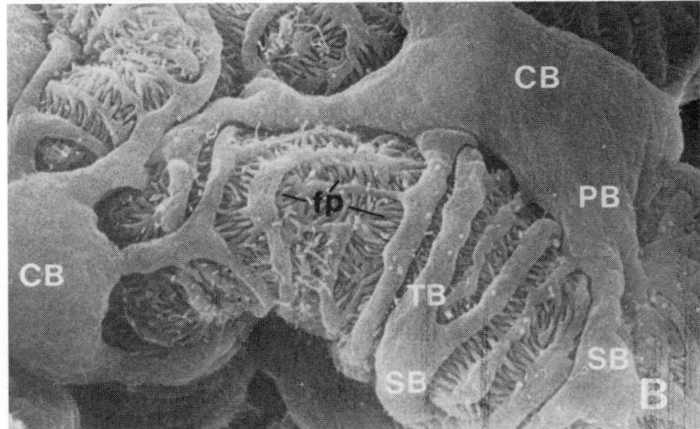

FIG. 1–12. A, Section of renal cortex shows Bowman's capsule (BC), Bowman's space between the glomerulus and Bowman's capsule (CS), visceral epithelial cell bodies (PC), and cytoplasmic branches of visceral epithelial cell bodies (arrows). **B,** A visceral epithelial cell body (CB) with primary (PB), secondary (SB), and tertiary (TB) cytoplasmic branches. The terminal foot processes (fp) of the visceral epithelial cells (so-called podocytes) interdigitate on the outer aspect of glomerular basement membranes. (Courtesy of Dr. Robert F. Hammer, University of Minnesota.)

cationic macromolecules, and impede passage of anionic macromolecules.

(e). The GBM appears to impede passage of larger uncharged macromolecules, whereas slit-pore membranes impede passage of somewhat smaller molecules.

(f). Visceral epithelial cells may also recover proteins that leak through the filters.

(g). The mesangium reconditions and unclogs the filtration barriers by removing and disposing of filtration residues that accumulate on the endothelial side of the GBM.

(8). Loss of the negative charge (charge selective barrier) of glomerular capillary walls or damage to the GBM or slit-pore membranes (size selective barriers) as a result of various disease processes may alter the selective semipermeability of glomeruli and result in varying degrees of proteinuria. Disorders that cause proliferation and hypertrophy of mesangial cells and/or an increase in mesangial matrix may result in cellular and matrix encroachment on glomerular capillary lumen size. If generalized and severe, increase in the mesangium may lead to reduced perfusion of glomerular capillaries, reduction in glomerular filtration rate, and retention of metabolites normally filtered by glomeruli (urea, creatinine, and phosphorus).

e. Bowman's capsule

(1). A glomerulus and corresponding Bowman's capsule are called a renal corpuscle (Figs. 1–6, 1–8, and 1–12 through 1–14).

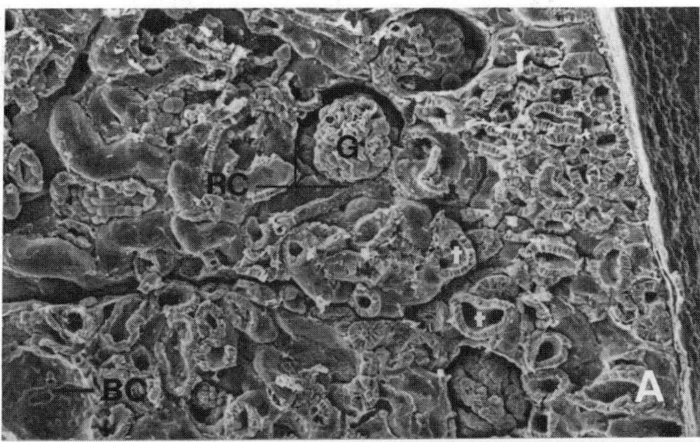

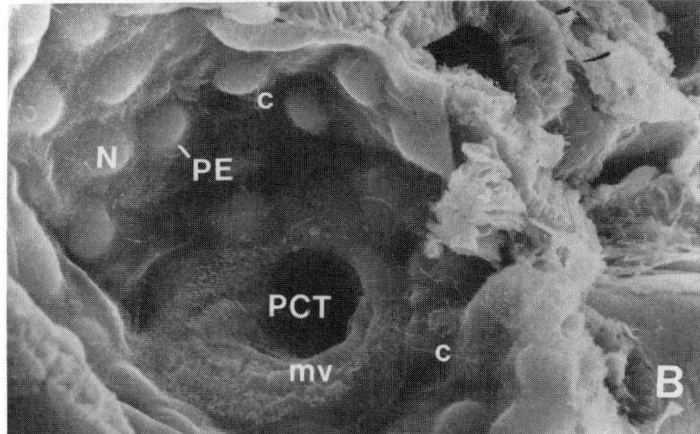

FIG. 1–13. A, Cut surface of the renal cortex reveals renal corpuscles (RC) with glomeruli (G), profiles of transected tubules (t), and an empty Bowman's capsule (BC). **B,** Parietal epithelium (PE) of Bowman's capsule with nucleated portion (N) of cells, each with a single cilium (c). The origin of the proximal convoluted tubule (PCT) is surrounded by microvilli (mv) of proximal tubular epithelial cells. (Courtesy of Dr. Robert F. Hammer, University of Minnesota.)

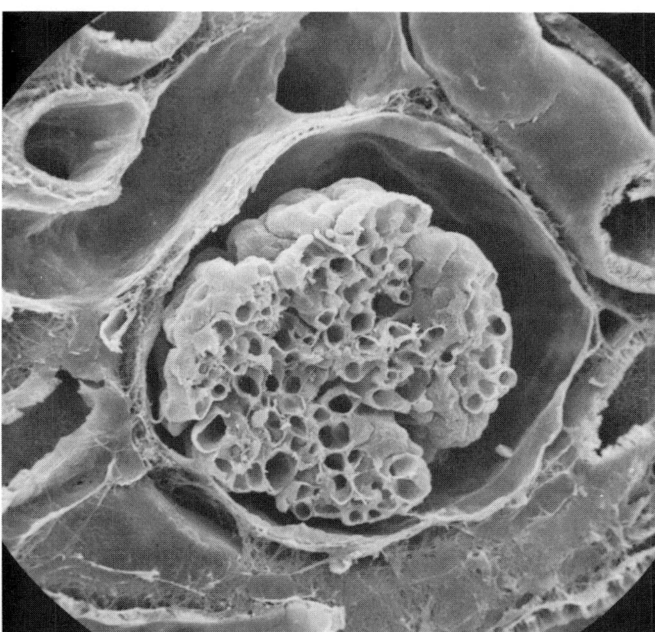

FIG. 1–14. Scanning electron micrograph of a cross section of a glomerulus of an adult dog illustrates the relationship of glomerular capillaries to Bowman's space, and of Bowman's capsule to adjacent renal tubules. Note the scant quantity of interstitial tissue between renal tubules. (Courtesy of Dr. Robert F. Hammer, University of Minnesota.)

(2). Bowman's capsule is composed of a collagenous membrane lined by flattened squamous epithelium called parietal epithelium (see Figs. 1–6 and 1–8). The parietal epithelium of Bowman's capsule is continuous with the visceral epithelium covering glomerular capillaries. Parietal epithelial cells are also continuous with those lining the proximal tubules.

(3). Bowman's capsule has generally been assumed to function as a passive container for glomerular filtrate, which is then passed on to proximal tubules.

(4). Although passage of material through the wall of Bowman's capsule may be of little quantitative significance under physiologic conditions, it may become functionally significant under pathologic conditions.[67]

(5). Proliferation of parietal epithelial cells may result in formation of multiple layers of cells surrounded by varying quantities of collagen-like material that protrude into Bowman's space. Because proliferation of these cells results in concentric layers of cells and intracellular material, they are commonly called crescents. Progressive enlargement of crescents may encroach on the glomerulus and ultimately lead to adhesions and eventual tuft collapse. The general concensus is that crescents represent a reaction of parietal epithelium to macromolecules that have escaped into the urinary space as a result of severe damage to glomerular capillary walls.[67] When present in large numbers of renal biopsy samples, crescents indicate severe and often irreversible glomerular damage.

f. Proximal tubules

(1). Proximal tubules collect glomerular filtrate from Bowman's space (see Fig. 1–13).

(2). Classically, the beginning portion of the proximal tubule is called the pars convoluta because it has a convoluted configuration that pursues a meandering path through the renal cortex. It joins the straight portion called the pars recta, which descends toward the renal medulla. On the basis of morphologic characteristics, however, the proximal tubule of dogs has been divided into four distinct anatomic segments.[11]

(3). Proximal tubules are lined by a single layer of columnar to cuboidal epithelial cells that facilitate active and passive reabsorption of almost 75% of the glomerular filtrate.

(a). The luminal borders of proximal tubular epithelial cells are completely covered with a well-developed "brush-border" formed by numerous elongated microvilli (Figs. 1–13 and 1–15).

(b). These microvilli increase the luminal reabsorptive surface area of proximal tubules (by a factor greater than 35× in rabbits) in a fashion analogous to that of the microvilli in the small intestine.[88]

(4). Feline kidneys contain more lipid in proximal tubular epithelial cells than do kidneys of other common domestic species of animals.

(a). The quantity of lipid present is influenced by several factors.[28]

1′). Kittens and immature cats have less fat than adults.

2′). Sexually inactive males have more fat than sexually active males.

3′). Castration of male cats results in an increase in renal lipid content within 3 weeks.

4′). The quantity of renal lipid is influenced by the stage of the estrous cycle of females.

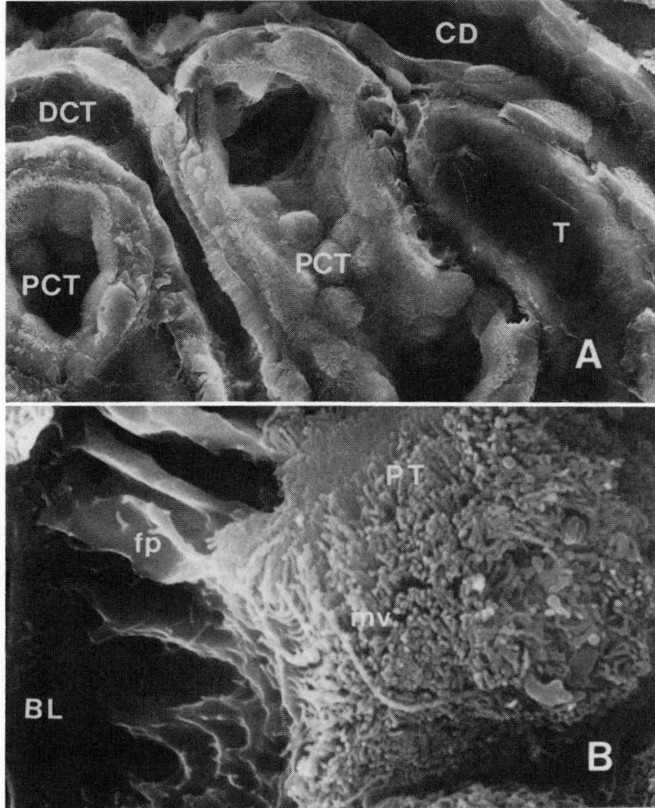

FIG. 1–15. A, Cross section of kidney reveals a distal convoluted tubule (DCT) coursing between two proximal convoluted tubules (PCT). A collecting duct (CD) and the basal lamina of an uncut tubule (T) are also present. **B,** Microvilli (mv) from a proximal tubule (PT) seen from the luminal surface. Lateral projections from the epithelial cells (fp) project down to the basal lamina (BL). (Courtesy of Dr. Robert F. Hammer, University of Minnesota.)

(b). These characteristics should be considered when the morphology of cats' kidneys is being evaluated.

g. Loops of Henle

(1). Filtrate modified by proximal tubules drains into loops of Henle, which are tubular structures that traverse a hairpin pathway as they move toward and then away from the renal pelvis.[11] The descending and ascending limbs of the loops of Henle run in opposite directions, but in close proximity to each other. In dogs, the pars recta of proximal tubules joins the thin descending limb of the loop of Henle near the corticomedullary junction.[11] The initial segments of the ascending limb of the loop of Henle are lined by narrower epithelial cells (thin portion) than subsequent segments (thick portion) that eventually join with the distal tubules (see Fig. 1–18).

(2). Loops of Henle play a major role in generating a hyperosmotic gradient of solute concentration within the medullary interstitium. Maintenance of high solute concentration in the renal medulla is essential for concentration of urine.

(a). Lengths of loops of Henle depend on the location of corresponding glomeruli within the renal cortex. Nephrons with glomeruli in the outer cortex have the shortest loops of Henle, which extend to the outer zone of the medulla. Nephrons with glomeruli located near the corticomedullary junction have the longest loops of Henle, extending deep into the inner zone of the medulla. Nephrons arising in the central portion of the renal cortex have loops of Henle that extend approximately halfway into the medulla. Varying ability of different species to maximally concentrate urine (man = ± 1.035; dog = ± 1.060; cat = ± 1.080) may be related, at least in part, to the ratio of shorter to longer loops, and to the actual length of loops.[77]

(b). Other anatomic factors may also be involved in formation of concentrated urine.[76]

h. Distal tubules (see Fig. 1–15)

(1). The thick ascending limbs of loops of Henle lie in close proximity to arterioles and glomeruli to which they are attached.

(2). The distal tubule begins in the vicinity of its own glomerulus.

(a). In that location, the distal tubular lumen is somewhat dilated, and tubular cells adjacent to juxtaglomerular cells of afferent arterioles become narrower and taller.

(b). These specialized tubular epithelial cells form the macula densa, a component of the juxtaglomerular apparatus.

(c). The macula densa arbitrarily marks the beginning of the distal convoluted tubule.

(d). Cells lining remaining portions of distal tubules are lower than those of proximal tubules and contain only a few luminal microvilli.

(3). The distal segment of the distal tubule is convoluted, and is contained entirely within the renal cortex.

3. Collecting ducts (see Figs. 1–15 and 1–18).

a. Distal convoluted tubules drain into collecting ducts.

b. Although initial portions of collecting ducts are

continuous with distal tubules, traditionally they are not included as components of nephrons.

c. As they traverse the renal parenchyma toward the renal pelvis, collecting ducts begin to join one another. The largest segments of collecting ducts that enter the renal pelvis are often called papillary ducts.

d. Two distinct cell types line collecting ducts.
   (1). The major cell type is called a "light cell" because it contains relatively few cytoplasmic organelles.
   (2). Dark (intercalated) cells located in the cortical segments of collecting ducts contain large numbers of mitochondria and other cytoplasmic organelles.

e. Cells lining loops of Henle, distal tubules, and collecting ducts have been shown by immunofluorescent techniques to have the capacity to secrete a mucoprotein called Tamm-Horsfall mucoprotein.[44]

4. Interstitial tissue.
   a. Interstitial tissue surrounds glomeruli, tubules, vessels, and nerves. It is normally scant in quantity, but progressively increases from cortex to medulla (Fig. 1–14).
   b. Normal interstitial tissue is composed of stellate cells, fibroblasts, collagen, and mononuclear cells.
   c. The predominant cell type (stellate cell) in the renal medulla contains lipid. Although the renal medulla is a major site for prostaglandin synthesis, a direct relationship between the lipid droplets within interstitial cells and prostaglandin synthesis is thought to be unlikely.[83]

5. Vascular Supply
   a. Macrocirculation[10,57]
      (1). Each kidney is usually supplied by one main renal artery. The left renal artery is completely double in structure in approximately 13% of dogs[3,73,80]; double renal arteries occur in 10% of cats.[74] On occasion three renal arteries may occur.
         (a). Evaluation of normal dogs by renal angiography revealed that the renal arteries originated from the aorta at the region adjacent to the caudal one third of the 2nd lumbar vertebrae, and the intervertebral space between the 2nd and 3rd lumbar vertebrae.[3]
         (b). The left renal artery usually originates from the aorta one third of a vertebral segment caudal to the origination of the right renal artery.
      (2). The primary renal artery divides into two branches, each of which subdivide into five to seven so-called interlobar arteries (Fig. 1–16).[34] These arteries pass adjacent to, but outside of, the renal pelvis. Evagination of the renal pelvis around the interlobar vessels results in formation of renal pelvic diverticulae (Fig. 1–17).
      (3). Following penetration of the renal parenchyma at the corticomedullary junction, interlobar arteries give rise to arcuate arteries.

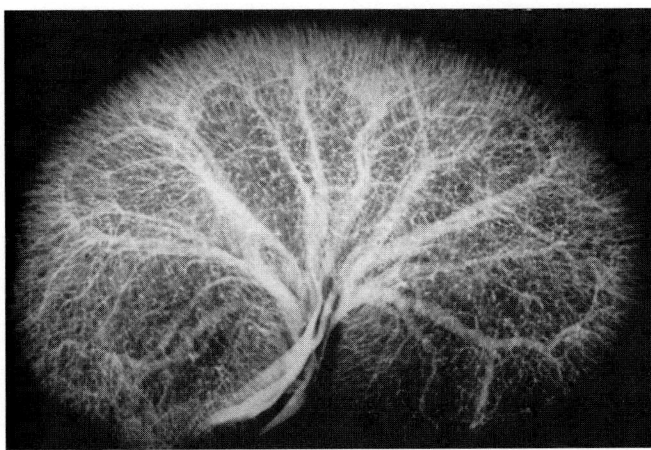

FIG. 1–16. High-resolution angiogram of the kidney of a normal young adult mixed-breed dog illustrates the arborizing architecture of interlobar, arcuate, and interlobular arteries. (Courtesy of Dr. James W. Wilson.)

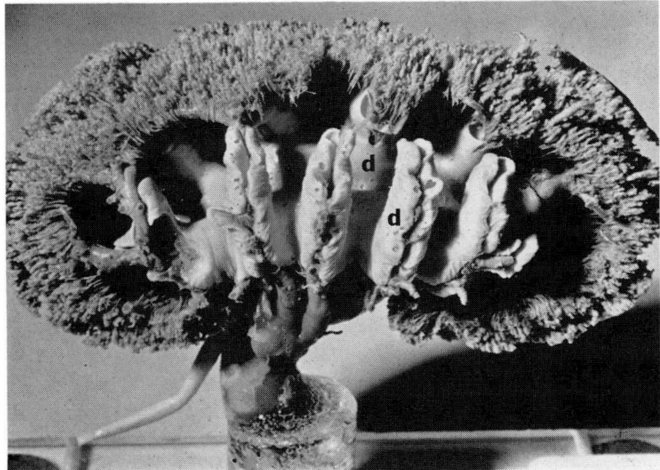

FIG. 1–17. Vinyl corrusion cast of venous vasculature of a normal adult canine kidney. Polymerized perfusion medium fills the lumens of renal veins and the lumens of the renal pelvis and ureter. The renal parenchyma was dissolved in an acid solution. Portions of the venous vasculature have been removed to expose the renal pelvis with pelvic diverticulae (d). Reprinted with permission from Osborne, C.A., et al. Urinary system: pathophysiology, diagnosis, and treatment. *In* General Small Animal Surgery. New York: J.B. Lippincott, 1985.

(4). Arcuate arteries radiate toward the periphery of the cortex and branch into interlobular arteries; the smallest vessels are identified by angiography.[6] Interlobular arteries in turn give rise to afferent arterioles. Afferent arterioles provide comparatively less resistance to blood flow, and thus transmit blood at relatively high hydrostatic pressure to glomeruli. Afferent arterioles divide into numerous capillaries to form glomeruli, the sites for filtration of blood (Figs. 1–4, and 1–5). Glomerular capillaries subsequently reunite to form one or more efferent arterioles capable of high resistance to blood flow.[34]

Coordination of vasomotor activity and vascular resistance to blood flow in afferent and efferent arterioles maintains renal blood flow at a relatively stable and high hydrostatic pressure despite wide variations in mean systemic arterial pressure (80 to 180 mm Hg).[72] This phenomenon is called "autoregulation." If renal artery perfusion pressure declines, renal vessels dilate. Below approximately 60 mm Hg, further vasodilation does not occur, and renal blood flow declines in proportion to reduction in perfusion pressure. Consult Chapter 2 on applied renal physiology for additional details about autoregulation.

(5). Renal arteries are considered to be "end arteries" without significant collateral blood supply.

(a). The clinical relevance of this observation is that sudden occlusion of any portion of the renal arterial tree by thrombosis or embolism would be followed by infarction of parenchyma perfused by the vessel distal to the obstructed site.

(b). Studies recently performed in normal and experimental dogs have revealed collateral arterial connections between interlobar or arcuate arteries and extrarenal arteries (i.e., phrenicoabdominal, spermatic, deep circumflex iliac, ureteral, caudal mesenteric, lumbar, and adrenal arteries).[17] In diseases associated with gradual occlusion of the main renal artery or its major branches, these collateral arterial connections may undergo sufficient hypertrophy to maintain significant renal function.

(6). Multiple renal veins are common in cats,[74] but are rare in dogs.[73]

(a). In both species, venous vessels anastomose at several levels (see Fig. 1–17).

(b). Both dogs and cats have well-developed cortical venous systems.[4,7]

(c). The outer cortical veins in cats form a prominent subcapsular network that extends around the surface of the kidney to join the renal vein at the hilus. Inner cortical and medullary venous return is thought to occur via intrarenal veins.[64]

(d). In dogs and cats, the left gonadal vein (ovarian or spermatic) drains the left renal vein. The right renal vein drains directly into the caudal vena cava.

(7). The kidneys contain extensive lymphatic vessels. In dogs, lymphatic drainage is continuous from the renal capsule, through the cortex, and into the hilar region.[83]

b. Microcirculation

(1). The structure and function of glomeruli have been described under the section entitled "The Nephron" in this chapter.

(2). The microcirculation of the renal cortex and that of the medulla are different.

(3). The efferent arterioles divide into capillaries of different structure and function depending on their location within the renal cortex.[7]

(a). Efferent arterioles derived from glomeruli in outer portions of the cortex form a peritubular capillary network that perfuses tubules and interstitial tissue primarily in the renal cortex. An association between efferent arterioles and corresponding tubules of the same nephron only exists for proximal tubules of the superficial cortex.[7] Perfusion of corticomedullary tubules originating from glomeruli located deeper in the cortex is dissociated from perfusion of postefferent vessels of the same nephron, in that perfusion may be derived from vessels originating from several unrelated nephrons.[4,5] Whereas superficial cortical microcirculation patterns can be highly localized, perfusion patterns of the juxtamedullary cortex and medulla are derived from several sources. This microvascular organization provides a plausible explanation for the patchy and seemingly unpredictable pattern of tubular epithelial cell and basement membrane destruction commonly associated with acute ischemic renal failure.[7]

(b). Efferent arterioles that arise from glomeruli located adjacent to the medulla form vessels called vasa recta that loop deep into the renal medulla before returning to the cortex (Fig. 1–18). Multiple vasa recta arise from a single efferent arteriole.[34] Their hairpin configuration is similar to the loops of Henle. Vasa recta are a vital component of the countercurrent system. They remove the excess water from the medullary interstitium that might otherwise reduce solute concentrated there.

(4). Hydrostatic pressure in peritubular capillaries is reduced to a value significantly below that in glomerular capillaries by efferent arteriolar tone and capillary surface area. Whereas the high hydrostatic pressure in glomerular capillaries favors glomerular filtration, the much reduced hydrostatic pressure in peritubular capillaries favors reabsorption of solute and water from tubular lumens.[7]

(5). Peritubular capillaries depend on blood flow through glomeruli. This dependency provides a plausible explanation of one mechanism whereby diseases of glomeruli may result in secondary diseases of tubulo-interstitial structures. Interruption of blood flow through glomeruli results in a corresponding reduction in perfusion of peritubular capillaries. The potential consequence is ischemic atrophy and/or necrosis of tubulo-interstitial structures.

(6). In a review, renal circulation was described as a composite of several microcirculations, each having a specialized role.[7] Although nephrons comprise the accepted functional units of the kidney, they cannot function independently of vascular perfusion. The microcirculation in different regions of the kidney has structural organizational and functional properties uniquely suited to specific exchange processes that facilitate production of urine of required volume and composition. The glomerular circulation is specialized for filtration, the first step in urine formation; the cortical peritubular capillary network is specialized for reabsorption of fluid and solutes from tubules; the medullary circulation is specialized to facilitate urine concentration and dilution. Abnormalities of these specialized microcirculations play important roles in the pathophysiology of renal disease. Selective damage to glomerular capillaries leads to decreased glomerular filtration rate and/or proteinuria. Similarly, destruction of medullary microcirculations impairs urine concentration and/or dilution.

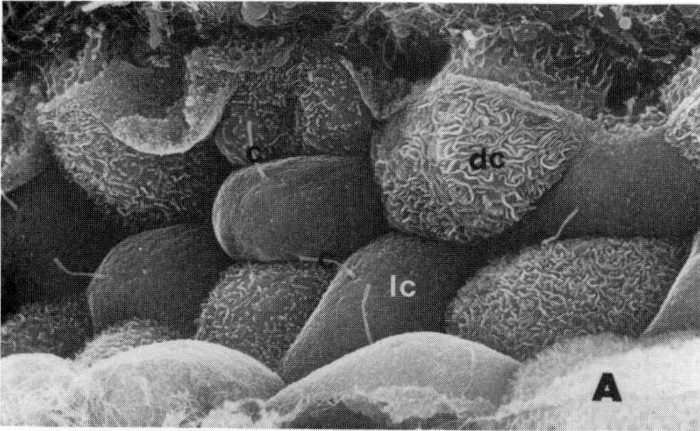

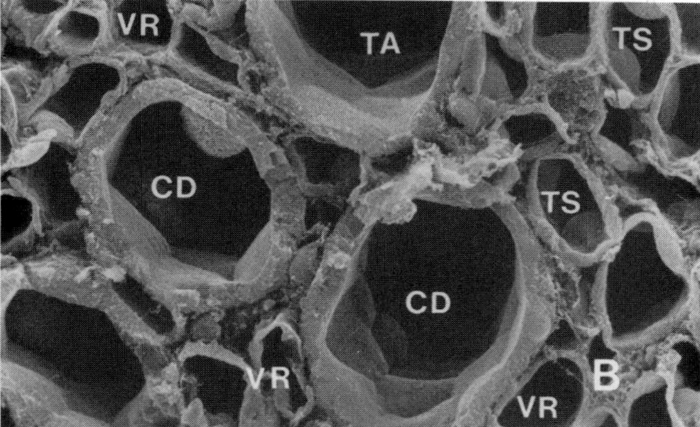

FIG. 1–18. A, Dark cells (dc) of the collecting duct have an elaborate pattern of microfolds on their luminal border. Light cells (lc) have a smooth surface with a single cilium (c). **B,** Thin segments (TS) and the thick ascending limb (TA) of the loop of Henle located in the renal medulla. Cross sections of collecting ducts (CD) and vasa recta (VR) are also present. (Courtesy of Dr. Robert F. Hammer, University of Minnesota.)

6. Innervation
   a. The kidneys contain adrenergic and cholinergic nerve fibers.
   b. The nerve supply generally follows arterial vessels.
   c. Adrenergic and cholinergic nerve fibers have been observed in vascular walls of canine kidneys to the level of afferent arterioles.[59,60]
   d. In dogs and other species, extensive innervation of efferent arterioles of juxtamedullary glomeruli eventually forms afferent vasa recta.[59,83]

II. RENAL PELVIS

A. Gross and microscopic appearance.

1. The renal pelvis, located at the hilus of the kidney, is a thin-walled distensible funnel-shaped structure that surrounds the renal crest (innermost portion of the medulla).
   a. In dogs and cats, it is almost completely surrounded by renal parenchyma, making it inaccessible to surgical incision (pyelotomy) in normal animals (see Fig. 1–17).

b. There is no precise junction between the renal pelvis and the proximal ureter. The renal pelvis is an expanded portion of the proximal ureter that is elongated in its craniocaudal axis and narrow in its dorsoventral axis.

c. The wall of the renal pelvis consists of three layers that are identical to, but less well developed than, those of the ureter:

(1). An external connective tissue adventitia.

(2). A thin smooth muscle layer.

(3). A mucous membrane featuring transitional epithelium (sometimes called urothelium).

2. The appearance of the renal pelvis during routine intravenous urography is similar to that of an open umbrella.

a. When distended with contrast media, several paired (five to seven) diverticulae may be seen extending from the pelvis into the renal parenchyma (see Fig. 1–17).[10]

(1). These paired diverticulae form as a result of reflection of the pelvic wall around the second (interlobar)- and third-order branches of the renal artery and renal vein (see Fig. 1–17).

(2). Detection of alterations in shape of these diverticulae by contrast radiography is often helpful in localizing inflammatory, infectious, or obstructive disorders of the urinary tract to the kidney(s).

b. The optimum time to evaluate the length and width of the renal pelvis and its diverticulae in dogs with normal renal function is 20 to 40 minutes after intravenous injection of sodium iothalamate given at a dose of 400 mg of iodine per pound of body weight.[25]

B. Function.

1. The renal pelvis collects urine from the papillary ducts and channels it into the ureters.[90]

a. In dogs, the renal pelvis has been estimated to hold less than 8 mL of urine.[32]

b. The renal pelvis contains one or more "pacemakers" that initiate peristaltic contraction of the smooth muscle of the upper urinary tract at regular intervals.[41,86]

(1). The pacemakers are apparently activated by mechanical (pressure and volume) and perhaps chemical stimuli.[9,48,86,89]

(2). During contraction, the shape of the renal pelvis may change.

(3). Contraction of the pelvic wall does not normally generate high intraluminal pressure.

(a). It varies from less than 10 cm H_2O in the resting state to 20 to 40 cm H_2O during contraction.[40]

(b). Resting intraluminal pressure of ureters is approximately 0 to 5 cm H_2O, but may reach 80 cm H_2O during contraction of the ureteral wall.[23]

2. From a functional standpoint, the renal pelvis and ureter comprise a single unit and, with the kidneys, are collectively referred to as the upper urinary tract.

a. Their primary function is to transport urine produced by the kidney to the urinary bladder for storage.

b. They do not significantly alter the composition of urine produced by nephrons and collecting ducts, although they may produce substances that prevent microbial adherence to, and colonization of, their urothelial lining.

III. URETERS

A. Gross appearance and position.

1. The ureters are thick-walled fibromuscular ducts that connect the renal pelves with the urinary bladder.

a. They are highly compliant and deformable structures that lie directly beneath the peritoneum adjacent to the post cava and aorta in the dorsal part of the abdomen.

b. The right ureter is longer than the left because of the more cranial position of the right kidney. The actual length of the ureters varies with body size, but is 12 to 16 cm in a 16-kg dog.[24]

c. The width of the ureteral lumens of normal dogs evaluated by contrast urography was reported to be 0.07 (± 0.018) times the length of the 2nd lumbar vertebra visualized on ventrodorsal views.[25]

2. The distal portions of the ureters are surrounded by the reflected layers of peritoneum that form the lateral ligaments of the urinary bladder. In male dogs, the ductus deferens loop around each ureter about 2 cm from the junction of the ductus deferens with the urinary bladder neck.

3. Ureters enter the dorsolateral aspect of the urinary bladder cranial to its neck, and open at a location that comprises the cranial border of the trigone (see Figs. 1–1 and 1–2).

a. The ureters turn almost 180 degrees from a caudal to a cranial direction as they approach and enter a distended urinary bladder of dogs.[14] When the bladder is empty and assumes a more caudal position within the abdomen, the curvature of the distal ureters lessens.

b. After entering the bladder wall, the submucosal portion of the ureters passes obliquely through the thickness of the bladder wall.

c. The fact that the ureters do not form a straight pathway adjacent to and within the bladder wall is of importance in evaluation of radiographic studies, ureteral catheterization, and reconstructive ureteral surgery.

d. The ureteral openings have a slit-like appearance in the bladder mucosa. They are horseshoe shaped in dogs.[14]

4. Anatomic ureterovesical sphincters are not present.

a. The segment of ureter within the bladder wall is several millimeters long (4 to 15 mm in dogs and 3 to 7 mm in cats) and pursues an oblique course through the muscular layers before opening into the bladder lumen at the trigone.[38] The submucosal portion of the ureters of dogs is long and thin when the bladder is distended. The intramuscular portion is more prominent when the bladder is empty.[14]

b. The oblique and relatively long course of the ureters through the bladder wall facilitates mechanical closure of the distal ureter by pressure when the bladder is distended with urine.[14-16]

(1). This arrangement represents a one-way flap valve, which normally prevents retrograde flow of urine from the bladder into the ureters (vesicoureteral reflux).

(2). The ureterovesical valves protect the renal pelves and kidneys from abnormal retrograde pressure and from contamination with microbes in patients with infections of the lower urinary tract.

5. The trigone is an internally evident triangular area of the dorsal wall of the bladder neck.

a. It is located immediately adjacent to the proximal urethra.

b. The apex of the trigone is at the urethral orifice, and its base is formed by transverse ureteric musculature that connects the two ureteral openings.

B. Structural organization.

1. Like the renal pelvis, urinary bladder, and urethra, the wall of the ureter is composed of external adventitia, a multilayered smooth muscle coat, and an inner layer of mucosa.

a. The adventitia is composed primarily of loose connective tissues that blend with the muscular layers and surrounding retroperitoneal tissues.

(1). It contains small blood vessels, lymphatic vessels, and nonmyelinated nerve fibers.

(2). As the ureter passes obliquely through the bladder, its adventitia persists as a connective tissue sheath that separates the ureter from muscle fascicles of the adjacent vesical wall.

b. The smooth muscle has been reported to be organized into an inner and an outer longitudinal layer, and a middle layer with an orientation that varies from circular (transverse) to oblique.[2,24,33] This arrangement, however, has been disputed.[82]

(1). One investigator divided the canine ureter into three different segments on the basis of the architectural organization of smooth muscle layers.[2]

(a). The middle segment has circular fibers in its center layer of smooth muscle.

(b). The junctions between the middle and the upper and lower segments are marked by a change in the orientation of the middle layer fibers from circular to oblique.

(c). It has been hypothesized that this anatomic configuration facilitates adaptation of the ureter to different rates and volumes of urine flow.[2]

(2). Immediately adjacent to the urinary bladder, smooth muscle fascicles from the bladder are reflected on the adventitial surface of the ureter and thereby are incorporated into the external longitudinal muscle layer. Likewise, smooth muscle from the ureteral wall continues into the trigone of the inner part of the dorsal bladder wall.

c. The mucosa of the ureters lies adjacent to the submucosa and consists of transitional epithelium (urothelium), which is three to six cells deep.

2. When a cross section of the ureter is examined in an empty state, its lumen has a stellate appearance bounded by collapsed mucosa.[2,85]

a. The expansion capacity of the mucosa allows the ureter to accommodate to wide variations in luminal volume.

b. During peristalsis associated with transport of urine, the outline of the expanded ureteral lumen changes from stellate to square or circular.[52]

c. The diameter of a distended ureter in the dog has been reported to be 0.6 to 0.9 cm.[24]

3. The ureters receive pain stimuli as a result of sympathetic and parasympathetic innervation.[84]

C. Vascular supply.

1. Ureteral vessels are derived from several sources.

a. The upper portion of the ureter is perfused with blood supplied by branches of the renal arteries (cranial ureteral artery).

b. The lower portion of the ureter receives branches from the prostatic or vaginal artery (caudal ureteral artery).

c. There is extensive anastomoses of these vessels at the level of the adventitia of the ureteral wall, facilitating considerable mobilization of the ureters during surgery.

2. The ureteral arteries have venous counterparts that drain into the renal and ultimately the prostatic or vaginal veins.

3. Lymphatics are also located adjacent to ureteral arteries.

a. Proximal lymphatics drain into para-aortic lymph nodes.

b. Distal lymphatics drain into internal iliac lymph nodes.

D. Innervation.

1. Pain afferents are activated by ureteral distention.

2. The ureters receive autonomic nerve fibers. Be-

cause ureteral peristalsis is myogenic in origin, the function of autonomic innervation is not yet known. It may affect the force of ureteral contraction.[40,86]

E. Function.

1. The primary function of the ureters is to propel urine from the kidney to the urinary bladder.
2. Ureteral function has been evaluated with the aid of radiographic techniques, measurements of intraluminal pressure, and electromyography of ureteral muscle.[40,48]
3. The primary functional unit of the ureter is the smooth muscle cell.[87]
   a. Peristaltic activity is initiated in proximal portions of the collecting system (probably the renal pelvis).
      (1). From that site, electrical impulses are conducted distally from one smooth muscle cell to another across gap junctions.
      (2). This gives rise to peristaltic contractions, which propel boluses of urine to the bladder.[86]
   b. Distention of any portion of the ureter with a bolus of urine may stimulate peristaltic activity that moves toward the urinary bladder.[87] Thus, if urine remains within a ureter following passage of a peristaltic wave from the renal pelvis, production of another peristaltic wave from within the ureter may expel the residual urine.
   c. Peristaltic waves that originate below the renal pelvis may also travel toward the renal pelvis. Thus, a bolus of urine entering the distal ureter in patients with vesicoureteral reflux may cause retrograde peristalsis.[87]
   d. Like detrusor smooth muscle of the urinary bladder, each smooth muscle cell of the ureter does not contain a neuromuscular junction.[87]
      (1). Ureteral smooth muscle cells are joined by gap junctions that permit spread of excitation from one muscle cell to another. Consequently, ureteral peristalsis may persist after transplantation, and normal antegrade propagation of the ureteral impulse occurs after reversal of a segment of ureter in situ.[87]
      (2). Damage to gap junctions of ureteral smooth muscle cells may alter ureteral peristalsis.
   e. Even though the ureters can function without innervation, the autonomic system may influence its activity.
      (1). Ureters contain alpha-excitatory and beta-inhibitory adrenergic receptors, which may affect the force of ureteral contraction.[40,46]
      (2). The role of the parasympathetic system in modulating ureteral peristalsis is less well understood.
4. For the ureters to propel urine effectively, the contraction wave must completely encircle ureteral walls.
   a. This phenomenon accounts for the observation that the entire length of the normal ureter is uncommonly filled with radiopaque contrast medium during intravenous urography.
   b. Normal ureteral contractions occur 2 to 6 times per minute in humans,[23] and 3 to 6 times per minute in dogs[2,41] at a velocity of 2 to 5 cm/second.[12]
   c. The frequency of ureteral peristaltic waves increases as urine flow rate increases up to a maximum.[86]
   d. After maximum frequency is attained, further increases in mean urine flow occur by an increase in bolus volume.
      (1). As bolus volumes increase, they coalesce. As a result, the ureters become filled with urine and dilate.
      (2). In addition to impaired outflow of urine, diuresis (physiologic, pathologic, or pharmacologic) may cause stasis of urine and dilatation of the ureteral lumen.[87]
5. Transection and subsequent anastomosis of the canine ureter prevents ureteral peristalsis from crossing the site of anastomosis for about 2 weeks.
   a. Distention of the distal portion of the transected ureter initiates a peristaltic wave that migrates to the urinary bladder.
   b. Because of interruption of coordinated peristalsis following transection and anastomosis of ureters, urinary diversion via percutaneous nephrostomy tubes is sometimes used.
   c. After 2 weeks, conduction of peristaltic waves across the anastomotic site of an otherwise normal ureter returns, and coordinated contractions along the entire length of the ureter resume.

IV. URINARY BLADDER

A. Gross appearance.

1. For descriptive purposes, anatomists often divide the urinary bladder (urocyst) into three sections.[33]
   a. The cranial portion has been called the apex. In humans, it is also called the dome.
   b. The narrow caudal portion that joins with the urethra is called the neck of the bladder. It is shorter in cats than in dogs.[20]
   c. The extensive region between the apex and the neck is called the body of the bladder.
   d. From a functional standpoint, the urinary bladder is best considered as a body and an outlet (see section on function of the lower urinary tract in this chapter).
2. The triangular area formed by the ureteral openings and the beginning of the urethral orifice is commonly called the trigone (trigonon = Latin for "triangle"), because it contains a triangular ar-

rangement of musculature that helps to anchor the ureters to the bladder.

a. The musculature outlining the trigone appears to be an expansion of muscle fibers from the ureters. Longitudinal fibers from each ureter extend transversely to form the base of the trigone and caudally to form the side and apex of the trigone, including the urethral crest in the dorsal wall of the urethra.[82]

b. The trigone is the thickest and least distensible portion of the bladder.[54] The mucosa covering the trigone is smooth and tightly adhered to the muscle coat.

B. Position.

1. The location of the urinary bladder is influenced by the volume of urine it contains.
   a. When empty or slightly distended, it is a teardrop- or pear-shaped organ that lies just ahead of the bony pelvis or within the pelvic inlet.
   b. When distended, it becomes almost spherical in shape and moves to a more cranioventral position within the abdominal cavity.
   c. Because of a long preprostatic urethra, the urinary bladder of male cats is often located farther forward in the abdominal cavity than in dogs.
   d. The location of the bladder may also be influenced by changes in size and/or position of adjacent organs, especially the prostate gland.
2. The mobility of the bladder is limited by its attachment to the urethra and three peritoneal ligaments.
   a. These ligaments are composed of double layers of peritoneum between which are blood vessels, nerves, lymphatics, and adipose tissue.[33,36]
   b. The median ligament reflects from the ventral surface of the bladder and extends from the proximal urethra along the ventral midline of the abdominal wall to the umbilicus. In the fetus, the median umbilical ligament contains the urachus.
   c. The lateral ligaments of the bladder connect the lateral surfaces of the bladder to the lateral aspects of the pelvic canal. They enclose the ureters, ductus deferens, and umbilical arteries.

C. Structural organization.

1. The entire urinary bladder of dogs and cats is covered by visceral peritoneum.
2. The wall of the urinary bladder is comprised of primarily a muscle coat lined by submucosa and mucosa. The bladder wall is of uniform thickness when distended.
   a. The multilayered smooth muscle coat of the bladder wall is referred to as the detrusor muscle (detrusor = Latin for "to push down").
      (1). Unlike the smooth muscle layers of the ureters, smooth muscle fibers of the urinary bladder are arranged in a meshwork without consistent layers. Many smooth muscle bands traverse a direction that is oblique to the longitudinal axis of the bladder.[33]
      (2). At the junction of the body of the bladder with its neck, muscle bands are organized into deep and superficial longitudinal layers. When the detrusor muscle contracts, longitudinal muscle fascicles can dilate the lumen of the relaxed neck and proximal urethra.
   b. The submucosa contains loose fibrous connective tissue that surrounds blood vessels, nerve fibers, and an occasional reticuloendothelial cell. Subepithelial capillaries lie in close proximity to the transitional epithelial cells. When the bladder is not distended with urine, the mucosal surface forms longitudinal folds. The anatomic structure of the mucosa and submucosa allows the bladder to adapt to substantial changes in urine volume without corresponding increases in intravesical pressure.
   c. The transitional epithelium (urothelium) that lines the mucosal surface of the bladder is typically three to four cell layers thick and, in the undistended state, is separated from muscle layers by an abundant coat of submucosa.[55]
      (1). Transitional cell epithelium is not comprised of a homogeneous population of cells.
         (a). Small relatively undifferentiated cells are located adjacent to the mucosal basement membrane, whereas large highly differentiated cells are located at the surface.
         (b). Cells between basal and surface layers are intermediate in differentiation.
      (2). Tight junctions and desmosome junctions that interconnect surface cells act in conjunction with luminal membranes of cells to form a diffusion barrier between extracellular fluids and urine (which may attain extremely high osmolality).[42]
         (a). The ability of transitional epithelium to prevent absorption of various components of urine from the bladder lumen is remarkable when one considers that the bladder mucosa must be capable of considerable expansion.
         (b). No other epithelium is known to offer a satisfactory substitute as a permeability barrier between tissue fluids and urine. The mucosa lining the ileum and rectum allows reabsorption of varying quantities of water, electrolytes, and nitrogenous wastes.[43]

(c). Undifferentiated neoplastic bladder epithelium may become more permeable to fluid than are normal cells.[43]

D. Vascular supply.

1. The bladder receives blood from branches of the internal iliac arteries.
   a. The cranial portion (apex) of the bladder is supplied by cranial vesical arteries, which are branches of the umbilical artery.
   b. The bladder is primarily vascularized by caudal vesical arteries, which are branches of the urogenital artery (prostatic or vaginal artery).
   c. Examination of the luminal surface of the bladder by cystoscopy reveals numerous superficial blood vessels, thereby providing a logical explanation for the ease with which hematuria is induced by trauma.
2. The veins of the urinary bladder are satellites of the arteries.
3. Urinary bladder lymphatics drain into the hypogastric and lumbar lymph nodes.

E. Innervation.

1. The detrusor muscle of the urinary bladder is supplied by sympathetic and parasympathetic nerve fibers.
   a. Sympathetic nerve fibers travel in the hypogastric nerve (spinal segments = L-1–L-4 in dogs and L-2–L-5 in cats).
   b. Parasympathetic fibers arrive from the pelvic nerve (spinal segments = S1–S3).
   c. The pelvic and hypogastric nerves reach the bilateral pelvic plexus located retroperitoneally and lateral to the rectum. Branches from each plexus reach the bladder by passing through the lateral ligaments along with the caudal vesical arteries.
2. Smooth muscle of the urinary bladder has several unique characteristics that are essential for its dual role as a storage receptacle (storage phase of micturition) and as a high-pressure pump (voiding phase of micturition).
   a. The detrusor muscle is relatively insensitive to quick stretch.
   b. The detrusor muscle is activated by nerves.
   c. Coordinated detrusor muscle maintains tone, but accommodates to being stretched during the urine storage phase of micturition. Thus, intravesicular pressure remains relatively constant while bladder volume expands.
3. All smooth muscle cells of the detrusor are not directly innervated.[65]
   a. Smooth muscle cells are activated by transmitter chemicals (so-called neurotransmitters) released from nerve varicosities. These neurotransmitters reach smooth muscle cells by diffusion.
   b. Some detrusor muscle cells might possibly serve as "pacemaker" cells.
      (1). Impulses within stimulated pacemaker cells travel to adjacent cells through specialized adaptations of smooth muscle cell walls called gap junctions, thereby stimulating the cells to contract.
      (2). Impulses generated in these cells are then transmitted to adjacent cells.
      (3). A gap junction consists of contacts between rosettes of membrane proteins from two adjacent cells to form a single channel that has a low resistance to impulse transmission.
         (a). Overdistention of the bladder may disrupt gap junctions and inhibit spread of a wave of detrusor excitation.
         (b). The result is impaired detrusor contraction, impaired ability to void, and retention of urine.

F. Concepts of micturition.

1. Definitions
   a. We define urination as formation and elimination of urine from the body. Although some use the term as a synonym for micturition, urination also encompasses formation of urine by the processes of glomerular filtration, tubular reabsorption, and tubular secretion (Table 1–1).
   b. We define micturition as a two-phase process of storage of urine in the bladder lumen and intermittent voiding of urine to the exterior. We do not use the term to describe the process of urine formation.
      (1). Micturition is a reflex involving parasympathetic, sympathetic, and somatic neurons; the activity of these neurons is organized in the brain stem and spinal cord.
         (a). Normal, complete voiding requires a functional pons and intact pathways

TABLE 1–1
OVERVIEW OF URINE FORMATION AND ELIMINATION

Organ	Functions
1. Kidneys	Glomerular filtration Tubular reabsorption Tubular secretion
2. Renal pelves	Urine collection under involuntary control Ureteral peristalis initiation
3. Ureters	Urine transport under involuntary control
4. Urinary bladder	Urine storage and voiding under voluntary and involuntary control
5. Urethra	Urine transport or retention under voluntary and involuntary control

between the pons and sacral spinal cord.

(b). Micturition is inhibited by forebrain centers.

(2). Internal and external urethral sphincters are controlled by spinal reflex. The external (striated) sphincter is subject to voluntary initiation.

2. Overview
   a. From a functional standpoint, the urinary bladder and urethra serve as an interdependent unit involved in two reciprocal phases of micturition.
      (1). Storage of urine.
      (2). Intermittent appropriate voiding of urine.
   b. These two phases of micturition depend on a complex neural control system for coordination.
3. Storage Phase of Micturition
   a. During the storage phase of micturition, the urinary bladder becomes a low-pressure expansible reservoir, whereas the bladder neck (dog), or the bladder neck and proximal urethra (cat), act as a high-resistance outflow valve (internal sphincter mechanism). Urinary continence is maintained provided intraurethral resistance exceeds intravesical pressure.
   b. As will be reviewed in further detail, the external urethral sphincter also contributes urethral resistance to urine outflow during the storage phase of micturition, especially when a sudden increase in intravesical pressure occurs.
   c. Other properties of the urethra that contribute to intraluminal resistance include fibroelastic elements of the urethral wall and pressure in submucosal venous sinus.
4. Voiding Phase of Micturition
   a. During the voiding phase of micturition, the urinary bladder becomes a high-pressure pump, which normally is activated by distention of the bladder wall.
      (1). Filling of the bladder lumen ultimately stimulates volume and tension receptors, which initiate sustained contraction of the detrusor muscle and expulsion of urine from the bladder.
      (2). Simultaneous inhibition of the internal and external urethral sphincters causes the urethra to become a low-resistance conduit that channels urine stored in the bladder to the exterior.
      (3). Voiding associated with detrusor contraction is normally so efficient that only 0.2 to 0.4 mL of urine per kilogram of body weight remains in the bladder lumen.[62]
5. Concepts of Reciprocal Innervation
   a. It is conceptually useful to consider innervation of effector organs of the lower urinary tract, and to become familiar with the distribution of neurotransmitters. The effector organs of the lower urinary tract are:
      (1). The detrusor muscle of the urinary bladder.
      (2). The internal sphincter mechanism of the bladder neck and proximal urethra.
      (3). The external urethral sphincter, which surrounds distal portions of the urethra.[49,68]
   b. It is important to recall that the terms parasympathetic and cholinergic are often used synonymously. Likewise, the terms sympathetic and adrenergic are often used synonymously.
      (1). Stimulation of acetylcholine receptors of the lower urinary tract causes smooth muscle contraction.
      (2). Stimulation of alpha-adrenergic receptors of the lower urinary tract by norepinephrine causes smooth muscle contraction.
      (3). Stimulation of beta-adrenergic receptors of the lower urinary tract causes smooth muscle relaxation.
      (4). Beta-adrenergic receptors are stimulated by low concentrations of epinephrine; alpha-adrenergic receptors are stimulated by high concentrations of norepinephrine.[22,31]
   c. The body and apex of the bladder, which constitute the detrusor muscle, primarily contain cholinergic receptors, but also contain some beta-adrenergic receptors.[49,62] The detrusor does not contain a functional quantity of alpha-adrenergic receptors.
      (1). During the storage phase of micturition, the parasympathetic system is inhibited and the sympathetic system is stimulated.
      (2). During the voiding phase of micturition, the parasympathetic system is activated and the sympathetic system is inhibited. These neurologic events cause the detrusor muscle to expel urine.
   d. The proximal internal urethral sphincter mechanism contains primarily alpha-adrenergic neuroreceptors.[49] It contains substantially fewer beta-adrenergic receptors. It does not contain a functional quantity of cholinergic neuroreceptors.
      (1). During the storage phase of micturition, the sympathetic system is active, thereby causing increased sphincter muscle tone and high resistance to urine outflow. The parasympathetic system contributes little to urethral resistance to urine outflow.
      (2). During the voiding phase of micturition, the sympathetic system is inhibited, thereby reducing urethral resistance and facilitating urine outflow.

e. Receptors in striated muscle fibers of the external urethral sphincter are activated by acetylcholine.
   (1). The external urethral sphincter (primarily the urethralis muscle) provides some intraurethral resistance during the storage phase of micturition, although urinary continence can be maintained even if it is denervated.
   (2). In the event of a rapid increase in intravesical pressure associated with a rapid increase in intra-abdominal pressure caused by barking, coughing, or vomiting, involuntary stimulation of the external urethral sphincter by the sympathetic system results in a further increase in intraurethral pressure. This reflex prevents urinary incontinence under the circumstances described.
   (3). During the voiding phase of micturition, activity in the external urethral sphincter is inhibited, at least partially, by connecting interneurons in the spinal cord. Inhibition is also influenced by the cerebellum.
   (4). Rhythmic contractions of striated musculature of the membranous urethra have been observed in male dogs during the voiding phase of micturition.[63]
   (5). The external urethral sphincter may also be voluntarily activated during voiding, with the result that urine outflow is suddenly interrupted.

f. In summary, current data indicate that the effector organs of the lower urinary tract are integrated by a phenomenon sometimes called reciprocal innervation.
   (1). During the storage phase of micturition, the sympathetic system plays the primary role.
   (2). During the voiding phase of micturition, the parasympathetic system plays the primary role.
   (3). Activation of the sympathetic system during the voiding phase of micturition may cause functional outflow obstruction (detrusor urethral reflex dyssynergia).

V. URETHRA

A. Basic structure.

1. The urethras of female dogs and cats are qualitatively similar, but those of male dogs and cats are different. Differences in urethral morphology among species are of clinical significance because they imply differences in urethral function, in diagnostic evaluation, and in the choice of medical and surgical therapy.
2. The urethra consists of a distensible fibromuscular tube lined by a continuous layer of mucosa.
3. The length and diameter of the urethra vary with species, body size, gender, and stage of micturition (storage or voiding).
4. All species have a proximal involuntary smooth muscle internal sphincter mechanism and a distal voluntary striated external urethral sphincter (primarily the urethralis muscle). The location and size of these sphincters vary between species and gender.[18-21]
5. The innervation of the urethra is similar in dogs and cats.
   a. It receives:
      (1). Sympathetic nerve fibers via the hypogastric nerve.
      (2). Somatic nerve fibers via the pudendal nerve.[65]
      (3). To a lesser extent, parasympathetic nerve fibers via the pelvic nerve.
   b. The involuntary internal sphincter mechanism is stimulated primarily by sympathetic nerve fibers, whereas the voluntary external urethral sphincter is innervated primarily by somatic nerve fibers.

B. Male dogs (Fig. 1–19).

1. For descriptive purposes, the urethra of male dogs is often divided into three macroscopic parts. Unlike male cats, male dogs lack a distinctive preprostatic urethra.
   a. The short section of prostatic urethra extends from the neck of the urinary bladder to the

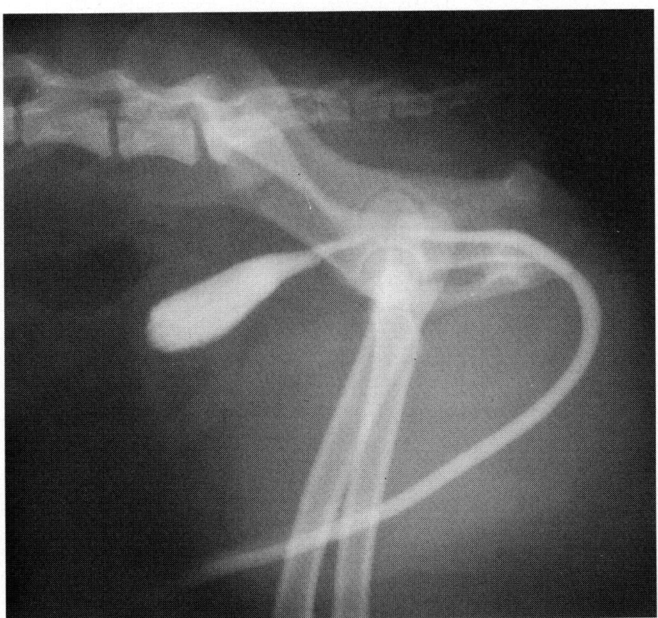

FIG. 1–19. Normal retrograde urethrogram of a normal adult male dog. A Swan-Ganz catheter was used to prevent reflux of radiopaque contrast material out of the distal end of the urethra. The urinary bladder is only partially distended with contrast medium. (Courtesy of Dr. Gary R. Johnston, University of Minnesota.)

caudal end of the prostate gland. It passes through and is completely surrounded by the prostate gland.

b. The membranous (postprostatic) urethra extends from the caudal aspect of the prostate gland to the urethral bulb of the penis. Unlike cats, male dogs do not have bulbourethral glands at the end of the membranous urethra.
c. The penile urethra begins at the root of the penis (level of the ischial arch), and extends to the tip of the penis.
   (1). The urethral groove of the os penis surrounds approximately two thirds of the dorsolateral circumference of the canine penile urethra.
   (2). The urethral groove of the os penis limits expansion of the penile urethra.

2. Microstructure.
   a. Transitional epithelium lining the proximal portion of the urethra changes to columnar or stratified cuboidal epithelium in distal portions of the urethra.[8,61] At the level of the body of the prostate gland, the mucosal surface of the dorsal urethral wall contains an elongated protrusion called the seminal hillock or colliculus seminalis. The ductus deferens and prostatic ductules empty into the urethra at the seminal hillock.
   b. The submucosa of the pelvic urethra contains a rich vascular plexus that is continuous with the corpus spongiosum penis.
   c. In the proximal portion of the urethra, the urethral muscle is composed of an inner layer of longitudinal smooth muscle fibers and an outer layer of longitudinal muscle fascicles derived from the urinary bladder.[33] Between these layers, circular muscle fascicles contribute functionally to the internal urethral sphincter of the bladder neck.
      (1). The internal urethral sphincter is not an anatomically conspicuous structure, but rather consists of smooth muscle in the neck of the bladder and, to a minor degree, the proximal urethra.
      (2). The proximal (prostatic) urethra contains substantial quantities of elastic fibers that facilitate closure of the urethral lumen.[33]
   d. The body of the prostate gland disrupts the muscle coat of the proximal urethra. Smooth muscle in this location blends with connective tissue stroma of the prostate gland and is inconspicuous in the midprostatic urethra.[19] Thus, there apparently is no mechanism for active closure of the lumen of this portion of the urethra.
      (1). During the storage phase of micturition, the prostatic urethra closes passively as a result of elastic fibers in the adjacent urethral wall.
      (2). During spontaneous micturition and during maximum distention retrograde urethrocystography, the diameter of the prostatic urethral lumen is often larger than adjacent portions of the urethra.
      (3). Passive distention of the fibroelastic tissue surrounding the prostatic urethral lumen in response to pressure generated by contrast material may account for this normal variation in urethral appearance.[46,47]
   e. The striated urethralis muscle comprises the primary component of the external urethral sphincter.
      (1). The urethralis muscle begins at the caudal border of the prostate gland and extends to the level of the bulbospongiosus muscle at the root of the penis.[33] It comprises more than 50% of the wall of the membranous urethra,[19] and undoubtedly plays an important role in voluntary interruption of micturition by male dogs for territorial marking.
      (2). Transection of the pudendal nerve, which supplies the urethralis muscle, does not result in urinary incontinence because of the function of the internal urethral sphincter.

3. Vascular Supply.
   a. The prostatic urethra is supplied with blood from the prostatic artery, which in turn is derived from the internal pudendal artery.
   b. The membranous portion of the urethra is supplied by small urethral arteries, which branch off the prostatic artery.
   c. The penile urethra is supplied with blood from the artery of the bulb of the penis.
   d. The urethral veins are satellites of the arteries and drain into the pudendal vein.
   e. Lymphatics drain into the iliac, hypogastric, superficial inguinal, and sacral lymph nodes.

C. Female dogs (Figs. 1–20 and 1–21).

1. The urethra of female dogs is shorter than that of males, and has a larger and more uniform diameter.
   a. It originates from the neck of the urinary bladder and terminates in an orifice located in the floor of the vestibule on a small ridge-like elevation called the urethral tubercle.
   b. The urethral tubercle is located cranial to the clitoris, about 4 to 5 cm from the ventral commissure of the vulva.
   c. The dorsal aspect of the urethra lies in close proximity to the ventral wall of the vagina.
2. The smooth muscle of the urethra of female dogs is composed of outer and inner longitudinal layers and a middle circular layer.
3. Immediately cranial to the external urethral orifice, the vagina and urethra are surrounded by the striated urethralis muscle. This muscle is under

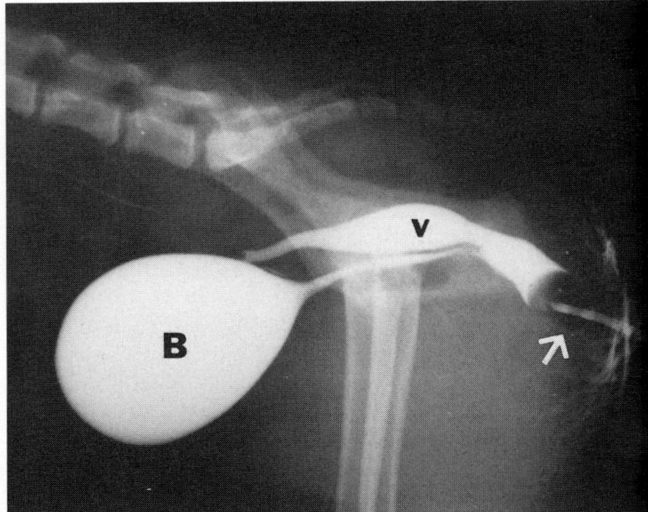

FIG. 1–20. Retrograde vaginourethrocystogram of a normal adult female dog. The inflated balloon of a Foley catheter is visible in the urethra (arrow). V = vagina; B = urinary bladder. The urethral lumen is not maximally distended with contrast medium.

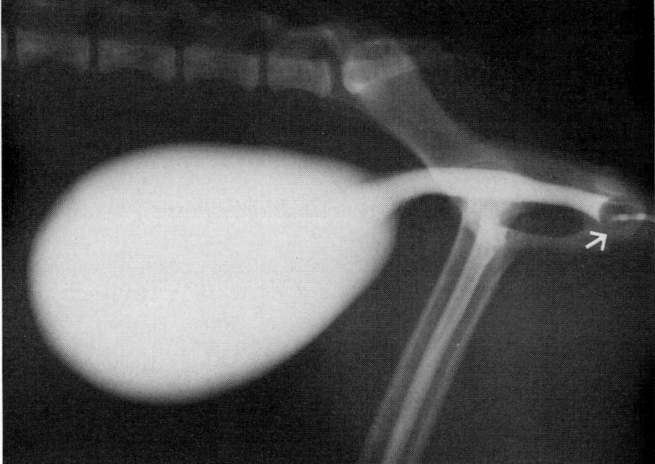

FIG. 1–21. Retrograde urethrocystogram of a normal adult female dog. The distended balloon of a Swan-Ganz catheter is visible in the distal urethra (arrow). Compare to Figure 1–20. (Courtesy of Dr. Gary R. Johnston, University of Minnesota.)

voluntary control and comprises the primary component of the external urethral sphincter.[18]

4. The proximal portion of the urethra in a female dog is lined by transitional epithelium, but changes to stratified cuboidal or stratified columnar epithelium in distal portions.[8] The submucosa is highly vascular.
5. The blood supply to the urethra of a female dog is derived from the caudal vesical branches of the vaginal artery.[24]
6. Lymphatic drainage is similar to that of male dogs.

D. Male cats (Fig. 1–22). The urethra of male cats may be divided into four segments for descriptive purposes.

1. The preprostatic urethra extends from the neck of the urinary bladder to the prostate gland.
   a. The prostate gland of cats is located 3 to 4 cm caudal to the bladder neck.
   b. The preprostatic urethra contains smooth muscle.
2. The prostatic urethra traverses the prostate gland. The postprostatic (membranous) urethra extends from the prostate gland to the paired bulbourethral glands, which are located at the level of the ischial arch of the bony pelvis on the dorsolateral surface of the urethra.
   a. This segment of the urethra contains functionally insignificant smooth muscle.
   b. It is surrounded by a thick layer of striated muscle (urethralis muscle). The urethralis muscle of male cats is thicker but shorter than the same muscle in dogs.[20]
   c. The submucosa of the postprostatic urethra contains so-called "disseminate" prostate glands, which may produce mucus.[20]
3. The penile urethra extends from the level of the bulbourethral glands to the tip of the penis.
   a. It lies along the dorsal surface of the penis embedded in the corpus spongiosum penis (Fig. 1–23).

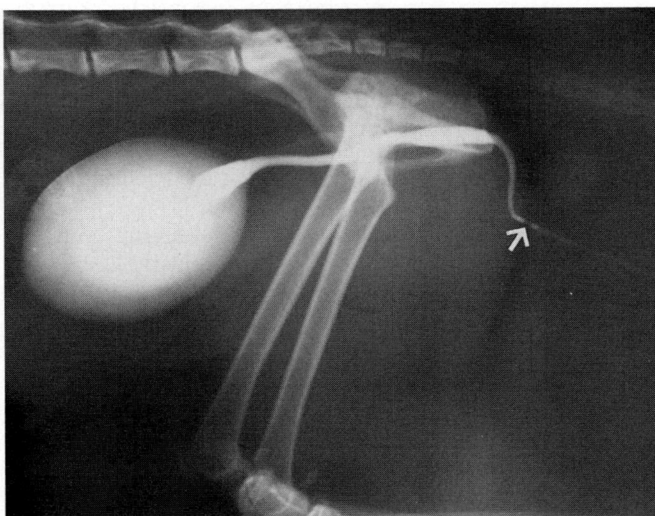

FIG. 1–22. Normal retrograde contrast urethrocystogram of an adult male domestic short-haired cat. The distended balloon of a Swan-Ganz catheter is visible in the distal urethra (arrow). Compare to Figure 1–1. (Courtesy of Dr. Gary R. Johnston, University of Minnesota.)

b. The os penis, when present, is not grooved to accommodate the penile urethra.
c. The diameter of the penile urethra becomes progressively smaller toward the external urethral orifice.

4. The prostate gland in cats is much less developed than that in dogs, and the prostatic urethra of cats is correspondingly shorter (Fig. 1–24).
   a. The prostate gland of male cats does not surround the ventral portion of the prostatic urethra.
   b. Although this section of the prostatic urethra is short, it is occasionally seen as a narrowed region in the midpelvic area of contrast urethrograms.[46] The mucosal lining of the urethra in a male cat is similar to that of the dog.
   c. The penile urethra is lined by stratified columnar epithelium.
   d. The postprostatic (membranous) urethra is lined by stratified columnar and transitional epithelium.[8]

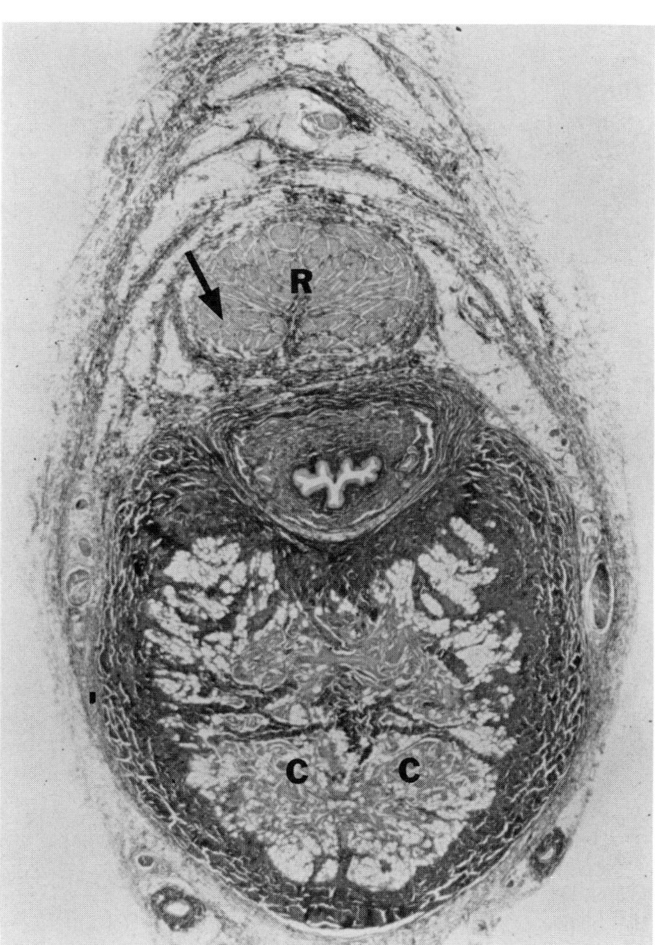

FIG. 1–23. Cross section of the penis of a male cat. R = retractor penis muscle; C = corpus cavernosum penis; arrow = urethral lumen. (Magnification, 12×.) (Courtesy of Dr. W.C. Cullen.)

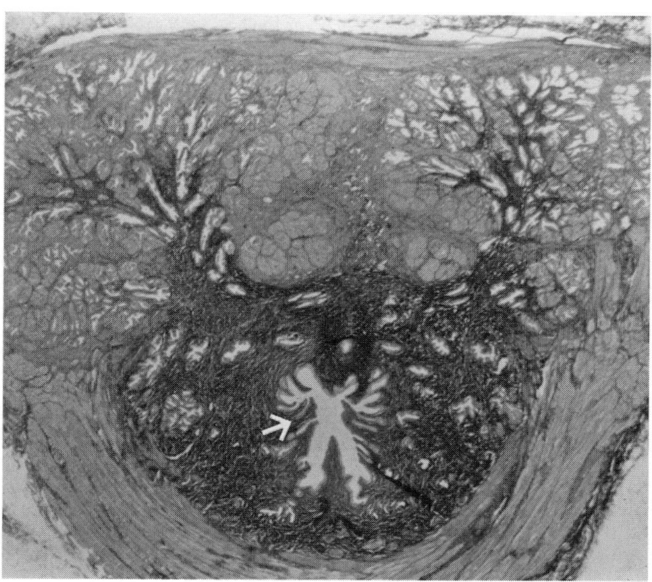

FIG. 1–24. Cross section of the prostatic urethra of a male cat illustrates the anatomic relationship of the prostrate gland dorsal to the urethra. Arrow = urethral lumen. (Magnification, 12×.) (Courtesy of Dr. W.C. Cullen.)

5. The preprostatic urethra is lined by transitional epithelium.
6. The blood supply to the urethra of a male cat is derived from the urogenital (prostatic) artery and the internal pudendal artery.

E. Female cats (Fig. 1–25).

1. The urethra of the female cat is similar in structure and location to that of the female dog.
   a. It extends from the urinary bladder between the vaginal wall and floor of the bony pelvis to the caudal portion of the vagina, where it opens in a groove in the floor of the vestibule.
   b. It is shorter in length and larger in diameter than the urethra of male cats.
2. As was the situation in dogs, the vagina and urethra immediately cranial to the vestibule are surrounded by the striated urethralis muscle. This muscle is proportionately smaller in female cats than in female dogs.[21]
3. The distal and midportion of the urethra are lined by stratified cuboidal or columnar epithelium, which changes to transitional epithelium near the urinary bladder.[8]
4. The blood supply to the urethra is derived from the vaginal (urogenital) artery.

F. Function.

1. The urethra plays a key role in maintaining urinary continence during the storage phase of micturition by virtue of its internal sphincter and external sphincter mechanisms. During the voiding phase of micturition, it provides a low-resistance conduit, which channels urine to the exterior.

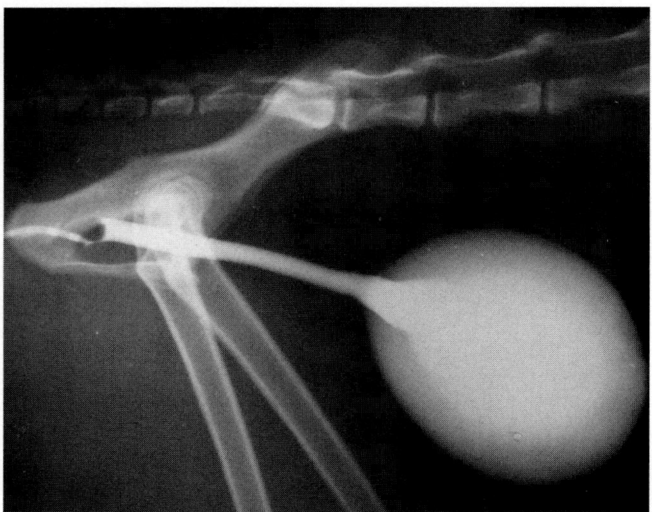

FIG. 1–25. Normal retrograde contrast urethrocystogram of an adult female domestic short-haired cat. The distended balloon of a Swan-Ganz catheter can be seen in the distal urethra. Compare to Figure 1–2. (Courtesy of Dr. Gary R. Johnston, University of Minnesota.)

2. The urethra contains an integrated anatomic and functional defense system that prevents retrograde passage of pathogens and semen into proximal portions of the urinary tract.[69]
3. In males, the urethra transports contents produced in the genital system to the exterior.
4. The frequency with which male cats develop urethral obstruction prompts questions about the functional purpose of the anatomic configuration of the male urethra.
   a. Perhaps the mechanism facilitates urine spraying to mark their domain.
   b. It may also be important in copulation because male cats produce only a small volume of ejaculate (less than 1 mL).[81]
   c. The fluid dynamics of the urethra of male cats appear to be a prototype of the garden hose with adjustable nozzle.

REFERENCES

1. Anderson, A.C.: Renal system. *In* The Beagle as an Experimental Dog. Edited by A.C. Anderson and L.S. Good. Ames, IA, Iowa State University Press, 1970.
2. Bannigan, J.: The structure and function of the ureter in the dog. Ir. J. Med. Sci., 144:426-436, 1975.
3. Barber, D.L.: Renal angiography in veterinary medicine. J. Am. Vet. Rad. Soc., 1975; 16:187-205.
4. Beeuwkes, R.: Efferent vascular patterns and early vascular-tubular relations in the dog kidney. Am. J. Physiol., 221:1361-1374, 1971.
5. Beeuwkes, R., and Bonaventure, J.V.: Tubular organization and vascular tubular relations in the dog kidney. Am. J. Physiol., 229:695-713, 1975.
6. Beeuwkes, R.: The vascular organization of the kidney. Annu. Rev. Physiol., 42:531-542, 1980.
7. Beeuwkes, R., Ichikawa, I., Brenner, B.M.: The renal circulations. *In* The Kidney, 2nd Edition. Vol. 1. Edited by B.M. Brenner and F.C. Rector. Philadelphia, W.B. Saunders, 1981.
8. Bharadwaj, M.B., and Calhoun, M.L.: Histology of the urethral epithelium of domestic animals. Am. J. Vet. Res., 20:841-851, 1959.
9. Boyarsky, S., and Labay, P.: Principles of ureteral physiology. *In* The Ureter, 2nd Edition. Edited by H. Bergman. New York: Springer-Verlag, 1981.
10. Brodsky, S.L., Dure-Smith, P., Zimskind, P.D.: Gross and radiologic anatomy of the canine kidney. Invest. Urol., 14:356-360, 1977.
11. Bulger, R.E., Cronin, R.E., Dobyan, D.C.: Survey morphology of the dog kidney. Anat. Rec., 194:41-66, 1979.
12. Butcher, H.R., and Sleator, W.: A study of electrical activity of intact and partially mobilized human ureters. J. Urol., 73:970, 1955.
13. Caulfield, J.P., and Farquhar, M.G.: Distribution of anionic sites in glomerular basement membranes: Their possible role in filtration and attachment. Proc. Natl. Acad. Sci., 73:1646, 1976.
14. Christie, B.A.: The ureterovesical junction in dogs. Invest. Urol., 9:10-15, 1971.
15. Christie, B.A.: Incidence and etiology of vesicoureteral reflux in apparently normal dogs. Invest. Urol., 9:184-194, 1971.
16. Christie, B.A.: Vesicoureteral reflux in dogs. J. Am. Vet. Med. Assoc., 162:772, 1973.
17. Christie, B.A.: Collateral arterial blood supply to the normal and ischemic canine kidney. Am. J. Vet. Res., 41:1519-1525, 1980.
18. Cullen, W.C., Fletcher, T.F., Bradley, W.E.: Histology of the canine urethra. I. Morphometry of the female urethra. Anat. Rec., 199:177-186, 1981.
19. Cullen, W.C., Fletcher, T.F., Bradley, W.E.: Histology of the canine urethra. II. Morphometry of the male pelvic urethra. Anat. Rec., 199:187-195, 1981.
20. Cullen, W.C., Fletcher, T.F., Bradley, W.E.: Morphometry of the male feline pelvic urethra. J. Urol., 129:186-189, 1983.
21. Cullen, W.C., Fletcher, T.F., Bradley, W.E.: Morphometry of the female feline urethra. J. Urol., 129:186-189, 1983a.
22. DeGroat, W.C., and Booth, A.M.: Physiology of the urinary bladder and urethra. Ann. Intern. Med., 92:212-315, 1980.
23. Edmond, P., Ross, J.A., Kirkland, I.S.: Human ureteral peristalsis. J. Urol., 104:670-674, 1970.
24. Evans, H.E., and Christenson, G.C.: Anatomy of the Dog, 2nd Edition. Philadelphia, W.B. Saunders, 1979.
25. Feeney, D.A., et al.: Normal canine excretory urogram: Affects of dose, time, and individual dog variation. Am. J. Vet. Res., 40:1596-1604, 1979.
26. Feeney, D.A., et al.: Normal canine excretory urogram: Effects of dose, time, and individual dog variation. Am. J. Vet. Res., 40:1596-1604, 1981.
27. Finco, D.R.: Kidney function. *In* Clinical Biochemistry of Domestic Animals, 3rd Edition. Edited by J.J. Kaneko. New York, Academic Press, 1980.
28. Finco, D.R., Barsanti, J.A., Crowell, W.A.: The urinary system. *In* Feline Medicine. Edited by P.W. Pratt. Santa Barbara, CA, American Veterinary Publications, 1983.
29. Finco, D.R., and Duncan, J.R.: Relationship of glomerular number and diameter to body size of the dog. Am. J. Vet. Res., 33:2447-2450, 1972.
30. Finco, D.R., et al.: Radiologic estimation of kidney size in the dog. J. Am. Vet. Med. Assoc., 159:995-1000, 1971.
31. Finkbeiner, A.E., and Bissada, N.K.: Drug therapy for lower urinary tract dysfunction. Urol. Clin. North Am., 7:3-16, 1980.
32. Fischer, C.P., and Sonda, L.P.: Cryoprecipitate: Its use and effects in canine coagulum pyelolithotomy. Invest. Urol., 16:266-269, 1979.

33. Fletcher, T.E.: Anatomy of pelvic viscera. Vet. Clin. North Am., 4:471-486, 1974.
34. Fourman, J., and Moffat, D.B.: The Blood Vessels of the Kidney. Philadelphia, Blackwell Scientific Publications, F.A. Davis, 1971.
35. Gillette, E.L., Thrall, D.E., Label, J.L., Corwin, L.A.: Veterinary Radiology. Philadelphia, Lea & Febiger, 1977.
36. Gordon, N.: Surgical anatomy of the bladder, prostate gland, and urethra. J. Am. Vet. Med. Assoc., 136:215-221, 1960.
37. Grandage, J.: Some effects of posture on the radiographic appearance of the kidneys of the dog. J. Am. Vet. Med. Assoc., 166:165-166, 1975.
38. Gruber, C.M.: A comparative study of the intra-vesical ureters in man and experimental animals. J. Urol., 21:567-581, 1929.
39. Hall, V.E., and MacGregor, W.W.: Relation of kidney weight to body weight in the cat. Anat. Rec., 69:319-331, 1937.
40. Hanna, M.K.: Clinical application of hydrodynamics of the ureter and renal pelvis. *In* The Ureter, 2nd Edition. Edited by H. Bergman. New York, Springer-Verlag, 1981.
41. Hannappel, J., and Golenhofen, K.: Comparative studies on normal ureteral peristalsis in dogs, guinea-pigs, and rats. Pflugers Arch., 348:65-76, 1974.
42. Hicks, R.M.: The permeability of rat transitional epithelium. J. Cell Biol., 28:21-31, 1966.
43. Hicks, R.W., and Wakefield, J.S.: Experimental tumors. *In* Scientific Foundation of Urology. Vol. 2. Edited by D.I. Williams and G.D. Chisholm. Chicago, Year Book Medical Publishing, 1976.
44. Hoyer, J.R., and Seiler, M.W.: Kidney Int., 16:279-289, 1979.
45. Jackson, B., and Capiello, V.P.: Ranges of normal organ weight of dogs. Toxicol. Appl. Pharmacol., 6:664-668, 1964.
46. Johnston, G.R., Feeney, D.A., Osborne, C.A.: Urethrography and cystography in cats. Part I. Techniques, normal radiographic anatomy, and artifacts. Comp. Cont. Ed., 4:823-836, 1982.
47. Johnston, G.R., Feeney, D.A., Osborne, C.A.: Urethrography and cystography in cats. Part II. Abnormal radiographic anatomy and complications. Comp. Cont. Ed., 4:931-946, 1982.
48. Kal, F.: Physiology of the renal pelvis and ureter. *In* Campbell's Urology, 4th Edition. Vol. 1. Edited by J.H. Harrison. Philadelphia, W.B. Saunders, 1978.
49. Khanna, O.P.: Disorders of micturition. Neuropharmacologic basis and results of drug therapy. Urology, 8:316-328, 1976.
50. Kneller, S.K.: Role of the excretory urogram in the diagnosis of renal and ureteral disease. Vet. Clin. North Am., 4:843-861, 1974.
51. Kunkel, P.A.: The number and size of glomeruli in the kidney of several mammals. Bull. Johns Hopkins Hosp., 47:285-291, 1930.
52. Lapides, J.: The physiology of the intact human ureter. J. Urol., 59:501, 1948.
53. Lee, R., and Leowijuk, C.: Normal parameters in abdominal radiology of the dog and cat. J. Small Anim. Pract., 23:251, 1982.
54. Lich, R., Howerton, L.W., Amin, M.: Anatomy and surgical approach to the urogenital tract in the male. *In* Campbell's Urology, 4th Edition. Edited by J.H. Harrison, et al. Philadelphia, W.B. Saunders, 1978.
55. Lloyd-Davies, W.R., Hayes, T.L., Hinman, F.: Urothelial microcontour. I. Scanning electron microscopy of normal resting and stretched urethra and bladder. J. Urol., 105:236, 1971.
56. Lord, P.F., Scott, R.C., Chan, K.F.: Intravenous urography for evaluation of renal disease in small animals. J. Am. Anim. Hosp. Assoc., 10:139-152, 1974.
57. Ludders, J.W., Wilson, J.W., Ribble, G.A.: Microangiography and correlated histology: A research technique for examining renal microcirculation. Am. J. Vet. Res., 46:2536-2538, 1985.
58. Macfarlane, W.V.: Water and electrolytes in domestic animals. *In* Veterinary Physiology. Edited by J.W. Phillis. Philadelphia, W.B. Saunders, 1976.
59. McKenna, O.C., and Angelakos, E.T.: Adrenergic innervation of the canine kidney. Circ. Res., 22:345, 1961.
60. McKenna, O.C., and Angelakos, E.T.: Acetylcholinesterase-containing nerve fibers in the canine kidney. Circ. Res., 23:645, 1968.
61. Mooney, J.K., and Hinman, F.: Surface differences in cells of proximal and distal canine urethra. J. Urol., 111:495, 1974.
62. Moreau, P.M.: Neurogenic disorders of micturition in the dog and cat. Comp. Cont. Ed., 4:2-21, 1982.
63. Mygind, T., and Hald, T.: Radiological analysis of urethral morphology and function in male dogs. Invest. Radiol., 1:301-305, 1966.
64. Nissen, O.I., and Galskov, A.: Direct measurement of the superficial and deep venous flow in the cat kidney. Circ. Res., 30:82-96, 1972.
65. Oliver, J.E., and Lorenz, M.D.: Handbook of Veterinary Neurologic Diagnosis. Philadelphia, W.B. Saunders, 1983.
66. Osborne, C.A., Finco, D.R., Low, D.G.: Pathophysiology of renal disease, renal failure, and uremia. *In* Textbook of Veterinary Internal Medicine. Edited by S.J. Ettinger. Philadelphia, W.B. Saunders, 1983.
67. Osborne, C.A., et al.: The glomerulus in health and disease: A comparative review of domestic animals and man. Adv. Vet. Sci. Comp. Med., 21:207-285, 1977.
68. Osborne, C.A., and Klausner, J.S.: War on urolithiasis: Problems and their solutions. South Bend, IN, 1978 Scientific Proceedings AAHA, 1978.
69. Osborne, C.A., Klausner, J.S., Lees, G.E.: Urinary tract infections: Normal and abnormal host defense mechanisms. Vet. Clin. North Am., 9:587-609, 1979.
70. Osborne, C.A., and Low, D.G.: Size, adequacy and artifacts of canine renal biopsy samples. Am. J. Vet. Res., 32:1865-1871, 1971.
71. Osborne, C.A., Low, D.G., Finco, D.R.: Canine and feline urology. Philadelphia, W.B. Saunders, 1972.
72. Pitts, R.F.: Physiology of the Kidney and Body Fluids, 3rd Edition. Chicago, Year Book Medical Publishing, 1974.
73. Reis, R.H., and Tepe, P.: Variations in the patterns of renal vessels and their relation to the type of posterior vena cava in the dog. Am. J. Anat., 99:1-55, 1956.
74. Rieck, A.F., and Reis, R.H.: Variations in patterns of renal vessels and their relation to the type of posterior vena cava in the cat. Am. J. Anat., 93:457-474, 1953.
75. Rytand, D.A.: The number and size of mammalian glomeruli as related to kidney and to body weight, and methods for their enumeration and measurement. Am. J. Anat., 62:507-520, 1938.
76. Schmidt-Nielsen, B.: Urinary concentrating processes in vertebrates. Yale J. Biol. Med., 52:545-561, 1979.
77. Schmidt-Nielsen, B., and O'Dell, R.: Structure and concentrating mechanism in the mammalian kidney. Am. J. Physiol., 200: 1119-1124, 1961.
78. Sellwood, R.V., and Verney, E.B.: Enumeration of glomeruli in the kidney of the dog. J. Anat., 89:63-68, 1955.
79. Sherwood, T., Lavender, J.P., Greenspan, R.H.: Renal magnification angiograms in the dog. Br. J. Radiol., 42:241-246, 1969.
80. Shively, M.J.: Origin and branching of renal arteries in the dog. J. Am. Vet. Med. Assoc., 173:986-989, 1978.
81. Sojka, N.J.: Feline semen collection, evaluation, and artificial insemination. *In* Current Therapy in Theriogenology. Edited by D.A. Morrow. Philadelphia, W.B. Saunders, 1980.
82. Tanagho, E.A.: Development of the ureter. *In* The Ureter, 2nd Edition. Edited by H. Bergman. New York, Springer-Verlag, 1981.
83. Tisher, C.C., and Madsen, K.M.: Anatomy of the kidney. *In* The

Kidney, 3rd Edition. Vol. 1. Edited by B.M. Brenner and F.C. Rector. Philadelphia, W.B. Saunders, 1986.
84. Velardo, J.T.: Histology of the ureter. *In* The Ureter, 2nd Edition. Edited by H. Bergman. New York, Springer-Verlag, 1981.
85. Weinberg, S.L.: Ureteral function. III. The catheter and the geometry of the ureter (canine). Invest. Urol., 13:339, 1976.
86. Weiss, R.M.: Ureteral function. Urology, 12:114-133, 1978.
87. Weiss, R.M.: Clinical implications of ureteral physiology. J. Urol., 121:401-413, 1979.
88. Welling, L.W., and Welling, D.J.: Surface areas of brush border and lateral cell walls in the rabbit proximal nephron. Kidney Int., 8:343-348, 1975.
89. Wendel, R.M., and King, L.R.: Ureteral peristasis (dog). Invest. Urol., 10:354-358, 1973.
90. Zimskind, P.D.: The renal pelvis and calyces. *In* Urodynamics. Edited by S. Boyarsky, et al. New York, Academic Press, 1971.

CHAPTER 2

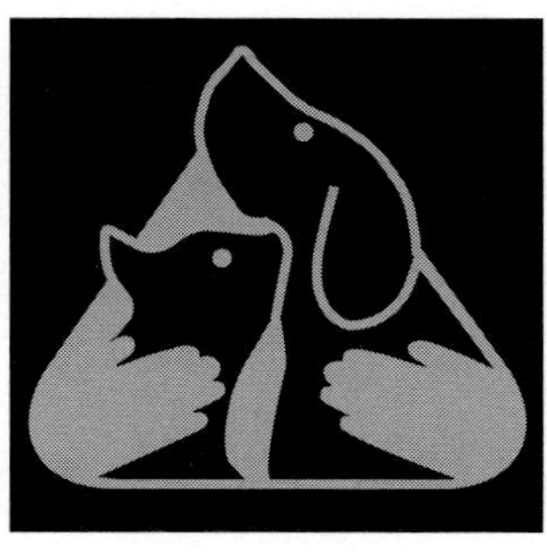

Applied Physiology of the Kidney

DELMAR R. FINCO

I. OVERVIEW OF URINE FORMATION AND ELIMINATION

A. The kidneys play an essential role in life by eliminating metabolic wastes from the body and by maintaining electrolyte and acid-base homeostasis. An understanding of formation and elimination of urine is an essential prerequisite for diagnosis, prognosis, and treatment of disorders of the urinary system.

B. The functional unit of the kidney is the nephron, which is composed of a glomerulus, proximal tubule, loop of Henle, distal tubule, and collecting duct (Fig. 2–1). In each nephron, formation of urine results from three basic processes: glomerular filtration, tubular reabsorption, and tubular secretion. These mechanisms are modified by several hormones of renal and nonrenal origin.

C. Nearly all blood going to the kidneys via the renal arteries enters the glomerular capillaries (Fig. 2–2). The walls of glomerular capillaries are porous to water and other small-molecular-weight molecules. About one fourth to one third of plasma water escapes from the glomerular capillary lumens into Bowman's spaces. The massive volume of filtrate formed is reduced in volume as it passes from Bowman's spaces through the nephrons. The force for filtration is hydraulic (hydrostatic) pressure that is generated by contraction of the heart. Because water and small molecules pass through the filter readily, they appear in filtrate in nearly the same concentrations as they exist in plasma. However, the barrier to passage of material through the capillary wall increases as molecular size increases. Generally, compounds with a molecular weight greater than 70,000 daltons cannot pass through glomerular capillary pores. For compounds with approximately this molecular weight, electrical charge and shape are additional factors affecting filtration. During filtration, blood cells and most plasma proteins are retained in the glomerular capillary lumens and leave the glomerular capillaries via the efferent arteriole (see Fig. 2–2).

D. The renal tubule modifies filtrate by reducing its volume and altering its composition. Major objectives of this modification include:

1. Maintenance of water balance.
2. Maintenance of electrolyte balance, particularly with regard to sodium, potassium, phosphorus, magnesium, and chloride.
3. Acid-base homeostasis.
4. Excretion of nitrogenous wastes.

E. Tubular functions are influenced by several factors, including glomerular function (glomerulotubular balance), blood composition, and

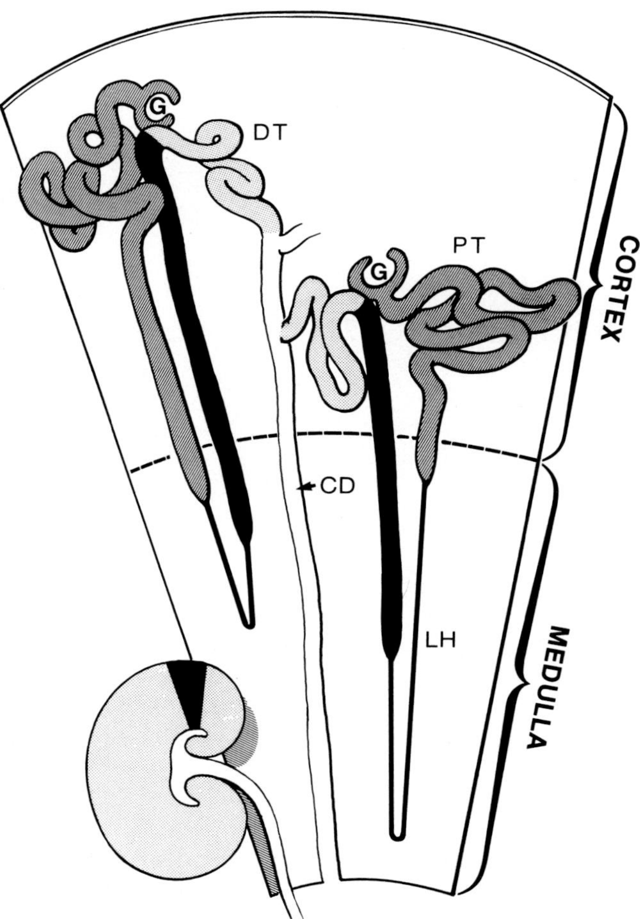

FIG. 2–1. Schematic representation of two nephrons. Glomerulus (G), proximal tubule (PT), distal tubule (DT), and part of the collecting duct (CD) and loop of Henle are located in the cortex; the remaining loop of Henle (LH) and part of the CD are medullary.

responses to hormones released by other body organs.

1. Tubular reabsorption returns needed components to the body after their passage into the tubule lumen following glomerular filtration. The route of this return is tubule lumen, tubule cell or intercellular paths, renal interstitium, peritubular capillaries, renal venous system, and finally the systemic circulation (Fig. 2–3).
2. Tubular secretion adds materials to the tubule lumens. Materials not filtered by glomeruli pass on to the peritubular capillary network by way of efferent glomerular arteries. Depending on protein binding and the permeability of peritubular capillary walls, substances may diffuse into the renal interstitium, where they become available at the basolateral membrane of tubule cells for transport into the tubular lumen.

F. The kidneys produce or modify hormones, respond to hormones, and degrade hormones.

1. Hormones produced or modified by the kidneys include:
   a. Erythropoeitin.
   b. Calcitriol—25-OH vitamin is hydroxylated at C-1 to form the most active form of vitamin D, 1,25-$(OH)_2$ vitamin D (calcitriol).
   c. Renin—required both for intrarenal and systemic generation of angiotensin II.
2. Hormones to which the kidney responds include atrial natriuretic peptide, aldosterone, antidiuretic hormone (ADH), parathyroid hormone (PTH), thyroid hormone, growth hormone, and others.
3. The kidneys degrade and eliminate hormones, including PTH, thyroid hormone, insulin, and thyrotropic hormone.

G. The collection and unidirectional transport of urine from the renal pelvis to the bladder and the elimination of urine by micturition complete the excretory process. Urine that accumulates in the renal pelvis initiates peristaltic movement of pelvic and then ureteral smooth muscle. As a result, boluses of urine are propelled through the ureteral lumen to the urinary bladder. Anatomic ureterovesical sphincters are not present, but the oblique course of

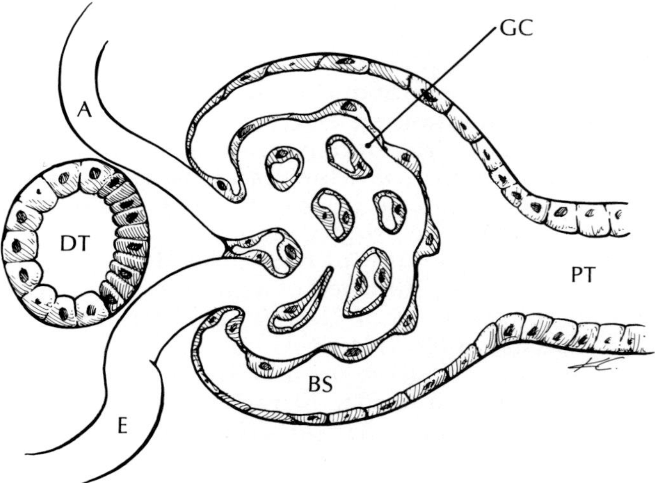

FIG. 2–2. Schematic drawing of a glomerulus and surrounding structures. Blood enters the glomerular capillaries (GC) via the afferent arteriole (A). Fluid forced through the capillary walls moves into Bowman's space (BS) before entering the proximal tubule (PT). Blood cells and unfiltered fluid leave via the efferent arteriole (E). Located between the arterioles is the distal tubule (DT); the arteriolar arrangement with the DT facilitates the operation of tubuloglomerular feedback (see text). Resistance (tone) in the A and E modulates glomerular filtration rate by influencing blood flow, and thus hydraulic pressure, in the GC.

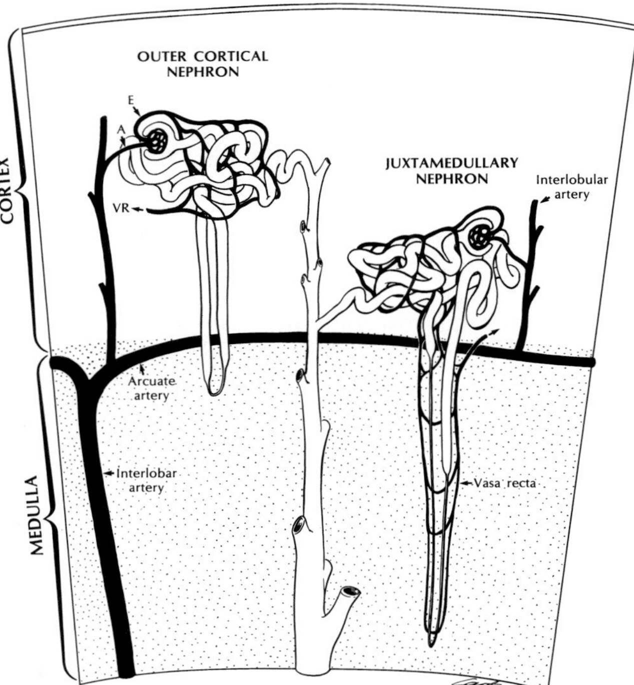

FIG. 2–3. Circulation of blood in the kidney. Efferent arterioles (E) from outer cortical and midcortical (not shown) glomeruli divide into a peritubular capillary network that provides for blood-tubule exchange in the cortex. Juxtamedullary efferent arterioles give rise to vasa recta, which course into the medulla and then return to the cortex. Slow blood flow through the vasa recta allows maintenance of medullary hypertonicity, which is essential for urine concentration. A = afferent arteriole; VR = vasa recta.

the ureters through the bladder wall at the trigone forms a flap valve that normally prevents retrograde flow of urine from the bladder. Ureterovesical valves protect the kidneys from abnormal retrograde pressure and from reflux of bladder urine.

H. Micturition is the act of expelling urine from the urinary bladder via the urethra. Micturition is a reflex facilitated and inhibited by higher brain centers. Like defecation, it is subject to voluntary initiation and inhibition. (See Chapter 14, Tests of Lower Urinary Tract Function in Dogs and Cats.)

II. REQUIREMENTS FOR NORMAL KIDNEY FUNCTION

A. Adequate perfusion of the kidneys.

1. The kidneys of the dog normally receive 10 to 20% of cardiac output.[31] This translates into a renal blood flow (RBF) of about 20 ml per minute per kg of body weight, or a renal plasma flow (RPF) of about 12 mL per minute per kilogram of body weight.
2. Adequate blood flow through the kidneys depends on two factors:
   a. Delivery of blood at appropriate pressures to the kidney.
   b. A suitable state of intrarenal vascular tone that allows blood to enter the kidneys rather than being diverted away.
3. Adequate RBF is a prerequisite for normal renal function.
   a. Most excretory functions of the kidney depend on glomerular filtration. As subsequently reviewed, the rate of glomerular filtration (GFR) depends on intraglomerular hydrostatic pressure. Hydrostatic pressure is a function of arteriolar resistances and RBF.
   b. Although less than needed for filtration, blood flow is also required to provide nutrients and O_2 to renal cells so that their metabolism can be maintained.
4. Extrarenal factors that may alter RBF include:
   a. Cardiac output.
   b. Circulatory volume.
   c. Systemic vascular resistance.
5. Intrarenal vascular factors that may alter RBF include:
   a. Anatomic patency of renal vessels.
   b. Vascular tone, particularly of the afferent and efferent arterioles (see Fig. 2–2). Vascular tone is modified by several hormones produced extrarenally (angiotensin II, catecholamines, ADH), by renal sympathetic innervation, and by substances produced intrarenally (prostaglandins, angiotensin II, nitric oxide).
6. Inadequate RBF may lead to functional abnormalities, the extent of which is related to the degree and duration of the decreased RBF.
   a. Azotemia is defined as the abnormal accumulation of nitrogenous wastes (urea nitrogen and creatinine) in blood. Azotemia is said to be prerenal when decreased RBF impairs glomerular filtration, but perfusion is still adequate for renal cells to remain viable.
   b. If RBF is decreased severely and for a sufficiently long time, renal cell ischemia occurs. This condition (renal ischemia) is one cause of acute renal failure. (See Chapter 22, Acute Renal Failure: Ischemia and Chemical Nephrosis.)
7. Some causes of prerenal azotemia are:
   a. Decreased cardiac output (cardiac valvular insufficiency or stenosis, myocardial disease, arrhythmias, congenital anomalies, dirofilariasis, cardiac tamponade).
   b. Decreased circulatory volume (dehydration, shock, adrenocortical insufficiency, reduced colloid osmotic pressure resulting from severe hypoalbuminemia).

c. Decreased autoregulatory function (see Section III-A of this chapter).

8. Prerenal azotemia causes clinical signs identical to those of azotemia of other causes to be reviewed subsequently. Laboratory evaluation of blood urea nitrogen (BUN) and serum creatinine concentrations and their ratios are not of value in differentiating prerenal and primary renal azotemia in dogs.[15] However, renal concentrating ability is usually present with prerenal azotemia, but may be impaired with primary renal failure. (See Chapter 10, Evaluation of Renal Functions.)

B. Normal renal function also requires a sufficient quantity of functional renal tissue. Inadequate functional renal tissue causes primary renal azotemia.

1. The kidneys have considerable functional reserve; signs of renal failure do not occur until two thirds to three fourths of both kidneys are nonfunctional. (See Chapter 16, Pathophysiology of Renal Failure and Uremia.)
2. A decrease in the quantity of functional renal tissue below one fourth of normal is associated with primary renal failure and uremia. If the loss of functional tissue is gradual, however, compensatory changes often permit survival with much less than one fourth of the total functional renal tissue. (See Chapter 16, Pathophysiology of Renal Failure and Uremia.)

C. Patent and functional urine outflow tract.

1. A small amount of the hydraulic pressure that causes glomerular filtration forces the filtrate through the lumens of the renal tubules into the renal pelvis. Once in the renal pelvis, urine accumulation stimulates smooth muscle contraction of the pelvis and a peristaltic contraction of the ureter. This action forces the urine into the urinary bladder. A functional bladder and patent urethra are necessary for subsequent elimination of urine from the body.
2. Obstruction to urine flow anywhere in the outflow system may lead to postrenal azotemia. Azotemia occurs primarily because glomerular filtration is opposed by backpressure that develops proximal to the site of obstruction. (See Chapter 42, Obstructive Uropathy and Hydronephrosis.)
3. Because common tests of renal function are relatively insensitive, outflow obstruction does not cause detectable azotemia unless it affects both kidneys.
4. Tests of renal function do not distinguish between postrenal azotemia and other types of azotemia.
5. Some causes of postrenal azotemia are:
   a. Urethral obstruction from any cause (e.g., calculi, displacement of the urinary bladder, urethral or prostatic neoplasia).
   b. Obstructive lesions of the bladder trigone, or other lesions that impair urine outflow from both ureters.
   c. Rupture of both ureters, the bladder, or the proximal urethra.

III. MECHANISMS OF KIDNEY FUNCTION

A. RBF and autoregulation.

1. Renal functions depend on adequate flow of blood through the kidney and adequate formation of glomerular filtrate. Recall that 10 to 20% of cardiac output normally perfuses the kidneys.
2. Intrarenal control of blood flow exists in health to keep RBF (and thus GFR) constant over a range of blood pressures from about 70 to 180 mm Hg. This phenomenon is called autoregulation (Fig. 2–4).
3. Two major theories have emerged to explain autoregulation.
   a. Myogenic theory. The preglomerular vessels (afferent arteriole and more proximal arteries) may alter their tone in direct response to blood pressure to achieve constant RBF and GFR.[40]
   b. Tubuloglomerular feedback theory.[51]
      (1). The ascending limb of the loop of Henle passes between the afferent and efferent arterioles, adjacent to the glomerulus (see Fig. 2–2). These anatomic structures are referred to as the juxtaglomerular apparatus.
      (2). Contents of the lumen of the ascending limb of the loop of Henle may initiate a signal that is transmitted to the arterioles.

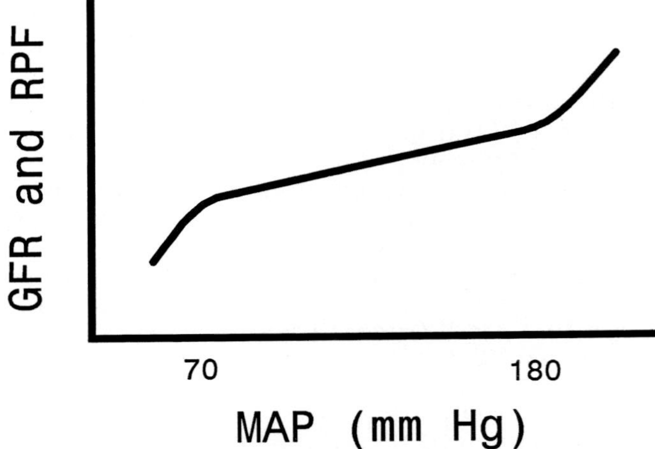

FIG. 2–4. Autoregulation. Between systemic blood pressure values of 70 to 180 mm Hg, glomerular filtration rate (GFR) and renal plasma flow (RPF) are maintained relatively constant because afferent arteriole resistance is modulated to prevent changes in glomerular capillary hydraulic pressure. Ability to autoregulate is blunted during renal failure, as well as some other diseases or states. MAP = mean arterial pressure.

Chloride transport and osmolality have been described as the signals.

(3). The response to the signal is a modification of arteriolar muscle tone that in turn affects RBF and GFR.

4. Autoregulation occurs normally, but it does not necessarily persist with disease. Loss of autoregulatory capacity may account for azotemia in some clinical states.

B. Glomerular filtration.[2,5,18,37]

1. Movement of fluid through the glomerular capillary walls into Bowman's space occurs as the net effect of several factors.
2. These factors are given in the following equation and illustrated in Figure 2–5.

$$GFR = K \times (P_{GC} - P_T) - ({}_{GC} - {}_{T})$$

a. K = effective permeability

b. P_{GC} = hydraulic (hydrostatic) pressure in the capillary lumen

c. P_T = hydraulic pressure in Bowman's space

d. ${}_{GC}$ = COP (colloid osmotic pressure) in the capillary lumen

e. ${}_{T}$ = COP in Bowman's space

3. The major force pushing fluid from the capillary lumen into Bowman's space is hydraulic pressure (P_{GC}).

a. Measurements in dogs indicate that hydraulic pressure in glomerular capillaries is about 60 mm Hg.[60]

b. The COP in Bowman's space has the potential to enhance filtration, but the protein concentration in fluid here is so low (0.1 to 10.0 mg/dL) that COP of filtrate is not normally a factor in filtration.

4. Forces opposing filtration are plasma COP (${}_{GC}$) and hydraulic pressure in Bowman's space (P_T).

a. Plasma COP is about 28 mm Hg at the beginning of the glomerular capillary bed. Because the plasma proteins become more concentrated as fluid moves out of the capillary, COP is 36 mm Hg at the end of the capillary bed.

b. Pressure in Bowman's space is 18 mm Hg.

5. The difference between opposing forces can be summarized as follows: Outward force minus inward forces equals net filtration pressure, or 60 – (28 to 36 + 18) = 6 to 14 mm Hg (net filtration pressure).

6. Any factor altering these forces may modify filtration rate. For example:

a. A decrease in hydraulic pressure (i.e., shock, hypovolemia, dehydration) can decrease GFR if blood pressure falls below the autoregulation range or if autoregulation fails.

b. An increase in plasma COP (i.e., severe dehydration) decreases GFR.

c. An increase in hydrostatic pressure in tubules (i.e., ureteral or urethral obstruction) decreases GFR.

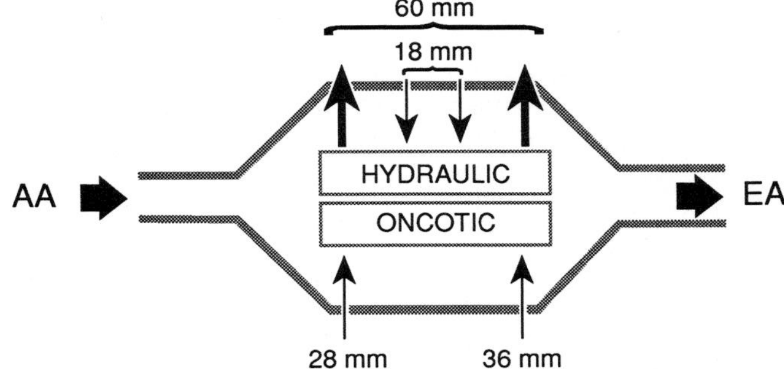

FIG. 2–5. Schematic illustration of forces operating in the process of glomerular filtration. Capillary hydraulic pressure (60 mm Hg) induces filtration, whereas colloid oncotic pressure (28 to 36 mm Hg) and Bowman's space hydraulic pressure (18 mm Hg) oppose filtration. AA = afferent arteriole; EA = efferent arteriole.

7. The effective permeability of the glomerular capillaries (K) depends on surface area and porosity.

a. Surface area.

(1). The surface area of a glomerulus can be altered by mesangial cells.

(2). Mesangial cells contain actin and are capable of contracting in response to certain stimuli, such as angiotensin II and ADH.

(3). Mesangial cell contraction decreases surface area and GFR.

(4). Diseases in which glomeruli are obliterated result in a decrease in total kidney glomerular capillary surface area and thus a decrease in GFR.

b. Porosity. Although the porosity of the glomerular filter is difficult experimentally to distinguish from that of its surface area, evidence has shown that the two factors may change independent of one another.

8. Normally about one fourth to one third of the blood plasma flowing through glomerular capillaries becomes filtrate. This is referred to as the filtration fraction. The filtration fraction can be calculated as follows from values for RPF and GFR.

$$\text{filtration fraction} = \frac{\text{glomerular filtration rate (GFR)}}{\text{renal plasma flow (RPF)}}$$

9. Passage of small molecules into filtrate.

a. Glomerular capillary walls are much more porous to water and other small molecules than are other body capillaries.

b. Water and other small-molecular-weight compounds pass into filtrate in essentially the same proportions, and thus the concentration of electrolytes, glucose, amino acids, and other small molecules is the same in plasma water as in glomerular filtrate, except for the following two factors.

(1). Plasma protein binding of particles.

(a). Plasma proteins, particularly albumin, may bind some charged particles.

(b). The physicochemical factors significant in binding are complex and cannot be predicted accurately.

(c). Empiric trials indicate that sodium and potassium are not protein bound, whereas nearly 50% of plasma calcium and a lesser percentage of magnesium are bound.

(d). Many drugs are protein bound.

(e). The percent of small molecules that are protein bound depends on affinity between the small molecule and the plasma protein. It also depends on the concentration of small molecules in blood, because binding sites on the protein molecules are limited in number.

(f). Small molecules bound to proteins cannot escape into filtrate.

(2). Gibbs-Donnan equilibrium.

(a). At the pH of blood, albumin molecules have a net negative charge.

(b). Because essentially all albumin normally is restricted from passing into filtrate, negatively charged molecules are retained in the plasma.

(c). These negative particles provide some attraction to positively charged particles, such as sodium, potassium, magnesium, and calcium.

(d). Thus, plasma water has slightly higher concentrations of these positively charged particles than do filtrates, and slightly lower concentrations of negatively charged diffusible particles, such as chloride and bicarbonate.

(e). The magnitude of the differences in concentrations between plasma water and filtrate is small, and thus is of rare clinical significance.

10. Glomerular filtration of macromolecules.[6,8,11]

a. The glomerulus functions as a sieve. As the size of molecules increases, likelihood that they will pass through the filter lessens (Table 2–1). Cells, many plasma proteins, and lipoproteins are restricted to the plasma because of their size.

b. Factors that influence the passage of macromolecules through the pores in these sieves include:

TABLE 2–1
INFLUENCE OF SIZE ON MOVEMENT OF MOLECULES THROUGH GLOMERULAR CAPILLARY WALLS INTO BOWMAN'S SPACE.

Substance	Molecular Weight	Relative Permeability
Water	18	1.0
Electrolytes	23–95	1.0 (unless protein-bound)
Inulin	5,500	0.98
Myoglobin	17,000	0.75
Hemoglobin	65,000	0.03
Albumin	69,000	< 0.0001

(1). RPF and hydrostatic pressure.

(2). The molecular weight and size of proteins.

(3). The electrical charge of proteins.

(4). The shape of proteins.

c. RPF and hydraulic pressure

(1). Increased intraglomerular hydrostatic pressure seems to increase the passage of protein into filtrate.

(2). With progression of glomerular lesions in proteinuric patients, the severity of proteinuria may decrease, presumably because of reduced GFR.

d. Molecular weight and size of proteins.

(1). Proteins with a molecular weight of 70,000 daltons or greater are usually excluded from glomerular filtrate.

(2). Binding of smaller proteins, such as hemoglobin, to larger proteins, such as haptoglobin, results in the formation of a large complex that prevents loss of hemoglobin in urine. However, hemoglobinuria occurs when the binding capacity of haptoglobin is exceeded.

(3). Investigators have postulated that, once proteins are in the pores of the glomerular sieve, further movement may be hindered by friction between protein molecules and the adjacent stationary layer of fluid along the pore wall. This phenomenon is called "viscous drag."

e. Electrical charge.

(1). The outer components of the glomerular capillary walls (sialoproteins) are negatively charged; this negative charge plays an important role in repelling circulating anionic macromolecules, such as albumin. This phenomenon has been called "electrical hindrance."

(2). Conversely, the negatively charged components of glomerular capillary walls slightly enhance filtration of circulating cationic macromolecules.

f. Shape of proteins.

(1). Proteins of similar size and molecular weight but with different shapes (i.e., one elongated, as albumin, and one spherical, as hemoglobin) may not pass through pores of the glomerular sieve at equal rates.

(2). For the elongated protein (with a long axis that is greater than the diameter of the pores) to gain entrance to the pore, it must have proper orientation toward the pore. Restriction of filtration of molecules through glomerular capillary walls as a result of a nonspherical shape of the molecule is called stearic hindrance.

11. Measurement of GFR is a valuable index of renal function because passage of many substances through the glomerular filter represents their sole method of removal from the body.

a. Measurements of blood urea or creatinine concentrations are used to crudely evaluate renal function because of their simplicity, but they lack sensitivity.

b. Clearance is defined as the volume of plasma from which a substance is completely removed by the kidney per unit time.

c. Inulin is a fructose polymer that freely passes through the glomerular filter, but it is neither secreted nor reabsorbed by the tubules. These properties are essential for its use to measure GFR. Inulin also fulfills other criteria (not metabolized, not stored in kidney, not protein bound, not toxic, no effect on filtration rate) considered essential for valid measurements of GFR.[53]

d. Inulin clearance (GFR) is measured by infusing inulin to achieve a constant blood concentration. Measurement of the blood concentration and the urine content of inulin allows calculation of GFR using the clearance formula.

$$C = \frac{U_C \times U_V}{P_C} = \text{mL/min}$$

C = clearance; U_c = urine concentration; U_v = urine volume; and P_c = plasma concentration.

e. See Chapter 10, Evaluation of Renal Functions, for a review of clinical tests used to estimate GFR.

f. Normal GFR is approximately 4 mL per minute per kilogram of body weight in the dog and cat.[14,53]

C. Tubular reabsorption.

1. Tubular reabsorption of many substances (sodium, potassium, phosphate, glucose, amino acids, and others) is an active process that requires energy.

a. The sodium-potassium-ATPase pump consumes a substantial quantity of the energy generated by the kidney.

b. Glucose and amino acids are reabsorbed by cotransport mechanisms that depend on the sodium-potassium-ATPase system.[58]

2. Passive reabsorption of water occurs in many parts of the nephron secondary to osmotic gradients created by active transport of solutes.

3. Passive reabsorption of solutes may occur as a result of concentration gradients, electrical gradients, or the net effect of these factors as mathematically described by the Nernst equation.[20]

4. Other organs produce hormones that influence tubular reabsorption of specific substances. Examples follow:

a. ADH released from the posterior pituitary gland alters water permeability of cells of the distal tubules and collecting ducts.

b. Aldosterone released from the adrenal glands stimulates sodium reabsorption and potassium secretion by the renal tubules.

c. PTH from the parathyroid glands promotes calcium reabsorption and inhibits phosphorous reabsorption by the tubules.

D. Tubular secretion.

1. Tubular secretion refers to transfer of materials from the peritubular area into the lumen of the tubules.

2. Tubular secretion occurs in both cats and dogs; however, its role in the nitrogen excretory processes is less important in mammals than in birds, reptiles, amphibians, and fish.

3. Tubular secretion is important in acid-base balance, potassium excretion, and secretion of certain organic ions.

4. The pars recta of the proximal tubule is a site of active renal secretion of naturally occurring organic anions and of certain drugs, including penicillin.

5. The distal tubule and collecting duct are important sites for proton (H^+) and potassium secretion.

E. Tubular maximum concept.[53]

1. The quantities of substances that are reabsorbed or secreted by tubules depend on several factors, including:

a. The physiologic capacity of the tubules.

b. The needs of the body for the substance in question.

c. Functional alterations that occur as a result of renal disorders.

2. Many substances are subject to tubular reabsorption or secretion by active transport or in association with an active transport mechanism. Glucose, amino acids, water-soluble vitamins, and sodium are examples of such substances.

3. The maximal rate at which a tubular transport system can operate is described as the tubular transport maximum (T_m) for the system.
4. Tubular reabsorption of filtered glucose is used as an example to illustrate T_m.
   a. If the plasma concentration of glucose is 100 mg/dL and GFR is 4 mL per minute per kilogram, then about 4 mg of glucose per minute per kilogram of body weight appears in filtrate and is delivered to the tubules. Essentially all the glucose is reabsorbed; none can be detected in the urine by clinical methods of measurement (Fig. 2–6A).
   b. If blood glucose concentration is increased, more appears in filtrate, and the tubules must reabsorb the additional amount if glucosuria is to be avoided (Fig. 2–6B).
   c. A progressive increase in blood glucose concentration causes an increased delivery of glucose to tubules, and the tubular cell capacity to reabsorb glucose is eventually exceeded (Fig. 2–6C). Glucosuria occurs in normal dogs and cats when blood glucose concentration exceeds about 180 mg/dL. This value may vary, because a rapid rate of passage of filtrate through the tubule decreases efficiency of reabsorption.
   d. The point at which the glucose transport mechanism is maximally operating is referred to as the tubular maximum, or T_mG (G = glucose). An increase in glucose reabsorption above that amount cannot occur regardless of blood glucose concentration.

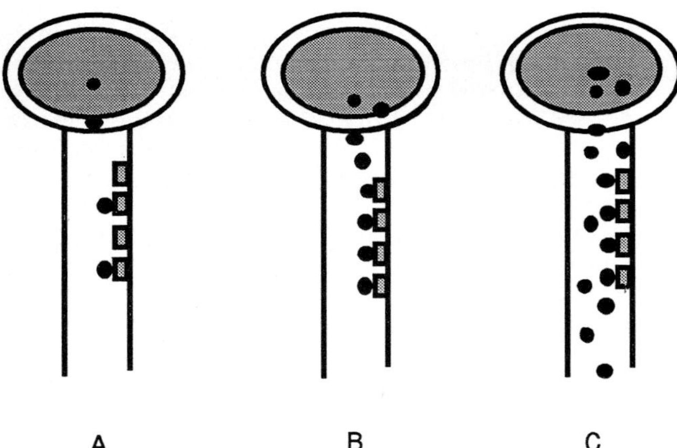

FIG. 2–6. Schematic illustration of tubular maximum (T_m) concept. When a fixed number of transporters operate, a maximum transport capacity exists. Below saturation of transporters **(A),** all filtered glucose is reabsorbed, with transporters to spare. At T_m **(B),** all transporters are saturated at any instant, but glucosuria is prevented because of a fortuitous match between transporter numbers and glucose to be transported. Above T_m, **(C)** glucosuria ensues because glucose is presented in excess of tubule transport capacity for reabsorption.

   e. Thus, glucosuria can occur because of two distinct mechanisms.
      (1). An increase in blood glucose concentration (and thus amount of glucose delivered to tubules) so that T_mG is exceeded. This occurs during diabetes mellitus.
      (2). An abnormally low T_mG, which allows loss of glucose at normal or marginally elevated blood glucose concentrations. A low T_mG can occur with a variety of diseases. In some, only the glucose transport system is abnormal, whereas in others, multiple proximal tubule transport defects exist. The diseases with multiple defects for proximal tubule reabsorption are referred to as Fanconi syndrome.
   f. Significant glucosuria rarely occurs as a manifestation of naturally occurring primary renal failure because decreased tubular function is paralleled by decreased GFR. (See Chapter 16, Pathophysiology of Renal Failure and Uremia.)
   g. Renal tubular transport of glucose is unaffected by insulin.

IV. RENAL REGULATION OF BLOOD ELECTROLYTES

A. Sodium.

1. The amount of sodium appearing in filtrate each day is massive. About 99% of the sodium in filtrate is reabsorbed throughout the tubule without regard for body need. Adjustments in reabsorption of the remaining 1% are required to maintain body sodium balance.
   a. In usual circumstances of health, excess sodium is ingested. Renal regulation results in elimination of sodium in the urine, the quantity depending specifically on intake.
   b. With anorexia or extrarenal sodium loss (i.e., vomiting, diarrhea), the kidneys conserve sodium to the limit of their ability. If affected patients have normal renal function, little sodium exists in the urine.
2. Several factors influence renal regulation of sodium balance.[34,46] These include:
   a. The filtered load of sodium. With hypernatremia, more sodium is excreted.
   b. Aldosterone
      (1). This adrenal hormone enhances the tubular reabsorption of sodium and tubular excretion of potassium.
      (2). Stimuli for aldosterone secretion include angiotensin II, hyponatremia, and hyperkalemia.
   c. Physical factors (peritubular colloid osmotic pressure). This force enhances reabsorption of all components of filtrate, including sodium.
   d. The role of other factors in sodium homeostasis is less certain. These factors include:
      (1). The sympathetic nervous system

(2). Prostaglandins
(3). Atrial natriuretic hormone

e. Ablation of renal sympathetic innervation leads to natriuresis (sodium loss) in some experimental models of study, but not in others.[22]
f. Renal prostaglandins cause natriuresis under some conditions, but not under others.
g. Natriuretic hormone
(1). A natriuretic factor produced in and released from the atrium of the heart has been isolated, chemically identified, and produced synthetically. It is referred to as atrial natriuretic factor (ANF).[35]
(2). Specific biologic effects of this peptide hormone are still being studied, but they include natriuresis, increased GFR, diuresis, and increased urinary potassium excretion.
(3). More studies are required to determine the importance of ANF in sodium homeostasis.

3. Extracellular water (ECW) content and sodium intake.
a. Homeostatic mechanisms do not operate perfectly to keep body content of water and sodium constant at varying levels of sodium intake.
b. Consequently, water and sodium retention occurs when sodium intake is increased (Fig. 2–7).
(1). An abrupt increase in sodium intake is not matched by a comparable increase in urinary excretion for 2 to 3 days. Sodium retention is accompanied by water retention during this time.
(2). ECW volume increases progressively for 2 to 3 days until urinary sodium excretion again matches dietary intake.
(3). The increase in ECW volume is maintained as long as daily intake of sodium remains high.
(4). The body content of sodium and water reverts to original lower levels when sodium restriction is reinstituted (Fig. 2–7). Such restriction is practiced in such conditions as hypertension and congestive heart failure in which the patient benefits from contraction of circulatory volume.
c. Authorities have theorized that in most areas of the world, sodium is ingested in excess of need: sodium intake near zero is satisfactory in health because of excellent renal conservation of this ion.[28]

4. Dogs with chronic renal failure have a reduced population of nephrons with which to maintain sodium balance.
a. If dietary intake of sodium remains constant during progressive nephron loss, residual nephrons must increase sodium excretion if body balance is to be maintained. This adaptation occurs.[50]
b. However, once adapted, a sudden decrease in sodium intake is not associated with an immediate renal response to conserve sodium. As a result, a negative sodium balance and contracted extracellular fluid volume may occur.[7]
c. Most dogs with chronic renal failure appear to be able to adapt to moderate fluctuations in dietary sodium intake, but because the ability to adapt is blunted, sudden changes in sodium intake should be avoided.

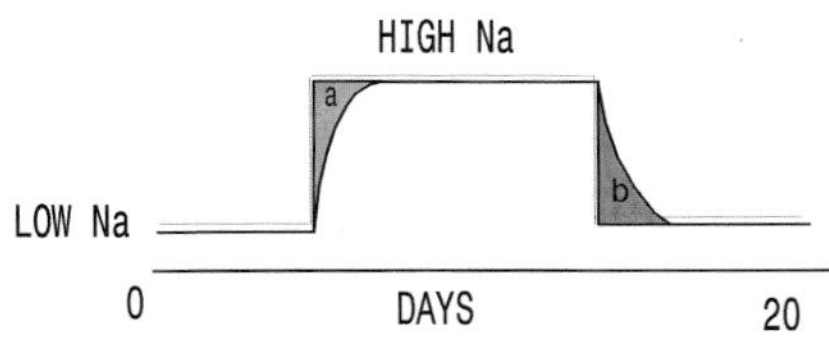

FIG. 2–7. Sodium balance under conditions of low and high sodium intake. Abrupt change from low to high intake (dotted line) is not matched by urinary sodium excretion (solid line), and a positive sodium balance (hatched area a) ensues. After a few days of adaptation, daily balance is restored, but sodium earlier retained (hatched area a) causes water retention and increased extracellular volume. Return to a low-sodium diet causes a transient negative sodium balance (hatched area b) and return of body sodium content and extracellular volume to original values.

B. Potassium.

1. Potassium, like sodium, is freely filtered by glomeruli. Loss of filtered potassium would quickly deplete extracellular stores if tubular reabsorption did not occur.
2. Most potassium (65 to 80%) is reabsorbed in the proximal tubules; additional reabsorption occurs in the thick ascending limb of the loop of Henle.[21]
3. Potassium is secreted by distal tubule cells to adjust plasma potassium concentration. Potassium in the blood (peritubular capillaries) diffuses into the renal interstitium. From there it is actively transported into distal tubule cells by the sodium-potassium-ATPase system. Potassium in these cells then diffuses into the tubule lumen for excretion. Although the diffusion is passive, it is controlled so that homeostasis prevails.
4. Several factors enhance potassium secretion in the distal tubule.[19] These factors include:
a. Aldosterone.
b. Increased delivery of fluid to the distal tubule.
c. Unreabsorbable anions in the distal tubule (i.e., $SO_4^{=}$).
5. Several other factors probably contribute to overall potassium homeostasis.[12,52,54] These include:
a. Glucocorticoids may influence potassium excretion by altering renal hemodynamics and

hence the rate of fluid delivery to the distal tubules.

b. Suppression of ADH may blunt potassium excretion that might otherwise occur during conditions of water diuresis.

c. Catecholamines and insulin enhance potassium uptake by extrarenal cells and thus influence the plasma potassium concentration to which the kidney must respond.

6. Normal kidneys adapt to increased potassium intake.
   a. This phenomenon occurs in isolated perfused kidneys and thus is independent of extrinsic factors.[52]
   b. The sodium-potassium-ATPase activity necessary for secretion is increased during adaptation independent of changes in aldosterone secretion.[27,28]
7. Remnant kidneys have increased levels of sodium-potassium-ATPase, and this factor likely plays a role in potassium adaptation during decreased renal mass. In dogs and cats with renal failure, renal adaptation to potassium loading is impressive. Hyperkalemia usually does not occur until GFR is so low that oliguria exists.

C. Calcium.

1. Plasma calcium concentration is primarily under the control of the parathyroid glands rather than the kidneys. However, the kidneys participate in calcium homeostasis.
2. The kidney handles calcium as follows.[9,56]
   a. Only the ionized and complexed portions of plasma calcium appear in glomerular filtrate; the protein-bound portion cannot pass through the filter.
   b. The renal handling of calcium roughly parallels that of sodium until the distal tubule is reached. Thereafter, some divergence occurs.
      (1). Calcium reabsorption occurs throughout the tubule, with the possible exception of the thin portion of the loops of Henle.
      (2). At major sites of reabsorption (proximal tubule, thick ascending limb of loop of Henle), much of the calcium is reabsorbed secondary to sodium reabsorption.
      (3). Independent calcium reabsorption also occurs at these sites, as well as in the distal tubule.
      (4). Several factors influence tubular reabsorption of calcium.
         (a). Parathyroid hormone enhances reabsorption in the thick ascending limb of the loop of Henle, in the distal tubule, and in the collecting duct.
         (b). Hypocalcemia, metabolic alkalosis, and hyperphosphatemia enhance calcium absorption.
         (c). Hypercalcemia, metabolic acidosis, phosphate depletion, and hypermagnesemia inhibit calcium reabsorption.
3. When calcium ingestion is increased, fecal calcium excretion increases markedly, and a small increase in urinary calcium occurs. Although the influence of diet on urinary excretion is minor, it may influence formation of uroliths containing calcium.
4. The kidney has an effect on intestinal absorption of calcium via its role in metabolism of vitamin D. (See Section VIII of this chapter.)
5. Hypercalcemia resulting from several causes may occur and persist in animals that initially have normal renal function. This emphasizes the lack of direct control by the kidneys on serum calcium concentration. (See Chapter 21, Canine and Feline Hypercalcemic Nephropathy.)

D. Phosphates.[4,9,25,32,38]

1. Plasma inorganic phosphates ($HPO_4^=$, $H_2PO_4^-$) are commonly referred to as phosphorus or inorganic phosphorus.
2. The kidneys provide the major control of plasma phosphate concentration.
3. Phosphates are present in glomerular filtrate in nearly the same concentration as in plasma water. At blood pH, they exist as four molecules of $HPO_4^=$ to one of $H_2PO_4^-$.
4. They are reabsorbed primarily in the proximal tubules by a mechanism also involving sodium transport.
5. Parathyroid hormone appears to be a major factor involved in renal control of phosphate homeostasis. This hormone inhibits proximal tubular phosphate reabsorption via an adenyl cyclase, cyclic AMP system.
6. However, parathyroidectomized animals are capable of modifying renal excretion of phosphate in the appropriate direction, apparently because of an intrinsic ability of renal tubular cells to adjust to body phosphate needs.[4]
7. Other factors influencing renal phosphate excretion are:
   a. Acid-base abnormalities. Metabolic alkalosis increases urinary phosphate reabsorption and chronic metabolic acidosis decreases it.
   b. Vitamin D and growth hormone increase renal phosphate reabsorption.
   c. Volume expansion decreases phosphate reabsorption.

E. Chloride.

1. Chloride is freely filtered; most chloride present in tubular lumens is reabsorbed passively throughout many parts of the nephrons secondary to active transport of cations.
2. An interrelationship may exist between plasma chloride and plasma bicarbonate concentrations. In acidosis, decreased plasma bicarbonate con-

centration is sometimes accompanied by increased plasma chloride concentration, apparently for maintaining electroneutrality. An undefined renal mechanism maintains the higher plasma concentration of chloride in cases of acidosis accompanied by a normal anion gap.

F. **Magnesium.**[45]

1. About 80% of plasma magnesium is freely filtered; apparently the other 20% is protein bound.
2. Tubular handling of magnesium is unique compared to that of other electrolytes.
   a. Only 20 to 30% of filtered magnesium is reabsorbed in the proximal tubules.
   b. The major site of reabsorption under normal conditions is the loop of Henle, especially the thick ascending portion.
   c. About 10% of filtered magnesium is absorbed more distally.
3. Major renal control of magnesium homeostasis resides in the thick ascending loop of Henle. Parathyroid hormone may influence magnesium absorption, but it is not required for magnesium homeostasis.

V. RENAL REGULATION OF ACID-BASE BALANCE[23,24,33]

A. **In health, extracellular fluid pH is maintained within relatively narrow limits. Arterial blood pH is usually near 7.4. To maintain this pH, the lungs and the kidneys each function to adjust certain blood components.**

1. The lungs control P_{CO_2} and thus carbonic acid content of blood.
   a. Decreasing P_{CO_2} provides a quick mechanism for correcting a metabolic acidosis, but it does not provide a permanent solution to the problem, because hydrogen ions (H^+) are not lost from the body during respiratory compensation.
   b. Once P_{CO_2} is restored to its normal level, H^+ reappear according to the equation

$$CO_2 + H_2O \leftrightarrow H_2CO_3 \leftrightarrow H^+ + HCO_3^-$$

2. The kidneys must provide the final defense for metabolic acidosis by excretion of H^+ and by conservation of existing bicarbonate and synthesis of new bicarbonate.

B. **Reclamation of filtered bicarbonate.**

1. Bicarbonate passes freely into glomerular filtrate and would be lost if not reclaimed by the tubules.
2. The renal tubules normally reabsorb bicarbonate to maintain plasma concentrations in the range of about 22 to 28 mEq/L in dogs.[43]
3. When alkali, or foods giving alkali as a product of metabolism, is ingested so that plasma bicarbonate concentration is increased, tubular reabsorption of filtered bicarbonate is incomplete and bicarbonaturia occurs.
4. If plasma bicarbonate concentration is decreased, all filtered bicarbonate is reabsorbed, and more is synthesized by the renal tubular cells.
5. Bicarbonate reabsorption depends on the secretion of H^+.
   a. Bicarbonate, as such, cannot be transferred through the luminal membrane of the tubule.
   b. Instead, filtered bicarbonate and H^+ secreted from tubule cells into the tubular lumens react to form carbonic acid.
   c. Carbonic anhydrase in the brush border of the cells catalyzes carbonic acid breakdown to carbon dioxide and water. The carbon dioxide diffuses from the lumens into the cells, where the process is reversed to generate bicarbonate. The bicarbonate then moves into the interstitium and into the peritubular capillaries.
6. Most bicarbonate is reabsorbed in the proximal tubule, but absorption may occur more distally in the nephron as well.
7. The medullary collecting duct may secrete bicarbonate; this mechanism may facilitate bicarbonate excretion during metabolic alkalosis.

C. **Synthesis of new bicarbonate.**

1. Plasma bicarbonate is available to buffer H^+ that are ingested or that are produced as a consequence of metabolism.
   a. In buffering H^+, bicarbonate is converted to carbonic acid (H_2CO_3). Thus, plasma bicarbonate concentrations could decrease as bicarbonate is neutralized.
   b. Renal mechanisms exist for generation of new bicarbonate to replace that used to buffer H^+.
2. Metabolic processes in proximal tubule cells result in CO_2 production. This CO_2 and water yield H_2CO_3, which dissociates into HCO_3^- and H^+.
3. The H^+ is secreted by proximal tubule cells into the tubular lumens and is excreted in the urine.
4. The HCO_3^- is transported from the tubular cell into the systemic circulation via the basolateral cell surface and the peritubular capillary network.

D. **Renal H^+ secretion.**

1. Large quantities of H^+ are secreted into the lumens of proximal tubules in association with bicarbonate reabsorption. However, no net H^+ secretion occurs during bicarbonate reabsorption because of the overall mechanism involved.
   a. In the tubular lumen, the following reaction occurs.

$$HCO_3^- + H^+ \leftrightarrow H_2CO_3 \leftrightarrow CO_2 + H_2O$$

   b. The CO_2 that forms diffuses into the cell, and then the preceding reaction is reversed.
   c. Thus, for every bicarbonate reabsorbed, a H^+ is first secreted into the tubular lumen, but then is regenerated in the cell.
2. A small net secretion of H^+ into the lumens of

proximal tubules can occur. However, the H^+ pump cannot attain a high lumen-cell H^+ differential. The H^+ secretion stops when a luminal pH of 6.8 is reached.

3. By contrast, the H^+ pump of cells of the distal tubules and collecting ducts can secrete against a concentration gradient of 1000 to 1. Therefore, if need exists for removal of H^+ from the body, the H^+ can be pumped into luminal fluid until a pH of about 4.5 is attained. This pH value represents the maximum capacity of the kidney for acidification of urine.

E. Role of urine buffers in H^+ excretion.

1. Because H^+ secretion by tubular cells is limited by the luminal concentration of H^+, any mechanism that eliminates H^+ activity facilitates excretion of more H^+ into the tubule lumen. Buffers that accept H^+ perform this function.
2. Several buffers are present in blood. Of these, phosphates are freely filtered and can accept H^+ in the tubule lumen to facilitate H^+ secretion, according to the reaction:

$$H^+ + HPO_4^{=} <-> H_2PO_4^-$$

3. In addition, an intrarenal mechanism for H^+ utilization occurs.
   a. Normal renal tubular cells can deaminate several amino acids, particularly glutamine.
   b. An older idea was that the NH_3 generated from deaminations provided a molecule for H^+ uptake, with the subsequent renal excretion of NH_4^+.
   c. A newer hypothesis is that the metabolism of the deaminated carbon skeleton of the amino acid results in H^+ consumption.[24]
      (1). The product of deamination of glutamine is alpha-ketoglutarate, a negatively charged molecule that is converted into neutral end products of metabolism (glucose, or carbon dioxide and water).
      (2). The H^+ are consumed during the metabolism of alpha-ketoglutarate.
   d. The deamination process by the kidney results in NH_4^+ production, rather than NH_3 as previously proposed. This NH_4^+ must be excreted in the urine if any alkalinizing effect of alpha-ketoglutarate metabolism is to occur. If the NH_4^+ were transported to the liver for urea synthesis, alkalinization would not occur because conversion of ammonium to urea consumes bicarbonate.
   e. Several days following an acidosis stimulus are required for maximum glutamine metabolism to occur.
4. Titratable acidity
   a. Urine pH is a measure of free hydrogen ions (H^+).
   b. Because the quantity of buffer (and thus the amount of bound H^+) in urine may vary, urine pH does not measure the total amount of H^+ being excreted.
   c. Titration of urine back to the pH of blood with alkali is a more meaningful measurement of H^+ secretion, because buffer-bound H^+ is measured by this procedure.
   d. This value is referred to as titratable acidity.
5. Total H^+ secretion by the kidney is the sum of titratable acidity and H^+ excreted as NH_4^+, minus HCO_3^- excreted.
6. Defects in acid-base balance.
   a. In generalized renal failure, proximal tubule bicarbonate reabsorption, H^+ secretion, and renal genesis of ammonia all may be impaired.
   b. More specific defects in renal regulation of acid-base balance also may exist with other disorders.[44]
      (1). Proximal renal tubular acidosis occurs as a consequence of impaired bicarbonate reabsorption in the proximal tubules.
      (2). Distal renal tubular acidosis occurs as a consequence of impaired H^+ excretion of the distal portions of the nephron.

VI. RENAL REGULATION OF WATER BALANCE[23,30,48]

A. Body balance of fluids.

1. The sum of water intake and metabolic water produced must equal output if body water balance is to be maintained.
2. Water input includes oral intake (drinking water and water in food) and water formed during metabolism. In health, the volume of metabolic water formed is small compared to volumes ingested.
3. Water output occurs via the gastrointestinal, respiratory, integumentary, and urinary systems. Loss from the first three systems occurs without regard for body need; the kidneys correct imbalances caused by gain or loss of water via these systems.
4. The kidneys conserve water in times of need and excrete it in times of excess. Their capacity to perform these functions is large but not infinite. Extrarenal factors may modify kidney responses to body fluid status. Thus, overhydration and dehydration may occur even when renal function is normal.

B. Mechanisms of urine concentration and dilution.

1. Although all details of this process have not been elucidated, the general scheme that operates for urine concentration (conservation of water) and urine dilution (excretion of water) is known.
2. The mammalian kidney is a high filtration system. A normal 10-kg dog has a GFR of nearly 60 L per 24 hr, but a urine volume of about 0.5 L per

24 hr. Clearly, survival depends on efficient conservation of glomerular filtrate by renal tubules.

3. Water transfer is passive, occurring secondary to hydrostatic or osmotic forces; active transport of water does not occur in mammals. Reabsorption of glomerular filtrate occurs secondary to osmotic differences between tubular luminal fluid and the peritubular luminal environment. Active transport of particles by tubular cells provides the osmotic gradient for water reabsorption.
4. The approximate percentages of glomerular filtrate reabsorbed by various segments of the nephron during states of negative water balance and antidiuresis are:[20]

a. Proximal tubule	75%
b. Loop of Henle	5%
c. Distal tubule	15%
d. Collecting duct	≥4%
	>99%

5. During all states of body water content, the values for water reabsorption are the same in the proximal portions of the nephron. Thus, more than 99% of glomerular filtrate is reabsorbed regardless of body need.
6. Adjustments in water reabsorption needed to maintain body water balance are conducted by manipulation of the water remaining in the tubule lumens in the latter parts of the distal tubules and in the collecting ducts. These adjustments are under the control of ADH.
   a. Characteristics of the ADH system are:
      (1). ADH (vasopressin) is synthesized by neurons of the hypothalamus that are located in the supraoptic and paraventricular nuclei.
      (2). ADH flows via axons in the hypothalamo-hypophyseal tract to the posterior pituitary gland.
      (3). Release of ADH is controlled primarily by osmoreceptors in the anterior hypothalamus. Changes in plasma osmolality of the magnitude of 2% may stimulate or inhibit release from the posterior pituitary gland. Volume receptors in the atria and large vessels may also control ADH release; ADH is secreted when blood volume decreases by 7%.
      (4). ADH has a short biologic half-life (about 20 minutes) because of renal and hepatic elimination.
   b. In times of antidiuresis, water reabsorption is facilitated by action of ADH on the distal tubules and collecting ducts. ADH receptors exist on the peritubular borders of the cells. When ADH is fixed to receptors, cellular changes occur that make luminal membranes water permeable. Water then passes from the tubule lumen into the cell and then into the hypertonic interstitium.
   c. In times of water excess, ADH secretion ceases and the same cells are nearly impermeable to water. Thus, the water in the tubules is not reabsorbed and is eliminated as urine.
7. The countercurrent mechanism explains how water can be reabsorbed passively in the distal nephron secondary to osmotic factors.
8. The essential parts of the nephron responsible for the countercurrent mechanism are depicted in Fig. 2–8. They include the loop of Henle, distal tubule, and collecting duct. The medullary portions of the nephrons are in intimate contact with capillary loops (vasa recta), which supply the medulla with blood and remove materials passing from tubule lumens to the interstitium.
9. Hyperosmotic renal medulla.
   a. The renal medullary interstitium becomes progressively more hyperosmotic from the outer portion of the medulla to the papillary tip.
   b. The genesis of this hyperosmolality is reviewed later. Of immediate importance is the concept that the portions of the nephron residing in the medulla are exposed to an osmolality greater than those portions residing in the cortex.
10. Descending loop of Henle.
   a. Fluid entering the descending limb from the proximal tubule is isosmotic to plasma (approximately 300 mOsm/L).
   b. The cells of the thin descending limb are very permeable to water. They have limited per-

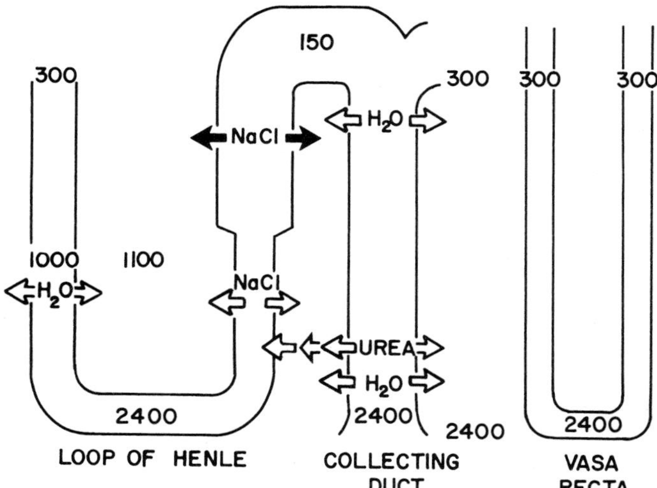

FIG. 2–8. Schematic drawing of anatomic relationship of renal components responsible for the operation of the countercurrent system of urine concentration and dilution. See text for a description of the system.

meability to other small molecules, such as sodium and urea.
 c. As fluid descends within the tubules, water is extracted from their lumens by the high interstitial osmolality.
 d. Removal of water concentrates remaining particles so that osmolality of intratubular fluid increases. At the turn of the loop, the osmolality of intraluminal and interstitial fluids is the same.

11. Ascending limb, loop of Henle.
 a. The entire ascending limb is impermeable to water regardless of ADH levels in plasma, but is permeable to many other molecules.
 b. Because more sodium is in the tubule lumen than in the medullary interstitial space, sodium passively diffuses from the lumen into the interstitium from the thin portion of the ascending limb.
 c. Because of active transport in the thick ascending portion, chloride and sodium are pumped from the tubular lumen into the interstitium.
 d. Some urea enters the lumen of the ascending limb from the interstitium.
 e. The effect of the outward movement of sodium chloride and the restriction of water is a decrease in osmolality of fluid in the ascending limb, so that values of 50 to 150 mOsm exist at the beginning of the distal tubule.
12. Distal tubule.
 a. Sodium, chloride, and water are reabsorbed from the proximal portions of the distal tubules independent of ADH concentration in plasma.
 b. In the dog, intraluminal fluid osmolality remains hyposmolar until the terminal portion of the distal tubule is reached.
 c. In the cat, the fluid becomes isosmolar before the terminal portions are reached.
 d. The terminal portion of the distal tubule responds in the same manner as subsequently described for the outer medullary collecting duct.
13. Collecting duct.
 a. Reabsorption of water in the collecting duct requires the presence of ADH.
 b. In the absence of ADH, only minimal absorption can occur, and the bulk of intraluminal fluid is voided as urine.
 c. In the outer medulla, ADH facilitates diffusion of water, but not urea, into the interstitium.
 d. In the inner medulla, ADH facilitates diffusion of both water and urea into the interstitium, further reducing urine volume.
  (1). Water diffuses out of the tubule lumen because of high interstitial osmolality.
  (2). Urea diffuses out of the tubule lumen because of high intraluminal concentrations. This is a consequence of:
   (a). Filtration of urea with subsequent concentration secondary to removal of water from the nephron lumen.
   (b). Passage of urea from the interstitium into the ascending limb of the loop of Henle.
14. Role of vasa recta.
 a. Vasa recta (see Fig. 2–3) provide nutrition to the medulla.
 b. Because blood flow through the vasa recta is slow, the high concentration of solutes within the medulla is not "washed out."
  (1). Blood osmolarity increases progressively as blood flows through the descending limbs of vasa recta because of water extraction and solute addition by the hyperosmolar interstitial environment.
  (2). Blood osmolarity decreases as it courses through the ascending vasa recta and is nearly isosmolar as it leaves the medulla.
 c. The excess of materials (e.g., water, salts) that would otherwise accumulate in the interstitium subsequent to diffusion from the loops of Henle and collecting ducts is removed by the vasa recta.
15. Origin and maintenance of the hyperosmolar medullar environment.
 a. The sodium chloride pump in the thick ascending limb of the loops of Henle transfers these ions from the lumen to the interstitium and creates the high concentration of sodium in the outer medulla.
 b. Passive transfer of sodium chloride out of the thin ascending limb contributes to the interstitial hyperosmolality of the inner medulla.
 c. Urea contributes to inner medullary hyperosmolality as it diffuses from the inner medullary collecting duct into the interstitium.
16. The net effect of the countercurrent system is the generation of a hyperosmotic environment in the renal medulla that permits movement of water out of the lumen of the distal tubules and collecting ducts into the interstitium and out of the medulla via the vasa recta.
 a. Substantial water reabsorption at these sites depends on ADH.
 b. Conservation of water in the lower portion of the nephrons would not be possible without hypertonicity of the medullary interstitium, even in the presence of ADH.

C. Defects in the urine concentration mechanism fall into three categories.

1. Impermeability of the collecting duct cells to water may be associated with:

a. Lack of ADH (central or pituitary diabetes insipidus).
b. Lack of tubular response to ADH (renal diabetes insipidus).
(1). ADH has its effect on basal membranes of tubule cells. It stimulates adenyl cyclase for transfer of information via the cyclic AMP system.
(2). Cellular responses to calcium, magnesium, prostaglandin E, adrenal corticosteroids, and adrenergic agents are important in the biologic expression of ADH effects. Cells may not respond to ADH when cellular concentrations of these factors are altered.[26]

2. Lack of the medullary osmotic gradient, which may be caused by:
a. Interference with the sodium chloride pump in the loop of Henle.
b. "Washout" via rapid blood flow through vasa recta or fluid flow through the tubules.
3. Maintenance of particles with osmotic activity in lumens of tubules (osmotic diuresis). Examples include:
a. Administration of mannitol.
b. Glomerular filtration of endogenously produced or exogenously administered glucose in excess of T_m levels.
c. Lack of reabsorption of constituents of glomerular filtrate. Osmotic diuresis caused by this factor is significant in polyuria of renal failure (consult Chapter 16, the Pathophysiology of Renal Failure and Uremia for further details about obligatory osmotic diuresis).

VII. EXCRETION OF NITROGENOUS WASTES

A. Urea.

1. The origin, distribution, and nonrenal fate of urea in the body are summarized elsewhere (see Chapter 10, Evaluation of Renal Functions).
2. Urea (MW = 60 d) appears in filtrate in the same concentration as in plasma.
3. Active transport of urea has not been detected in mammals; movement occurs secondary to concentration gradients.
4. Some parts of the nephron are permeable to urea.
a. Urea diffuses from the interstitium into the lumen of the thin ascending limb of the loop of Henle.
b. In the presence of ADH, urea diffuses from the lumen of the collecting duct into the medullary interstitium.
5. Under the usual conditions of urine flow in the dog, about 60% of the urea filtered is reabsorbed.[43]
6. The amount of urea reabsorbed is decreased, and the amount excreted is increased, by increasing urine flow rate (Fig. 2–9).
7. As a result, a decrease in BUN may occur without a change in GFR following induction of polyuria by administration of parenteral fluids or diuretics.

B. Creatinine.

1. See Chapter 10, Evaluation of Renal Functions, for information on the origin, distribution, and nonrenal excretion of creatinine.
2. Creatinine (MW = 113 d) appears in filtrate in the same concentration as in plasma.
3. No tubular reabsorption of creatinine occurs.
4. A weak tubular secretory mechanism exists for creatinine in the male, but not in the female, dog.[39,57]
5. Tubular secretion of creatinine does not occur in the cat.[13]
6. Creatinine clearance may be used to estimate GFR, but certain reservations must be applied. (See Chapter 10, Evaluation of Renal Functions.)

C. Other nitrogenous compounds.

1. With rare exceptions, dogs other than dalmations, as well as cats, excrete allantoin as the end product of purine metabolism.
2. Dalmations excrete both allantoin and uric acid in their urine.
3. Proteins and amino acids are usually conserved rather than excreted because of their value to the animal. An exception is the excretion of the amino acid felinine by cats. This sulfur-containing amino acid is present in cat urine at a concentration of 100 to 180 mg/dL.[3,59]
4. Generation of NH_3 with subsequent excretion of NH_4^+ was reviewed in Section V, Part E, of this chapter.
5. Minor quantities of other nitrogenous compounds appear in urine, but the amounts are rarely measured unless an inborn error of metabolism is suspected.

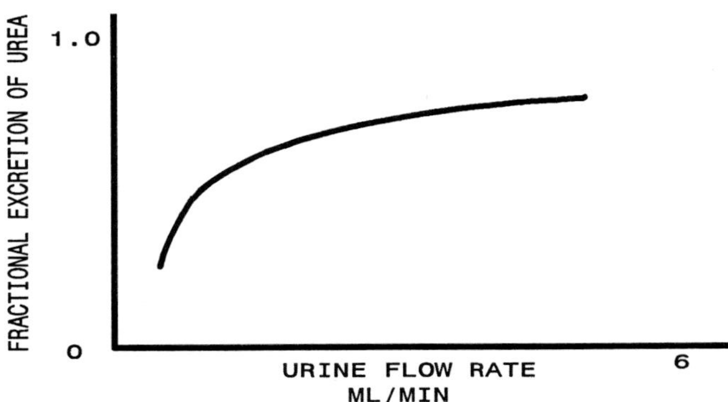

FIG. 2–9. Notice that increased urine flow rate increases urea excretion. Clinically, the change in fractional excretion (FE) for urea with flow rate must be considered when interpreting BUN values from patients receiving fluid therapy.

VIII. THE KIDNEY AS AN ENDOCRINE ORGAN

A. Erythropoietin.[10,16]

1. Erythropoietin is a circulating glycoprotein that stimulates bone marrow stem cells at several stages of maturation to produce erythrocytes.[1]
2. Renal hypoxia appears to be the major stimulus for erythropoietin production. Other factors that may play a role include:[10]
   a. Renal artery constriction.
   b. Intrarenal vascular injury.
   c. Renal cysts.
   d. Hydronephrosis.
   e. Renal neoplasms or extrarenal neoplasms that autonomously produce erythropoietin.
   f. Vasoactive agents.
   g. Hormones, including androgens, thyroxin, and adrenocortical steroids.
3. Cloning of the human erythropoietin gene and commercial production of human erythropoietin have been achieved.[29] (See Chapter 29, Medical Management of the Anemia of Chronic Renal Failure).

B. Renin-angiotensin.[41,42]

1. The renin-angiotensin system involves several organs, including the kidney.
2. Renin is a glycoprotein produced by cells of afferent and efferent glomerular arterioles. However, some proteolytic enzymes with renin-like activity are produced extrarenally.
3. Renin cleaves the terminal 10 amino acid segment from a plasma protein that is produced by the liver.
4. This decapeptide, named angiotensin I, has little biologic activity until transformed into an octapeptide, angiotensin II, by angiotensin-converting enzyme (ACE). Several organs produce ACE, but the lungs are a major source.
5. Angiotensin II is a potent vasoconstrictor. It also stimulates adrenal release of aldosterone. Production of angiotensin II in many organs has local effects.[47]
6. Angiotensin III is a heptapeptide that is a breakdown product of angiotensin II. It is present in low levels in the blood, has high affinity for adrenal receptors, and is the most potent form of angiotensin for aldosterone stimulation.
7. Stimuli for renin production include:
   a. Renal ischemia (a renal baroreceptor exists that responds to changes in arteriolar wall tension).
   b. Renal sympathetic nerve stimulation.
   c. Renal prostaglandins (prostaglandin inhibitors inhibit renin release).
   d. An intrarenal single nephron feedback loop (so-called tubuloglomerular feedback).
      (1). Events occurring in a tubule may modify filtration by the glomerulus of that nephron.
         (a). As flow rates through the ascending limb of the loop of Henle and initial portion of the distal tubule increase, glomerular filtration in the same nephron decreases. Conversely, a reduction in flow of tubular filtrate at these sites results in an increase in GFR.
         (b). This phenomenon helps to maintain the rate of flow through nephrons within normal limits.
      (2). The sensor for tubuloglomerular feedback is apparently the macula densa (see Fig. 2–2). The stimulus is not defined with certainty, but may be the rate of chloride reabsorption at this site.
         (a). Increased reabsorption of chloride results in increased renin secretion, constriction of the afferent arteriole, and reduced GFR.
         (b). Decreased reabsorption of chloride results in decreased renin secretion, dilation of the afferent arteriole, and increased GFR.
8 Function of the renin-angiotensin system.
   a. Maintenance of extracellular fluid volume is an important function of the angiotensin-aldosterone system. Increased aldosterone secretion results in increased renal retention of sodium and water.
   b. An intrarenal system for generation of angiotensin II exists, and it affects renal functions, including renal blood flow, GFR, and tubular reabsorption of sodium.[47]
      (1). Administration of angiotensin II antagonists may result in decreased GFR.
      (2). Intrarenally generated angiotensin II apparently can maintain GFR via efferent arteriole constriction, which increases intracapillary pressure.
   c. Other organs are capable of generating angiotensin II, and some of its properties include:
      (1). Dipsogenic properties.
      (2). Modulation of sympathetic function.
9. Renin-dependent hypertension can be produced in dogs by partial occlusion of the renal arteries bilaterally. The role of the renin-angiotensin system in naturally occurring hypertension in the dog is not known at present.

C. Vitamin D.[17]

1. Vitamin D is relatively impotent prior to hydroxylation of the molecule in the 1 and 25 positions.
2. After 25-hydroxylation by the liver, the normal kidney performs 1-hydroxylation in renal cell mitochondria to yield 1,25-dihydroxy vitamin D (calcitriol).
3. This compound is released by the kidney and has effects on the intestines and bones.

a. Calcium absorption by the small intestines is stimulated by calcitriol.
b. Bone remodeling depends on calcitriol.

4. Renal regulation of the hydroxylation of 25-hydroxy vitamin D is modulated by inorganic phosphate either directly or via parathormone (PTH).
5. Renal vitamin D hydroxylation may be impaired with kidney disease. Impairment of hydroxylation may affect both intestinal absorption of calcium and bone metabolism. Moderate to severe renal failure usually must exist before impaired vitamin D hydroxylation is clinically significant.
6. Extrarenal locations for 1-hydroxylation of 25-hydroxy vitamin D synthesis exist (placenta, monocytes), but quantities produced at these sites are normally inadequate for body needs.
7. PTH secretion is primarily influenced by plasma ionized calcium concentration, but also is influenced by calcitriol. Calcitriol inhibits PTH secretion by direct effects on the parathyroid glands. If plasma calcitriol concentrations are reduced because of advanced renal failure, both hyperphosphatemia and low plasma concentrations of calcitriol contribute to renal secondary hyperparathyroidism.

D. Prostaglandins.[49]

1. Prostaglandins are a family of 20-carbon unsaturated fatty acids with a 5-carbon cyclic structure.
2. They are produced locally in the tissues from phospholipids of cell membranes.
3. Most function locally in the tissue in which they are produced, differing from classic hormones in this respect.
4. Biologic effects of prostaglandins vary depending on their molecular configuration and concentration. Prostaglandins often appear to be one of several components of a renal regulatory mechanism.
5. Several alterations in renal function can be produced by prostaglandins. These include:
   a. Modulation of renal blood flow.
   b. Natriuresis.
   c. Suppression of ADH activity.
6. Their roles in various renal physiologic and pathophysiologic mechanisms are being elucidated.
7. One concept is that renal prostaglandins serve in a cytoprotective role. Thus, during euvolemic states, the inhibition of their production has little effect. However, when renal function is altered by fluid imbalance or renal disease, their presence is important for adaptation.[49] In such circumstances, administration of drugs that inhibit prostaglandin production, such as nonsteroidal anti-inflammatory agents, may cause adverse effects.

IX. RENAL PROTEIN METABOLISM

A. Mechanism.

1. As previously indicated, molecular properties relevant to glomerular filtration of proteins are their size, shape, and surface charge.
2. Many proteins pass through the normal glomerular filter and appear in the tubular lumen. In general, these proteins have molecular weights of less than 70,000 daltons.
3. Their quantity in filtrate is sufficiently low so that nearly all are removed from luminal fluid by cellular pinocytosis in proximal tubules. Most are then degraded by lysosomal enzymes, and the products of degradation are returned to the blood.[36]

B. Significance.

1. The normal kidney is a major organ for the degradation of some polypeptides.
2. For example, a significant quantity of insulin, growth hormone, and lysozyme is removed from the blood by the kidneys.
3. In conditions in which glomerular leakage of albumin is increased, a considerable amount is reabsorbed by proximal tubular cells. A T_m for protein reabsorption exists. Once saturated, additional albumin appears in the urine.[55]
4. Thus, protein loss from blood caused by glomerular disease is not restricted to that which is measured in urine. Amino acids of proteins reabsorbed by pinocytosis do remain in the body, however.

REFERENCES

1. Anagnostou, A., and Kurtzman, N.A.: Hematologic consequences of renal failure. *In* The Kidney. Edited by B.M. Brenner and F.C. Rector. Philadelphia, W.B. Saunders, 1986.
2. Arendhorst, W.J., and Gottschalk, C.W.: Glomerular ultrafiltration dynamics: historical perspective. Am. J. Physiol., 248: F163-F174, 1985.
3. Avizonis, P.V., and Wriston, J.C.: On the biosynthesis of felinine. Biochem. Biophys. Acta, 34:279-281, 1959.
4. Bonjour, J.P., Troehler, U., Preston, C., Fleisch, H.: Parathyroid hormone and renal handling of P_i: Effect of dietary P_i and diphosphonates. Am. J. Physiol., 234:F497-F505, 1978.
5. Brenner, B.M., Dworkin, L.D., Ichikawa, I.: Glomerular filtration. *In* The Kidney. Edited by B.M. Brenner and F.C. Rector. Philadelphia, W.B. Saunders, 1986.
6. Brenner, B.M., Hostetter, T.H., Humes, H.D.: Molecular basis of proteinuria of glomerular origin. N. Engl. J. Med., 298:826-833, 1978.
7. Bricker, N.S.: Sodium homeostasis in chronic renal disease. Kidney Int., 21:886-897, 1982.
8. Deen, W.M., Bohrer, M.P., Robertson, C.R., Brenner, B.M.: Determinants of the transglomerular passage of macromolecules. Fed. Proc., 36:2614-2618, 1977.
9. Dennis, V.W., Stead, W.W., Myers, J.L.: Renal handling of phosphate and calcium. Annu. Rev. Physiol., 41:257-271, 1979.
10. Erslev, A.J., and Caro, J.: Pathophysiology of erythropoietin. *In* Current Concepts in Erythropoiesis. Edited by C.D. Dunn. New York, John Wiley & Sons, 1983.

11. Fang, L.S.: Light-chain nephropathy. Kidney Int., 27:582-592, 1985.
12. Field, M.J., and Giebisch, G.J.: Hormonal control of renal potassium excretion. Kidney Int., 27:379-387, 1985.
13. Finco, D.R., and Barsanti, J.A.: Mechanism of urinary excretion of creatinine by the cat. Am. J. Vet. Res., 43:2207-2209, 1982.
14. Finco, D.R., Coulter, D.B., Barsanti, J.A.: Simple, accurate method for clinical estimation of glomerular filtration rate in the dog. Am. J. Vet. Res., 42:1874-1877, 1981.
15. Finco, D.R., and Duncan, J.R.: Evaluation of blood urea nitrogen and serum creatinine concentration as indicators of renal function. A study of 111 cases and a review of related literature. J. Am. Vet. Med. Assoc., 168:593-601, 1976.
16. Fischer, J.W.: Erythropoietin: Pharmacology, biogenesis, and control of production. Pharmacol. Rev., 24:459-508, 1972.
17. Fraser, D.R.: Regulation of the metabolism of vitamin D. Physiol. Rev., 60:551-613, 1980.
18. Fried, T.A., and Stein, J.H.: Glomerular dynamics. Arch. Intern. Med., 143:787-791, 1983.
19. Gabow, P.: Disorders of potassium metabolism. *In* Renal and Electrolyte Disorders. Edited by R.W. Schrier. Boston, Little, Brown, 1976.
20. Ganong, W.F.: Review of Medical Physiology. Los Altos, CA, Lange Medical Publication, 1979.
21. Gennari, F.J., and Cohen, J.J.: Role of the kidney in potassium homeostasis: lessons from acid-base disturbances. Kidney Int., 8:1-5, 1975.
22. Gottschalk, C.W.: Renal nerves and sodium excretion. Annu. Rev. Physiol., 41:229-240, 1979.
23. Guyton, A.C.: Textbook of Medical Physiology. Philadelphia, W.B. Saunders, 1986.
24. Halperin, M.L., and Jungas, R.L.: Metabolic production and renal disposal of hydrogen ions. Kidney Int., 24:709-713, 1983.
25. Haramati, A., Haas, J.A., Knox, F.G.: Adaptation of deep and superficial nephrons to changes in dietary phosphate intake. Am. J. Physiol., 244:F265-F269, 1983.
26. Hays, R.M., and Levine, S.D.: Vasopressin. Kidney Int., 6:307-322, 1974.
27. Hayslett, J.P., and Binder, H.J.: Mechanism of potassium adaptation. Am. J. Physiol., 243:F103-F112, 1982.
28. Hollenberg, N.K.: Setpoint for sodium homeostasis: Surfeit, deficit, and their implications. Kidney Int., 17:423-429, 1980.
29. Reference deleted.
30. Jamison, R.L., and Oliver, R.E.: Disorders of urinary concentration and dilution. Am. J. Med., 72:308-322, 1982.
31. Kaihara, S., Rutherford, R.B., Schwentker, E.P., Wagner, H.N.: Distribution of cardiac output in experimental hemorrhagic shock in dogs. J. Appl. Physiol., 27:218-222, 1969.
32. Knox, F.G.: The intrarenal metabolism of phosphate. Physiologist, 20:25-31, 1977.
33. Kurtzman, H.A., Arruda, A.L., Westenfelder, C.: Renal regulation of acid-base homeostasis. Contrib. Nephrol., 14:1-13, 1978.
34. Lifschitz, M.D., and Stein, J.H.: Hormonal regulation of renal salt excretion. Semin. Nephrol., 3:196-204, 1983.
35. Maack, T., et al.: Atrial natriuretic factor: structure and functional properties. Kidney Int., 27:607-615, 1985.
36. Maack, T., et al.: Renal filtration, transport, and metabolism of low-molecular-weight proteins: a review. Kidney Int., 16:251-270, 1979.
37. Marchand, G.R.: Direct measurement of glomerular capillary pressure in dogs. Proc. Soc. Exp. Biol. Med., 167:F163-F174, 1985.
38. Mizgala, C.L., and Quamme, G.A.: Renal handling of phosphate. Physiol. Rev., 65:431-466, 1985.
39. O'Connell, J.B., Romeo, J.A., Judge, G.H.: Renal tubular secretion of creatinine in the dog. Am. J. Physiol., 203:985-990, 1962.
40. Ofstad, J., and Aukland, K.: Renal circulation. *In* The Kidney: Physiology and Pathophysiology. Edited by D.W. Seldin and G. Giebisch. New York, Raven Press, 1985.
41. Peach, M.J.: Renin-angiotensin system: Biochemistry and mechanisms of action. Physiol. Rev., 57:313-369, 1977.
42. Peart, W.S.: Renin-angiotensin system. New Engl. J. Med., 292:302-306, 1975.
43. Pitts, R.F.: Physiology of the Kidney and Body Fluids. Chicago, Year Book, 1974.
44. Pohlman, T., Hruska, K.A., Menon, M.: Renal tubular acidosis. J. Urol., 132:431-436, 1981.
45. Quamme, G.A., and Dirks, J.H.: Renal magnesium transport. Rev. Physiol. Biochem. Pharmacol., 97:69-110, 1983.
46. Raymond, K.H., Reineck, J., Stein, J.H.: Sodium metabolism and maintenance of extracellular fluid volume. *In* Fluid Electrolyte and Acid-Base Disorders. Edited by A.I. Arieff and R.A. De Fronzo. New York, Churchill-Livingstone, 1985.
47. Reid, T.A.: The renin-angiotensin system and body function. Arch. Intern. Med., 145:1475-1579, 1985.
48. Roy, D.R., and Jamison, R.L.: Countercurrent system and its regulation. *In* The Kidney: Physiology and Pathophysiology. Edited by D.W. Seldin and G. Giebisch. New York, Raven Press, 1985.
49. Schlondorff, D.: Renal prostaglandin synthesis. Am. J. Med., 81(Suppl. 2B):1-11, 1986.
50. Schmidt, R.G., Bourgoigne, J.J., Bricker, N.S.: On the adaptation in sodium excretion in chronic uremia. The effect of proportional reduction of sodium intake. J. Clin. Invest., 53:1736-1741, 1974.
51. Schnermann, J., and Briggs, J.: Function of the juxtaglomerular apparatus: local control of glomerular hemodynamics. *In* The Kidney: Physiology and Pathophysiology. Edited by D.W. Seldin and G. Giebisch. New York, Raven Press, 1985.
52. Silva, P., Brown, R.S., Epstein, F.H.: Adaptation to potassium. Kidney Int., 11:466-475, 1977.
53. Smith, H.W.: The Kidney: Structure and Function in Health and Disease. New York, Oxford University Press, 1951.
54. Sterns, R.H., Cox, M., Feig, P.U., Singer, I.: Internal potassium balance and the control of the plasma potassium concentration. Medicine, 60:339-354, 1981.
55. Strober, W., and Waldmann, T.A.: The role of the kidney in the metabolism of plasma proteins. Nephron, 13:35-66, 1974.
56. Sutton, R.A.: Disorders of renal calcium excretion. Kidney Int., 23:665-673, 1983.
57. Swanson, R.E., and Hakim, A.A.: Stop-flow of creatinine excretion in the dog. Am. J. Physiol., 203:980-984, 1962.
58. Ulbrich, K.J.: Sugar, amino acid, and Na^+ cotransport in the proximal tubule. Annu. Rev. Physiol., 41:181-195, 1979.
59. Westall, R.G.: The amino acids and other ampholytes of urine. Biochem. J., 55:244-248, 1953.
60. Youngberg, S.P., et al.: Filtration dynamics in dogs: glomerular capillary pressure. Fed. Proc., 36:2609-2613, 1977.

PART II

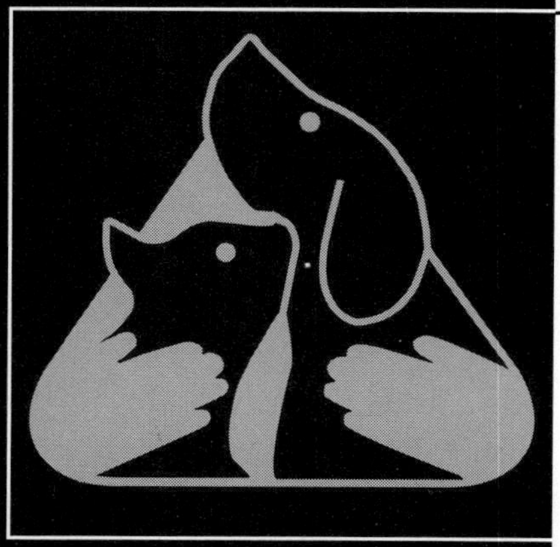

CLINICAL EVALUATION OF THE URINARY SYSTEM

CHAPTER 3

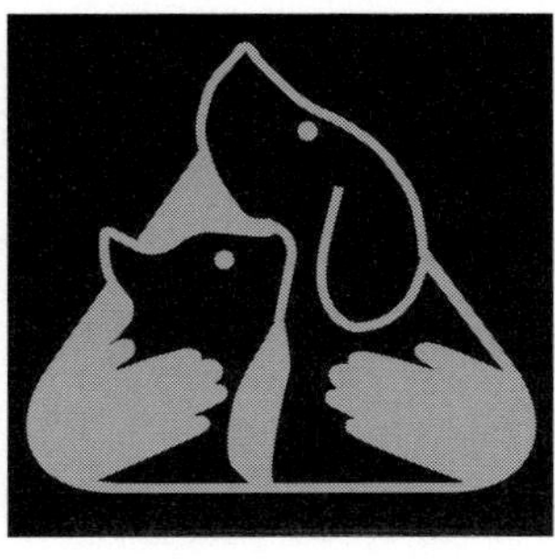

Fundamentals of the Practice of Veterinary Nephrology and Urology

GEORGE E. LEES

I. USING CLINICAL SYNDROMES TO PRACTICE VETERINARY NEPHROLOGY AND UROLOGY

A. Care of patients with disorders of the urinary system is facilitated by categorizing them according to the basic clinical syndrome(s) that they exhibit.

B. Each basic clinical syndrome has several fundamental characteristics.

1. Affected patients have similar clinical and pathophysiologic features, which permit the syndrome to be readily recognized near the outset of clinical investigation.
2. Diagnostic issues and therapeutic objectives are similar for affected patients.

C. The rationale underlying use of syndromes to guide clinical activities in the practice of veterinary nephrology and urology is that:

1. All patients with disease of the urinary system are affected by at least one basic clinical syndrome that is readily identified.
2. Identification of a basic clinical syndrome also identifies:
   a. Relevant diagnostic issues and methods of investigation.
   b. Therapeutic goals and criteria of outcome assessment.
   c. General probability of possible clinical outcomes.
3. Thus, a unique set of general rules exists for each syndrome. These form a template for clinical decision making about each syndrome, which makes patient care more efficient and effective.

D. Clinical syndromes are useful in problem-oriented veterinary practice.

1. The syndrome name is an informative initial problem statement.
2. The syndrome's unique general rules lead directly to initial diagnostic plans (i.e., common causes to rule in or rule out), therapeutic plans (i.e., priorities and goals of treatment), and client education (i.e., explanation of illness and prognosis).
3. Additional findings may permit refinement of the problem statement to a major syndrome subdivision with particular implications, or to a more highly specific etiopathogenic entity.
4. Therapeutic interventions are coupled to the problem statement. Unrefined problems may be managed with symptomatic and supportive therapy; problem refinement, on the other hand, may lead to use of specific therapy.
5. Comparison of clinical course with general expectations permits refinement of therapeutic plans and prognosis.

E. The basic clinical syndromes of veterinary nephrology and urology are: acute renal failure, chronic renal failure, nephrotic syndrome, renal tubular defects, urinary retention, urinary tract infection, urolithiasis, abnormal micturition, and subclinical urinary abnormalities.

II. BRIEF DESCRIPTIONS OF BASIC CLINICAL SYNDROMES OF URINARY SYSTEM DISEASE

A. Acute renal failure.

1. Acute renal failure (ARF) exists when azotemia is caused by renal parenchymal disease or injury that has occurred recently (i.e., less than a week ago).
   a. Because of their recent development, potentially reversible renal lesions have not had sufficient time to resolve or be repaired.
   b. Functional adaptations to compensate for loss of nephrons affected by irreversible renal lesions also have not had time to fully develop.
   c. With lesion repair and adaptation by surviving nephrons, substantial improvement of intrinsic renal function is possible in patients with acute renal failure.
2. Development of ARF usually is heralded clinically by the abrupt onset of oliguria, azotemia, or both.
   a. Some animals with ARF are not oliguric.
   b. In animals that already have azotemia due to some other cause (e.g., prerenal azotemia, chronic renal failure), onset of ARF may be signaled by an abrupt further increase in the severity of azotemia.
3. Signs of uremia generally develop rapidly in animals with ARF.
   a. Although signs typically develop quickly, it is the rapid change in renal lesions and kidney function that actually differentiates ARF from chronic renal failure.
   b. Notable clinical signs often appear to develop abruptly in animals with chronic renal failure as well as in those with ARF.
4. ARF has numerous possible causes.
   a. ARF usually is caused by renal hypoperfusion or a nephrotoxin (e.g., nephrosis).
      (1). Common causes of inadequate renal perfusion are shock and hypotension of any cause, thrombosis of renal arteries, and hyperthermia (heat stroke).
      (2). Nephrotoxins often encountered include antimicrobial drugs (e.g., aminoglycosides, amphotericin B), ethylene glycol (antifreeze), and hypercalcemia; however, a variety of other substances occasionally cause ARF.
   b. ARF sometimes is caused by severe or rapidly progressive inflammatory renal lesions (e.g., nephritis).
      (1). Glomerulonephritis, interstitial nephritis, and pyelonephritis are examples of such lesions.
      (2). Inflammatory lesions that cause acute renal failure often are part of a polysystemic illness (e.g., systemic lupus erythematosus, bacterial endocarditis, leptospirosis).
5. Diagnosis of ARF is based on a combination of findings.
   a. Begin by excluding nonrenal causes of azotemia and oliguria.
      (1). Prerenal azotemia, which is characterized by physiologic oliguria (i.e., formation of a small volume of highly concentrated urine).
      (2). Postrenal azotemia (see section on Urinary Retention).
   b. Prompt diagnosis of ARF requires a high index of suspicion arising from knowledge of existing environmental or medical factors that might lead to ARF.
   c. With appropriate historical clues, diagnosis of ARF is confirmed by finding pathologic oliguria (i.e., formation of a small volume of urine that is not highly concentrated) together with a constellation of biochemical and clinical derangements that occur because of inability to form and excrete urine adequately (i.e., azotemia and uremia).
   d. Urinalysis sometimes gives evidence of the etiologic cause of ARF, but when the urinalysis is not helpful, investigation of the specific cause of ARF is focused more on scrutinizing the history than on performing diagnostic tests.
   e. Renal biopsy sometimes is required for definitive diagnosis of ARF.
6. Therapeutic objectives for patients with ARF are similar regardless of the cause of the problem.
   a. Minimize further renal injury by restoring and maintaining adequate tissue perfusion and by stopping use of potentially nephrotoxic drugs, if possible, or modifying their dosage appropriately.
   b. Combat derangements of extracellular fluid volume and composition (i.e., electrolytes and acid-base balance).
   c. Promote diuresis once extracellular fluid deficits are corrected.
   d. Give supportive care by combatting uremic gastropathy and vomiting and potential infection, and providing for nutritional requirements.
   e. Consider use of peritoneal dialysis or hemodialysis to remove retained solutes and thus preserve the life of persistently oliguric patients with potentially reversible renal lesions.
   f. When recovery begins, carefully manage fluid, electrolyte, and nutritional balances until adequate renal function is restored.
7. Prognosis for ARF largely depends on the severity of renal injury.
   a. When the renal injury is less severe, the nadir of renal function and the peak severity of azotemia and uremia are limited, oliguria is less likely, and the time that elapses before functional recovery commences is reduced.
   b. Short-term survival depends upon whether the

animal can live through the worst period of an episode of ARF.

(1). Persistent oliguria and a protracted period of severe renal dysfunction are difficult to survive; a variety of life-threatening complications commonly develop in patients with such severe disease.

(2). Expert medical care, albeit mainly symptomatic and supportive, permits some animals that would otherwise die to survive the worst of their illness.

c. Long-term prognosis generally is fair to good for animals that are so fortunate as to survive the nadir of renal function and begin to experience functional recovery.

B. Chronic renal failure.

1. Chronic renal failure (CRF) exists when azotemia is caused by renal parenchymal disease or injury that has developed over an extended period (i.e., usually several months or more).
   a. Because they are long-standing, renal lesions already have exhausted their potential for repair and resolution.
   b. Surviving nephrons already have adapted their function to compensate for antecedent nephron loss.
   c. Intrinsic renal function will not improve; if renal function changes in the future (and it usually does), it deteriorates.
2. Development of CRF usually is characterized by insidious onset and progressive deterioration of renal function leading to polyuria, then azotemia, and eventually to uremia.
   a. The rate of progressive deterioration of renal function varies greatly in different animals; however, rate of deterioration often is fairly constant in a given individual.
   b. In CRF, onset of clinical signs can seem abrupt (mimicking ARF) because early mild signs are not noticed or because some event precipitates a uremic crisis.
3. CRF has many possible causes.
   a. The primary renal lesion in animals with CRF usually is a glomerulopathy or an inflammatory tubulointerstitial disease.
   b. However, specific cause(s) of CRF often are numerous, multifactorial, and impossible to determine at the end stage of disease when the condition is diagnosed.
4. Diagnosis of CRF usually is based on a combination of findings.
   a. Identification of CRF often is aided by discovery of tell-tale signs of chronic renal disease in animals with azotemia or azotemia and uremia. These signs include a prior history of polyuria and polydipsia, existence of a hypoproliferative anemia, indications of renal osteodystrophy, evidence of small, misshapen kidneys, and stable or progressive azotemia documented over several weeks or more.
   b. Once CRF is identified, further diagnostic evaluation has two utilitarian goals:
      (1). Discovery of any potentially treatable cause of further renal injury (e.g., infection, chronic partial obstruction, subacute or chronic toxicity).
      (2). Characterization of the type and severity of functional impairments as a guide to therapy and as a basis for subsequent evaluation of disease progression and/or response to treatment.
5. General therapeutic objectives for patients with CRF are similar regardless of the cause of the problem.
   a. Minimize prerenal and postrenal adversities that might further compromise renal function, and avoid stress or iatrogenic disease.
   b. Regulate (supplement or limit) the dietary intake of nutrients as needed to compensate for impaired renal conservation and elimination. Nutrients of particular interest include water, nonprotein calories (carbohydrates and fats), protein, phosphate, sodium, calcium, and water-soluble vitamins.
   c. In addition to dietary phosphate restriction, use intestinal phosphate binders as needed to control hyperphosphatemia.
   d. In addition to dietary sodium restriction, use drugs as needed to control hypertension.
   e. Consider administration of hormones to correct endocrine deficiencies arising from inadequate renal production of erythropoietin and/or calcitriol.
   f. Emphasize optimum management of factors that may affect the rate of progression of chronic renal failure. Present evidence suggests that these factors include dietary protein intake, phosphate balance, and hypertension among other possibilities.
6. Short-term and long-term prognosis for CRF should be considered independently.
   a. In the short term, the physiologic and clinical status of an animal having a uremic crisis of CRF usually can be improved substantially with fluid therapy and supportive care.
   b. Depending on the degree of renal dysfunction, many animals with CRF can be medically assisted so that they can live adequately despite their disability.
   c. The length of time that an animal with CRF can be managed successfully is variable and not highly predictable.
   d. In the long term, most animals with CRF experience further progressive deterioration of their renal function, become more difficult to manage successfully, and eventually do not have sufficient renal function to sustain their lives.

C. Nephrotic syndrome.

1. Nephrotic syndrome exists when an animal has proteinuria, hypoalbuminemia, hypercholesterolemia, and excessive fluid accumulation in tissues or body cavities.
2. The massive urinary protein loss that is necessary to produce the nephrotic syndrome is always caused primarily by glomerular renal disease.
   a. The main categories of glomerular lesions associated with the nephrotic syndrome are glomerulonephritis and amyloidosis.
   b. Glomerular renal diseases usually occur secondary to some other disease process in the animal.
      (1). Glomerulonephritis usually is caused by immune-mediated events that can be secondary to numerous other diseases.
      (2). Amyloidosis usually is the reactive type (amyloid A) that occurs secondary to a variety of other diseases.
3. The glomerular renal diseases, with the potential to cause the nephrotic syndrome, often do not cause affected patients to develop the nephrotic syndrome. That is, many animals with significant proteinuria of glomerular origin do not have (and never develop) the nephrotic syndrome. These patients are properly categorized in other syndromes.
   a. Many have renal failure; usually it is CRF, but sometimes it is ARF.
   b. Some proteinuric animals have neither renal failure nor the nephrotic syndrome. Such animals fit in the Subclinical Urinary Abnormalities syndrome (see later section).
4. Diagnostic evaluation of animals with the nephrotic syndrome should address several issues.
   a. Investigation of the renal disease is appropriate.
      (1). Characterize the proteinuria (i.e., quantitative and qualitative features of the urinary protein loss).
      (2). Characterize the renal lesion, which requires evaluation of kidney biopsy specimens for definitive morphologic diagnosis of the renal disease.
   b. Investigation of the underlying primary disease is needed, because most glomerulopathies are secondary disorders.
      (1). Many animals have an identifiable underlying illness such as infection (e.g., bacterial, fungal, rickettsial, viral, or parasitic), disordered immune regulation, neoplasia, or miscellaneous other diseases.
      (2). Potentially treatable underlying illnesses are the most important to discover.
      (3). In some animals, an underlying illness that might be the cause of the glomerulopathy cannot be identified.
   c. Evaluation of the functional consequences and complications of the animal's nephrotic syndrome also is important. Common problems include perturbations of fluid balance, deficient protein balance, and thrombotic complications.
5. Treatment of animals with the nephrotic syndrome is mainly symptomatic and supportive. Specific therapeutic maneuvers that beneficially modify the anatomic or functional characteristics of glomerular lesions in animals with spontaneous glomerulopathies have not yet been adequately proved. Effective specific therapy often is not available.
   a. Combat fluid retention by restricting sodium intake and using diuretics judiciously while providing unlimited water intake.
   b. Provide an appropriate diet containing ample quantities of nonprotein calories. Protein intake should be sufficient for maintenance and replacement of basal urinary losses; however, further supplementation of protein intake tends to accelerate urinary protein loss rather than building body protein stores.
   c. Minimize stress and iatrogenic disease, and consider administration of an anabolic steroid hormone.
   d. Treat accordingly components of the animal's underlying disease that are amenable to specific therapy.
6. Prognosis for the nephrotic syndrome depends on many variables.
   a. In animals with the nephrotic syndrome, the renal disease and proteinuria rarely resolve completely, regardless of therapy. In fact, the underlying renal disease most often progresses.
      (1). Amyloidosis is more predictably progressive than is glomerulonephritis.
      (2). The magnitude of associated proteinuria may actually abate while the underlying renal disease progresses.
   b. The clinical course of the nephrotic syndrome is variable and unpredictable.
      (1). Clinically apparent fluid retention (i.e., formation of edema or ascites) sometimes ceases spontaneously or following a period of symptomatic and supportive therapy.
      (2). Fluid retention that persists usually can be successfully managed with medical strategies so long as the animal maintains an adequate glomerular filtration rate.
   c. Azotemia may or may not be associated with the nephrotic syndrome, but the underlying glomerular disease commonly progresses to CRF over a variable period.
   d. Most animals with the nephrotic syndrome eventually die of causes related to their renal disease.
      (1). Many develop renal failure that becomes unmanageable.

(2). Some develop fatal thrombotic complications.

D. Renal tubular defects.

1. There are two distinctly different types of renal tubular defects:
   a. Anatomic renal tubular abnormalities, which produce cystic or polycystic kidneys.
   b. Functional renal tubular abnormalities, which produce defective secretion or reabsorption of solutes or water.
2. Overall, renal tubular defects constitute a clinical syndrome of minor importance because these diseases occur infrequently.
3. Anatomic renal tubular defects may be recognized in several ways.
   a. These are uncommon congenital abnormalities and are found predominantly in young animals.
   b. When affected animals develop clinical signs, the signs usually are of another syndrome (e.g., CRF).
   c. Some instances of polycystic kidney disease produce marked renal enlargement, making affected kidneys readily palpable.
   d. Cystic or polycystic kidneys sometimes are discovered incidentally by radiography, ultrasonography, exploratory surgery or necropsy.
4. Functional renal tubular defects also may be recognized in a number of different ways.
   a. These also are uncommon abnormalities, but they may be either congenital or acquired lesions.
   b. Defective transport of solutes or water by renal tubular cells may have several clinical manifestations:
      (1). Polyuria and compensatory polydipsia.
      (2). Excessive urinary concentrations of specific substances.
         (a). Substances that readily dissolve in urine (e.g., glucose, bicarbonate) only cause polyuria.
         (b). Substances that do not readily dissolve in urine (e.g., cystine, uric acid) may form urinary calculi.
      (3). Serum biochemical abnormalities arising from excessive urinary loss of substances that should be conserved.
5. Diagnosis, treatment, and prognosis of renal tubular defects are highly variable, depending on the condition.
   a. Anatomic defects cannot be corrected. Clinically ill animals usually have chronic renal failure, and the principles for managing that syndrome are applied.
   b. Except for conditions associated with urolithiasis, diagnosis and treatment of disorders caused by functional renal tubular defects are a very small and highly specialized part of veterinary nephrology/urology. Acquired lesions (e.g., drug-induced defects) may resolve, but congenital abnormalities will persist.

E. Urinary retention.

1. Urinary retention exists when an abnormality affecting the renal pelves, ureters, urinary bladder, urethra, or adjacent structures prevents normal flow of urine through the excretory pathway and out of the animal.
2. Urinary retention is recognized either by finding abnormal or inappropriate distention of the excretory pathway by urine or by discovering leakage of urine from the excretory pathway.
   a. Physical examination findings often are sufficient for recognition of this syndrome.
   b. Urethral obstruction, a common cause of urinary retention, often is recognized partly because difficulty is encountered in passing a urethral catheter.
   c. When physical diagnostic methods are inconclusive, contrast radiographic procedures usually are employed to verify or exclude suspected urinary retention.
3. Inappropriate urine retention has many possible causes, including:
   a. Obstruction (i.e., abnormal resistance to normal urine flow)
      (1). Intraluminal abnormality (e.g., urolith, blood clot)
      (2). Intramural lesion (e.g., neoplasia, fibrotic stricture)
      (3). Extraurinary lesion (e.g., prostatic disease, entrapment in a hernia, reflex dyssynergia)
   b. Perforation of the excretory pathway (e.g., puncture, laceration, rupture)
4. Clinical signs associated with urinary retention are highly variable.
   a. Obstruction produces diverse signs depending on the site of obstruction, whether the obstruction is partial or complete, and whether it is acute (recent) or chronic (protracted).
   b. Perforation produces diverse signs depending on whether urine leakage is retroperitoneal, intraperitoneal, or into pelvic or perineal tissues, as well as on the amount and duration of urine leakage.
5. Acute, complete urinary retention (i.e., due to obstruction or perforation) produces a metabolic and clinical illness that sometimes has been classified as a type of ARF. Because renal parenchyma is *not* the principal site of disease or damage, however, it seems more accurate to classify this illness as "postrenal azotemia/uremia."
6. For animals with urinary retention, two sets of diagnostic concerns arise. These are:
   a. Characterization of the site and nature of the abnormality producing urine retention
      (1). Ordinarily, survey and contrast radio-

graphic studies are the mainstays of this investigation.
    (2). Other diagnostic techniques that may be useful include ultrasonography, endoscopy, cytology, biopsy, and urodynamic testing.
  b. Assessment of the consequences of urine retention that have developed in the animal
    (1). These often include the constellation of polysystemic clinical and metabolic disturbances of azotemia/uremia.
    (2). Occasionally, sequelae include anatomic or functional changes in the urinary tract (e.g., hydronephrosis, CRF), particularly in cases of chronic obstruction or severe overdistention.
7. Many elements of treatment of urinary retention are similar, regardless of the cause of the condition.
  a. Because it is a potentially life-threatening condition, the immediate therapeutic issue for patients with urine retention is management of postrenal azotemia/uremia when present. The general sequence of treatment efforts needed for postrenal azotemia/uremia is:
    (1). Correct deficits and excesses of extracellular fluid volume and composition.
    (2). Restore urine flow or otherwise relieve urine retention.
    (3). Maintain patency of some route for urine flow out of the animal.
    (4). Continue fluid therapy and supportive care while the physiologic consequences of urinary retention abate.
    (5). Proceed with remaining diagnostic and therapeutic steps that may be required to restore the animal's health.
  b. Specific therapy for lesions causing urinary retention depends on the site and nature of the abnormality.
8. Prognosis for urinary retention depends on numerous factors.
  a. With timely diagnosis and proper treatment, the short-term prognosis for animals with acute urinary retention usually is very good.
  b. In cases of chronic partial obstruction, prognosis generally relates to the degree of irreversible structural or functional damage, which may be minimal, severe, or anything in between.
  c. In all cases, long-term prognosis is determined mainly by the biologic behavior of the excretory pathway lesion causing urinary retention.
    (1). Lesions that can be repaired or completely resolved (e.g., ruptured urinary bladder, urethral obstruction by urolith) usually have an excellent long-term prognosis.
    (2). Progressive, incurable lesions (e.g., malignant neoplasia) usually have a poor, long-term prognosis.

F. Urolithiasis.

1. Urolithiasis exists when one or more crystalloid concretions form in the excretory pathway.
2. Recognition of urolithiasis usually is straightforward.
  a. Uroliths usually are detected in the urinary tract by physical diagnosis (e.g., palpation, catheterization) or by imaging studies (e.g., radiography, ultrasonography).
  b. Uroliths occasionally are found when they pass from the urinary tract.
3. Uroliths (urinary calculi) have distinctive characteristics.
  a. Uroliths are rigid structures composed of organic or inorganic crystalloids and a small amount of organic matrix.
  b. Uroliths are usually named and classified according to their crystalloid composition.
  c. Uroliths vary greatly in size and shape, as well as in their number, in an affected animal.
4. Because uroliths may be located anywhere in the excretory pathway, clinical signs associated with urolithiasis are diverse.
  a. In dogs and cats, most uroliths are found in the bladder or urethra.
    (1). Females typically have bladder stones that may cause changes in patterns of micturition (e.g., pollakiuria, dysuria) but do not cause obstruction.
    (2). Males typically come to medical attention because of urethral stones causing complete or partial obstruction. Such animals often have bladder stones as well. Altered patterns of micturition (e.g., pollakiuria, dysuria, strangury, paradoxic incontinence) are commonly seen.
  b. Signs associated with uroliths in the renal pelves or ureters are highly variable.
5. The syndrome of urolithiasis overlaps other syndromes of urinary disease in many patients.
  a. Because uroliths so often affect the bladder and urethra, disorders of micturition are common in animals with urolithiasis.
  b. Uroliths are a common cause (in dogs, they are the single most common cause) of urinary retention.
  c. Urinary tract infection (UTI) often is associated with urolithiasis. Urinary calculi predispose the animal to development of infection, and certain infections can cause formation of uroliths.
  d. Consequences of obstruction or infection associated with urinary calculi can lead to renal failure.
6. Several general principles govern the management of urolithiasis in all affected patients.
  a. Locate all the calculi in the urinary tract.
  b. Detect, characterize, and correct (or plan correction of) any complicating abnormalities that may exist, including:

(1). Abnormalities arising from effects of urolithiasis (e.g., postrenal azotemia/uremia, UTI).
(2). Preexisting abnormalities that predispose the patient to development of urolithiasis (e.g., portosystemic vascular shunts, diseases causing hypercalciuria, UTIs, defects that may have led to UTI).

c. Remove all calculi from the urinary tract.
(1). Various surgical procedures (e.g., nephrotomy, cystotomy, urethrotomy) have been used for this purpose.
(2). Recent development of methods for in situ fragmentation or dissolution of urinary calculi has added nonsurgical alternatives for stone removal in many cases.

d. Determine the composition of any calculi that are passed or removed from the urinary tract.

e. Based on knowledge of the stone type and its pathogenesis, use appropriate strategies to minimize recurrent stone formation.

7. In general, urolithiasis itself has a very good to excellent prognosis because an episode of urolithiasis usually can be resolved by dissolution or removal of the calculi. Factors that may diminish the prognosis for patients with urolithiasis are:
a. Complications arising from the effects of the calculi (e.g., structural or functional changes that are not completely reversible, infections that are not easily eradicated).
b. Inherent causes or predispositions for urolith formation that cannot be corrected or effectively offset by preventative measures. This leads to recurrent urolithiasis and diminishes long-term prognosis. Examples include some portosystemic vascular shunts and inborn errors of metabolism leading to excessive urine content of insoluble substances (e.g., cystine, uric acid).

G. Urinary tract infection.

1. UTI exists whenever microbes have colonized any portion of the urinary system that is normally sterile (i.e., the kidneys and all of the excretory pathway except the terminal portion of the urethra).

2. The etiologic agents of UTI usually are aerobic bacteria (e.g., enterobacteria, staphylococci, streptococci) that have ascended the excretory pathway; however, other microbes, anaerobic bacteria, fungal organisms, or viruses, or other routes of infection (e.g., through vascular channels or by extension from adjacent sites) are involved occasionally. Because the normal urinary tract is highly resistant to infection, occurrence of some noninfectious abnormality of the urinary system often precedes development of infection.

3. UTI may be manifested in many ways.
a. Inflammation often develops in infected tissues, and illness may be expressed as manifestations of this inflammation and associated exudation.
(1). Clinical signs due to inflamed tissues or organs (e.g., pollakiuria and dysuria due to urethrocystitis, renal pain due to pyelonephritis) may be seen.
(2). Abnormal laboratory findings (e.g., pyuria, hematuria, and proteinuria due to exudation into the urinary space) are commonly observed.
(3). In some cases, the inflammation associated with UTI is so mild or limited in extent that clinical signs are not apparent (i.e., subclinical UTI); however, laboratory indications of urinary tract inflammation generally are seen in these cases.
b. Virtually any other urinary disease can predispose to development of UTI, which may then exacerbate or modify the clinical signs and laboratory abnormalities exhibited by the animal. Examples include many causes of urinary incontinence, many causes of urinary retention, urolithiasis, neoplasia of the bladder or urethra, and renal failure.
c. UTI can cause other urinary diseases, with the illness then being mainly or entirely due to manifestations of a disorder which is actually a complication of infection.
(1). Infection of the kidneys may impair function sufficiently to cause renal failure (acute or chronic).
(2). UTI is a common cause of struvite (magnesium ammonium phosphate) urolithiasis in animals that do not develop clinical signs (i.e., they have subclinical UTI) until calculi form and grow large enough to cause signs.
d. UTI can lead to infection in extraurinary sites, with clinical manifestations then attributable to such disorders as septicemia, discospondylitis, prostatitis, epididymitis, or orchitis.

4. Diagnosis of UTI has several elements.
a. UTI usually is initially suspected because of clinical signs, laboratory findings, or discovery of some other disease with which UTI often is associated.
b. Definitive diagnosis of UTI, however, requires the demonstration of viable organisms in urine or urinary tissues that are obtained and processed so that contaminants are either excluded or distinguished from true evidence of infection.
(1). This usually is accomplished by performing bacterial cultures of urine because most urinary infections are caused by bacterial organisms that proliferate in the urine of affected patients.
(2). Occasionally, culture or microscopic inspection of urine or urinary tissues for

other types of infectious agents is necessary.

c. Identification of the anatomic distribution of infection within the urinary tract (i.e., localization of the infection) also is an important diagnostic issue.
   (1). Localization is important because appropriate therapeutic plans and accurate assessment of prognosis are greatly affected by the anatomic extent of infection.
   (2). Localization usually is based on clinical criteria, laboratory findings, and response to treatment; however, imaging studies and invasive tests (e.g., biopsy) are needed sometimes.
   (3). Methods for localizing urinary infections in animals are not highly sensitive or specific; therefore, diagnostic uncertainty often prevails. This makes careful monitoring of response to treatment especially important.

5. Management of patients with urinary infections is guided by their clinical categorization on the basis of apparent localization and coexistence of other urinary tract abnormalities. Clinical forms of UTI include:
   a. Complicated infections, which are those associated with other urinary abnormalities impairing host defenses against infection. This group may be further subdivided according to site of infection or type of complicating disease.
   b. Uncomplicated urethrocystitis, which is an infection associated with lower urinary tract (bladder and urethra) signs when other abnormalities impairing host defenses are not apparent.
   c. Uncomplicated pyelonephritis, which is an infection associated with upper urinary tract (renal pelvis and parenchyma) signs when other abnormalities impairing host defenses are not apparent.
   d. Subclinical infections, which are those in patients that lack clinical signs referable to infection and do not have apparent abnormalities impairing host defenses.
   e. Recurrent infections, which are any of the aforementioned forms exhibiting a chronic, intermittent course. Patterns of bacteriuria that may be associated with recurrent UTI include persistence, relapse, and reinfection.

6. Treatment of UTI has two general goals. These are to combat (hopefully eradicate) the existing infection as risk of subsequent infection or sequelae.
   a. Eradicating existing infection depends on proper antimicrobial therapy, which usually is the main method of treatment, and on ancillary therapy, which is especially important in complicated infections.
   b. Minimizing subsequent infections and complications usually depends on correction of reversible abnormalities that predispose to the development of UTI , but it sometimes depends on a judicious use of antimicrobial drugs to prevent or suppress clinically important infections associated with irreversible abnormalities.

7. Prognosis for UTI depends on several factors.
   a. Patients with acute, uncomplicated UTI generally have an excellent prognosis with proper treatment.
   b. Factors that diminish the prognosis for patients with UTI include:
      (1). Protracted duration of infection, which permits structural and functional changes associated with chronic inflammation to increase.
      (2). Extension of infection into tissues where attaining effective levels of antimicrobial agents is difficult. Important examples include the renal medullae and the prostate gland.
      (3). Existence of complicating abnormalities, in which case prognosis depends greatly on the type, severity, and potential for cure of the associated disease.
   c. In some patients, UTI cannot be cured.

H. Abnormal micturition.

1. Abnormal micturition exists whenever the ability of the bladder and urethra to accomplish normal storage and voiding of urine is altered by disease.
2. Abnormal micturition may be related to other syndromes of urinary disease.
   a. Altered patterns of micturition often are observed in animals in which one of the other syndromes of urinary disease can be identified as the primary problem. In such cases, proceeding with evaluation and treatment of the primary syndrome usually is the most effective approach. Examples include:
      (1). Altered frequency of otherwise normal voiding caused by increased (polyuria) or decreased (oliguria) rate of urine formation in animals with renal failure.
      (2). Increased frequency of voiding without increased rate of urine formation (pollakiuria), evidence of discomfort associated with urination (dysuria), excessive straining in attempts to pass urine (strangury), or combinations of these abnormalities in animals with urinary retention, urolithiasis, or UTI.
   b. Patients with altered patterns of micturition that cannot readily be attributed to another syndrome should be evaluated and treated according to principles for the syndrome of abnormal micturition.

3. Causes of abnormal micturition include:
   a. Disorders of the storage phase of micturition.
      (1). Anatomic abnormalities permitting urine flow to bypass normal sphincters. These usually are congenital anomalies (e.g., ectopic ureter, patent urachus), but can be acquired lesions (e.g., ureterovaginal fistula).
      (2). Functional abnormalities associated with noninfectious primary lesions of the bladder or urethra (e.g., feline idiopathic hemorrhagic cystitis, neoplasia, fibrosis).
      (3). Functional abnormalities not associated with evident primary lesions of the bladder or urethra. These usually are deficiencies of urethral contraction (e.g., urethral incompetence) but can be due to the inability of the bladder to fill normally (e.g., detrusor instability).
   b. Disorders of the voiding phase of micturition.
      (1). Disruption of the micturition reflex arc (i.e., upper and lower motor neuron deficits in neurologic control of the bladder and urethra).
      (2). Excessive resistance to urine flow from the bladder through the urethra (see the aforementioned section on causes of inappropriate urine retention [E, 3]).
4. Manifestations of abnormal micturition largely depend on the phase of micturition that is affected.
   a. Disorders of the storage phase of micturition usually are characterized by urinary incontinence (involuntary passage of urine), but urine retention may also occur in some cases.
   b. Disorders of the voiding phase of micturition typically cause some degree of urine retention, but urinary incontinence may also occur, particularly in animals with neurogenic disorders.
5. Diagnosis and treatment of abnormal micturition should be pursued in an orderly fashion.
   a. Paradoxic incontinence (leakage of urine past a partial obstruction) usually can be excluded by careful examination.
   b. Neurologic examination is used to exclude or identify neurogenic disorders of micturition.
      (1). Investigation and management of the primary disease then should be based on the principles of neurology.
      (2). Supportive care of animals with neurologic disease often requires attention to relief of urine retention, improving effectiveness of voiding, and prevention or treatment of urinary infection.
   c. Developmental anomalies usually are suspected on the basis of the animal's signalment and history.
      (1). Contrast radiographic studies usually are employed to verify the diagnosis, more fully characterize the lesion, and discover other associated abnormalities.
      (2). Treatment usually consists of surgical correction.
   d. Acquired primary lesions of the bladder and urethra are discovered by combining physical examination, routine laboratory testing, and imaging studies (e.g., survey and contrast radiography, ultrasonography).
      (1). Following their discovery, such lesions are investigated using whatever diagnostic techniques (e.g., cytology, endoscopy, surgical exploration, biopsy, urodynamic testing) are appropriate.
      (2). Treatment depends on the cause and severity of the lesion.
   e. Functional abnormalities are identified when morphologic abnormalities cannot be found in animals with dysfunction.
      (1). Urodynamic studies (e.g., cystometry, urethral pressure profilometry) may be used to further characterize the condition.
      (2). Therapeutic trials are conducted to discover whether such conditions are pharmacologically manageable.
6. Prognosis for animals with abnormal micturition is highly variable (that is, excellent to hopeless) and depends almost entirely on the cause, severity, and prospects for successful treatment of the condition producing abnormal micturition.

I. Subclinical urinary abnormalities.

1. Subclinical urinary abnormalities exist when there is evidence of disease of the urinary system in patients that do not have clinical signs of illness.
2. This syndrome designation is used for seemingly healthy animals that are found to have diseases of the urinary system on the basis of:
   a. Laboratory test results (e.g., proteinuria, hematuria, inability to concentrate urine normally).
   b. Imaging studies (e.g., radiography or ultrasonography showing abnormal renal size, shape, or echogenicity).
   c. Miscellaneous other findings (e.g., seeing a renal lesion while performing abdominal surgery).
3. The clinical importance of subclinical abnormalities often is uncertain.
   a. Subclinical abnormalities usually require surveillance, but exhaustive investigation of their cause may not be necessary or productive.
   b. Subclinical abnormalities often either resolve spontaneously or progress until they can be classified in a more specific syndrome.
4. Persistent or progressive abnormalities usually warrant diagnostic investigation, at least as needed to exclude potentially treatable conditions. For some abnormalities (e.g., proteinuria,

hematuria, polyuria), systematic investigative approaches (i.e., algorithms) have been developed to guide diagnostic evaluation.

5. Treatment and prognosis for subclinical urinary abnormalities vary greatly depending on the cause of disease.

III. OVERVIEW OF INVESTIGATION OF DISORDERS OF THE URINARY SYSTEM

A. Introduction.

1. In the practice of veterinary nephrology/urology, management of each case can be somewhat arbitrarily divided into three phases: beginning, middle, and end. In general, the focus of clinical activity shifts from investigation to intervention as the case passes through these phases.
2. Diagnostic investigation generally proceeds in a stepwise fashion along a path marked by two conceptual scales. One scale is the sequence of progressive steps in the investigation of a clinical problem. These steps are to verify the problem's existence, to localize its origin, to characterize its salient features, to identify its specific cause, and finally to monitor its temporal course. The second scale governing diagnostic investigations is the degree of invasiveness and risk of harm to the patient. Noninvasive procedures usually have no risk and are performed before minimally invasive procedures, which have minor risk. Invasive procedures, which usually have some potential for causing harm, generally are done last.
3. Formulation of treatment also proceeds along a general path marked by two conceptual scales. The first of these scales is the type of therapeutic intervention (i.e., symptomatic, supportive, or specific). The second scale is the priority for therapeutic intervention, such as:
   a. Emergency: eventual outcome of the case is likely to be adversely affected by delay of treatment.
   b. Urgent: eventual outcome is unlikely to be changed by delay, but prompt relief of some condition (e.g., patient pain or distress) is needed.
   c. Necessary: treatment that is required (albeit not needed as urgent or emergency treatment) for the patient to recover, improve, or do satisfactorily.
   d. Optional: treatment that is not required to obtain a satisfactory outcome, or treatment with uncertain benefit.
4. In the beginning of a case, diagnostic investigation is the main focus of attention. Except for treatments of emergency or urgent priority, therapeutic intervention usually is deferred until the cause and present status of the animal's illness are adequately defined.
   a. Investigation starts with noninvasive procedures, which often are sufficient for verification and localization of the animal's problem(s).
   b. Initial investigation often is extended by using minimally invasive procedures. These tests sometimes are needed for problem verification and localization; however, they are often used to begin problem characterization as well.
   c. Even when emergency or urgent treatment is needed, starting the clinical investigation properly is important also.
5. Culmination of diagnostic investigation and commencement of therapeutic intervention generally overlap in the middle of a case.
   a. Specialized tests and invasive diagnostic procedures are used as needed to adequately characterize a problem or to pin down its specific cause.
   b. Treatment usually begins with application of symptomatic and supportive therapy, which often can be rationally formulated even when the pathogenesis or specific cause of the problem is still poorly understood. In many patients, benefits of such therapy are needed before they are subjected to specialized tests or invasive procedures.
   c. As more fundamental understandings of the patient's problem(s) emerge, the specificity of therapeutic interventions generally increases.
   d. In some cases, a single invasive procedure (e.g., surgery) is used for both diagnostic and therapeutic purposes.
6. In the end phase of case management, orchestration of appropriate interventions is the main focus of attention. Diagnostic testing in this phase is used mostly to monitor the course of illness or response to treatment.
   a. Interventions may be intended to accomplish any of several goals, including to control clinical signs, to eradicate or cure the condition, to prevent or minimize its progression, or to prevent or minimize its recurrence.
   b. One or more interventions may be chosen from any of several categories, including dietary alterations, pharmacologic manipulations, or surgical corrections.
   c. As the animal's condition changes, whether spontaneously or in response to treatment, therapeutic endeavors commonly need to be adjusted, reformulated, or discontinued.
   d. Renewed diagnostic evaluation sometimes is made necessary by the occurrence of an unexpected clinical course or by the lack of an anticipated response to therapy.

B. History-taking.

1. History-taking is a crucially important, noninvasive method of clinical investigation.
2. History-taking should follow several general principles.
   a. Use a systematic approach to obtain a descrip-

tion of the present illness, review the animal's past history, and appraise the animal's environment and husbandry.

b. Discover the important characteristics of any signs that are reported by asking pertinent additional questions.

c. Determine the temporal relations of events and observations to build an understanding of the development and present status of the animal's problem(s).

3. Specific aspects of an animal's medical history that often relate to urinary system disease include:
   a. General patient status (e.g., attitude, activity, and appetite).
   b. Disturbances of gastrointestinal tract function (e.g., vomiting, diarrhea, and weight loss).
   c. Indicators of fluid balance (e.g., polyuria, polydipsia, and oliguria or anuria).
   d. Patterns of micturition (e.g., pollakiuria, dysuria, strangury, and incontinence).
   e. Abnormalities of urine (e.g., unusual color, clarity, and odor).
4. Refer to the section in Chapter 4 regarding minimum data bases for history and physical examination for additional details.

C. Physical examination.

1. Physical examination is another noninvasive method of clinical investigation having crucial importance.
2. General principles.
   a. Physical examination techniques that are useful for evaluation of the urinary system are observation, inspection, and palpation.
   b. Thorough, systematic physical examination of all accessible portions of the urinary tract is necessary whenever disease of any portion of the urinary system is suspected.
3. Examination of anatomic areas of interest.
   a. The kidneys may be examined by abdominal palpation. Both kidneys usually can be palpated in cats. In many dogs, neither kidney is palpable; however, one (the left) or both kidneys sometimes can be felt. During palpation, note the number, size, shape, position, contour, consistency, and sensitivity of the kidneys.
   b. Ureters ordinarily are not evaluated by physical examination techniques.
   c. Examination of the urinary bladder is by abdominal palpation and occasionally by digital rectal palpation. Evaluate the size, shape, position, contour, consistency, sensitivity, wall thickness, and contents of the bladder.
   d. The prostate gland of male dogs is examined by digital rectal palpation combined with simultaneous abdominal palpation. During palpation, note the size, shape, position, contour, consistency, and sensitivity of the prostate gland.
   e. Examination of the urethra is by digital rectal palpation, palpation and inspection of the perineal area (in males), and inspection of the external urethral orifice. Evaluate the position, contour, consistency, sensitivity, and contents of the urethra.
4. Refer to the section in Chapter 4 regarding minimum data bases for history and physical examination for additional details.

D. Cystocentesis and urinary catheterization.

1. These are minimally invasive physical procedures that are frequently used in the investigation of urinary diseases.
2. Cystocentesis usually is performed to obtain urine for diagnostic testing (e.g., analysis or culture) because specimens obtained in this way yield test results that are most likely to indicate in vivo conditions. Cystocentesis sometimes is used to decompress the urinary bladder when the urethra is obstructed.
   a. Most dogs and cats tolerate cystocentesis at least as well as, and often better than, they tolerate jugular venipuncture.
   b. Cystocentesis is a procedure that is quite safe, provided that a few common-sense precautions are observed.
   c. Refer to Chapter 5, Techniques of Urine Collection and Preservation, for additional details.
3. Urinary catheterization is performed for numerous diagnostic and therapeutic purposes.
   a. Diagnostic purposes for catheterization include collection of urine specimens for analysis or culture; detection of obstacles (e.g., uroliths) in the urethral lumen; measurement of urine formation rate; collection of accurately timed volumes of urine for renal function studies; instillation of contrast medium for radiographic studies of the bladder, urethra, or prostate gland; catheter biopsy of urethral, prostatic, or bladder lesions; and measurement of postmicturition residual urine volume.
   b. Therapeutic uses of catheterization include relief of urethral obstruction or urine retention, instillation of medications into the urinary bladder, and facilitation of surgery of the bladder, urethra, or surrounding structures.
   c. Urinary catheterization may be single or repeated brief catheterizations, or it may be indwelling catheterization.
   d. Adverse effects of catheterization may include physical injury (i.e., trauma) to the urinary tract and catheter-induced UTI.
   e. Urinary catheter usage always should be carefully planned and performed to minimize potential harm to the patient.
   f. Refer to the section in Chapter 5 regarding collection of urine for additional details.

E. Laboratory testing of specimens.

1. Laboratory testing of urine, blood, or other specimens obtained using minimally invasive methods

is a common and often crucial element of investigating disorders of the urinary system.

2. Urinalysis.
   a. Among methods for investigation of urinary disease, only history-taking and physical examination are more often useful or critically important than careful examination and analysis of a fresh urine specimen.
      (1). Findings of a complete urinalysis are needed to detect or to adequately characterize most urinary disorders.
      (2). Evaluation of renal function is most logically approached by combining urinalysis with serum chemistry testing. Renal function creates the difference between the composition of plasma and the composition of urine; therefore, comparison of urine with plasma yields direct evidence regarding renal function.
   b. A complete urinalysis requires both macroscopic and microscopic examinations. Macroscopic evaluations include appearance, volume, concentration, and reagent-strip tests for pH and abnormal quantities of various urine constituents (e.g., protein, glucose, blood, and others). Microscopic examination of urine sediment is used to identify and estimate the abundance of formed elements in the urine (e.g., erythrocytes, leukocytes, casts, crystals, epithelial cells, bacteria, and others).
   c. General implications of common urinalysis findings should be determined (refer to the section in Chapter 7, A Clinician's Analysis of Urinalysis, regarding interpretation of urinalysis for additional details).
      (1). Appearance
         (a). Abnormal urine constituents sometimes alter the gross appearance of the urine.
         (b). A visible change in urine color or clarity may be the first sign of disease, and it generally warrants further investigation.
         (c). A complete urinalysis usually identifies the entity causing the abnormal appearance.
      (2). Urine volume and concentration
         (a). Diseases that disrupt normal renal regulation of the volume and composition of extracellular fluid often are manifested by perturbations of urine formation rate (urine volume) and urine concentration.
         (b). Impaired urine-concentrating ability is a hallmark of both acute and chronic renal failure.
         (c). In acute renal failure (ARF), urine formation rate usually is reduced (i.e., oliguria or anuria), but sometimes is normal or increased.
         (d). In chronic renal failure (CRF), urine formation rate usually is increased (i.e., polyuria), but sometimes is normal or decreased.
         (e). Urine volume influences the apparent concentration or density of urine constituents that are assessed by semiquantitative methods. This influence, which is roughly proportional to urine concentration, must be considered when interpreting urinalysis results.
      (3). Urine pH.
         (a). Urine pH influences the solubility of calculogenic crystalloids in urine, and therefore is important to consider in the investigation of urolithiasis.
         (b). A highly alkaline urine pH often is associated with bacterial UTI caused by organisms (e.g., staphylococci, *Proteus* spp.) that produce the enzyme urease.
         (c). Inability to form acidic urine appropriately can be a sign of renal tubular dysfunction.
      (4). Proteinuria.
         (a). Marked proteinuria is the hallmark of glomerular renal lesions and is one of the identifying characteristics of the nephrotic syndrome.
         (b). Renal or excretory pathway lesions causing exudation or hemorrhage into the urinary space also are frequent causes of proteinuria. Proteinuria attributable to these causes typically is associated with hematuria, pyuria, or both.
         (c). Mild, transient renal proteinuria can be caused by functional changes in the healthy kidneys of patients with fever, passive renal congestion, or a variety of other conditions.
         (d). Besides being a marker for or a characteristic of many urinary diseases, proteinuria may occur when urinary tract lesions do not exist.
            1′). Proteinuria sometimes occurs because abnormal plasma proteins pass through the normal glomerular filtration barrier.
            2′). Proteinuria also sometimes occurs because of contamination arising from the genital tract or external genitalia.
         (e). The magnitude, source, and cause of proteinuria often must be thoroughly investigated. Refer to Chapter 9, Urinary Protein Loss, for additional details.

(5). Glucosuria
(a). Glucosuria usually is caused by hyperglycemia, such as that associated with diabetes mellitus, rather than by urinary disease.
(b). Glucosuria that is not attributable to hyperglycemia is an indication of renal tubular dysfunction.
(6). Cylindruria
(a). Urinary casts form in renal tubules and therefore are indicators of events occurring in the kidneys.
(b). Identifying the type(s) of casts seen, particularly when their cellular contents (e.g., tubular epithelial cells, erythrocytes, leukocytes) can be recognized, helps to characterize renal disease processes.
(7). Hematuria
(a). Finding blood in the urine indicates that hemorrhage or hemorrhagic inflammation is associated with a lesion somewhere in the urinary tract.
(b). Because blood contains proteins as well as cells, hematuria usually is accompanied by proteinuria.
(c). Hematuria most often arises from excretory pathway lesions; however, renal lesions occasionally cause hematuria.
(d). In male dogs, hematuria may also be associated with disease of the prostate gland.
(e). Hematuria is an important, but generally nonspecific, indicator of urinary disease.
(8). Pyuria
(a). Finding leukocytes in the urine generally indicates that suppurative inflammation is associated with a lesion somewhere in the urinary tract.
(b). Because exudates contain proteins and leukocytes, pyuria usually is accompanied by proteinuria.
(c). Pyuria most often arises from excretory pathway lesions; however, renal lesions occasionally cause pyuria.
(d). Because bacterial UTI is a common cause of hemorrhagic and suppurative inflammation in the excretory pathway, the combination of proteinuria, hematuria, pyuria, and bacteriuria occurs frequently.
(e). Frequent association with bacterial infection makes pyuria a more specific finding than hematuria, but noninfectious inflammatory lesions in the urinary tract also can produce pyuria.
(9). Bacteriuria
(a). As a urinalysis finding, bacteriuria is a microscopic observation of bacterial organisms in urine sediment or in stained smears of urine.
(b). Identification of bacteriuria by urinalysis is much less reliable than its identification by bacteriologic methods such as quantitative culture of a properly collected urine specimen.
(c). Whether the evidence is obtained from urinalysis or from urine culture results, bacteriuria demonstrated by a method that clearly indicates that it was present in vivo is the pathognomonic feature of bacterial UTI.
(10). Crystalluria
(a). Some of the substances excreted by the kidneys are sparingly soluble in urine and tend to precipitate from solution, forming crystals which are seen during microscopic examination of urine sediment.
(b). The type and number of crystals that are observed are influenced by numerous factors.
(c). Generally, crystalluria is important either because of its relation to urolithiasis or because it indicates a metabolic aberration (or both).
(d). In an animal with urolithiasis, identification of crystals in the urine can be a clue to the composition of the uroliths; however, crystalluria in such patients does not always match the stone type.
(e). Crystalluria is sometimes an important clue to the diagnosis of metabolic disorders such as ethylene glycol toxicity (oxalate crystals) or portosystemic vascular shunts (urate crystals).

3. Hematologic studies.
a. Many urinary diseases do not produce notable changes in the patient's hemogram, or they produce nonspecific changes. Consequently, routine hematologic studies often do not play an important role in the investigation of urinary diseases.
b. In patients suspected of having urinary disease, routine hematologic studies often are performed mainly to screen for evidence of disorders affecting other organ systems.
c. General implications of common hematologic findings are as follows:
(1). Anemia
(a). Hypoproliferative (nonregenerative) anemia is so common in animals with CRF that finding an anemia of this

type is an important clue suggesting chronicity in patients with renal failure.

(b). Anemia arising from excessive blood loss or hemolysis (i.e., regenerative anemias) and anemia arising from bone marrow suppression that is not attributable to CRF can be a feature of a variety of nonurinary or polysystemic diseases that may cause or complicate urinary disorders.

(c). Anemia rarely is caused by excessive bleeding solely from the urinary tract.

(2). Polycythemia

(a). Relative polycythemia that is due to hemoconcentration may be associated with urinary diseases that produce dehydration of animals that are not already anemic (e.g., some patients with ARF).

(b). Absolute polycythemia is occasionally associated with a renal disease that causes excessive production of erythropoietin.

(3). Leukocytosis

(a). Finding an increased white blood cell count generally indicates the presence of inflammation, which may have an infectious or a noninfectious cause.

(b). Even in patients with urinary disease, leukocytosis often is mainly due to inflammation in one or more other organ systems. That is, inflammatory nonurinary or polysystemic diseases can cause or be complicated by urinary disease processes that do not contribute substantially to the leukocytosis.

(c). When leukocytosis is caused by inflammation within the urinary system, the site of inflammation generally is in parenchymal tissue rather than in the excretory pathway. That is, leukocytosis is associated with nephritis or prostatitis, but not with cystitis or urethritis.

(4). Disorders of hemostasis

(a). Thrombocytopenia, when found in a patient with urinary disease, generally is associated with a nonurinary or polysystemic component of the animal's illness.

(b). Bleeding that is due to a congenital or acquired disorder of hemostasis can be the cause of hematuria.

(c). Evidence of disseminated intravascular coagulation is sometimes found in patients with severe polysystemic illnesses that become complicated by ARF.

(d). A hypercoagulable state, which predisposes to thrombus formation, develops in some animals with the nephrotic syndrome.

4. Serum chemistry tests.

a. In order of general importance for investigation of urinary diseases, serum chemistry testing ranks just behind urinalysis among laboratory evaluations.

(1). Results of serum chemistry tests often are crucial for the detection and/or characterization of diseases of the urinary system, particularly those affecting the kidneys.

(2). Evaluation of renal function using serum chemistry test results is greatly aided by also performing a urinalysis on a specimen obtained at about the same time that the blood specimen is drawn.

b. General implications of common serum chemistry findings are as follows:

(1). Azotemia (refer to Chapter 10, Evaluation of Renal Functions, for additional details).

(a). Azotemia is an abnormally high serum or plasma concentration of urea nitrogen (BUN), creatinine, or (most frequently) both.

(b). The principal method by which both urea and creatinine are removed from extracellular fluids is glomerular filtration. This renal function, however, depends on the integrity and function of prerenal and postrenal components. Because the driving force for filtration is provided by the left ventricle of the heart, the prerenal component is the cardiovascular system's provision of cardiac output, blood pressure, and patent vessels leading to and from the kidneys. Because the urine formed by the kidneys must be discharged from the body, the postrenal component is provided by an intact and unobstructed excretory pathway for urine.

(c). Causes of azotemia are classified as prerenal, renal, or postrenal perturbations. Prerenal causes include increased influx of nitrogenous waste (e.g., increased ureagenesis) and any cardiovascular disruption of adequate perfusion of the kidneys (e.g., dehydration, hypovolemia, hypotension, vascular occlusion). Postrenal causes are lesions of the excretory pathway that obstruct the flow of urine (leading to a decline of filtration caused by backpressure) or permit urine to leak into tissues or body cavities (from which sites the urea and creatinine are reabsorbed). Renal causes of azotemia are lesions of kidney parenchyma that reduce glomerular filtration rate. The existence of renal failure is defined by discovery of azotemia that is attributable to renal lesions.

(d). Whenever azotemia is discovered, categorizing its cause(s) as prerenal, renal, or postrenal has high priority in the initial phase of diagnostic investigation. Postrenal azotemia generally is recognized by finding direct evidence of excretory pathway obstruction (e.g., unproductive efforts to urinate, inability to pass a urinary catheter) or perforation (e.g., accumulation of urine in the peritoneal cavity or in periurethral tissues). Prerenal azotemia generally is recognized by virtue of its coexistence with formation of urine that is highly concentrated in a patient affected by some condition impairing renal perfusion. Renal azotemia generally is recognized by exclusion of postrenal and prerenal causes and by its coexistence with formation of urine that is not well concentrated.

(2). Hyperphosphatemia

(a). Hyperphosphatemia often accompanies azotemia because glomerular filtration rate also is a major determinant of phosphate excretion. Degree of hyperphosphatemia associated with azotemia tends to be greatest when the condition has an abrupt onset and azotemia develops rapidly (e.g., ARF, complete urethral obstruction).

(b). Compared with urea and creatinine-excretion, phosphate excretion is subject to a much greater degree of renal tubular regulation. This regulatory control permits chronically failing kidneys to sustain phosphate excretion to a much better degree than would otherwise be possible with a given decrement in filtration. For this reason, hyperphosphatemia accompanying chronic renal failure generally is less severe (in proportion to the azotemia) than the hyperphosphatemia that accompanies ARF.

(c). Hyperphosphatemia and the regulatory responses that compensate for impaired phosphate excretion are closely coupled to disturbances of calcium regulation in patients with CRF. Additionally, pathophysiologic processes associated with disturbed phosphate regulation may contribute to progressive deterioration of remnant kidney function. For these reasons, medical strategies for monitoring and controlling hyperphosphatemia have a prominent role in the management of patients with CRF.

(3). Serum calcium abnormalities

(a). Disturbances of calcium regulation are associated with a number of disorders of the urinary system.

(b). Hypercalcemia, which may arise by several possible mechanisms, is an important cause of ARF.

(c). Hypocalcemia develops in some patients with ARF, especially those with ethylene glycol toxicity.

(d). In patients with CRF, hypocalcemia tends to develop for a number of reasons, including inadequate renal synthesis of calcitriol. However, many patients with CRF have normal serum calcium levels, and hypercalcemia occasionally develops in these patients.

(e). In patients with the nephrotic syndrome, hypoproteinemia often is associated with hypocalcemia that can be attributed to decreased plasma protein-bound calcium levels. The biologically active, unbound fraction of serum calcium usually is regulated normally in these patients.

(4). Acid-base disturbances

(a). The kidneys normally have an important role in the regulation of acid-base balance; therefore, some urinary disorders produce acid-base disturbances.

(b). Inadequate renal acid excretion often leads to metabolic acidosis in patients with postrenal azotemia/uremia and in those with a uremic crisis due to ARF or CRF. The degree of metabolic acidosis generally is proportional to the severity of the animal's azotemia and uremia; however, gastrointestinal loss of hydrogen ion due to vomiting sometimes ameliorates the acidosis.

(c). Metabolic acidosis also is a characteristic of some types of functional renal tubular defects (e.g., renal tubular acidosis).

(5). Electrolyte disturbances
(a). Hyperkalemia is a characteristic and potentially life-threatening component of the biochemical derangement that develops in patients with anuria or oliguria due to postrenal lesions (e.g., obstruction or perforation of the excretory pathway) or ARF.
(b). In addition to hyperkalemia, hyponatremia typically develops in patients with leakage of urine into the peritoneal cavity (e.g., with a ruptured bladder).
(c). Unless potassium intake is augmented appropriately, hypokalemia often develops in patients experiencing marked diuresis (e.g., during periods of intravenous fluid therapy following relief of obstruction or in the early recovery phase of ARF), especially when the animal is not yet eating well. Hypokalemia is a common finding in cats with chronic polyuric renal failure.
(6). Hypoproteinemia
(a). Hypoalbuminemia is one of the defining features of the nephrotic syndrome.
(b). Hypoalbuminemia also can be an indication of protein malnutrition in CRF patients on protein-restricted diets.
(7). Hypercholesterolemia: patients with the nephrotic syndrome typically exhibit hypercholesterolemia.

5. Microbiologic studies.
a. As their initial goal, microbiologic studies generally are intended to discover whether the pathogenesis of a given animal's disease of the urinary system includes infectious agents.
(1). Attempting to grow pathogens from specimens obtained from affected areas in the patient is most often used to find evidence of an infectious agent. Other methods that are sometimes employed include using various types of microscopy to directly demonstrate organisms in appropriate specimens, and serologic techniques to provide indirect evidence of infection.
(2). Microbiologic investigation of urinary disorders most often focuses on infectious agents that cause disease after migrating up the excretory pathway. The great majority of such pathogens are aerobic bacteria that are abundant in the urine of affected animals. These organisms are not fastidious; therefore, they usually can be grown from a suitable urine specimen with ease.
b. Once an infectious agent that can be incriminated as a pathogen is isolated, additional microbiologic studies usually are focused on identifying and characterizing the agent. Characteristics that have implications for prognosis and therapy (e.g., susceptibility to various antimicrobial drugs) are especially important.
c. Bacterial urine culture (refer to the section in Chapter 8, Diagnostic Urine Culture, regarding microbiologic investigation of urinary disorders for additional details.)
(1). Bacterial urine culture generally entails aerobic incubation of appropriate media inoculated with urine.
(a). The culture method must permit a quantitative or semiquantitative assessment of the density of bacteriuria in the original urine specimen because proper interpretation of urine culture results depends partially on this information.
(b). The culture method also should permit isolation of the infecting organisms in pure culture so that bacterial identification and antimicrobial drug susceptibility testing can be performed when needed.
(2). Depending on the way in which specimens are collected and handled, urine obtained from animals that do not have UTI may contain bacteria (even in large numbers).
(a). This "insignificant" bacteriuria generally arises because of contamination of the specimen with bacteria from the distal urethra, adjacent genital structures, or extraneous sites. Regardless of precautions taken to minimize contamination, specimens obtained by voiding or catheterization have some risk of contamination from the urethra. Such contamination can be avoided by obtaining urine for culture by cystocentesis.
(b). In properly collected specimens, the magnitude of bacteriuria that is due to contamination generally is less than the magnitude of bacteriuria that is due to untreated infections; however, some specimens obtained from uninfected animals by catheterization or voiding will have a high magnitude of bacteriuria similar to that expected from infected animals. In addition, the conditions of specimen transportation and storage can permit a few contaminants to grow to misleadingly large numbers before the specimen is cultured.

(c). For these reasons, urine culture results must be interpreted in light of the specimen collection and preservation techniques used.

(3). Properly interpreted urine culture results can be used to guide the diagnosis and treatment of animals with bacterial UTI in a variety of ways, including:

(a). To verify or exclude bacterial infection as a pathogenic component of an animal's urinary disease.

(b). To aid formulation of predictably effective drug treatment plans based on identity of the infecting organisms or on their in vitro susceptibility to antimicrobial agents.

(c). To verify eradication of bacteriuria during and/or following antimicrobial drug treatment.

(d). To detect recurrent bacteriuria and provide a basis for categorizing its cause as relapse (recrudescence of the same infection) or reinfection (development of a new infection).

6. Cytologic evaluations.

a. Characterization of the cellular elements of specimens obtained from diseased tissues or organs is a simple and inexpensive yet powerful diagnostic method. With the assistance of appropriate stains, microscopic evaluation of cellular specimens can be highly informative.

(1). Specimens that are useful for cytologic evaluation can be obtained in a variety of ways. Secretions, exudates, scrapings, washings, and fine-needle aspirates can be smeared directly on glass microscope slides for staining and examination. Specimens that are not highly cellular (e.g., some secretions and washings) can be concentrated by various techniques to make finding and examining the cells more efficient.

(2). Although findings are not always conclusive, cytologic evaluations may yield a variety of categorical or more specific interpretations (e.g., normal, hypertrophy, hyperplasia, inflammation, neoplasia).

b. Common uses in investigation of urinary diseases include the following:

(1). Much of the microscopic examination of urine sediment during a complete urinalysis is a form of cytologic evaluation. However, cells rapidly deteriorate in urine, and critical cytologic evaluation of cells found in urine sediment often is impossible.

(2). Cytology plays a prominent role in the evaluation of dogs with prostatic disease. Fluid specimens, which often are informatively cellular, can be obtained by ejaculation or by massage of the gland followed by aspiration or washing to recover the specimen from the prostatic portion of the urethra. Depending on the size and position of the gland, fine-needle aspirates can be obtained using one of several approaches.

(3). Most bladder and urethral neoplasms are of epithelial origin, and they often will readily exfoliate malignant cells when their surfaces are abraded with a urinary catheter. Recovery of the specimen in sterilized saline (i.e., not in urine) helps to preserve cellular detail. The cytology of bladder washings must be interpreted cautiously, however, because inflammation of the urinary bladder can stimulate reactive epithelial hyperplasia, with the production of many cells having characteristics that often are associated with malignancy.

(4). Fine-needle aspirates sometimes can be used to evaluate the kidneys, especially when they are enlarged by parenchymal infiltration. In cats with renal lymphoma, for example, the diagnosis often can be readily made by examining fine-needle aspirates from their kidneys.

(5). When surgical procedures are used to biopsy lesions in the urinary tract, cytologic examination of impression smears or scrapings from the excised tissue (before it is immersed in fixative) often will give a sufficient indication of the nature of the lesion to guide the surgeon in making any intraoperative decisions that might be required.

F. Diagnostic imaging methods.

1. Obtaining images that demonstrate or represent morphologic changes in urinary tract organs or adjacent structures often is a crucial component of the diagnostic investigation of patients with urinary disorders.

a. Diagnostic imaging sometimes is the means by which the existence of urinary disease first becomes recognized.

b. Imaging methods sometimes produce findings that are sufficiently distinctive to permit the making of highly specific diagnoses of urinary tract diseases.

c. Even when imaging methods yield nonspecific findings, the morphologic changes that they reveal generally are highly useful for localizing and characterizing diseases of the urinary system.

d. Conversely, absence of expected morphologic changes often is important evidence against existence of a urinary disorder that is under consideration.

2. Diagnostic imaging techniques range from relatively simple, noninvasive procedures such as ultrasonography and survey radiography to more complex and invasive procedures such as contrast radiography.
   a. Noninvasive imaging techniques are most often used in the initial phases of diagnostic investigations.
      (1). Survey radiography is frequently used to screen for changes in the size, shape, position, or radiodensity of urinary tract organs near the outset of investigation.
      (2). While noninvasive imaging techniques are useful and sometimes highly informative screening methods, they lack diagnostic sensitivity and specificity for a great many urinary tract lesions and disorders.
   b. Invasive imaging techniques are most often used to further characterize lesions or conditions that have been discovered and partially characterized by results of preceeding noninvasive and minimally invasive tests.
3. Obtaining optimum value from diagnostic imaging procedures requires careful planning and coordination of the imaging studies with one another as well as with other parts of the investigation.
   a. The medical imaging methods that are the mainstays of contemporary practice of veterinary nephrology and urology are survey radiography, a variety of contrast radiographic procedures, and ultrasonography.
      (1). Each of these studies has different capabilities and limitations, and each often produces findings that complement the others. Integration and correlation of results from several different imaging studies often yields a more complete composite picture of the problem than could be obtained otherwise.
      (2). Invasive imaging techniques can affect results of other tests or lead to the development of new problems; therefore, they must be fitted into the rest of the animal's diagnostic investigation and treatment with some care.
   b. Rapid development of new technology for medical imaging is occurring. Increased availability and use of methods such as scintigraphy, computed tomography, and magnetic resonance imaging can be anticipated for the future. Adding these imaging modalities will make the challenges of selecting the best studies to perform and properly integrating the results of multiple studies much greater.
4. Refer to Chapter 11, Diagnostic Imaging of the Urinary Tract, for additional details.

G. Ancillary diagnostic methods for diseases of the urinary system.

1. Overview.
   a. A variety of special procedures are sometimes used to investigate disorders of the urinary system. Each procedure is focused on evaluating a very specific area or function in depth, and most are invasive. Consequently, these procedures are employed in the final phases of diagnostic investigations to answer important questions that remain after history-taking, physical examination, laboratory testing, and imaging studies have been performed and interpreted. They are rarely appropriate in the initial phases of clinical investigations.
   b. Common categories of special diagnostic procedures include renal function studies, urodynamic studies, endoscopy, exploratory surgery, and biopsy.
2. Renal function studies.
   a. In general, these procedures are used to measure specific renal functions for the purpose of:
      (1). Detecting or characterizing certain renal diseases.
      (2). Evaluating severity of functional impairment as a guide to prognosis, formulation of therapy, and/or evaluation of response to treatment.
   b. Special renal function studies are of two basic types:
      (1). Those that evaluate glomerular function.
      (2). Those that evaluate tubular secretion and/or absorption.
   c. Special tests of glomerular function include:
      (1). Direct measurement of glomerular filtration rate (GFR), such as by determination of inulin clearance, endogenous or exogenous creatinine clearance, or clearance of certain radiopharmaceuticals. Refer to Chapter 10, Evaluation of Renal Functions, for additional details.
      (2). Measurement of proteinuria and other indicators of altered glomerular permeability such as urine protein:creatinine ratio (which actually is a minimally invasive evaluation that often is used early in the investigation of proteinuria) or quantitative analysis of daily urine protein loss. Refer to Chapter 9, Urinary Protein Loss, for additional details.
   d. Special tests of renal tubular function include the following (refer to Chapter 10, Evaluation of Renal Functions, for additional details):
      (1). Urine-concentrating ability demonstrated in response to water deprivation (iatrogenic dehydration), which essentially is an endogenous antidiuretic hormone (ADH) release and response test, or to the admin-

istration of antidiuretic hormone (i.e., an exogenous ADH response test).

(2). Urine-acidifying ability in response to administration of a defined acid load.

(3). Clearance ratios, which are expressions of the tubular handling (i.e., fractional excretion) of filtered solutes.

3. Urodynamic studies.
   a. In general, these procedures measure fluid pressure and flow relationships in the bladder and/or urethra during storage and/or voiding phases of micturition to evaluate lower urinary tract function.
   b. Specific urodynamic tests include:
      (1). Urethral pressure profile, which demonstrates the pressures observed along the length of the urethral lumen during the storage phase of micturition.
      (2). Cystometrogram, which demonstrates the pressures observed in the bladder lumen while the bladder is filled with fluid (i.e., storage phase) until a micturition reflex is stimulated and detrusor contraction occurs (i.e., voiding phase). Although the voiding phase of micturition is included, a urinary catheter in the urethra (which is used to fill the bladder and measure intravesical pressures) alters the urodynamics of natural voiding.
      (3). Micturition study, which is a technique combining a cystometry performed with bladder catheters placed through the abdominal wall (rather than through the urethra) with measurement of fluid flow through the urethra (uroflowmetry). The entire micturition cycle (storage, micturition reflex, and voiding) is evaluated.
   c. Refer to Chapter 14, Tests of Lower Urinary Tract Function in Dogs and Cats, for additional details.
4. Endoscopy.
   a. In general, endoscopy is used to visualize the lumen of internal organs or body cavities for the purpose of identifying and characterizing lesions and performing biopsies of affected tissues.
   b. Access to areas of interest may be obtained by:
      (1). Passing a suitable endoscope up the excretory pathway (i.e., through the external urethral orifice or a urethrostomy).
      (2). Passing a suitable endoscope through the wall of the urinary tract (e.g., percutaneous antepubic cystoscopy using a laparoscope).
      (3). Using a laparoscope to examine the kidneys in their retroperitoneal locations.
   c. Refer to Chapter 13, Endoscopy, for additional details.
5. Surgical exploration.
   a. In general, surgical procedures are used to gain access to the organs of the urinary tract for the purposes of:
      (1). Identifying and characterizing lesions.
      (2). Obtaining tissues or other specimens for microscopic examination or other special evaluations.
      (3). Performing surgical treatments such as removing undesirable contents, excising abnormal tissues, repairing injuries, and/or reconstructing damaged organs.
   b. Most of the urinary tract is accessible through a midline celiotomy incision from the pubis to the level of the kidneys, but a variety of other surgical approaches can be used to advantage, depending on the anatomic area(s) of interest.
   c. Exploratory surgery has the advantage of being within the expertise and equipment available in most veterinary practices, whereas some of the other diagnostic procedures (e.g., ultrasonography, endoscopy) require expertise and/or equipment that is not as widely available.
6. Biopsy.
   a. Definitive diagnosis of renal or prostatic parenchymal lesions or of infiltrative/proliferative lesions of the excretory pathway often requires microscopic examination of tissue obtained from the affected area to characterize the pathologic process.
   b. Specific procedures include the following:
      (1). Endoscopically guided biopsy, usually with an instrument passed through the endoscope.
      (2). Percutaneous techniques using special biopsy instruments that are guided by rectal or abdominal palpation, digital palpation through small "keyhole" incisions, or ultrasonography (e.g., various techniques used for biopsy of kidney or prostate gland).
      (3). Intraoperative excision of tissues for further examination during surgical procedures that have obtained full visual exposure of the area(s) of interest (e.g., exploratory celiotomy, cystotomy, nephrotomy).
   c. Refer to Chapter 12, Canine and Feline Renal Biopsy, for additional details.

CHAPTER 4

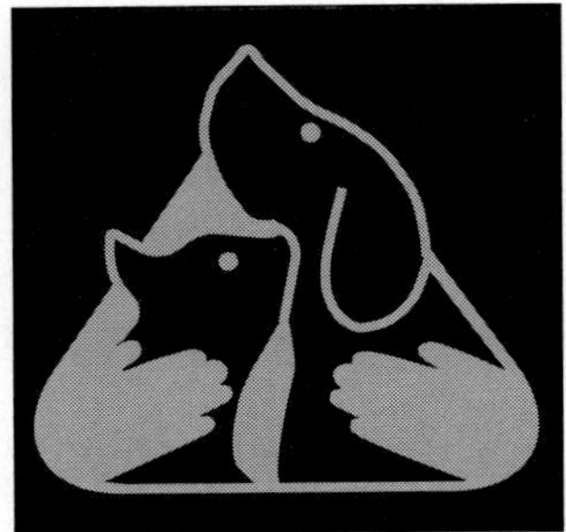

Clinical Algorithms and Data Bases for Urinary Tract Disorders

Outline

I. Concepts - priorities of clinical investigation
II. Data bases
  A. Defined data base
  B. Minimum data base
  C. Problem-specific data base
III. Algorithms
IV. Tables and figures
  A. General overview
    1. Table 4–1. General priorities for clinical evaluation
    2. Table 4–2. Defining problems at an appropriate level of refinement
    3. Table 4–3. Properly refined versus overstated problems
    4. Table 4–4. DAMN IT acronym of pathophysiology
    5. Fig. 4–1, **A.** Schematic of a decision tree for a clinical problem
    6. Fig. 4–1, **B.** Illustration of a decision tree for the clinical problem of bacteriuria
  B. Urinary tract disorders
    1. Table 4–5. Outline of minimum data base for diagnosis of urinary tract disorders
    2. Disorders related to diseases of the upper urinary tract
      a. Problem-specific data base
        i. Table 4–6. Outline of problem-specific data base for renal failure
        ii. Figure 4–2. Algorithm for the diagnosis of renal failure
      b. Clinical signs
        i. Figure 4–3. Algorithm for the diagnosis of polyuria
        ii. Table 4–7. Problem-specific data base for persistent vomiting
        iii. Figure 4–4. Algorithm for the diagnosis of anorexia
        iv. Figure 4–5. Algorithm for the diagnosis of weight loss
        v. Table 4–8. Clinical significance of kidney size
      c. Laboratory data
        i. Figure 4–6. Algorithm for the diagnosis of proteinuria
        ii. Table 4–9. Problem-specific data base for protein-losing glomerulopathy
        iii. Figure 4–7. Algorithm for the diagnosis of glucosuria
        iv. Figure 4–8. Algorithm for the diagnosis of anemia in dogs
        v. Figure 4–9. Algorithm for the diagnosis of anemia in cats
        vi. Figure 4–10. Algorithm for the diagnosis of hyperkalemia
        vii. Figure 4–11. Algorithm for the diagnosis and treatment of hypokalemia
        viii. Figure 4–12. Algorithm for the diagnosis and treatment of hypernatremia
        ix. Figure 4–13. Algorithm for the diagnosis of hyponatremia
        x. Figure 4–14. Algorithm for the diagnosis of hypercalcemia
        xi. Figure 4–15. Algorithm for the diagnosis of hypocalcemia
        xii. Figure 4–16. Algorithm for the diagnosis of increased serum activities of amylase and lipase
        xiii. Figure 4–17. Algorithm for the diagnosis of

abnormalities in serum total protein and albumin concentrations

d. Radiography
   i. Figure 4–18. Algorithm for the interpretation of the radiographic appearance of the kidneys following intravenous injection of radiopaque contrast media

3. Disorders related to diseases of the upper and lower urinary tracts
   a. Clinical signs
      i. Figure 4–19. Algorithm for the diagnosis of red, brown, or black colored urine
      ii. Table 4–10. Probable localization of gross hematuria
      iii. Figure 4–20. Algorithm for the diagnosis of abdominal distention
   b. Laboratory data
      i. Table 4–11. Problem-specific data base for urinary tract infections
      ii. Figure 4–21. Algorithm for the treatment of bacterial urinary tract infections
      iii. Figure 4–22. Algorithm for the diagnosis and treatment of fungal urinary tract infections
      iv. Table 4–12. Problem-specific and therapeutic-specific data base for the diagnosis and management of urolithiasis
4. Disorders related to diseases of the lower urinary tract
   a. Clinical signs
      i. Figure 4–23. Algorithm for the diagnosis of dysuria and pollakiuria
      ii. Table 4–13. Problem-specific data base for urinary incontinence
      iii. Figure 4–24. Algorithm for the diagnosis of urinary incontinence
   b. Laboratory data
      i. Figure 4–25. Algorithm for the treatment of urate urocystoliths in dogs
      ii. Figure 4–26. Algorithm for the prevention of urate urocystoliths in dogs
      iii. Figure 4–27. Algorithm for the prevention of calcium oxalate urocystoliths in dogs

I. Conceptually, minimum data bases, defined data bases, problem-specific data bases, and algorithms are used to prioritize consistently efficient and effective management of patients.[1]
   A. The first step in the diagnostic process must be to define and verify clinical problems (Table 4–1).
      1. Problems must be defined before they are solved.
      2. Errors made in identification and verification of clinical problems may not only lead to fruitless pursuit of nonexistent disorders, they may result in a costly and time-consuming series of diagnostic and therapeutic plans before errors are identified.
   B. Following accurate definition and verification of problems from data collected from the history, physical examination, and laboratory or radiographic procedures when appropriate, a complete problem list should be constructed.
      1. Problems should be stated at their highest level of refinement and should be defined in such a way that their refinement can be defended with reasonable certainty on the basis of current knowledge about the patient.
      2. Listed from the lowest to the highest level of refinement, problems may be defined as: a subjective clinical sign (such as red urine); an objective diagnostic finding (such as azotemia, hematuria, bacteriuria, and bilateral renomegaly); a pathophysiologic syndrome (such as primary renal failure); and a specific diagnostic entity (such as bacterial pyelonephritis).
      3. Disciplined thought is required to construct a meaningful problem list (Tables 4–2 and 4–3).
      4. When integrating problems to their highest degree of refinement, it is important to consider that clinical manifestations of disease are usually a combination of signs induced by the disease, such as obligatory polyuria associated with bacterial infection of the urinary tract, and the body's compensatory response to these problems, such as compensatory polyuria and inflammation designed to eradicate bacteria and repair damaged tissues.
   C. Localization of problems should follow their definition and verification (see Table 4–1).
   D. Following localization of problems to a body system or organ, it is useful to think of basic pathophysiologic mechanisms when trying to determine probable (rather than possible) causes of each problem.
      1. The acronym DAMN IT may be useful for this purpose (Table 4–4).[2]
      2. One of the most frequent errors made by diagnosticians is the premature consideration of specific disease entities without: a) verifying the existence of problems, especially those identified by owners; b) localizing problems to the appropriate body system or organ; and c) considering basic pathophysiologic disease mechanisms that might be involved.
   E. Following establishment of the most probable causes of a problem, appropriate diagnostic tests and procedures should be performed to prove (rule in) or disprove (rule out) them.
II. A data base is defined as a large collection of data organized so that it can be expanded, updated, and retrieved rapidly for various uses.
   A. The defined data base is based on the premise that data collection cannot be infinite; it is in reality finite.[1]
      1. If an examination were complete, the medical history could be infinitely long, the physical examination could last for hours, and the laboratory examination could require weeks for completion.
      2. Such fanatic thoroughness is medically unnecessary and economically unsound.[3]
      3. In the context of the problem-oriented system of diagnosis, the defined data base includes a defined history and a defined (rather than complete) physical examination, and may include laboratory and/or other procedures (including urinalysis, hemogram, etc.).
      4. Defined data bases need not be confined to information obtained from the medical history and physical examination.
      5. The composition of defined data bases, including minimum data bases and problem-specific data bases, is established prior to evaluation of patients.
   B. The term minimum data base is often used synonymously with the term defined data base.[1]
      1. The minimum data base represents the minimum amount of information used to define what at least is evaluated before a system(s) or organ(s) is considered to be normal (Table 4–5); it is typically a screening diagnostic tool.
      2. Rarely is initial collection of data confined to the

minimum data base.

3. If an abnormality is detected by history, physical examination, and laboratory procedures, more data may be (and usually is) required to evaluate it than originally specified in the minimum data base.

C. A problem-specific data base represents a more defined data base formulated for a specific clinical problem (Tables 4–6 through 4–13).[1]
   1. A problem-specific data base is more detailed than a minimum data base; it is typically a searching diagnostic tool.
   2. All of the data requested in problem-specific data bases should be collected from each patient with the problem in question.

III. Algorithms are special diagrams designed to facilitate solving specific problems.[4–6]
   A. Algorithms are represented graphically by a detailed step-by-step decision tree for solving problems (Figure 4–1).
      1. Algorithms are reported to have first been used by computer scientists to represent the computer's stepwise solution to a problem.
      2. Clinical algorithms are organized sets of rules of procedures for solving diagnostic or therapeutic problems.
         a. Clinical algorithms represent a sequence of clinical decisions that guide patient care.
            i. Each algorithm is a branching network of decision points.
            ii. Each point branches into at least two paths, each path leading to successive decision points that in turn branch into at least two more points until a defined endpoint is reached.
            iii. The endpoint is unique to the pathway leading from the point of origin.
         b. Properly constructed algorithms concisely, clearly, and consistently inform users about which procedures to perform and the sequence in which various procedures are to be performed; they represent a "given this, do that" scheme of action.
   B. Use of algorithms facilitates consistency of clinical evaluation and therapy (Figures 4–2 through 4–27).[4,6,7]
      1. Algorithms may save time by eliminating the need for paramedical personnel to ask certain questions.
      2. Algorithms can be constructed to connect specific decisions to scientific literature that documents the decisions' validity or explains the rationale for the decisions.
      3. Algorithms facilitate teaching.
      4. Algorithms provide a format that facilitates thought and recall about clinical problems.
      5. Algorithms minimize the time required by medical personnel to reconstruct diagnostic and therapeutic plans.
      6. Algorithms developed by systems or discipline specialists enable primary care veterinarians to manage problems that are otherwise beyond their level of competency.
      7. Algorithms can be constructed to emphasize preconceived priorities or probabilities.
   C. Clinical algorithms are not the ultimate answer for consistent delivery of quality patient care.
      1. Algorithms cannot ensure accuracy of observations, and they have no judgment.
      2. Unlike decision analysis (which specifies the probability that a particular clinical state exists and quantitates the value of the outcome of the decision), the innate structure of an algorithm does not specify probability of outcome.
      3. If terms and directions are not carefully chosen and explained by their designer, different meanings may be conveyed to different users.
      4. Algorithms must be interpreted in the context of relevant probabilities.
         a. Algorithms may not apply only to a specific patient.
         b. No algorithm can be applied to a patient until the patient, who is always unique, has been carefully examined.
         c. An algorithm can be used only when it is determined that a patient's problem suits the problem defined in an algorithm.
         d. The clinical decision regarding whether or not the patient fits the algorithm has to be repeated at each point at which the algorithm defines a clinical problem.
         e. The algorithm enables the practice of a defined standard of care.
      5. Algorithms rarely encompass all probabilities.
      6. Minor exceptions do not negate the general rule.
      7. An inability to understand algorithms denotes an inability to solve practical problems systematically by using branching logic.
   D. Construction of an algorithm requires careful planning and a thorough understanding of the topic.[4,7]
      1. Clinical algorithms are branching decision trees.
         a. At each branching point, one of three outcomes may occur: i) a problem is identified; ii) a diagnostic decision must be made; or iii) a therapeutic decision must be made.
         b. When a problem is identified, a course of action must be chosen.
         c. When a diagnostic or therapeutic decision is made, the consequences of the choice may be predicted; however, consequences may also occur by chance.
         d. Decision analysis rests on the theory of how patients ought to behave in the face of uncertainty; it is not a theory of how patients actually behave.
         e. A "good" decision may, because of the uncertainty, lead to a "bad" outcome; therefore, the quality of a decision cannot be judged by its outcome.
         f. The quality of the process by which the choice was made can be judged, however, and if the choice had the highest expected value of any choice available, then given the particular probabilities and values, it was, in decision analytic terms, the best choice, regardless of the outcome.
         g. In decision analysis, the process of choosing is emphasized, not the choice itself.
      2. Algorithms are constructed in a stepwise fashion.
         a. Identify the topic that requires problem definition and solution.
         b. Define the problem to be solved.
         c. Specify who will solve the problem.
            i. This will influence the terminology used.
            ii. This will influence the degree of complexity of the algorithm.
         d. Develop a first draft of decisions that connect the starting point with the outcome.

i. At this phase, one must define specific methods that facilitate solution of the problem.
ii. Use of case examples may be very helpful at this phase of development.

e. Evaluate and, if necessary, revise the algorithm until graphic reliability is attained.
f. Test, and, if necessary, revise the algorithm until performance effectiveness is attained.
   i. It may be useful to consult with a systems, discipline, or species specialist when validating the reliability of the algorithm.
   ii. Once algorithms are designed, they must be evaluated for reliability and safety before being adopted for routine use.

E. Algorithmic pathways frequently must be supplemented with additional information.
   1. Algorithms are rarely designed to be consistently reliable in circumstances in which two or more different disorders interact in the same patient.
   2. Clinical algorithms typically require judgment in the absence of certainty.
   3. If pertinent new clinical data become available after an algorithmic decision has been made, the algorithm may be reapplied to the entire collection of clinical data.

REFERENCES

1. Klausner JS, Osborne CA. The urinary tract: Minimum and problem-specific data bases. *Vet Clin North Am Small Anim Pract.* 1981;11:523.
2. Osborne CA. The transition of quality patient care from art to a science. The problem-oriented concept. *J Am Anim Hosp Assoc.* 1975;11:250.
3. Hurst JW: How does one develop a defined data base? Who collects the data? In: Hurst JW, Walker HK, eds. *The Problem-Oriented System.* New York, NY: Medcom Press; 1972.
4. Osborne CA. Clinical algorithms: Tools that foster quality patient care. In: Kirk RW, ed. *Current Veterinary Therapy X.* Philadelphia, Pa.: WB Saunders Co; 1989.
5. Margolis CZ. Uses of clinical algorithms. *JAMA.* 1983;249:627.
6. Hadorn DC, McCormick K, Koikno A. An annotated algorithm approach to clinical guideline development. *JAMA.* 1992;267:3311.
7. Gorry GA. New perspectives on the art of clinical decision making. *Am J Clin Pathol.* 1980;75(supplement):483.

TABLE 4–1
GENERAL PRIORITIES FOR CLINICAL EVALUATION*

Collect Information
- A. Define data to be collected
  - 1. Minimum data base
  - 2. Problem-specific data base
  - 3. Clinical algorithms

Define Problem(s)
- A. Refine to highest degree of refinement
- B. Do not overstate problems

Formulate Diagnostic Plans
- A. Verification of problem(s) is first priority
  - 1. Especially important for historical problems such as hematuria, polyuria, dysuria
  - 2. Also of significance for transient or intermittent problems
- B. Localization of problem(s) to body system(s) or organ(s) is second priority
- C. Consider probable cause(s) as third priority
  - 1. Pathophysiology first (DAMN IT, Table 4–4)
  - 2. Specific cause(s) next

Formulate Prognosis
- A. Short-term versus long-term
- B. With therapy versus without therapy

Formulate Therapeutic Plans
- A. Specific
- B. Supportive
- C. Symptomatic
- D. Palliative

Formulate Follow-up Plans

*Modified from Osborne CA, Finco DR. Diagnostic procedures in urology: Use and misuse. In: *Scientific Proceedings of the American Animal Hospital Association.* South Bend, Ind: American Animal Hospital Association; 1978.

TABLE 4–2
DEFINING PROBLEMS AT AN APPROPRIATE LEVEL OF REFINEMENT

Unrefined	Refined
1. Palpable bladder mass 2. Hematuria 3. Dysuria 4. Proteinuria 5. Pyuria 6. Significant bacteriuria	Disease of the urinary bladder associated with: 1. Palpable mass 2. Primary or secondary infection of the urinary tract (significant bacteriuria) 3. Dysuria 4. Inflammation of the urinary tract (pyuria, proteinuria, hematuria)

TABLE 4–3
PROPERLY REFINED VERSUS OVERSTATED PROBLEMS

Unrefined Problem	Proper Definition	Overstated Problem
1. Dysruia 2. Abnormal urine odor 3. Bacteriuria 4. Pyuria 5. Hematuria 6. Proteinuria	Disease of the urinary tract associated with: Primary or secondary bacterial infection (significant bacteriuria) Inflammation of the urinary tract (proteinuria, pyuria, hematuria)	Bacterial cystitis

TABLE 4–4
DAMN IT ACRONYM OF PATHOPHYSIOLOGY*

D — Degenerative disorders
    Dementia
A — Anomalies
    Autoimmunity
M — Metabolic Disorders
N — Neoplasia
        Benign
        Malignant
  — Nutritional disorders
I — Inflammation (infectious or noninfectious)
  — Immune disorders
  — Iatrogenic disorders
  — Idiopathic disorders
T — Toxicity (endogenous or exogenous)
  — Trauma (external or internal)

*Modified from Osborne CA. The transition of quality patient care from an art to a science: The problem-oriented system. *J Am Anim Hosp Assoc.* 1975;11:250.

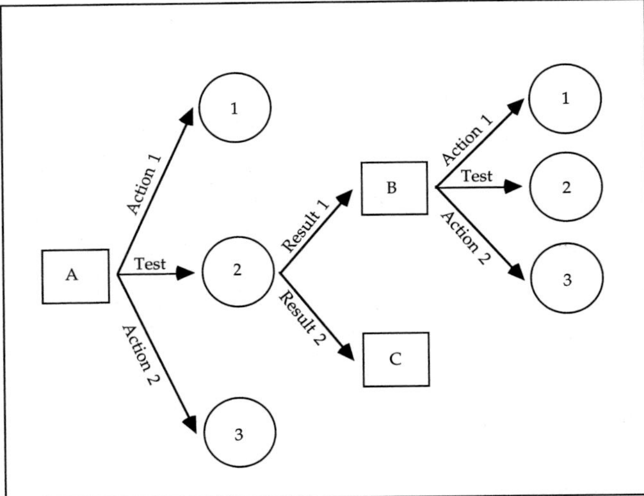

FIG. 4–1, A. Schematic of a decision tree for a clinical problem. Key: □ = points where the decision maker must choose a particular action; ○ = points where outcomes of decisions (consequences) are influenced by chance.

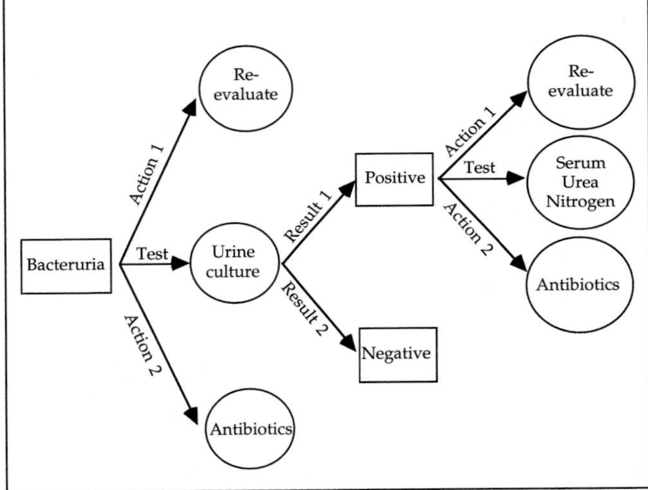

FIG. 4–1, B. Illustration of a decision tree for the clinical problem of bacteriuria. Key: □ = points where the decision maker must choose a particular action; ○ = points where outcomes of decisions (consequences) are influenced by chance.

TABLE 4–5
OUTLINE OF MINIMUM DATA BASE FOR DIAGNOSIS OF URINARY TRACT DISORDERS

History

A. Diet: type(s), frequency of feeding, duration of feeding, diet, supplements, treats?
B. Water consumption: increased, decreased, no change, unknown?
C. Duration of problem(s)?
D. Recurrence of problems, and intervals involved?
E. Person who observes?
F. Previous illness or injury?
G. If other pets at home, are they normal or abnormal?
H. Exposure to other animals, potential toxins, etc.?
I. Micturition
  1. Character, frequency, quantity?
  2. Pollakiuria (dysuria, tenesmus)?
  3. Polyuria (polydipsia)?
  4. Oliguria?
  5. Anuria?
  6. Urinary incontinence?
  7. Micturition in unusual locations?
  8. Change in urine color
    a. Red (hematuria, hemoglobinuria, myoglobinuria)?
    b. Brown, black, green, etc.?
  9. Uroliths voided during micturition?
J. Change in odor of urine?
K. Licking vulva or prepuce?
L. Association with other signs not directly related to urinary system
  1. Vomiting?
  2. Diarrhea?
  3. Anorexia?
  4. Weight loss?
  5. Others?
M. Are problem(s) increasing in severity, decreasing in severity, or static?
N. Medication: type, dose, duration, response?

Physical Examination

A. Temperature, pulse rate, respiratory rate?
B. Body weight?
C. Skin pliability?
D. Mouth
  1. Mucosal ulcers?
  2. Discoloration of tongue?
  3. Pallor of mucous membranes?
  4. Evidence of vomitus?
  5. Loose or missing teeth?
  6. Enlargement of maxillary tissues?
  7. Xerostomia?
  8. Uremic breath?
E. Rectal examination
  1. Feces normal or abnormal?
  2. Palpation of urethra and periurethral tissues?
F. Kidneys
  1. Both palpable? Bilaterally symmetric?
  2. Position in abdominal cavity?
  3. Shape, consistency, and surface contour?
  4. Size (Table 4–8)?
  5. Pain?
G. Urinary bladder
  1. Position?
  2. Size, shape, consistency?
  3. Grating or nongrating masses or adjacent to bladder lumen*? (If present, is location constant or variable?)
  4. Pain?
  5. Thickness of bladder wall?
H. Prostate gland
  1. Position?
  2. Size, shape, consistency?
  3. Pain?
I. Urethra
  1. In male dogs and cats, urethral or preputial discharge?
  2. Examination of perineal urethra in male dogs?
  3. Rectal examination of urethra
    a. Position?
    b. Size, shape, and consistency?
    c. Periurethral abnormalities?
J. Micturition
  1. Normal storage and voiding phases of micturition?
  2. Results of neurologic examination?
  3. Ease of inducing voiding by palpation?
  4. Residual urine following voiding?
  5. Evidence of incontinence?

Laboratory Data

A. Complete blood count
B. Urinalysis

*If overdistention with urine interferes with palpation of lumen, repalpate following removal of an appropriate quantity of urine.

TABLE 4–6
OUTLINE OF PROBLEM-SPECIFIC DATA BASE FOR RENAL FAILURE*

Minimum Data Base

A. Medical History Checklist
   1. Age?
   2. Breed?
   3. Duration of illness?
   4. Previous illness or injury?
   5. Past history of renal disease? Recent evaluation indicating adequate renal function?
   6. Exposure to possible nephrotoxins?
   7. Recent trauma, surgery, or anesthesia?
   8. Diet: Type? Frequency of feeding? Supplements? Recent diet changes? Preferences?
   9. Water consumption: Increased, decreased, unknown, or no change? If change noted, when?
   10. Micturition? Frequency? Quantity? Color? Odor? Changes? Urinary incontinence? Micturition in abnormal locations?
   11. Detection of signs not directly referable to the urinary tract:
       Anorexia? Weight loss? Vomiting?
       Constipation? Diarrhea? Others?
   12. Are clinical signs increasing in severity, decreasing in severity, or remaining the same?
   13. Medication history: Medications given? When given? Dose? Duration? Response? Tolerance?

B. Physical Examination Checklist
   1. Temperature, pulse, and respiratory rate?
   2. Hydration status (skin pliability, xerostomia, etc.)?
   3. Body weight?
   4. Mouth: Mucosal ulcers? Discoloration of tongue? Pallor of mucous membranes? Loose or missing teeth? Enlargement of maxillary tissue?
   5. Cardiovascular system: Pulse rate and character? Mucous membrane color? Capillary refill time? Heart sounds? Venous distention? Arterial blood pressure (if available)?
   6. Kidneys: Both palpable? Bilaterally symmetric? Position? Size (Table 4–8)? Shape? Consistency? Contour? Pain?
   7. Urinary bladder: Size (before and after micturition)? Shape? Consistency? Position? Pain? Wall thickness? Intraluminal masses (consistency? attached? grating sensation?)?
   8. Urethra (if possible): Position? Size? Shape? Consistency? Intraluminal masses (consistency? attached? grating sensation?)?
   9. Penis, prepuce, vulva: Shape? Consistency? Discharge? Pain?
   10. Ophthalmoscopic examination of fundus for evidence of hypertension: Retinal detachment? Hemorrhage? Others?

C. Laboratory Data Checklist
   1. Urinalysis, including urine sediment
   2. Kidney function tests (serum creatinine and urea nitrogen)
   3. Hematocrit, total plasma protein concentration (CBC?)

Further Diagnostic Consideration

A. Serum biochemical profile (Na, Cl, K, P, TCO_2, Ca, albumin, others to identify associated complications and extrarenal causes of azotemia [i.e., hypoadrenocorticism, hyponatremia, others])
B. Urine culture (especially if microburia, dysuria, or hematuria is detected)
C. Survey abdominal radiography (to verify kidney number, size, shape, and position)
D. Urine protein creatinine ratio (to quantify protein loss in patients with proteinuria)
E. Arterial blood pressure
F. Intravenous urography
G. Renal ultrasonography
H. Renal biopsy

*Modified from Lulich JP, Osborne CA, O'Brien TD, Polzin DJ. Feline renal failure: Questions, answers, questions. *Compen Cont Educ.* 1992;14:127.

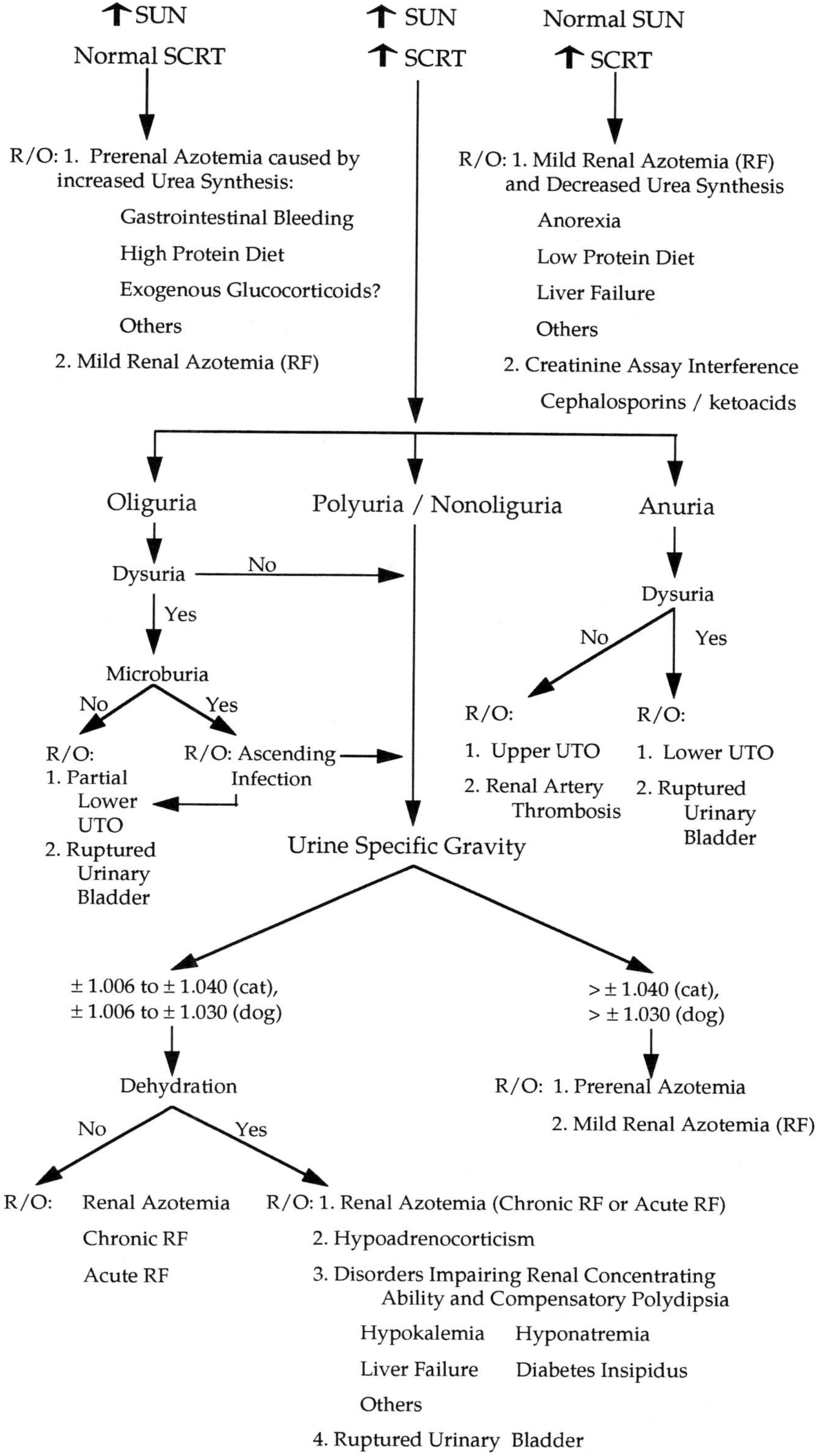

FIG. 4–2. Algorithm for the diagnosis of renal failure. Modified from Lulich JP, Osborne CA, O'Brien TD, Polzin DJ. Feline renal failure: Questions, answers, questions. *Compen Cont Educ.* 1992;14:127. Key: SUN = serum urea nitrogen concentration; SCRT = serum creatinine concentration; R/O = rule out; RF = renal failure; UTO = urinary tract obstruction.

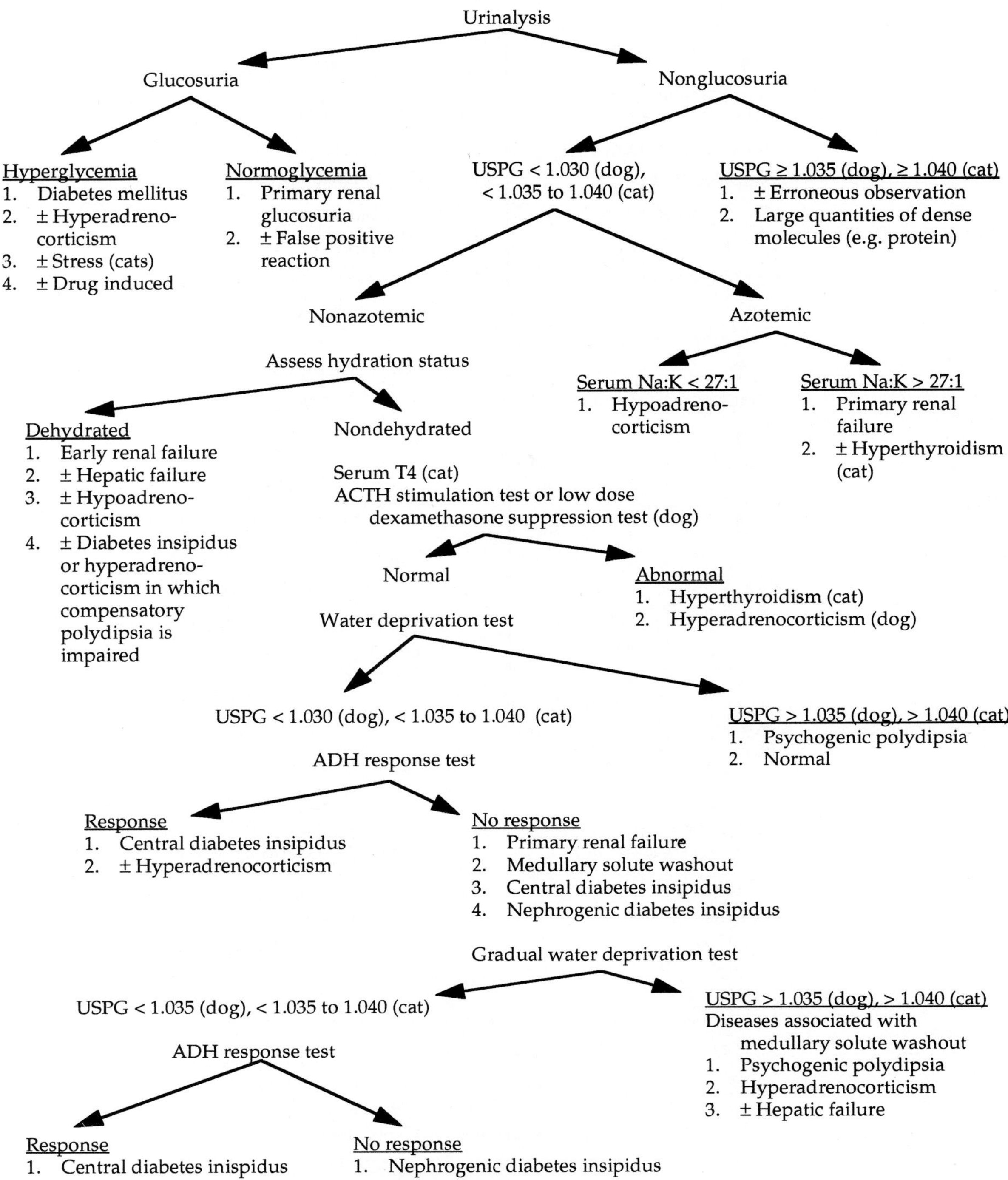

FIG. 4–3. Algorithm for the diagnosis of polyuria. Modified from Osborne CA. Clinical algorithms: Tools that foster quality patient care. In Kirk RW, ed. *Current Veterinary Therapy,* Vol IX, pp. 26–33. Philadelphia, Pa: WB Saunders Co; 1989. Key: USPG = Urine specific gravity.

TABLE 4–7
PROBLEM-SPECIFIC DATA BASE FOR PERSISTENT VOMITING*

A. History
  1. Observed by whom?
  2. Previous illness or injury?
  3. Other pets at home? Normal or abnormal? Duration?
  4. Association with other signs (polydipsia, polyuria, diarrhea, etc.)?
  5. Character, quantity, frequency?
  6. Any change: better, worse, same?
  7. Associated with eating?
  8. Exposure to toxins, foreign bodies, etc.?
  9. Medication given? Type? Dose? Response?

B. Physical examination
  1. Temperature, pulse, respiration, body weight?
  2. Skin pliability?
  3. Examine mouth?
  4. Visualize and palpate thoracic inlet?
  5. Visualize respiration and auscultate chest?
  6. Palpate abdomen in different positions; use sedation if necessary?
  7. Rectal examination; examine feces on glove?

C. If hospitalization is required:
  1. Verify emesis and characterize vomitus
  2. Hemogram
  3. Serum biochemical analysis ± thyroxine concentration in cats and freeze extra serum
  4. Urinalysis
  5. Examine feces for quantity and quality
  6. Survey abdominal radiography

D. If causes of emesis are localized to gastrointestinal tract:
  1. ±Contrast gastroenterography
  2. ±Gastroduodenoscopy and biopsy
  3. ±Laparoscopy and biopsy
  4. ±Exploratory laparotomy and biopsy

*Modified from Klausner JS, Osborne CA. The urinary tract: Minimum and problem-specific data bases. *Vet Clin North Am.* 1981;11:523.

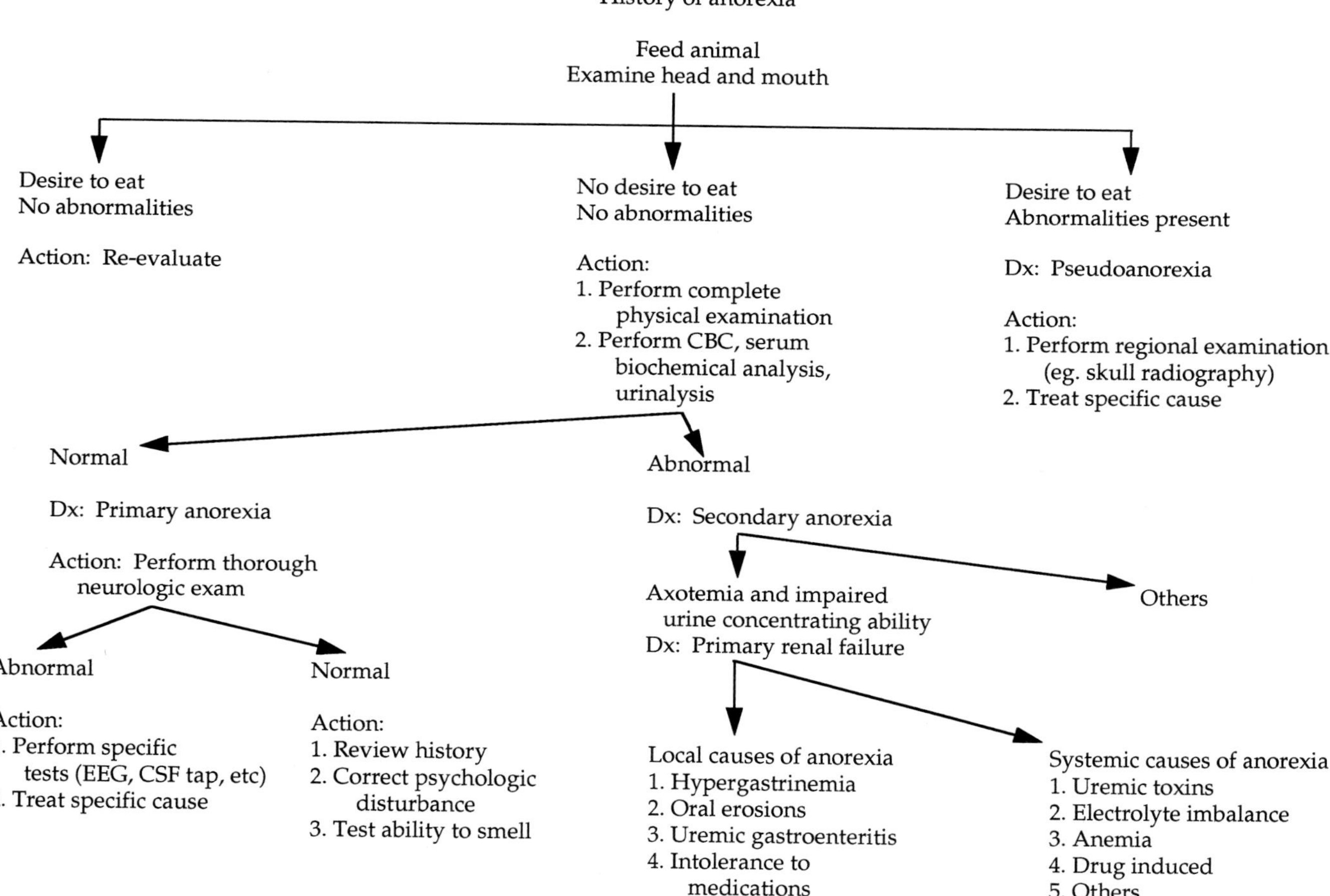

FIG. 4–4. Algorithm for the diagnosis of anorexia. Modified from Lorenz MD, Cornelius LM. *Small Animal Medical Diagnosis.* Philadelphia, Pa: JB Lippincott Co; 1987: p. 31. Key: Dx = diagnosis; CBC = cell blood count; EEG = electroencephalogram; CSF = cerebrospinal fluid.

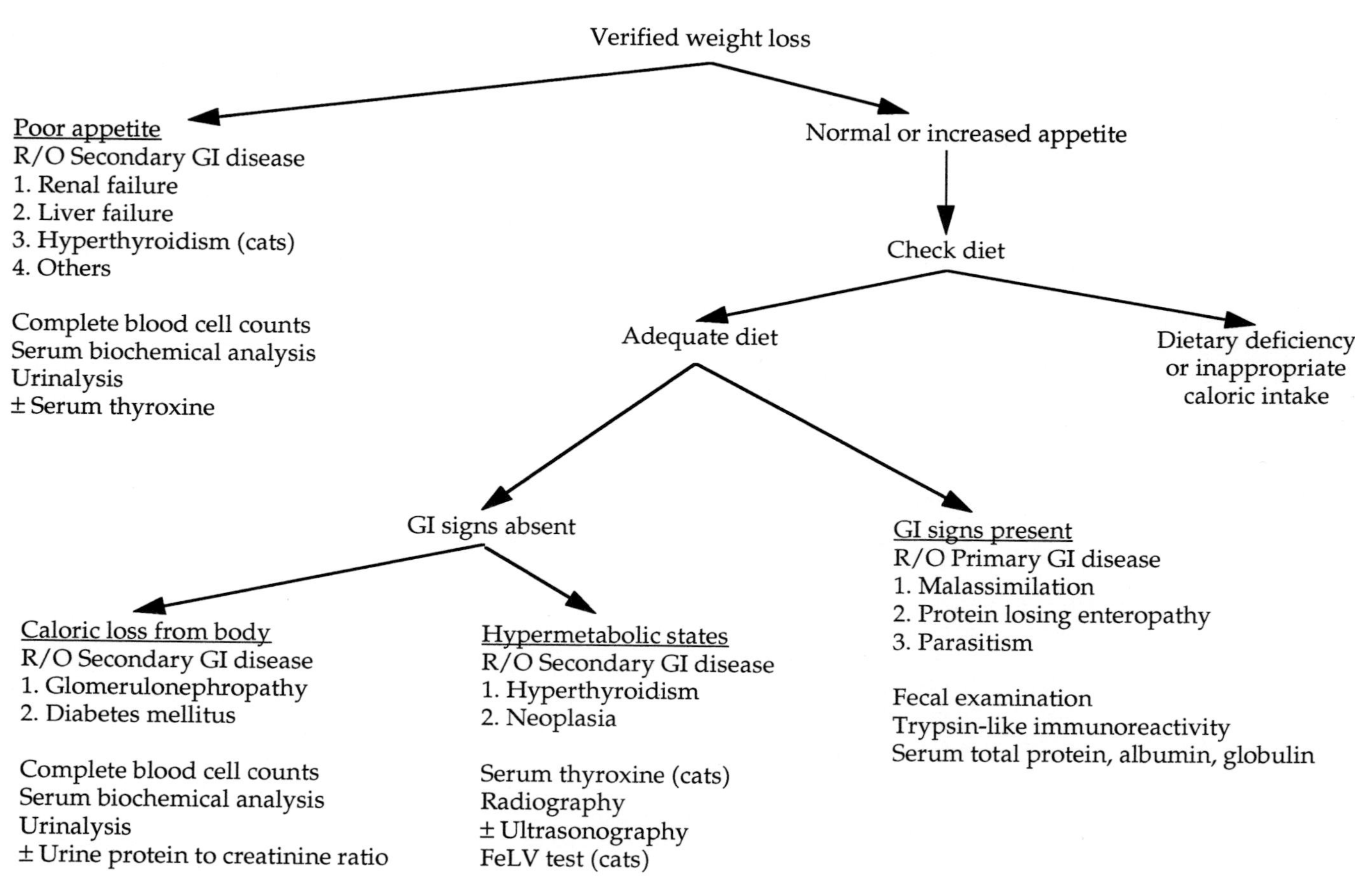

FIG. 4–5. Algorithm for the diagnosis of weight loss. Modified from Lorenz MD, Cornelius LM. *Small Animal Medical Diagnosis.* Philadelphia, Pa: JB Lippincott Co; 1987. Key: R/O = rule out; GI = gastrointestinal; ± = sometimes; FeLV = feline leukemia virus.

TABLE 4–8
CLINICAL SIGNIFICANCE OF KIDNEY SIZE*

Kidney Size	Possible Cause	Kidney Size	Possible Cause
Absent	Failure to evaluate patient by contrast urography Congenital aplasia Nephrectomy Obstruction of renal artery Marked or total obstruction of urine outflow High rate of solute and water excretion by affected kidney	Normal†	All diseases except congenital hypoplasia
		Slight to moderate	Swelling Acute nephritis, nephrosis Hydronephrosis (bilateral)‡ Polycystic kidneys (irregular contour) Subcapsular or pericapsular hemorrhage
Small	Chronic inflammation Infection (i.e., pyelonephritis) Ischemia (i.e., amyloid, glomerulonephritis) Infarction Congenital hypoplasia	Marked enlargement	Hydronephrosis (unilateral smooth contour)‡ Neoplasia (irregular contour) Polycystic kidneys (irregular contour)

*Modified from Osborne CA, Johnston GR, Feeney DA. A compendium of survey and contrast uroradiography. In: 1979 Scientific Proceedings of the American Animal Hospital Association, Annual Meeting, South Bend, Indiana, 1979.

†The normal length of canine kidneys is 2.5 to 3.5 times the length of the second lumbar vertebrae. The normal length of feline kidneys is 2.4 to 3.0 times the length of the second lumbar vertebrae.

‡Marked enlargement of both kidneys will not occur in patients with bilateral hydronephrosis because they die of uremia before extensive changes have time to develop.

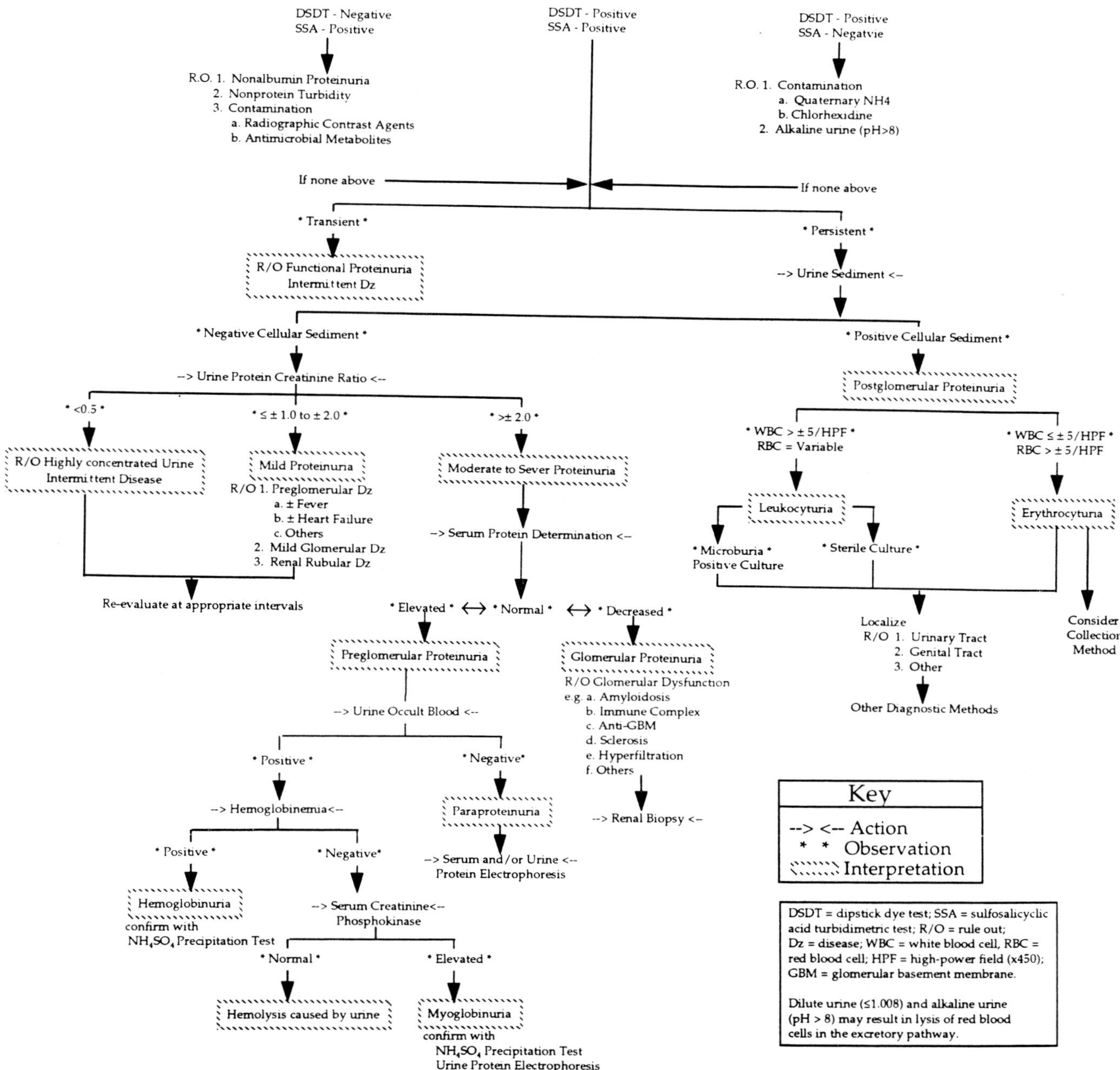

FIG. 4–6. Algorithm for the diagnosis of proteinuria. Modified from Lulich JP, Osborne CA. Interpretation of urine protein–creatinine ratios in dogs with glomerular and nonglomerular disorders. *Compen Cont Educ.* 1990;12:59.

TABLE 4–9
PROBLEM-SPECIFIC DATA BASE FOR PROTEIN-LOSING GLOMERULOPATHY*

A. Medical history and physical examination (Table 4–5)
B. Urinalysis
C. Quantitative measures of proteinuria
    1. Urine protein-creatinine ratio
    2. 24–hour protein excretion
D. Serum total protein, albumin, and globulin concentrations
E. Kidney function tests
    1. Serum urea nitrogen
    2. Serum creatinine concentration
    3. Consider endogenous creatinine clearance determination for nonazotemic patients
F. Serum cholesterol concentration (triglycerides?)
G. Complete blood count (including cytologic examination of blood cells)
H. Serum (or plasma) electrolyte and acid-base profile
    1. Sodium, potassium, and chloride concentrations
    2. Bicarbonate or total carbon dioxide concentrations
    3. Calcium and phosphorus concentrations
I. Serum alanine aminotransferase, alkaline phosphatase, amylase, and lipase activities (R/O hepatic and pancreatic disease)
J. Blood pressure determination (R/O systemic hypertension)
K. Consider:
    1. Freezing aliquots of serum (or plasma) and urine for additional diagnostic determinations that may be desired later (e.g., titers against infectious agents, toxicologic studies, etc.)
    2. Survey radiographs of thorax and abdomen (to identify/localize infectious, inflammatory, or neoplastic processes)
    3. Knott test, occult heartworm test—R/O dirofilariasis
    4. Immune panel—R/O immune-mediated diseases
        a. Coombs' test
        b. Antinuclear antibody test
        c. Lupus erythematosus preparation
        d. Joint taps?
        e. Serum protein electrophoresis
        f. Others?
    5. Fundic examination—R/O hypertensive lesions, infectious diseases
    6. Screening for infectious diseases
        a. R/O feline leukemia virus—FeLV test
        b. R/O bacterial endocarditis—blood cultures, echocardiogram
        c. R/O borreliosis-specific antibody titers
        d. R/O brucellosis-specific antibody titers
        e. R/O ehrlichiosis-specific antibody titers
    7. Coagulation studies—particularly antithrombin III and fibrinogen levels
    8. Renal biopsy to identify morphologic lesion
        a. Light microscopy
        b. Immunofluorescence microscopy
        c. Electron microscopy

*Modified from Polzin DJ, Osborne CA, O'Brien TD. Diseases of the kidneys and ureters. In: Ettinger SJ, ed. *Textbook of Veterinary Internal Medicine.* 3rd ed. Philadelphia, Pa: WB Saunders Co; 1989:2015.
Key: R/O = rule out.

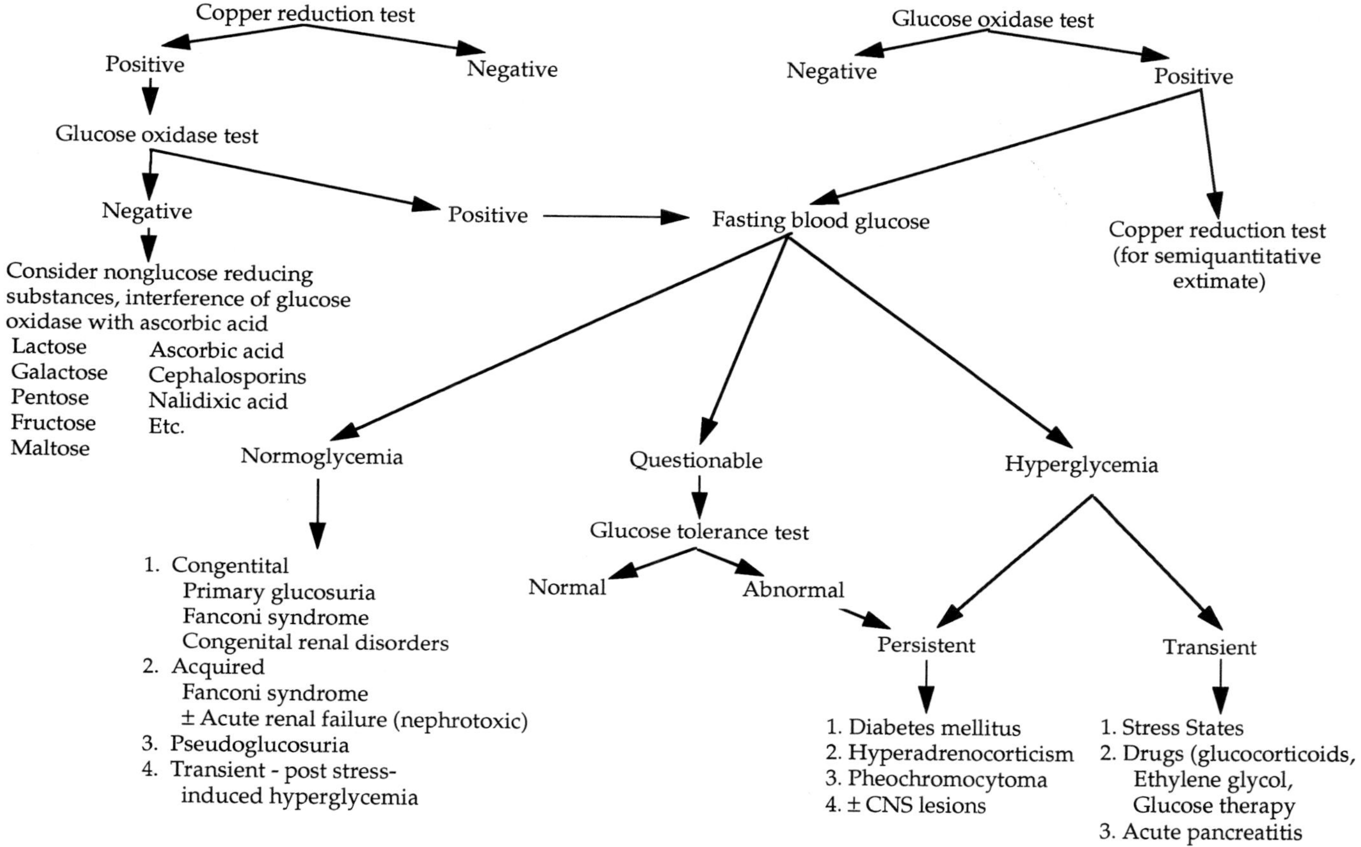

FIG. 4–7. Algorithm for the diagnosis of glucosuria. Modified from Osborne CA. Clinical algorithms: Tools that foster quality patient care. In: Kirk RW, ed. *Current Veterinary Therapy IX.* Philadelphia, Pa: WB Saunders Co; 1989. Key: ± = sometimes; CNS = central nervous system.

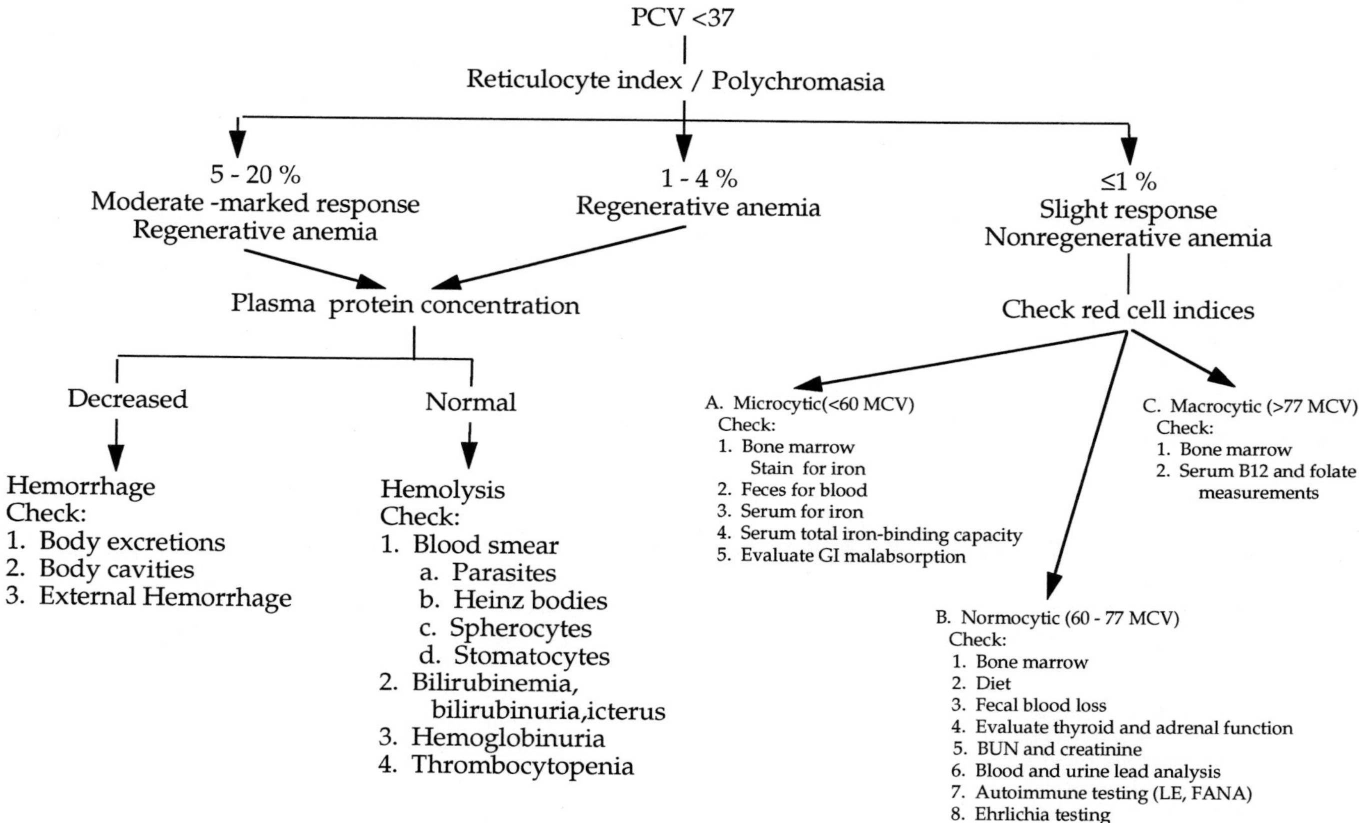

FIG. 4–8. Algorithm for the diagnosis of anemia in dogs. Modified from Meyer DJ, Coles EH, Rich LJ. *Veterinary Laboratory Medicine.* Philadelphia, Pa: WB Saunders Co; 1992. Key: PCV = packed cell volume; MCV = mean corpuscular volume; GI = gastrointestinal; BUN = blood urea nitrogen; LE = lupus erythematosus; FANA = fluorescent antinuclear antibody.

PCV <27

Reticulocyte index / Polychromasia

3 - 4%
Marked response
Definitely regenerative anemia

0.5 - 2%
Moderate response
Probably regenerative anemia

≤0.4%
Slight response
Nonregenerative anemia

Plasma protein concentration

FeLV test

Decreased

Hemorrhage
Check:
1. Body excretions
2. Body cavities
3. External Hemorrhage

Normal

Hemolysis
Check:
1. Blood smear
   a. Parasites
   b. Heinz bodies
   c. Spherocytes
   d. Stomatocytes
2. Associated findings
   a. Bilirubinemia, bilirubinuria, icterus
   b. Hemoglobinuria
   c. Thrombocytopenia

Positive

FeLV - related bone marrow diseases
Check:
1. Bone marrow

Negative

FeLV - latent infection
Non - FeLV causes
Check:
1. Bone marrow
2. Drug therapy
3. Toxins
4. Immune - mediated disease

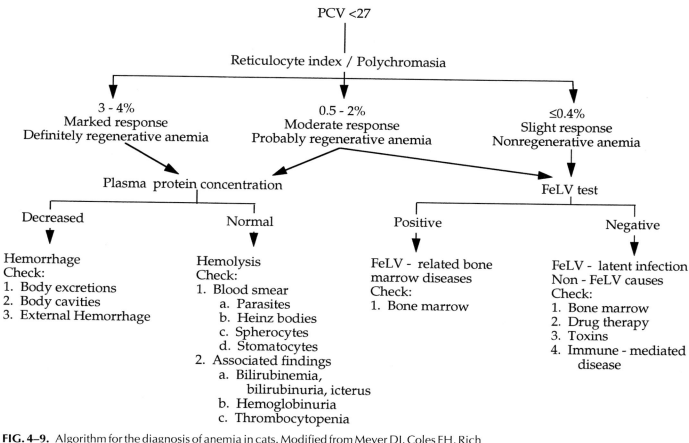

FIG. 4–9. Algorithm for the diagnosis of anemia in cats. Modified from Meyer DJ, Coles EH, Rich LJ. *Veterinary Laboratory Medicine.* Philadelphia, Pa: WB Saunders Co; 1992. Key: PCV = packed cell volume; FeLV = feline leukemia virus.

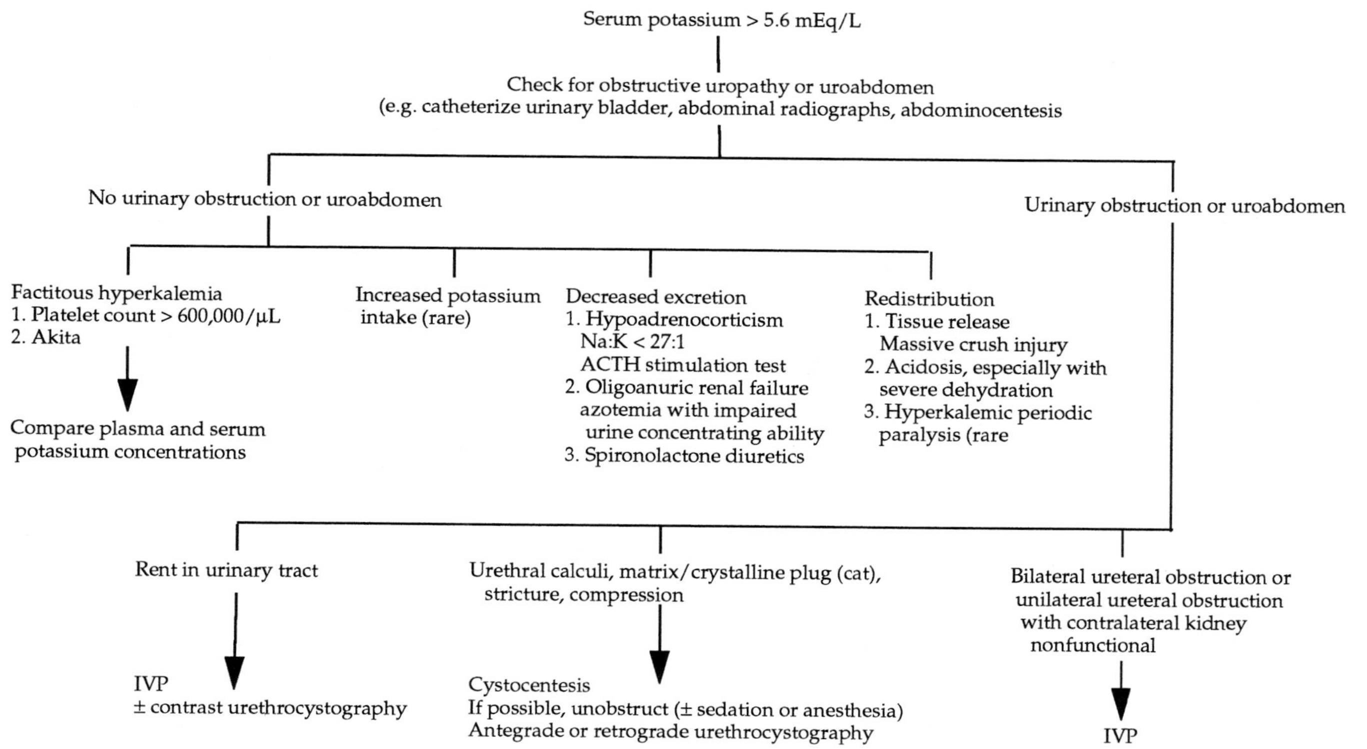

FIG. 4–10. Algorithm for the diagnosis of hyperkalemia. Key: IVP = intravenous pyelography; ACTH = adrenocorticotropic hormone; ± = sometimes.

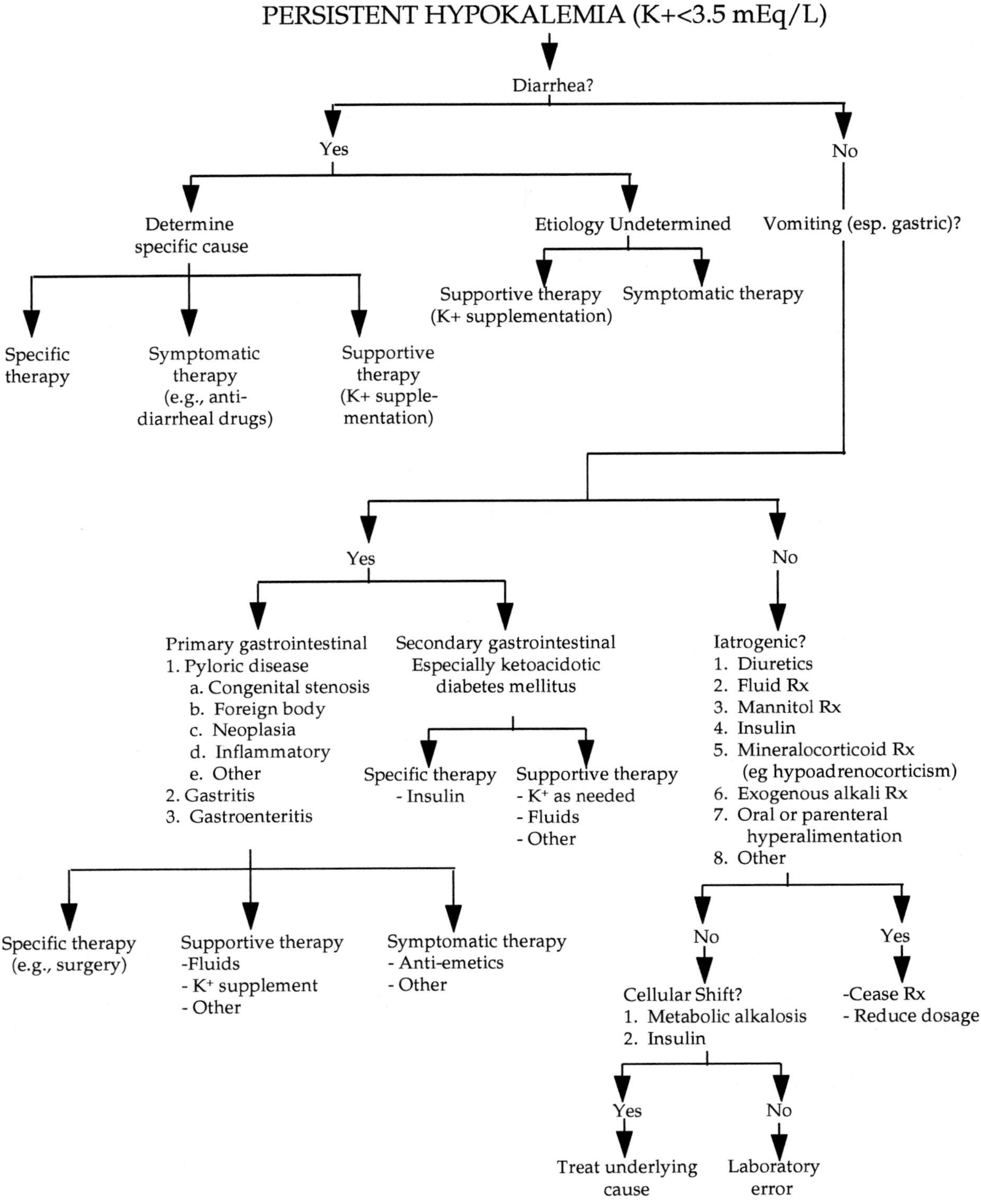

FIG. 4–11. Algorithm for the diagnosis and treatment of hypokalemia. Modified from Bell FW, Osborne CA. Treatment of hypokalemia. In: Kirk RW, ed. *Current Veterinary Therapy IX.* Philadelphia, Pa: WB Saunders Co; 1992. Key: Rx = treatment.

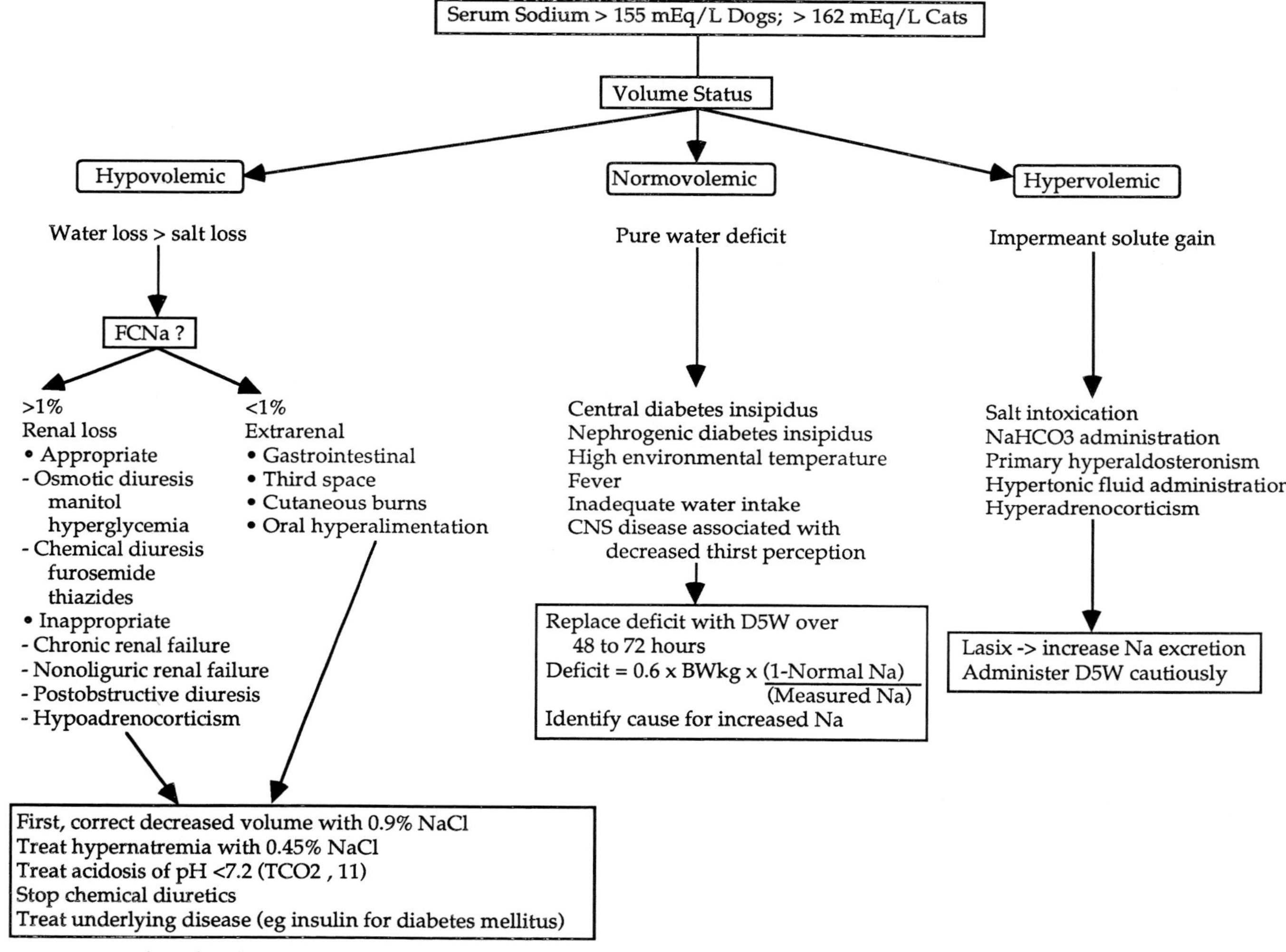

FIG. 4–12. Algorithm for the diagnosis and treatment of hypernatremia. Modified from Hardy RM. Hypernatremia. *Vet Clin North Am.* 1989;19:231 and DiBartola SP. Disorders of sodium and water: Hypernatremia and hyponatremia. In: DiBartola SP, ed. *Fluid Therapy in Small Animal Practice.* Philadelphia, Pa: WB Saunders Co; 1992. Key: CNS = central nervous system; D_5 = 5% dextrose in water; bw = body weight; ± = sometimes.

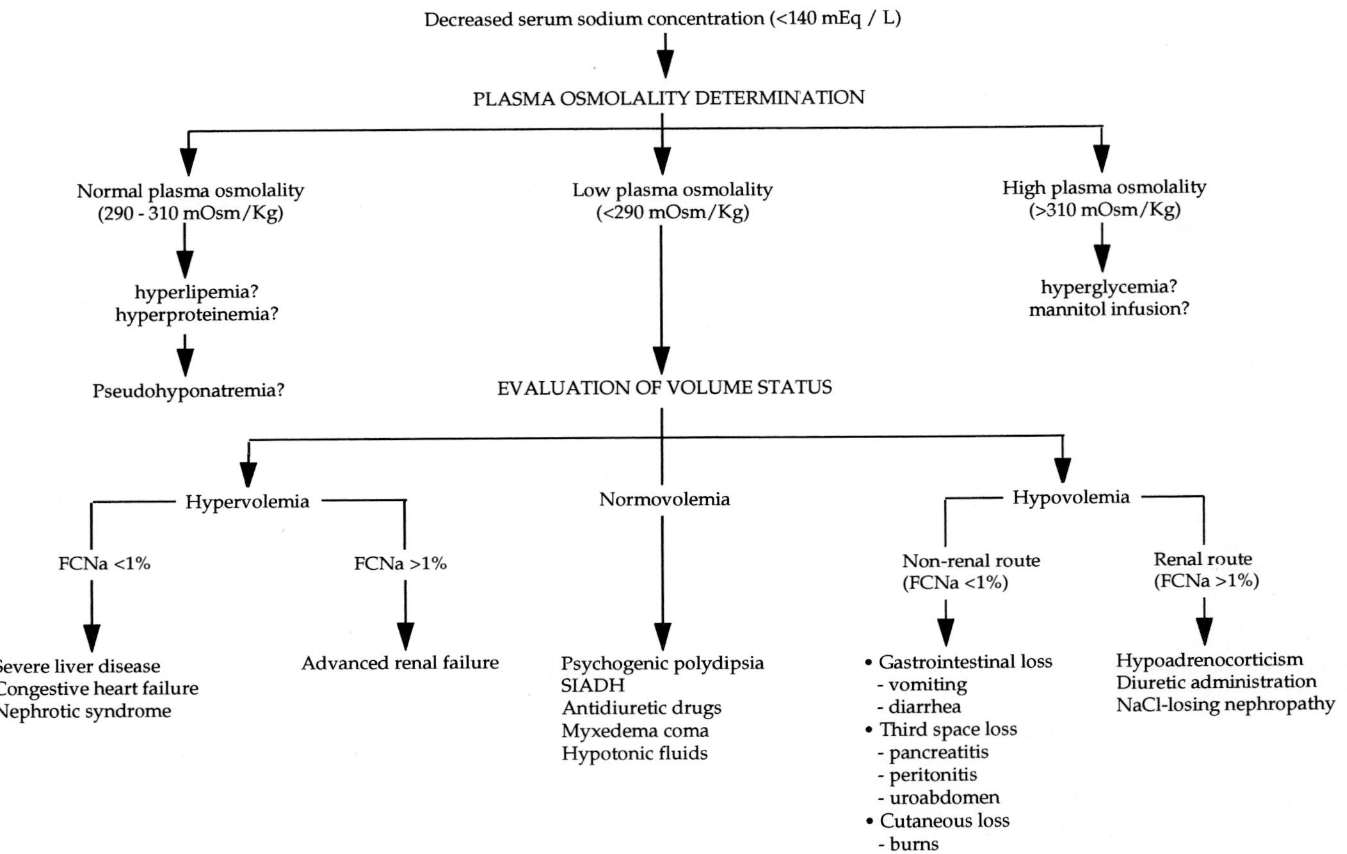

FIG. 4–13. Algorithm for the diagnosis of hyponatremia. Modified from DiBartola SP, ed. *Fluid Therapy in Small Animal Practice.* Philadelphia, Pa: WB Saunders Co; 1992. Key: SIADH = syndrome of inappropriate secretion of antidiuretic hormone.

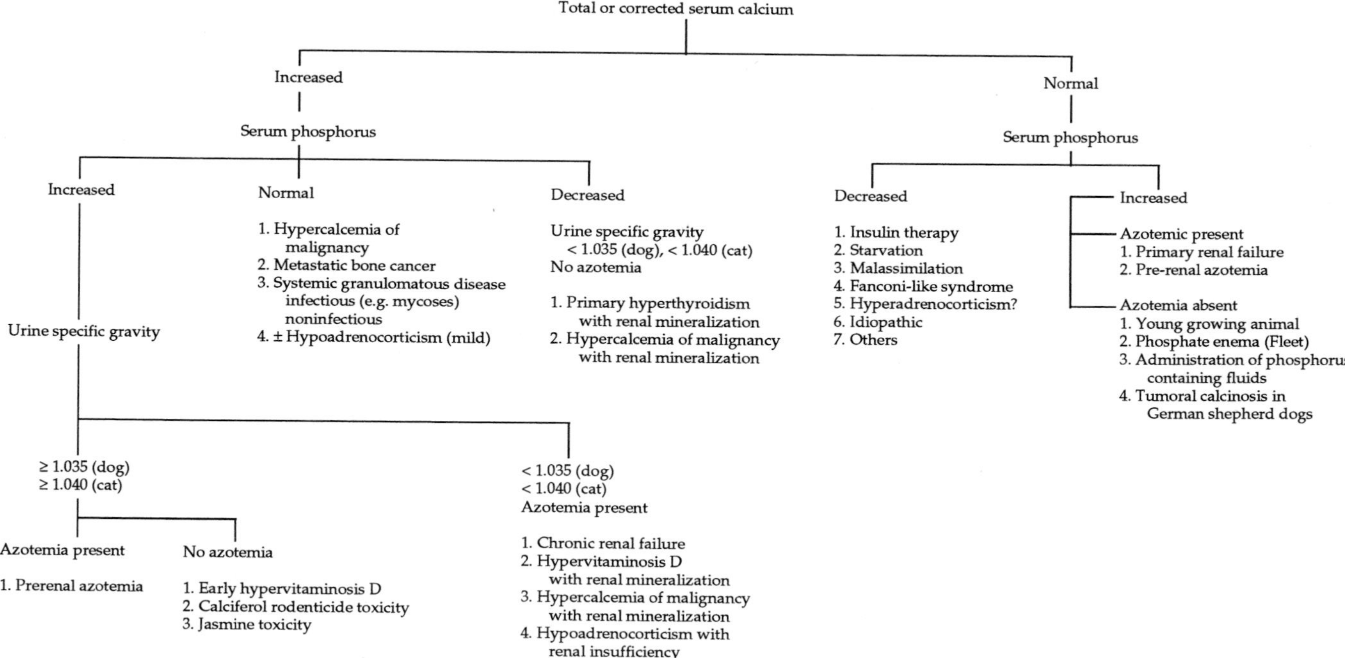

FIG. 4–14. Algorithm for the diagnosis of hypercalcemia. Modified from Meyer DJ, Coles EH, Rich LJ. *Veterinary Laboratory Medicine.* Philadelphia, Pa: WB Saunders Co; 1992. Note: corrected $Ca^{2+} = Ca^{2+}_{measured} + [3.5 - albumin_{measured}]$. Key: ± = sometimes.

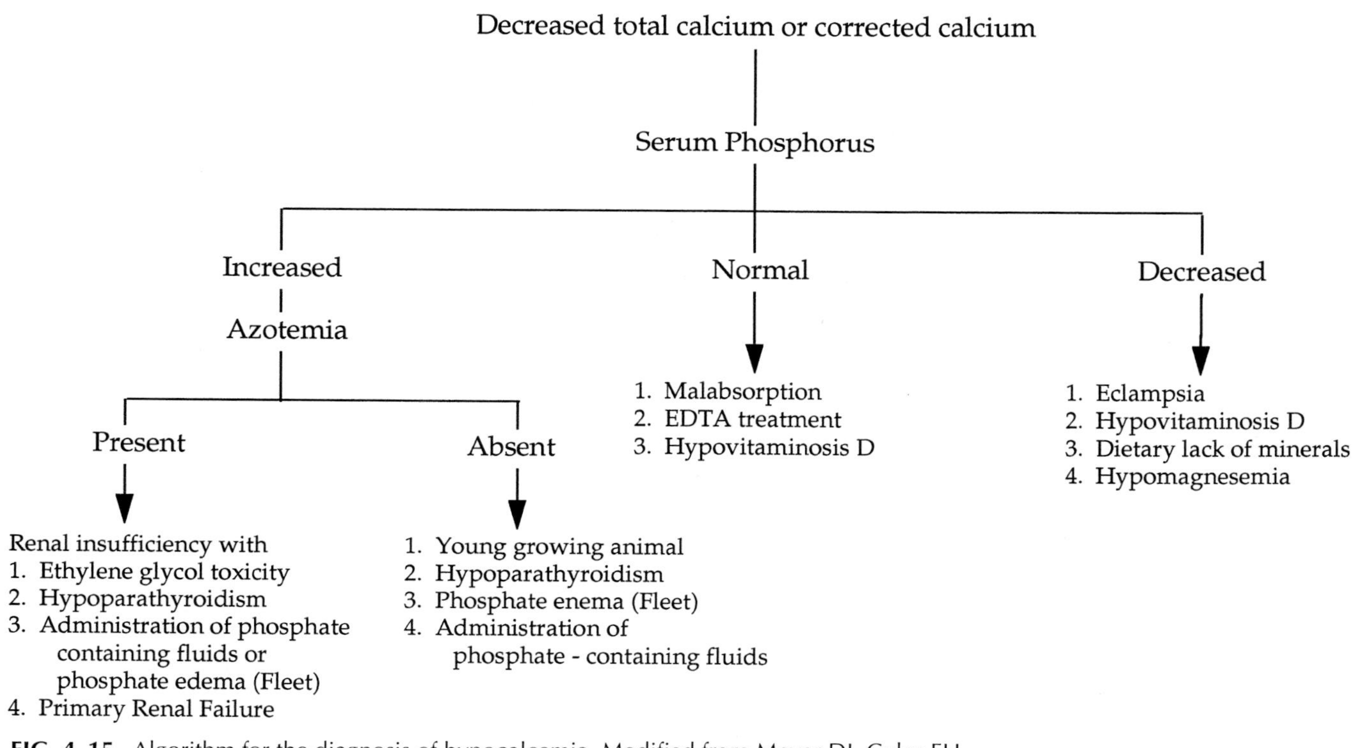

FIG. 4–15. Algorithm for the diagnosis of hypocalcemia. Modified from Meyer DJ, Coles EH, Rich LJ. *Veterinary Laboratory Medicine.* Philadelphia, Pa: WB Saunders Co; 1992. Note: corrected $Ca^{2+} = Ca^{2+}_{measured} + (3.5 - albumin_{measured})$. Key: EDTA = ethylenediaminetetraacetic acid.

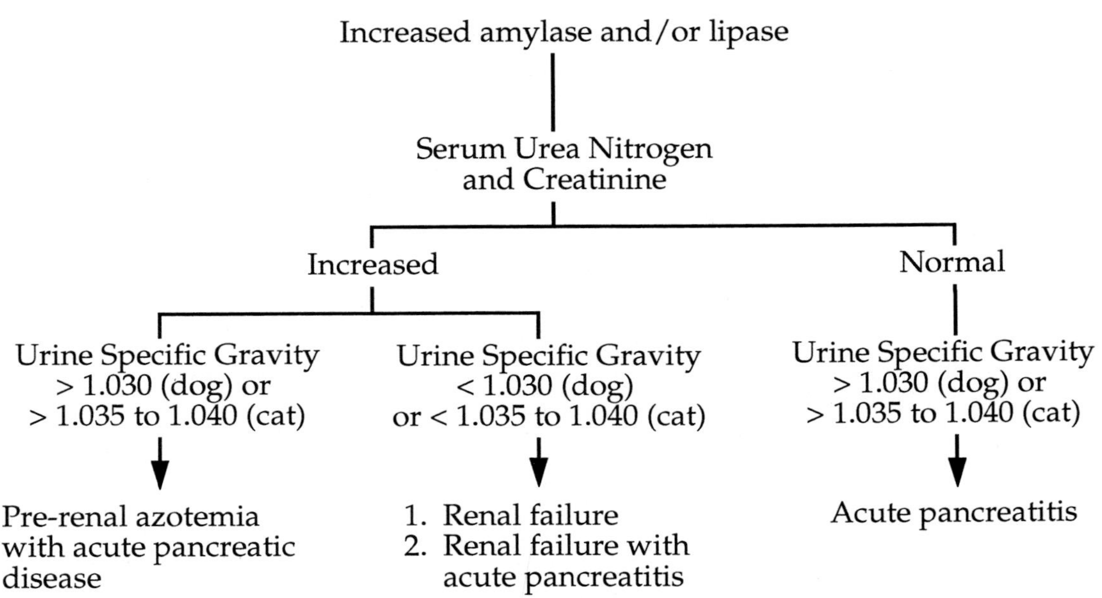

FIG. 4–16. Algorithm for the diagnosis of increased serum activities of amylase and lipase. Modified from Meyer DJ, Coles EH, Rich LJ. *Veterinary Laboratory Diagnosis.* Philadelphia, Pa: WB Saunders Co; 1992.

Total serum protein

- Increased
  - Albumin
    - Increased
      - Globulins increased or normal
        - Dehydration usually accompanied by PCV increase(unless animal also anemic)
    - Normal or decreased
      - Globulins increased
        - Electrophoresis
          - Polyclonal
            1. Antigen stimulation (inflammation, Infections, neoplasia)
          - Monoclonal
            1. Ehrlichiosis, confirm with serology
            2. Plasma cell myeloma
            3. Lymphosarcoma
            - Bone marrow examination
              - if many plasma cells = myeloma
              - If many lymphocytes =lymphosarcoma
- Normal
  - Albumin
    - Normal
      - Globulins decreased
        1. Lack of colostrum in suckling
        2. Immunodeficiency
    - Decreased
      - Globulins
        - Increased
          1. Inflammation
          2. Plasma cell tumor or lympho-sarcoma
        - Normal
          - Low albumin caused by:
            1. Liver insufficiency
            2. Malassimilation
            3. Protein-losing nephropathy
- Decreased
  - Albumin
    - Normal
      - Globulins decreased
        1. Young animals (less than 4 mo)
        2. Immunodeficiency
    - Decreased
      - Globulins
        - Normal (A/G decreased)
          1. Albumin loss (glomerulo-nephropathy, enteropathy)
          2. Lack of albumin production
             a. Liver insufficiency
             b. Chronic severe malnutrition
        - Decreased (A/G normal)
          1. Blood loss
          2. Fluid therapy
          3. Protein-losing enteropathy

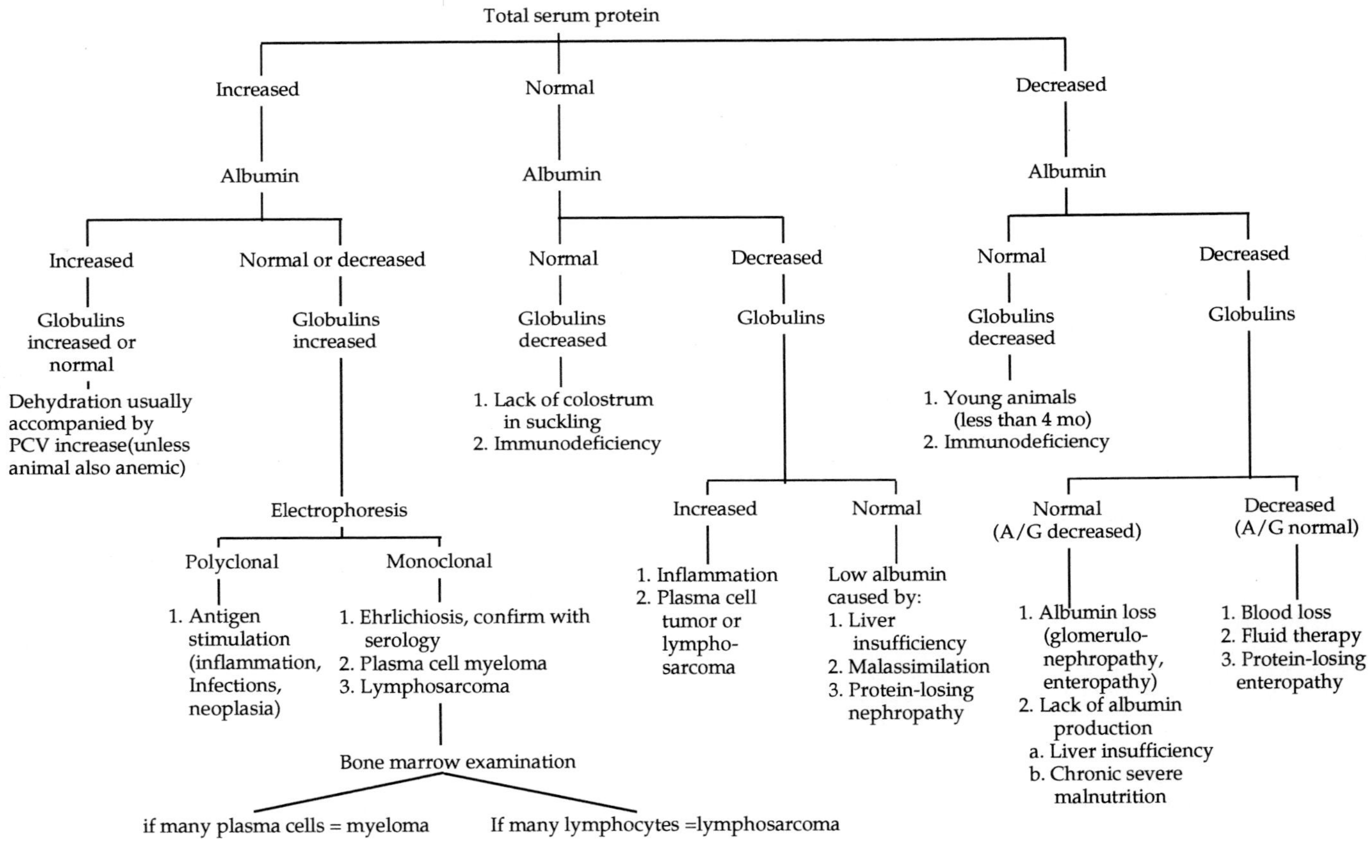

FIG. 4–17. Algorithm for the diagnosis of abnormalities in serum total protein and albumin concentrations. Modified from Meyer DJ, Coles EH, Rich LJ. *Veterinary Laboratory Medicine.* Philadelphia, Pa: WB Saunders Co; 1992. Key: PCV = packed cell volume; A/G = albumin/globulin.

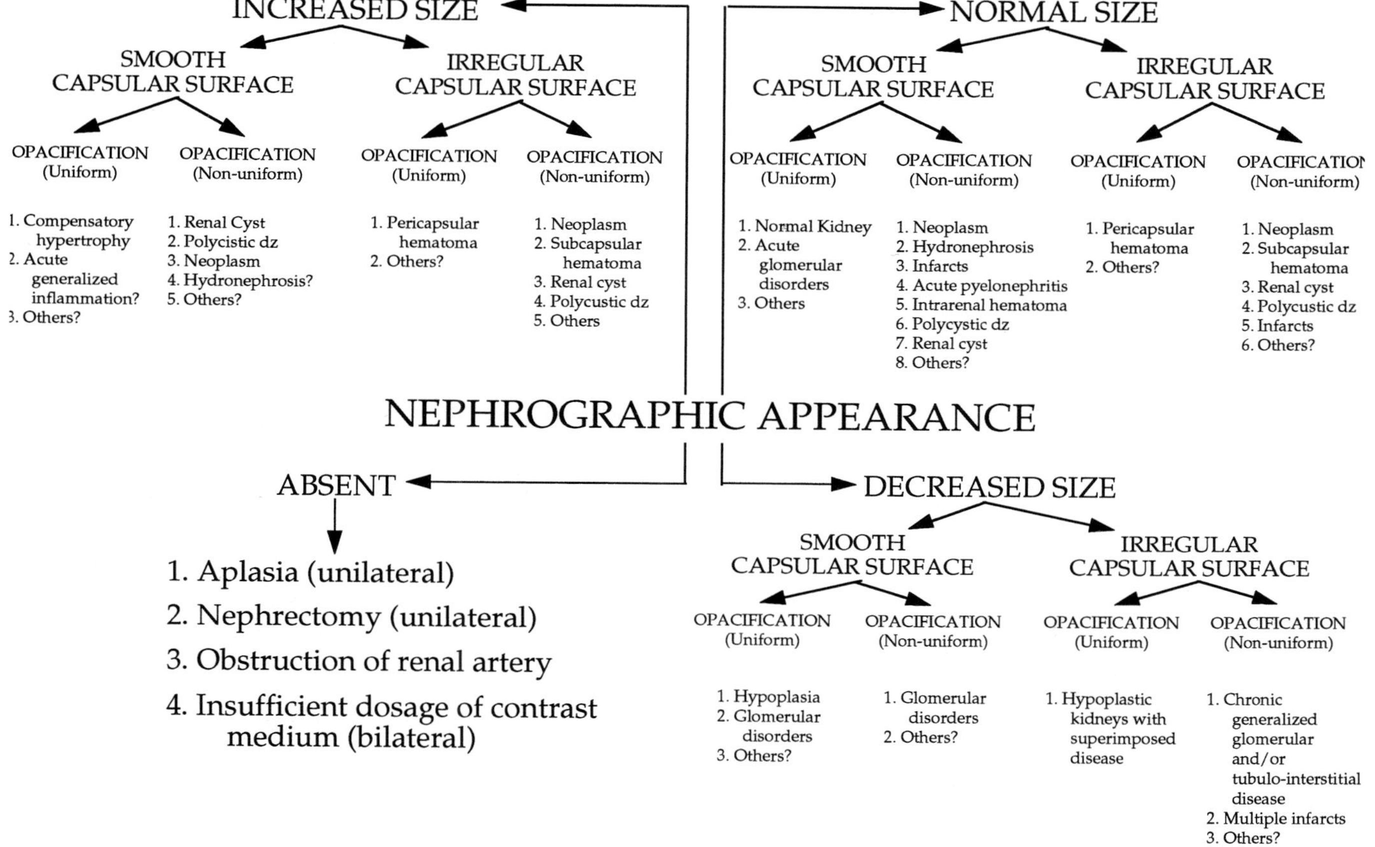

FIG. 4–18. Algorithm for the interpretation of the radiographic appearance of the kidneys following intravenous injection of radiopaque contrast media. Feeney DA, Barber DL, Osborne CA. Advances in Canine Excretory Urography. Gaines Veterinary Symposium, Corvallis, Oregon. Gaines, White Plains, NY, 1981.

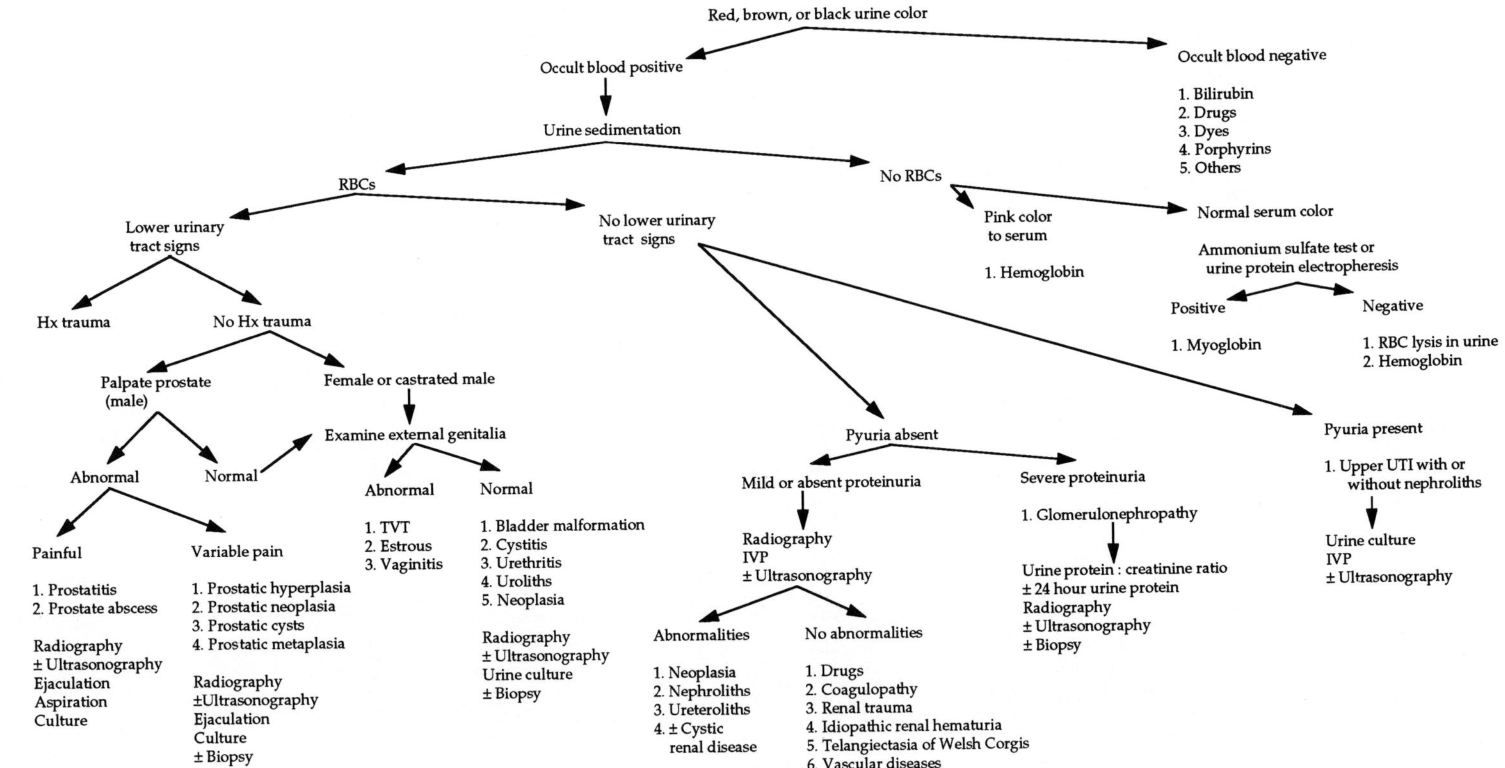

FIG. 4–19. Algorithm for the diagnosis of red, brown, or black colored urine. Key: IVP = intravenous pyelogram; TVT = transmissible venereal tumor; RBC = red blood cell; Hx = history; ± = sometimes; UTI = urinary tract infection.

TABLE 4–10
PROBABLE LOCALIZATION OF GROSS HEMATURIA*

Hematuria Throughout Micturition
R/O Renal disorder
  Dx Abdominal palpation; survey and contrast radiography; ultrasonography; biopsy; exploratory surgery
R/O Diffuse bladder lesions
  Dx Abdominal palpation; examination of urine sediment; survey and contrast radiology; ultrasonography; catheter biopsy; cystoscopy and biopsy; exploratory surgery
R/O Focal ventral or ventrolateral bladder lesions in active patients
  Dx Abdominal palpation; examination of urine sediment; survey and contrast radiology; ultrasonography; catheter biopsy; cystoscopy and biopsy; exploratory surgery
R/O Severe prostatic or urethral lesions
  Dx Rectal and abdominal palpation; survey and contrast radiology; ultrasonography; catheter biopsy; aspiration biopsy; exploratory surgery
R/O Hemoglobinuria
  Dx Examination of urine sediment for red blood cells; hemogram
R/O Systemic clotting defect
  Dx Clotting profile, platelet count; evaluation of other body systems for hemorrhage
Hematuria Independent or at the Beginning of Micturition
R/O Urethral lesions
  Dx Rectal and abdominal palpation; comparison of analysis of urine samples collected by voiding and cystocentesis; survey and contrast radiology; catheter biopsy; exploratory surgery
R/O Genital disease
  Dx Abdominal, rectal, and vaginal palpation; vaginal cytology; comparison of analysis of urine samples collected by voiding and cystocentesis; survey and contrast radiography; ultrasonography; endoscopy; exploratory surgery
Hematuria at End of Micturition
R/O Focal ventral or ventrolateral lesions in inactive patients
  Dx Abdominal palpation, examination of urine sediment; survey and contrast radiography; ultrasonography; catheter biopsy; cystoscopy and biopsy; exploratory surgery
R/O Renal disorder with intermittent hematuria in inactive patients
  Dx Abdominal palpation; survey and contrast radiography; biopsy; exploratory surgery; ultrasonography

*Modified from Osborne CA, Klausner JS. A problem-specific data base for urinary tract infections. *Vet Clin North Am.* 1979;9:783.
Key: R/O = rule out; Dx = diagnosis.

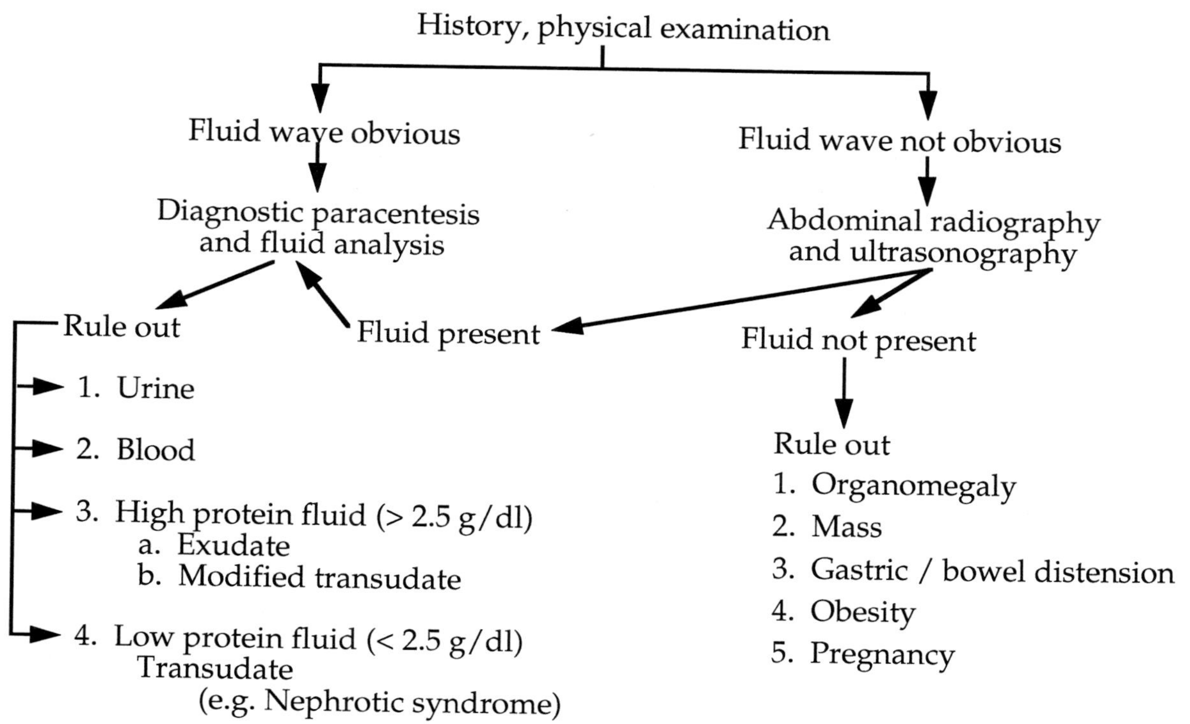

FIG. 4–20. Algorithm for the diagnosis of abdominal distention.

TABLE 4–11
PROBLEM-SPECIFIC DATA BASE FOR URINARY TRACT INFECTIONS*

I. History Checklist
   A. Micturition
      1. Character, frequency, quantity?
      2. Pollakiuria (dysuria, tenesmus)?
      3. Polyuria (polydipsia), oliguria, anuria?
      4. Urinary incontinence?
      5. Micturition in unusual locations?
   B. Calculi voided during micturition?
   C. Hematuria (Table 4–10)
      1. Throughout micturition?
      2. Beginning of micturition?
      3. Independent of micturition?
      4. End of micturition?
   D. Change in urine color?
   E. Change in urine odor?
   F. Licking vulva or penis?
   G. Vomiting?
   H. Medication given? Type? Dose? Duration? Response?
II. Physical Examination Checklist
   A. Physical examination of the urinary system is limited to inspection and palpation. Abdominal and rectal palpation are especially important because they often permit localization of a disease process in the urethra, urinary bladder, or kidneys. Application of gentle digital pressure through the abdominal wall and systematic tracing of palpable structures within the abdominal cavity are essential. If the patient resists abdominal palpation by tensing its abdominal muscles, tranquilization or anesthesia should be considered.
   B. Kidneys
      1. Size (Table 4–8)?
      2. Shape, surface contour, consistency?
      3. Pain?
      4. Both palpable? Bilateral symmetrical?
   C. Urinary bladder
      1. Position, size, shape, consistency?
      2. Grating or nongrating masses within or adjacent to bladder lumen? If present, constant or variable location?
      3. If overdistention interferes with palpation of lumen, repalpate following removal of an appropriate quantity of urine?
      4. Thickness of bladder wall?
      5. Pain?
   D. Prostate gland
      1. Position, size, shape, consistency?
      2. Pain?
   E. Urethra
      1. Examination of prepuce and penis of male dogs and cats? Examination of perineal urethra of male dogs?
      2. Rectal examination of urethra for position, size, shape, and consistency, and periurethral abnormalities?

*Modified from Osborne CA, Klausner JS. A problem-specific data base for urinary tract infections. *Vet Clin North Am.* 1979;9:783.

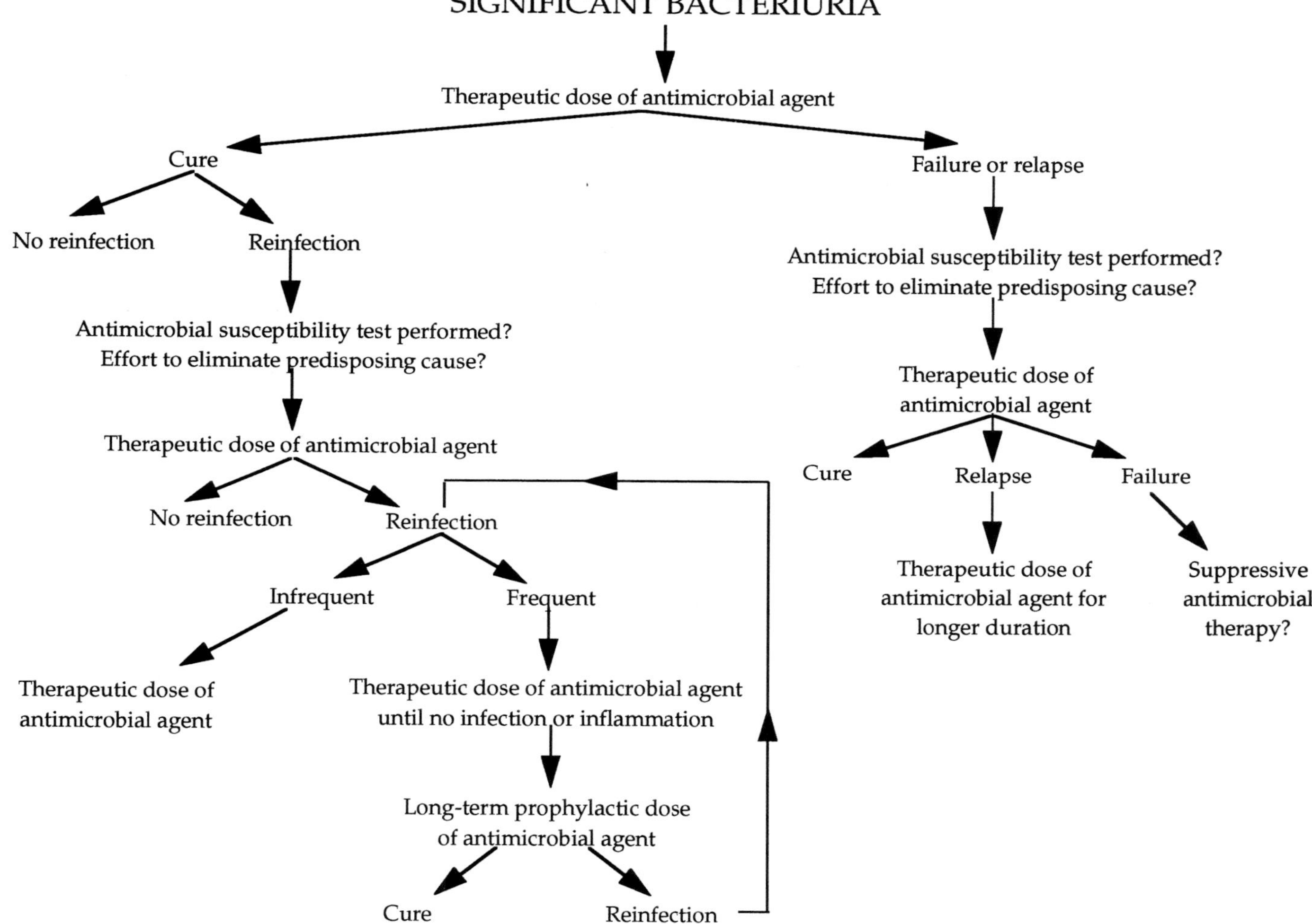

FIG. 4–21. Algorithm for the treatment of bacterial urinary tract infections. Modified from Osborne CA. Clinical algorithms: Tools that foster quality patient care. In: Kirk RW, ed. *Current Veterinary Therapy IX*. Philadelphia, Pa: WB Saunders Co; 1989.

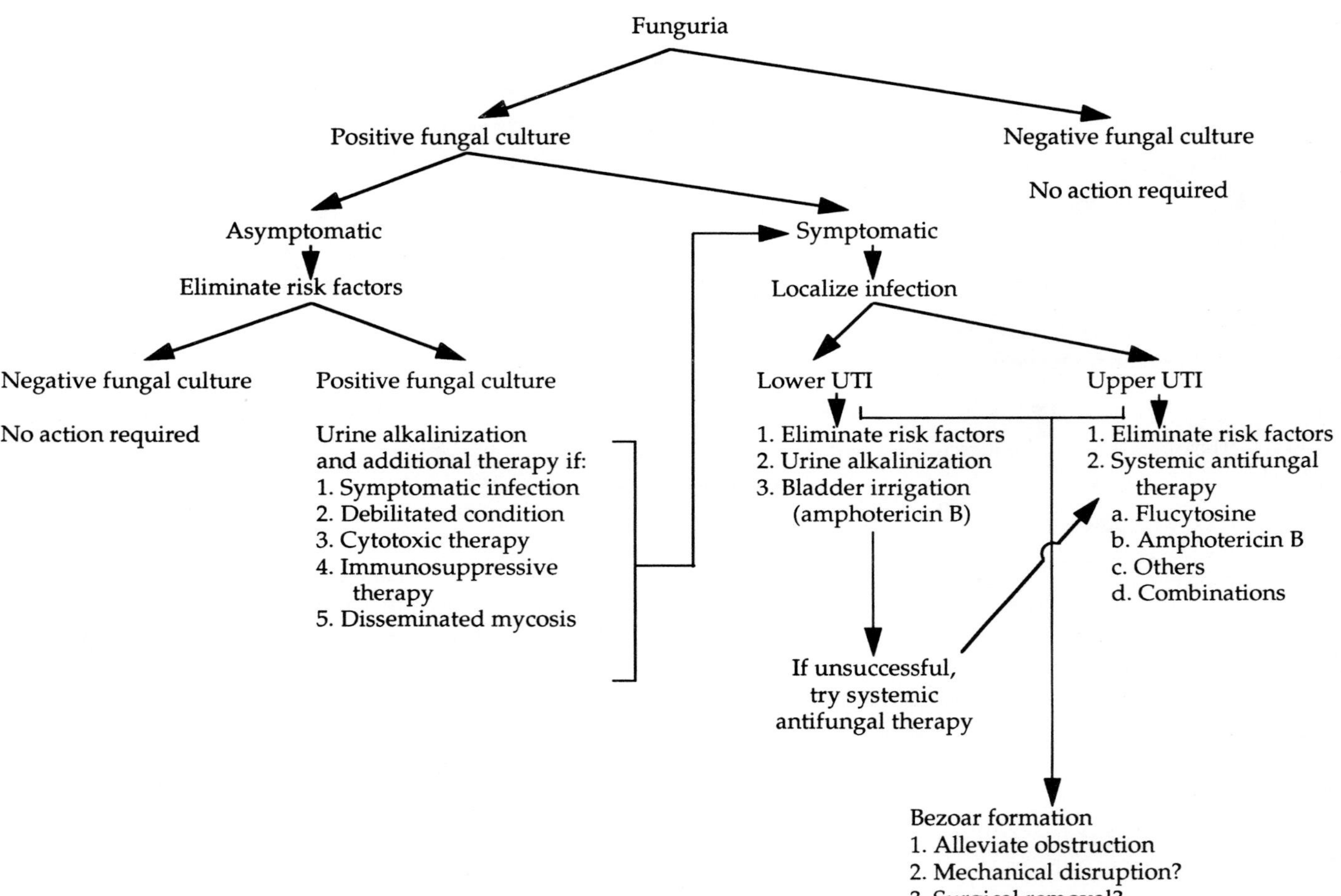

FIG. 4–22. Algorithm for the diagnosis and treatment of fungal urinary tract infections. Modified from Lulich JP, Osborne CA. Fungal urinary tract infections. In: Kirk RW, Bonagura JD, eds. *Current Veterinary Therapy XI*. Philadelphia, Pa: WB Saunders Co; 1992.

TABLE 4–12
PROBLEM-SPECIFIC AND THERAPEUTIC-SPECIFIC DATA BASE FOR THE DIAGNOSIS AND MANAGEMENT OF UROLITHIASIS

1. Obtain appropriate history and perform physical examination, including rectal examination of urethra.
2. Perform complete urinalysis; save aliquot for possible determination of mineral concentration.*
3. Obtain quantitative urine culture and determine urine urease activity; test for antimicrobial susceptibility if bacterial pathogens are identified. Consider attempts to isolate Ureaplasma if urease-positive urine is bacteriologically sterile.
4. Perform complete blood cell count.
5. Freeze aliquot of serum collected at time of venipuncture to obtain complete blood cell count for possible determination of urea nitrogen, creatinine, calcium and/or uric acid concentrations.
6. Obtain radiographs.
   a. Take survey radiographs of entire urinary system.
   b. Consider IV urography for patients with renal or ureteral uroliths.
   c. Consider IV urography or contrast cystography for patients with bladder uroliths.
   d. Consider contrast urethrography for patients with urethral uroliths.
   e. Ultrasonography is recommended if equipment is available
7. Determine mineral composition of uroliths.
   a. Do a quantitative analysis of uroliths passed during micturition or retrieved during diagnostic procedures.
   b. Use results obtained from history, physical examination, laboratory examination, and radiography to determine probable mineral composition of uroliths.
8. Initiate therapy to eradicate UTI, if present.
9. Initiate therapy for urolithiasis.
   a. Initiate therapy to promote dissolution of uroliths if amenable to medical therapy.
      i. Formulate follow-up protocol to monitor dissolution of uroliths.
      ii. Formulate alternative treatment options if uroliths do not dissolve or if problems such as recurrent outflow obstruction occur.
   b. Remove uroliths by voiding urohydropropulsion.
   c. Use nephrotomy or cystotomy to remove uroliths.
      i. During surgical procedure, remove bladder or kidney biopsy specimens for microscopic examination.
      ii. Correct any anatomic defects, if present.
      iii. Compare number of uroliths removed during surgery with number identified by radiography.
      iv. Postsurgical radiographs should be obtained to evaluate completeness of urolith removal.
      v. Submit uroliths for quantitative analysis.
10. Once uroliths have been surgically removed or medically dissolved, initiate therapy to prevent recurrence of uroliths.
11. Formulate follow-up protocol with clients.

*The patient's diet should be the same as when the uroliths formed. Alternatively, a standard diet designed to promote reproducible excretion of minerals in the urine of normal animals may be used.
Key: UTI = urinary tract infection.

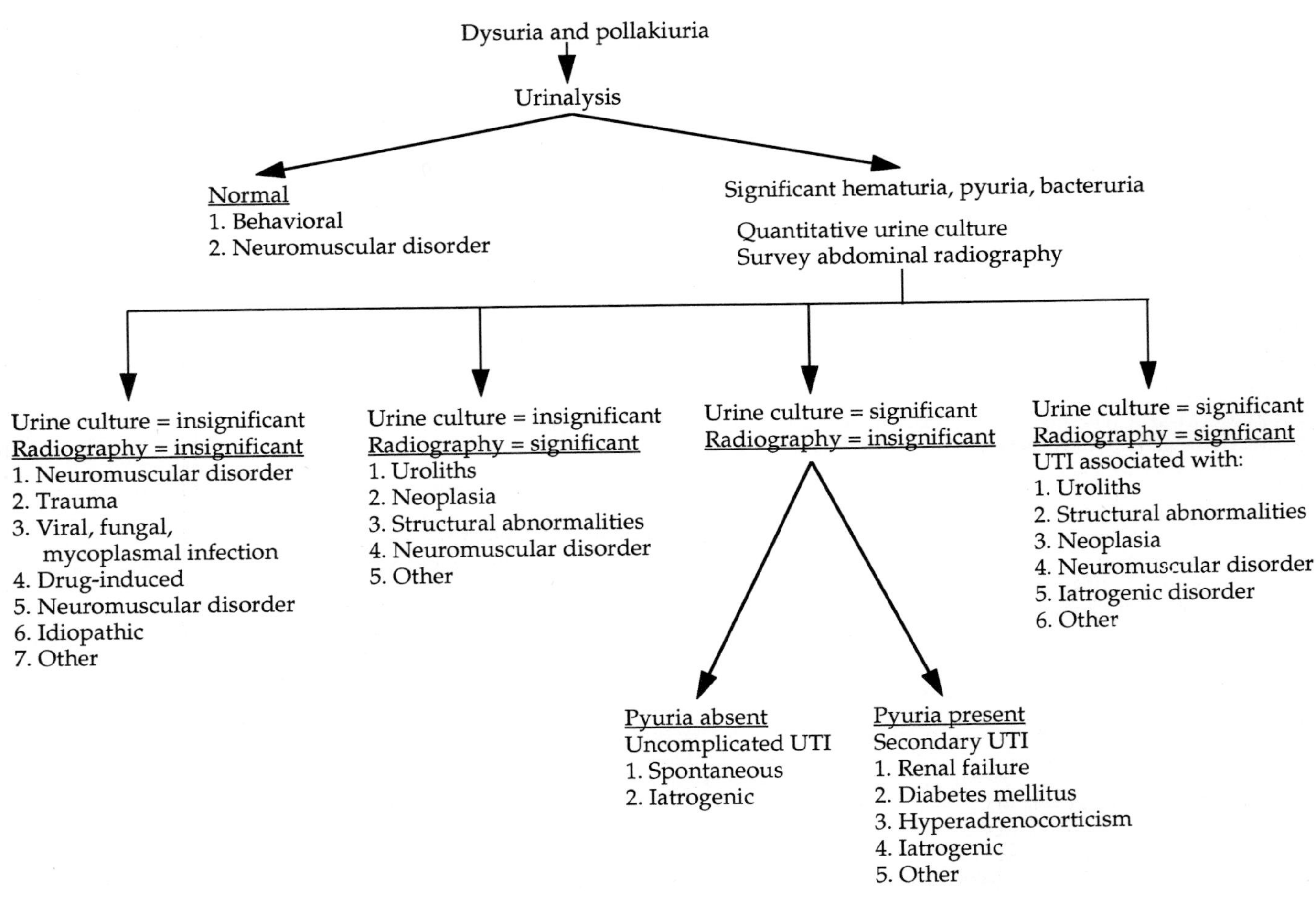

FIG. 4–23. Algorithm for the diagnosis of dysuria and pollakiuria. Modified from Osborne CA. Clinical algorithms: Tools that foster quality patient care. In: Kirk RW, ed. *Current Veterinary Therapy IX*. Philadelphia, Pa: WB Saunders Co; 1989. Key: UTI = urinary tract infection.

TABLE 4–13
PROBLEM-SPECIFIC DATA BASE FOR URINARY INCONTINENCE*

A. Owner's definition of incontinence
   1. Constant or intermittent?
   2. Positional?
   3. Nocturnal?
   4. Exertional?
B. Micturition
   1. Character, frequency, quantity?
   2. Pollakiuria (dysuria, tenesmus)?
   3. Polyuria (polydipsia)?
   4. Oliguria?
   5. Micturition in unusual locations?
   6. Change in urine color
      a. Red (hematuria, hemoglobinuria, myoglobinuria)?
      b. Brown, black, green, etc.?
C. Duration of incontinence?
D. Age of onset of incontinence?
E. Status of reproductive tract and relationship to incontinence?
F. Medications given? Type? Dose? Duration? Response?
G. Verification of incontinence?
H. Evaluation of bladder size
   1. Before micturition?
   2. After micturition?
I. Results of neurologic examination?
J. Results of urinalysis?
K. Evaluation of survey abdominal radiographs?
L. Catheterization to evaluate patency of urethral lumen if patient is dysuric or if urine cannot be easily expelled from the bladder by manual compression?
   Contrast radiography
M. 1. ±Retrograde contrast urethrocystography
   2. ±Retrograde vaginography
   3. ±High-dose intravenous urography
   4. ±Intravenous urography combined with pneumocystography ± fluoroscopy of ureters, if available

*Modified from Osborne CA, Oliver JE, Polzin DJ. Non-neurogenic urinary incontinence. In: Kirk RW, ed. *Current Veterinary Therapy,* 8th ed. Philadelphia: WB Saunders Co; 1980:1122–1127.

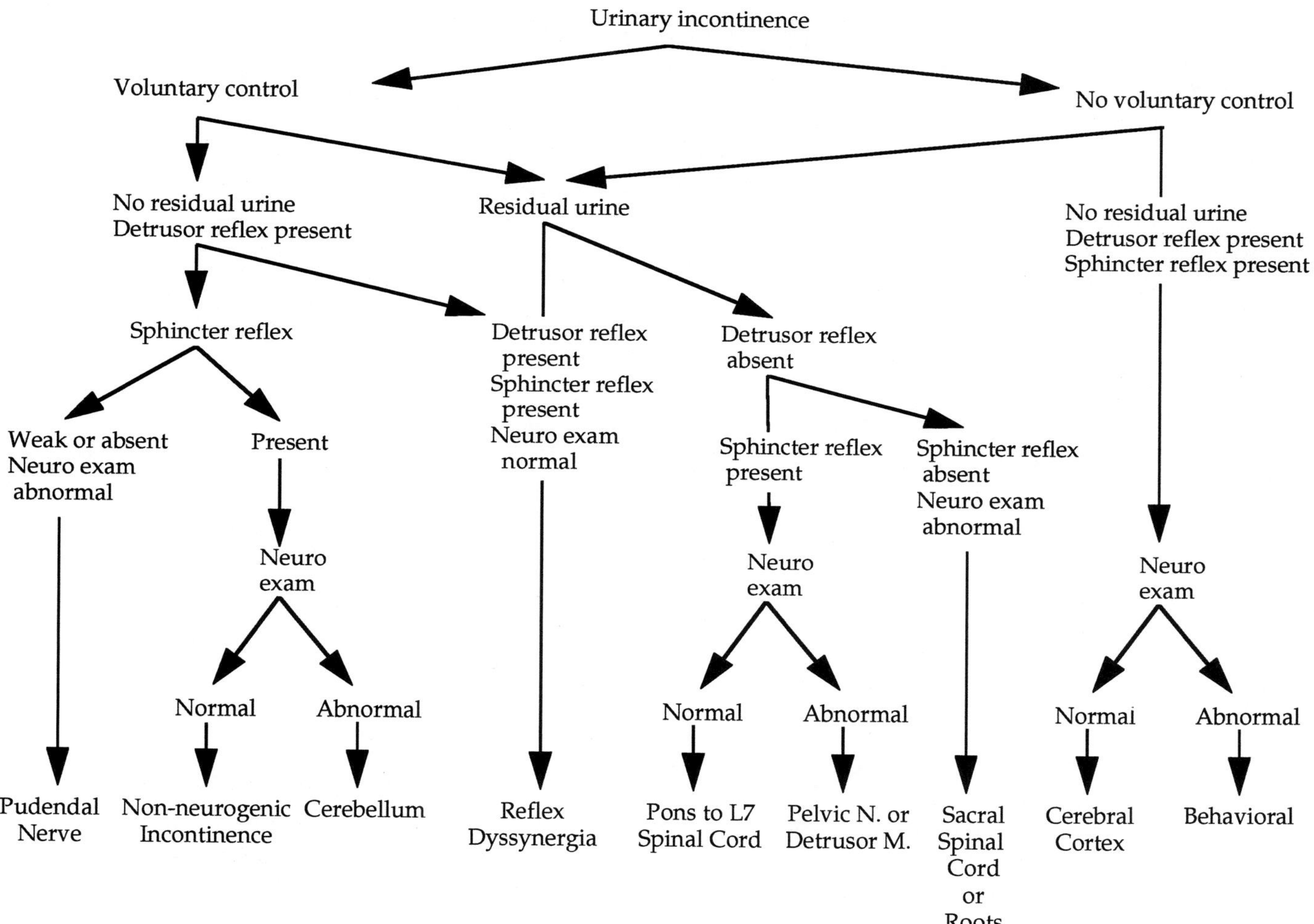

FIG. 4–24. Algorithm for the diagnosis of urinary incontinence. Modified from Oliver JE, Osborne CA. Neurogenic urinary incontinence. In: Kirk RW, ed. *Current Veterinary Therapy VII.* Philadelphia, Pa: WB Saunders Co; 1980.

Dysuria, pollakiuria, hematuria

No urethral obstruction
- double contrast cystography
- urethrography

urethral obstruction
- retrograde urohydropropulsion

urocystolith size and number

less than distended urethral diameter
- voiding urohydropropulsion

urocystoliths greater than distended urethral diameter

cystotomy and post operative double contrast cystography

all uroliths retrieved
- refer to prevention algorithm

all uroliths not retrieved

- diet: restricted purine and urine alkalinizing
- allopurinol: ~15 mg/kg PO q 12hr

all uroliths not retrieved

all uroliths retrieved
- refer to prevention algorithm

4 weeks:
- urinalysis
- double contrast cystography

urocystoliths not present
- refer to prevention algorithm

urocystoliths present

no change or increase in size and/or number of urocystoliths

decrease in size and/or number of urocystoliths
- continue therapy

urocystoliths not retrieved
- cystotomy
- double contrast cystography

urocystoliths retrieved and analyzed

xanthine

urate
- increase allopurinol dose by 10 to 25%

uroliths present

no uroliths
- refer to prevention algorithm

stop allopurinol, continue diet, wait 1 to 2 months, repeat double contrast cystogram, retrieve uroliths and analyze. If urate, begin allopurinol at 25% dosage reduction

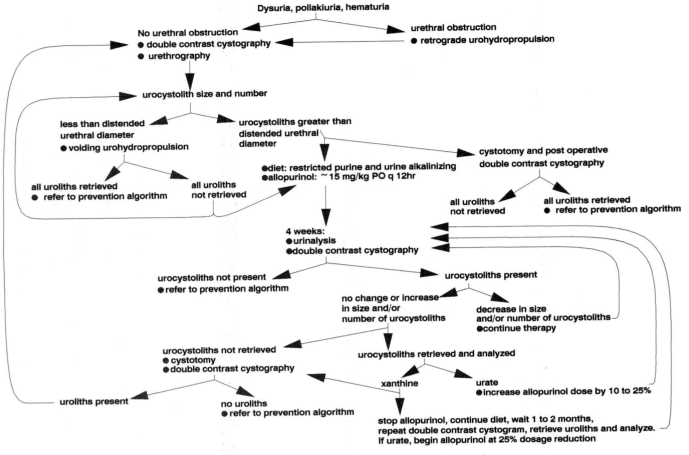

FIG. 4–25. Algorithm for the treatment of urate urocystoliths in dogs. Key: p.o. = by mouth; q = every.

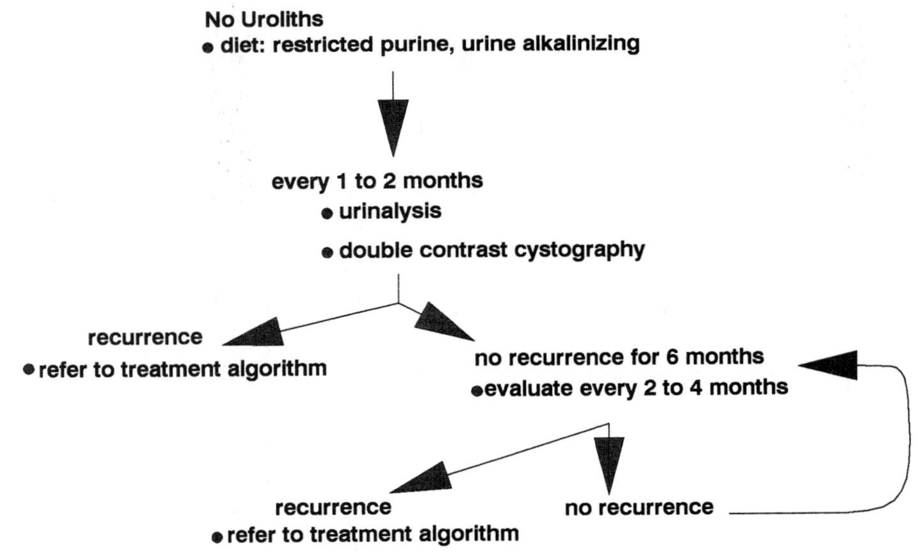

FIG. 4–26. Algorithm for the prevention of urate urocystoliths in dogs.

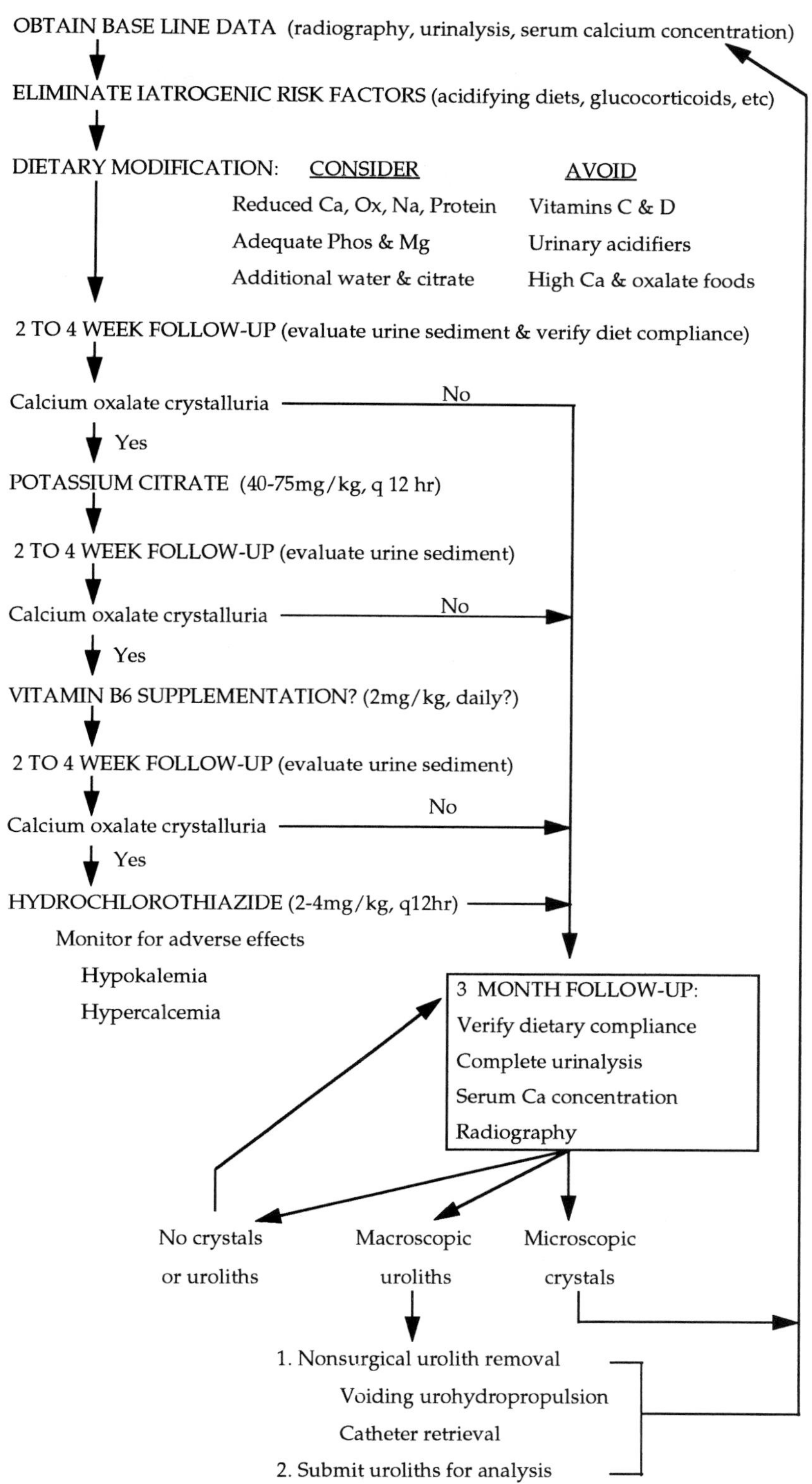

FIG. 4–27. Algorithm for the prevention of calcium oxalate urocystoliths in dogs. Modified from Lulich JP, Osborne CA, Felice LJ, et al. *Calcium Oxalate Urolithiasis.* Sixteenth Annual Waltham/OSU Symposium, Columbus, Ohio. Kal Kan Foods Inc, Vernon, Ca, 1992. Key: Ox = oxalic acid; p.o. = by mouth; q = every.

CHAPTER 5

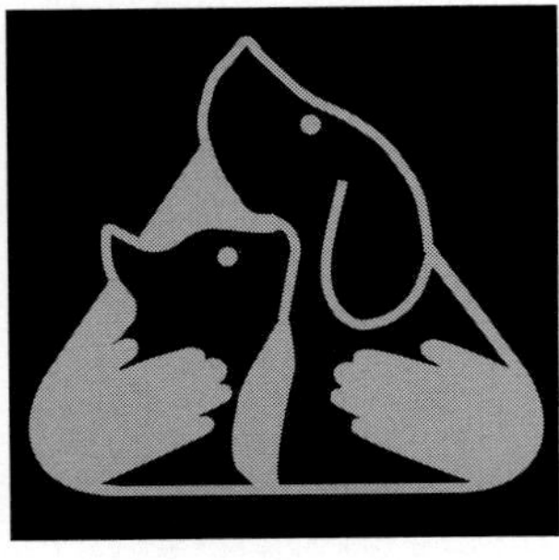

Techniques of Urine Collection and Preservation

CARL A. OSBORNE

I. OVERVIEW

A. Urinalysis is one of the most important diagnostic tools available to veterinarians. All veterinarians in clinical practice should master laboratory techniques and interpretation of urinalysis.

B. In addition to techniques of analysis and interpretation of results, collection of urine is an integral part of urinalysis. The method of collection and the collection container itself may influence test results and their interpretation.

C. Patients should be protected from iatrogenic complications associated with collection techniques, including trauma to the urinary tract and urinary tract infection.

D. Every effort should be made to collect a sample whose in vitro characteristics are similar to its in vivo characteristics.

1. The collection container should be selected with care.
2. Because drugs may alter laboratory test values by a variety of pharmacologic, physical, and/or chemical mechanisms, urine samples should always be collected prior to the administration of diagnostic or therapeutic agents.
   a. Withholding the administration of fluids prior to sample collection is especially important since oral or parenteral fluids may significantly alter urine specific gravity.
   b. The significance of sterile urine bacterial culture obtained from a patient that has been receiving antibiotics should be ascertained.
   c. Erroneous conclusions formulated on the basis of erroneous laboratory data may result in incorrect diagnosis.

II. COLLECTION CONTAINERS

A. Disposable and reusable containers designed specifically for collection of urine from human beings may be obtained from a variety of medical supply houses.

B. We routinely use disposable plastic cups.[a]

1. These cups are clean, readily available, inexpensive, and have tight-fitting lids.
2. They may be sterilized with ethylene oxide gas.

C. Use of containers improvised by owners are not recommended since they often contain contaminants (detergents, food, cosmetics, and so on) that may interfere with enzymatic and chemical tests.

D. Use of transparent containers made of glass or plastic facilitate observation of macroscopic characteristics of urine. If urinalysis cannot be performed within 30 min following collection, however, opaque containers should be considered to minimize photochemical degradation of urine constituents by bright light.

[a]Available from Nebco Distributing, 4150 Berkshire Lane, Plymouth, Minnesota 55446.

E. Urine obtained for bacterial culture must be collected in sterilized syringes or sterilized containers with tight-fitting lids. Sterilized containers may be obtained by:

1. Sterilizing disposable plastic cups in ethylene oxide gas.
2. Sterilizing glass or metal drinking cups in an autoclave.
3. Purchasing them from commercial manufacturers.

III. COLLECTION OF TABLE-TOP URINE SAMPLES

A. Patients with lower urinary tract disease often have reduced bladder capacity and urge incontinence. As a result, collection of urine into a cup during the voiding phase of micturition, or by cystocentesis, is difficult. Frequently, small quantities of urine are voided before they can be collected.

B. Collection of urine for analysis from smooth clean table tops with the aid of a needle and syringe may be facilitated by the use of two rectangular microscopic slides. The goal is to use the edges of the microscopic slides to form a deeper pool of urine that can more readily be aspirated.

1. The long edges of two microscopic slides should be placed flat on the table surface so that the small sample of urine is between them. The slides should be parallel to each other, and tilted away from the urine sample at an angle.
2. With the edges of the slides in close contact with the table, the slides should be advanced toward each other (Fig. 5–1). This will cause the urine to pool along the edges of the slides. During this time, an assistant with a syringe and needle should aspirate the urine as it pools in front of the microscopic slides. When the slides meet, they will form a V-shaped trough, from which most of the voided urine may be collected.

C. Urine samples collected in this fashion are satisfactory for screening urinalysis provided they are analyzed soon after collection. The value of the results will be influenced by the cleanliness of the table from which the sample was collected.

IV. COLLECTION TECHNIQUES

A. Urine may be removed from the bladder by one of four methods:

1. Natural voiding.
2. Manual compression of the urinary bladder.
3. Transurethral catheterization.
4. Cystocentesis.

B. Regardless of the method used:

1. Proper technique should be used to prevent iatrogenic trauma to the urethra and urinary bladder.
2. Proper technique must be used to prevent iatrogenic urinary tract infection.

C. Additional comments.

1. Early morning samples are preferred because they are most likely to be concentrated. Since consumption of water is likely to be greatest during the daytime, urine is more likely to be less concentrated during the daytime.
   a. Knowledge that urine is adequately concentrated provides important information about the status of renal function.
   b. Dilute urine (i.e., specific gravity below approximately 1.008) will lyse formed elements such as red and white blood cells.
   c. Voiding of large volumes of dilute urine tends to reduce the concentration of all substances present in the sample.
2. The significance of debris, cells, or organisms in urine sediment should always be interpreted with knowledge of the method of collection. This should be included on the form used to record urinalysis results.

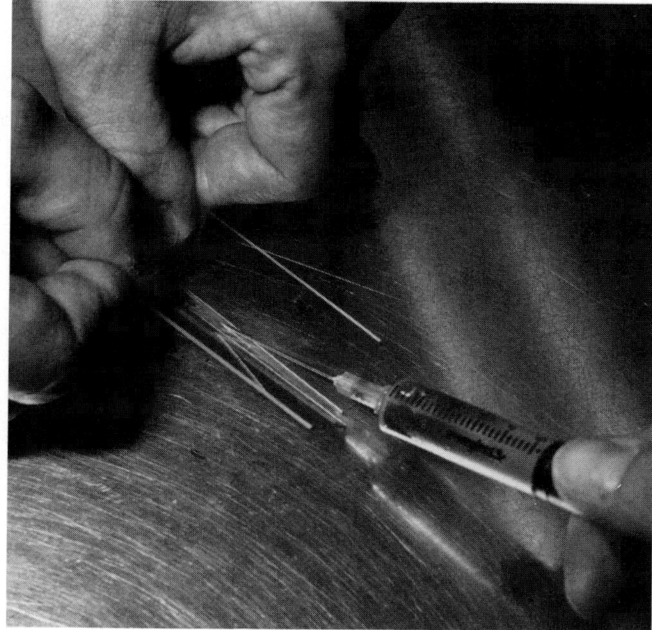

FIG. 5–1. Position of two microscope slides to facilitate aspiration of pooled urine voided on a table. As the tilted slides are advanced toward each other, the pooled urine is aspirated through a hypodermic needle into a syringe.

V. NORMAL VOIDING

A. The primary advantages of this technique are that:

1. It is not associated with any risk of complications to the patient.
2. It can be used by clients.

B. The primary disadvantages of this method are:

1. Samples are frequently contaminated with cells, bacteria, and other debris located in the genital tract or on the skin and hair. Voided samples are usually unsatisfactory for culture of urine for bacteria.
2. Samples may be contaminated by substances in the external environment.

3. The patient will not always void at the will of the veterinarian.

C. Voided samples are satisfactory for routine urinalysis obtained to screen patients for abnormalities of the urinary tract and other body systems. Depending on specific circumstances, however, it may be necessary to repeat analysis of a urine sample collected by cystocentesis. Voided samples are also satisfactory for serial evaluation of various chemical tests (glucose, ketones, bilirubin, and so on).

D. Comparison of abnormal results in voided urine samples to urinalysis results collected by cystocentesis or catheterization may aid in localization of the underlying cause(s) of the abnormal results (e.g., is the disorder proximal and/or distal to the urinary bladder).

E. When possible, the first portion of the urine stream should be excluded from the sample submitted for analysis because it is often contaminated during contact with the genital tract, skin, and hair. In order to facilitate this recommendation, two cups may be used to collect the sample.

1. The portion of the sample collected in the second cup, when available, represents a midstream sample; the beginning portion of the sample in the first cup may be discarded, or used to localize hemorrhage or inflammatory disease to the urethra or genital tract.
2. If technical difficulties prevent collection of the sample in two cups, the sample in the first cup is still available for analysis.

VI. MANUAL COMPRESSION OF THE URINARY BLADDER

A. Induction of micturition by application of digital pressure to the urinary bladder through the bladder wall may be used to collect urine samples from dogs and cats.

B. The primary advantages of this procedure are:

1. The risk of iatrogenic lower urinary tract infection and iatrogenic trauma is minimal.
2. Urine samples may be collected from patients with distended urinary bladders at the convenience of the clinician.

C. The primary disadvantages of this procedure are:

1. The urinary bladder may be traumatized if excessive digital pressure is used. This is not only detrimental to the patient, the associated hematuria may interfere with interpretation of results.
2. The urinary bladder may not contain a sufficient volume of urine to facilitate this technique.
3. Samples are frequently contaminated with cells, bacteria, and other debris located in the genital tract, or on the skin and hair. Therefore, they are unsatisfactory for bacterial culture (see section V., Normal Voiding).
4. Micturition may be difficult to induce in some patients, especially male cats.
5. Bladder urine contaminated or infected with bacteria may be forced into the prostate gland, ureters, renal pelves, and kidneys.[4] Unlike normal micturition where detrusor contraction is associated with a coordinated relaxation of voluntary and involuntary urethral sphincters, manual compression of the bladder increases intravesical pressure, but may not be associated with simultaneous relaxation of the urethral sphincters. Application of digital pressure to the urinary bladder for a prolonged period to initiate the urine voiding is associated with a greater risk of reflux than application of digital pressure for a transient period.
6. It is unsatisfactory for use during the immediate postoperative phase of cystotomies.

D. Technique.

1. Outline the urinary bladder by abdominal palpation. As a generality, this technique will not be successful in the conscious patient unless the bladder contains at least 10 to 15 ml of urine.
2. The patient may be in a standing or recumbent position.
3. Gradually exert moderate digital pressure over as large an area of the bladder as possible with the fingers and thumb of one hand, or with the fingers of both hands (Fig. 5–2).
   a. Try to direct the force toward the neck of the urinary bladder.

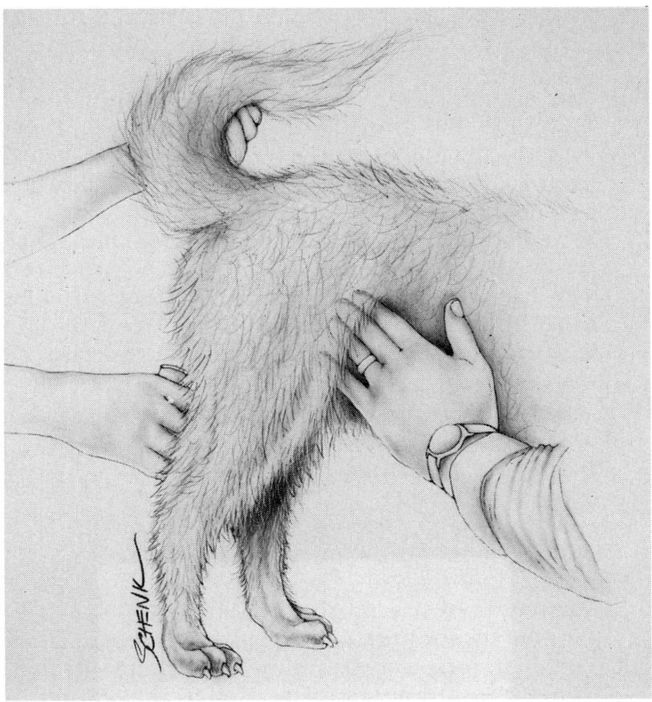

FIG. 5–2. Collection of urine by manual compression of the urinary bladder. The fingers of both hands are used to gradually exert moderate digital pressure over as large an area of the bladder as possible. Illustration by Michael P. Schenk.

b. A gradual but steady increase in pressure should be applied rather than forced intermittent squeezing motions.
c. Avoid vigorous palpation and/or excessive pressure since the latter is invariably associated with iatrogenic hematuria caused by trauma.
d. Sustain moderate digital pressure until the urethral sphincters relax and urine is expelled from the bladder. Several minutes of digital pressure may be required before micturition is induced.
e. Never use excessive pressure.

4. If the bladder is overdistended with urine because of partial obstruction to urine outflow, caution must be used not to rupture the bladder or urethra.
5. Although diuretics such as furosemide have been recommended by some investigators to facilitate collection of urine samples by increasing urine formation, alteration of urine specific gravity is a notable drawback of this procedure. Use of diuretics to enhance urine collection by augmenting urine flow is therefore best suited for serial urine sample collections when quantitative information about urine specific gravity and semiquantitative information about chemical tests and structures found in urine sediment are not significant.
6. If voiding does not occur following application of digital pressure to the urinary bladder, return the patient (cat) to the ward with a container of plastic litter, or walk the patient (dog) outside.[8] If the bladder contains a sufficient volume of urine, the patient will often voluntarily void it at that time.

VII. TRANSURETHRAL CATHETERIZATION

A. Overview.

1. Avoid unnecessary catheterization
2. Catheterization should be performed in an atraumatic and aseptic fashion by persons familiar with correct procedure. Because of the risks of trauma and bacterial urinary tract infection, it is not a technique that should be delegated to inadequately trained personnel unaware of these consequences.

B. Indications.

1. Indications for transurethral catheterization of the urinary bladder may be categorized as diagnostic or therapeutic (Table 5–1).
2. The purpose(s) of catheterization largely determines which of three general types of catheterization will be useful. Single brief catheterization is appropriate when the need for a catheter can be accomplished in a few hours or less. However, when need for catheterization spans longer periods, intermittent or indwelling catheterization is required.

C. Size, composition and types of catheters.

1. Size.
   a. The scale of measurement commonly used for calibrating the diameter of catheters is the French scale (commonly abbreviated as F).
      (1). Each French unit is equivalent to ⅓ mm; thus, French units may be converted to millimeters by dividing by 3.
      (2). A 9F catheter has an external diameter of 3 mm.
   b. Catheters are available in a variety of diameters and lengths.
2. Composition.
   a. Urinary catheters are fabricated from a variety of materials including rubber, plastic, metal, nylon, latex, and woven silk.
   b. Catheters impregnated with radiopaque material are of value when used in conjunction with radiographic evaluation of the urinary system.
   c. Catheters impregnated with antimicrobial agents have been recommended to minimize iatrogenic infection in human beings.
3. Types (Figs. 5–3 to 5–6).
   a. A wide variety of catheters are available for use in human and veterinary medicine; each is designated to serve a particular need (Figs. 5–3 to 5–6).
   b. The openings adjacent to the tips of catheters are commonly called "eyes."
      (1). Catheters may have as few as one or as many as six eyes.
      (2). The edges of eyes of polypropylene catheters are often rough and, as a consequence, irritate the mucosa of the bladder and urethra.
   c. On the basis of the site of their insertion, human catheters are classified as urethral or ureteral catheters.

TABLE 5–1
INDICATIONS FOR TRANSURETHRAL CATHETERIZATION OF THE URINARY BLADDER

DIAGNOSTIC
Collection of a urine sample for analysis or bacterial culture
Collection of accurately timed volumes of urine for renal function studies
Measurement of urine output
Measurement of postmicturition residual urine volume
Instillation of contrast material for radiographic studies of the bladder, urethra, or prostate gland
Verification and localization of urethral obstruction
Catheter aspiration biopsy of urethral, prostatic, or bladder lesions

THERAPEUTIC
Relief of urethral obstruction to urine flow
Relief of urine retention
Instillation of medications into the urinary bladder
Facilitation of surgery of the bladder, urethra, or surrounding structures

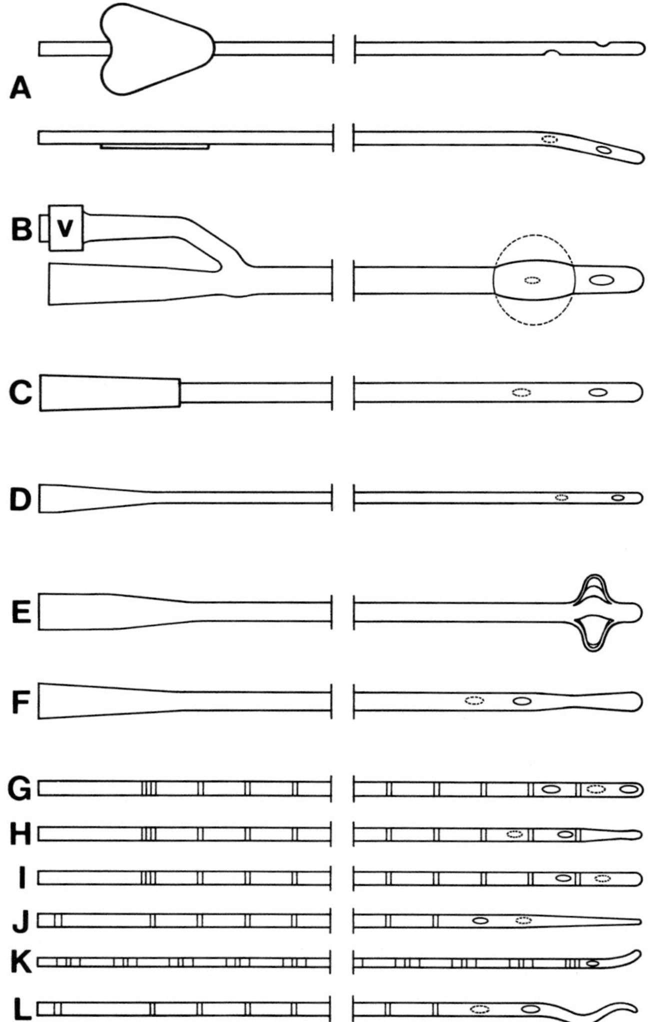

FIG. 5–3. Different types of catheters available for urine collection. Key: A = rigid metal canine female urethral catheter; B = Foley self-retaining catheter with valve (v) for injection of air to inflate balloon (dotted circle); C = human urethral catheter with round tip; D = canine flexible urethral catheter; E = Malecot self-retaining four-winged catheter; F = olive-tip human urethral catheter; G = whistle-tip human ureteral catheter; H = olive-tip human ureteral catheter; I = round-tip human ureteral catheter; J = Blasucci flexible-tip human ureteral catheter; K = coudé-tip human ureteral catheter; L = Blasucci human ureteral catheter with flexible spiral filiform tip.

(1). Human urethral catheters are usually too large (and sometimes too short) for routine use in veterinary medicine.

(2). Human ureteral catheters are commonly used to catheterize male and female dogs.

(3). Urethral catheters with inflatable balloons are called Foley catheters (Figure 5–6).[b]

(a). By inflating the balloon following insertion of the catheter into the bladder, the tip of the catheter cannot migrate out of the bladder lumen.

(b). Foley catheters are designed to be used as indwelling (or retention) catheters.

[b]Available from Rusch, Inc., 2450 Meadowbrook Parkway, Duluth, Georgia 30136.

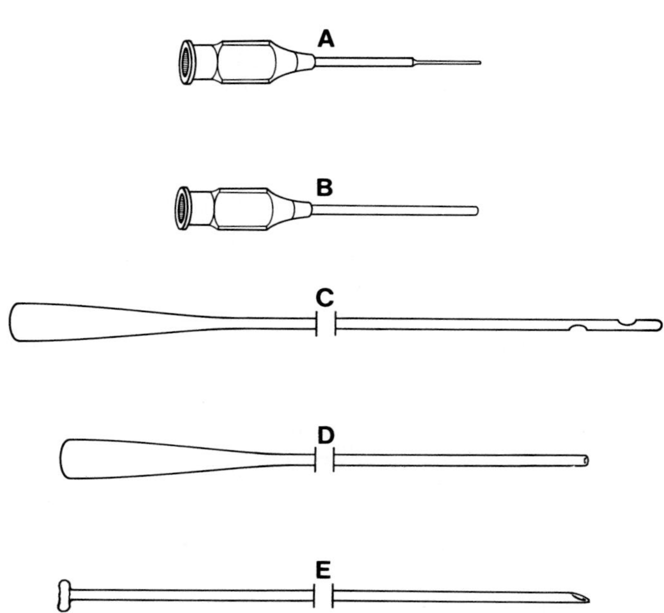

FIG. 5–4. Catheters used to collect urine and/or backflush the urethra of cats. Key: A = rigid metal lacrimal cannula; B = silver abscess cannula; C = tomcat catheter; D = open-end tomcat catheter; E = intradermic polyethylene tubing with one end flared.

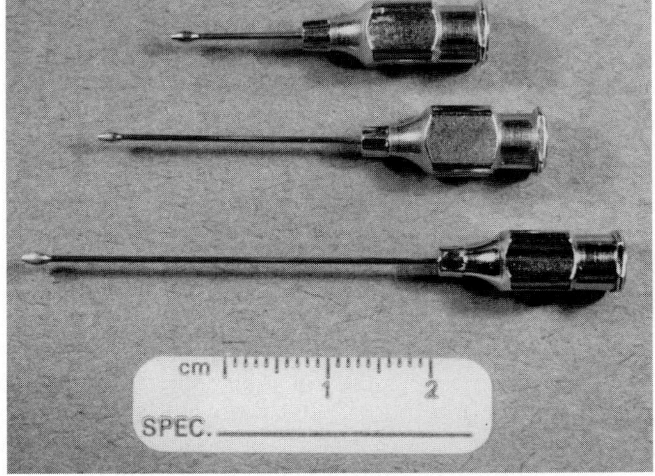

FIG. 5–5. Minnesota olive-tip urethral catheters, available in 22-gauge 0.5-, 1.0-, and 1.5-in. lengths from E JAY International, Glendora, CA 91740.

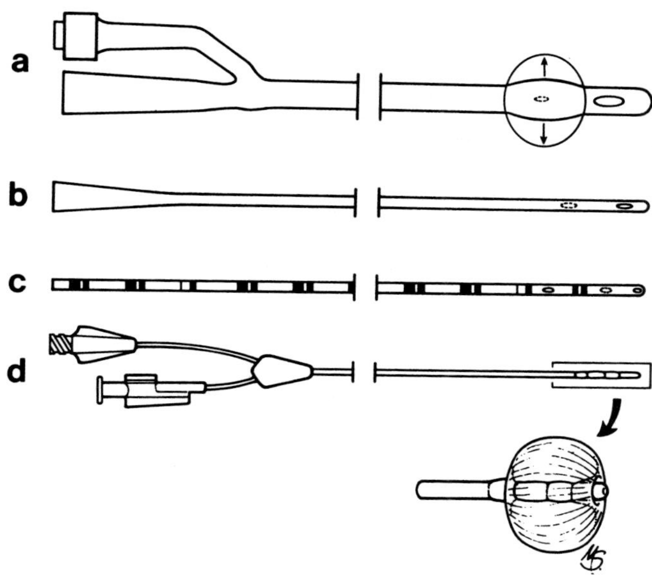

FIG. 5–6. Drawings of catheters used for retrograde contrast urethrocystography, retrograde contrast vaginography, and various types of collection of urine from the urinary bladder. Key: a = pediatric Foley catheter—air injected through the upper arm of the catheter will inflate the balloon (arrows); b = polypropylene urethral catheter with two eyes; c = whistle-tip ureteral catheter; d = Swan Ganz flow-directed balloon catheter; air injected into the valve (lower arm) will inflate the balloon (insert). Illustration by Michael P. Schenk.

(c). Foley catheters are sometimes used for retrograde contrast urethrography and retrograde vaginography.

(4). Angiographic catheters with inflatable balloons (Swan-Ganz flow-directed balloon catheters) may be used for retrograde urethrocystography (see Fig. 5–6).[c]

d. Canine urinary catheters

(1). Flexible plastic[d] and rubber[e] catheters similar in diameter and length to human ureteral catheters may be used to catheterize male or female dogs. In our experience, polypropylene catheters frequently traumatize the urethra of male dogs as it curves around the ischial arch because they are relatively inflexible.

(2). Metal catheters designed for use in female dogs are not recommended because their rigid structure frequently is the cause of iatrogenic trauma to the mucosa of the urethra and urinary bladder.

(3). Swan-Ganz flow-directed balloon catheters designed for human angiography are very useful for collection of quantitative urine specimens from dogs (and cats) (Fig. 5–6).[3]

e. Feline urinary catheters

(1). Disposable polypropylene tom cat catheters (3½ to 5 French) are available from commercial manufacturers (Fig. 5–4).[f]

(2). Infant feeding tubes[e] and polyethylene tubing may also be used to catheterize cats.

(3). Minnesota olive tip feline urethral catheters[g] and silver abscess cannulas[h] are often used to remove plugs from the distal urethra of male cats. They are too short to reach the lumen of the bladder (see Figs. 5–4 and 5–5).

(4). The use of rigid metal tom cat catheters is not recommended since they often cause trauma to the urethral and bladder mucosa.

(5). Wysong urethral catheters[i] constructed of a silicone elastomer are designed for indwelling use in male cats.[11]

(6). Jackson cat catheters[j] are also designed for indwelling use in male cats. However, their relatively rigid construction may cause trauma to the urinary bladder as it contracts.

f. Filiforms and followers

(1). Filiforms and followers are instruments commonly used in human medicine to locate and dilate ureteral strictures.

(2). Filiforms are solid structures made of pliable woven silk or plastic material. They have a variety of different types of tips (i.e., coudé and corkscrew).

(3). Followers are made of woven silk or metal. They may be solid or hollow. Hollow followers permit catheterization.

g. Sounds

(1). Sounds are special instruments made of solid metal that may be used instead of catheters to explore the urethra for stenoses and to dilate the urethra and bladder neck.

(2). Sounds are available in a wide variety of designs for use in man.

(3). Consult human textbooks of urology for

[c]Available from Baxter-Edwards Laboratories, Inc., P.O. Box 11150, Santa Ana, California 92711.

[d]Polypropylene catheters, Sherwood Medical Industries, Inc., St. Louis, Missouri 63103.

[e]Sterile disposable feeding tube and urethral catheter, Sherwood Medical Industries, Inc., St. Louis, Missouri 63103.

[f]Tom cat catheter, Sherwood Medical Industries, Inc., St. Louis, Missouri 63103.

[g]Available from Enjay International, Inc., P.O. Box 1835, Glendora, California 91740.

[h]Available from Becton Dickenson Co., Rutherford, New Jersey.

[i]Available from Wysong Medical Corporation, 4925 Jefferson Ave., Midland, Michigan 48640.

[j]Available from Arnold's Veterinary Products Ltd., 14 Tessa Road, Richfield Avenue, Reading, England RG1 8NF.

specific details about filiforms, followers, and sounds.

h. It is recommended that a special drawer in the hospital be designated as a catheter drawer (analogous to a tool box).
   (1). Sterilized catheters of all sizes, composition, and types should be stored in this drawer so that they will be readily available when needed.
   (2). Speculums and light sources may also be stored in the catheter drawer.

D. Care of urinary catheters.

1. Only sterilized catheters that are in excellent condition should be used.
   a. Catheters weakened during use or abuse may break apart while in the patient.
   b. The "eye" is the weakest part of flexible catheters.
   c. Catheters that have a rough external surface may damage the mucosa of the urethral and urinary bladder. Not only are they detrimental to the patient, iatrogenic hematuria may interfere with interpretation of the urinalysis.
2. Catheters should be individually packaged prior to use. Use of transparent packages that may be sterilized with ethylene oxide[k] aids in storage and selection since it permits visualization of the catheter.
3. Nonsterilized catheters should never be used because:
   a. They may cause iatrogenic infection of the urinary system.
   b. They may contaminate urine that is collected for bacterial culture.
4. Sterilization.
   a. Catheters must be thoroughly cleaned prior to sterilization. Cleansing solutions should be thoroughly rinsed from them since they may interfere with enzymatic and chemical tests.
   b. Repeated autoclaving of nonmetal catheters may reduce their longevity.
   c. Ethylene oxide sterilization is excellent.
   d. Microwave ovens may be used to sterilize catheters.[2]
      (1). A technique utilizing microwave ovens to sterilize urinary catheters has been described.
      (2). Basically, the technique involved placing flexible urinary catheters in reusable freezer bags and placing them in a microwave oven. Along with the catheter, a beaker with water must be placed in the oven to absorb excessive heat. The microwave oven was set at 12 min (high power). The authors emphasized the need to avoid "cold areas" in the microwave oven.
      (3). We recommend that this procedure be validated with each hospital's microwave before using it to stabilize urinary catheters. This may be accomplished by culturing contaminated urinary catheters for bacteria before and after microwaving them.
   e. Chemical sterilizing solutions containing quaternary ammonia compounds may be used, but are less effective than sterilization by autoclaving or ethylene oxide gas. In addition, if residual antiseptic solutions are not thoroughly rinsed from catheters, they may:
      (1). Irritate the mucosa of the urethra or urinary bladder.
      (2). Interfere with growth of bacteria.
      (3). Alter chemical and enzyme tests.
   f. Disposable catheters which are prepackaged in sterilized wrappers may be obtained from commercial manufacturers.

E. Potential complications of transurethral catheterization.

1. Urinary catheters may produce two general types of adverse effects:
   a. Trauma to the urinary tract caused by insertion or continued presence of the catheter.
   b. Initiation of bacterial urinary tract infection (UTI).
   c. The risk of these adverse effects varies from patient to patient because it is affected by numerous factors.
2. Status of the urinary tract.
   a. Foremost among the variables which affect the risk of catheter-induced complications is the physical and functional status of the patient's urinary tract (especially the urethra and bladder) during and following catheterization. When diseases of the urinary tract make catheterization mechanically difficult, poor technique which leads to bacterial contamination and urinary tract trauma are likely.
   b. Local urinary tract defense mechanisms are usually compromised by urinary tract diseases. Thus, animals with urinary tract disorders have greater risk of catheter-induced complications. Unfortunately, it is these patients for which catheterization is most often indicated. Consult Chapter 40, Bacterial Infections of the Canine and Feline Urinary Tract, for additional details.
3. Patient profile.
   a. Risk of catheter-induced complications is also associated with species, sex, size, temperament, and general health status.
      (1). Cats are generally more difficult to catheterize than dogs. However, dogs may be more susceptible to UTI than cats. Regardless of species, males are more easily catheterized than females. Perhaps this and other sex-related factors are associ-

[k]Available from Baxter Scientific, 1210 Waukegan Road, McGaw Park, Illinois 60085.

ated with the greater risk of catheter-induced UTI in females as compared to male dogs.

(2). Because veterinary patients vary greatly in size and cooperativeness, equipment and techniques that work optimally for some are less satisfactory for others. Failure to use methods that are appropriate for each patient can be detrimental.

(3). Catheter-induced UTI can lead to episodes of bacteremia, particularly when a catheter is removed from an infected urinary tract.

b. General health status and concomitant disorders can influence the risk of catheter-associated complications.

(1). Dogs with Cushing's syndrome, diabetes mellitus, and renal failure have increased susceptibility to UTI.

(2). Patients with valvular cardiac disease have increased risk of developing bacterial endocarditis as a result of such bacteremia.

4. Techniques.

a. Techniques of catheterization influence the frequency and nature of adverse sequelae. Abrasion, contusion, laceration, and even puncture of the urethra and bladder can occur during catheterization. Prevention of these undesirable effects, in addition to control of catheter-induced UTI, is dependent on selection and careful use of an appropriate catheter.

b. Frequency and duration of catheterization also influence the risk of catheter-induced complications. Iatrogenic infection is least likely to occur as a consequence of a single brief catheterization. Studies of repeated intermittent brief catheterization have revealed that the risk of inducing infection is similar following each catheterization. Thus, the cumulative risk of catheter-induced UTI is proportional to the number of catheterizations.

c. Risk of iatrogenic infection is greatest during indwelling catheterization, especially when the portion of catheter protruding from the urethra is not connected to a receptical (i.e., it is open).[5,7] In general, the risk of infection during indwelling catheterization is proportional to the duration of catheterization.[1,5,7] When there is need for long term catheterization, intermittent catheterization is often safer because it is less likely to induce UTI than indwelling catheterization. In addition, indwelling catheters may cause continuous trauma to the urinary tract, and may elicit a foreign body reaction in surrounding tissue.[6] In some situations, however, risk of urethral trauma caused by repeated insertion of a catheter is sufficient to make indwelling catheterization the safer alternative.

d. Because of the risk of inducing infection of the bladder as a result of catheterization, indiscriminate use of this technique is condemned. This generality must be kept in perspective, however. When necessary for diagnostic or therapeutic purposes, carefully performed transurethral catheterization of the urinary bladder should be performed without hesitation.

e. Procedures which may be used to prevent and/or treat catheter-induced bacterial UTI include the following:

(1). Avoid unnecessary catheterization, especially in patients with increased risk for bacterial UTI and its sequelae. They include patients with:

(a). Urinary disease, especially of the lower urinary tract

(b). Hyperadrenocorticism

(c). Diabetes mellitus

(d). Polyuria

(2). Urinary catheterization should only be performed by properly trained personnel.

(3). If the need for catheterization spans more than a few hours, consider intermittent catheterizations as well as indwelling catheterization.

(4). If a single brief catheterization is required for a high-risk patient, consider an antibiotic excreted in high concentration in urine and administer it 8 to 12 hrs before and 8 to 12 hrs after catheterization.

(5). Avoid overinsertion of catheters, to minimize damage to bladder mucosa.

(6). If indwelling urethral catheters are required, strive to maintain a closed system.

(7). Select indwelling urethral catheters constructed of materials least likely to cause irritation and inflammation of the adjacent mucosa.

(8). Consider administering antibiotics during indwelling urethral catheterization only if evidence of infection is detected. This minimizes the likelihood of infection with bacteria resistant to antimicrobial agents. If catheter-induced infection develops and remains asymptomatic, treat the infection following removal of the catheter.

(9). Periodically perform urinalysis and bacterial culture during the period of indwelling urethral catheterization, and always at the time the catheter is removed.

F. Technique—generalities for male and female dogs and cats.

1. Regardless of the specific procedure employed, meticulous aseptic and gentle "feather touch" technique should be used to prevent damage to the delicate tissues of the genital tract, urethra, and urinary bladder.

2. Only well-trained individuals who comprehend the potential consequences of iatrogenic trauma and UTI should be given the responsibility to catheterize the urethra and urinary bladder.
3. Conscious patients should be restrained by an assistant in order to minimize contamination of the catheter as well as trauma to the urethra.
4. Animals should be gently restrained in a comfortable position in order to minimize the possibility of sudden unexpected movement which may result in contamination of the catheter or trauma to the urinary tract. Some type of sedation may be required for male cats and is usually required for female cats. Appropriate caution should be used so as not to use a drug that alters the diagnostic, physical, or chemical composition of urine.
5. Use the smallest diameter catheter which will permit the objective of catheterization. Few patients will tolerate the passage of large catheters without some form of sedation.
6. Catheters with flared ends are recommended, especially if the length of the catheter is similar to the length of the urethra (see Figs. 5–3 to 5–6).
   a. If the end is not flared, the catheter may migrate into the urethra to a point where it cannot be manually removed. In this event, insertion of a Swan-Ganz flow-directed balloon catheter inside the lumen of the damaged catheter, followed by distention of the balloon, may be used to withdraw it.
   b. Many commercially prepared catheters have flared ends which will accommodate the tip of a syringe.
7. If a stylet is used in the catheter, it should be lubricated before it is inserted into the lumen of the catheter. If it is not lubricated, difficulty may be encountered in removing the stylet after the catheter is placed in the patient (especially male dogs).
8. If necessary, structures adjacent to the external urethral orifice should be cleansed with germicidal soap, water, and sterilized sponges. The soap and water mixture should be thoroughly removed by rinsing to prevent contamination of the urine sample. Soapy water may:
   a. Impart a cloudy appearance to the sample.
   b. Inhibit bacterial growth.
   c. Cause lysis of cells.
   d. Interfere with chemical and enzyme tests.
9. The distance from the external urethral orifice to the beginning of the lumen of the bladder lumen should be "guesstimated" and mentally transposed to the catheter.
   a. This step will reduce the likelihood of traumatizing the bladder mucosa due to overinsertion of the catheter.
   b. It will also prevent the catheter from reentering the urethra.
10. The tip of the catheter and adjacent portions should be liberally lubricated with sterilized aqueous lubricant.
   a. Proper lubrication of the catheter will minimize discomfort to the patient and catheter-induced trauma to the urethra.
   b. In man, filling and coating the catheter with a large quantity of water soluble lubricant containing an antibacterial agent has been reported to decrease the number of bacteria pushed into the bladder lumen.
11. Although usually unnecessary, local anesthesia may be induced with a topical anesthetic such as lidocaine hydrochloride.[1]
12. Asepsis must be maintained throughout the procedure.
   a. The catheter should not be allowed to contact the hair or skin of the patient or clinician.
   b. The catheter may be manipulated:
      (1). Through the packaging material in which it is contained.
      (2). With the aid of a sterilized pediatric hemostat.
      (3). With sterilized surgical gloves.
      (4). By holding the distal end only.
13. Never force the catheter through the urethra.
   a. If difficulty is encountered in inserting the catheter through the urethra, withdraw the catheter for a short distance and insert it again with a gradual rotating motion. If difficulty persists, reevaluate the diameter of the catheter.
   b. Injection of a sterilized mixture of aqueous lubricant, whose viscosity has been diluted with sterilized water or saline, through the lumen of the catheter may be of value.
   c. If these steps are unsuccessful, a smaller diameter catheter should be used.
14. The tip of the catheter should be positioned so that its eyes are located just beyond the junction of the neck of the bladder with the urethra. In most instances, this may be accomplished by inserting the catheter approximately one inch beyond the point at which urine flows through the catheter lumen.
   a. This position may be verified by injection of a known quantity of air through the catheter into an otherwise empty bladder lumen. Inability to remove most of the air indicates improper positioning of the catheter. The catheter should be repositioned until the quantity of air injected into the bladder lumen can be readily aspirated into the syringe.
   b. Proper positioning of catheters facilitates removal of all of the urine from the bladder and

[1]Anestacon, Conal Pharmaceuticals, Inc., Chicago, Illinois 60640. Xylocaine 2% Jelly, Astra Pharmaceutical Products, Inc., Westborough, Massachusetts 01581. Uro-Jet Delivery System (2% lidocaine HCl Jelly), International Medications Systems Ltd., 1886 Santa Anita Ave., South Elmonte, California 91733.

minimizes the possibility of catheter-induced trauma.

15. Urine may be aspirated from the bladder with the aid of a syringe.
    a. Aspiration must be gentle in order to prevent trauma to the bladder or urethral mucosa as a result of sucking it into the eyes of the catheter.
    b. Attempts to force urine through the catheter by application of digital pressure to the bladder is not recommended as a routine procedure since it increases the likelihood of catheter-induced damage to the bladder mucosa.
    c. Use of a 2-way or 3-way valve will minimize inadvertent injection of bacteria into the bladder.
16. Unless desired for specific study, the first several milliliters of urine obtained via the catheter should be discarded since it may be contaminated with bacteria, debris, and cells from the genital tract and urethra.
17. In patients with a high risk of developing iatrogenic infection as a result of catheterization:
    a. Sterilized solutions of antimicrobial drugs may be injected into the bladder lumen as a prophylactic measure. However, local instillation of antimicrobial agents should not be used as a substitute for orally or parenterally administered antimicrobial agents if the risk of iatrogenic bacterial UTI warrants antimicrobial therapy.
    b. Follow-up urinalyses or bacterial cultures should be considered several days later in an attempt to detect iatrogenic infection at a subclinical stage.

G. Transurethral catheterization of the urinary bladder of male dogs (Fig. 5–7).

1. Refer to general discussion about catheterization.
2. The length and diameter of the catheter will vary with the size of the patient.
    a. Four to ten French catheters are satisfactory for most dogs.
    b. The length of human ureteral and veterinary ureteral catheters usually does not vary.
3. The external urethral orifice should be exposed by reflecting the prepuce away from the penis. To retract the prepuce, apply caudal pressure with the index finger at the point where the prepuce reflects onto the ventral abdomen. Grasp the penis through the prepuce with the other hand, and push it cranially.
    a. Once exposed, the tip of the penis and the external urethral orifice should be thoroughly cleansed with soap and water.
    b. Once reflected, the prepuce must not be allowed to contact the catheter as it is being advanced through the urethral lumen.
4. Difficulty in advancing the catheter through the urethral lumen may be encountered at the level of the os penis and at the site where the urethra curves around the ischial arch. Resistance encountered at the level of the os penis may be minimized by grasping the penis through the prepuce and pushing it forward along the ventral body wall. Resistance of the catheter at the ischial arch may be minimized by application of digital pressure over the top of the catheter as it is slowly advanced.
5. Care must be used not to insert an excessive length of the catheter because it may follow the curvature of the bladder wall, double back on itself, and reenter the urethral lumen (Fig. 5–8). As the catheter is withdrawn, the loop of the catheter becomes progressively smaller until a point is reached where the wall of the catheter bends. The catheter often bends at the eye since it is the weakest point of the catheter wall (Fig. 5–9). As the bent catheter is withdrawn, it usually lodges at the caudal end of the os penis. If a catheter does become lodged in the wall of the urethra as a result of bending on itself, the following procedures, listed in order of priority, should be considered.[9]
    a. Advance the catheter back into the bladder lumen with the objective of releasing the tight bend in the catheter wall.
    b. Apply a liberal quantity of sterilized lubricant to the outside wall of the catheter, and insert a dilute solution (2 parts lubricant to 1 part water) of sterilized lubricant into the catheter

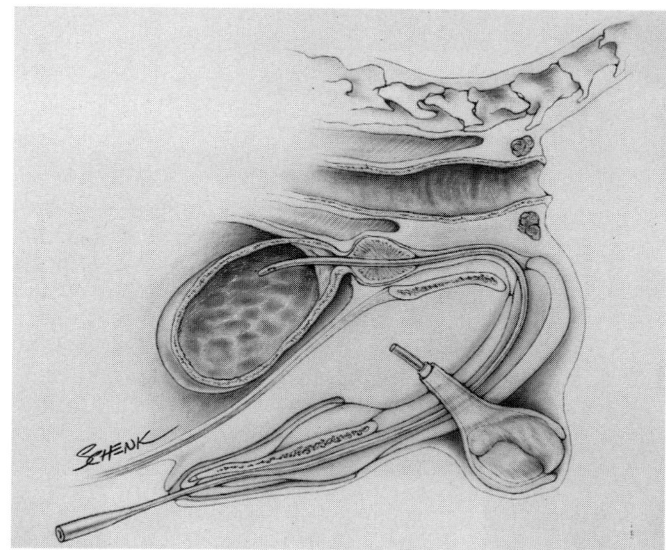

FIG. 5–7. Proper position of tip of flexible catheter in the lumen of the urinary bladder of a male dog. Rigid plastic catheters are often unsatisfactory because they may cause trauma and pain during passage through the curved portion of the perineal urethra. Reprinted with permission from Osborne CA, Schenk MP. Techniques of urine collection. In: *Forty-fourth Annual Proceedings of the American Animal Hospital Association.* Denver, Colo., American Animal Hospital Association; 1977, pp. 431–442.

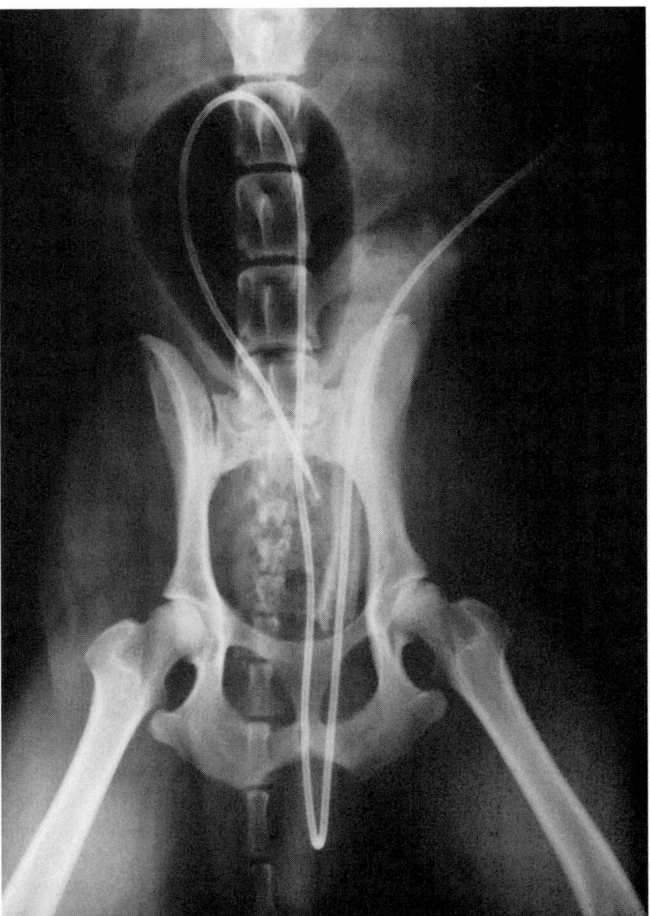

FIG. 5–8. Overinsertion of a flexible catheter into the urinary bladder of a 9-year-old mixed-breed dog: The tip of the catheter has reentered the urethra.

lumen. Apply gentle, steady traction to the catheter with the objective of dilating the urethral lumen ventral to the os penis and withdrawing the catheter (Fig. 5–10). Do not apply traction of such force as to tear the urethral mucosa.

c. If the catheter cannot be removed by steady traction, inject a liberal quantity of dilute sterilized aqueous lubricant through and around the catheter. An assistant should then occlude the lumen of the pelvic urethra by applying digital pressure against the ischium through the ventral wall of the rectum. Next, a teat cannula (or similar catheter), with attached syringe loaded with sterilized saline, should be placed in the penile urethra via the external urethral orifice (Fig. 5–11). The external urethral orifice should be compressed around the teat cannula and catheter by digital pressure. As a result of these maneuvers, a portion of the urethra from the external urethral orifice to the bony pelvis becomes a closed system (Fig. 5–11). Saline should then be injected into the urethra until a definite rebound is perceived through the syringe plunger. This rebound should be associated with a palpable increase in the diameter of the pelvic urethra. At this point, another assistant should grasp the catheter and attempt to remove it with gentle but steady pressure. If the portion of the urethral lumen ventral to the os penis dilates sufficiently, the catheter may be removed from the patient.

d. Inject aqueous organic iodinated material into and around the catheter with the objective of visualizing the exact nature of the problem via contrast radiography. Anesthetize the patient and repeat step b or c. Stretching the urethral lumen with the catheter will induce a lesser degree of injury than a urethrotomy.

e. If all of the above steps are unsuccessful, the catheter must be removed by urethrotomy.

H. Transurethral catheterization of the urinary bladder of female dogs (Figs. 5–12 to 5–16).

1. Equipment

   a. Flexible veterinary urethral or human ureteral catheters identical to those used for male dogs are recommended. Rigid metal catheters are not recommended for routine use because they have a tendency to traumatize the mucosa of the vagina, urethra, and urinary bladder.

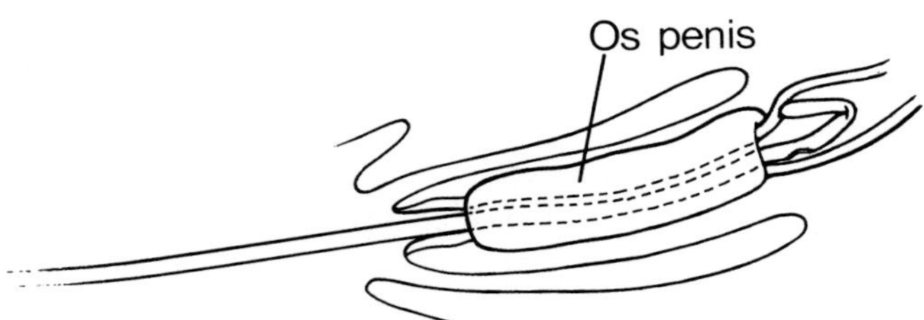

FIG. 5–9. Illustration of the consequences of overinsertion of a catheter into the urinary bladder to the extent that the catheter tip curved around the bladder vertex and reentered the bladder neck and urethra. Withdrawal of the overinserted catheter resulted in its bending and kinking on itself at one of the "eyes." Further withdrawal of the folded catheter resulted in it becoming lodged behind the os penis.

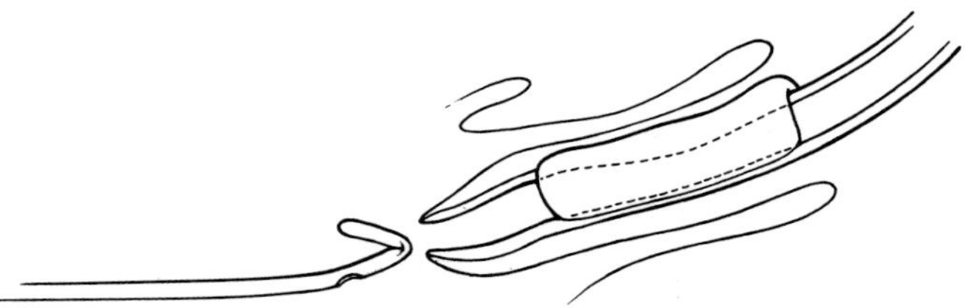

FIG. 5–10. Removal of an overinserted catheter from the urethra by steady traction (see Figs. 5–8 and 5–9).

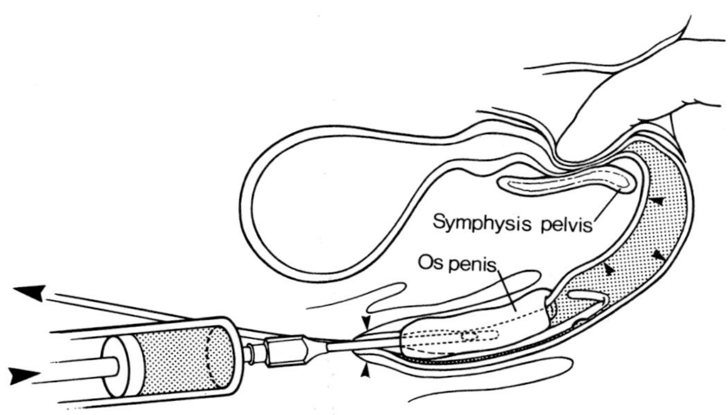

FIG. 5–11. Dilation of the segment of urethral lumen containing a kinked catheter by digital compression of the distal urethra, digital compression of the pelvic urethra against the bony pelvis, and injection of sterile saline. When the urethral lumen is distended, the kinked catheter may be removed by steady traction (see Figs. 8 and 9).

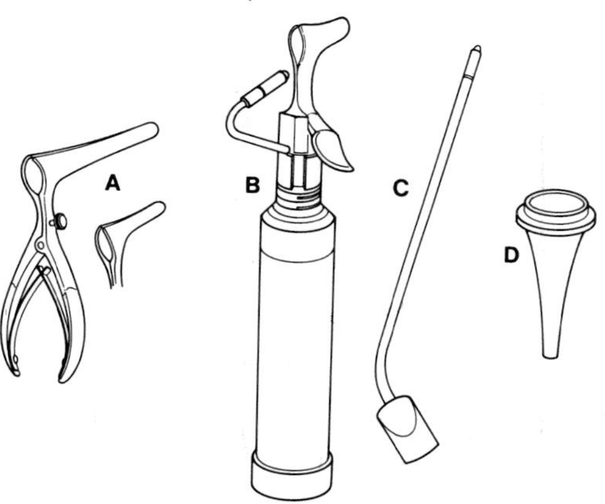

FIG. 5–12. Instruments that may be used as vaginal endoscopes. Reprinted with permission from Osborne CA, Stevens JB. *Handbook of Canine and Feline Urinalysis.* St. Louis, Mo.: Ralston Purina Co.; 1981. Key: A = nasal specula with blades of different lengths; B = nasal speculum with attached light source; C = transilluminator (without handle containing power source); D = otoscope head.

b. A variety of endoscopes (Fig. 5–12) may be used in the vagina to aid visualization of the external urethral orifice, including:
   (1). Human nasal specula
   (2). Brincker-Hoff's human rectal speculum (small size)
   (3). Specula fashioned from disposable Monoject syringe cases (Fig. 5–13)
   (4). Pyrex test tubes from which the end has been removed and the edge fire-polished
   (5). Otoscope cones
   (6). Laryngoscopes
   (7). Cystoscope sheaths

c. Transilluminator (Welch-Allen) and light sources for otoscopes.

2. Refer to the general discussion about catheterization.
3. If necessary, remove excessive hair from around the vulva. Cleanse the perivulvar skin and vulva with germicidal soap, water, and sterilized sponges.
4. If necessary, flush the lumen of the vagina with sterilized water or saline injected through a sy-

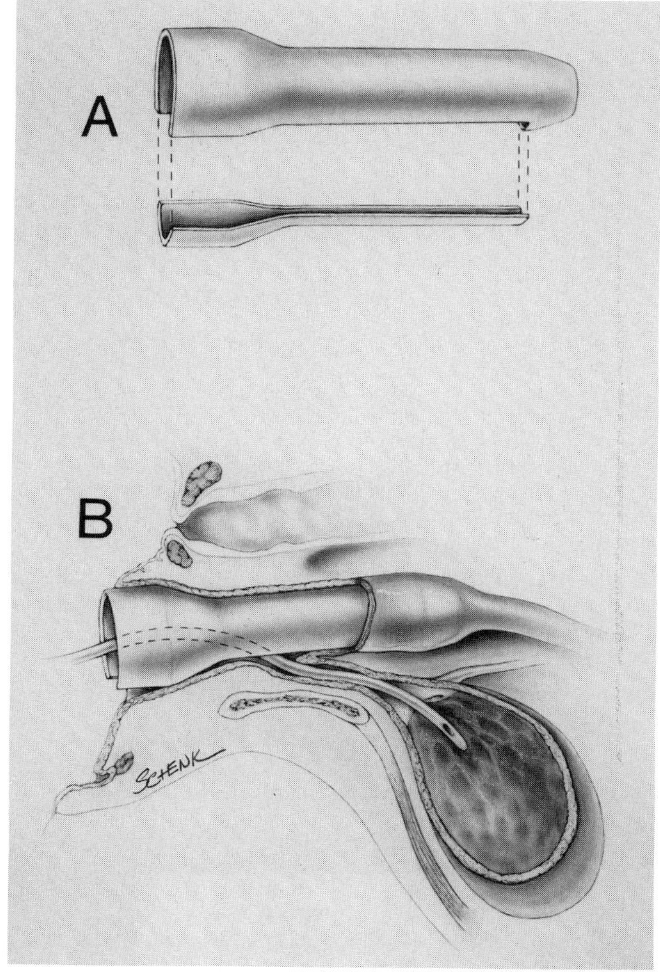

FIG. 5–13. Catheterization of a female dog with the aid of an endoscope made from a Monoject disposable syringe container (Sherwood Medical Industries). The endoscope was made by removing a rectangular section from the side of the syringe case (A). Following insertion of the endoscope into the vagina with the open side positioned ventrally, a catheter can readily be directed into the external urethral orifice (B). Reprinted with permission from Osborne CA, Schenk MP. Techniques of urine collection. In: *Forty-fourth Annual Proceedings of the American Animal Hospital Association.* Denver, Colo., American Animal Hospital Association; 1977, pp. 431–442.

ringe. Lidocaine jelly may be injected into the distal lumen of the vagina.

5. The external urethral orifice is located on a small tubercle in the ventral wall of the vagina.
   a. In mature small to medium-sized dogs, the external urethral orifice is approximately 3 to 5 cm cranial to the ventral commissure of the vulva.
   b. The clitoral fossa lies just caudal to the external urethral orifice. Catheters and endoscopes inserted into the vagina must be carefully directed above and past this structure.
6. Catheterization via endoscopy (Figs. 5–12 to 5–14)
   a. Good restraint, a good light source, and a comfortable position for both patient and clinician are important considerations.
   b. Having the dog in a standing position is recommended because it facilitates anatomical orientation required to locate the external urethral orifice.
   c. Ideally, the speculum must be large enough to remove the folds of the vaginal wall by distending its lumen.
   d. Injection of air into the vagina sometimes is of value in promoting dilatation of the lumen.
7. Foley catheter technique.
   a. For patients too small to permit visualization of the external urethral orifice with the aid of an endoscope, an 8 to 10 French Foley catheter may permit catheterization.
   b. Insert the Foley catheter into the vagina as far as possible and inflate the balloon.
   c. Insert a small nasal speculum into the vagina and open the blades.
   d. Gently pull the Foley catheter outward.
   e. The ureteral orifice may be visualized as a small opening in the ventral midline of the vaginal floor.
   f. Insertion of the urethral catheter is usually not hindered by the Foley balloon. If it is, however, the balloon should be deflated.
8. Digital technique (Fig. 5–15).
   a. Female dogs large enough to permit digital palpation of the vagina may be catheterized without the need of direct visualization. This technique is more likely to be associated with

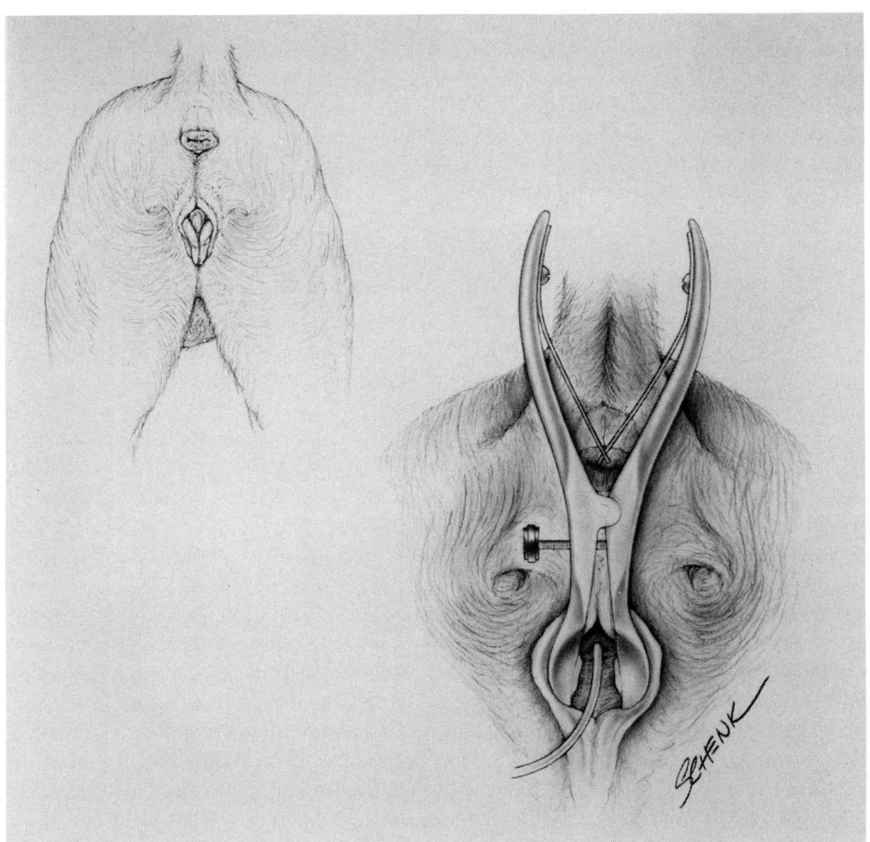

FIG. 5–14. Preferred position of nasal speculum used as vaginal endoscope to permit visualization of the external urethral orifice of female dogs. Reprinted with permission from Osborne CA, Stevens JB. *Handbook of Canine and Feline Urinalysis.* St. Louis, Mo.: Ralston Purina Co.; 1981, p. 29.

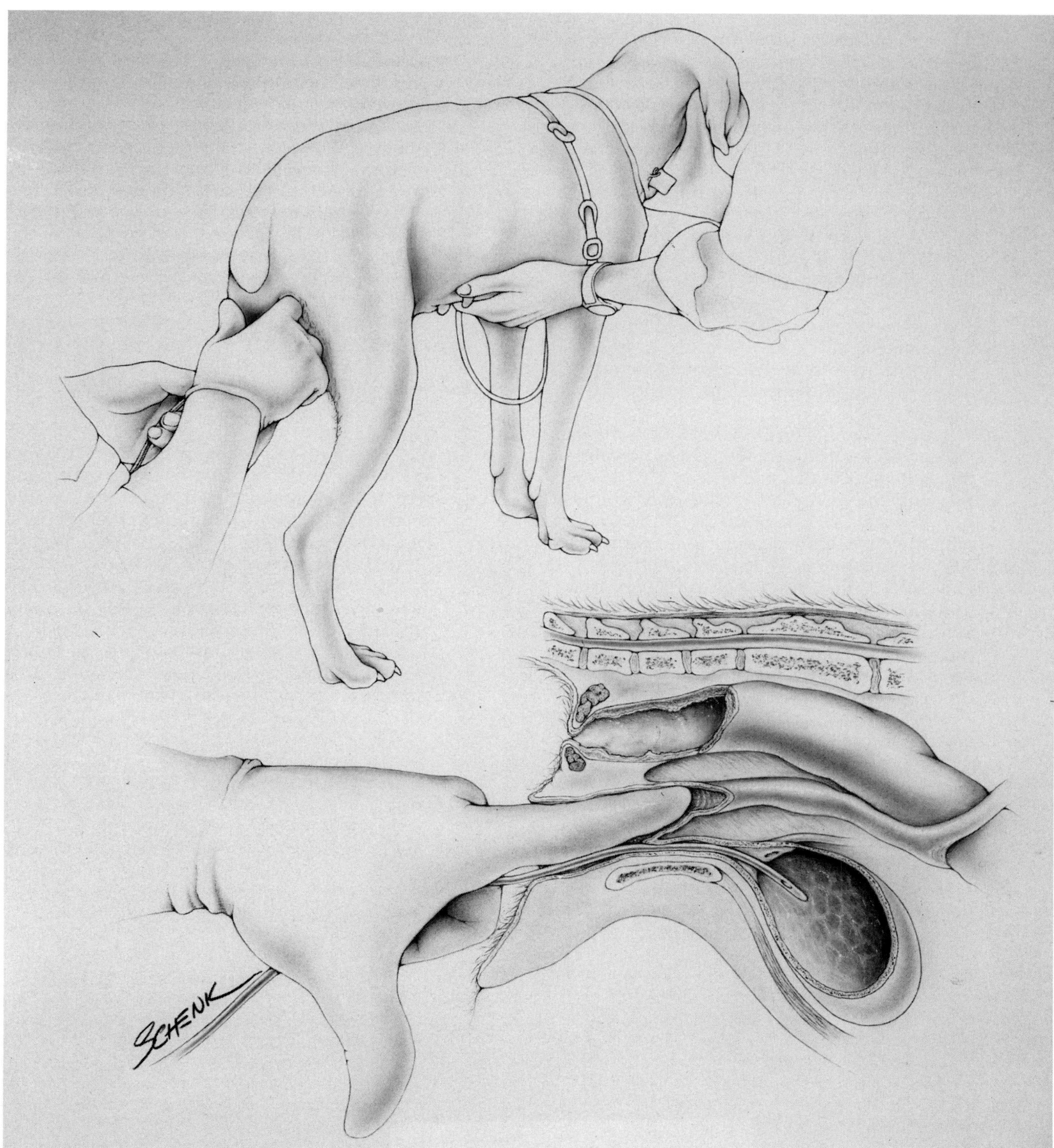

FIG. 5–15. Illustration depicting correct techniques of guiding flexible catheter into the external urethral orifice of a female dog. Keeping the patient in a standing position aids in anatomical orientation during blind digital palpation of the vaginal lumen. Illustration by Michael P. Schenk.

bacterial contamination of the urinary tract than use of endoscopy to directly visualize the external urethral orifice.

b. The dog should be standing because this facilitates anatomical orientation. The external urethral orifice is located on the ventral midline of the vaginal floor.
c. Using sterilized gloves, a finger should be lubricated and gently inserted into the vagina.
d. A sterilized flexible catheter should be inserted into the lumen of the vagina, dorsal to the clitoral fossa, and guided along the midline of the vaginal floor toward the external urethral orifice.
e. Although the external urethral orifice cannot be palpated, entry of the catheter into the urethra can readily be determined when the tip of the catheter disappears into the floor of the vagina.
f. The most common error of individuals inexperienced with this technique is overinsertion of the catheter into the vagina.
g. For those inexperienced with this technique, a catheter may be first placed into the urethra with the aid of an endoscope and light source. After the catheter is in place, remove the endoscope. Then insert a gloved index finger into the vaginal lumen and palpate the catheter at the site of the external urethral orifice. Next, pull the catheter out just far enough so that the tip of the catheter is just distal to the external urethral orifice. Practice reinserting the catheter into the urethra with the aid of the index finger.

9. Blind catheterization (Fig. 5–16).
   a. This technique is more difficult than the methods described above.
   b. Blind catheterization may be useful when visualization or digital palpation of the external urethral orifice is not feasible because patients are uncooperative, have a small vulvar orifice, or have vaginal strictures.
   c. Because the position of the portion of the catheter within the vagina cannot be visualized, caution must be used to prevent trauma to the genital tract.
   d. With the patient in a standing position to facilitate anatomical orientation, the lips of the vulva should be parted.
   e. A sterilized, lubricated catheter should be inserted into the vagina and directed above the clitoral fossa.
   f. With the long axis of the catheter directed in a cranioventral direction with respect to the long axis of the vagina, the tip of the catheter should be slowly advanced along the ventral midline of the vaginal floor.
   g. Detection of increased resistance to advancement of the catheter indicates that it has encountered the vaginal ornix. In this situation, the catheter should be withdrawn to a position just cranial to the clitoral fossa and the procedure should be repeated.
   h. Successful entry into the bladder may be de-

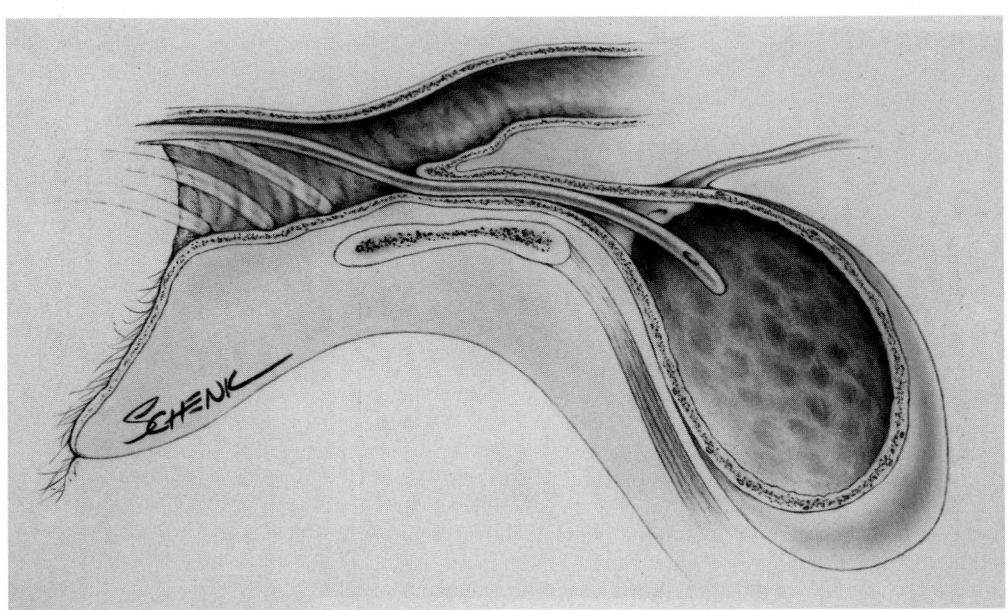

FIG. 5–16. Schematic drawing illustrating proper direction and curvature of a flexible catheter during blind advancement through the vaginal lumen into the external urethral orifice of a female dog. Illustration by Michael P. Schenk.

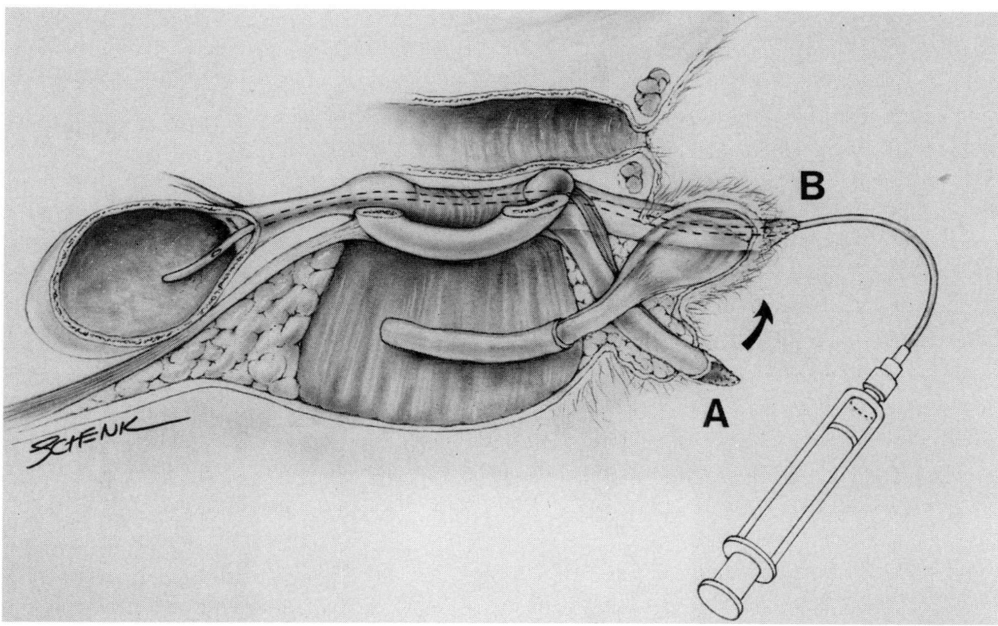

FIG. 5–17. Catheterization of a male cat. The penis has been extended from the preputial sheath by pulling it in a caudal position (A). The natural curvature of the caudal portion of the urethra is then minimized by displacing the extended penis in a dorsal direction with the objective of aligning the long axis of the urethra with the long axis of the vertebral column (B). Reprinted with permission from Osborne CA, Schenk MP. Techniques of urine collection. In: *Forty-fourth Annual Proceedings of the American Animal Hospital Association.* Denver, Colo., American Animal Hospital Association; 1977, pp. 431–442.

tected by lack of resistance to advancement of the catheter, and/or by passage of urine through the lumen.

I. Transurethral catheterization of the urinary bladder of male cats (Fig. 5–17).

1. Equipment
   a. Commercially prepared flexible catheters that are 3 to 5Fr in diameter are usually satisfactory.
   b. Catheters made from polyethylene tubing may be prepared by cutting one end at a 45-degree angle, and flaring the other end with heat (Bunsen burner, match, and so on).
   c. Rigid metal catheters should be avoided for transurethral catheterization of the urinary bladder as they often induce trauma to the urethral and vesical mucosa.
2. Refer to general discussion about catheterization.
3. Although manual restraint by an assistant is usually satisfactory, sedation may be required for uncooperative cats. Appropriate caution should be used in selection of sedatives in order to prevent alterations of diagnostic, physical, and chemical components of urine.
4. Extend the penis from the preputial sheath by pulling it in a caudal direction.
5. Wash the end of the penis with germicidal soap, water, and sterilized sponges.
6. Displace the extended penis in a dorsal direction until the long axis of the urethra is approximately parallel to the vertebral column. This maneuver will facilitate atraumatic catheterization by reducing the natural curvature of the caudal portion of the urethra.
7. Gently insert the tip of the catheter into the external urethral orifice and advance it to the lumen of the urinary bladder.
8. Variable degrees of resistance may be encountered in normal cats because of the curvature of the urethra adjacent to the bony pelvis, and/or voluntary contraction of skeletal muscle that surrounds the distal urethra. Resistance may be minimized by:
   a. Advancing the catheter with a gradual rotating motion.
   b. Injecting a small quantity of sterilized isotonic fluid to distend the urethral lumen (caution—injection of fluids may alter test results).
9. Use care not to overinsert the catheter into the bladder lumen.

J. Transurethral catheterization of the urinary bladder of female cats.

1. Equipment
   a. Flexible catheters used for catheterization of male cats are satisfactory.

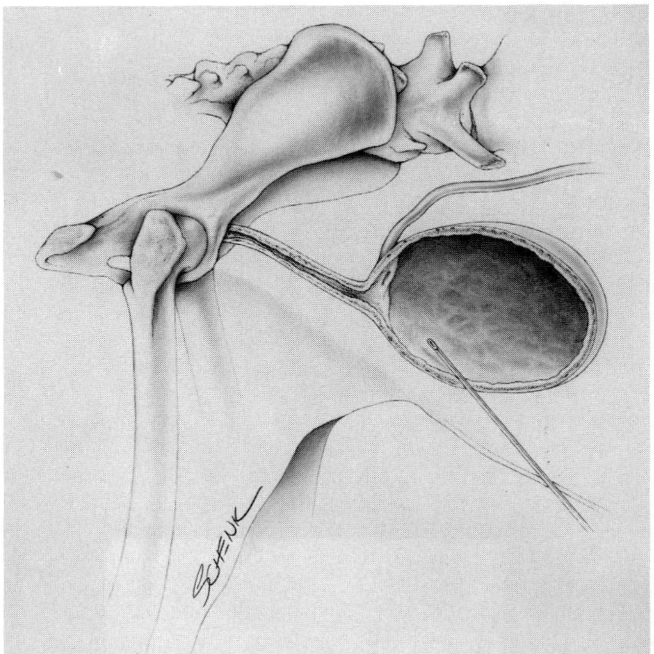

FIG. 5–18. Schematic illustration of cystocentesis in a cat. A 22-gauge 3-in. spinal needle has been inserted through the ventral wall of the urinary bladder at an oblique angle. The point of insertion is several centimeters cranial to the junction of the bladder with the urethra. Reprinted with permission from Osborne CA, Schenk MP. Techniques of urine collection. In: *Forty-fourth Annual Proceedings of the American Animal Hospital Association.* Denver, Colo., American Animal Hospital Association; 1977, pp. 431–442.

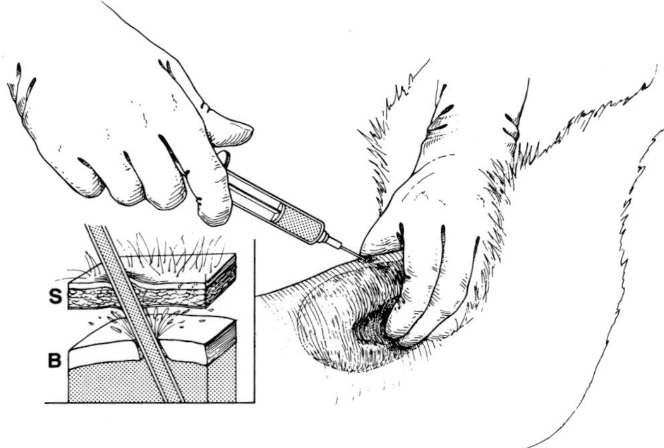

FIG. 5–19. Schematic drawing illustrating escape of urine through the bladder wall adjacent to the needle tract as a result of excessive digital pressure used to localize and immobilize the bladder. Key: S = skin of abdominal wall; B = wall of urinary bladder. Reprinted with permission from: Osborne CA, et al. Cystocentesis. In: Kirk RW, ed. *Current Veterinary Therapy VII.* Philadelphia: W.B. Saunders Co.; 1980, pp. 1150–1153.

b. Otoscope cones provide satisfactory vaginal endoscopes.

2. Refer to the general discussion about catheterization.
3. Some form of pharmacologic restraint is often required.
4. Carefully insert the tip of the catheter into the slit-like external urethral orifice located in the midline of the vaginal floor, and advance it to the lumen of the urinary bladder.

K. Indications for indwelling transurethral catheters.

1. Indwelling catheters should generally be reserved for use:
   a. During intensive care of critically ill patients when continuous measurement of urine production is required, and
   b. During the initial management period following relief of urethral obstruction. In this situation, the purpose of the catheter is to assure urethral patency and prevent continued urine retention. The three main indications for use of indwelling catheters following initial relief of urethral obstruction are:
      (1). Lack of a relatively normal urine stream.
      (2). Persistence of intraluminal material or extraluminal compression likely to cause reobstruction.
      (3). Loss of detrusor muscle contractility and overdistention of the bladder that has induced ineffective micturition despite urethral patency.
   c. If these abnormalities do not exist following relief of urethral obstruction, indwelling catheterization is usually unnecessary and should be avoided!
2. If indwelling catheters are employed, closed drainage systems should be used. Even if an antimicrobial drug is administered, UTI may still develop. Therefore, the catheter should be removed as soon as it has served its purpose and bacterial urine culture should be obtained to detect iatrogenic infection.
3. Urine retention caused by neurogenic disorders of urinary tract function (e.g., spinal cord disease, reflex dyssynergia, etc.) is optimally managed by manual compression of the bladder to expel the urine, or by intermittent catheterization. Indwelling catheterization is the least desirable method of combating urine retention in these situations because of the likelihood of iatrogenic infection and trauma.

VIII. CYSTOCENTESIS (FIGS. 5–18 AND 5–19)

A. Cystocentesis is a form of paracentesis consisting of needle puncture of the urinary bladder for the purpose of removing a variable quantity of urine by aspiration. Extensive clinical experience has revealed that properly performed

cystocentesis is of great diagnostic and therapeutic value. This technique is usually associated with a smaller risk of iatrogenic infection than catheterization and is often better tolerated by patients (especially cats and female dogs) than catheterization.

B. Indications.

1. Diagnostic cystocentesis may be indicated to:
   a. Prevent contamination of urine samples with bacteria, cells, and debris from the lower urogenital tract.
   b. Aid in localization of hematuria, pyuria, and bacteriuria.
   c. Minimize iatrogenic UTI caused by catheterization especially in patients with diseases that predispose them to bacterial UTI (consult Chapter 40, Bacterial Infections of the Canine and Feline Urinary Tract, for further details).
2. Therapeutic cystocentesis may be employed to provide temporary decompression of the excretory pathway of the urinary system when urethral obstruction or herniation of the urinary bladder prevents normal micturition. It is frequently used to decompress the urinary tract of obstructed male cats and dogs prior to reverse flushing or other nonsurgical techniques designed to restore patency of the urethral lumen (consult Chapter 35, Disorders of the Feline Lower Urinary Tract, and Chapter 41, Canine and Feline Urolithiases, for further details).

C. Contraindications.

1. The main contraindications to cystocentesis are an insufficient volume of urine in the urinary bladder and patient resistance to restraint and abdominal palpation. Blind cystocentesis performed without digital localization and immobilization of the urinary bladder is usually unsuccessful, and may be associated with damage to the bladder or adjacent structures. Cystocentesis of patients with recent cystotomy incisions should be performed with appropriate caution.
2. In our experience, collection of urine by cystocentesis from patients with bacterial UTI has not been associated with a detectable spread of infection outside the urinary tract. In fact, collection of a urine sample for bacterial culture that has not been contaminated by passage through the urethra and genital tract is a frequent reason for performing cystocentesis.
3. The major diagnostic limitation of cystocentesis is that it is frequently associated with varying degrees of microscopic hematuria. The magnitude of hematuria induced by cystocentesis is greatest in patients with inflammation and/or congestion of the urinary bladder. Therefore, cystocentesis is not recommended for monitoring remission of microscopic hematuria originating from the urinary bladder following diagnosis.

D. Equipment.

1. We routinely use 22-gauge needles. Depending on the size of the patient and the distance of the ventral bladder wall from the ventral abdominal wall, 1.5-in. hypodermic or 3-in. spinal needles[m] may be selected.
2. Small-capacity ($2\frac{1}{2}$- to 12-mL) syringes are usually employed for diagnostic cystocentesis, while large-capacity (20- to 60-mL) syringes separated from the hypodermic needle by an intravenous extension set and a 2-way or 3-way valve[n] are used for therapeutic cystocentesis.

E. Site.

1. Careful planning of the site and direction of needle puncture of the bladder wall will minimize risk to the patient. Although some clinicians recommend insertion of the needle into the dorsal wall of the bladder to minimize gravity-dependent leakage of urine into the peritoneal cavity following withdrawal of the needle, we recommend that the needle be inserted in the ventral or ventrolateral wall of the bladder in order to minimize the chance of trauma to the ureters and major abdominal vessels (Fig. 5–18).
2. If therapeutic cystocentesis is to be performed, we recommend insertion of the needle a short distance cranial to the junction of the bladder with the urethral rather than at the vertex of the bladder. This will permit removal of the urine and decompression of the bladder without need for reinsertion of the needle into the bladder lumen. If the needle is placed in, or adjacent to, the vertex of the bladder, it may not remain within the bladder lumen as the bladder progressively decreases in size following aspiration of urine.
3. We also recommend that the needle be directed through the bladder wall at approximately a 45 degree angle so that an oblique needle tract will be created (see Fig. 5–18). By directing the needle through the bladder wall in an oblique fashion, the elasticity of the vesical musculature and the interlacing arrangement of individual muscle fibers will provide a better seal of the small pathway created by the needle when it is removed. In addition, subsequent distension of the bladder wall as the lumen refills with urine will tend to force the walls of the needle tract into apposition in a fashion somewhat analagous to the flap valve of the ureterovesical junction.

F. Precystocentesis considerations.

1. Because insertion and withdrawal of a 22-gauge needle through the walls of the abdomen and bladder are associated with little discomfort, tran-

[m]Yale Spinal Needles, available from Becton Dickenson Company, Rutherford, New Jersey 07070.

[n]Available from Pharmaseal, Inc., Toa Alta, Puerto Rico 00758.

quilization, general anesthesia, and local anesthesia are rarely required for diagnostic or therapeutic cystocentesis.

2. If the urinary bladder does not contain a sufficient volume of urine to permit digital localization and immobilization, the patient may be given oral fluids or a diuretic. Although diuretics such as furosemide may be used to facilitate collection of urine samples by increasing urine formation, alteration of urine specific gravity and urine pH are notable drawbacks of this procedure. Even the quantity of bacteria per milliliter of urine may be significantly reduced, altering results of quantitative urine cultures. Use of diuretics to enhance urine collection by augmenting urine flow is therefore best suited for serial urine sample collection when information about urine specific gravity, urine pH, and semiquantitative evaluation of routine test components is not significant.

G. Techniques of cystocentesis.

1. In order to minimize risk to the patient, careful planning of the site and direction of needle puncture is essential. The bladder must contain a sufficient volume of urine to permit immobilization and localization by palpation. Excessive hair should be removed with scissors or clippers. The ventral abdominal skin penetrated by the needle should be cleansed with an antiseptic solution each time cystocentesis is performed. Appropriate caution should be used to avoid iatrogenic trauma and/or infection of the urinary bladder and surrounding structures.
2. In cats, it is usually easiest to perform the procedure with the patient in lateral or dorsal recumbency. In large dogs, the procedure may also be performed when the patient is standing. In order to enhance recovery of crystalline material that may have gravitated to the dependent portion of the bladder lumen, urine within the bladder may be gently agitated via abdominal palpation just prior to cystocentesis. Elevating the rear of the dog by lifting with the legs (wheelbarrow position) may be helpful.
3. Following localization and immobilization of the urinary bladder, the needle should be inserted through the ventral abdominal wall and advanced to the caudoventral aspect of the bladder. The precise location of entry of the needle into the bladder wall is not critical. The needle should be inserted through the bladder wall at an oblique angle. If a large quantity of urine is to be aspirated, the needle should be directed so that it will enter the bladder lumen a short distance cranial to the junction of the bladder with the urethra. While the needle and bladder are immobilized, urine should be gently aspirated into the syringe.
4. Excessive digital pressure should not be applied to the bladder wall while the needle is in its lumen in order to prevent urine from being forced around the needle into the peritoneal cavity (see Fig. 5–19). Use of a 3-in. spinal needle rather than a 1.5-in. hypodermic needle when the ventral surface of the bladder wall is more than 1 to 1.25 in. from the ventral abdominal wall permits immobilization of the urinary bladder without pulling it toward the ventral abdominal wall.
5. An appropriate quantity of urine for analysis and/or bacterial culture should be aspirated into the syringe. If disease of the bladder wall or virulence of urinary pathogens is a likely cause of complications associated with loss of urine into the peritoneal cavity, the bladder should be emptied as completely as is consistent with atraumatic technique. These potential complications have not been a problem in our patients.

H. Post-cystocentesis considerations.

1. The need for prophylactic antibacterial therapy following cystocentesis must be determined on the basis of the status of the patient and retrospective evaluation of technique. In most instances, it is not required.
2. In order to minimize contamination of the peritoneal cavity with urine, unnecessary digital pressure should not be applied to the urinary bladder immediately following cystocentesis.

I. Post-cystocentesis complications.

1. Other than hematuria, we have not observed antemortem postbiopsy complications. Potential complications include damage to the bladder wall or adjacent structures with the needle, local or generalized peritonitis, vesicoperitoneal fistulas, and adhesion of adjacent structures to the bladder wall.
2. We have encountered a few instances in which penetration of a loop of intestine by the needle resulted in false positive significant bacteriuria. Varying degrees of microscopic hematuria might be expected for a short period of time following cystocentesis.

IX. SAMPLE PRESERVATION[10]

A. The objective of all preservation procedures is to prevent alterations from occurring in the physical and chemical properties of urine, and to prevent degenerative changes in cellular elements and casts from occurring. Preservations are used in an attempt to provide samples whose in vitro characteristics are similar to their in vivo characteristics.

1. There is no universal preservative which is satisfactory for routine urinalysis procedures.
   a. Bacteriostatic and bacteriocidal agents often interfere with one or more chemical tests.
   b. Changes in pH induced by acid preservatives may alter cellular and crystalline elements.
   c. Freezing urine may destroy cellular elements.
2. A fresh urine sample is the most desirable.
   a. Freshly voided urine is not always synonymous with newly formed urine.

(1). Bladder atony from neurological disease may prevent micturition.
(2). Dehydration from any cause normally results in the formation of a small volume of urine. Lack of urine volume in the bladder may be associated with infrequent micturition.

b. Microorganisms are normal inhabitants of distal portions of the urethra. In addition, bacteria normally inhabit the vaginal vault and labia of females and prepuce of males.
(1). Urine may be a good culture media for some microorganisms.
(2). Microorganisms may alter the chemical characteristics of urine.
(3). Large numbers of microorganisms alter physical characteristics by causing:
(a). Cloudy urine
(b). An ammoniacal odor

3. Some form of preservation is indicated if urinalysis cannot be performed within 30 min after collection (especially 24-hour collections).

a. Refrigeration at 5° C will preserve urine specimens for approximately two to three hours and possibly overnight.
(1). Urine samples should be warmed to room temperature before analysis.
(a). Enzyme-based tests (glucose oxidase) require that urine be at room temperature.
(b). Specific gravity of cold urine is higher than warm urine.
(2). Avoid freezing the sample.

b. Protect the specimen from exposure to light, especially sunlight.
(1). Bilirubin, as detected by diazo tests, will become undetectable within one hour following exposure to sunlight.
(2). Amber glass containers will protect samples from light.

c. Short term preservation of casts and cellular elements can be effected by acidification of urine.
(1). Casts and cellular elements (i.e., RBC, WBC, epithelial cells, and so on) tend to dissolve in alkaline urine.
(2). Acidification procedure
(a). Determine pH of urine specimen.
(b). If alkaline, add 0.1 normal hydrochloric acid dropwise until the pH is on the acid side of neutrality.
(c). Crystals normally found in alkaline urine will tend to dissolve after acidification, while crystals found in acid urine will tend to form. Hence, the sediment will be altered by this procedure.

d. Many types of chemical preservations are available; each alters the characteristics of urine. Two general categories of preservatives exist. One group prevents microbial growth, while the other prevents chemical changes (such as the addition of ascorbic acid to prevent oxidation of bilirubin).
(1). Formaldehyde prevents microbial growth and aids in the preservation of casts and cellular elements.
(a). One drop of 40% formalin per 30 mL of urine is adequate.
(b). Formaldehyde interferes with the detection of glucosuria.
(2). Thymol is primarily an antimicrobial agent.
(a). Thymol is added to urine as a 10% (w/v) solution in isopropanol. Five to 10 mL is sufficient to preserve a 24-hour urine collection from an average-size dog.
(b). Thymol will cause false positive reactions for protein when either sulfosalicylic acid or Exton's reagent is used.
(3). Toluene prevents microbial proliferation when added in sufficient quantities to saturate the urine.
(a). A quantity sufficient to form a film over the top of the urine is adequate.
(b). Toulene will help to prevent loss of acetone, but will alter the quantity of acetone detected since acetone is half as soluble in toluene as in water.
(c). The portion of the urine specimen to be examined should be collected from beneath the surface film of toluene.
(4). Chloroform is an antimicrobial preservative when added in sufficient quantities to saturate urine. Five ml of chloroform is adequate to preserve a 24-hour urine sample obtained from an average-size dog.
(5). Boric acid at a concentration of 0.8% (one-fourth saturation) has been reported to be superior to formaldehyde, chloroform, and toluene in preventing bacterial growth.
(a). One gram of boric acid is adequate to preserve a 24-hour urine sample.
(b). Urine preserved with boric acid can be used for analysis of:
(1′). Androsterone
(2′). Chorionic gonadotropin
(3′). Dehydroepiandrosterone
(4′). 17-Ketogenic steroids
(5′). Pituitary gonadotropins
(6′). Pregnanediol
(7′). Pregnanetriol
(8′). 5-Hyroxyindole acetic acid
(9′). Vanillyl mandelic acid

(6). Hydrochloric acid (HCl) may be used to preserve chemical constituents in urine.
   (a). A sufficient quantity of HCl is added to bring the specimen to a pH of 1 to 2 (usually 1 mL HCl per 100 mL urine).
   (b). For 24-hour collections, the collection container should contain approximately 10 mL HCl.
   (c). Urine preserved with hydrochloric acid can be used for analysis of:
      (1′). delta-amino-levulinic acid
      (2′). Catecholamines
      (3′). Estradiol
      (4′). Estrogen
      (5′). Estrone
      (6′). Hydroxyproline
   (d). Preservation of urine for amino acid analysis may be accomplished by adding drops of one normal hydrochloride until a pH of 3 is reached. The sample should then be frozen.

(7). Sodium fluoride may be used to preserve glucose in urine.
   (a). Sodium fluoride prevents enzymatic degradation of glucose.
   (b). Sodium fluoride will inhibit enzymatic tests for glucose including the commonly used dipsticks.°
   (c). Because sodium fluoride is not a good antibacterial agent, thymol is usually also added.
   (d). Ten mg sodium fluoride plus 1 mg thymol is used per ml of urine.

(8). Metaphosphoric acid (HPO_3) is used to preserve ascorbic acid (Vitamin C).
   (a). An aqueous solution of 10% metaphosphoric acid is used.
   (b). One volume of acid is added to 5 volumes of urine.

B. All forms of preservation alter the urine specimen.

1. The volume of the specimen is altered with the addition of fluid preservatives such as metaphosphoric acid solution.
2. Preservation of one constituent may prevent detection of another.
   a. Ascorbic acid in concentrations of 100 mg per 100 ml will prevent oxidation of bilirubin.
   b. Ascorbic acid in concentrations of 20 mg per 100 ml will inhibit enzymatic tests used to detect glucose.
3. Because of these problems, it is advisable to:
   a. Consult laboratory manuals about the specific constituent to be measured for additional information on the effects that preservatives have on the detection procedures.
   b. Consult the laboratory that is to perform the special test for specific instructions on which preservative (if any) to use.

°Available from Ames Co., Elkhart, Indiana 46515.

X. SAMPLES FOR QUANTITATIVE VERSUS QUALITATIVE ANALYSIS

A. Urine samples collected without regard to rate of urine formation (i.e., number of milliliters per unit of time) are only suitable for qualitative and semiquantitative evaluation of substances because the concentration of any solute will vary with the quantity of water being excreted at that time. Samples for routine analysis are usually collected in this fashion.

B. Collection of urine specimens during a specified period of time is required for quantitative analysis.

1. Quantitative renal function tests (glomerular filtration rate, clearances of various analytes, and so on) require collection of all urine formed during a known period of time.
2. A metabolism cage to collect all urine formed during a 24-hour interval is frequently used to determine the quantity of electrolytes or hormones (cortisol metabolites, and so on) excreted per day.
3. For best results, two or more 24-hour collections should be performed after the patient has had one or more days to adapt to the metabolism cage.
4. For best results, the urinary bladder should be emptied with the aid of a urinary catheter at the beginning and at the end of each timed collection period.

C. Oral or parenteral administration of appropriate antimicrobial agents at least 8 hours prior to catheterization, and for 2 to 3 days following catheterization will minimize the likelihood of catheter-induced bacterial urinary tract infections.

D. Normal 24-hour urine volume is variable.

1. It is influenced by:
   a. Water consumption
   b. Dietary moisture
   c. Dietary ingredients that affect urine concentrating capacity
   d. Environmental conditions
   e. Activity of the patient
2. Normal dogs produce approximately 12 to 30 mL of urine per pound of body weight per 24 hours.
3. Normal cats produce approximately 4.5 to 9.0 mL of urine per pound of body weight per 24 hours.

REFERENCES

1. Barsanti JA, Blue J, Edmunds J. Urinary tract infection due to indwelling bladder catheters in dogs and cats. *J Am Vet Med Assoc.* 1985;187:384–388.
2. Douglas C, Burke B, Kessler DL, et al. Microwave: Practical cost-effective method for sterilizing urinary catheters in the home. *Urology.* 1990;35:219–222.
3. Garner D, Laks MM. Technique for the performance of repeatable urine clearances in the conscious male dog. *Nephron.* 1976;16:143–147.

4. Feeney DA, Osborne CA, Johnson GR. Vesicoureteral reflux induced by manual compression of the urinary bladder of dogs and cats. *J Am Vet Med Assoc.* 1983;182:795–797.
5. Lees GE, Osborne CA, Stevens JB, et al. Adverse effects of open indwelling urethral catheterization in normal male cats. *Am J Vet Res.* 1981;42U:825–833.
6. Lees GE, Osborne CA, Stevens JB, et al. Adverse effects caused by polypropylene and polyvinyl feline urinary catheters. *Am J Vet Res.* 1980;41:1836–1840.
7. Lees GE, Osborne CA. Use and misuse of indwelling urinary catheters in cats. *Vet Clin North Am.* 1984;14:599–608.
8. Matandos CK, Franz DR. Collection of urine from caged laboratory cats. *Lab Anim Science.* 1980;30:562–564.
9. Osborne CA, Low DG, Finco DR. *Canine and Feline Urology.* Philadelphia, Pa: WB Saunders; 1972.
10. Osborne CA, Stevens JB. *Handbook of Canine and Feline Urinalysis.* St. Louis, Mo: Ralston Purina Co.; 1981.
11. Wysong RL. A new indwelling tomcat urethral catheter. *Vet Med, Small Anim Clin.* 78:703–708.

CHAPTER 

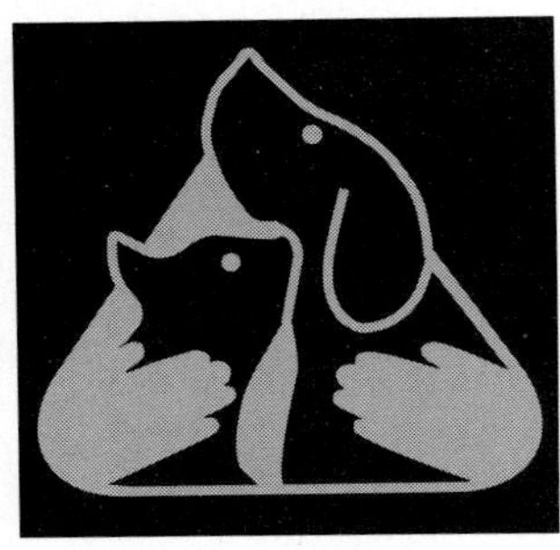

Collection and Analysis of Prostatic Fluid and Tissue

JEANNE A. BARSANTI

I. INTRODUCTION

A. Dog versus cat.

1. The prostate gland is the only accessory sex gland in the male dog. Diseases of the canine prostate gland have been widely recognized and are fairly common. Diagnostic testing of prostatic fluid and of tissue often are necessary to establish a definitive diagnosis.
2. In contrast, male cats have two accessory sex glands: the prostate gland and the bulbourethral glands. Diseases are not commonly recognized and have not been studied in any depth. Almost nothing is known of prostatic fluid composition in cats because ejaculates are difficult to collect and very small in volume (<0.25 mL).[27]
3. For these reasons, this chapter will deal only with prostatic fluid and tissue analysis in dogs.

B. Relationship of the canine prostate gland to the urinary tract.

1. The prostate gland encircles the urethra at the neck of the bladder (see Chapter 1, Applied Anatomy of the Urinary System with Clinicopathologic Correlation).
2. The acini within the prostate gland produce a fluid that comprises the last and largest fraction of the ejaculate.
3. Prostatic fluid enters the urethra and refluxes into the bladder, mixing with urine, when ejaculation is not occurring.[13]
4. In addition, urine can enter prostatic ducts during urination (at least in humans).[20]

C. Indications for collection of prostatic fluid.

1. Anytime one suspects that a clinically significant prostatic disease may be present, evaluation of prostatic fluid is indicated to determine whether and what type of prostatic disease exists. The initial suggestion that prostatic disease may be present usually arises from the history or the physical examination.
   a. Historical findings that strongly suggest prostatic disease include:
      (1). A urethral discharge independent of urination
      (2). Straining to defecate.
   b. Other findings that may indicate prostatic disease are hematuria, dysuria, caudal abdominal or skeletal pain, urinary incontinence, fever, and weight loss.
   c. Physical findings that strongly suggest prostatic disease include prostatomegaly, prostatic asymmetry, and change in prostatic consistency.
2. Finding hematuria, pyuria, and/or bacteriuria in a urinalysis in a male dog should also prompt consideration of prostatic disease. Examination of prostatic fluid often is necessary to localize the site of origin of hemorrhage, inflammation, or infection to the prostate gland.

D. Indications for collection of prostatic tissue.

1. If noninvasive clinical testing, including history, physical examination, urinalysis, complete blood count, prostatic fluid evaluation, radiography, and, when available, ultrasonography, has provided inconclusive results for diagnosis of prostatic disease, aspiration and possibly biopsy are indicated.
2. If a presumptive diagnosis has been made based on noninvasive tests, but response to therapy has not been as expected, aspiration and biopsy are indicated.
3. Evaluation of both prostatic fluid and prostatic tissue is necessary in many cases of prostatic disease because the information gained is often different. For example, prostatic fluid samples originate from all functional acini and thus sample a larger part of the gland than a single aspirate. On the other hand, aspirates and biopsies permit visualization of cells infiltrating the interstitium of the prostate. Aspiration also provides a method of sampling fluid from cysts that may not be communicating with the urethra.

II. COLLECTION AND ANALYSIS OF PROSTATIC FLUID

A. Urethral discharge.

1. A urethral discharge must be distinguished from a preputial discharge.
2. The most common cause of a urethral discharge in dogs is disease of the prostate gland. With prostatic disease, the fluid comprising the urethral discharge is prostatic fluid that is being produced in sufficient volume to flow down the urethra as well as to reflux into the bladder. Not all cases of prostatic disease are characterized by a urethral discharge. In addition, urinary incontinence and urethral diseases should also be considered potential causes of a urethral discharge.
   a. Urinary incontinence can be ruled out by comparing the appearance, pH, specific gravity, dipstick findings, and microscopic characteristics of the urethral discharge to urine collected from the bladder by cystocentesis or catheterization.
   b. Urolithiasis and neoplasia are the most common urethral diseases which might result in a urethral discharge. (See Chapter 38, Urethral Diseases of the Dog and Cat.) Urethral diseases are often accompanied by dysuria, which is uncommon with prostatic disease in the absence of severe prostatomegaly. However, a thorough radiographic or endoscopic evaluation of the urethra may be needed to exclude the possibility of urethral disease.
3. If a urethral discharge is present, it should be collected for microscopic examination.
   a. The penis should be extruded from the sheath. Any preputial exudate should be gently removed with moistened gauze sponges.
   b. The discharge should then be collected on a microscope slide, dried, stained, and examined (Fig. 6–1).
4. In general, a urethral discharge is not cultured for bacteria because of potential contamination by the normal resident bacterial flora of the distal urethra and prepuce. (See Chapter 40, Bacterial Infections of the Canine and Feline Urinary Tract, for a description of the normal urethral flora.) Samples collected by ejaculation are preferred. However, if the discharge is purulent and an ejaculate collection cannot be collected, culture of a urethral discharge may be informative.
   a. The penis should be extruded from the sheath, gently cleansed with dilute hexachlorophene soap or chlorhexidine solution, and gently rinsed and dried with a sterile gauze sponge.
   b. The discharge should be allowed to drip freely into a sterile container (such as a sterile urine cup or syringe case) without the container touching the penis.
   c. Quantitative bacterial culture should always be performed because of the presence of the normal urethral flora.[24]
   d. Any organism isolated by culture could be either a contaminant from the normal urethral flora or a cause of infection. Both possibilities always should be considered. The organism is more likely to be a cause of infection if:
      (1). It is also isolated from urine collected by cystocentesis;

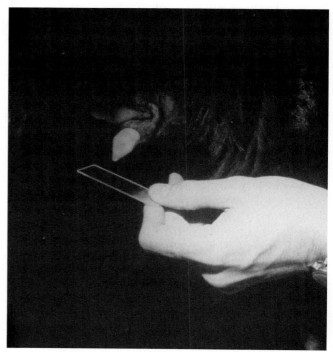

FIG. 6–1. Collecting a sample of a urethral discharge for cytology. The prepuce has been retracted so the urethral discharge can drip directly onto the slide without preputial contamination.

(2). It is present in large numbers (>100,000/mL); and/or

(3). Cytology on the same fluid suggests active inflammation.

B. Ejaculate.

1. Composition.

a. An ejaculate is valuable in assessing prostatic disease since prostatic fluid is the largest component of semen volume (greater than 95% in dogs).[17,22]

b. In dogs, semen is composed of three fractions (Fig. 6–2). The first fraction (presperm) is clear and small in volume (0.1 to 2 mL). The origin of this fraction has traditionally been considered to be the urethra[34]; however, recent work suggests that the fluid may originate in the prostate gland.[11] The second fraction is white and cloudy due to the large number of sperm. The volume of the second fraction is 0.1 to 4 mL. Both the first and second fractions are ejaculated over 1 to 3 minutes.[5] The third fraction is prostatic fluid. This fraction (1 to 16 mL) is normally clear and is ejaculated over 3 to 35 minutes.[5,34]

2. Technique (Fig. 6–3).

a. To collect an ejaculate, the dog should be handled quietly, gently, and calmly throughout the collection, as the dog's willingness to cooperate is essential!

b. In a quiet, familiar area, have an assistant gently hold the dog's head with a leash. The assistant should stand or squat quietly without petting or disturbing the dog, but gently preventing the dog from turning toward the collector.

(1). If the dog is confident and sexually experienced, the sample can usually be collected by manual stimulation alone.

(2). If the dog is timid or inexperienced, a teaser is used. The bitch may be one in estrus or an anestrus bitch to whom the dog pheromone methyl-*p*-hydroxybenzoate* is applied to the vulva.[15] This compound is supplied as a powder. A small amount of the powder is suspended in water; the powder is insoluble and will not dissolve.

(3). Samples from timid, inexperienced dogs are often not initially collectible. Such dogs will often cooperate on a later attempt as they become more familiar with the situation.

(4). Dogs which are in pain as a result of prostatic disease often will not ejaculate.

c. An ejaculate can be collected with or without using a sterile artificial vagina.

(1). It is easier to collect the entire sperm-rich fraction using the artificial vagina.[18]

(2). An artificial vagina is unnecessary if the ejaculate is being evaluated for prostatic disease rather than fertility. The prostatic fraction can be easily collected directly into a sterile container without the artificial vagina.

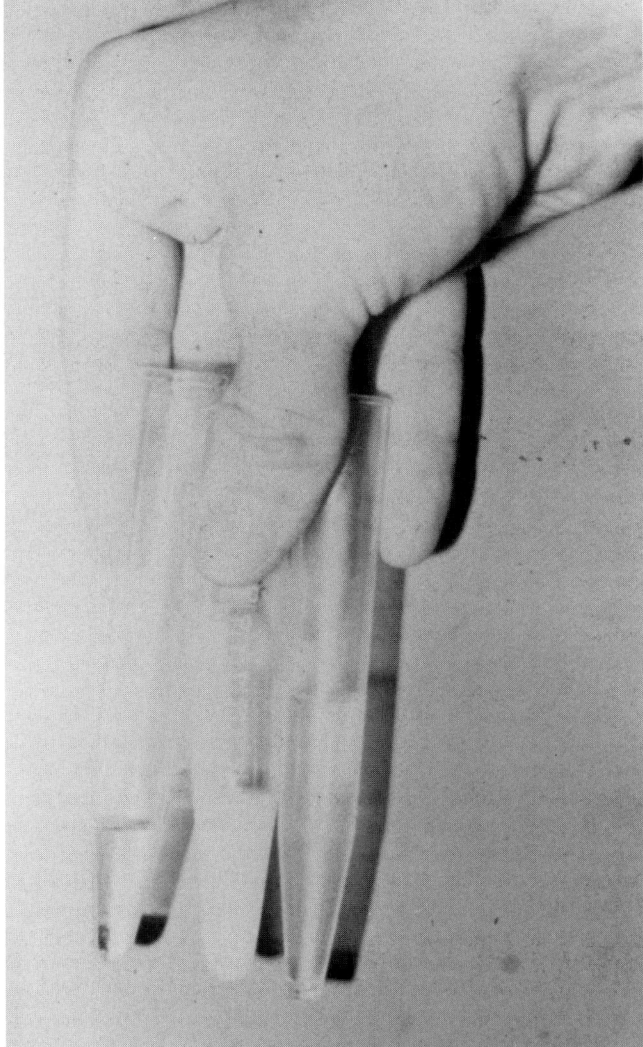

FIG. 6–2. The three fractions of the normal canine ejaculate are a small-volume, clear pre-sperm fraction; the milky sperm-rich fraction; and the clear, larger-volume prostatic fraction.

d. If right-handed, the collector approaches the dog from the left side. Using the thumb and forefinger, the collector places gentle pressure on the dog's penis through the sheath just behind the bulbus glandis. Stimulation of the penis involves gentle, moderate pressure with gentle, short massage at the back of the glans. When erection begins, the collector's other hand is used to gently push the prepuce back over the penis, being careful to avoid touching the penis directly. The sheath should be withdrawn to a point caudal to the bulbus glandis so

*methyl-*p*-hydroxybenzoate, Eastman Kodak Co., Rochester, New York 14850.

that the swollen bulbis is outside and not within the sheath. Although some dogs will ejaculate with the bulbus within the sheath, others seem to find this painful and will lose their erection. During the movement of the sheath with one hand, the other hand maintains gentle but firm pressure behind the bulbus glandis.

e. As the penis protrudes from the sheath, it should be examined for any preputial exudate on the surface. If exudate is noted, and if it could drip into the collection device, it must be removed. A gauze sponge moistened with warm water is used; removal must be gentle to prevent the dog from losing its erection.

f. Pulsations will be felt as the dog begins to ejaculate. The fluid ejaculated is collected using a sterile funnel and test tube, a sterile syringe case, or a sterile urine cup. The more narrow the opening of the container, the less likelihood of environmental contamination, but the more difficult to collect the sample. The sample should be caught in the container as the fluid squirts or drips from the urethral orifice without the container touching the penis. Contamination with preputial discharge, or debris or dust from the environment, should be avoided. This is difficult in some dogs who move about during ejaculation. If one suspects that the sample has become contaminated, a new container should be substituted for the original one.

g. After thrusting, the dog will usually attempt to step one leg over the collector's arm so that the penis is directed caudally (similar to the position of the "tie" in natural mating). The collector should continue to maintain gentle pressure behind the bulbis glandis throughout collection.

h. For assessment of prostatic disease, collection of the last fraction of the ejaculate is most important. Normally, the prostatic fraction of the ejaculate is clear and follows the milky sperm-rich fraction so that the two are easily separated (Fig. 6–2). In normal dogs, the volume of the last fraction of the ejaculate varies from 1 to 16 mL with an average of 4 mL.[5] For diagnostic purposes, 2 to 3 mL is adequate. The prostatic fraction is the easiest part of the ejaculate to collect cleanly, as it drips from the urethral orifice for at least several minutes after the dog completes any thrusting motion.

3. Abnormal appearance of ejaculate.
   a. In some dogs with prostatic disease, the entire ejaculate appears to be abnormal. In these cases, testicular or epididymal diseases as well as prostatic disease may exist.
   b. The testicles and epididymes should be carefully palpated. However, lack of palpable abnormalities does not exclude disease.
   c. If the ejaculate appears to be abnormal, it cannot be divided into fractions, and the entire sample is used for analysis.
4. Both cytology and culture results must be assessed for accurate diagnosis. Quantitative culture is essential since the distal urethra has a normal bacterial flora.[24]
5. Assessment of results.
   a. Cytology
      (1). Normal[4]—Prostatic fluid from normal dogs has occasional red and white blood cells. Squamous cells also may be found (Fig. 6–4). Contaminating bacteria may be seen occasionally. The bacteria may be within squamous cells. The pH of normal canine ejaculates is 6.0–6.7.[4-6]
      (2). Abnormal
         (a). Large numbers of white blood cells (WBC) indicate inflammation (Fig. 6–5).
         (b). Large numbers of red blood cells indicate recent hemorrhage. Hemosiderin-containing macrophages indicate chronic hemorrhage.
         (c). Bacteria, especially if within white blood cells or macrophages, suggest infection.
         (d). Abnormal epithelial cells suggesting neoplasia are rarely found in ejaculates.
   b. Bacterial culture
      (1). Normal[4]
         (a). Normal ejaculates often contain bacteria due to contamination with urethral organisms.
         (b). Contaminant bacteria usually number less than 100,000/mL and are usually gram-positive.
         (c). With contamination, more than one species of bacteria often are cultured.
      (2). Abnormal
         (a). High numbers (>100,000/mL) of a single species of gram-negative organism suggest infection.
         (b). High numbers of gram-positive organisms with large numbers of WBC on cytology also suggest infection if obvious preputial contamination did not occur.
         (c). Lower numbers of gram-negative or gram-positive organisms must be correlated with clinical signs, results of urinalysis and urine culture, and ejaculate cytology in order to determine their significance.[3]
         (d). The significance of mycoplasma/ureaplasma in canine ejaculates is not known. These organisms are part of the normal urethral and preputial flora,[7,10,24,26] but some researchers

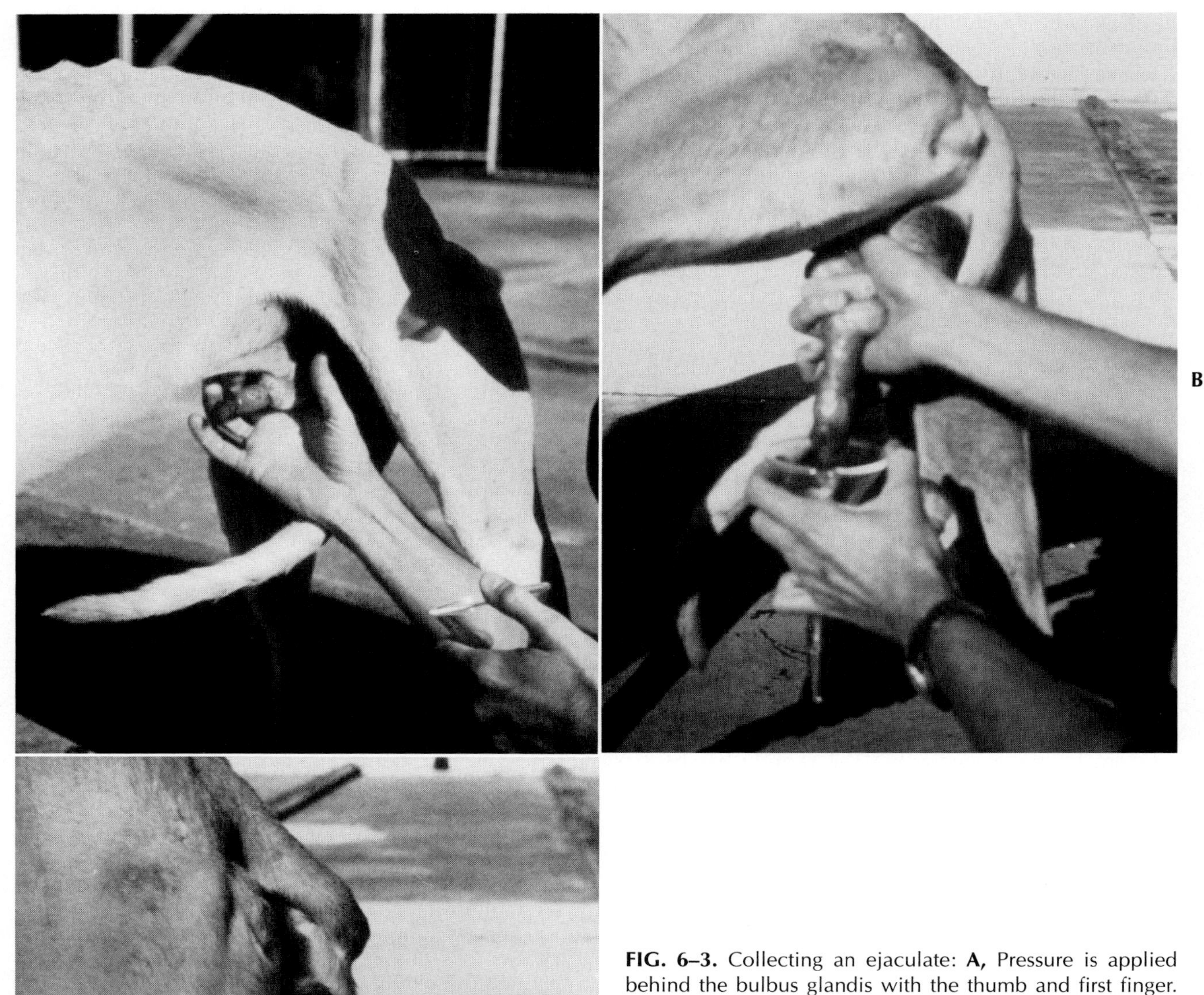

FIG. 6–3. Collecting an ejaculate: **A,** Pressure is applied behind the bulbus glandis with the thumb and first finger. Gentle massage may also be used. As erection develops, the sheath is gently brought back behind the bulbus glandis. **B,** During ejaculation, the dog will step over the collector's hand. Note that the collector maintains pressure behind the bulbus glandis. This collector is using a funnel and tube for collection, but other containers such as a sterile plastic syringe case are acceptable when collecting prostatic fluid. **C,** Prostatic fluid is the last component of the ejaculate and will drip or squirt from the urethral orifice for 3 to 30 minutes after the sperm-rich fraction. This usually occurs after the dog has stepped over the collector's arm, as in the "tie" in natural mating.

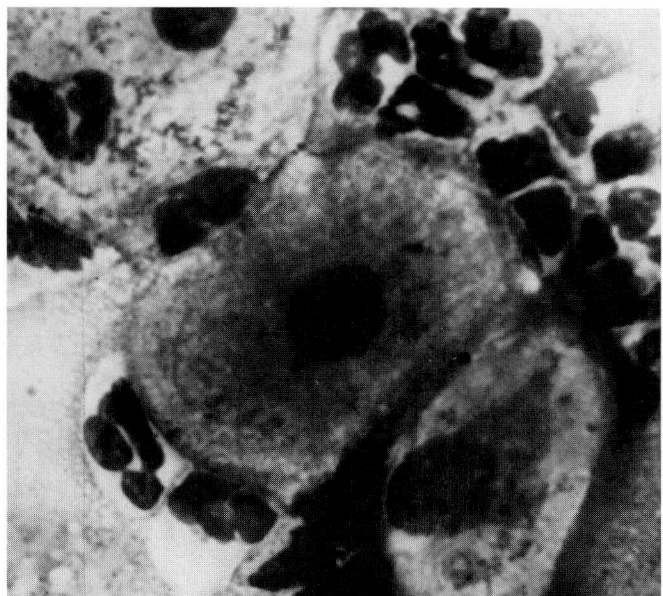

FIG. 6–4. Cytology of an ejaculate showing squamous cells and white blood cells. Although a few squamous cells and white blood cells can be found normally in ejaculates, the number in this sample was excessive. The dog was found to have a Sertoli cell tumor with squamous metaplasia of the prostate gland and chronic inflammation. (With appreciation to Dr. Keith Prasse, Department of Pathology, College of Veterinary Medicine, University of Georgia.)

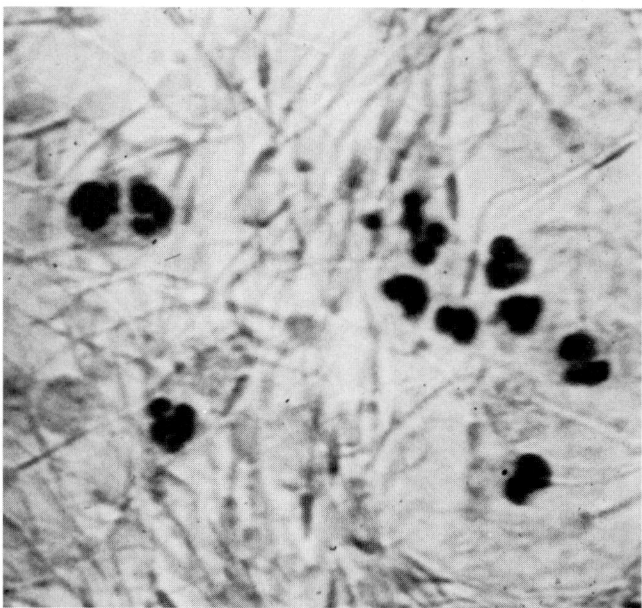

FIG. 6–5. Cytology of an ejaculate containing numerous sperm and a moderate number of white blood cells. If this number of white blood cells is consistent throughout the slide, it is consistent with inflammation. (With appreciation to Dr. Keith Prasse, Department of Pathology, College of Veterinary Medicine, University of Georgia.)

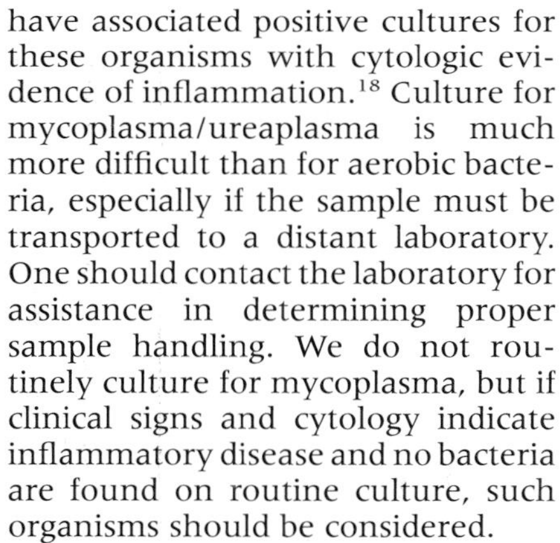

have associated positive cultures for these organisms with cytologic evidence of inflammation.[18] Culture for mycoplasma/ureaplasma is much more difficult than for aerobic bacteria, especially if the sample must be transported to a distant laboratory. One should contact the laboratory for assistance in determining proper sample handling. We do not routinely culture for mycoplasma, but if clinical signs and cytology indicate inflammatory disease and no bacteria are found on routine culture, such organisms should be considered.

(e). Likewise, anaerobic bacteria are uncommon causes of prostatic infection, except in a few cases of abscessation. Culturing for anaerobic bacteria is only performed if evidence for inflammatory disease is present and cultures for aerobic bacteria are negative.

c. An abnormality in the ejaculate does not localize the problem to the prostate, since the testicles, epididymides, deferent ducts, and urethra also contribute to or transport the ejaculate. As noted previously, the fraction of the ejaculate examined, the physical examination findings in the urinary and reproductive tracts, and the possibility of sample contamination must be considered when interpreting the results.

d. Use of a urethral swab† (Fig. 6–6) has been advocated to rule out urethral contamination as a cause of a positive ejaculate culture.[22,23]

(1). With this technique, the penis is cleaned and dried, and a sterile swab is advanced approximately 5 cm into the distal urethra. The swab is moved back and forth several times and withdrawn. The swab and a short portion of the shaft are dropped into 3 mL of sterile saline or lactated Ringer's solution and agitated. The saline is then cultured quantitatively. This sample is collected prior to or independently from collecting an ejaculate.

(2). Correct interpretation of the results of the culture of the urethral swab can be difficult.

(a). It is recommended that larger numbers of organisms in the ejaculate than from the urethral swab by a

†Calgiswab Type IV, American Can Co., Glenwood, Illinois 60425.

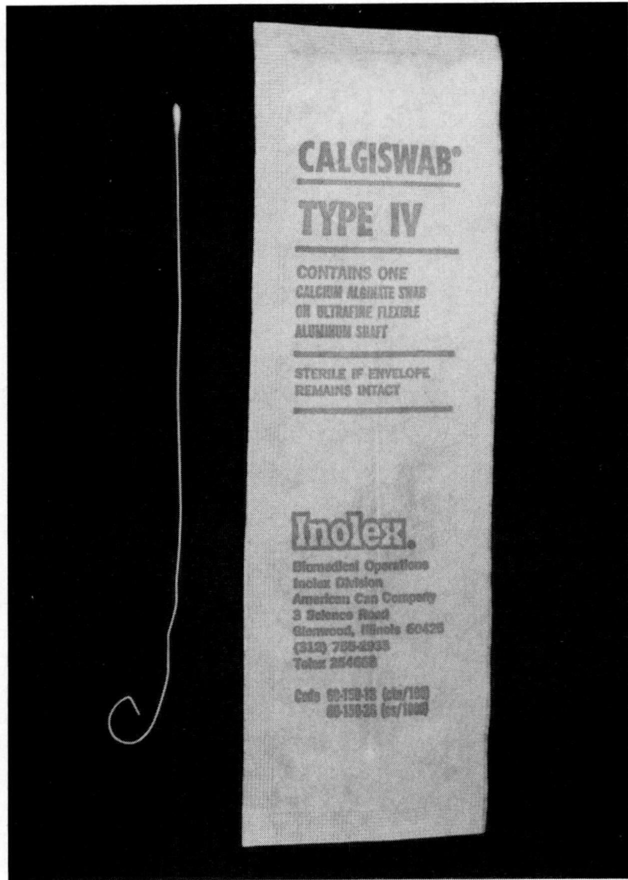

FIG. 6–6. Swab that can be used to determine the bacterial flora of the urethra. Reproduced with permission from Barsanti JA, Finco DR. Canine prostatic disease. In: Ettinger SJ, ed. *Veterinary Internal Medicine*. Philadelphia, Pa: WB Saunders; 1989:1859–1880.

factor of 10^2 is indicative of prostatic infection.[22]

(b). However, in dogs with prostatitis, some dogs without prostatic infection had higher numbers of organisms in the ejaculate than in the urethral swab, and some dogs with urinary tract infection and prostatic infection had high numbers of the same organism in the urethral swab sample.[3,23]

(c). These problems indicate that results from urethral swabs may be misleading in some cases. The ejaculate culture alone is accurate in the diagnosis of prostatic infection approximately 80% of the time.[3,23] An accuracy of 80% was also found using the urethral swab.[23] With these problems and no increase in accuracy, it is probably best to utilize the swab primarily in dogs without urinary tract infection and with questionable numbers of organisms in the ejaculate to determine the distal urethral flora of that particular dog for comparison to the suspected infecting agent.

C. Prostatic massage.

1. Indications.
   a. Because of a dog's pain, inexperience, or temperament, it is not possible to collect semen on all dogs with suspected prostatic disease. Prostatic massage is an alternative technique for collecting prostatic fluid.[4]
   b. In cases of suspected prostatic neoplasia with invasion of the prostatic urethra, specimens from prostatic massage are more likely to contain abnormal cells than ejaculates.[1] The reason is that prostatic massage involves aspiration directly from the prostatic urethra.
2. Technique[4] (Fig. 6–7).
   a. The dog is allowed to urinate first to empty the bladder.
   b. A urinary catheter is passed to the bladder using an aseptic technique. (See Chapter 5, Techniques of Urine Collection and Preservation.) The bladder is emptied, residual urine volume determined, and a sample of urine saved for urinalysis and urine culture.
   c. The bladder is flushed several times with sterile saline to ensure that it is empty. The last flush of 5 to 10 mL is saved as the preprostatic massage sample.
   d. The catheter is retracted distally to the prostate as determined by rectal palpation.
   e. The prostate is massaged rectally or per abdomen, or both, for 1 to 2 minutes.
   f. Sterile physiologic saline (5 to 10 mL) is injected slowly through the catheter, with the urethral orifice manually occluded around the catheter to prevent reflux of the fluid out the urethral orifice.
   g. While continuously aspirating gently, especially in the prostatic urethra, the catheter is slowly advanced to the urinary bladder. The majority of the fluid will be aspirated from the bladder.
   h. In cases in which involvement of the prostatic urethra is suspected (such as in the presence of dysuria or suggestive radiographic findings), a urinary catheter biopsy[25] or urethral brush technique[19] can be combined with prostatic massage. Such techniques are especially useful in cases of neoplasia of either prostatic or transitional epithelial cell origin.[16] The urinary catheter biopsy technique utilizes supplies commonly available in veterinary practices.
      (1). Prostatic massage is performed as described, except that after placing the urinary catheter in the prostatic urethra by

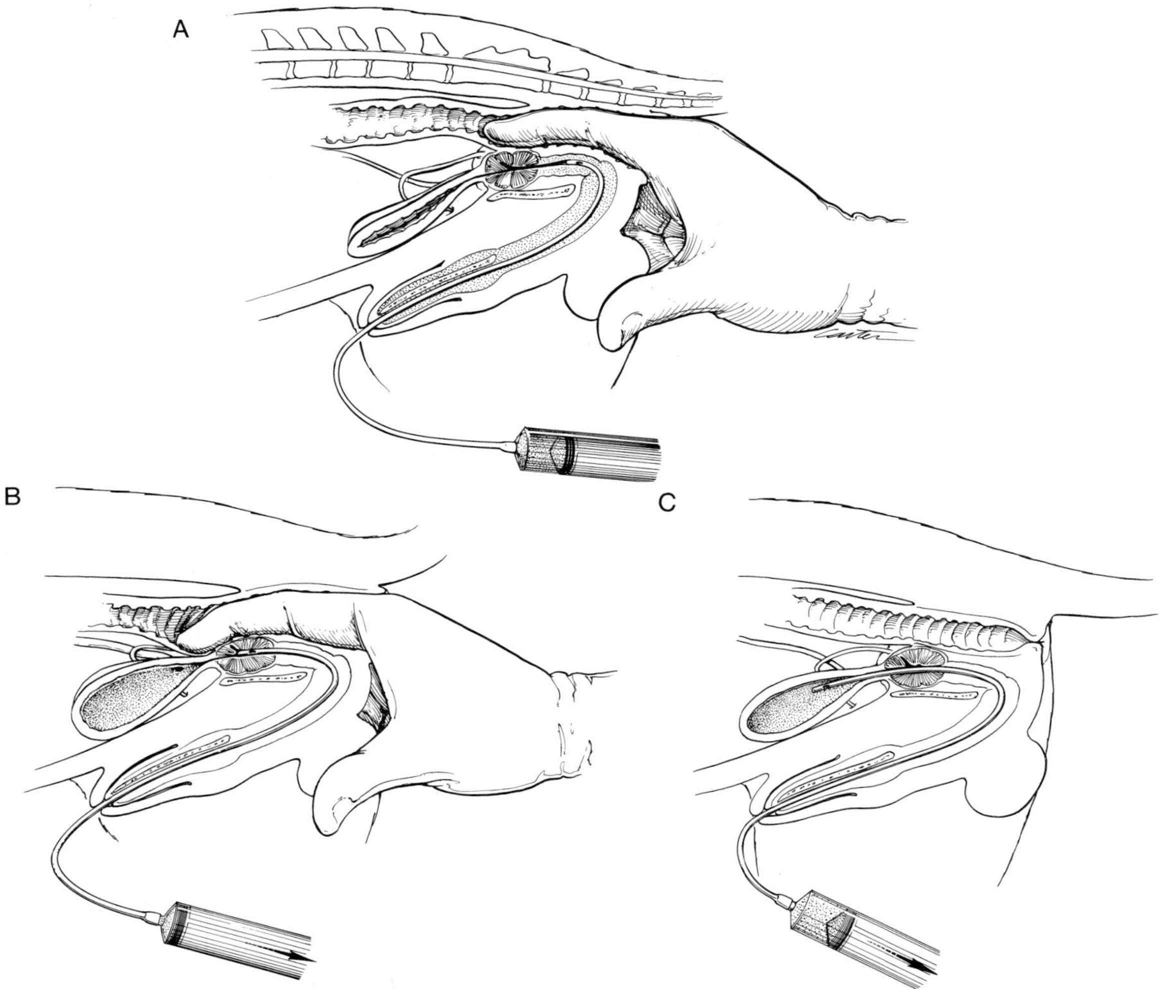

FIG. 6–7. When performing prostatic massage, the bladder is emptied and flushed with collection of a premassage sample (see text). The rest of the procedure is as follows: **A,** The prostate is massaged per rectum, per abdomen, or both, depending on prostatic location, for 1 to 2 minutes. The urinary catheter is positioned distal to the prostate gland. **B,** Five ml of sterile saline or lactated Ringer's solution is injected through the catheter with occlusion around the urethral orifice. The catheter is then advanced to the prostatic urethra via rectal guidance. Negative pressure is applied to the syringe. **C,** The catheter is then advanced to the bladder, where most of the fluid is retrieved. The catheter is then withdrawn.

rectal palpation, the urinary catheter is moved rapidly back and forth while applying negative pressure. Negative pressure is maintained as the catheter is advanced to the bladder for retrieval of fluid.

(2). Alternatively, urinary catheter biopsy can be used independently of prostatic massage.[25] Approximately 5 mL of sterile saline is placed in a 12-mL syringe attached to the catheter. The catheter is guided by rectal palpation into the prostatic urethra. Approximately 4 mL of the saline is injected through the catheter, leaving 1 ml remaining in the syringe. While maintaining negative pressure on the syringe, the catheter is moved rapidly back and forth and then withdrawn.

(3). Slides for cytology are prepared from the material collected. If a sufficiently large sample of tissue is collected, an impression smear can be made and the remaining sample fixed and submitted for histologic study.

3. Sample handling.
   a. The urine and the pre- and post-massage samples are examined microscopically and by quantitative culture.
   b. It is very important to compare the post-

massage sample to the pre-massage sample to differentiate prostatic from bladder or urethral disease.

4. Assessment of results.
   a. Normal results[4]
      (1). Cytology—Macroscopically, the sample appears clear. Microscopically, only a few red blood, white blood, squamous, and transitional epithelial cells (which may be binucleate) are seen.[4] It is uncommon to find prostatic epithelial cells.
      (2). Culture—Cultures are usually negative or contain low numbers of organisms (<1000/mL) consistent with urethral contamination associated with urethral catheterization.[8,9]
   b. Abnormal results—Diagnosis of disease of the prostate gland is dependent on finding more severe abnormalities in the post-massage sample than in the pre-massage sample.
      (1). Cytology
         (a). Macroscopically, the post-massage sample may appear hemorrhagic or cloudy as compared with the pre-massage sample (Fig. 6–8).
         (b). Microscopically, the post-massage sample may contain red blood cells indicating recent hemorrhage, hemosiderin-laden macrophages indicating chronic hemorrhage, white blood cells and macrophages indicating inflammation, free or phagocytized bacteria suggesting infection, or abnormal-appearing epithelial cells suggesting neoplasia or squamous metaplasia.[31] Normal prostatic epithelial cells are uniform in size and appearance, with a round to oval nucleus with a single small nucleolus. Their cytoplasm is basophilic and vacuolated[31,34] (Fig. 6–9). Cytologic characteristics typical of neoplasia are variability in cell size, with some cells larger than normal. The cells have anisokaryosis, with large nuclei and numerous, prominent nucleoli. Some cells may have multiple nuclei, and some may be in mitosis (Fig. 6–10). A diagnosis of neoplasia is difficult on the basis of cytology alone, as both transitional and prostatic epithelial cells can become variable in size and shape with inflammation or hyperplasia. All clinical findings should be considered, and a biopsy is often necessary for a definitive diagnosis.
      (2). Culture
         (a). If the number of bacteria in the post-massage sample is greater than the number in the pre-massage sample (some bacterial species), prostatic infection is probable.
         (b). One problem in interpreting results of prostatic massage is difficulty in detecting increases in bacterial numbers in the post-massage sample when urine is infected.[3] In these

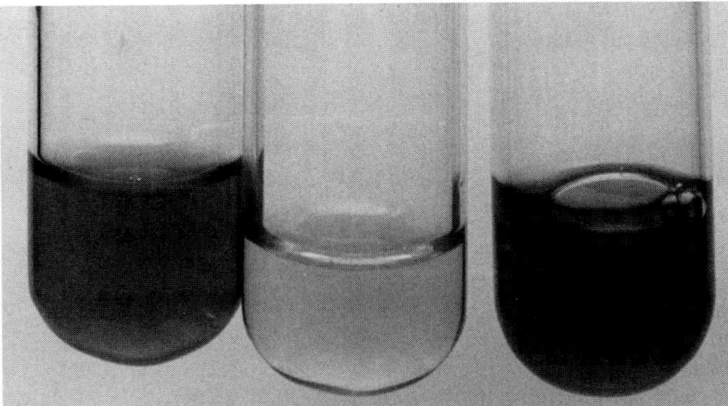

FIG. 6–8. Samples collected during prostatic massage in a dog with hematuria of unknown origin. Samples from left to right are urine, the preprostatic massage sample, and the postprostatic massage sample. Blood was most predominant in the postmassage sample, suggesting prostatic disease as the origin of the hematuria. Cystic hyperplasia was identified by prostatic biopsy. Reprinted with permission from: Barsanti JA, Finco DR. Canine prostatic disease. In: Ettinger SJ, ed. *Veterinary Internal Medicine.* Philadelphia, Pa: WB Saunders; 1989:1859–1880.

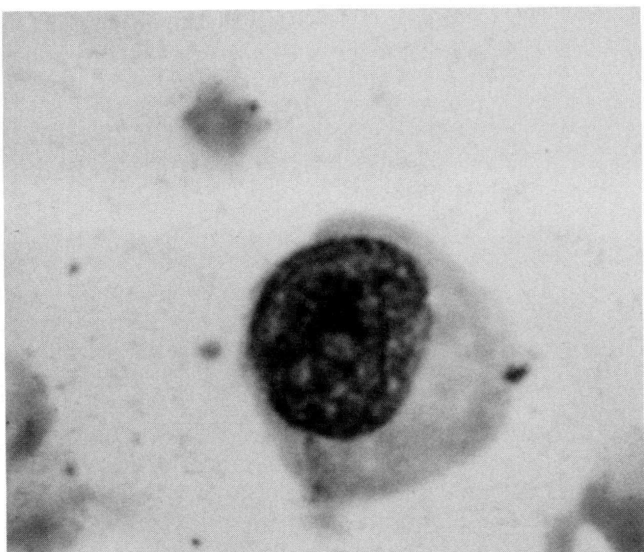

FIG. 6–9. A normal prostatic epithelial cell. (With appreciation to Dr. Keith Prasse, Department of Pathology, College of Veterinary Medicine, University of Georgia.)

cases, the urine often contains $>10^5$ bacteria/mL, the highest number reported by most laboratories, and the pre-massage sample will contain the same large number of organisms, despite bladder lavage.

(c). There are two potential solutions to this problem.

(1′). One can eliminate the urinary tract infection with appropriate antibiotic therapy and then perform the massage.

(2′). One can administer antibiotics which enter the urine but do not enter prostatic fluid (e.g., ampicillin)[12,29,33] for 1 day prior to massage.[3] The samples obtained must be cultured immediately so that the antibiotic in the urine does not kill any bacteria in the prostatic fluid after collection.[12] In experimental infection, this method identified 3 of 6 cases, but in 2 of 6 dogs all cultures became negative in spite of continuing prostatic infection.[3] When antibiotics are being given, even low counts of bacteria may be significant.[12]

(d). Cytologic evidence of inflammation is highly correlated with prostatic infection[3] and is often helpful in determining whether inflammatory prostatic disease exists in cases in which culture results are ambiguous.

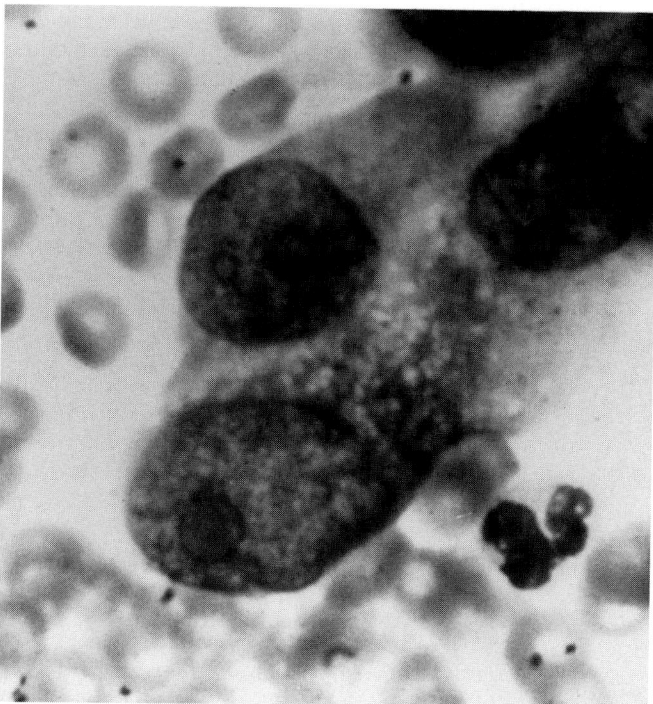

FIG. 6–10. Two prostatic epithelial cells that appear abnormally large in size with prominent nucleoli and chromatin. Numerous similar cells were found, suggestive of neoplasia, but such a diagnosis should be based on all clinical findings since epithelial cells can be variable in appearance. Red blood cells and a few white blood cells are also seen. A biopsy confirmed prostatic carcinoma in this dog. (With appreciation to Dr. Keith Prasse, Department of Pathology, College of Veterinary Medicine, University of Georgia.)

D. Aspiration.

1. If the prostate gland contains fluid-filled spaces, the fluid can be obtained by aspiration. If an abscess is likely, aspiration may be contraindicated (see the following section, Collection of Prostatic Tissue).
2. In order to determine that the prostate contains such spaces, prostatic ultrasonography is required. Ultrasonography can also be used to guide the needle into the areas containing fluid.[28] (See Chapter 11, Diagnostic Imaging of the Urinary Tract.)
3. Based on ultrasonographic findings, either a transabdominal or a transperineal route for aspiration is chosen. The chosen site is prepared as for surgery.
4. A small-gauge (18 or 20 g), long (8 to 15 cm) spinal needle is usually used for aspiration.
5. Percutaneous aspiration without ultrasound guidance may occasionally result in the collection of fluid. This technique will be described in the next section, Collection of Prostatic Tissue.
6. If prostatic fluid is obtained by aspiration, it should be examined microscopically and cultured for aerobic bacteria. Culture for anaerobic bacteria also should be considered if available.
7. Obtaining fluid by aspiration is considered abnormal, since significant amounts of fluid cannot be collected from normal prostate glands by this technique.
   a. Cytologic examination should include evaluation for hemorrhage (RBC), purulence (WBC), or neoplasia (abnormal-appearing epithelial cells) (Fig. 6–11).
      (1). As noted under prostatic massage, one must be cautious in diagnosing neoplasia from cytology alone, as epithelial cells can vary in appearance.
      (2). The fluid from noninfected prostatic cysts is often light yellow, resembling urine. It is often necessary to compare this fluid to urine collected at the same time to be sure one has not inadvertently punctured the bladder during aspiration. This comparison should include specific gravity, pH, dipstick analysis, and microscopic evaluation, and could include measurement of urea and creatinine.

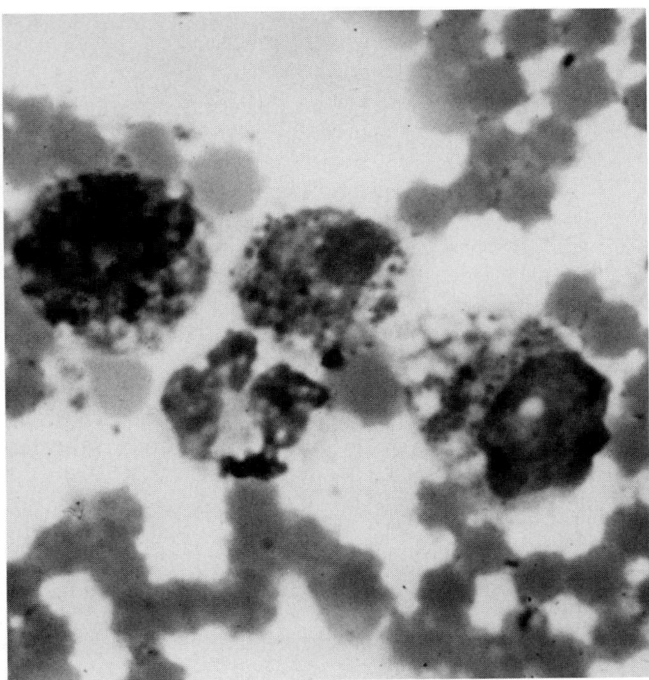

FIG. 6–11. Cytology of fluid aspirated from a prostatic cyst showing largely red blood cells with a few neutrophils and macrophages. (With appreciation to Dr. Keith Prasse, Department of Pathology, College of Veterinary Medicine, University of Georgia.)

(3). Normal-appearing prostatic epithelial cells are occasionally found in fluid aspirated from prostatic cysts.

b. The prostate gland is normally sterile, so culture of any bacteria is considered abnormal as long as contamination during collection and processing does not occur. It is possible to penetrate the colon during percutaneous aspiration. When this occurs, usually a wide variety of organisms is found on culture. In contrast, most prostatic infections are caused by a single species of organism.

III. COLLECTION OF PROSTATIC TISSUE

A. Aspiration.

1. Indication: Aspiration is indicated when noninvasive tests (history, physical examination, complete blood count, urinalysis, blood chemistry profile, radiography, ultrasonography, and prostatic fluid evaluation) have failed to identify a likely etiology of a problem related to prostatic disease.
2. Contraindication.
   a. Needle aspiration should be avoided in dogs with abscessation since large numbers of bacteria may be seeded along the needle tract, or localized peritonitis may develop, causing fever, pain, and vomiting.[2]
   b. The presence of an abscess is suggested by fever and leukocytosis in the presence of purulent prostatic fluid. Aspiration should be performed in such cases only if it is deemed necessary for case management, and only if potential adverse effects are recognized.
   c. If an abscess is suspected on the basis of laboratory work and ultrasonography but an aspirate is deemed necessary, the aspirate should be performed only after results of urine and/or prostatic fluid culture are returned. The dog should be placed on appropriate therapy prior to, during, and after aspiration. The drug is administered intravenously during and 24 hours after aspiration to treat potential bacteremia.
   d. In spite of avoiding aspiration in dogs with fever and leukocytosis, occult abscesses may be present. Ultrasonography to detect cystic lesions may help identify such abscesses and may help guide needle aspiration. If an abscess is aspirated inadvertently, intravenous antibiotics should be begun immediately and continued for at least 24 hours, followed by oral antimicrobial therapy.
3. Technique.
   a. Needle aspiration is most easily done in the dog by the perirectal or transabdominal routes, depending on the location of the prostate gland.
   b. The procedure is done aseptically using a long needle with a stylet such as a spinal needle.
   c. In the perirectal approach, the needle is guided by rectal palpation (Fig. 6–12).
   d. In the transabdominal approach, the needle can be guided by palpation or via ultrasound.[28] The procedure can be performed in most dogs with mild tranquilization.
4. Normal results.[4]
   a. On cytology, normal prostatic epithelial cells are found, which are cuboidal to columnar; of uniform size (10-15 μm in diameter); with central to basilar, round to oval nuclei; and finely granular, basophilic cytoplasm (Fig. 6–10).[31] They are differentiated from transitional cells in that transitional cells are larger with prominent chromatin and less granular cytoplasm.[31]
   b. Culture for bacteria should be negative.
5. Abnormal results—These are similar to those discussed under the section on aspiration of prostatic fluid.
6. Complications are rare and usually related to the inadvertent penetration of abscesses as described above. Occasionally, mild transient hematuria lasting less than 4 days has been noted.[4]

B. Prostatic biopsy.

1. Indication—Obtaining prostatic tissue is necessary for precisely determining the type of disease present. It is necessary when less-invasive clinical

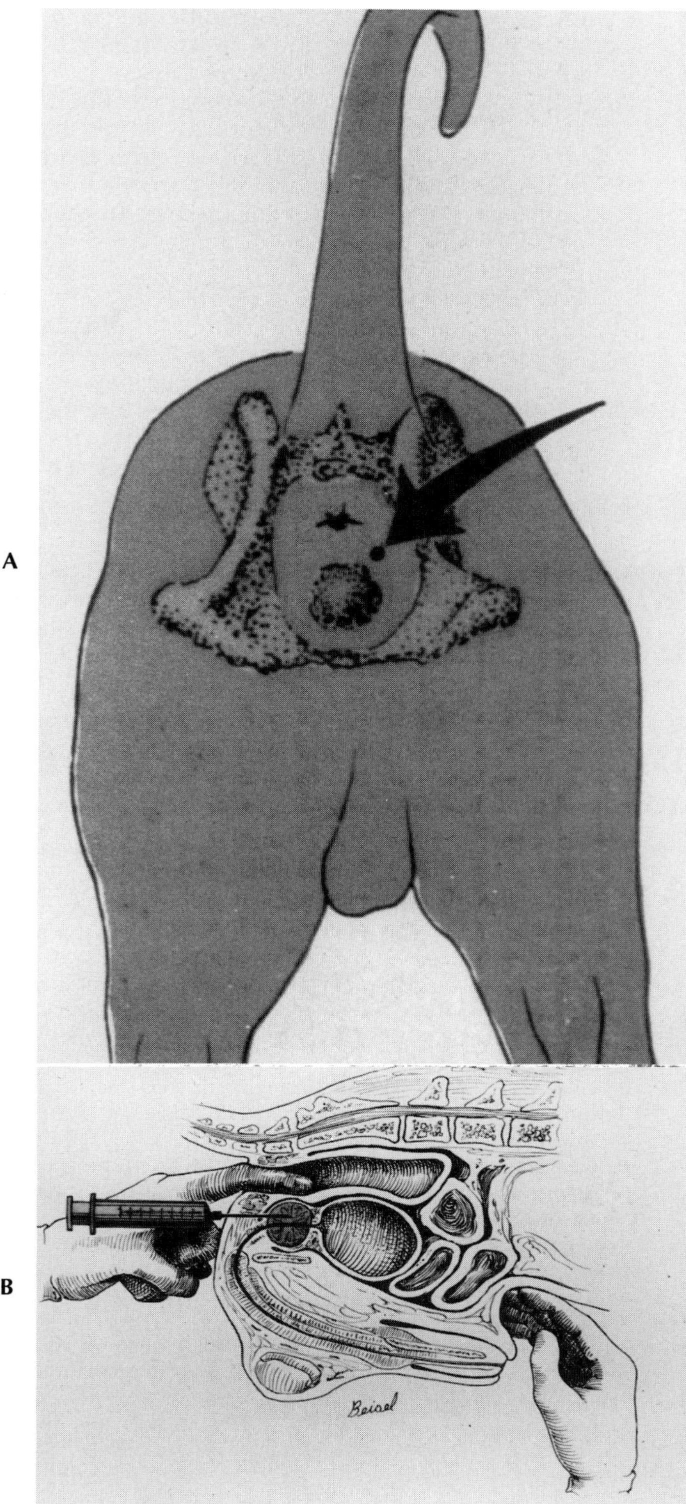

FIG. 6–12. A, Site of needle insertion for aspiration of the prostate gland via the perirectal approach. **B,** Schematic of perirectal aspiration of the prostate gland. The needle is guided into the prostate gland via digital rectal palpation. Reprinted with permission from Barsanti JA, Finco DR. Canine prostatic disease. In: Ettinger SJ, ed. *Veterinary Internal Medicine.* Philadelphia, Pa: WB Saunders; 1989:1859–1880.

findings do not indicate a probable diagnosis, when response to therapy for the suspected underlying disease is not successful, or when the most probable diagnosis is a serious illness, such as neoplasia or abscessation, which requires immediate and extensive therapy if confirmed.

2. Samples obtained by biopsy can be used for bacterial culture and cytology (impression smears). Tissue can be fixed and processed for histologic examination.
3. Contraindications.
   a. Acute, septic inflammation is a contraindication to biopsy because of the possibility of inducing septicemia or peritonitis and because acute bacterial prostatitis is usually responsive to antibiotic therapy.
   b. Prostatic abscess is a contraindication to a percutaneous biopsy.
   c. In parenchymal cystic lesions identifiable by ultrasound, aspiration should always be performed rather than biopsy.
4. There are two methods for prostatic biopsy: percutaneous and surgical.
5. Percutaneous (closed) prostatic biopsy.
   a. Caution—Because of the possibility of an occult prostatic abscess, aspiration should always precede a blind biopsy technique.

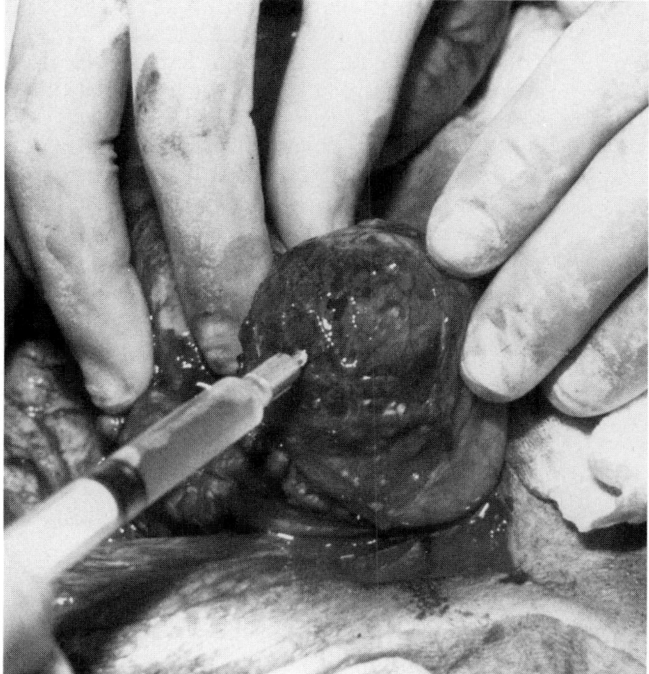

FIG. 6–13. Aspiration of fluid from a paraprostatic cyst at surgery. Reprinted with permission from: Barsanti JA, Finco DR. Canine prostatic disease. In: Ettinger SJ, ed. *Veterinary Internal Medicine.* Philadelphia, Pa: WB Saunders, 1989:1859–1880.

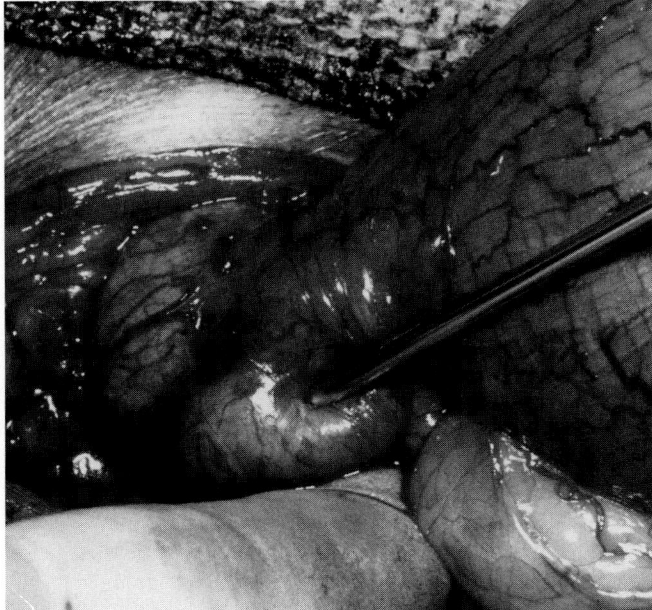

FIG. 6–14. Tru-Cut needle biopsy of the prostate gland by way of caudle celiotomy. The prostate gland appears normal. Reprinted with permission from: Barsanti JA, Finco DR. Canine prostatic diseases. In: Morrow DA, ed. *Current Therapy in Theriogenology.* Philadelphia, Pa: WB Saunders; 1986:553–560.

b. Percutaneous prostatic biopsy can be performed perirectally or transabdominally with tranquilization and local anesthesia.[4,14,32]

c. The biopsy needle‡ can be guided by palpation, as in aspiration (Fig. 6–12), or by use of ultrasound.[28]

d. Dogs should be observed closely for several hours after biopsy to detect any complications.
   (1). The most common complication reported is mild hematuria,[4,21] although significant hemorrhage is possible, as with any biopsy procedure.
   (2). Orchitis and scrotal edema were reported in one dog.[32]

6. Surgical biopsy.
   a. Caution—Cystic or potentially abscessed areas should always be aspirated before taking a biopsy (Fig. 6–13).
   b. The surgical approach is through a parapreputial abdominal incision. Surgery textbooks should be consulted for technique.[30]
   c. The biopsy from an area which appears abnormal may be taken with a biopsy needle, such as a Tru-Cut needle‡ (Fig. 6–14), or by removal of a wedge of prostatic parenchyma with a scalpel blade. Multiple sites can be sampled, depending on visual and palpable abnormalities detected, since prostate glands can be affected simultaneously with multiple disease processes.
   d. With a needle biopsy, no suturing is required, but with a wedge biopsy, the site should be apposed with 4–0 absorbable suture material in a mattress pattern through the parenchyma. Surgery texts should be consulted for further detail.[30]
   e. Potential complications
      (1). Hemorrhage
      (2). Dissemination of infection or neoplasia
      (3). Trauma to the urethra—If the urethra is potentially in the area of a wedge biopsy, a urethral catheter should be passed into the prostatic urethra prior to biopsy so that the location of the urethra can be precisely determined and the urethra avoided.

‡Tru-Cut Needle, Travenol Laboratories Inc., Deerfield, Illinois 60015.

REFERENCES

1. Barsanti JA, Finco DR. Evaluation of techniques for diagnosis of canine prostatic diseases. *J Am Vet Med Assoc.* 1984; 185:198.
2. Barsanti JA, Finco DR. Canine prostatic diseases. 3rd ed. In: Ettinger SJ, ed. *Textbook of Veterinary Internal Medicine.* Philadelphia, Pa: WB Saunders Co; 1989.
3. Barsanti JA, Prasse KW, Crowell WA, et al. Evaluation of various techniques for diagnosis of chronic bacterial prostatitis in the dog. *J Am Vet Med Assoc.* 1983; 183:219.
4. Barsanti JA, Shotts EB, Prasse K, et al. Evaluation of diagnostic techniques for canine prostatic diseases. *J Am Vet Med Assoc.* 1980; 177:160.
5. Boucher JH, Foote RH, Kirk RW. The evaluation of semen quality in the dog and the effects of frequency of ejaculation upon semen quality, libido, and depletion of sperm reserves. *Cornell Vet.* 1958; 48:67.
6. Branam JE, Keen CL, Ling GV, Franti CE. Selected physical and chemical characteristics of prostatic fluid collected by ejaculation from healthy dogs and from dogs with bacterial prostatitis. *Am J Vet Res.* 1984; 45:825.
7. Bruchim A, Lutsky I, Rosendal S. Isolation of mycoplasmas from the canine genital tract: a survey of 108 healthy dogs. *Res Vet Sci.* 1978; 25:243.
8. Carter JM, Klausner JS, Osborne CA, Bates FY. Comparison of collection techniques for quantitative urine culture in dogs. *J Am Vet Med Assoc.* 1978; 173:296.
9. Comer KM, Ling GV. Results of urinalysis and bacterial culture of canine urine obtained by antepubic cystocentesis, catheterization, and the midstream voided methods. *J Am Vet Med Assoc.* 1981; 179:891.
10. Doig PA, Ruhnke HL, Bosu WTK. The genital mycoplasma and ureaplasma flora of healthy and diseased dogs. *Can J Comp Med.* 1981; 45:233.
11. England GC, Allen WE, Middleton DJ. An investigation into the origin of the first fraction of the canine ejaculate. *Res Vet Sci.* 1990; 49:66.
12. Fair WR. Diagnosing prostatitis. *Urology.* 1984; 24(suppl):6.
13. Farrell JI. The newer physiology of the prostate gland. *J Urol.* 1938; 39:171.
14. Finco DR. Prostate gland biopsy. *Vet Clin North Am.* 1974; 4:367.
15. Goodwin M, Gooding KM, Regnier F. Sex pheromone in the dog. *Science.* 1979; 203:559.
16. Holt PE, Lucke VM, Brown PJ. Evaluation of a catheter biopsy

technique as a diagnostic aid in lower urinary tract disease. *Vet Rec.* 1986; 118:681.

17. Huggins C, Masina MH, Eichelberger LE, Wharton JD. Quantitative studies of prostatic secretion. *J Exp Med.* 1939; 70:543.
18. Johnston SD. Performing a complete canine semen evaluation in a small animal hospital. *Vet Clin North Am Small Anim Pract.* 1991; 21:545.
19. Kay ND, et al. Cytological diagnosis of canine prostatic disease using a urethral brush technique. *J Am Anim Hosp Assoc.* 1989; 25:517.
20. Kirby RS, Lowe D, Bultitude MI, Shuttleworth KED. Intraprostatic urinary reflux: an aetiological factor in abacterial prostatitis. *Br J Urol.* 1982; 54:729.
21. Leeds EB, Leav I. Perineal punch biopsy of the canine prostate gland. *J Am Vet Med Assoc.* 1969; 154:925.
22. Ling GV, Branam JE, Ruby AL, Johnson DL. Canine prostatic fluid: techniques of collection, quantitative bacterial culture, and interpretation of results. *J Am Vet Med Assoc.* 1983; 183:201.
23. Ling GV, et al. Comparison of two sample collection methods for quantitative bacteriologic culture of canine prostatic fluid. *J Am Vet Med Assoc.* 1990; 196:1479.
24. Ling GV, Ruby AC. Aerobic bacterial flora of the prepuce, urethra, and vagina of normal adult dogs. *Am J Vet Res.* 1978; 39:695.
25. Melhoff T, Osborne CA. Catheter biopsy of the urethra, urinary bladder, and prostate gland. In: Kirk RW, ed. *Current Veterinary Therapy VI.* Philadelphia, Pa: WB Saunders Co; 1977.
26. Rosendal S. Canine mycoplasmas: their ecologic niche and role in disease. *J Am Vet Med Assoc.* 1982; 180:1212.
27. Sojka NJ. Management of artificial breeding in cats. In: Morrow DA, ed. *Current Therapy in Theriogenology 2.* Philadelphia, Pa: WB Saunders Co; 1986.
28. Smith S. Ultrasound-guided biopsy. *Vet Clin North Am.* 1985; 15:1249.
29. Stamey TA, Meares EM, Winningham DG. Chronic bacterial prostatitis and the diffusion of drugs into prostatic fluid. *J Urol.* 1970; 103:187.
30. Stone EA, Barsanti JA. *Small Animal Urologic Surgery.* Philadelphia, Pa: Lea & Febiger; 1992.
31. Thrall MA, Olson PN, Freenmyer FG. Cytologic diagnosis of canine prostatic disease. *J Am Anim Hosp Assoc.* 1985; 21:95.
32. Weaver AD. Transperineal punch biopsy of the canine prostate gland. *J Small Anim Pract.* 1977; 18:573.
33. Winningham DG, Nemoy NJ, Stamey TA. Diffusion of antibiotics from plasma into prostatic fluid. *Nature.* 1968; 219:139.
34. Wright PJ, Parry BW. Cytology of the canine reproductive system. *Vet Clin North Am Small Anim Pract.* 1989; 19:851.

CHAPTER 

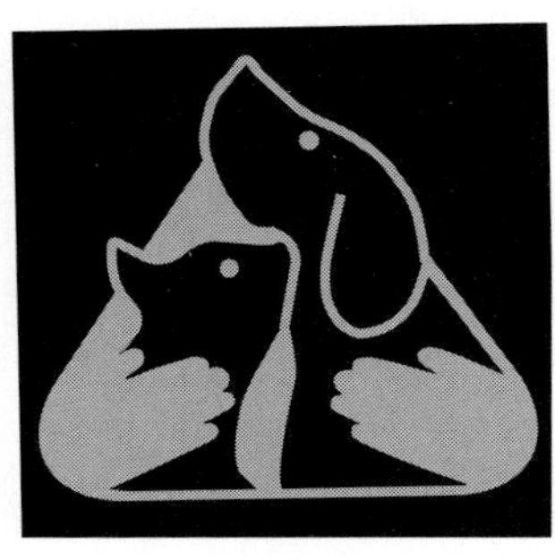

A Clinician's Analysis of Urinalysis

CARL A. OSBORNE
JERRY B. STEVENS
JODY P. LULICH
LISA K. ULRICH
KATHLEEN A. BIRD
LORI A. KOEHLER
LAURA L. SWANSON

I. QUALITATIVE, SEMIQUANTITATIVE, AND QUANTITATIVE URINALYSES

A. Because the concentration of solutes and cells varies with the quantity of water being excreted at a particular time, urine samples collected without regard to rate of urine formation (i.e., number of milliliters per unit of time) are only suitable for qualitative and semiquantitative determinations.

1. Daily variation in urine volume and composition influenced by eating, drinking, metabolism, and various diseases must be considered when interpreting test results.
2. Erroneous precision implied by urine specific gravity values conventionally measured in thousands of a unit (i.e., 1.001 to 1.080+) and by solutes (e.g., glucose, protein) listed as mg/dl should not be overinterpreted.
3. Randomly collected urine samples are usually suitable for diagnostic screening; however, measurement of substances in urine obtained during timed intervals or comparison of excretion rates of such substances as protein to excretion rates of creatinine (urine protein/creatinine ratio) may be subsequently required to clarify the significance of questionable results.

B. Collection of urine specimens during a specified time period is required for quantitative determination of excretion rates of some endogenous and exogenous substances.

1. For quantitation of endogenous substances (e.g., uric acid, hormones, electrolytes), 24-hour urine collections are usually preferred because they eliminate diurnal variations in urine excretion. Twenty-four hour urine collections may also be used to verify the existence of and/or to determine the magnitude of polyuria.
   a. A metabolism cage is frequently used to collect all urine formed during a 24-hour interval. In some situations, a shorter time interval may be used; values may be prorated to a 24-hour interval. For best results, the urinary bladder should be emptied and the urine discarded at the beginning of the collection period. It should be emptied again at the end of the procedure, but the urine should be included in the calcu-

lation. For quantitation of endogenous substances, the bladder lumen may be flushed with a known volume of saline and/or air, and the flushed contents may be added to the collection vial.

b. When possible, the patient should be allowed to acclimate to the environment of the metabolism unit for a day or so before the beginning of the study. This facilitates more precise measurements.

c. Reproducible 24-hour collections are notoriously difficult to obtain. The best data are usually obtained by measuring and comparing urine output (and water intake) for each of 2 or 3 days.

d. Quantitation of substances in urine may be obtained by measuring the quantity in a representative aliquot of the 24-hour sample, and correcting this value for the 24-hour volume.

2. For quantitation of exogenous substances, exogenous creatinine clearance, and urinary excretion of phenolsulfonphthalein dye, shorter time intervals are commonly used.
   a. Inability of most animals to cooperate in timing of voiding usually requires use of urinary catheters.
   b. Swan-Ganz flow-directed balloon catheters are recommended for timed urine collections (refer to review of urinary catheters in Chapter 5, Techniques of Urine Collection and Preservation.

C. Fractional clearance of filtered substances, such as electrolytes, may be measured in "spot" urine samples. Collection of a timed urine sample is unnecessary.

1. The concept of a fractional clearance is related to the fact that the quantity of a filtered substance that ultimately appears in urine is influenced by the net effect of tubular reabsorption and tubular secretion.
   a. Using creatinine to measure glomerular filtration rate, the fractional excretion of a filtered substance is calculated by dividing the measured clearance of that substance by the measured clearance of creatinine.
   b. The formula for the fractional clearance of a substance, x, is:

$$FCx = \frac{UxV/Px}{UcrV/Pcr} = \frac{Ux\ Pcr}{Ucr\ Px}, \text{ where:}$$

FC = fractional clearance
Ux = urine concentrations of substance x
Px = plasma concentration of substance x
V = urine volume in milliliters
Ucr = urine concentration of creatinine
Pcr = plasma concentration of creatinine

2. In normal animals, the fractional excretions of electrolyte are substantially less than 1 because they are conserved to varying degrees following filtration.
3. Consult Chapter 16, Pathophysiology of Renal Failure and Uremia.

D. Comparison of urine substances to urine creatinine concentration.

1. Urine protein/urine creatinine ratios provide a reliable estimate of 24-hour urine protein excretion.[59] Collection of a timed urine sample is unnecessary. (See Chapter 9, Urinary Protein Loss, for additional details.)
2. Comparison of other substances in urine to urine creatinine concentration has not consistently proved to be a reliable index of their 24-hour urine excretion.

II. DIAGNOSTIC PERSPECTIVE

A. When urinalyses are indicated.

1. A complete urinalysis should be considered for all patients suspected of having disease of the urinary system; collected data help to verify or eliminate diagnostic possibilities formulated on the basis of observations obtained from the history and physical examination. Examples of some findings associated with some urinary diseases include:
   a. *Primary renal failure:* varying degrees of impaired ability to concentrate and dilute urine in response to appropriate stimuli, low pH, sometimes proteinuria, sometimes glucosuria.
   b. *Renal disease:* sometimes casts, proteinuria, hematuria, pyuria, bacteriuria, and glucosuria.
   c. *Urinary tract infection:* significant bacteriuria typically associated with varying degrees of pyuria, hematuria, and proteinuria.
   d. *Renal tubular acidosis:* impaired ability to acidify urine or conserve bicarbonate in response to appropriate stimuli.
   e. *Fanconi syndrome:* normoglycemia, glucosuria, amino-aciduria, proteinuria, and renal tubular acidosis.
   f. *Cystinuria:* precipitation of cystine crystals, especially in acid urine.
   g. *Neoplasia:* sometimes presence of exfoliated neoplastic cells in urine sediment.
2. Evaluation of urinalyses is also particularly helpful in problem definition and problem verification in patients with nonurinary disorders. Like complete blood counts, the results of urinalyses provide information about the integrity of many body systems. For this reason, we include urinalyses and hemograms as a part of the initial evaluation (so-called minimum data base) of all patients with illness of unknown cause that requires hospitalization (or frequent evaluation as an outpatient if hospitalization is not feasible). Detection of abnormal findings by urinalysis may dictate the need for further evaluation. Because the results often indicate the body system(s) or organ(s) affected, they often influence selection of additional diagnostic tests or procedures. Examples of findings in uri-

nalyses that may be associated with extraurinary diseases include:

a. *Diabetes mellitus:* hyperglycemia, glucosuria, sometimes ketonuria, sometimes evidence of bacterial urinary tract infection.
b. *Central diabetes insipidus:* hyposthenuria.
c. *Hepatic disease:* bilirubinuria; sometimes ammonium urate, tyrosine, and other crystals.
d. *Severe hemolytic disease:* hemoglobinuria, hyperurobilinogenuria.
e. *Prerenal azotemia:* formation of concentrated urine (also called baruria or hypersthenuria).
f. *Systemic acidosis (acidemia):* frequently the formation of acidic urine.

B. Normal versus abnormal results.

1. Results of urinalysis provide information that helps to evaluate the integrity of the urinary and other body systems. The value of test results that indicate an abnormality is obvious. Results of tests that indicate normalcy are also of great value. Normal findings indicate that selected physiologic processes governing formation of urine (including selective permeability of glomeruli, tubular reabsorption of some metabolites, and tubular secretion of others) are functioning adequately. Knowledge that physiologic processes are functioning adequately provides objective information with which to exclude them as a cause of clinical signs.
2. Whether a particular value is normal or abnormal is often influenced by the diet consumed, the condition of the patient at the time the sample was collected, the method of collection, the type (if any) of preservation used, the laboratory method used, and whether or not diagnostic or therapeutic agents were given prior to sample collection. Therefore, appropriate consideration of these variables is extremely important in interpreting test results.

C. Serial urinalyses.

Single determinations of most laboratory tests indicate the status or functional competence of the organ or body system at the time the tests are performed. Single evaluation of many laboratory tests, including urinalyses, is analogous to obtaining a patient's temperature once. In either situation, it cannot be determined whether an abnormality is remaining static or is increasing or decreasing in severity, nor can the rate at which change is occurring be determined. Re-evaluation of appropriate components of urinalyses often indicates the trend of the abnormality. Detection of remission or exacerbation of abnormal test results by serially performed tests often provides a reliable index of prognosis and/or the efficacy of treatment.

III. LABORATORY CONSIDERATIONS

A. Overview.

1. Urinalyses may provide a great wealth of diagnostic information. Because of the complex nature of normal and abnormal urine, however, and because of rapid and unpredictable changes in urine composition that may occur following collection, analysis of this golden liquid is not a "routine" task that should be relegated to improperly trained personnel who have neither a perspective of the need for standardization and precision in technique and for quality control, nor an understanding of the conceptual difference between observations and interpretations. Although diagnostic analysis of urine is comparatively rapid and inexpensive, incorrect technique and overinterpretation or underinterpretation of test results may seriously hinder diagnostic efforts. Erroneous diagnostic information is often a greater stumbling block than is lack of diagnostic information because such errors tend to eliminate the search for correct information. The unfortunate outcome may be misdiagnosis, erroneous prognoses, and administration of ineffective or contraindicated therapy.
2. Like all laboratory tests, results of urinalyses are helpful, but not infallible. Their value is directly proportional to the diagnostician's ability to interpret them. Because the results of urinalyses are significantly influenced by biologic as well as technical factors, results should be interpreted in combination with available findings from the history and physical examination and from data from radiographic, ultrasonographic, biopsy, and other laboratory procedures when available.

B. Procedure for routine screening urinalysis.

1. Warm sample to room temperature if refrigerated.
2. Thoroughly mix sample.
3. Transfer a standard volume (5 mL) to a conical-tip centrifugal tube. The remainder of the urine sample should be saved until all procedures are completed so that any of the tests may be repeated, if necessary, or other special tests can be performed.
4. Evaluate color and turbidity in the transparent centrifuge tube.
5. Immerse test portions of reagent strips into the well-mixed urine sample and rapidly remove. Gently tap edge of strips on the edge of collection container to remove excess urine. Compare color of various reagent pads to the color scale provided by the manufacturer at the proper time intervals.
6. Determine urine specific gravity.
7. Centrifuge 5 ml of urine in a conical-tip centrifuge tube for 3 to 5 minutes at 1500 to 2000 rpm.
   a. Remove the supernatant by decanting or using a rubber-topped disposable pipette, and save it for potential chemical analysis. Allow a standard volume (approximately ½ mL) of supernatant to remain in the test tube.
   b. Thoroughly resuspend the urine sediment in the remaining supernatant by agitation of the tube or "finger-flipping" of the tube.

c. Use a rubber-topped disposable pipette to transfer a drop of reconstituted sediment to a microscope slide, and place a coverslip over it.
d. Subdue the intensity of the microscope light by lowering the condenser and closing the iris diaphragm (or use a phase-contrast microscope).
e. Systematically examine the entire specimen under the coverslip with the low-power objective, assessing the quality and type (casts, cells, crystals) of sediment.
f. Examine the sediment with the high-power objective to identify the structure of elements and to detect microbes.

8. If the uncentrifuged urine specimen was visibly bloody or very turbid, repeat the dipstick analysis on the supernatant.
9. Record the results.

C. Drug-induced errors of routine urinalyses.

1. Overview
   a. Because drugs may alter laboratory test values by a variety of pharmacologic, physical, and/or chemical mechanisms, urine samples should be collected prior to administration of diagnostic and therapeutic agents.
   b. If therapy has been given prior to sample collection, the time and sequence of therapy and sampling should be recorded to facilitate meaningful interpretation of results.
2. Fluids and diuretics.
   a. Oral or parenteral administration of fluids or diuretics may alter urine specific gravity and osmolality.
   b. Therapeutic dosages of furosemide may cause urine to become acid.
   c. Increased urine volume may suppress positive test results by dilution of reactants.
   d. Dilute urine (urine specific gravity <1.008) often causes varying degrees of cell lysis.
   e. Administration of parenteral solutions containing glucose may cause varying degrees of glucosuria and diuresis.
3. Antimicrobial agents.
   a. Urine for diagnostic culture should be collected prior to administration of antimicrobial agents. When diagnostic culture is needed following initiation of antimicrobial therapy, we suggest that such therapy be withdrawn for 3 to 5 days before samples for culture are collected.
   b. Large dosages of carbenicillin and benzylpenicillin may cause an increase in urine specific gravity in human beings.[100]
   c. Release of formaldehyde from methenamine may inhibit glucose oxidase and peroxidase systems utilized in some glucose and occult blood, hemoglobin, and myoglobin determinations. Formaldehyde may also interfere with tests for urobilinogen.
   d. Large dosages of penicillin, cephaloridine, and sulfisoxazole have been reported to give a false-positive reaction for protein detected by sulfosalicylic acid.[10]
4. Acidifiers and alkalinizers.
   a. Administration of acidifiers or alkalinizers may alter crystal composition in addition to urine pH.
   b. Highly alkaline urine samples may induce false-positive reactions for protein detected by commonly used reagent strips, and false-negative reactions for protein detected by sulfosalicylic acid.
   c. Ascorbic acid may cause a false-positive reaction for glucose detected by copper reduction methods, and a false-negative reaction for glucose detected by glucose oxidase methods.
   d. Ascorbic acid may also inhibit reduction of nitrate to nitrite, and chemical tests for red blood cells (RBC), hemoglobin, and myoglobin.
5. Radiopaque contrast agents.
   a. Commonly used tri-iodinated radiopaque contrast agents may alter urine specific gravity and osmolality.[30,31]
      (1). With respect to tri-iodinated contrast agents given intravenously, if the preadministration urine sample has a specific gravity below approximately 1.040, the specific gravity will typically rise following urinary excretion of radiopaque contrast agents. If the preadministration urine sample has a specific gravity above approximately 1.040, the specific gravity will typically fall following urinary excretion of radiopaque contrast agents (possibly as a result of osmotic diuresis).
      (2). If tri-iodinated radiopaque contrast agents are directly injected into the urinary tract via a catheter, urine specific gravity will increase.
   b. Tri-iodinated radiopaque contrast agents may induce false-positive reactions for protein detected by sulfosalicylic acid.
   c. Radiopaque contrast agents may also alter the structure of cells in urine sediment, and they may alter survival rates of some bacterial pathogens.
   d. Radiopaque contrast agents have been reported to cause crystalluria, although in our experience this phenomenon is uncommon.[31]

D. Timing of analysis.

1. Urine obtained at any time may be satisfactory for screening analysis; however, the composition of urine may vary considerably throughout the day.
2. There are advantages to collection of urine for analysis during specific periods.
   a. Early morning (or fasting) samples.
      (1). Advantages.
         (a). Most likely to be concentrated when obtained from indoor animals, and

therefore facilitates evaluation of tubular capacity to concentrate urine without special techniques.

(b). Most likely to contain higher yield of cells, casts, and bacteria because:

(1′). Of duration of formation.

(2′). Likely to be acid (an acid pH tends to prevent dissolution of proteinaceous structures).

(3′). Of concentration. Dilute urine promotes lysis of cells.

(2). Disadvantages.

(a). Less likely than a 1- to 3-hour postprandial sample to reveal hyperglycemic glucosuria.

(b). Cytologic detail of cells likely to be altered by prolonged exposure to wide variations in pH and osmolality and to waste products.

b. Recently formed sample.

(1). Advantages.

(a). Cytologic detail often superior to that of samples stored in bladder for several hours.

(b). Fastidious bacteria inhibited by urine may be easier to detect.

(2). Disadvantages.

(a). Sample may not be sufficiently concentrated to permit evaluation of tubular function.

(b). Dilute samples may cause lysis or distortion of cells (especially RBC and WBC).

E. Do's and dont's in technique and interpretation.

1. DO make every effort to collect and analyze a urine specimen that has *in vitro* characteristics similar to its in vivo characteristics. If analysis cannot be performed within 30 minutes from the time of collection, refrigerate the sample.
2. DON'T administer diagnostic or therapeutic agents prior to collection of urine for screening diagnostic tests.
3. DON'T rely on a contaminated sample.
4. DO minimize variations in results for your laboratory by consistently performing all steps in analysis of urine in a standard fashion.
5. DO rewarm refrigerated urine to room temperature before analysis.
6. DO store commercial reagents in a cool dry place (not a refrigerator).
7. DO keep reagents away from moisture, direct sunlight, heat, acids, alkalis, and volatile fumes.
8. DO evaluate test results at times specified by the manufacturer.
9. DON'T prepare urine sediment by centrifugation at excessive speeds.
10. DO record test results in an orderly fashion immediately after they are obtained.
11. DO consider the method of urine collection and urine specific gravity before interpreting the significance of test results.
12. DO use caution in interpretation of results. Remember, the reliability and specificity of many commercially manufactured tests for human beings have not been evaluated in animals under controlled conditions.

IV. PHYSICAL PROPERTIES OF URINE

A. Volume.

1. Normal (see Table 7–11)

a. Normal urine volume is influenced by several variables, including:

(1). Species.

(2). Body weight and size.

(3). Diet and ingredients that affect urine concentration capacity.

(4). Fluid intake.

(5). Fluid loss by gastrointestinal tract.

(6). Physical activity.

(7). Environmental factors, such as temperature and humidity.

(8). Urinary solute excretion.

b. Estimates suggest that normal adult dogs in a normal environment produce approximately 20 to 40 ml of urine per kilogram of body weight per 24 hours (1.0 to 2.0 mL per kilogram of body weight per hour).

c. In one study, normal adult cats produced an average of 28 mL of urine per kilogram of body weight per 24 hours.[99]

d. Normal daily urine volume for kittens has been estimated to range between 5 and 60 mL per kilogram of body weight per 24 hours.[19]

2. Indications for determination of urine volume include:

a. Verification of an observation of polyuria or oliguria.

b. Quantitation of substances excreted in urine (such as protein).

c. Evaluation of renal perfusion in patients with shock.

3. Measurement.

a. Guesstimation of urine volume by observation of micturition is unreliable.

b. Use of metabolism cages provides more accurate data. (See Section I this chapter, Qualitative, Semiquantitative, and Quantitative Urinalyses.)

c. Urine volume may be inferred from urine specific gravity.

(1). When the urine specific gravity of nonglucosuric urine samples is greater than 1.030 (dog) or 1.035 (cat), polyuria seldom exists. A specific gravity of this magnitude indicates that water is being reabsorbed from glomerular filtrate in excess of solute.

(2). When the urine specific gravity is less than 1.030 (dog) or 1.035 (cat), any of the following might be present:

(a). The patient could have physiologic polyuria.
(b). The patient could have pathologic polyuria.
(c). The patient could have pathologic oliguria.

4. Polyuria
   a. Polyuria is defined as the formation and elimination of large quantities of urine.
      (1). Depending on the body's need to conserve or eliminate water and/or solutes, polyuria may be normal (physiologic) or abnormal (pathologic). (See Chapter 4, Clinical Algorithms and Data Bases for Urinary Tract Disorders.)
      (2). The significance of polyuria without knowledge of additional information (e.g., history, physical examination, results of urinalysis) cannot be determined.
   b. Physiologic polyuria.
      (1). The most common cause of polyuria is physiologic polyuria.
      (2). Physiologic polyuria usually occurs as a compensatory response to increased fluid intake.
      (3). Proper evaluation of a patient with physiologic polyuria often requires a water deprivation or vasopressin response test.
   c. Pharmacologic polyuria may occur:
      (1). Following ingestion of sufficient quantities of salt to increase thirst.
      (2). Following administration of diuretic agents.
      (3). In dogs, following administration of glucocorticoids (apparently a species-specific phenomenon).
      (4). Following parenteral administration of fluids.
   d. Pathologic polyuria.
      (1). Polyuria may be classified into water diuresis or solute diuresis categories on the basis of examination of urine and blood.
      (2). Water diuresis.
         (a). In general, water diuresis is characterized by a urine specific gravity (SG) and osmolality (Osm) below (SG = 1.001 to 1.006; Osm = 50 to ±150 mOsm/kg H_2O) those of glomerular filtrate (SG = 1.008 to 1.012; Osm = ±300 mOsm/L).
         (b). Water diuresis results from lack of antidiuretic hormone (ADH) (central diabetes insipidus), decreased renal tubular response to adequate concentrations of ADH (renal diabetes insipidus), or excessive water consumption (psychogenic polydipsia).
      (3). Solute diuresis.
         (a). In general, solute diuresis is characterized by a urine specific gravity and osmolality greater than those of glomerular filtrate.
         (b). Solute diuresis results from excretion of solute in excess of tubular capacity to absorb it (i.e., glucose in diabetes mellitus), impaired tubular reabsorption of one or more solutes (i.e., urea, creatinine, phosphorus, and other solutes in primary renal failure), and/or abnormal reduction in medullary solute concentration that impairs the countercurrent system.
         (c). Disorders associated with pathologic polyuria and solute diuresis include chronic primary renal failure, the diuretic phase of acute renal failure, postobstructive diuresis, hyperadrenocorticism, and some hepatic disorders (Table 7–1).
         (d). Polyuria that occurs in association with clinical dehydration (caused by vomiting, diarrhea) indicates that the

TABLE 7–1
CHARACTERISTIC URINE VOLUMES AND URINE SPECIFIC GRAVITY ASSOCIATED WITH DIFFERENT TYPES OF AZOTEMIA IN DOGS AND CATS‡

Prerenal Azotemia
Physiologic oliguria
Dogs: $U_{SG} > 1.030$
Cats: $U_{SG} > 1.035$*
Primary Acute Ischemic or Nephrotoxic Azotemia
Initial oliguria or nonoliguric phase
Dogs: U_{SG} = 1.006 to ~ 1.029
Cats: U_{SG} = 1.006 to ~ 1.034*
Subsequent Polyuric Phase
Dogs: U_{SG} = 1.006 to ~ 1.029
Cats: U_{SG} = 1.006 to ~ 1.034*
Obstructive Postrenal Azotemia
Initial oliguria or anuria
Diuresis and polyuria following relief of obstruction
Primary Chronic Azotemia
Polyuria
Dogs: 1.006 to ~ 1.029
Cats: 1.006 to ~ 1.034*†
Terminal nonpolyuric phase
Usg = 1.007 to ~ 1.013
Reversible oliguria may be caused by onset of nonrenal disorder that induces prerenal azotemia.
Dogs: Usg = 1.006 to ~ 1.029
Cats: Usg = 1.006 to ~ 1.034*

*Some cats with primary renal azotemia may concentrate urine to 1.045 or greater.

†Urine specific gravity may become fixed between approximately 1.007 and 1.013 if sufficient nephron function is altered. The specific gravity of glomerular filtrate is approximately 1.008 to 1.012.

‡Modified from Osborne CA, et al: Pathophysiology of renal disease, renal failure, and uremia. In: Ettinger SG, ed. *Textbook of Veterinary Internal Medicine.* 2nd ed. Philadelphia, Pa: WB Saunders Co; 1982; 2:1758.

kidneys are unable to conserve water in spite of the body's need for water.

(1′). If renal function were normal, physiologic oliguria would be expected to occur as a compensatory response of the body to restore fluid balance.

(2′). Diseases that commonly, but not invariably, are associated with polyuria, vomiting, and clinical dehydration include primary renal failure (regardless of cause), diabetic ketoacidosis, some cases of pyometra, and, in some instances, liver disorders.

(3′). Although polyuria, polydipsia, and dehydration may be associated with central diabetes insipidus, nephrogenic diabetes insipidus, hyperadrenocorticism, and primary polydipsia, these diseases are not typically associated with severe vomiting.

5. Oliguria.

a. The term oliguria has been used to describe:

(1). States associated with decreased urine formation by kidneys.

(2). States associated with decreased elimination of urine from the body.

b. Oliguria associated with formation of a reduced quantity of urine is related to renal function, and may be physiologic or pathologic in nature.

(1). Physiologic oliguria.

(a). Physiologic oliguria occurs when normal kidneys conserve water in excess of solute to maintain or restore normal body fluid balance. Physiologic oliguria is characterized by the formation of a small volume of urine in high specific gravity.

(b). Urine production in patients with prerenal azotemia is a notable example of physiologic oliguria.

(1′). Prerenal azotemia is caused by abnormalities that reduce renal function by reduce renal perfusion with blood (i.e., dehydration, shock, cardiac disease, hypoadrenocorticism). Because blood pressure provides the force necessary for glomerular filtration, marked decrease in blood pressure results in reduction of glomerular filtrate. As a result, a variable degree of retention of substances normally filtered by glomeruli (e.g., urea, creatinine, phosphorus) results. To combat low perfusion pressure and reduced blood volume, the body secretes ADH to promote conservation of water filtered through glomeruli. Production of urine of high specific gravity, high osmolality, and low volume results.

(2′). Prerenal azotemia implies structurally normal kidneys that are initially capable of quantitatively normal function provided the prerenal cause is rapidly removed. If the prerenal cause is allowed to persist, primary ischemic renal disease may develop.

(2). Pathologic oliguria.

(a). Pathologic oliguria may occur during the early phase of acute primary renal failure caused by generalized ischemic or nephrotoxic tubular disease.

(1′). The exact pathophysiology involved in the production of oliguria in patients with acute renal failure has not been established, although different mechanisms may be associated with different causes.

(2′). Available clinical and experimental evidence has been interpreted to suggest that marked renal vasoconstriction and decreased glomerular permeability are important factors. Obstruction of tubular lumens and abnormal reabsorption of filtrate through damaged tubular walls may also be involved in some cases.

(3′). The oliguria usually persists for hours to days, but in some instances, its duration is so transient that it is not detected. In some patients, particularly those with drug-induced nephrotoxicity, the term "nonoliguric" is used to reflect a constant urine volume intermediate between oliguria and polyuria. (See Chapter 22, Acute Renal Failure: Ischemia and Chemical Nephrosis.)

(4′). The specific gravity of urine (regardless of volume) obtained from patients with acute renal failure reflects impaired concentrating capacity if a sufficient quantity of nephrons has been damaged.

(b). An oliguric state may occur in a patient with primary polyuric renal failure if some prerenal abnormality (e.g., vomiting, decreased water consumption, cardiac decompensation) develops. If the prerenal cause is removed and/or if proper fluid balance is restored, polyuria will resume.

(c). Oliguria or a nonpolyuric state may develop as a terminal event in patients with chronic progressive generalized renal disease.

c. Oliguria associated with elimination of decreased volume of urine from the body is associated with diseases of the lower urinary system (ureters, urinary bladder, urethra) that impair flow of urine through the excretory pathway. Examples of such diseases include:

(1). Neoplasms, strictures, or uroliths that partially occlude the urethral lumen.

(2). Herniation of the urinary bladder that partially obstructs urine outflow through the urethra or urine inflow from the ureters.

6. Anuria

a. The term anuria has been used to indicate the absence of urine formation by the kidneys and absence of elimination of urine from the body.

b. Although anuria could result from complete shutdown of renal function caused by lack of renal perfusion or primary renal failure, anuria is usually associated with obstructive uropathy or rents in the lower urinary tract.

B. Color.

1. Because of ease and lack of expense, determination of urine color is included in the routine complete urinalysis.

a. Caution must be used not to overinterpret the significance of urine color. Care should be used to differentiate color from transparency.

(1). Significant disease may exist when urine is normal in color.

(2). Abnormal colors of the same type are caused by several endogenous or exogenous pigments. Although they indicate an abnormality, they provide relatively nonspecific information.

b. Knowledge of urine color may also be of importance since it may induce varying degrees of interference with colorimetric test results.

c. Because the intensity of colors is dependent on the quantity of water in which associated pigments are excreted, it should be interpreted in light of urine specific gravity.

d. Detection of abnormal urine color should prompt questions related to diet, administration of medications, and environment.

e. Causes of abnormal colors should be substantiated with appropriate laboratory tests and examination of urine sediment.

2. Normal urine color.

a. Normal urine is typically transparent, light yellow, yellow, or amber (Table 7–2).

b. The yellow coloration is imparted primarily by two pigments.

(1). Urochrome is a sulfur containing oxidation product of the colorless urochromogen.

(2). Urobilin is a degradation product of hemoglobin.

c. Because the 24-hour urinary excretion of urochrome is relatively constant, highly concentrated urine will be amber in color, while dilute urine may be transparent or light yellow in color.

d. Increased quantities of urochrome may be excreted as a result of fever or starvation.

3. Abnormal urine color (consult Table 7–2 and see Chapter 4, Clinical Algorithms and Data Bases for Urinary Tract Disorders).

C. Odor.

1. Normal urine has a characteristic odor that varies between species and between gender within species.

2. Detection of abnormal urine odors indicates the need for further evaluation.

a. Detection of abnormal urine odors is rarely of specific diagnostic significance.

b. In man, abnormal urine odors in newborn infants are sometimes associated with metabolic defects and urinary tract infections.

c. Excretion of drugs, such as ampicillin, may be associated with abnormal and sometimes characteristic odors.

d. The cause of abnormal urine odor is best determined by evaluation of a complete urinalysis. Depending on the cause, additional laboratory tests and/or clinical investigation may be required.

3. Ammoniacal (NH_3) odors.

a. An ammoniacal odor is a common abnormality of urine.

(1). NH_3 imports the characteristic odor; NH_4^+ and urea are odorless.

(2). Fresh normal urine at room temperature does not have an ammoniacal odor because it contains an insignificant quantity of NH_3. It contains large quantities of urea, however, and may contain a large quantity of NH_4^+.

b. Potential causes of ammoniacal odor include:

(1). Urea that has been degraded to NH_3 by urease-producing bacteria.

(a). Urease-producing bacteria may be pathogens or contaminants.

(b). Freshly voided urine with an ammoniacal odor suggests (but does not prove) infection of the urinary tract with urease-producing bacteria.

(2). NH_4^+ transformed to NH_3 by endogenous or exogenous heat.

c. A putrid odor indicates bacterial degradation of a large quantity of protein and is abnormal.

d. Ketonuria has been reported to impart a characteristic odor to urine.

(1). Many individuals are unable to detect this odor.

(2). Laboratory tests provide a more reliable index of ketonuria.

D. Transparency—turbidity.

1. In most species, freshly voided urine is transparent (see Table 7–2).
   a. Concentrated urine is more likely to be turbid than is dilute urine.
   b. In vitro alterations, especially changes in temperature and pH, may cause varying degrees of loss of transparency.
2. The degree of turbidity is commonly estimated by reading newspaper print through a clear container filled with urine.
3. The cause of urine turbidity is usually best explained by evaluation of urine sediment.[4]
4. Potential causes of urine turbidity include one or more of the following:
   a. Crystals.
   b. RBC, WBC, and/or epithelial cells.
   c. Semen.
   d. Bacteria, yeasts.

TABLE 7–2
SOME CAUSES OF DIFFERENT URINE COLORS

1. Pale Yellow, Yellow, or Amber
   a. Normal urochromes
   b. Urobilin
2. Deep Yellow
   a. Highly concentrated urine
   b. Quinicrine (Atabrine); following acidification*
   c. Nitrofurantoin*
   d. Phenacetin*
   e. Riboflavin (large quantities)*
   f. Phenolsulfonphlalein (acid urine)
3. Blue
   a. Methylene blue
   b. Indigo carmine and indigo blue dye*
   c. Indicans*
   d. *Pseudomonas* infections*
4. Green (mixture of blue plus yellow)
   a. Methylene blue
   b. Dithiazanine iodide (Dizan)
   c. Indigo blue*
   d. Evan's blue*
   e. Biliverdin
   f. Riboflavin*
   g. Thymol*
5. Orange-Yellow
   a. Highly concentrated urine
   b. Excess urobilin
   c. Bilirubin
   d. Phenazopyridine (Pyridium; Azo Gantrisin)
   e. Salicylazosulfapyridine (Azulfidine)*
   f. Fluorescein sodium*
6. Red, Pink, Red-Brown, Red-Orange, or Orange
   a. Hematuria
   b. Hemoglobinuria
   c. Myoglobinuria (red-brown)
   d. Porphyrinuria
   e. Congo red
   f. Phenosulfonphthalein (following alkalinization)
   g. Neoprontosil
   h. Warfarin (orange)*
   i. Rhubarb*
   j. Carbon tetrachloride*
   k. Phenazopyridine
   l. Phenothiazines*
   m. Diphenylhdantoin*
   n. Bromsulphalein (following alkalinization)
7. Brownish
   a. Methemoglobin
   b. Melanin
   c. Salicylazosulfapyridine (Azulfidine)*
   d. Nitrofurantoin*
   e. Phenacetin*
   f. Naphthalene*
   g. Sulfonamides*
   h. Bismuth*
   i. Mercury*
8. Yellow-Brown, Green-Brown
   a. Bile pigments
9. Brown to Black (Brown or Red-Brown when viewed in bright light or in thin layer)
   a. Melanin
   b. Methemoglobin
   c. Myoglobin
   d. Bile pigments
   e. Thymol*
   f. Phenolic compounds (ingested or from decomposed protein)*
   g. Nitrofurantoins*
   h. Nitrites*
   i. Naphthalene*
   j. Chlorinated hydrocarbons*
   k. Analine dyes*
   l. Homogentisic acid*
10. Colorless
    a. Very dilute urine
11. Milky white
    a. Chyle
    b. Pus
    c. Phosphate crystals

*Reported in human beings.

e. Contaminants from the collection container.
f. Lipid droplets (tend to rise to surface).
g. Contamination with feces.

5. Crystals are a common cause of turbidity.
   a. The solubility of most crystals is influenced by temperature. Hence, crystals may form as urine at body temperature cools to room temperature. If crystals interfere with microscopic examination of sediment, their dissolution may be promoted by warming the sample in a 37°C water bath.
   b. Precipitation of crystals may also be influenced by pH. (See Section VII C for further information.)
6. Hematuria versus hemoglobinuria.
   a. Hematuria typically results in brownish to red (occasionally black) turbid urine.
   b. Hemoglobinuria (and myoglobinuria) results in brownish to red (occasionally black) transparent urine.

V. DETERMINATION OF SOLUTE CONCENTRATION OF URINE BY OSMOLALITY, SPECIFIC GRAVITY, AND REFRACTIVE INDEX

A. Indications.

There are two major indications for routine evaluation of specific gravity of all urine samples analyzed.

1. Interpretation of other results of the urinalysis depends on knowledge of specific gravity (or osmolality) because such data provide information regarding the ratio of solutes to solvent (water).
   a. Tests of routine urinalyses are typically performed on a relatively small sample of urine without regard to the rate of formation of urine or to total urine volume. Semiquantitative interpretation of results is infeasible in such samples without knowledge of specific gravity.
   b. Protein is used as an example. A 2+ proteinuria at a specific gravity of 1.010 reflects a much greater loss of protein than does a 2+ proteinuria at 1.030. The same concept is applicable to interpretation of the significance of glucose, bilirubin, and constituents in urine sediment.
2. Urine specific gravity and/or osmolality are used to assess the ability of the renal tubules to concentrate (i.e., remove water in excess of solute) or dilute (i.e., remove solute in excess of water) glomerular filtrate. Knowledge of urine specific gravity is extremely helpful when attempting to localize azotemia (see Table 7–1).

B. Methodology.

1. Osmolality
   a. Applied physics.
      (1). Dissolution of one or more substances (or solutes) in a solvent (water) change four mathematically interrelated physical characteristics (known as colligative properties): osmotic pressure, freezing point, vapor pressure, and boiling point. These properties are all directly related to the total number of solute particles within the solution and are independent of the homogeneity or nonhomogeneity of molecular species, molecular weight, and molecule size.
      (2). As solute is added to solvent:
         (a). Osmotic pressure increases.
         (b). Freezing point decreases.
         (c). Vapor pressure decreases.
         (d). Boiling point increases.
      (3). Changes in these colligative properties depend on the number of particles of solute in solution, and *not* on other characteristics, such as molecular weight, electrical charge, chemical nature, or shape of dissolved particles.
      (4). Although osmometers provide a measurement of the number (or concentration) of osmotically active particles in solution, they do not indicate the type(s) of solute present.
   b. Applied physiologic chemistry.
      (1). The unit of osmotic concentration is the *osmole.*
         (a). One osmole of an ideal solution in 1 kg of water has a freezing point of −1.86°C compared to pure water.
         (b). Because the *osmole* represents a large mass of solute, the *milliosmole* has been developed for clinical use.
            (1′). 1 milliosmole (mOsm) = 0.001 osmole.
            (2′). Use of milliosmoles eliminates the necessity of using fractions when evaluating osmolality of biologic fluids.
         (c). For osmolality, the unit of solvent measurement is mass (kg), and therefore osmolality is expressed as mOsm/kg of solution. For osmolarity, the unit of solvent measurement is volume (L), and therefore osmolarity is expressed as mOsm/L of solution. The numeric difference between osmolality and osmolarity values of biologic fluids is usually small, and therefore the values are commonly used interchangeably.
      (2). Osmotic activity in the body.
         (a). Sodium, chloride, and bicarbonate account for approximately 90% of the osmotic activity of extracellular fluid. Nonelectrolytes, such as urea, proteins, and glucose, account for the remainder of the osmotic activity.
         (b). Sodium, chloride, and urea account for most of the osmotic activity in urine.
         (c). The difference between the osmolality (or specific gravity) of uncentri-

fuged urine and that of the supernatant of centrifuged urine is usually insignificant because cells and casts do not contribute significantly to osmotic pressure.

(d). The difference between serum and plasma osmolality is insignificant because fibrinogen does not exert a significant osmotic effect. The quantity and type of anticoagulant used to obtain plasma may be of significance, however. For example, EDTA may contribute 5 to 20 mOsm/kg H_2O to plasma osmolality, depending on the amount of blood in a 2-ml Vacutainer (Becton Dickenson) tube.

(e). The osmotic concentration of plasma, serum, interstitial fluid, transcellular fluid, and intracellular fluid is approximately 280 to 310 mOsm/kg H_2O. The osmotic concentration of glomerular filtrate is about 300 mOsm/kg H_2O.

(f). Normally, the osmotic concentration of urine is variable, depending on the fluid and electrolyte balance of the body and the nitrogen content of the diet. Species differences in the ability to concentrate urine are also significant (Table 7–3 and Table 7–11).

(g). The ratio of urine osmolality (U_{osm}) to plasma osmolality (P_{osm}) is a good clinical index of the ability of the kidneys to concentrate or dilute glomerular filtrate.[8]

(1′). A U_{osm}/P_{osm} ratio greater than 1 indicates that the kidneys are concentrating urine above plasma and glomerular filtrate. Following water deprivation, the U_{osm}/P_{osm} of normal dogs may be 7 or more.[44]

(2′). A U_{osm}/P_{osm} ratio of approximately 1 indicates that water and solute are being excreted in a state that is iso-osmotic with plasma.

(3′). A U_{osm}/P_{osm} ratio significantly less than 1 indicates that the tubules are capable of absorbing solute in excess of water (i.e., they are diluting glomerular filtrate).

2. Specific gravity

a. Definition and characteristics.

(1). Urine specific gravity is a measurement of the density of urine compared to pure water. Stated in another way, urine specific gravity is the ratio of the weight of urine to the weight of an equal volume of water, both measured at the same temperature:

$$SG = \frac{\text{wt. of urine}}{\text{wt. of water}}$$

(a). The specific gravity of water is 1.000 under conditions of standard temperature and pressure.

(b). Urine is more dense than water because it is composed of water and various sources of different densities.

(2). The relationship between specific gravity and total solute concentration is only approximate.[56] In addition to the number of molecules of solute, specific gravity is influenced by other factors, including molecular size and molecular weight of solutes. Therefore, each species of solute has its own characteristic effect on the specific gravity of urine.

(a). Urine samples with equivalent numbers of solute molecules per unit volume may have different specific gravity values if different mixtures of solutes are present.

(b). Equal numbers of molecules of urea, sodium chloride, albumin, globulin, fibrinogen, and glucose all have a

TABLE 7–3
OSMOLALITY AND SPECIFIC GRAVITY VALUES FOR ADULT DOG, CAT, AND HUMAN URINE

	Species		
Factor	**Dog**	**Cat**	**Human**
Range of normal SG	1.001 to ± 1.065	1.001 ± 1.080+	1.001 to ± 1.035+
Usual SG—normal hydration	1.015 to 1.045	1.035 to 1.060	1.015 to 1.025
Range of normal osmolality (mOsm/kg)	50 to 2700	50 to 3200+	50 to 1500

different quantitative effect on specific gravity.

(c). Addition of any of the following substances to 100 ml of urine increases specific gravity by 0.001.

(1′). 0.147 g of sodium chloride.

(2′). 0.36 g of urea.

(3′). 0.27 g of glucose.

(4′). 0.4 g of albumin.

(3). Urine specific gravity is affected by temperature.

(a). Although the weight of urine remains constant regardless of its temperature, the density of urine decreases with an increase in temperature. Conversely, the density of urine increases with a decrease in temperature.

(b). For precise work, the temperature of urine should be compared with the reference temperature of the instrument used to determine specific gravity.

(4). Urine specific gravity is a direct, but not proportional, function of the number of solute particles in urine.

(a). Urine specific gravity varies with the kind of solute present, whereas urine osmolality is independent of the types of solute present.

(b). Urine specific gravity provides only an estimation of osmolality.[56] It is useful as a screening procedure, but may be unsuitable in some circumstances requiring more precise evaluation of renal tubular concentration and diluting capacity.

b. Methodology—urinometers

(1). The precision of urinometers is not great.

(2). Urinometers are calibrated at a reference temperature, which should be considered when measuring urine specific gravity.

(3). Consult reference material for details.

3. Refractive index.[75]

a. Definition and characteristics.

(1). Refractive index is defined as the ratio of the velocity of light in air to the velocity of light in a solution. Aqueous solutions, such as urine, contain substances that absorb various wavelengths of light and, as a consequence, "bend" light rays. The degree of "bending" may be measured by an instrument called a refractometer.

(2). Like specific gravity, the refractive index of urine is related to the quantity of solutes present and to the characteristics of the solutes present. It therefore provides an estimate of osmotic concentration.

b. Methodology—refractometers.

(1). Small hand-held refractometers calibrated to determine urine specific gravity are available. The instruments may also be calibrated to provide results in terms of refractive index or total solids.

(2). The variability in the quality and cost of refractometers is considerable. We have confidence in the Goldberg refractometer because it typically provides reproducible results, has an adjustable scale, and contains a built-in mechanism for temperature correction (from 60 to 100°F). Improvements in newer models have also increased reproducibility of results.

(3). Refractometers are calibrated at a reference temperature. Within limits, however, their design permits temperature compensation.

(a). Because the temperature of the small drop of urine required to obtain a measurement with refractometers rapidly equilibrates with temperature of the instrument, a temperature-corrected result may be obtained provided the temperature of the instrument is near the reference temperature. Caution should be used to prevent significant alterations in the temperature of the instruments by holding them for prolonged periods and storing them adjacent to heating vents.

(b). Goldberg refractometers and some other models have a built-in temperature-compensating mechanism.

4. Specific gravity reagent strips.

a. This test is based on the pKa change of certain pretreated polyelectrolytes in relation to ionic concentration.[17] The reagent strip actually measures ionic concentration of the urine, which is related to its specific gravity.

b. Because the highest value that these reagent strips can detect is approximately 1.025 to 1.030, they are unsatisfactory to detect adequate renal concentrating capacity in dogs or cats.

5. Osmometers versus refractometers versus urinometers.

a. Osmometers provide a more accurate assessment of osmolality of individual urine samples than do refractometers or urinometers and, therefore, should be used when errors in assessment of renal function are of significant consequence (i.e., in conjunction with water deprivation and vasopressin response tests.) Vapor pressure osmometers are preferable to freezing point osmometers when assessing urine samples with high osmolality.

b. Refractometry is entirely satisfactory for routine screening by urinalysis.
c. Refractometers are recommended rather than urinometers for determination of urine specific gravity because:
(1). They provide more reproducible results.
(2). They require a small sample size.
(3). They are temperature compensated.
(4). They are technically easy to use.

C. Interpretation.

1. Normal (Table 7–3 and Table 7–11) (See also Chapter 4, Clinical Algorithms and Data Bases for Urinary Tract Disorders.)
a. The specific gravity of urine of normal dogs and cats is variable, depending on the fluid and electrolyte balance of the body, the composition of the diet, and other variables related to species and individuals. The urine specific gravity often fluctuates widely from day to day and within the same day.
b. Urine specific gravity may range from 1.001 to 1.065 or greater in adult normal dogs, and from 1.001 to 1.080 or greater in adult normal cats. Depending on the requirements of the body for water and/or solutes, any specific gravity value within these ranges may be normal. Therefore, the concept of an average normal specific gravity is misleading because it implies that values greater than or less than the average may not be normal.
c. Randomly collected urine samples from normal adult dogs and cats often have a specific gravity that encompasses a narrower range than that just mentioned, but an individual urine sample with a specific gravity outside these values is not reliable evidence of renal dysfunction (Table 7–3).[4,8,44]
d. Maximum and minimum specific gravity values for infant and immature dogs and cats have apparently not been evaluated.
(1). In newborn infants, the kidneys can only concentrate urine to a maximum of 700 to 800 mOsm/kg at the time of birth, but can dilute urine to values as low as 40 mOsm/kg.[27,41] The time of maturation of various renal functions in immature dogs and cats is unknown.
(2). In a study of kittens consuming a maintenance dry cat food, urine osmolality ranged from 618 to 2680 (mean = 1424) in those 4 to 6 weeks old, 1214 to 3474 (mean = 2432) in those 7 to 12 weeks old, 1408 to 3814 (mean = 2797) in those 13 to 19 weeks old, and 918 to 3384 (mean = 2383) in those 20 to 24 weeks old.[19,48]
(3). In another study, measurement of urine specific gravity values of canine fetuses prior to birth revealed values that ranged from 1.008 to approximately 1.025.[84] Randomly collected urine samples from dogs that were 2 days old had an osmolality approximately 2 times that of plasma, but the ratio was approximately 7 times that of plasma when the pups were 77 days old.[47] These observations suggest that kidneys of newborn puppies can concentrate urine to some degree and that concentration capacity improves with age.[34]
(4). Appropriate caution must be used when interpreting the significance of urine specific gravity and osmolality values in immature animals because they apparently have different average and minimum and maximum values than those of mature animals.
e. A urine specific gravity similar to that of glomerular filtrate (1.008 to 1.012) may be observed in individuals with normal renal function because the ability of normal kidneys to influence specific gravity encompasses these values. Because such values may be normal or abnormal, they should be viewed as presumptive evidence of an abnormality. Further data are required, however, to prove or disprove this presumption.
f. The ability of patients to excrete urine with a specific gravity significantly greater than that of glomerular filtrate (1.008 to 1.012) depends on an intact system for production and release of ADH, a sufficient population of functional nephrons to generate and maintain a high solute concentration in the renal medulla, and a sufficient population of functional tubules to respond to ADH. Data obtained from experimental studies in dogs suggest that only about one third of the nephrons of both kidneys are required to concentrate urine to 1.025 or greater.[46] Stated another way, significant impairment of the ability of the kidney to concentrate (or dilute) urine is usually not detected until at least two thirds of the total renal functional parenchyma has been impaired. In general, patients with at least one third of the total nephron population functional have adequate renal function to prevent clinical signs of primary renal failure.
g. Significance of urine specific gravity of 1.025 in man, dogs, and cats.
(1). The ability of dogs to concentrate urine to a specific gravity of 1.025 was at one time generally accepted as evidence of "adequate" renal concentrating capacity (i.e., at least one third of the total nephron population if functional) to maintain homeostasis.
(2). The urine specific gravity end point of 1.025 was extrapolated from human data. Because human beings can concentrate their urine to a maximum of 1.035 to

1.040, whereas values for dogs may reach 1.060 or more, and values for cats may reach 1.080 or more, concentration of urine to 1.025 implies better renal tubular function in man than in cats or dogs.

(3). Clinical observations in dogs indicate that detection of a urine specific gravity of 1.030 or greater indicates an adequate population of nephrons to prevent clinical signs associated with primary renal failure.

(a). A significant degree of renal disease may exist in dogs able to concentrate their urine to a specific gravity of 1.025.

(b). In 1 study, the maximal urine specific gravities of 3 partially nephrectomized dogs (⅔ of total nephrons removed) subjected to 48 hours of water deprivation were 1.023, 1.018, and 1.027.[46]

(4). Experimental studies of cats have revealed that animals with less than 25% functional nephrons could concentrate their urine significantly higher than a specific gravity of 1.040.[2,61,85] Although we commonly use a specific gravity value of 1.035 to 1.040 to indicate adequate urine concentrating capacity for cats, further studies are required to determine the urine specific gravity value that best indicates an adequate population of functional nephrons to prevent clinical signs associated with primary renal failure.

h. Because metabolic work is required to dilute glomerular filtrate (SG = 1.008 to 1.012) by removing solute in excess of water, a urine specific gravity significantly below 1.008 indicates that a sufficient number of functional nephrons (commonly estimated to be at least one third of the total population) are present to prevent clinical signs associated with primary renal failure. Dilution of urine is an appropriate compensatory response to overhydration.

i. Although the minimum number of nephrons required to dilute canine or feline urine to a specific gravity of 1.005 or less has not been determined, the number has been assumed to be similar to that required for urine concentration (i.e., about one third of the total nephron population). However, normal dilution ability may be maintained with fewer functional nephrons than normal concentration ability.[78]

2. Abnormal.

a. Interpretation of urine specific gravity values of randomly obtained samples depends on knowledge of the patient's hydration status, the plasma or serum concentration of urea nitrogen or creatinine, and knowledge of drugs or fluids that have been administered to the patient. Knowledge of urine volume and water consumption may also be helpful. In some instances, interpretation may require knowledge of urine and plasma osmolality.

b. Consult Section IV A of this chapter for additional information related to physiologic and pathologic polyuria and physiologic and pathologic oliguria. Knowledge of urine specific gravity (or osmolality) is of great value in localizing the source of abnormal urine volume.

c. Varying degrees of impaired ability to concentrate or dilute glomerular filtrate are a consistent finding in all forms of primary renal failure.

(1). Because the kidneys have tremendous reserve capacity, impairment of their ability to concentrate or dilute urine may not be detected until at least two thirds (dogs) or more (cats) of the total population of nephrons has been damaged.

(2). Complete inability of the nephrons to modify glomerular filtrate typically results in formation of urine with a specific gravity that is similar to that of glomerular filtrate (1.008 to 1.012). This phenomenon has been commonly called "fixation of specific gravity."

(3). Total loss of the ability to concentrate and dilute urine (SG = 1.008 to 1.012) often does not occur as a sudden event, but may develop gradually. For this reason, when urine specific gravity values between approximately 1.007 to 1.029 in dogs and 1.007 to 1.034 in cats are associated with clinical dehydration and/or azotemia, they are highly suggestive of primary renal failure.

(4). Once the urine specific gravity reflects impaired ability to concentrate or dilute urine, it is more an index of nephron function than of distal tubular and collecting duct function, because in addition to generalized tubular lesions, this abnormality may occur as a result of factors not specifically related to tubular damage. These factors include:

(a). Compensatory increase in glomerular filtration that occurs as a result of a decrease in the quantity of functional nephrons. Increased production of glomerular filtrate floods the distal tubules and collecting ducts. It is associated with decreased fractional tubular reabsorption of sodium and phosphorus by viable nephrons.

(b). A decrease in the number of functioning nephrons that impairs maintenance of a high osmotic gradient normally present in renal medulla.

(c). Increased glomerular filtration of solutes retained in plasma (e.g., urea, creatinine, phosphorus), which induces an osmotic diuresis. This accentuates the degree of obligatory polyuria.

(5). Once the ability to concentrate or dilute urine has been permanently destroyed, repeated evaluation of specific gravity is not of aid in evaluation of progressive deterioration of renal function. Therefore, serial evaluation of urine specific gravity is of greatest aid in detecting functional changes earlier during the course of primary renal failure or in monitoring functional recovery associated with reversible renal diseases.

(6). If sufficient clinical evidence is present to warrant examination of the patient's renal function by determining the serum concentration of creatinine or blood urea nitrogen, the urine specific gravity (or osmolality) should be evaluated at the same time.

(a). As previously emphasized, an adequately concentrated urine sample associated with an abnormal elevation in serum creatinine or urea nitrogen concentration suggests the probability of *prerenal azotemia*.

(b). If nonazotemic patients have impaired ability to concentrate urine, causes of pathologic polyuria should be explored. Determination of urine specific gravity or osmolality may allow one to determine whether a disorder characterized by water (1.001 ± 1.006) or solute (±1.008 or greater) diuresis is probable. (See Section IV A of this chapter.)

(c). Azotemia associated with a specific gravity of 1.007 to ±1.029 in dogs and of 1.007 to 1.034 in cats indicates the probability of primary renal failure, although on occasion hypoadrenocorticism may induce similar findings.

(d). If a *nondehydrated, nonazotemic* patient suspected of having pathologic polyuria does not have a urine specific gravity that indicates that the kidneys can definitely concentrate urine, further tests are required before any meaningful conclusions can be established about the capacity of the kidney to concentrate urine.

(1′). In the nonazotemic, nondehydrated patient deprived of water for an appropriate period of time, ADH normally is released from the posterior pituitary gland as a compensatory response to hydropenia.[32,34,44] ADH enhances fluid reabsorption from the distal tubules and collecting ducts by increasing tubular cell permeability to water.

(a′). Clinical experience has revealed that the results of water deprivation tests are often difficult to reproduce. Boundary values have been established above which renal function is assumed to be adequate and below which it is assumed to be impaired. A zone of doubt exists in between.

(b′). Uncontrolled clinical observations indicate that dogs with "adequate" renal function excrete urine with a high specific gravity (≥1.030), high osmolality, and relatively small volume (physiologic oliguria).

(c′). Studies of dogs with completely normal renal function were interpreted to indicate 95% of normal dogs subjected to water deprivation sufficient to produce a slight degree of dehydration should have a urine specific gravity of at least 1.048, a urine osmolality of at least 1787 mOsm/kg, and a U_{osm}/P_{osm} ratio of at least 5.7/1.[44] If such values are not obtained, nephron dysfunction may exist. The degree of dysfunction, however, may not be severe enough to be associated with clinical signs.

(2′). Patients unable to concentrate urine following appropriately conducted water deprivation tests should be evaluated for diseases that cause medullary solute washout, central diabetes insipidus, and/or renal diabetes insipidus.

(7). Formation of dilute urine (SG < 1.007)

(especially in patients who need to conserve water) may represent an abnormality associated with several diseases, including:

(a). Central or renal diabetes insipidus.

(b). Hyperadrenocorticism.

(c). Hypercalcemia.

(d). Pyometra.

(e). Liver disorders.

(f). Psychogenic water consumption.

d. Urine specific gravity and localization of azotemia.

(1). Although the following generalities apply to dogs and cats, we emphasize that some azotemic cats with primary renal failure retain comparably greater urine concentrating capacity than do dogs.

(a). In dogs with primary renal failure, azotemia usually follows loss of the ability to concentrate urine to a specific gravity of at least 1.030.

(b). In some cats with primary renal failure, azotemia may precede loss of the ability to concentrate urine to values of 1.035 to 1.045.[2,61,85]

(2). Prerenal azotemia.

(a). Pathogenesis and causes.

(1′). Extraurinary diseases may cause varying degrees of alteration in glomerular filtration as a result of reduction of renal blood flow. Inadequate perfusion of normal glomeruli with blood, regardless of cause (dehydration, cardiac disease, shock, hypoadrenocorticism, decreased plasma colloidal osmotic pressure) may cause prerenal azotemia (Tables 7–1 and 7–4).

(2′). Prerenal azotemia is initially associated with structurally normal kidneys that are capable of quantitatively normal renal function, provided compromised renal perfusion is corrected prior to the onset of ischemic nephron damage. Development of primary renal failure resulting from ischemia prolongs and reduces the likelihood of complete recovery.

(3′). A diagnosis of prerenal azotemia should be considered if abnormal elevation in the serum or plasma concentration of urea nitrogen and creatinine is associated with adequately concentrated urine (SG ≥ 1.030 in dogs; SG ≥ 1.035 in cats) in patients with no specific evidence of generalized glomerular disease.

(a′). Detection of adequate concentrated urine in association with azotemia indicates that a sufficient quantity of functional nephrons is present to prevent primary renal azotemia. Significant elevations in the serum or plasma concentration of urea nitrogen or creatinine as a result of primary renal failure cannot be detected in dogs until approximately 70 to 75% of the nephron population is nonfunctional.

(b′). Elevation in urine specific gravity associated with prerenal azotemia probably reflects a compensatory response by the body to combat low perfusion pressure and blood volume by secreting ADH (and possibly other substances) to conserve water filtered through glomeruli.

TABLE 7–4
CLASSIFICATION OF ALTERED GLOMERULAR FILTRATION AND AZOTEMIA

Cause	Classification of Azotemia
Decreased blood volume	Prerenal
Decreased blood pressure	Prerenal
Decreased colloidal osmotic pressure	Prerenal
Decreased number of patent vessels	Primary renal
Decreased glomerular permeability	Primary renal
Increased renal interstitial pressure	Primary renal
Increased intratubular pressure	Primary renal (tubular obstruction)
Increased intratubular pressure	Postrenal (obstruction of ureters, bladder, urethra)

(c′). Restoration of renal perfusion by appropriate volume replacement therapy is typically followed by a dramatic drop in the concentration of serum urea and creatinine to normal in approximately 1 to 3 days.

(4′). Another form of potentially reversible prerenal azotemia may develop in glomerulonephritic patients with severe hypoproteinemia. At the level of the glomerulus, hypoalbuminemia enhances glomerular filtration rate as a result of a reduction in colloidal osmotic pressure. However, decreased renal blood flow and decreased glomerular filtration, which occur in association with marked reduction in vascular volume secondary to a reduction in colloidal osmotic pressure, result in a proportionate degree of retention of substances normally cleared by the kidneys (e.g., creatinine, urea) (Tables 7–4 and 7–5).

(a′). Therefore, the significance of an abnormal increase in the serum concentration of urea nitrogen or creatinine (or a reduction in creatinine clearance) must be carefully defined in hypoproteinemic nephrotic patients.

(b′). Azotemia cannot be accepted as indisputable evidence of severe primary glomerular lesions because it may be associated with a potentially reversible decrease in renal perfusion caused by hypoalbuminemia.

(b). Diagnosis of prerenal azotemia

(1′). Elevation of serum urea nitrogen or creatinine concentration.

(2′). Oliguria.

(3′). High specific gravity (≥1.030 in dogs; ≥1.035 to 1.040 in cats) or osmolality.

(4′). Detection of underlying cause.

(5′). Dramatic correction of azotemia following administration of appropriate therapy to restore renal perfusion.

(c). Prognosis.

(1′). Depends on reversibility of primary cause.

(2′). Favorable for renal function if perfusion rapidly restored.

(3′). *Complete* loss of renal perfusion for more than 2 to 4 hours results in generalized ischemic renal disease. With the exception of shock, this degree of reduced renal perfusion is uncommon. Thus, the onset of generalized renal disease is expected to require a longer period of altered renal perfusion.

(3). Postrenal azotemia.

(a). Pathogenesis.

(1′). Diseases that prevent excretion of urine from the body may cause postrenal azotemia.

(2′). Initially the kidneys are structurally normal and capable of quantitatively normal function provided the underlying cause is corrected.

(3′). If the underlying cause is allowed to persist, death from alterations in water, electrolyte, acid-base, and endocrine balance, in addition to accumulation of metabolic waste prod-

TABLE 7–5
DIFFERENTIATION OF PRERENAL AZOTEMIA FROM PRIMARY AZOTEMIA ASSOCIATED WITH GLOMERULOTUBULAR IMBALANCE

Factor	Prerenal Azotemia	Glomerulotubular Imbalance and Primary Renal Azotemia
Serum urea nitrogen	Increased	Increased
Creatinine	Increased	Increased
Urine specific gravity	≥1.030 dog ≥1.035 cat*	1.030-1.035 dog 1.035-1.040 cat
Proteinuria	Usually negative	Positive
Prerenal cause	Present	Absent
Response to correction of renal perfusion with fluids	Within 1 to 3 days	Minimal

*Some cats with primary renal azotemia may concentrate urine to 1.045 or greater.

ucts, will occur within a few days. If partial obstruction to urine outflow allows the patient to survive for a longer time, varying degrees of hydronephrosis may also occur.

(b). Causes.

(1′). Complete obstruction of urine outflow (i.e., obstruction in urethra, bladder, or both ureters) that persists for more than 24 hours usually results in postrenal azotemia.

(2′). Unilateral ureteral occlusion (an example of renal disease) is not associated with azotemia unless generalized disease of the nonobstructed kidney is also present.

(3′). Azotemia that occurs as a sequela to rupture of the excretory pathway (most commonly the bladder) is primarily related to absorption of urine from the peritoneal cavity. Unless damaged as a result of hypovolemic shock or trauma secondary to the underlying cause of rupture of the excretory pathway, the kidneys are structurally normal.

(c). Diagnosis of postrenal azotemia

(1′). Obstructive lesions are commonly associated with:

(a′). Elevation in serum urea nitrogen or creatinine concentration.

(b′). Oliguria or anuria, dysuria, tenesmus.

(c′). Detection of obstructive lesion(s) by physical examination (e.g., urethral plug, herniated bladder), radiography, and ultrasonography.

(2′). Rupture of the excretory pathway is commonly associated with:

(a′). Elevation in serum urea nitrogen or creatinine concentration.

(b′). Severe depression, painful abdomen, ascites.

(c′). History of trauma.

(d′). Inability to palpate bladder.

(e′). Paracentesis (modified transudate or exudate).

(f′). Abnormalities detected by retrograde contrast (positive or negative) cystography or urethrocystography.

(3′). Because of its variability, the urine specific gravity of patients with postrenal azotemia is not relied on for assessment of renal function to the same degree as it is in patients with primary renal and prerenal azotemia.

(d). Prognosis.

(1′). Obstructive lesions.

(a′). If the patient has total obstruction to urine outflow for a period of 3 to 6 days, death from uremia will occur. Death usually occurs before significant structural changes caused by obstruction have time to develop (i.e., hydronephrosis). Death is caused by alteration of fluid, acid-base, electrolyte, nutrient, and endocrine balance and by accumulation of metabolic waste products.

(b′). The prognosis is favorable for renal function if the obstructive lesion(s) is rapidly removed.

(c′). The long-term prognosis depends on the reversibility of the underlying cause.

(2′). Rupture of the excretory pathway.

(a′). If a rent in the excretory pathway is of sufficient magnitude to result in azotemia, the patient probably will die if it is not repaired.

(b′). The prognosis for renal function is favorable if the rent is repaired or heals.

(c′). The long-term prognosis depends on the reversibility of the underlying cause.

(4). Primary renal azotemia.

(a). Pathogenesis.

(1′). Primary azotemic renal failure may be caused by many disease processes that have in common destruction of approximately three fourths or more of the parenchyma of both kidneys.

(2′). Depending on the biologic behavior of the disease in question, primary renal failure may be reversible or irreversible, acute or chronic.

(b). Diagnosis.

(1′). In dogs, impairment of at least two thirds of the nephron mass is indicated if a dehydrated patient (that has not received fluid therapy) has impaired ability to concentrate urine.

(a′). Total loss of ability to concentrate and dilute urine does not always occur as a sudden event, but often develops gradually. For this reason, a urine specific gravity between approximately 1.007 to 1.029 for dogs, or 1.007 to 1.034 for cats, associated with clinical dehydration or azotemia is indicative of primary renal azotemia (Table 7–1).

(b′). Total inability of the nephrons to concentrate or dilute urine (so-called fixation of specific gravity or isosthenuria) results in the formation of urine with a specific gravity that is similar to that of glomerular filtrate (approximately 1.008 to 1.012).

(2′). Impairment of at least three fourths of the functional capacity of the nephron mass is indicated if a patient has an elevation in the serum or plasma concentration of urea nitrogen and creatinine and impaired ability to concentrate or dilute urine.

(3′). More definitive studies (e.g., ultrasonography, radiography, biopsy, exploratory surgery) are required to establish the underlying cause of primary azotemic renal failure.

(4′). Remember, uremic signs are not directly caused by renal lesions, but rather are related to varying degrees of fluid, acid-base, electrolyte, and nutrient imbalances, vitamin and endocrine alterations, and retention of waste products of protein catabolism, all of which develop as a result of damage to nephrons.

(5). Glomerulotubular imbalance.

(a). Abnormal elevation in the serum concentration of urea nitrogen or creatinine may occur in association with varying degrees of urine concentration in some patients with primary renal failure caused by generalized glomerular disease.

(1′). Caution should be used not to overinterpret the absolute value of the urine specific gravity in such patients because it may be slightly elevated by the effect of protein.

(2′). Addition of 40 mg of protein per 100 mL of urine increases the urine specific gravity by approximately 0.001.

(b). The renal lesion in such patients must be characterized by glomerular damage that is sufficiently severe to impair renal clearance of urea and creatinine, but that has not yet induced a sufficient degree of ischemic atrophy and necrosis of renal tubular cells to prevent varying degrees of urine concentration. Thus, glomerular filtrate that is formed may appear to be adequately concentrated.

(c). This group of patients may be differentiated from patients with prerenal azotemia by failure of a search for one of the extrarenal causes of poor perfusion, by the presence of persistent proteinuria, and by lack of response to restoration of vascular volume and perfusion with appropriate therapy (Table 7–5).

(6). Combination of primary renal azotemia, prerenal azotemia, and/or postrenal azotemia.

(a). Pathogenesis.

(1′). Severely diseased kidneys have impaired ability to compensate for stresses imposed by disease states, dietary indiscretion, and change in environment.

(2′). In patients with previously compensated primary renal disease, uremic crises are commonly precipitated or complicated by a variety of concomitant extrarenal factors.

(3′). Extrarenal mechanisms that may be associated with uremic crises include:

(a′). Factors that accelerate endogenous protein catabolism (anorexia, infection, extensive tissue necrosis, administration of catabolic drugs) increase the quantity of metabolic by-products in the body because the kidneys are incapable of excreting them. Protein by-products contribute significantly to the production of uremic signs in patients with renal failure.

(b′). Stress states (fever, infection, change of environment) are associated with release of glucocorticoids from the adrenal glands. Glucocorticoids stimulate conversion of proteins to carbohydrates (gluconeogenesis) and thus increase the quantity of protein waste products in the body.

(c′). Abnormalities that decrease renal perfusion (i.e., decreased water consumption, vomiting, diarrhea, shock, cardiac decompensation) cause prerenal uremia.

(d′). Administration of nephrotoxic drugs may precipitate a uremic crisis by damaging nephrons.

(b). Diagnostic considerations include:

(1′). Previous history of compensated primary renal failure.

(2′). Detection of primary extrarenal disease processes in addition to generalized renal disease.

(3′). Response to therapy or amelioration of signs because prerenal or postrenal causes are self-limiting. Whereas patients with uremic crises precipitated by reversible extrarenal disorders (e.g., pancreatitis, hepatic disease, gastroenteritis) may rapidly respond to supportive and symptomatic therapy, the therapeutic response of patients with uremic crises caused by progressive irreversible destruction of nephrons is usually slower.

VI. BIOCHEMICAL TESTS

A. Urine pH.

1. Indications.

a. Diagnostic.

(1). Urine pH may be used as a crude index of body acid-base balance. Caution: net urine pH is not always a reliable index of blood pH.

(a). Carnivores generally produce an excess of acid metabolites. The lungs regulate elimination of carbon dioxide (and therefore carbonic acid), whereas the kidneys regulate acid-base balance primarily via excretion of protons, ammonium ion, and phosphates.

(b). Diurnal variation in urine pH may be significant. Diet and disease may also induce considerable variation in urine pH. As was the situation with urine specific gravity, differentiation between normal and abnormal urine pH values is not possible without additional information. Both may fall within the same range.

(2). Knowledge of urine pH may aid in determination of the type of uroliths present prior to formulation of therapy.

(a). Calcium phosphate (apatite) and magnesium ammonium phosphate (struvite) uroliths tend to form in alkaline urine.

(b). Cystine, uric acid, and calcium oxalate uroliths tend to form in acid urine.

(c). Ammonium urate crystals may be flocculated by hydrogen ion (acid pH) or ammonium ion (alkaline pH).

(3). Urinary tract infections caused by urease-producing bacteria (primarily staphylococci and *Proteus* spp) frequently cause urine to become alkaline. Urinary tract infections are also commonly associated with acid urine because most bacterial pathogens do not produce urease.

(4). Knowledge of urine pH may be important in interpretation of findings in urine sediment. RBC, WBC, casts, and other proteinaceous structures tend to disintegrate in alkaline urine.

b. Therapeutic.

(1). Urine pH is commonly manipulated to dissolve or prevent recurrence of certain uroliths.

(a). Calcium phosphate and magnesium ammonium phosphate crystals are more soluble in acid urine.

(b). Cystine and uric acid crystals are more soluble in alkaline urine.

(c). Ammonium urate crystals are least likely to precipitate in urine that is not acidic.

(2). Because acid urine inhibits bacterial growth, urinary acidifiers are sometimes used as ancillary treatment of urinary tract infections.

(3). The therapeutic efficacy of some antimicrobial agents may be enhanced by alteration of urine pH. The solubility of some antimicrobial agents may also be pH dependent.

(4). Knowledge of urine pH is commonly used as a crude index of therapeutic response when attempting to correct states of systemic acidosis or alkalosis.

(5). Therapeutic manipulation of pH is also recommended in management of myoglobinuria.

2. Methodology.[75]

a. pH meters. pH meters provide excellent results, but are not commonly used for routine urinalyses because they are expensive and because of the technical ease provided by reagent strips.

b. Reagent strips.

(1). Urine pH can readily be determined by any one of several commercially available test strips impregnated with indicator dyes. The most reliable results are obtained by evaluation of fresh specimens.

(2). Wide-range hydrogen paper (pH 5.5 to 9) is satisfactory for routine urinalyses. It is available as LoBuff pH Paper from Microessential Labs, Inc., 4224 Avenue North, Brooklyn, NY 11210.

(3). Diagnostic strips produced by Ames Company (e.g., Multistix) and Bio-Dynamics, Inc. (e.g., Chemstrip) contain methyl red and bromthymol blue and are capable of monitoring change in urine pH from 5 to 9. According to many manufacturers, measured pH values are only accurate to within 0.5 pH units. Comparison of color reactions to the manufacturer's color standards should be performed in a properly illuminated area.

3. Interpretation.

a. Normal (see Table 7–11).

(1). The kidneys are capable of adjusting the pH of urine to between 4.5 to 5.0 and approximately 8.5, depending on the acid-base status of the body. Therefore, the pH of urine provides a reflection of the metabolic state of the body.

(a). Ingestion of dietary protein typically results in production of acid. The urine pH of dog and cat urine commonly lies between 6.0 and 7.5. In a study of 649 cats at the University of Minnesota, the mean urine pH was 6.6 (the range was 5.0 to 9.0).[56]

(b). Ingestion of low-protein diets primarily composed of vegetables and cereals typically results in production of more alkaline urine.

(2). Urine pH tends to vary throughout the day, in part because of events associated with eating and digestion.

(a). Urine of dogs and cats tends to become less acidic shortly following ingestion of food. This is commonly referred to as the "alkaline tide," and presumably is related to increased secretion of hydrochloric acid in the stomach.

(b). In an experimental study in cats fed a canned diet, urine pH increased from a value of 6 to 7.2 within 4 hours after feeding.[57]

(c). One can assume that the magnitude of change in urine pH following eating depends on the composition of the diet, the frequency of eating, the quantity of food consumed, and the pH of residual urine in the urinary bladder.

(d). Changes in urine pH at any instant in time may be masked by retained urine with a different pH value.

(3). In man, the pH of urine obtained following sleep for several hours tends to be more acidic, presumably a reflection of respiratory acidosis associated with decreased ventilation during sleep.

b. Abnormal.

(1). Abnormal (or inappropriate) urine pH values are similar to normal values. Meaningful interpretation may require knowledge of blood pH and P_{CO_2}, plasma bicarbonate (or T_{CO_2}) concentration, and response to controlled administration of acidifying or alkalinizing substances.

(2). The infrequency with which urine pH values less than 6.0 and greater than 7.5 occur in dogs should arouse suspicion of an abnormality when they are observed.

(3). The tendency to excrete acid urine may be associated with several disorders, including:

(a). Respiratory and metabolic acidosis (except some cases of vomiting).

(b). Diabetic ketoacidosis.

(c). Primary renal failure.

(d). Severe vomiting (so-called paradoxic acidosis of vomiting associated with chloride depletion).

(e). Severe diarrhea.

(f). Starvation.

(g). Pyrexia.
(h). Catabolism of endogenous or exogenous proteins.
(i). Oxygen debt.

(4). The tendency to excrete alkaline urine may be associated with several disorders, including:
(a). Urinary tract infections caused by urease-producing pathogens.
(b). Respiratory or metabolic alkalosis.
(c). Vomiting.
(d). Renal tubular acidosis. (More appropriately stated as an inability to acidify urine or reabsorb bicarbonate from glomerular filtrate in response to body need. The urine pH may be 6.5 or greater).
(e). Compensation for chronic metabolic acidosis by renal excretion of ammonium ions.

(5). Drugs that acidify urine include:
(a). Phosphate salts (sodium, potassium, or ammonium).
(b). d,1-Methionine.
(c). Ammonium chloride.
(d). Ascorbic acid, although studies in man and cats indicate that ascorbic acid is incapable of altering urine pH at commonly recommended therapeutic dosages.[16,70]
(e). Low dosages of furosemide.

(6). Drugs that alkalinize urine include:
(a). Sodium bicarbonate.
(b). Sodium lactate.
(c). Potassium citrate.
(d). Acetazolamide.
(e). Chlorothiazide.

c. Artifacts.
(1). Contamination of urine with urease-producing bacteria from the distal urethra, genital tract, or environment may result in alkalinization of urine.
(2). Loss of carbon dioxide from samples stored at room temperature tends to alkalinize urine samples.
(3). Detergents and disinfecting agents in collection containers may alkalinize urine.
(4). Administration of therapeutic dosages of furosemide tends to acidify urine.

B. Glucose.

1. Indications
a. Diagnostic.
(1). Although a small quantity of glucose is normally present in urine (2 to 10 mg/dl in man), the quantity is insufficient to be detected by screening tests commonly used as a part of routine urinalyses.
(2). Detection of glucosuria should prompt consideration of hyperglycemic and normoglycemic states, which may be physiologic or pathologic.
(3). Test strips have been designed to detect reduction of the quantity of glucose normally present in urine (2 to 10 mg/dl) as a result of consumption of bacterial pathogens.[51] These tests have been associated with many false-positive reactions in man, but have not been evaluated in dogs or cats.

b. Therapeutic.
(1). The dosage of insulin given to patients with diabetes mellitus was at one time commonly titrated by semiquantitative measurements of urine glucose. Although the concentration of urine glucose is related to the concentration of blood glucose, the relationship is variable. Therefore, serial measurement of blood glucose concentrations is recommended to titrate insulin dosage for patients with diabetes mellitus.
(2). Detection of urine glucose may be used as a qualitative index of response to therapeutic osmotic diuresis induced by parenteral administration of hypertonic dextrose (so-called intensive osmotic diuresis).

2. Methodology.[75]
a. Colorimetric tests are based on glucose oxidase activity. Dipsticks and reagent tapes impregnated with glucose oxidase and several other reagents are available from commercial sources.
(1). Although these enzymatic tests for detection of urine glucose are technically easy to perform, they involve interrelated enzymatic reactions that occur in stepwise fashion. Reliable results depend on adherence to the manufacturer's recommendations for use.
(2). Glucose oxidase enzyme reacts specifically with glucose; the enzyme does not react with nonglucose reducing substances. The tests incorporate colorimetric indicators that may react with nonglucose substances, however. Conversely, some substances may inhibit the test reaction.
(3). Glucose oxidase is a labile protein, and therefore, test strips do not have an indefinite shelf life, as indicated by an expiration date on their container.
(4). Test results may be influenced by temperature. Refrigerated samples should be warmed to room temperature before evaluation for glucose with enzyme-dependent tests requiring short reaction times (10 seconds).[77]

(5). The sensitivity of glucose oxidase tests is also influenced by pH and concentrations of inhibitors (e.g., ascorbic acid).
(6). Because many variables have the potential to affect the validity of the test, appropriate caution must be used in interpretation of semiquantitative results.

b. Colorimetric tests based on copper reduction. Copper reduction methods are based on color changes associated with reduction of cupric ions (blue) to cuprous oxide (orange-red). The color change from blue through green to orange depends on the concentration of reducing compounds (including glucose) in urine.

3. Interpretation (See Chapter 4, Clinical Algorithms and Data Bases for Urinary Tract Disorders.)
   a. Physiologic glucosuria.
      (1). Because of its molecular characteristics (MW = 180), glucose readily passes through glomerular capillary walls into glomerular filtrate. Almost all the glucose in glomerular filtrate is actively reabsorbed by the proximal tubules. Only a small quantity (2 to 10 mg/dl, or 100 to 200 mg/24 h in man) normally appears in urine. The quantity of glucose excreted in normal urine is insufficient to give a positive test strip result (see Table 7–11).
      (2). Physiologic glucosuria may occur any time the quantity of glucose in glomerular filtrate exceeds the transport capacity (so-called transport maximum or T_m) of the renal tubules for glucose. The T_m for urine glucose in dogs corresponds to a venous blood glucose concentration of approximately 180 to 220 mg/dl. The T_m for urine glucose in cats corresponds to a venous blood glucose of approximately 260 to 310 mg/dl.[53]
      (3). Physiologic glucosuria is usually transient in duration.
         (a). Hyperglycemic glucosuria may occur following significant stress, especially in cats. This phenomenon is usually associated with release of endogenous epinephrine and glucocorticoids and depends on mobilization of glycogen stored in the liver.
         (b). Hyperglycemic glucosuria has been reported in human beings following consumption of unusually large quantities of glucose. We have not observed this phenomenon in dogs or cats.
   b. Pharmacologic glucosuria.
      (1). Hyperglycemic glucosuria may occur following parenteral administration of solutions containing sufficient quantities of glucose.
      (2). Varying degrees of glucosuria may be induced by parenteral administration of glucocorticoids, but in our experience, this has been extremely uncommon in dogs and cats.
      (3). Other pharmacologic agents that have been reported to have the potential to induce glucosuria include:
         (a). Adrenocorticotropic hormone.
         (b). Glucagon.
         (c). Epinephrine.
         (d). Morphine.
         (e). Phenothiazines.
   c. Pathologic glucosuria.
      (1). Hyperglycemic glucosuria may be induced by several disorders, including:
         (a). Diabetes mellitus.
         (b). Acute pancreatitis (variable).
         (c). Hyperadrenocorticism (variable).
         (d). Central nervous system lesions (variable).
         (e). Pheochromocytoma.
         (f). Progesterone-associated hyperglycemia.
      (2). Normoglycemic glucosuria may be induced by several disorders, including:
         (a). Primary renal glucosuria.
         (b). Fanconi syndrome (amino-diabetes).
         (c). Congenital renal disorders.
         (d). Acute renal failure associated with significant tubular lesions (variable).

C. Ketones.

1. Indications.
   a. Definition. Ketones (sometimes called ketone bodies) include acetoacetic acid, acetone, and β-hydroxybutyric acid.
   b. Evaluation of urine for ketones in patients with diabetes mellitus is especially important because diabetic ketonuria suggests development of diabetic ketoacidosis.
   c. Evaluation of urine for ketones may aid in differentiation of a diabetic coma from therapeutically induced insulin shock.
   d. Occurrence of ketonuria in the absence of glucosuria suggests a derangement in carbohydrate metabolism characterized by excessive catabolism of lipids.
2. Methodology.[75] Most tests used as a part of routine complete urinalyses for detection of ketones are based on the reaction of acetoacetic acid and acetone with nitroprusside in an alkaline environment to produce a deep purple compound.
   a. Applied physiology.
      (1). During normal metabolism, fats are almost completely converted to carbon dioxide, water, and energy in the liver. In the process, however, small quantities of intermediary metabolites (acetoa-

cetic acid [also called diacetic acid], β-hydroxybutyric acid, and acetone) are formed. These intermediary metabolites are metabolized by peripheral tissues of the body at a limited rate. Some are filtered by glomeruli and are almost completely reabsorbed by the renal tubules. The T_m for tubular reabsorption of ketones is apparently easily saturated.

(2). Acetone is irreversibly formed from acetoacetic acid by nonreversible decarboxylation, whereas β-hydroxybutyric acid is reversibly formed from acetoacetic acid.

(3). Inadequate consumption of dietary carbohydrates and/or impaired endogenous utilization of carbohydrates for energy results in a shift to increased oxidation of fatty acids. When the proportion of fatty acids metabolized for energy becomes large, utilization becomes incomplete and excessive quantities of intermediary metabolites (acetoacetic acid and its conversion products [β-hydroxybutyric acid and acetone]) are formed. Catabolism of the amino acids leucine, tyrosine, and phenylalanine may also result in increased production of acetoacetic acid. When production of these metabolites exceeds the capacity of tissues to oxidize them, they accumulate in plasma (ketosis), are filtered by glomeruli, and exceed the capacity of the renal tubules to reabsorb them (ketonuria). Although ketones are excreted in urine in different relative proportions (78% β-hydroxybutyric acid, 20% acetoacetic acid, and 2% acetone), detection of one indicates the presence of the others.

b. Significance of ketonuria.

(1). Ketosis and ketonuria may be caused by any disorder associated with a significant shift of energy production from carbohydrates to fats.

(2). Uncontrolled diabetes mellitus is the most commonly encountered form of ketonuria in dogs and cats. Urinary excretion of ketones induces systemic electrolyte losses, including hyponatremia. The loss of sodium and ketones in urine contributes to the increased osmolality of the urine caused by glucose and, therefore, increases the magnitude of polyuria associated with diabetes mellitus.

(3). Starvation, low carbohydrate-high fat diets (ketogenic diets), and hypoglycemic syndromes (i.e., insulinomas) may also induce ketonuria.

(4). Immature animals are more likely to develop ketonuria as a result of starvation than are adults.

D. Bilirubin.

1. Indications.

a. Because detection of bilirubinuria by routine urinalysis may precede clinical recognition of jaundice, bilirubinuria may be an early indicator of naturally occurring disorders with the potential to induce jaundice.

b. Detection of abnormal quantities of bilirubin in urine may be used as a crude index of hepatotoxicity caused by potentially toxic therapeutic agents.

2. Methodology.[75]

Bilirubin is an unstable compound that may spontaneously oxidize to biliverdin, especially if allowed to stand at room temperature while being exposed to air. Biliverdin and photodegradation products do not react with commonly used tests for bilirubinuria. For this reason, urine should be ideally evaluated within 30 minutes from the time of collection or refrigerated (2 to 8°C) in a dark environment. Urine should not be filtered or centrifuged prior to examination for bilirubin because precipitates of calcium carbonate and calcium phosphate may absorb varying quantities of bilirubin.

3. Interpretation.[76]

a. Applied physiology.

(1). Bilirubin is derived primarily from the catabolism of the heme component of hemoglobin in reticuloendothelial cells of the body.

(2). Bilirubin formed as a result of degeneration of hemoglobin by reticuloendothelial cells is loosely bound to albumin and transported via the circulation of the liver. This form of protein-bound bilirubin is commonly called unconjugated bilirubin or indirect bilirubin. Because it is bound to protein, it cannot pass through glomerular capillary walls.

(3). The liver removes protein-bound bilirubin from the circulation and conjugates it with glucuronic and sulfuric acids. Conjugated bilirubin is water soluble and passes through glomerular capillary walls.

(4). Most of the conjugated bilirubin is transported to the intestinal tract in bile via the biliary system; however, a small amount escapes from the liver directly into the blood vascular system.

(a). Bilirubin excreted into the small intestine is converted to urobilinogen (a colorless pigment) by intestinal bacteria. Most of the urobilinogen is ultimately oxidized to urobilin, which imparts the characteristic dark color to feces. Some of the urobilinogen, however, is reabsorbed and excreted in urine.

(b). Conjugated bilirubin that escapes through glomeruli may appear in urine. The renal threshold for clearance of conjugated bilirubin apparently varies from species to species, but is low in dogs. The quantity of bilirubin excreted in normal urine is often insufficient to give a positive result, unless the urine is concentrated (see Table 7–11).

(5). At one time, the origin of bilirubin normally found in urine was thought to be primarily from effete RBC, with smaller quantities being derived from pre-erythroid bone marrow sources and bone marrow metabolism. Studies performed in dogs, however, have revealed that bilirubin may also be formed in the renal tubules following reabsorption of filtered hemoglobin. The capacity to form tubular-derived bilirubin from hemoglobin was found to be greater in males than females.[22] Because tubular epithelial cells of dogs have been shown to contain glucuronyl transferase, the capacity of these cells to conjugate bilirubin appears probable.

(6). Abnormal quantities of conjugated bilirubin in urine may be associated with:

(a). Increased production of conjugated bilirubin as a result of abnormal RBC destruction, hepatocellular disease, and/or bile duct obstruction.

(b). The combined occurrence of these disorders and renal dysfunction may lead to difficulties in quantitative interpretation of bilirubinuria because of alteration in the renal threshold for excretion of bile pigments.

(7). Abnormal quantities of unconjugated bilirubin would be expected to occur in conditions associated with hyperbilirubinemia (i.e., hemolytic disease) and alteration in the selective permeability of glomerular capillaries to proteins.

b. Significance.

(1). The magnitude of bilirubinuria should always be interpreted in light of urine specific gravity.

(2). Dogs.

(a). Small quantities of bilirubin are commonly observed in concentrated urine samples obtained from normal dogs (see Table 7–11).

(1′). This observation is commonly attributed to a low renal threshold for bilirubin. The low renal threshold for bilirubin is associated with low plasma concentrations of bilirubin.

(2′). Trace to mild reactions for bilirubin are relatively common when the urine specific gravity is 1.040 or greater.

(b). Detection of bilirubin in less concentrated urine samples or persistent bilirubinuria should prompt consideration of disorders characterized by prehepatic, hepatic, or posthepatic disorders of bile metabolism.

(1′). Bilirubinuria may precede hyperbilirubinemia.

(2′). A variable degree of bilirubinuria (usually mild) may be associated with starvation and/or fever.

(3′). A variable degree of bilirubinuria may be associated with intravascular hemolysis of sufficient magnitude to exceed the hemoglobin binding capacity of haptoglobin. In this situation, bilirubinuria may be associated with renal tubular cell production of bilirubin from hemoglobin. Although damage to glomeruli may be associated with subsequent loss of unconjugated bilirubin, this mechanism is unlikely to be of clinical significance because of the magnitude of proteinuria that would be required to deliver a detectable quality of bilirubin in urine.

(4′). Bilirubinuria of the greatest magnitude is usually associated with hepatocellular diseases (intrahepatic) or disorders that obstruct bile ducts (extrahepatic). A significant degree of liver disease can exist, however, in the absence of bilirubinuria.

(3). Cats.

(a). Retrospective evaluation of clinical cases admitted to the University of Minnesota Veterinary Hospital revealed that bilirubinuria was not a finding in normal cats, even when associated with highly concentrated urine samples (see Table 7–11).

(b). In the University of Minnesota series, feline bilirubinuria was associated with a variety of diseases, including primary hepatic diseases, diabetes mellitus, feline infectious peritonitis, and feline leukemia.[55,76]

E. Occult blood, hemoglobin, and myoglobin.

1. Indications.
   a. Chemical tests for RBC and hemoglobin may aid in identification of the underlying cause of abnormal urine color.
   b. These tests may be used to detect subvisual (occult) quantities of RBC, hemoglobin, or myoglobin in urine.
   c. Presence or absence of RBC, hemoglobin, or myoglobin may be of value in localizing the source of proteinuria.
   d. Chemical evaluation of urine for RBC may aid in interpretation of the significance of urine sediment. Because microscopic examination of urine sediment does not detect free hemoglobin released from lysed RBC, total reliance on sediment examination for semiquantitation of hematuria may result in underestimation of the degree of hematuria.
2. Methodology.[75]
   a. Commonly used chemical tests for rapid detection of RBC and hemoglobin are based on the pseudoperoxidase activity of the heme moiety of hemoglobin. Myoglobin (a heme-containing compound) also has pseudoperoxidase activity and causes a positive test reaction. Porphyrin does not react with these tests.
   b. The peroxidase activity of hemoglobin or myoglobin causes release of monomolecular oxygen from substrate (peroxide). Transfer of monomolecular oxygen to a suitable chromogen (often o-tolidine) induces a characteristic color change. The chromogen indicator system is often similar to that used in glucose oxidase-based tests for detection of urine glucose.
   c. Commonly used tests are all based on this phenomenon, but differ in the type of peroxide or chromogen used.
   d. For screening tests, evaluation should be performed on well-mixed, noncentrifuged samples.
3. Interpretation.
   a. Applied physiology.
      (1). RBC.
         (a). A few RBC are often present in the urine of normal dogs and cats.
         (b). Studies performed in human beings indicate that as many as 5 RBC/μL (5000/mL) are normal (so-called physiologic microhematuria). Similar quantitative determinations have apparently not been established for normal dogs, cats, or other animals.[75]
         (c). Refer to the review of RBC in Section VII C of this chapter.
      (2). Hemoglobin.
         (a). Hemoglobin is the oxygen-carrying pigment of RBC.
         (b). Normally, hemoglobin released into plasma is specifically bound to a carrier protein known as haptoglobin. The molecular characteristics of haptoglobin-hemoglobin complexes are such that they normally cannot pass through glomerular capillary walls into glomerular filtrate. Under normal conditions, plasma-derived hemoglobin does not escape into urine because the binding capacity of hemoglobin is not exceeded.
         (c). If abnormal intravascular hemolysis of sufficient magnitude to saturate the hemoglobin binding capacity of haptoglobin occurs (variably estimated to be approximately 50 to 250 mg/dL of hemoglobin in dogs, and 100 mg/dL of hemoglobin in man), the tetrameric form of hemoglobin (MW = 69,000) or its smaller dimers (MW = 32,000) may pass through glomerular capillary walls. At this concentration, the plasma is typically pink. If the quantity of filtered hemoglobin is in turn sufficient to exceed the reabsorptive capacity of the renal tubules, it will appear in urine.
         (d). The concentration of haptoglobin may vary considerably with different disease states.
         (e). Large quantities of free hemoglobin may also escape into urine if significant numbers of RBC undergo lysis within the excretory pathway. Hemolysis results when the urine specific gravity is lower than approximately 1.008 and increases in proportion to urine alkalinity (in vivo or in vitro).
      (3). Myoglobin.
         (a). Myoglobin is the oxygen-carrying pigment of muscle. Although similar to hemoglobin, it has distinctly different physical, chemical, and immunologic properties.
         (b). Myoglobinemia of sufficient magnitude to permit detectable myoglobinuria is not normal.
         (c). Myoglobinemia and myoglobinuria may occur as a result of traumatic, toxic, or ischemic injury and/or necrosis (rhabdomyolysis) to muscle cells.
         (d). Because of its molecular characteristics, myoglobin readily passes

through glomerular capillary walls (MW = 17,000). Unlike hemoglobin, it is not specifically bound to a plasma carrier protein. Therefore, detectable myoglobinuria may occur when the plasma concentration of myoglobin reaches 15 to 20 mg/dl. This concentration is insufficient to cause a color change in plasma.

b. Significance.
  (1). Always interpret test results in association with urine specific gravity.
  (2). Always interpret test results in association with microscopic evaluation of urine sediment.
  (3). A positive chemical test for blood associated with lack of identification of RBC in urine sediment might indicate:
    (a). Hemoglobinuria or myoglobinuria.
    (b). Generalized hemolysis following hematuria caused by dilute and/or alkaline urine.
    (c). A false-positive chemical reaction.
    (d). Mistaken identification of RBC in urine sediment.
  (4). A negative chemical test for blood associated with detection of RBC in urine sediment might indicate:
    (a). Use of outdated reagents.
    (b). Chemical evaluation of a poorly mixed or centrifuged urine sample.
    (c). Failure of small amounts of RBC to hemolyze.
    (d). Mistaken identity of RBC in urine sediment.
    (e). A false-negative chemical reaction.
  (5). Hematuria.
    (a). Hematuria is a nonspecific indicator of disease of the urinary tract. Once its presence has been verified, the next priority of clinical investigation is to localize its source.
    (b). Refer to the review of hematuria in Section VII C in this chapter.
  (6). Hemoglobinuria.
    (a). Hemoglobinuria may have a nonurinary or urinary origin.
    (b). Nonurinary hemoglobinuria is associated with hemoglobinemia and may be caused by:
      (1′). Transfusion reactions.
      (2′). Immune-mediated hemolytic anemia.
      (3′). Hemobartonellosis, babesiasis, ehrlichiasis, piroplasmosis, leptospirosis, or dirofilariasis (caval syndrome).
      (4′). Snake venom.
      (5′). Heat stroke.
      (6′). Hemolytic plant or chemical toxins.
      (7′). Severe hypophosphatemia.
      (8′). Disseminated intravascular coagulation.
      (9′). Phosphofructokinase deficiency (English springer spaniel).[38]
      (10′). Pyruvate kinase deficiency (in basenjis, beagles, and West Highland white terriers).[89]
      (11′). Drugs.
      (12′). Zinc-induced hemolytic disease.
    (c). Urinary hemoglobinuria is caused by extravascular hemolysis induced by dilute and/or alkaline urine.
  (7). Myoglobinuria.
    (a). Myoglobinuria has been an uncommonly encountered disorder in dogs and cats. This may be related, at least in part, to the fact that commonly used screening tests do not permit differentiation between myoglobinuria and hemoglobinuria.
    (b). Myoglobinuria should be interpreted in light of serum creatinine kinase activity.
    (c). Myoglobinuria may be caused by traumatic, toxic, or ischemic disorders of muscles. Examples include:
      (1′). Crush injuries.
      (2′). Heat stroke.
      (3′). Severe or prolonged muscular exertion.
      (4′). Snake bites.
      (5′). Electric shock.
      (6′). Idiopathic disorders.

F. PROTEIN

1. Indications.
  a. Definitions.[59,75]
    (1). *Proteinuria* is defined as the detection of protein in urine. Urine proteins are composed of variable quantities of plasma proteins, proteins derived from the urinary tract, and, depending on the method of collection, proteins derived from the genital tract. The term "proteinuria" is usually used to imply the presence of an abnormal quantity (>20 mg/kg/d) of protein in urine.[59] This laboratory finding is associated with a variety of causes. The term proteinuria is preferable to albuminuria because more than 40 proteins have been found in normal urine and may also be present in disease states associated with albuminuria.[6,79,80]
    (2). *Bence Jones proteinuria* is the presence of Bence Jones proteins in urine. These

small (MW = 22,000 to 44,000) proteins are named after the English physician Henry Bence Jones, who described their ability to precipitate when urine is gradually warmed (45 to 70°C) and subsequently to redissolve as urine is heated near boiling. Bence Jones proteins are identical to immunoglobulin light chains (compare with paraproteinuria) and may be observed in urine of patients with neoplastic disorders of plasma cells (multiple myeloma).[80]

(3). *Clinically significant proteinuria* warrants further investigation of its cause and biologic behavior. It is persistent and exceeds that associated with normal excretion.

(4). *Functional proteinuria* may occur in association with stress, exercise, fever, seizures, exposure to extremes of temperature, and venous congestion in the kidneys. Although glomerular function is temporarily altered, the process is rapidly reversible. The exact mechanisms are not clear but may be related to changes in glomerular blood flow or in the permeability of capillary walls of glomeruli. Although it must be differentiated from other forms of proteinuria, functional proteinuria has no apparent clinical significance.

(5). *Glomerular proteinuria* results from pathologic damage to various components of glomerular capillary walls. Glomerular proteinuria is typically persistent and usually involves albumin (66,000 daltons) and other proteins of high molecular weight (Table 7–6). Glomerular proteinuria may result in hypoalbuminemia.

(6). *Glomerular-overload proteinuria* (also called protein-overload proteinuria) has been experimentally induced in dogs by parenteral administration of large quantities of plasma proteins. As serum protein concentrations rise, large quantities of albumin and other proteins of high molecular weight are excreted in urine. Glomerular structure is reversibly altered during abnormal protein excretion. Glomerular-overload proteinuria should be considered as a cause of proteinuria in dogs with severe hyperproteinemia (>9 g/dl).[59]

(7). *Paraproteinuria* is a form of overload proteinuria that may occur when complete immunoglobulins, immunoglobulin fragments, macroglobulins, or cryoglobulins produced by neoplastic plasma cells reach abnormally high concentrations in plasma. If readily filtered through glomerular capillary walls, these proteins attain abnormally high concentrations in the urine.

(8). *Postglomerular proteinuria* results from protein loss arising within the urogenital tract but below the level of the glomerulus. Protein exudation is commonly the result of inflammatory, neoplastic, ischemic, or traumatic diseases. Examples include pyelonephritis, urocystitis, prostatitis, urolithiasis, acute tubular necrosis, and transitional cell carcinomas. Tubular proteinuria may also be considered a form of postglomerular proteinuria.

(9). *Preglomerular proteinuria* refers to proteinuria resulting from abnormalities in systems other than the urogenital tract. Examples include functional proteinuria and overload proteinuria.

TABLE 7–6
COMPARISON OF MOLECULAR WEIGHTS OR PLASMA PROTEINS INCLUDED IN AND EXCLUDED FROM GLOMERULAR ULTRAFILTRATE

Substance	Approximate Molecular Weight (daltons)	Presence in Glomerular Ultrafiltrate
Water	18	Present
Urea	60	Present
Creatinine	113	Present
Glucose	180	Present
β_2-microglobulin	11,800	Present
Lysozyme (muramidase)	14,400	Present
Myoglobin	17,600	Present
Bence Jones (monomer)	22,000	Present
α_1-microglobulin	27,000	Present
α_1-acid glycoprotein	40,000	Present
Bence Jones (dimer)	44,000	Present
Amylase	50,000	Present
Hemoglobin (tetramer)*	64,500	Sometimes present
Albumin	66,000	Sometimes present
Haptoglobin (monomer)	120,000	Absent
Immunoglobulin G	160,000	Absent
Immunoglobulin A (dimer)	300,000	Absent
Fibrinogen	400,000	Absent
α_2-macroglobulin	840,000	Absent
Immunoglobulin M	900,000	Absent

*Plasma hemoglobin is normally bound to haptoglobin. Once this binding capacity is saturated, dissociated hemoglobin readily passes through glomerular capillary walls as low-molecular-weight (32,000 daltons) dimmers.

(10). *Selective proteinuria* may occur in association with mild to moderate glomerular disease. Minimally damaged glomerular capillary walls allow passage of plasma proteins within a narrow range of molecular weights (approximately 60,000 to 80,000 daltons; Table 7–6). When glomerular lesions worsen, however, plasma proteins of all sizes and weights easily pass through the capillary walls (i.e., nonselective proteinuria).

(11). *Tubular proteinuria* is characterized by excretion of plasma proteins of low molecular weight (1500 to 45,000 daltons) as a result of defective resorption by proximal tubules. Protein electrophoresis may reveal prominent alpha and beta bands, which are characteristic of tubular proteinuria. In humans, excreted proteins typically include β_2-microglobulin, lysozyme, α-microglobulin, and α-acid glycoprotein in addition to many amino acids (Table 7–6).[80] Tubular diseases do not cause hypoalbuminemia.

(12). *Tubular-overload proteinuria* may be associated with excessive production of serum proteins of low molecular weight (<45,000 daltons). Such proteins easily pass through glomerular capillary walls and overload tubular resorptive mechanisms. The result is protein loss through the kidneys. Examples of this condition include hemoglobinuria, myoglobinuria, and paraproteinuria.

b. The quantity and composition of urine proteins vary in normal and abnormal states.

c. Evaluation of urine for protein is included as a part of complete routine urinalysis, because when interpreted in conjunction with other clinical and laboratory findings, test results often aid in detection, localization, and occasionally specific identification of underlying disorders.

2. Methodology.[74,75]

a. Overview.

(1). Urine proteins are more difficult to measure and identify than are serum proteins because:

(a). Urine proteins are often present in small quantities.

(b). The sample-to-sample variation in the amount and composition of urine protein is large.

(c). Protein in urine is derived from plasma, the urinary tract, and sometimes the genital tract.

(d). Protein degradation products are concentrated by the kidney and may be measured along with intact proteins.

(2). Qualitative, semiquantitative, and quantitative methods are available for analysis of protein.

(a). Most tests employed in conjunction with routine urinalyses provide qualitative and semiquantitative results.

(b). Methods to identify and quantify urine proteins, including protein electrophoresis, gel filtration, and immunochemical techniques, have been described.[80]

b. Sample collection.

(1). As with all tests of routine urinalyses, analyses should only be performed on samples collected prior to administration of diagnostic or therapeutic agents.

(2). Although screening tests for protein may be performed on uncentrifuged samples, the test should be repeated on the supernatant of centrifuged samples to eliminate positive results caused by proteinaceous material commonly found in urine sediment (e.g., RBC, WBC, epithelial cells, casts).

(3). Either fresh or refrigerated samples may be used. In one study, no significant change in protein concentration was detected in urine samples preserved by refrigeration at 4 to 10°C for 4 weeks.

c. Sulfosalicylic acid turbidometric test. This test is based on the fact that sulfosalicylic acid precipitates urine protein with resultant turbidity that is approximately equal to the quantity of protein present.

d. Dipstick colorimetric test. These tests are based on the phenomenon called the "protein error of pH indicator dyes." In simple terms, the test is based on the ability of amino groups of proteins to bind with and alter the color of some acid-base indicators even though their pH remains constant.

(1). Binding of the dye depends on the number of free amino groups of each protein.

(2). Albumin has more free amino groups than do globulins, hemoglobin, Bence Jones proteins, and mucoproteins. One study found that the development of the same color change as that caused by a certain albumin concentration required a globulin concentration two times as high and a mucoprotein concentration three times as high.[36]

(3). Because of reduced capacity to detect globulins and Bence Jones proteins, test results are semiquantitative.

e. Bence Jones proteinuria.
   (1). Electrophoretic and immunoelectrophoretic methods provide the best results.
   (2). The Bence Jones heat test is based on the unusual thermosolubility properties of Bence Jones proteins.
      (a). Albumin and globulins do not coagulate and precipitate out of solution until they are heated to a temperature of 56 to 70°C. The degree of turbidity may increase as the temperature rises.
      (b). Bence Jones proteins precipitate at 40 to 60°C and redissolve as the temperature rises to 85 to 100°C. As the temperature cools, Bence Jones proteins may reprecipitate at 40 to 60°C and redissolve at lower temperatures. Because of this unique heat solubility, Bence Jones proteins are sometimes called "pyroglobulins."

3. Interpretation (See Chapter 4, Clinical Algorithms and Data Bases for Urinary Tract Disorders.)
   a. Overview.
      (1). The interpretation of proteinuria depends on:
         (a). Knowledge of types and quantities of proteins normally present in urine.
         (b). Conceptual understanding of methods used to detect urine proteins.
         (c). The cause and pathophysiology of disorders associated with proteinuria.
      (2). Collect urine samples for detection of urine protein prior to the administration of diagnostic and therapeutic agents.
      (3). Because proteinuria may be transient and of little clinical significance, verify its existence and persistence before pursuing potentially costly and time-consuming diagnostic plans to determine its cause and before initiating therapy to control or correct it.
      (4). Always interpret qualitative and semiquantitative tests in light of urine specific gravity.
         (a). Most screening tests for proteinuria are performed on a small volume of urine without regard to the rate of formation of urine or total volume.
         (b). For example, mild proteinuria (1+) in the presence of a low specific gravity (i.e., SG = 1.005) implies a greater loss of protein than does mild proteinuria (1+) in a more concentrated sample (i.e., SG = 1.040).
      (5). Before considering the underlying cause of significant proteinuria, try to localize its source.
         (a). Localization is aided by knowledge of the method of urine collection.
         (b). Localization is aided by knowledge of the composition of urine sediment (Table 7–7).
      (6). Because of significant discrepancies among various laboratory tests for proteinuria, clinical significance of results should always be interpreted in association with other clinical and laboratory findings.
      (7). The absence of proteinuria does not eliminate the presence of renal disease or renal failure. Likewise, the severity of proteinuria is not a reliable index of the severity or reversibility of the underlying disorder.
   b. Specificity of tests.[74,75]
      (1). Sulfosalicylic acid turbidometric test.
         (a). Sulfosalicylic acid precipitates urine protein with resultant turbidity that is approximately equal to the quantity of protein present.
         (b). False-positive test results may be obtained if urine turbidity is caused by nonprotein substances. Positive test results may be overestimated if the degree of urine turbidity is augmented by nonprotein substances.
         (c). Radiopaque contrast agents that are excreted in urine give a false-positive reaction; radiopaque contrast agents also increase urine specific gravity.
         (d). Massive dosages of penicillin, cephalothin, cephaloridine, and sulfisoxazole (Gantrisin) have been reported to give a false-positive reaction for protein with sulfosalicyclic acid in man.
         (e). Highly buffered alkaline urine may give false-negative reactions (especially if a 3% rather than a 5% solution is used).
         (f). Because measurement of the degree of turbidity (i.e., 1+ to 4+) is not standardized, variability in test results between individuals and different laboratories may occur.
         (g). The preservative thymol may give a false-positive protein reaction with this test.
         (h). Unlike colorimetric tests, sulfosalicylic acid detects Bence Jones proteins in urine.
      (2). Dipstick colorimetric test.
         (a). Results are not affected by urine turbidity.

TABLE 7–7
EXAMPLES OF DIFFERENT CAUSES OF PROTEINURIA

	Cause				
Factors	**Normal Concentrated Sample**	**Contaminated with Hypaque***	**Glomerular Disease**	**Urinary Tract Infection**	**Hemorrhage**
Color	Yellow	Yellow	Yellow	Yellow	Reddish
Turbidity	Clear	Slightly Cloudy	Clear	Cloudy	Cloudy
Specific Gravity	1.058	1.068	1.024	1.020	1.030
pH	6.5	6.0	7.0	7.5	7.0
Glucose	Negative	Negative	Negative	Negative	Negative
Acetone	Negative	Negative	Negative	Negative	Negative
Bilirubin	Trace	Negative	Negative	Negative	Negative
Protein	1+	3+	4+	2+	2+
Occult Blood	Negative	Negative	Negative	3+	4+
RBC/HPF	1-3	0-1	Negative	100+	TNTC
WBC/HPF	0-2	None	1-3	TNTC	3-5
Casts/LPF	None	None	Occasionally Hyaline	None	None
Epithelial Cells	Occasionally	Occasionally	Occasionally	Many	Moderate
Bacteria	None	None	None	Many rods	None
Crystals	None	None	None	Struvite	Occasionally struvite

Key: HPF = high-power field; LPF = low-power field; RBC = red blood cells; WBC = white blood cells; TNTC = too numerous to count.
*Sulfosalicylic acid.

(b). The urine pH of all domestic animals is 4.5 to 5.0 or higher. Changes of pH within physiologic ranges of dilute urine usually do not affect test results. Highly alkaline urine samples, especially when concentrated, may induce false-positive results if the citrate buffer system is overcome and a shift in pH occurs. This problem may be corrected by reducing the pH of extremely alkaline or concentrated samples to 7 with an appropriate aliquot of acid reagent (HC1).

(c). False-positive results could occur if the strip was allowed to remain in the urine sample for a sufficient period for the citrate buffer to be leached out.

(d). As previously described, colorimetric reagents are more sensitive to albumin than to globulins, including hemoglobin. They may not detect Bence Jones proteins unless they are present in large quantities. Negative results are usually significant with the notable exception of pure Bence Jones proteinuria.

(e). False-negative results may occur if a sample is acidified following collection as the protein may precipitate out of solution.

(f). Benzalkonium (Zephiran, Winthrop), a cationic quaternary ammonium surface-acting antimicrobial agent, and chlorhexidine, may give false-positive results if sufficient residues remain in collection containers.[39]

(g). Phenazopyridine may cause false-positive reactions with Chemstrips.

(h). Infusion of polyvinylpyrrolidone as a plasma expander has been reported to cause false-positive reactions with Chemstrips in man.

c. Sensitivity of tests.

(1). Sulfosalicyclic acid turbidometric test.

(a). The range of sensitivity varies between trace (5 mg/dL) and 5000 mg/dL or greater.

(b). Consult Section VI, F, 3 of this chapter for additional information.

(2). Dipstick colorimetric tests.

(a). The range of sensitivity varies between trace (approximately 5 to 20 mg/dl) and 1000 mg/dL or greater. Consult Section VI, F, 3 of this chapter for additional information.

(b). Trace positive results are commonly encountered in concentrated urine samples obtained from normal dogs and cats.

(3). Reactions of 4+ detected by colorimetric dipstick and turbidometric tests may be as little as 0.5 to 1.0 g/dL. The quantity of protein present beyond this quantity cannot be estimated, however.

(a). We have evaluated dogs with generalized glomerular disease characterized by 4+ dipstick and sulfosalicylic test reactions that have excreted as little as 1 g and as much as 35 g of protein in their urine per 24 hours.

(b). Quantitation of 4+ screening test reactions for urine protein requires use of urine protein/creatinine ratios, or determination of the quantity of protein excreted in urine over 24 hours.

d. Applied physiology.

(1). Renal handling of protein.

(a). Although the precise mechanism by which proteins are handled by the kidneys is still not completely understood, the major variables involved are:

(1′). Glomerular selective permeability.

(2′). Tubular reabsorption and disposal of absorbed proteins.

(b). Glomerular permeability.

(1′). The capillary walls of glomeruli are semipermeable filters that retain most of the plasma proteins in the vascular compartment. Glomerular capillary walls are composed of the following three layers: capillary endothelial cells, noncellular basement membranes, and cytoplasmic processes (extensions) of renal epithelial cells (podocytes). The processes wrap around portions of capillary loops. Collectively, these three layers form the functional units (the so-called filtration barrier) of glomeruli.

(2′). As blood flows through a glomerulus, a large quantity of an acellular, low-protein ultrafiltrate is formed. The degree to which individual proteins are normally filtered through glomerular capillary walls is a function of their plasma concentration and their molecular size, shape, and charge.[20] In other words, the primary factors that influence the movement of proteins across glomerular capillaries are the size-selective properties of glomeruli, the charge-selective properties of glomeruli, and the hemodynamic forces operating across glomerular capillary walls.

(3′). In general, transport of protein molecules through glomerular capillary walls progressively diminishes as protein size (as estimated from molecular weight) increases (Table 7–6). Normally, proteins of high molecular weight (e.g., immunoglobulin M, which has a molecular weight of 900,000 daltons) do not appear in glomerular ultrafiltrate in detectable amounts.

(4′). Even though plasma contains high concentrations of albumin, small quantities of albumin are normally present in glomerular ultrafiltrate partly because albumin has a molecular weight of approximately 66,000 to 68,000 daltons. In addition, fixed negative charges on glomerular capillary walls impede the passage of negatively charged plasma molecules, such as albumin. Plasma proteins that have molecular weights of 1500 to 45,000 daltons pass through more readily but appear in urine in lower concentrations because of their relatively low concentrations in plasma and because of tubular recovery from glomerular filtrate.

(5′). Although hemoglobin has a small molecular size, it normally does not enter glomerular ultrafiltrate because it is usually bound to haptoglobin, which is a larger plasma protein (Table 7–6). This phenomenon is called protein binding.

(6′). Peptides (including several hormones) appear in glomerular ultrafiltrate, but are reabsorbed by the renal tubules.

(c). Tubular reabsorption and disposal of absorbed proteins.

(1′). Normally only a small quantity of protein is present in glomerular filtrate. In a study in dogs, the quantity of protein in proximal tubular fluid was 10 to 15 mg/dl or less.[24]

(2′). The proportion of filtered plasma proteins ultimately excreted in urine depends on the extent of resorption by renal tubules. Albumin constitutes approximately 40 to 60% of the total protein excreted in urine because it is not completely resorbed by renal tubule cells.[45,83] In contrast, plasma proteins of low molecular weight are actively resorbed from tubular filtrate, catabolized by proximal tubular cells, and returned to the blood as amino acids. The renal tubules also degrade a variety of peptide hormones, including parathormone, insulin, growth hormone, and thyrotropic hormone. Distal renal tubule cells secrete small amounts of protein (Tamm-Horsfall mucoprotein and possibly secretory immunoglobulin A), which add to the final urine protein concentration.[80,87]

(2). Proteins originating from the urinary tract.

(a). Forty to 60% of the proteins normally present in urine originate from the distal tubules and collecting ducts (Tamm-Horsfall mucoprotein), the epithelial lining of the lower urinary tract, and the genital tract.[10] Tamm-Horsfall protein has been reported at a concentration of 0.5 to 1.0 mg/dL in canine urine.[83]

(b). The urothelium may also secrete immunoglobulins, especially immunoglobulin A, as a part of local host defenses against ascending urinary tract infections.[80]

e. Normal urine protein concentration

(1). Few investigators have performed controlled studies of numerous dogs and cats to assess normal daily excretion of protein in urine (Table 7–8). Additional confusion concerning normal protein excretion exists because various methods used for protein determination give significantly different results. In one study, for example, the Coomassie brilliant blue method consistently yielded higher protein concentrations than were obtained by use of the trichloroacetic acid ponceau-S method on identical samples.[45] Differences were greater with higher protein concentrations.

(2). Likewise, two groups of investigators using the same method to determine urine protein concentration (Coomassie brilliant blue method) reported different values for normal dogs. Grauer and colleagues reported that young adult beagles excreted 0.6 to 5.1 mg/kg/d of protein.[40] This value is lower than that reported by McCaw and associates, who determined that normal canine outpatients ranging in age from 0.5 to 10 years excreted 1.8 to 22.4 mg/kg/d of protein.[64] Using the trichloroacetic acid Ponceau-S method for urine protein determination, Center and co-workers and White and colleagues found similar results (maximum protein excretion was 11.7 mg/kg/d).[14,98]

(3). Biewenga and associates evaluated 29

TABLE 7–8
DAILY URINE PROTEIN EXCRETION IN NORMAL CATS AND DOGS

Protein (mg/kg/d)				
Range	**Mean**	**Method of Analysis**	**Species**	**Number Evaluated**
0.6-5.1	2.3	Coomassie brilliant blue[40]	Canine	16
1.8-22.4	7.66	Coomassie brilliant blue[62]	Canine	14
0.2-7.7	2.45	Trichloroacetic acid ponceau-S[14]	Canine	19
1.9-11.7	4.76	Trichloroacetic acid ponceau-S[98]	Canine	8
2.7-23.2	6.6	Trichloroacetic acid ponceau-S[7]	Canine	29
4.55-28.3	13.9	Trichloroacetic acid ponceau-S[23]	Canine	17
2.99-8.88	4.93	Coomassie brilliant blue[1]	Feline	30

clinically normal dogs of various breeds, sexes, and ages and reported a range of 2.7 to 23.3 mg/kg/d of protein excretion.[7] Although the subjects were clinically and biochemically normal, immunofluorescent staining methodology revealed immune deposits of glomeruli in about half of the dogs. The significance of glomerular immune deposits in clinically normal dogs was not determined.

(4). Seventeen dogs (6 males and 11 females) evaluated by DiBartola and co-workers had urine protein excretion of 4.55 to 28.3 mg/kg/d.[23] Dogs with active urine sediment (more than five WBC per high-power field [HPF] or more than five RBC per high-power field [HPF] or both), however, were included in this group; their inclusion may account for protein excretion values higher than those reported by other investigators. The 24-hour urine protein excretion by male dogs (16.5 ± 10 mg/kg/d) was not significantly different from that of female dogs (12.4 ± 6.1 mg/kg/d) in the small sample of dogs evaluated.

(5). On the basis of these observations, we concluded that a urine protein concentration in adult dogs in excess of 20 mg/kg/d evaluated by either the Coomassie brilliant blue method or the trichloroacetic acid ponceau-S method is abnormal.[59] This value corresponds to a urine protein-creatinine ratio between 0.67 to 0.96, according to the linear regression equations established for dogs.[40,64,98]

(6). Hoskins and colleagues found that mean 24-hour urine protein excretion values for 4- to 30-week-old kittens (range, 2.54 ± 1.81 mg/kg at 4 weeks to 11.39 ± 7.61 mg/kg at 14 weeks) varied from week to week of age.[48] Urine protein was determined by the Coomassie brilliant blue dye-binding method.

(7). The sensitivity of commonly used tests for proteinuria is below the protein content of most normal urine samples.
   (a). Therefore, persistent proteinuria of sufficient quantity to be detected by usual laboratory tests should be investigated.
   (b). Trace and 1+ results are commonly observed with colorimetric dipstick tests used in concentrated urine samples obtained from normal dogs and cats (see Table 7–11). If reagent-strip tests are used as screening tests for proteinuria, positive findings may be confirmed with a test based on different biochemical reactions, such as the sulfosalicylic acid test.

f. Abnormal urine protein concentration
   (1). Proteinuria may be classified (localized) as preglomerular, glomerular, or postglomerular.[59]
   (2). Preglomerular proteinuria
      (a). Preglomerular proteinuria results from abnormalities of systems other than the urogenital tract. Preglomerular proteinuria can be further subdivided into functional proteinuria and overload proteinuria.
      (b). Functional proteinuria is sometimes associated with strenuous exercise, extremes of heat and cold, stress, fever, seizures, or venous congestion.[18] In humans, functional proteinuria apparently results from alterations in glomerular blood flow or in permeability of glomerular capillary walls.[21] Decreased tubular resorption of filtered proteins can also occur.[82] Although glomerular function is temporarily altered, the process is rapidly reversible. Functional proteinuria typically consists of mild, transient albuminuria.
      (c). Tubular-overload proteinuria is associated with excessive production of plasma proteins of low molecular weight (e.g., immunoglobulin fragments, myoglobin, or hemoglobin) or the reduction in available binding sites on carrier molecules (e.g., haptoglobin for hemoglobin).[28,38,71,94] When plasma concentrations of proteins that weigh less than 45,000 daltons (and that therefore easily pass through glomerular capillary walls) are increased, the resorptive mechanisms of the tubules become overloaded. Detectable quantities of protein then appear in urine.
      (d). Glomerular-overload proteinuria (also called protein-overload proteinuria) has been experimentally induced in dogs and rats by parenteral administration of large quantities of plasma proteins.[54,92,96] When plasma protein concentrations were greater than 9 g/dL, large quantities of albumin and other proteins of high molecular weight were excreted in urine. Alterations in glomerular structure were detected in rats during episodes of hyperproteinemia and proteinuria.[69,97] Glomerular abnormalities consisted of

numerous protein resorption droplets, as well as swelling and obliteration of the foot processes of epithelial cells. These changes completely reversed after resolution of hyperproteinemia and proteinuria. Glomerular-overload proteinuria should be considered as a cause of proteinuria in animals with severe hyperproteinemia (e.g., in animals with multiple myeloma or ehrlichiosis or after overzealous administration of plasma).[11,13,14,62,63,68,88,90]

(3). Glomerular proteinuria
   (a). Glomerular proteinuria is the most commonly recognized and potentially most severe form of proteinuria.
   (b). Glomerular proteinuria results from disease-induced alterations of glomerular capillary barriers, which normally prevent loss of larger plasma proteins into glomerular infiltrate. Damage can be characterized by loss of the fixed negative charges of glomerular capillaries. In addition, structural changes in filtration barriers may result from primary disorders (e.g., antiglomerular basement membrane disease, inflammation, or neoplasia) or secondary disorders (e.g., immune complex deposition, amyloidosis, hyperfiltration, or hyperadrenocorticism).
   (c). Protein in the urine of patients with these forms of glomerular dysfunction primarily consists of albumin and varying quantities of proteins of high molecular weight (e.g., immunoglobulins and coagulation proteins).
   (d). Although the origin of protein cannot be consistently predicted on the basis of the quantity of protein detected by urinalysis, persistent proteinuria in moderate to large quantities that occurs in the absence of hematuria or pyuria indicates generalized glomerular disease.

(4). Postglomerular proteinuria
   (a). In postglomerular proteinuria, plasma or tissue proteins gain access to urine after it has passed through the glomeruli.
   (b). Postglomerular proteinuria can result from normal genital secretions. It may also result if the epithelial linings of the urogenital tract are disrupted by inflammation, neoplasia, ischemia, or trauma.
   (c). Postglomerular proteinuria occasionally results from defects in proximal tubular resorption of proteins of between 1500 and 45,000 daltons; this condition is called tubular proteinuria.[43] In humans, almost 50 proteins, including enzymes, polypeptide hormones, immunoglobulin fragments, and microglobulins, have been identified in patients with tubular proteinuria.[80] This form of proteinuria is typically mild and may not be detected by qualitative screening tests for proteinuria. Familial (e.g., Fanconi syndrome) and acquired (e.g., gentamicin toxicity) causes of tubular proteinuria have occurred in dogs.[9,12,26]
   (d). Postglomerular proteinuria can usually be differentiated from glomerular proteinuria by evaluating clinical signs and urine sediment. Postglomerular proteinuria is often associated with leukocyturia or erythrocyturia or both; in the urine of patients with glomerular proteinuria, these cells are typically absent.
   (e). A combination of glomerular proteinuria and postglomerular proteinuria may be difficult to recognize. The combination may have been present if cell-free proteinuria persists after successful treatment of postglomerular inflammation or hemorrhage. If successful treatment of postglomerular proteinuria is not possible, detection of high concentrations of albumin in urine should prompt consideration of concurrent glomerular dysfunction, especially if hypoalbuminemia is also detected.

(5). Pseudoproteinuria (false proteinuria)
   (a). False-positive reactions for protein detected by colorimetric dipsticks include:
      (1′). Highly alkaline buffered urine as might result following administration of alkalinizing drugs or following degradation of urea to ammonia by urease-producing bacteria.
      (2′). Loss of citrate buffer from the dipstick as a result of prolonged immersion in the urine sample.
      (3′). Contamination of the sample with quaternary ammonium compounds.
   (b). False-positive reactions for protein detected by sulfosalicylic acid include:

(1′). Excessively turbid urine prior to initiation of the test.
(2′). Radiopaque contrast agents excreted in urine.[31]
(3′). Excretion of large quantities of penicillin, cephaloridine, or sulfisoxazole.
(4′). Contamination of the test sample with thymol, a urine preservative.
(5′). Coprecipitation of crystals caused by a change in urine pH induced by sulfosalicylic acid.

(6). False-negative proteinuria.
(a). False-negative reactions for protein detected by colorimetric dipsticks include:
(1′). Low to moderate amounts of Bence Jones proteins.
(2′). Examination of a urine sample that has been acidified following collection (protein precipitates as a result of acidity).
(b). False-negative reactions for protein detected by sulfosalicylic acid include:
(1′). Evaluation of highly buffered alkaline urine.
(2′). Inability to read the results because of urine turbidity prior to testing.

G. Nitrite.

1. In human beings, detection of reduction in urinary nitrate to nitrite by certain bacterial pathogens is used as a screening test for significant bacteriuria.
2. The nitrite reduction test does not detect significant bacteriuria in canine or feline urine samples. Ascorbic acid, a metabolite normally present in canine and feline urine, inhibits the nitrite test reaction.[51]

VII. URINE SEDIMENT

A. Indications.

1. The value of microscopic examination of urine sediment in the interpretation of urinalysis is comparable to microscopic examination of blood smears in the interpretation of hemograms. Meaningful interpretation of color, specific gravity, turbidity, protein, occult blood, and pH test results of routine analyses depends on knowledge of the composition of urine sediment. For example, a moderate degree of proteinuria in the absence of significant amounts of RBC and WBC usually indicates proteinuria of glomerular origin. In contrast, a moderate degree of proteinuria associated with hematuria and pyuria indicates an inflammatory response somewhere along the urinary and/or genital tracts. If proteinuria is detected without knowledge of hematuria and/or pyuria, the clinician may erroneously assume that protein has originated from lesions in glomeruli or tubules.
2. Examination of urine sediment may be considered as a form of biopsy (exfoliative cytology). Like other techniques of exfoliative cytology, the morphologic characteristics of cells, casts, crystals, and bacteria provide useful information, but frequently do not permit establishment of a specific diagnosis. Although disease states may be established on the basis of positive findings, they cannot always be eliminated by exclusion on the basis of negative findings. Therefore, the results of examination of urine sediment must be interpreted in combination with other clinical data, including the physical and chemical composition of urine.

B. Methodology.[75]

1. To minimize variations in sediment examination from sample to sample, we recommend that all steps in preparation be consistently performed in a standard fashion. Even with standardization of technique, reproducible semiquantitative results are often difficult to obtain.
2. The procedure to be followed in preparation of urine sediment for microscopic examination with a bright-field microscope is outlined in Table 7–9.
   a. Collection of specimen.
      (1). Every effort should be made to collect an uncontaminated urine sample in an appropriate container.

TABLE 7–9
PROCEDURE FOR PREPARATION OF URINE SEDIMENT

1. Collect urine specimen in appropriate container.
2. If analysis cannot be performed within 30 minutes from time of collection, refrigerate sample.
3. Thoroughly mix specimen, and transfer a standard volume (we prefer 5 mL) to a conical-tip centrifuge tape.
4. Centrifuge the sample for 3 to 5 minutes at 15000 to 2000 rpm.
5. Remove the supernatant with a rubber-topped disposable pipette or by decanting, and save it for chemical analysis. Allow a standard volume (approximately 1/2 mL) of supernatant to remain in the test tube.
6. Thoroughly resuspend the urine sediment in the remaining supernatant by agitation of the tube or "finger-flipping" of the tube.
7. Transfer a drop of reconstituted sediment to a microscope slide with a rubber-topped disposable pipette, and place a coverslip over it.
8. Subdue the intensity of the microscope light by lowering the condenser and closing the iris diaphragm.
9. Systematically examine the entire specimen under the coverslip with the low-power objective, assessing the quantity and type (casts, cells, crystals) of sediment.
10. Examine the sediment with the high-power objective to identify the structure of elements and to detect bacteria.
11. Record the results.

(2). Good test results cannot be obtained from poor samples.

(3). Consult Chapter 5, Techniques of Urine Collection and Preservation, for details.

b. Preservation of sample.

(1). Because the nature of urine sediment may be altered to a variable and unpredictable degree following elimination from the body, analysis of a freshly voided sample provides the most reliable results.

(2). One of the most detrimental alterations that occurs when urine is allowed to remain at room temperature following collection is a variable increase in pH secondary to proliferation of urease-producing bacterial contaminants and escape of CO_2 from urine into the atmosphere.

(a). Alkaline urine promotes disruption, fragmentation, or lysis of RBC, casts, and especially WBC, and may alter crystal composition as well.

(b). These changes may be minimized by the addition of preservatives, such as toluene or formaldehyde, but preservatives interfere with one or more results.

(3). Delay in examination may also result in loss of cellular detail caused by degenerative mechanisms.

(4). If urinalysis cannot be performed within 30 minutes following collection, the sample should be refrigerated to minimize changes caused by bacterial contaminants and autolysis. Refrigerated samples are suitable for examination several hours following collection.

(5). Consult Chapter 5, Techniques of Urine Collection and Preservation, for additional information.

c. Mix specimen and transfer to centrifuge tube.

(1). Failure to adequately mix a urine specimen before removing an aliquot for centrifugation may result in loss of formed elements that rapidly settle to the bottom of the container.

(2). Although some authors recommend the transfer of 10 to 15 mL of urine to a conical-tip centrifuge tube, the actual volume is not critical. More important is the use of a consistent volume of urine each time, so that the diagnostician can develop some perspective of normal and abnormal findings at that volume. We routinely use 5 mL of urine because of difficulties associated with consistently obtaining larger volumes from animals. The volume of urine should be recorded on the urinalysis results form.

(3). Although round-tip centrifuge tubes may be used, conical-tip tubes are recommended because they facilitate removal of the supernatant by decanting.

d. Centrifuge sample.

(1). The sample should be centrifuged at a relatively low rate of speed (1500 to 2000 rpm) for approximately 5 minutes. Centrifugation at high rpm or for prolonged periods may induce artifacts in cells, casts, and other structures.

(2). The duration of centrifugation is less important than the speed of centrifugation, although both should be standardized.

(3). If the urine is centrifuged at high speeds, the sediment may become distorted as a result of packing in the bottom of the tube. When the packed sediment is forcefully resuspended in the supernatant, the formed elements may fragment.

e. Remove the supernatant.

(1). The supernatant should be carefully removed from the test tube by decanting (invert the tube and pour off the supernatant) or with a rubber-topped disposable pipette and should be saved for chemical determinations. Care should be used not to disturb the sediment.

(2). Because the concentration of formed elements detected by microscopy is significantly influenced by the volume of supernatant allowed to remain in the test tube, every effort should be made to standardize this portion of the procedure. One-half milliliter is usually sufficient and usually remains following decanting of conical-tip centrifuge tubes.

f. Resuspend the sediment.

(1). This portion of the procedure is sometimes referred to as "reconstitution" of the sediment.

(2). Sediment may not be grossly visible. Whether or not a button of sediment in the bottom of the centrifuge is observed, the tube should be thoroughly mixed with the supernatant by flipping the tube with a finger or by gentle aspiration and discharge from a disposable pipette.

(3). If the sediment is not thoroughly reconstituted, heavy elements, such as casts, may remain in the bottom of the tube and escape detection.

(4). If special water-soluble stains, such as Sternheimer-Malbin stain or Sedistain, are to be used, they should be added to the sediment at this time. One drop of stain is usually mixed with one drop of sediment.

g. Preparation of microscopic slide.

(1). A drop of reconstituted sediment should be transferred to a clean microscope slide with a rubber-topped pipette. The drop to be examined should be sufficiently large to include the entire area covered by the coverslip, but not so large as to float the coverslip.

(2). A coverslip should then be placed over the preparation. The use of a glass coverslip is recommended because it:

(a). Promotes the formation of a uniformly thin layer of sediment.

(b). Prevents contact of the microscope objectives with the sediment.

(c). Permits examination of the sediment under oil immersion when necessary.

(d). Reduces the rate of evaporation of water.

(e). Minimizes movement of sediment.

(3). A short time should be allowed for heavier elements to gravitate to the surface of the microscope slide and for fat droplets to float to the undersurface of the coverslip.

h. Subdue the intensity of the bright-field microscope light.

(1). The refractive index of many formed elements in unstained urine sediment is similar to that of the surrounding medium. Therefore, the intensity of the microscope should be subdued to improve contrast.

(2). If necessary, the intensity of the light may be increased. If excessive light is used, however, many objects may be obscured.

(3). Reduced illumination may be accomplished by lowering the microscope condenser and/or closing the substage iris diaphragm.

(4). Visualization of formed and nonformed elements in the sediment also is aided by continuously varying the fine focus adjustment of the microscope while the sediment is being examined.

(5). Phase-contrast microscopy and polarized light microscopy may also be considered to enhance visualization of urine sediment.

i. Examination under low-power magnification.

(1). Initially the entire sample should be systematically scanned with the aid of the low-power objective (10X) to assess the quantity of sediment present and the suitability of the preparation.

(2). Good preparations are characterized by a relatively even distribution of elements without excessive overlapping.

(3). If the amount of material in the sediment appears to be excessive, it may be diluted with supernatant or physiologic saline solution. This dilution alters semiquantitative interpretation of results, however. If excessive quantities of RBC are still causing interference with evaluation of the sediment, addition of a 5% acetic acid solution will cause RBC hemolysis without destroying most other elements. However, it may alter urine crystals.

(4). Semiquantitation of the contents of the sediment may be obtained by counting structures in at least 10 fields and averaging the number of individual elements seen per low-power field (LPF) (same concept applies to counting per high-power field).

(5). Examination under low-power magnification aids in the detection of elements that may be present in only a few microscopic fields (i.e., casts, crystals, bile pigments).

(6). Heavier elements, especially casts, often accumulate near the edges of the coverslip when excess fluid is placed on the slide.

j. Examination under high-power magnification. Following examination of the specimen under low-power magnification, it should be examined under high-power magnification (40X). With the aid of increased magnification, the morphologic characteristics of cells (WBC, RBC, epithelial cells) and casts can often be seen. The presence of bacteria, yeasts, and lipid droplets may also be detected.

k. If the uncentrifuged urine specimen was visibly bloody or very turbid, repeat the dipstick chemical analysis on the supernatant.

l. Sources of technical error.

To obtain meaningful results, avoid the following:

(1). Examination of a contaminated sample.

(2). Examination of unrefrigerated stale urine.

(3). Failure to thoroughly mix the sample prior to examination.

(4). Allowing the sediment to dry on the microscope slide.

(5). Use of too much microscope light.

(6). Careless reconstitution of sediment following centrifugation.

(7). Centrifugation at excessive speeds.

(8). Use of dirty or scratched microscope slides and coverslips.

(9). Use of low-power or high-power magnification only.

m. Stains for urine sediment.

(1). Although with experience one can usually evaluate most details of formed elements in urine sediment in an unstained preparation with proper preparation and illumination, some elements may be more easily recognized following staining. Even with stains, however, all elements in urine sediment cannot be identified.

(2). Several stains have been recommended.

(a). For general use (wet stains):

(1′). Sternheimer-Malbin stain and modified Sternheimer-Malbin stain.[91]

(2′). Sedistain (Clay-Adams).

(b). For cellular elements (air-dried preparations):

(1′). New methylene blue.

(2′). Wright's stain.

(3′). Dif-Quick.

(c). For special needs:

(1′). Gram's stain (for confirmation and classification of bacteria).

(2′). Sudan III or IV, or oil Red O (for lipids).

(3). Consult textbooks of clinical pathology for specific recommendations concerning preparation of stains, fixation of specimens, and staining technique.

(4). If a sufficient quantity of sediment is available, a portion should be saved for unstained examination, and a portion saved for staining.

(5). Use of such stains as Sedistain or Sternheimer-Malbin stain dilute the sediment and alter semiquantitative evaluation of results.

(6). Some stains applied to air-dried films of sediment, such as Gram's or Wright's stain, may require special preparation, such as heat fixation or protein coating of slides. These procedures require several staining and washing steps and may result in loss of variable quantities of sediment from the slide.

C. Interpretation.

1. Overview.

a. Meaningful evaluation of urine sediment depends on recognition of cellular elements, casts, crystals, and other objects. Evaluation of urine sediment is often more difficult than evaluation of blood smears or cytologic preparations from other organs of the body, partly because cells may originate from the vascular system, interstitial tissue, or epithelial surfaces located in different areas of the urinary and/or genital tract. In addition, urine is an "unphysiologic" medium for most cells. Cells present in urine are subjected for varying periods to osmotic and pH changes that may be markedly different from levels in their normal environment. They may also be exposed to enzymes or toxic concentrations of other metabolites excreted in urine or produced by pathogenic organisms. As a result, they undergo changes in size, structure, and transparency.

b. To minimize degenerative changes caused by exposure of elements in sediment to urine, urine may be centrifuged as soon as possible after voiding, followed by immediate examination of the sediment. Alternatively, it may be maintained with an appropriate preservative.

c. Although with experience one can usually evaluate most details of formed elements in urine sediment in an unstained preparation with proper microscopic illumination, some elements may be more easily recognized by staining with Sternheimer-Malbin, new methylene blue, or Sedistain. Consult Section VIIB of this chapter for additional information.

d. Because knowledge of urine specific gravity provides useful information regarding the relative concentrations of water and elements in urine sediment, urine sediment results should always be interpreted in conjunction with urine specific gravity. In addition, dilute urine (SG = <1.008) may cause cell lysis.

e. The significance of cells, bacteria, and amorphous debris should always be interpreted with knowledge of the method of sample collection. Cells and bacteria in noncatheterized samples may originate from the urethra and/or genital tract, as well as from the bladder, ureters, or kidneys. RBC in catheterized samples or samples obtained by digital compression of the bladder may occur as a result of trauma induced by the collection technique. Knowledge of collection method is an important aid in localization of abnormalities.

f. Normal versus abnormal.

(1). Qualitative results (based on centrifugation of 5 mL of urine).

(a). Normal urine sediment may contain (see Table 7–11):

(1′). A few RBC (<5/HPF?)

(2′). A few WBC (<5/HPF?)

(3′). Transitional, squamous, and/or tubular epithelial cells.

(4′). A few hyaline casts.

(5′). A variety of crystals.

(6′). Spermatozoa.

(7′). Fat droplets.

(8′). Artifacts and contaminants.

(b). Identification of the following in urine sediment should be investigated:

(1′). More than a few RBC.

(2′). More than a few WBC.

(3′). Hyperplastic and/or neoplastic epithelial cells.

(4′). More than a few hyaline or granular casts.

(5′). Cellular (RBC, WBC, epithelial cell) casts, fatty casts, waxy casts, hemoglobin casts.

(6′). Cystine, tyrosine, and leucine crystals. (See Section VIIC.)

(7′). Parasite ova and microfilaria.

(8′). Bacteria in properly collected, transported, and prepared specimens.
(9′). Many yeast or hyphae.

(2). Quantitative results.
(a). Many variables alter the quantitative composition of urine sediment, thus making stringent quantitative interpretations meaningless.
(b). Quantitative sediment composition may be influenced by one or more of the following:
(1′). The volume of urine formed.
(2′). The method of urine collection.
(3′). Lysis of cells, crystals, and casts by changes in pH and/or the degree of dilution of the sample.
(4′). The volume of urine centrifuged.
(5′). The sedimentation force, which depends on speed of centrifugation (rpm), the radius of the centrifuge arm, and the duration of centrifugation.
(6′). The volume of urine in which the sediment is resuspended and the thoroughness of reconstitution of the sediment.
(7′). Dilution of the reconstituted sediment by addition of stains (e.g., Sedistain, Sternheimer-Malbin) or preservatives.
(8′). The quantity of sediment transferred to the microscope slide and subsequently examined (i.e., the thickness of the film of the slide preparation). The volume of urine covered by a standard 22-mm coverslip and scanned under 1 high dry objective field (570X) is about 1/30,000 mL.
(9′). Staining procedures that may result in loss of variable quanties of sediment during counterstaining and washing.
(10′). The ability to recognize various structures, and the ability to differentiate between various types of cells, casts, and crystals.

(3). Conventionally, the number of RBC and the number of WBC are counted in each of at least 10 to 15 microscopic fields, and are reported as the average number per high-power microscope field (HPF; 40X). Casts are conventionally reported as the average number per low-power field (LPF; 10X). Bacteria, parasites, crystals, sperm, and other elements are usually reported as few, occasional, frequent, or many. Because of the variables just described, the numbers of cells, casts, and other elements observed represent a crude semiquantitative value at best.

(4). As with all components of routine complete urinalyses, results of examination of urine sediment should be interpreted in combination with clinical observations and other laboratory, radiographic, or biopsy data.

2. Red Blood Cells (See Chapter 4, Clinical Algorithms and Data Bases for Urinary Tract Disorders.)
a. Hematuria may be gross or microscopic.
b. Gross hematuria.
(1). If gross hematuria has been observed, determining when during the process of micturition its intensity was most severe may be helpful in localizing the source of hemorrhage.
(2). Hematuria throughout micturition.
(a). Patients with persistent gross hematuria caused by renal disease often void urine that contains blood throughout the entire period of micturition. This occurs because the ureters enter the caudodorsal portion of the bladder and because boluses of urine are periodically discharged from the ureters into the bladder lumen.
(b). Patients with diffuse bladder lesions may also pass urine that contains blood throughout the entire period of micturition.
(c). Hematuria that occurs throughout micturition may also be observed when blood originating from severe prostatic or proximal urethral lesions refluxes from the prostatic urethra into the bladder.
(d). This pattern of hematuria could be observed in patients with systemic clotting defect.
(e). Caution must be used to distinguish hematuria from hemoglobinuria.
(3). Hematuria at the end of micturition.
(a). Blood observed predominantly at the end of micturition suggests a focal lesion in the ventral or ventrolateral aspect of the urinary bladder.
(b). This pattern of hematuria is frequently associated with large uroliths, and may be related to the fact

that uroliths in the dependent portion of the bladder continually traumatize this area. It may also be associated with polyps.

(c). It occurs in dogs that are sufficiently inactive to allow most of the RBC in the urine to remain in the dependent portion of the bladder lumen.

(d). Because urine contained in the uppermost portion of the bladder is forced into the urethra first, the bloody urine that has accumulated in the bottom of the bladder is voided last.

(e). This pattern of micturition could also be observed in dogs with *intermittent* gross hematuria of renal origin.

(4). Hematuria *independent* of micturition or that is most severe at the *beginning* of micturition usually indicates a hemorrhagic lesion in the urethra, vagina, or uterus of females or in the urethral or prostate gland of males.

c. Microscopic hematuria (Fig. 7–1 through 7–4).

(1). Hemolyzed RBC often cannot be detected by sediment evaluation.

(2). Reports state that RBC in urine with a specific gravity less than 1.010 are difficult to see; at a specific gravity less than 1.005, the cells disintegrate and cannot be detected.[37]

(3). Results of examination of sediment for RBC should be correlated with results of chemical evaluation of urine for blood. (See Section VI E of this chapter.) Reports state that, during centrifugation, only 50% of the RBC are recovered.[29]

(4). An occasional RBC in a high-power field (<5/HPF?) is often observed in the urine sediment of normal patients.

(5). More than occasional RBC in a high-power microscopic field indicate hemorrhage, inflammation, necrosis, trauma, or neoplasia somewhere along the urinary tract (or urogenital tract in voided samples).

(6). In man, some investigators have reported that erythrocytes of glomerular origin are often small, fragmented, and variable in size and shape, whereas RBC of nonglomerular origin are normal in size and shape. The explanation for this difference is that RBC apparently become deformed if they pass through the glomerular capillary wall.[93]

d. Disorders that may be associated with hematuria include:

(1). Strenuous exercise.

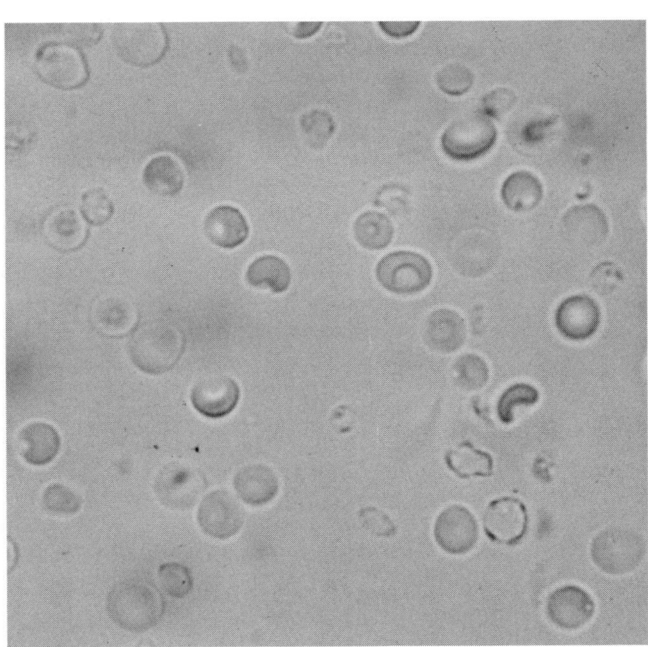

FIG. 7–1. Red blood cells in urine of a dog. Specific gravity was 1.029. An occasional white cell is also present. Unstained. (Magnification, 160X.) (From Osborne CA, Stevens JB. *Handbook of Canine and Feline Urinalysis*. St. Louis, Mo.: Ralston Purina Co; 1981.)

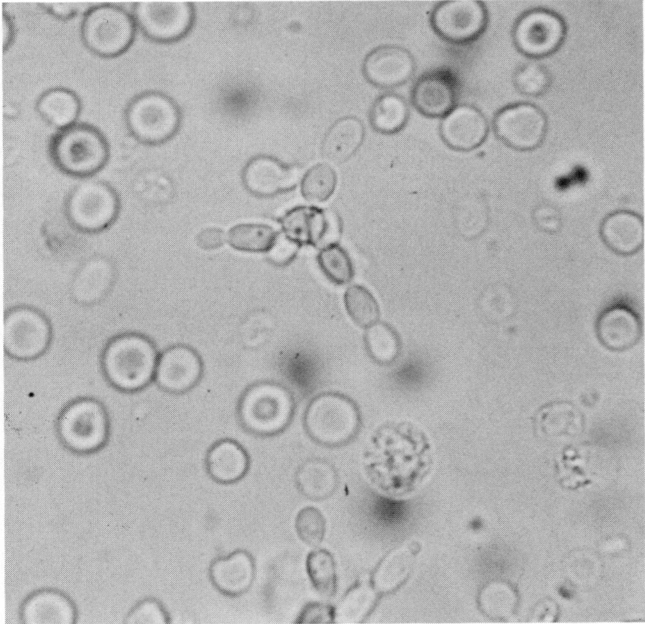

FIG. 7–2. Budding yeast in urine sediment of a cat, surrounded primarily by red blood cells. An occasional white cell is also present. Unstained. (Magnification, 60X.) (From Osborne CA, Stevens JB. *Handbook of Canine and Feline Urinalysis*. St. Louis, Mo.: Ralston Purina Co; 1981.)

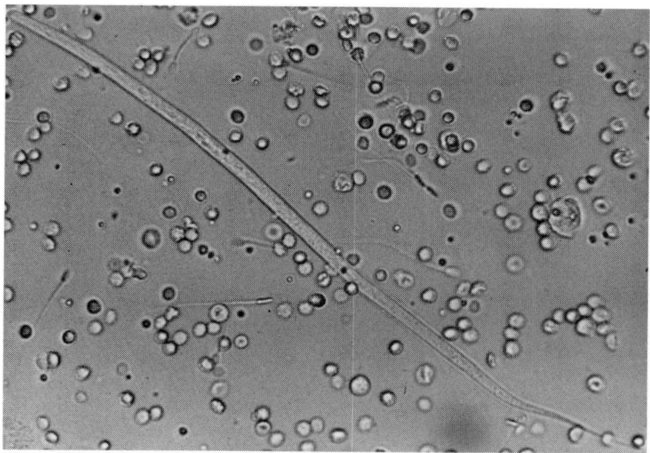

FIG. 7–3. Microfilaria of *Dirofilaria immitis* in urine sediment of a dog is surrounded by red blood cells, white cells, spermatozoa, and an occasional epithelial cell. Unstained. (Magnification, 40X.) (From Osborne CA, Stevens JB. *Handbook of Canine and Feline Urinalysis.* St. Louis, Mo.: Ralston Purina Co; 1981.)

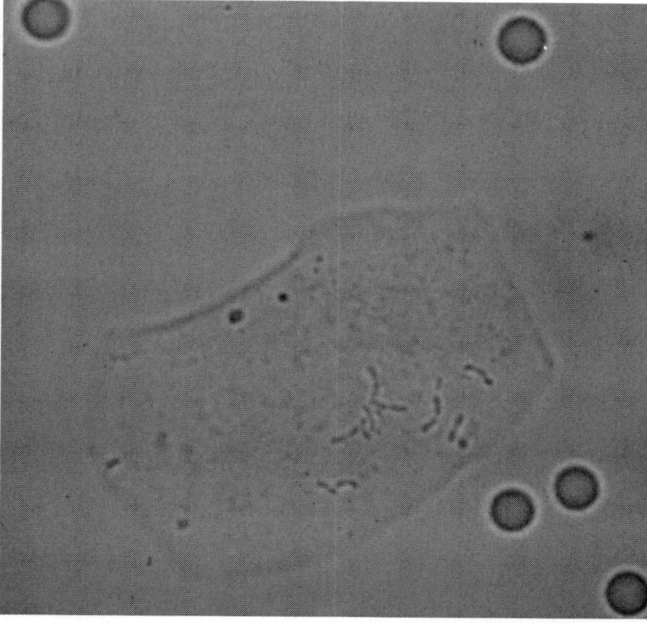

FIG. 7–4. Bacteria adhered to surface of a cornified squamous epithelial cell; red blood cells. Unstained. (Magnification, 160X.)

(2). Iatrogenic trauma associated with palpation of the kidneys or bladder, cystocentesis, or catheterization of the urinary bladder.
(3). Trauma.
(4). Uroliths in any location.
(5). Renal infarcts from any cause, including microthrombi associated with disseminated intravascular coagulation (associated with WBC, casts, and protein).
(6). Infection of any portion of the urinary system (also often associated with WBC, proteinuria, and bacteriuira).
(7). Benign or malignant neoplasms of any portion of the urinary system (or urogenital system in voided samples).
(8). Chronic passive congestion of the kidneys from any cause.
(9). Diseases with systemic hemorrhagic tendencies (i.e., thrombocytopenia, leptospirosis, warfarin toxicity, and hemophilia).
(10). Parasites *(Dioctophyma renale, Capillaria plica,* microfilaria of *Dirofilaria immitis).*
(11). Estrum.

3. White cells (Figs. 7–5 and 7–6)
   a. An occasional WBC in a high-power field (<5/HPF) may occur in normal patients.
   b. More than occasional WBC in a high-power field indicate an active inflammatory lesion anywhere along the urinary tract (or urogenital tract in voided samples).
      (1). The inflammatory response is typically, but not invariably, associated with varying amounts of RBC and proteinuria.
      (2). Bacteria in sufficient concentration to be visualized by microscopic examination of urine, and associated with hematuria, pyuria, and proteinuria, indicate that the inflammatory lesion has been caused or complicated by bacterial infection. (Consult Section VII C of this chapter for further information.)
      (3). Additional information is necessary to localize the site of the inflammatory process.
      (4). The possibility that pyuria has occurred as a result of passage of urine through the genital tract must be considered in noncatheterized and even catheterized samples of urine. When the origin of pyuria is questionable, a urine sample obtained by cystocentesis may help in localization.
   c. Absence of pyuria usually indicates that the urinary tract is not infected. We have occasionally encountered significant asymptomatic bacteriuria without pyuria in dogs and cats, however.
   d. Pyuria (leukocyturia) is a poor index of bacteriuria and therefore is not synonymous with urinary tract infection. Although pyuria

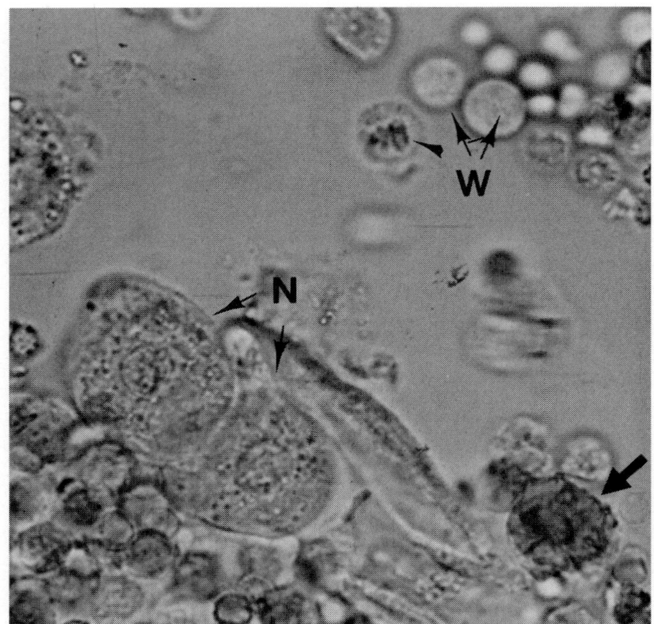

FIG. 7–5. Nucleated epithelial cells (N) surrounded by red cells, stained and unstained white cells (W), and cells of uncertain origin (arrows). Sedi-Stain. (Magnification, 160X.) (From Osborne CA, Stevens JB. *Handbook of Canine and Feline Urinalysis.* St. Louis, Mo.: Ralston Purina Co; 1981.)

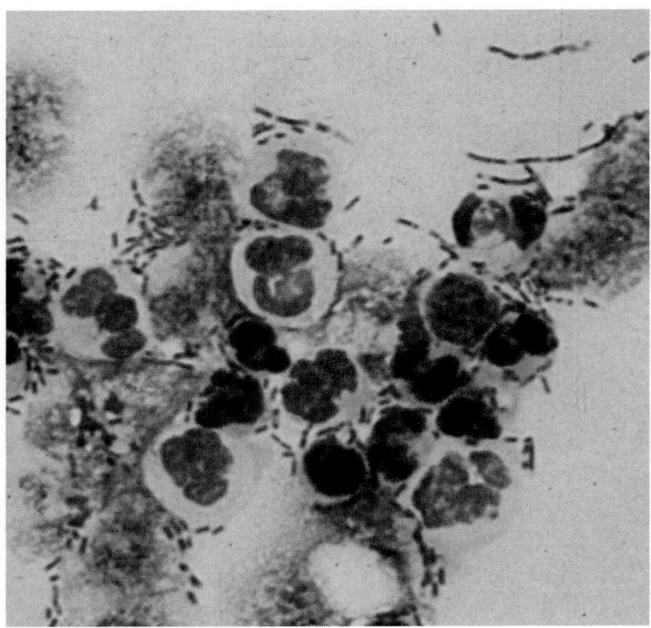

FIG. 7–6. Canine urine sediment containing bacteria in polymorphonuclear leukocytes undergoing varying stages of degeneration. New methylene blue stain. (Magnification, 400X.)

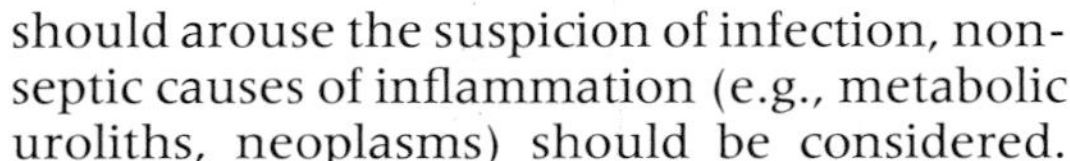

should arouse the suspicion of infection, nonseptic causes of inflammation (e.g., metabolic uroliths, neoplasms) should be considered.

e. The leukocyte esterase test strip commonly used to evaluate human urine has been found to be an insensitive method to detect pyuria in dogs.[95]

4. Epithelial cells (Figs. 7–7 through 7–9)
   a. Cuboidal epithelial cells from the renal tubules, transitional epithelial cells from the renal pelves, ureters, urinary bladder, and urethra, and squamous epithelial cells from the vagina and distal urethra are commonly in urine sediment obtained from normal dogs and cats. They are thought to occur as a result of normal attrition and exfoliation of epithelial cells.
   b. Accurate data regarding the number of epithelial cells that may normally be present in the urine of dogs and cats are not available. Although many cells may exfoliate as a result of disease, more reliable methods are available that should be used to confirm the presence of urinary lesions.
   c. Renal tubular epithelial cells:
      (1). Originate from the renal tubules.
      (2). Are normally found in urine in relatively small numbers.
      (3). Are not a reliable index of kidney disease because they are difficult, if not impossible, to differentiate from other types of epithelial cells (unless they are incorporated into casts).
   d. Transitional epithelial cells (Fig. 7–5)
      (1). Originate from the renal pelvis, ureters, urinary bladder, and/or urethra.
      (2). Are normally found in urine in relatively small numbers.
      (3). Exfoliate into urine in large numbers as a result of inflammation or neoplasia. In these instances, they may be hyperplastic.
   e. Squamous epithelial cells. (Figs. 7–7 and 7–8)
      (1). Originate from the genital tract.
      (2). Are commonly present in noncatheterized samples.
      (3). Are primarily of significance in relation to the fact that they indicate contamination of the urine sample with material from the genital tract.
   f. Neoplastic epithelial cells. (Fig. 7–9)
      (1). May be observed in patients with transitional cell carcinomas, rhabdomyosarcomas, and, less commonly, other types of neoplasms, but are not a consistent finding.
      (2). Are rarely encountered in patients with renal cell carcinomas.
      (3). Are often difficult to differentiate from nonneoplastic, hyperplastic transitional epithelial cells.
5. Casts (Figs. 7–10 through 7–22)

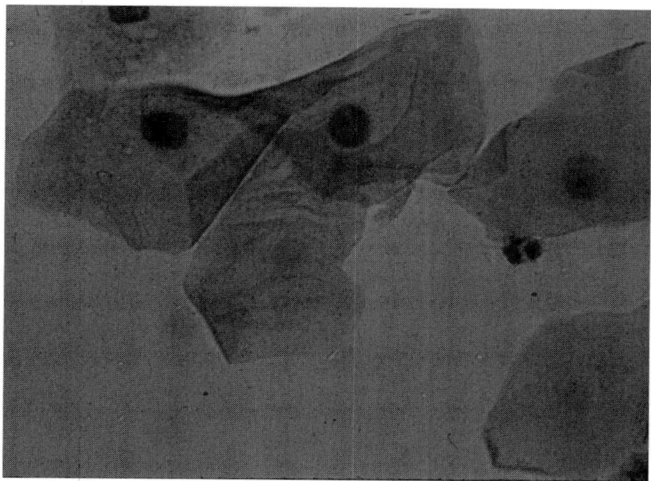

FIG. 7–7. Canine urine sediment containing cornified squamous epithelial cells. Unstained. (Magnification, 400X.) (From Osborne CA, Stevens JB. *Handbook of Canine and Feline Urinalysis.* St. Louis, Mo.: Ralston Purina Co; 1981.)

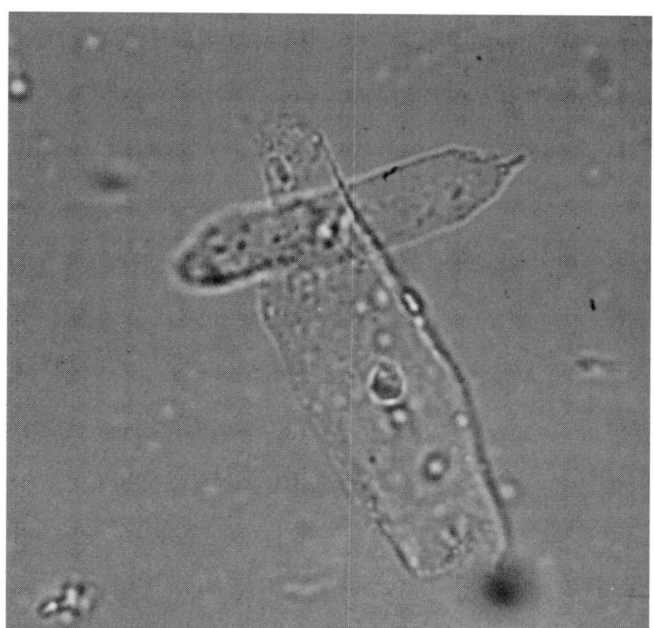

FIG. 7–8. Canine urine sediment containing squamous epithelial cells that resemble casts. Unstained. (Magnification, 160X.) (From Osborne CA, Stevens JB. *Handbook of Canine and Feline Urinalysis.* St. Louis, Mo.: Ralston Purina Co; 1981.)

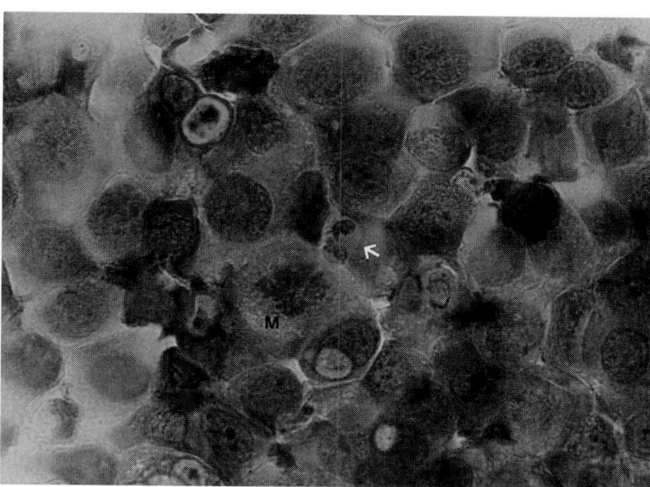

FIG. 7–9. Neoplastic transitional epithelial cells illustrate mitosis (M), nuclear enlargement, hyperchromasia, enlargement of nucleoli, and increased cell size. Compare to size of leukocyte (arrow). New methylene blue stain. (Magnification, 400X.) (From Osborne CA, Stevens JB. *Handbook of Canine and Feline Urinalysis.* St. Louis, Mo.: Ralston Purina Co; 1981.)

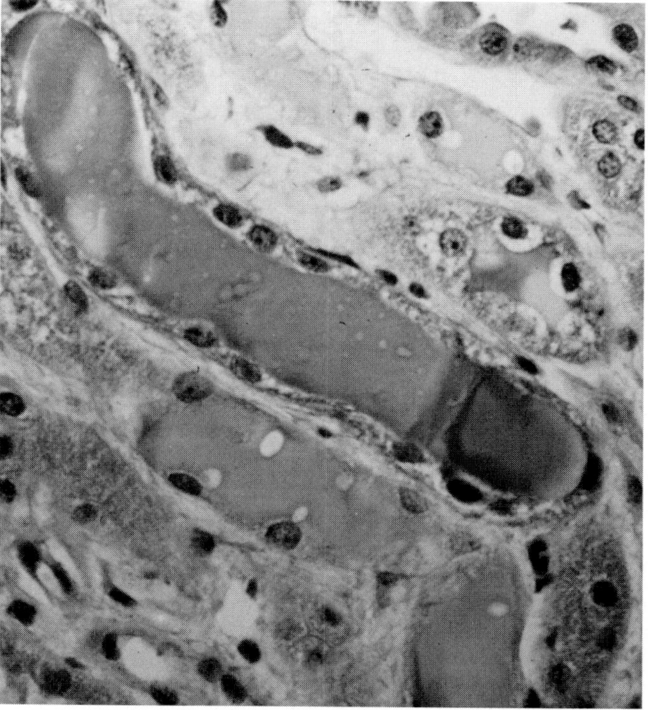

FIG. 7–10. Photomicrograph of a section of canine kidney illustrates a hyaline cast in a tubular lumen. H & E stain. (High-power magnification.)

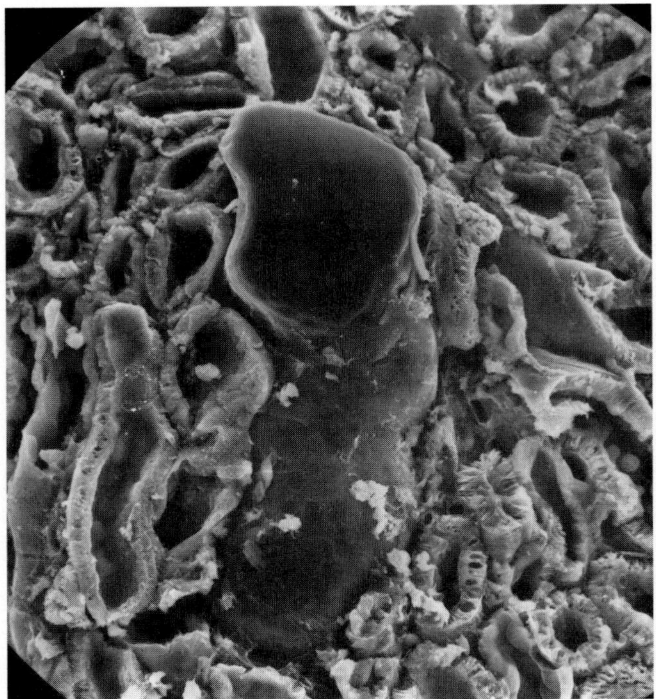

FIG. 7–11. Hyaline cast. Scanning electron microscopy. (Magnification, 360X.) (Courtesy of Dr. Robert F. Hammer, College of Veterinary Medicine, University of Minnesota.) (From Osborne CA, Stevens, JB. *Handbook of Canine and Feline Urinalysis.* St. Louis, Mo.: Ralston Purina Co; 1981.)

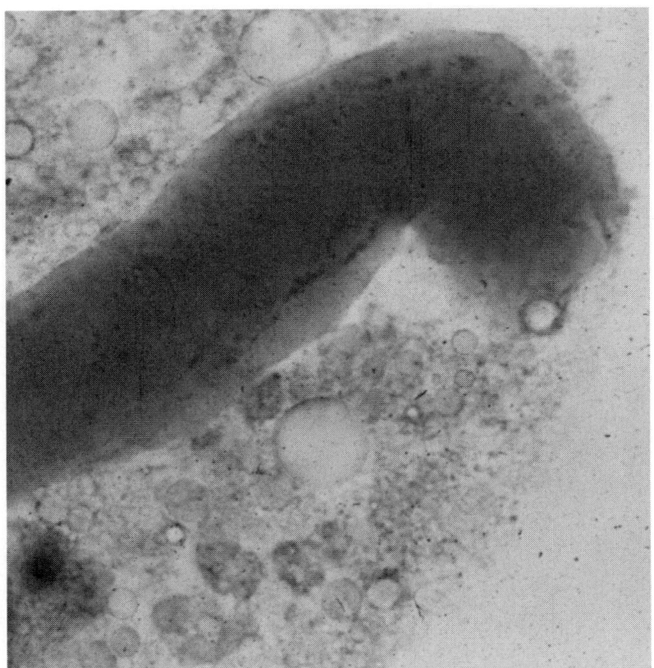

FIG. 7–12. Canine urine sediment containing hyaline cast surrounded by cellular material, debris, and lipid droplets. New methylene blue stain. (Magnification, 160X.) (From Osborne CA, Stevens JB. *Handbook of Canine and Feline Urinalysis.* St. Louis, Mo.: Ralston Purina Co; 1981.)

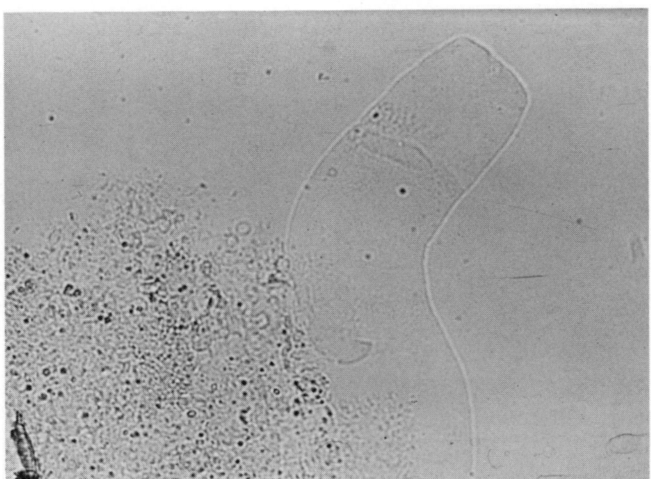

FIG. 7–13. Canine urine sediment containing broad hyaline cast adjacent to unidentified amorphous debris. Unstained. (Magnification, 160X.) (From Osborne CA, Stevens JB. *Handbook of Canine and Feline Urinalysis.* St. Louis, Mo.: Ralston Purina Co; 1981.)

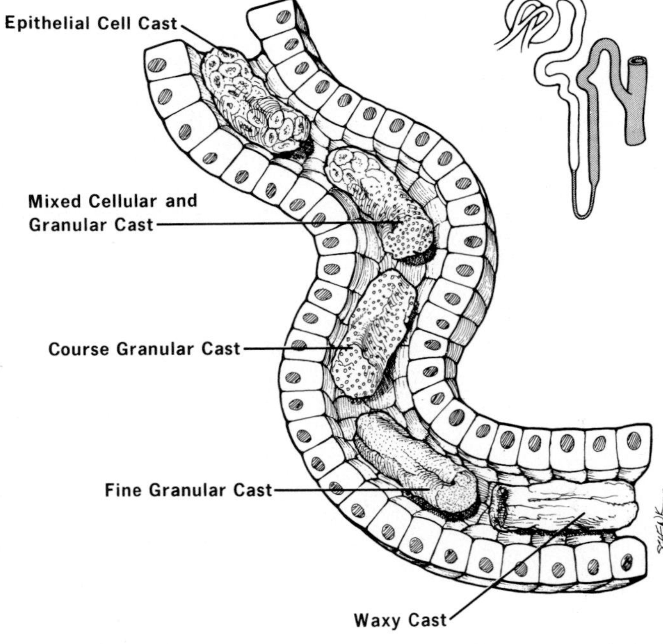

FIG. 7–14. Schematic illustration of transition between epithelial cell, coarse granular, and waxy casts formed in the loops of Henle, distal tubules, and collecting ducts (shaded area of nephron in upper right-hand corner). (From Osborne CA, Stevens JB. *Handbook of Canine and Feline Urinalysis.* St. Louis, Mo.: Ralston Purina Co; 1981.)

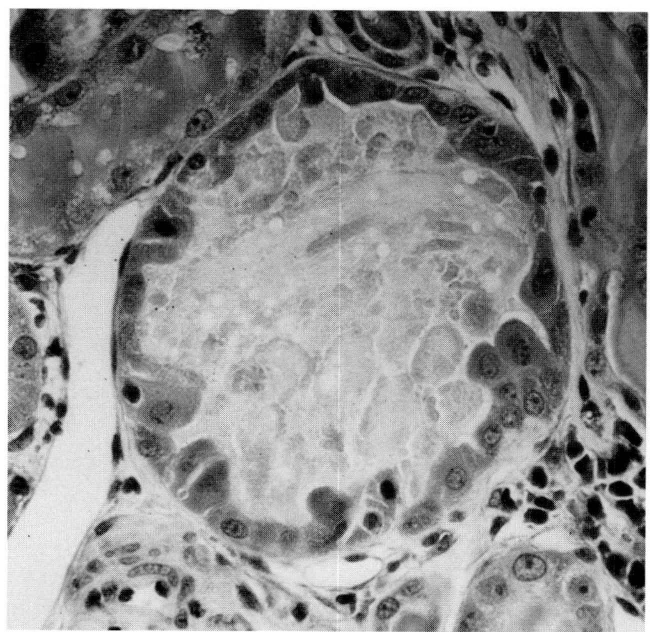

FIG. 7–15. Photomicrograph of a dilated renal tubule in a section of canine kidney illustrates sloughing and disintegration of epithelial cells. These cells may become trapped into a mucoprotein matrix to form epithelial, granular, or waxy casts. H & E stain. (High-power magnification.) (From Stevens JB, Osborne CA. Urinary casts: What is their significance? *Minn Vet.* 1978;18: 11-18.

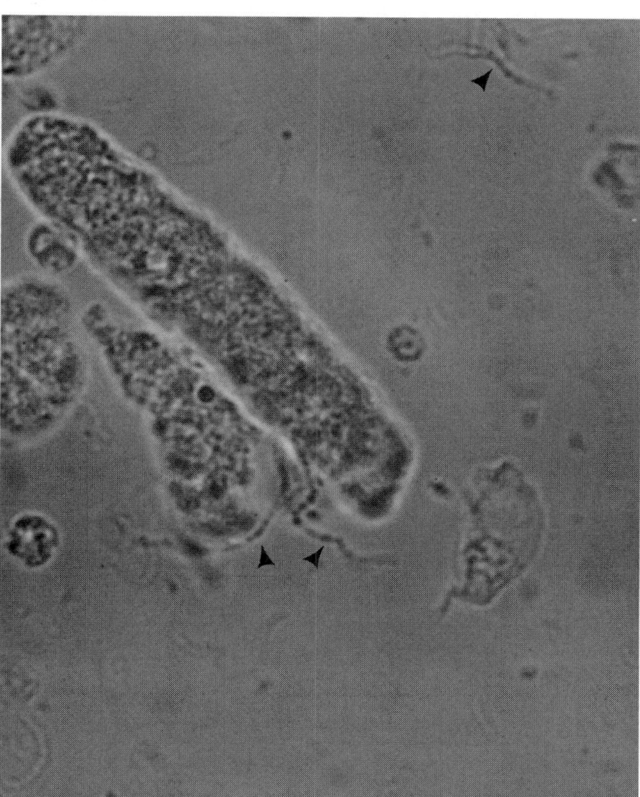

FIG. 7–16. Canine urine sediment containing a granular cast surrounded by bacteria (arrows) and granular epithelial cells. Unstained. (Magnification, 160X.)

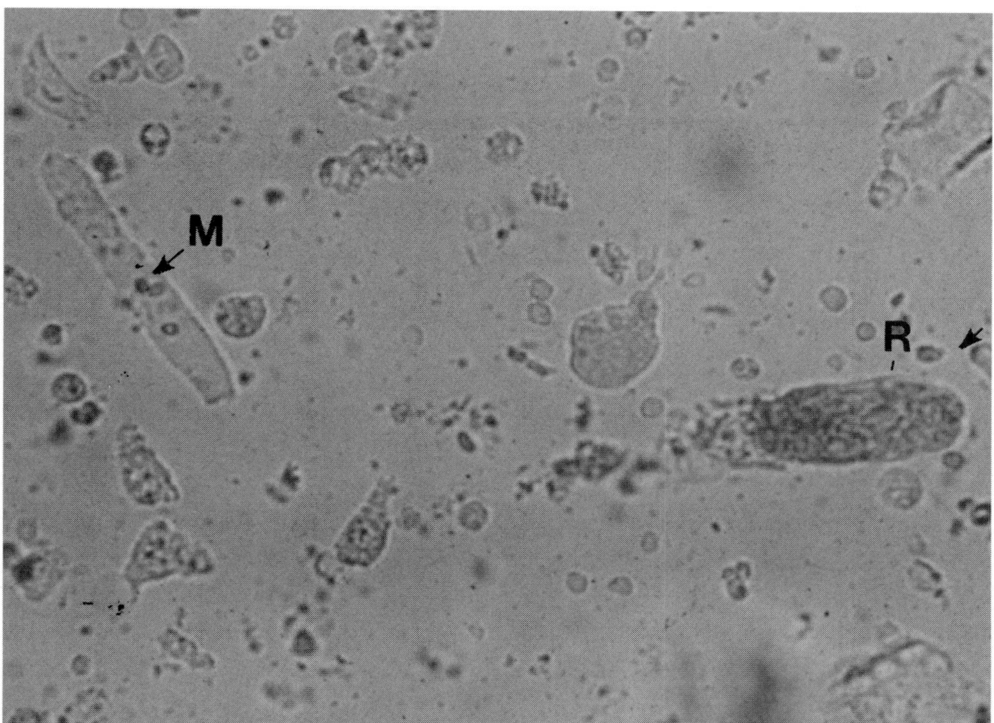

FIG. 7–17. Canine urine sediment containing red cell casts (R) and mixed granular and waxy cast (M). Unstained. (Magnification, 40X.) (From Osborne CA, Stevens JB. *Handbook of Canine and Feline Urinalysis.* St. Louis, Mo.: Ralston Purina Co; 1981.)

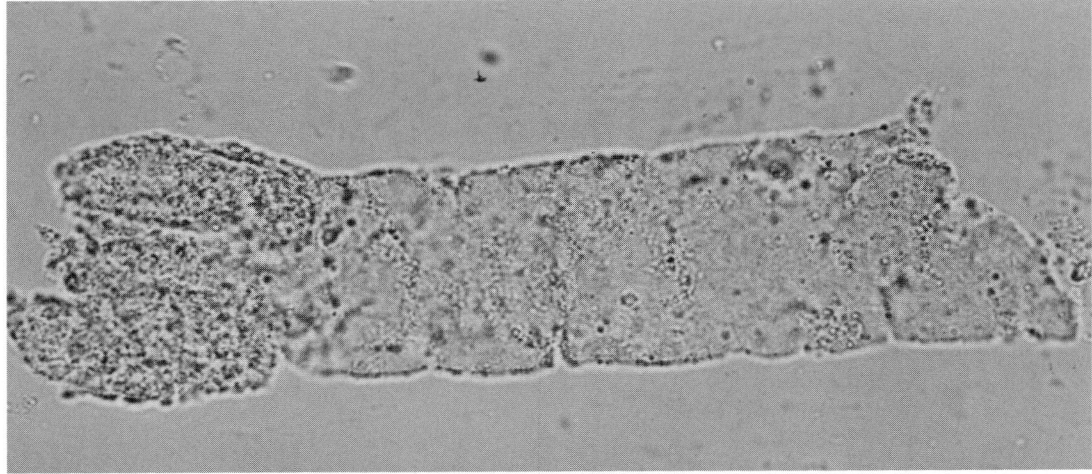

FIG. 7–18. Canine urine sediment containing a mixed granular and waxy cast. Unstained. (Magnification, 160X.) (From Osborne CA, Stevens JB. *Handbook of Canine and Feline Urinalysis.* St. Louis, Mo.: Ralston Purina Co; 1981.)

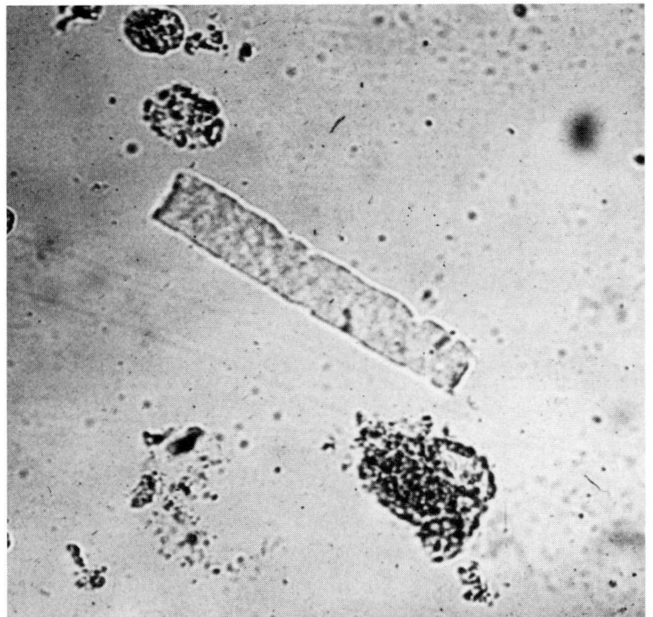

FIG. 7–19. Canine urine sediment containing a waxy cast. Unstained. (Lower-power magnification.)

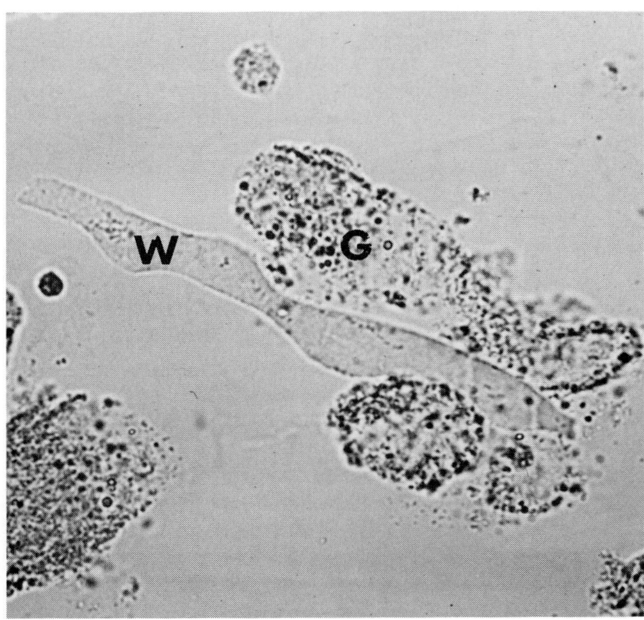

FIG. 7–20. Canine urine sediment with a waxy cast (W) adjacent to a granular cast (G). Unstained. (High-power magnification.)

a. Theories of formation.

(1). Casts are cylindric-shaped structures composed primarily of mucoprotein (called Tamm-Horsfall mucoprotein), which by scanning electron microscopy appears as a fibrillar protein meshwork.[49,86] Tamm-Horsfall mucoprotein is locally secreted by epithelial cells that line the loops of Henle, the distal tubule, and the collecting ducts.[65,81,87] Casts are not primarily composed of plasma proteins. Microdissection studies of renal tubules indicate that casts are formed in the loops of Henle, distal tubules, and collecting ducts. Although the mechanism(s) responsible for the precipitation of Tamm-Horsfall mucoprotein is not understood, cast formation in these areas of nephrons is thought to be related (at least in part) to the fact that the secretion of Tamm-Horsfall mucoprotein is limited to these sites.[67]

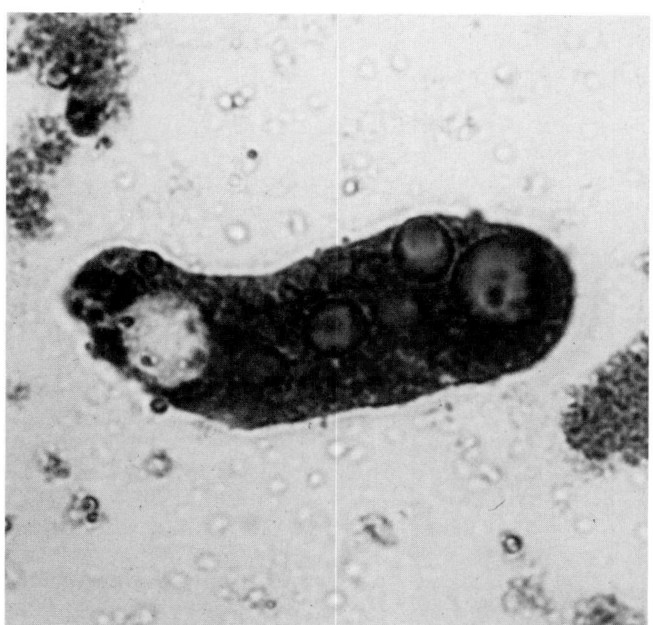

FIG. 7–21. Canine urine sediment containing a fatty cast. Sudan IV and new methylene blue stain. (Oil immersion magnification.)

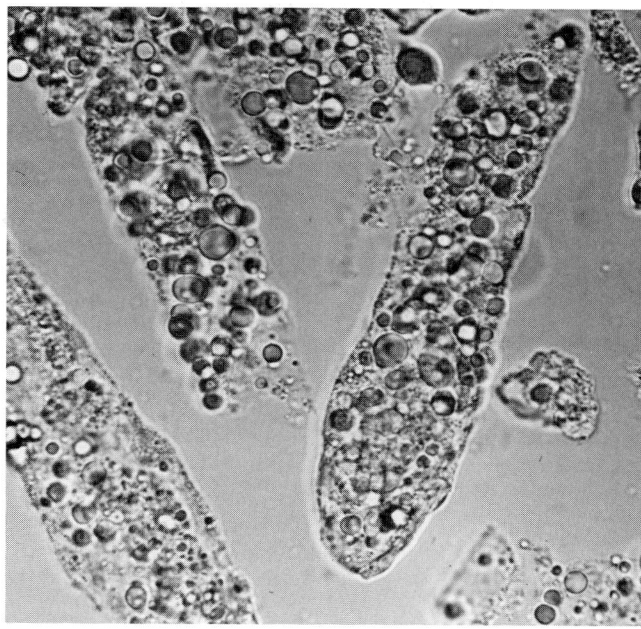

FIG. 7–22. Canine urine sediment containing fatty casts. Unstained. (Magnification, 82X.)

(2). A long-time and popular theory is based on the assumption that any material or object present within the lumen of tubules at the time Tamm-Horsfall mucoprotein gels become incorporated into the cast. Entrapment of cells and other structures in the precipitated mucoprotein matrix has been likened to entrapment of fruits and vegetables in gelatin salads.

(3). Another hypothesis states that casts may be formed by conglutination of cells and/or debris within tubular lumens.

(4). Studies of the surface ultrastructure of casts by scanning electron microscopy indicate that erythrocytes, leukocytes, and renal epithelial cells adhere to the surface of a fibrillar network of protein that subsequently surrounds the cells. The results of these structures corroborate the hypothesis that the hyaline cast is the primary structural unit of all casts.[42,58]

b. Appearance. (Figs. 7–10 to 7–22)

(1). Casts are cylindric-shaped structures formed in tubular lumens. They literally are a cast of the shape of tubular lumens.

(a). They may have round, square, irregular, or tapered ends.

(b). The width of casts is determined by the diameter of the tubular lumens in which they are formed. Casts formed in loops of Henle or distal tubules are not as wide as those formed in collecting ducts or abnormally dilated tubules.

(2). Accurate, precise identification of some casts by light microscopy may be difficult. Special stains, phase contrast microscopy, and interference contrast microscopy have been advocated by various investigators to avoid misinterpretation.

(3). Artifacts.

(a). Hyaline casts dissolve in neutral urine with a specific gravity of less than 1.003.

(b). There is an inverse relationship between the number of intact casts and urine pH. For this reason, casts are less commonly observed in alkaline urine.

(c). High-speed centrifugation and forceful reconstitution of urine may disrupt casts.

(4). Casts are commonly classified on the basis of their morphologic appearance as hyaline, epithelial, granular, waxy, fatty, RBC, WBC, hemoglobin, broad, bile-stained, and mixed casts. This classification is often of benefit in providing information about the type of lesion that is occurring in the kidneys.

(5). Hyaline casts (Figs. 7–10 through 7–13).

(a). Hyaline casts are primarily composed of Tamm-Horsfall mucoprotein; they contain no, or only a few, inclusions.[58,86]

(b). Because the refractive index of hyaline casts is similar to the refractive index of the surrounding medium, they are usually colorless, homogenous, and semitransparent in unstained sediment.

(c). They can be best detected in subdued light or following staining.

(6). Epithelial, fatty, granular, and waxy casts (Figs. 7–14 through 7–20)

(a). A popular, but unproven, hypothesis is that epithelial, fatty, granular, and waxy casts represent different stages of degeneration of epithelial cells in casts.

(b). Epithelial cell casts contain varying numbers of highly refractile desquamated tubular epithelial cells that have not yet disintegrated. Scanning electron micrographs have revealed that the epithelial cells are attached to a hyaline matrix by fibrin bands. The epithelial cells characteristically have a large round central nucleus.

(c). If lipid accumulates in the cytoplasm of cells prior to desquamation into tubular lumens, highly refractile fat droplets may be observed. Such casts are sometimes called fatty casts (Figs. 7–21 and 7–22). Verification of lipid in casts may be achieved by staining with Sudan III or Sudan IV or by examination with polarizing light microscopy.

(d). Once an epithelial cell cast has formed, its morphologic appearance does not remain static. As a result of being deprived of oxygen and metabolites, epithelial cells degenerate. With time, cell margins become indistinct, nuclear material begins to disintegrate, and coarse opaque granules appear, thereby forming a coarse granular cast. As the process of degeneration continues, fine granules are formed, and the casts are called fine granular casts. Distinction of coarse granular casts from fine granular casts is of no clinical significance.

(e). Further degeneration of the components of the epithelial cell results in the formation of a colorless, homogenous mass with a high refractive index, sharp borders, "broken off" ends, and a dull waxy appearance. They are called waxy casts.

(f). Because cellular degeneration of epithelial cells in casts occurs after cell death and desquamation, the degree (or stage) of disintegration of epithelial cells does not reflect the microscopic appearance of the tubules, but rather the duration of the disease process. Epithelial, fatty, granular, and waxy casts are usually associated with diseases that cause degeneration and necrosis of tubular epithelial cells.

(g). Granular casts may also occur as a result of degeneration of WBC in casts and as a result of aggregation of plasma proteins in Tamm-Horsfall mucoprotein matrix.[86]

(h). Apparently uncommon causes of granules within casts include packed bacteria, bacterial variants, some types of crystals, and precipitated hemoglobin secondary to severe intravascular hemolysis.[15]

(7). Cellular casts.

(a). As a result of degeneration of epithelial cells or WBC, cell types may be impossible to distinguish.

(b). Such casts are commonly called cellular casts or cellular granular casts.

(8). RBC casts (Fig. 7–17)

(a). RBC casts occur in association with hemorrhage into the renal tubules.

(b). In fresh urine they have a yellow-orange to orange-red color. This color often fades with time, and the RBC may disintegrate.

(c). Degeneration and lysis of RBC within a cast may result in a hemoglobin-induced golden-brown color and granularity.

(9). Hemoglobin and myoglobin casts.

(a). Hemoglobin casts may be observed following severe intravascular hemolysis and hemoglobinuria.

(b). Myoglobin casts may be associated with myoglobinuria.

(c). They are homogenous in consistency and have a reddish color.

(10). WBC casts.

(a). WBC casts are composed of WBC and Tamm-Horsfall mucoprotein matrix. They occur when the tubules and interstitium become involved in an inflammatory process.

(b). If the WBC degenerate before they are examined, granular casts may be formed.

(11). Broad casts (Fig. 7–13)

(a). The term broad cast refers to a wide cast formed in collecting ducts, abnormally dilated loops of Henle or distal tubules, or tubules that have undergone compensatory hypertrophy.

(b). Broad casts may be hyaline, granular, or waxy in appearance.

(c). At one time, broad casts were called renal failure casts, because when present in large numbers they were often associated with renal failure.

(12). Bile-stained casts represent any variety of cast that has become pigmented with bilirubin.

(13). Mixed casts (Figs. 7–17 and 7–18).

(a). Casts may be composed of a mixture of any of the types just described.

(b). For example, casts may contain cells and granular debris (cellular granular casts) or granular debris and waxy material (granular-waxy casts).

c. Significance.

(1). Because casts are formed in the loops of Henle, distal tubules, and collecting ducts, detection of significant numbers of casts in urine sediment (so-called cylinduria) indicates tubular involvement in an active pathologic process. Although classification of casts according to their morphologic appearance may reflect the character of the lesion in renal tubules, cast structure is rarely of specific diagnostic significance.

(2). Absence of casts does not rule out renal tubular disease.

(3). Casts may be eliminated in urine immediately after formation or may remain within tubules for varying periods undergoing varying degrees of degeneration.

(4). The number of casts is not a reliable index of the severity, duration, reversibility, or irreversibility of the underlying disease.

(a). For example, large or small numbers of casts may occur in patients with acute generalized renal disease because the casts tend to be discharged into the urine in intermittent showers.

(b). On the other hand, only a few casts may be observed in the urine of patients with chronic, progressive, generalized nephritis.

(c). Many casts always indicate active generalized renal disease, which is usually acute, but may be reversible or irreversible.

(d). Few casts may occur in patients with acute or chronic generalized renal disease.

(5). Clinical observations have revealed that a few hyaline or granular casts (<~1 to 2/LPF in moderately concentrated urine) in the sediment of otherwise normal patients is not a reliable index of significant renal damage.

(a). Under these circumstances, a few casts are of no apparent diagnostic or prognostic significance.

(b). Although casts indicate some pathologic change in the renal tubules, this change may be minor, transitory, and reversible.

(6). Hyaline casts.

(a). The general consensus has been that hyaline casts are commonly seen in association with renal and extrarenal causes of proteinuria. Some authors have proposed that albumin enhances the precipitation of Tamm-Horsfall mucoprotein.[66]

(b). They may be associated with mild or severe disease.

(7). Epithelial cell, fatty, granular, and waxy casts.

(a). These casts may be associated with diseases (e.g., infarction, ischemia, nephrotoxins) that cause degeneration and necrosis of tubular epithelial cells.

(b). Contrary to earlier reports, waxy casts are not a consistent finding in patients with amyloidosis and are not composed of amyloid.

(c). Granular casts may also arise from precipitation of plasma proteins in Tamm-Horsfall mucoprotein matrix, and as a result of degeneration of WBC.[86]

(d). Apparently uncommon causes of granules within casts include packed bacteria, bacterial variants, some types of crystals, and precipitated hemoglobin secondary to severe intravascular hemolysis.[15]

(8). RBC casts.

(a). RBC casts occur in association with hemorrhage into renal tubules.

(b). Although observation of RBC in urine sediment does not indicate the site of bleeding, observation of RBC casts indicates that the kidneys are involved.

(9). WBC casts.

(a). WBC casts occur in association with tubulo-interstitial inflammation.

(b). As was the situation with the RBC, observation of WBC in urine sediment does not indicate the site of inflammation. Observation of WBC casts indicates renal involvement in the inflammatory process.

(c). Absence of WBC casts does not exclude inflammation of the renal tubules.

(10). Broad casts.

(a). Broad casts indicate obstruction of more than one nephron if they originate in collecting ducts. At one time, they were called renal failure casts, because when present in large amounts, they were often associated with renal failure.

(b). Broad casts may originate in abnormally dilated tubules of nephrons.

(11). Bilirubin casts are associated with bilirubinuria. (See Section VI D of this chapter for additional information.)

6. Bacteria (Fig. 7–6)

a. Appearance.

(1). Bacterial rods and cocci may be observed in uncentrifuged urine or in urine sediment if present in sufficient amounts.[3,50]

(2). The sediment must be examined under high dry or oil immersion magnification.

(3). Single cocci are more difficult to identify than are rods and chains of cocci because single cocci are often mistaken for brownian movement of amorphous crystals, especially by unskilled observers.

(4). In vitro studies suggest that rod-shaped bacteria must be present in quantities equal to or greater than 10,000/mL before they can be reproducibly detected in unstained urine samples. Cocci are difficult to detect in unstained urine if their quantities are less than 100,000/mL.

(5). Because bacteria are apparently not affected by centrifugation at 1000 to 3000 rpm for 3 to 5 minutes in the same fashion as cells, crystals, and casts, either centrifuged or uncentrifuged samples may be examined. Centrifugation and examination of urine sediment may facilitate detection of bacteria in the cytoplasm of phagocytic inflammatory cells, however.

(6). Phase-contrast microscopy may facilitate detection of bacteria in unstained samples (see Figs. 7–29 and 7–58).

(7). A variety of stains (e.g., new methylene blue, Gram's stain) may facilitate detection and identification of rods and cocci in urine samples.

b. Significance.

(1). Microscopic examination of urine for bacteria should be used to complement rather than substitute for qualitative and quantitative urine culture.

(2). Bacteriuria may or may not be significant, depending on the method of urine collection and the length of time between collection and examination.

(3). Interpretation versus collection method.

(a). Normally, urine is sterile until it reaches the midurethra.

(b). The urethra of dogs and cats contains a resident population of bacteria that is greatest in quantity at the distal end of the urethra. Most of these organisms are gram positive.

(c). The significance of bacteria identified in voided or catheterized urine samples should be interpreted with caution, because samples collected by these methods may be contaminated with resident bacteria located in the distal urethra and genital tract.

(d). The concept of significant bacteriuria was introduced to allow differentiation between harmless bacterial contaminants of urine and pathogenic organisms causing infectious disease of the urinary system. The number of bacteria considered to be significant varies with the method of urine collection. (Consult Chapter 40, Bacterial Infections of the Canine and Feline Urinary Tract.)

(4). Interpretation versus length of time between collection and examination.

(a). The significance of detection of bacteria in urine samples allowed to incubate at room temperature prior to examination is unknown.

(1′). Pathogens and/or contaminants may continue to proliferate or may be destroyed.

(2′). In vitro bacteria growth or destruction is not synonymous with in vivo conditions.

(b). Detection of bacteria in improperly preserved samples warrants re-examination of a fresh specimen.

(5). Microscopic examination versus bacterial amounts.

(a). Rod-shaped bacteria may be seen in unstained preparations of urine when quantities are approximately 10,000/mL or greater. Larger amounts (100,000/mL) of cocci may be required to permit detection.

(b). The results of a study in dogs were interpreted to indicate that detection of bacteria in more than 1 oil immersion microscopic field was an indication of 100,000/mL or more.

(6). Significant bacteriuria is usually, but not invariably, associated with varying degrees of hematuria, pyuria, and proteinuria (i.e., an inflammatory response).

(7). Lack of detection of bacteria in urine sediment does not exclude their presence.

7. Yeasts and fungi (Figs. 7–2 and 7–23).
   a. Appearance.
      (1). Yeasts have an ovoid shape, are colorless, and often have characteristic budding forms. They are similar, but more variable, in size than RBC. Unlike RBC, they are insoluble in acid and alkali, and do not stain with eosin.
      (2). Fungi are usually characterized by distinct hyphae, which are often segmented. They must be differentiated from filamentous forms of bacteria.
      (3). Occasionally characteristic forms of deep systemic mycotic agents (e.g., blastomycosis, cryptococcosis) may be detected in urine sediment.
      (4). Gram's stain or new methylene blue stain can be used to highlight their appearance.
   b. Significance.
      (1). Yeasts and fungi usually represent contaminants.
      (2). Infections with *Candida albicans* and *Torulopsis* spp may occur, especially in patients with resistant urinary tract infections that have been unsuccessfully treated with a variety of antimicrobial agents for prolonged periods.[60]
      (3). On occasion, fungi (e.g., blastomycosis, cryptococcosis) may be observed in the urine sediment of patients with polysystemic fungal diseases that involve the urinary system (especially the kidneys).[60,75,90]
8. Parasites.
   a. *Dioctophyma renale.* (Fig. 7–24)
      (1). Eggs of *D. renale* are thickshelled, oval, and have characteristic surface mammilations, except at their poles.
      (2). Ova of *D. renale* may be observed in the urine sediment of animals (usually dogs)

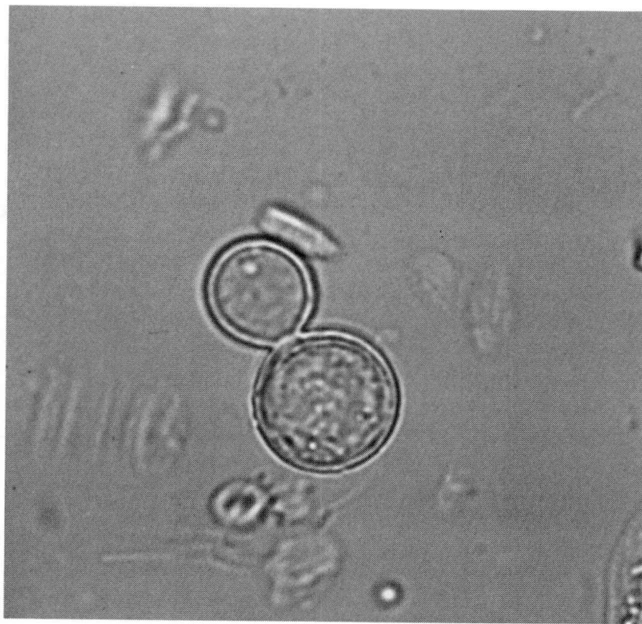

FIG. 7–23. Canine urine sediment containing budding yeast form of blastomycosis. Unstained. (Magnification, 160X.) (From Osborne CA, Stevens JB. *Handbook of Canine and Feline Urinalysis.* St. Louis, Mo.: Ralston Purina Co; 1981.)

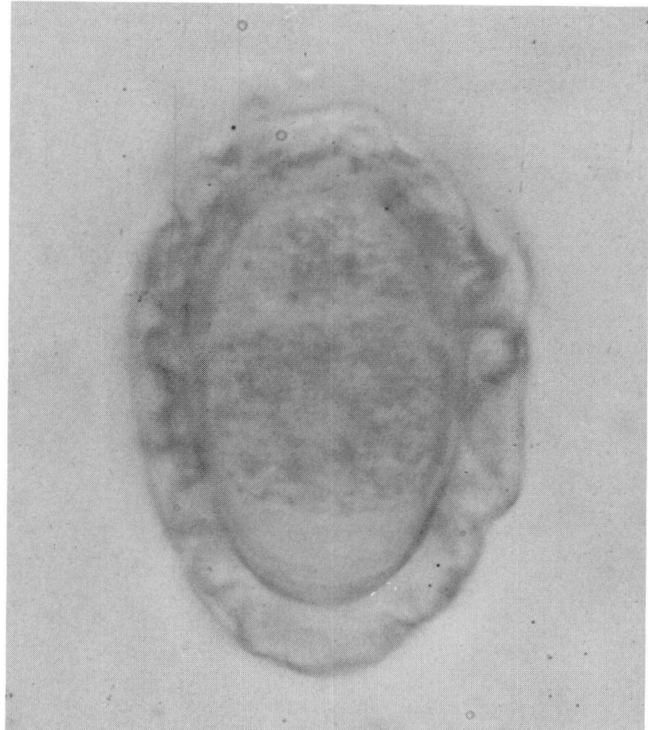

FIG. 7–24. *Dioctophyma renale* ovum in the urine sediment of a dog. Unstained. (High-power magnification.) (From Osborne CA, Stevens JB. *Handbook of Canine and Feline Urinalysis.* St. Louis, Mo.: Ralston Purina Co; 1981.)

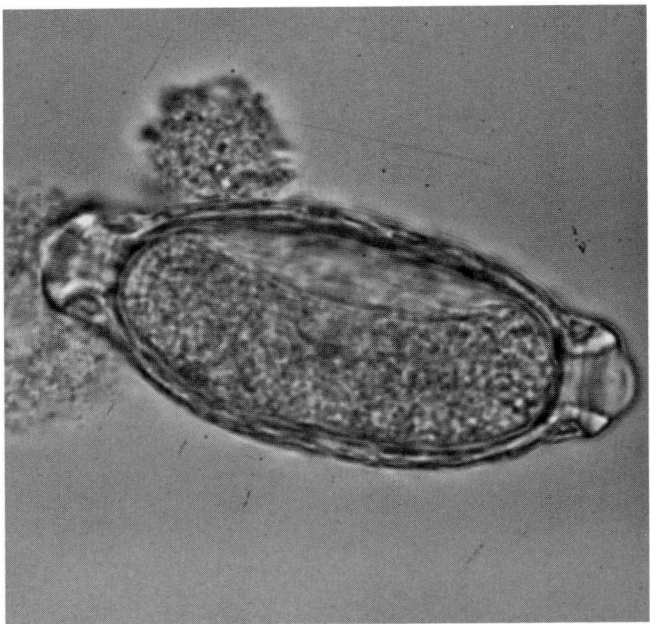

FIG. 7–25. *Capillaria plica* ovum in the urine sediment of a dog. Unstained. (Magnification, 160X.) (From Osborne CA, Stevens JB. *Handbook of Canine and Feline Urinalysis.* St. Louis, Mo.: Ralston Purina Co; 1981.)

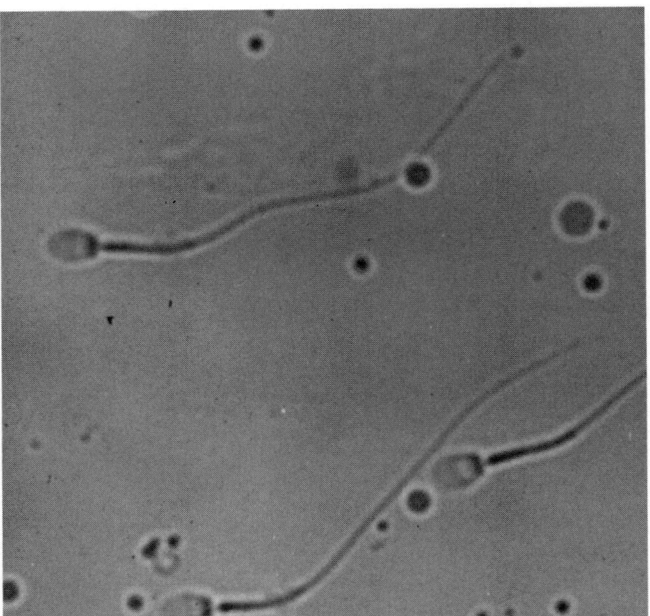

FIG. 7–26. Squad of spermatozoa surrounded by air bubbles. Unstained. (Magnification, 160X.)

infected with this parasite, provided a gravid female is present in the excretory pathway of the urinary system.

b. *Capillaria plica and Capillaria feliscati.* (Fig. 7–25)
   (1). Ova of *C. plica* and *C. feliscati* are oval in shape and have bipolar plugs. They are colorless and have a slightly pitted shell.
   (2). Care must be used to differentiate the ova of *Capillaria* spp from *Trichuris vulpus* ova that have appeared in urine as a result of fecal contamination.
c. Microfilaria of *Dirofilaria immitis* may be occasionally observed in the urine sediment of infected dogs, presumably as a result of hemorrhage into the excretory pathway of the urinary system. (Fig. 7–3).

9. Spermatozoa (Fig. 7–26).
   a. Spermatozoa are a normal finding in the urine of uncastrated male dogs and cats.
   b. They may be readily identified by their characteristic shape.
   c. They may be observed in bladder urine obtained by cystocentesis of male dogs and cats, apparently as a result of retrograde ejaculation and/or their motility.[25,33]
   d. On occasion, sperm are present as a contaminant in the urine of females following breeding.
10. Lipiduria (Fig. 7–12).
   a. Appearance.
      (1). Under low magnification with subdued light, lipid droplets appear as black, refractile spheres of variable size. As they float to the undersurface of the coverslip, they may move out of the plane of focus of other heavier elements in the sediment.
      (2). They have an orange to red color when stained with Sudan III or IV.
      (3). Lipid droplets that contain cholesterol typically have a bright maltese-cross light pattern when examined with the aid of polarization light microscopy.
   b. Significance.
      (1). The origin of fat droplets is often difficult to determine.
      (2). Fat droplets may originate as a result of physiologic attrition of tubular epithelial cells (especially in cats) and/or as a result of abnormal cytoplasmic degenerative changes in tubular epithelial cells.
      (3). Lipid-like droplets may occur as a result of contamination of urine with lubricants or the lining of some waterproof paper containers.
      (4). Apparently no correlation exists between lipemia and lipiduria.
11. Crystals.
   a. Overview.
      (1). The advent of effective medical protocols to dissolve and prevent uroliths in dogs

and cats has resulted in renewed interest in detection and interpretation of crystalluria. Evaluation of urine crystals may aid in: 1) detection of disorders predisposing animals to urolith formation, 2) estimation of the mineral composition of uroliths, and 3) evaluation of the effectiveness of medical protocols initiated to dissolve or prevent urolithiasis.

(2). Crystals form only in urine that is, or recently has been, supersaturated with crystallogenic substances. Therefore, crystalluria represents a risk factor for urolithiasis. However, detection of urine crystals is not synonymous with uroliths and clinical signs associated with them. Nor are urine crystals irrefutable evidence of a stone-forming tendency.

(a). For example, crystalluria that occurs in individuals with anatomically and functionally normal urinary tracts is usually harmless because the crystals are eliminated before they grow to sufficient size to interfere with normal urinary function.

(b). In addition, crystals that form following elimination or removal of urine from the patient often are of no clinical importance. Identification of crystals that have formed in vitro does not justify therapy.

(c). On the other hand, detection of some types of crystals (e.g., cystine and ammonium urate) in clinically asymptomatic patients, frequent detection of large aggregates of crystals (e.g., calcium oxalate or magnesium ammonium phosphate) in apparently normal individuals, or detection of any form of crystals in fresh urine collected from patients with confirmed urolithiasis may be of diagnostic, prognostic, or therapeutic importance.

(3). In patients with confirmed urolithiasis, microscopic evaluation of urine crystals should not be used as the sole criterion of the mineral composition of macroliths. Only quantitative urolith analysis can provide definitive information about the mineral composition of the entire stone. However, interpretation of crystalluria in light of other clinical findings often allows one to establish a tentative identification of the mineral composition of uroliths, especially their outermost layers. Subsequent reduction or elimination of crystalluria by therapy provides a useful index of the efficacy of medical protocols designed to dissolve or prevent uroliths.

b. Factors influencing urine crystal formation[72,73]

(1). In vivo and in vitro variables.

(a). Even though there is not a direct relationship between crystalluria and urolithiasis, detection of crystals in urine is proof that the urine sample is oversaturated with crystallogenic substances. However, oversaturation may occur as a result of in vitro events in addition to, or instead of, in vivo events. Therefore, care must be used not to overinterpret the significance of crystalluria.

(b). In vivo variables that influence crystalluria include:

1′). The concentration of crystallogenic substances in urine (which in turn is influenced by their rate of excretion and the volume of water in which they are excreted).

2′). Urine pH (Table 7–10).

3′). Solubility.

4′). Excretion of diagnostic agents (such as radiopaque contrast agents) and medications (such as sulfonamides).

(c). In vitro variables that influence crystalluria include:

1′). Temperature.

2′). Evaporation.

3′). pH.

4′). The technique of specimen preparation (e.g., centrifugation versus noncentrifugation and volume of urine examined) and preservation. We emphasize that in vitro changes that occur following urine collection may enhance formation or dissolution of crystals. Although in vitro changes may be used to enhance detection of certain types of crystals (e.g., acidification to cause precipitation of cystine), in vitro crystal formation may have no clinical relevance to in vitro formation of crystals in urine.

(d). When knowledge of in vivo urine crystal type is especially important, fresh specimens should be serially examined. The number, size, and structure of crystals should be

TABLE 7–10
COMMON CHARACTERISTICS OF SOME URINE CRYSTALS

		pH Where Commonly Found*		
Type of Crystal	**Appearance**	**Acidic**	**Neutral**	**Alkaline**
Ammonium urate	Yellow-brown spherulites; thorn apples	+	+	+
Amorphous urates	Amorphous or spheroid yellow-brown structures	+	±	–
Bilirubin	Reddish-brown needles or granules	+	–	–
Calcium carbonate	Large yellow-brown spheroids with radial striations, or small crystals with spheric ovoid or dumbbell shapes	–	±	+
Calcium oxalate dihydrate	Small colorless envelopes (octahedral form)	+	+	±
Calcium oxalate monohydrate	Small spindles, "hemp seed" or monohydrate dumbbells	+	+	±
Calcium phosphate	Amorphous, or long thin prisms	±	+	+
Cholesterol	Flat colorless plates with corner notch	+	+	–
Cystine	Flat colorless hexagonal plates	+	+	±
Hippuric acid	Four- to six-sided colorless elongated plates or prisms with rounded corners	+	+	±
Leucine	Yellow-brown spheroids with radial and concentric laminations	+	–	–
Magnesium ammonium phosphate	Three- to six-sided colorless prisms	±	+	+
Sodium urate	Colorless or yellow-brown needles or slender prisms, sometimes in clusters or sheaves	+	±	–
Sulfa metabolites	Sheaves of needles with central or eccentric binding; sometimes fan-shaped clusters	+	±	–
Tyrosine	Fine colorless or yellow needles arranged in sheaves or rosettes	+	–	–
Uric acid	Diamond or rhombic rosettes, or oval plates; structures with pointed ends; occasionally six-sided plates	+	–	–
Xanthine	Amorphous, spheroid, or ovoid structures with a yellow-brown color	+	±	–

*A + means crystals commonly occur at this pH; a ± means crystals may occur at this pH, but are more common at the other pH; and a – means crystals are uncommon at this pH.

evaluated, as well as their tendency to aggregate.

(2). Urine pH.

(a). The formation and persistence of several types of crystals are influenced by pH. Therefore, consideration of pH when interpreting crystalluria is often useful (Table 7–10).

(b). Different crystals tend to form and persist in certain pH ranges, although there are exceptions. Exceptions may be related to large concentrations of crystallogenic substances in urine or recent in vivo or in vitro changes in urine pH.

(3). Refrigeration.

(a). Refrigeration is an excellent method to preserve many physical, chemical, and morphologic properties of urine sediment. However, it must be used with caution when evaluating crystalluria from qualitative and quantitative standpoints.

(b). Although refrigeration of urine samples is likely to enhance formation of various types of crystals, this phenomenon may have no relationship to events occurring in the patient's body.

(4). Diet.

(a). Crystalluria may also be influenced by diet (including water intake).

(b). Dietary influence on crystalluria is of diagnostic importance because urine crystal formation that occurs while patients are consuming hospital diets may be dissimilar to urine crystal formation that occurs when patients are consuming diets fed at home.

(5). Drugs.

(a). Detection of unusual crystals in the urine of patients receiving medications should prompt consideration that the crystals may be drug metabolites.

(b). Drugs associated with crystalluria documented in dogs and cats include sulfadiazine and its metabolites.[73]

(c). Drugs associated with forms of crystalluria documented in man include ampicillin, ciprofloxacin, radiopaque contrast agents, primidone, 5-fluorocytosine, and 6-mercaptopurine.

(6). Combinations of crystals.

(a). Crystals form in a complex environment characterized by constant formation of urine of variable composition that traverses different components of the upper and lower urinary tract. More than one type of crystal may be observed in the same urine sample.

(b). Observation of a combination of brushite (calcium hydrogen phosphate dihydrate, a mineral precipitated in acid urine) and calcium apatite (calcium phosphate) crystals in human urine samples supports this hypothesis because brushite would not be expected to form in the alkaline environment required for precipitation of calcium apatite.

(c). Crystals of different composition may also form within the same location. For example, infection-induced magnesium ammonium phosphate crystals may form concomitantly with metabolic crystals (e.g., calcium oxalate, calcium phosphate, and ammonium urate).

c. Crystal habit.

(1). Habit is the term commonly used by mineralogists to refer to characteristic shapes of mineral crystals and is commonly used as an index of crystal composition. However, microscopic evaluation of the habits of urine crystals represents only a tentative indicator of their composition, because variable conditions associated with their formation, growth, and dissolution may alter their appearance. Therefore, definitive identification of crystal composition depends on optical crystallography, infrared spectrophotometry, thermal analysis, x-ray diffraction, electron microprobe analysis, or a combination of these. (See Chapter 41, Canine and Feline Urolithiases: Relationship of Etiopathogenesis to Treatment and Prevention.)

(2). If confirmation of the composition of microscopic crystalluria is desirable, an attempt to prepare a large pellet of crystals by centrifugation of an appropriate volume of urine in a cone-tipped centrifuge tube may be of value. Evaluation of the pellet by quantitative methods designed for urolith analysis may provide meaningful information about crystalluria associated with urolithiasis. However, the type of crystals identified by this method may only reflect the outer portions of uroliths.

d. Bilirubin crystalluria.

(1). Bilirubin may crystallize in urine to form yellow-red or reddish-brown needles or granules.

(2). Bilirubin crystals can be observed in highly concentrated urine from normal dogs. When observed in large numbers in serial samples of urine, they should arouse suspicion of an abnormality in bilirubin metabolism.

e. Calcium carbonate.

(1). Calcium carbonate may crystallize in the urine of horses, rabbits, guinea pigs, and goats to form large yellow-brown or colorless spheroids with radial striations, or smaller crystals with round, ovoid, or dumbbell shapes.

(2). Carbonate crystals have not been detected in canine or feline urine. If dumbbell-shaped crystals are observed in canine or feline urine, they are more likely to be calcium oxalate monohydrate than calcium carbonate.

f. Calcium oxalate. (Figs. 7–27 through 7–34)

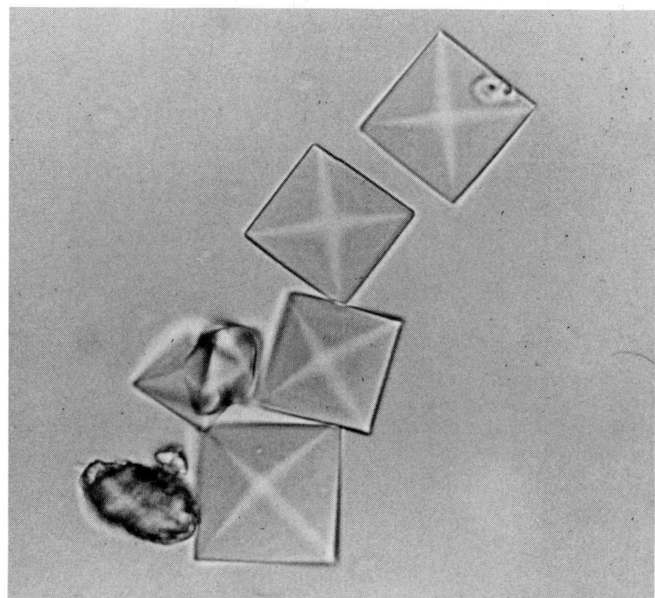

FIG. 7–27. Photomicrograph of urine sediment containing characteristic calcium oxalate dihydrate crystals. Unstained. (Magnification, 160X.)

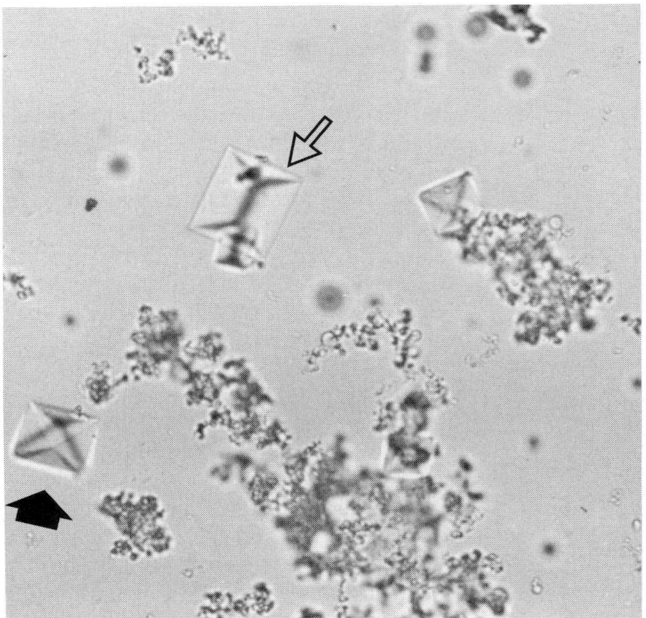

FIG. 7–28. Photomicrograph of urine sediment obtained from an adult female bichon frise containing calcium oxalate dihydrate (closed arrow), magnesium ammonium phosphate (open arrow), and amorphous calcium phosphate crystals. Unstained. (Magnification, 40X.)

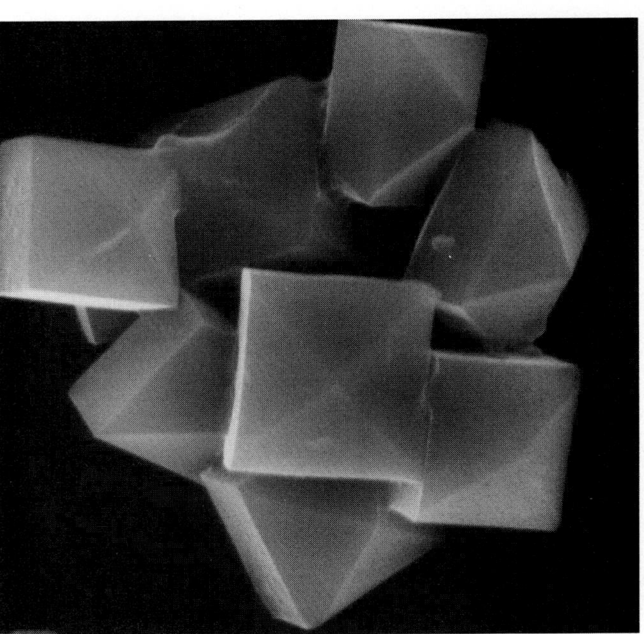

FIG. 7–29. Scanning electron micrograph of calcium oxalate dihydrate crystals in the urine sediment obtained from a 5-year-old female bichon frise. (Magnification, 7040X.) (From Osborne CA, et al.: Identification and interpretation of crystalluria in domestic animals: A light and electron microscopic study. *Vet Med.* 1990; 85:18-37.)

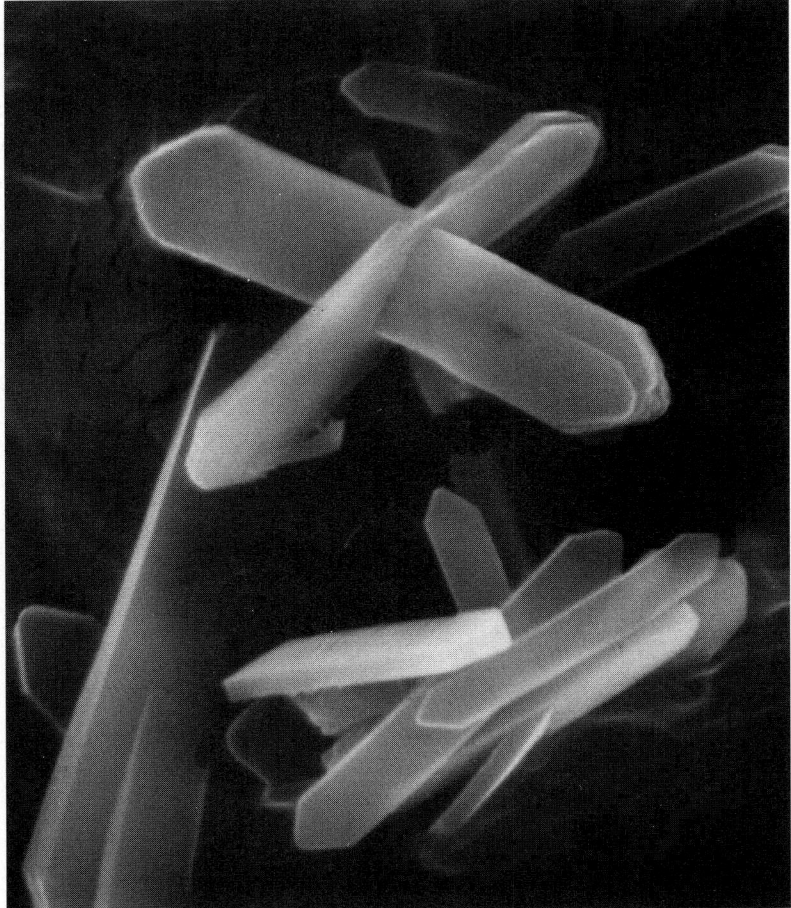

FIG. 7–30. Scanning electron micrograph of calcium oxalate monohydrate crystals in the urine sediment obtained from a 3-year-old female rottweiler with acute ethylene glycol toxicity. (Magnification, 10800X.) (From Osborne CA, et al.: Identification and interpretation of crystalluria in domestic animals: A light and electron microscopic study. *Vet Med.* 1990; 85:18-37.)

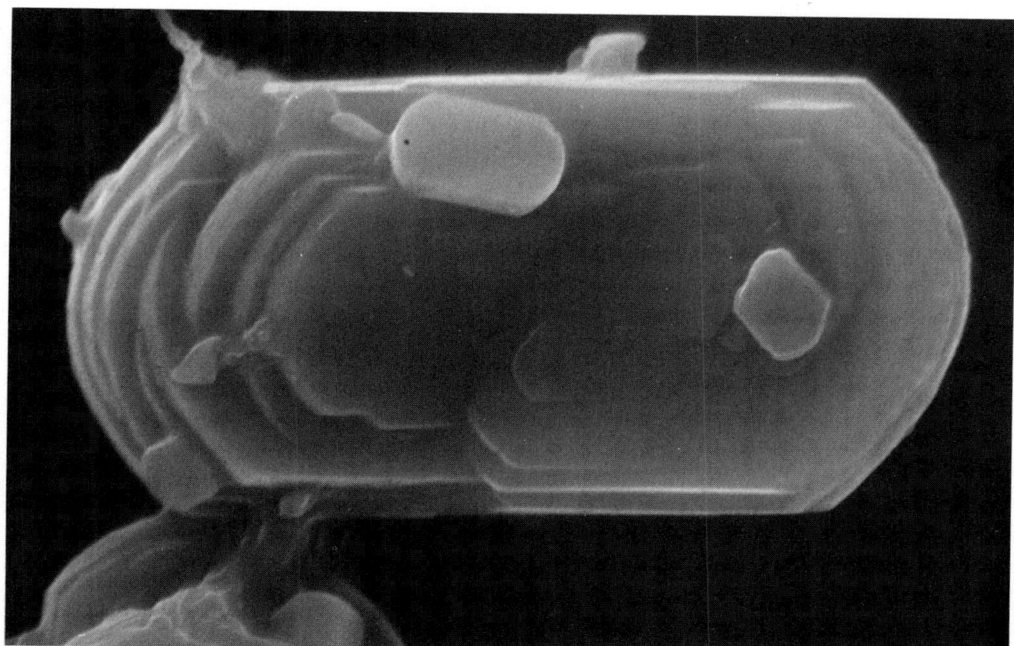

FIG. 7–31. Scanning electron micrograph of calcium oxalate monohydrate crystals in the urine sediment of a spayed female domestic short-haired cat. (Magnification, 5760X.) (From Osborne CA, et al.: Identification and interpretation of crystalluria in domestic animals: A light and electron microscopic study. *Vet Med.* 1990; 85:18-37.)

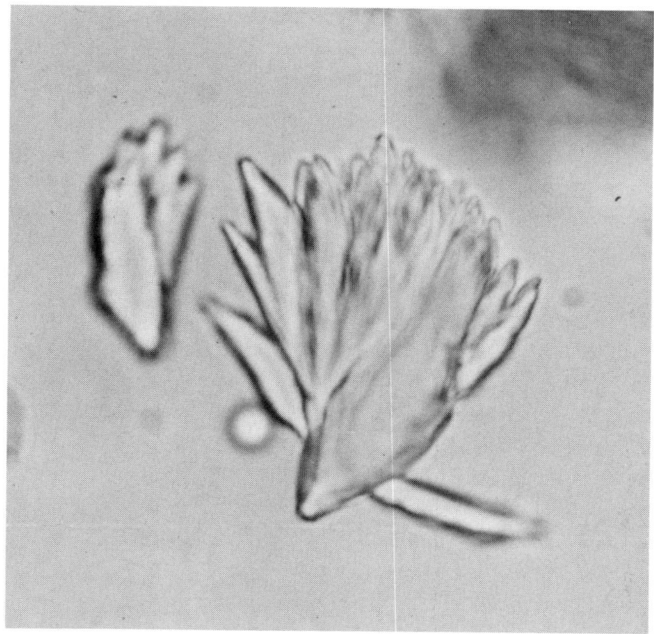

FIG. 7–32. Photomicrograph of an aggregate of calcium oxalate monohydrate crystals in the urine of a 7–year-old castrated male miniature schnauzer with calcium oxalate urocystoliths. Unstained. (Magnification, 250X.) (From Osborne CA, et al.: Identification and interpretation of crystalluria in domestic animals: A light and electron microscopic study. *Vet Med.* 1990; 85:18-37.)

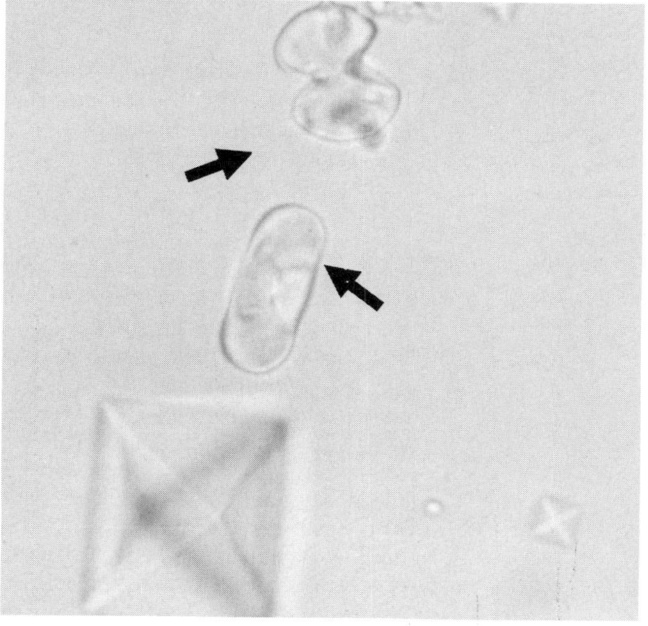

FIG. 7–33. Photomicrograph of urine sediment obtained from an adult spayed female miniature schnauzer illustrates calcium oxalate monohydrate (arrows) and calcium oxalate dihydrate crystals. Unstained. (Magnification, 100X.) (From Osborne CA, et al.: Identification and interpretation of crystalluria in domestic animals: A light and electron microscopic study. *Vet Med.* 1990; 85:18-37.)

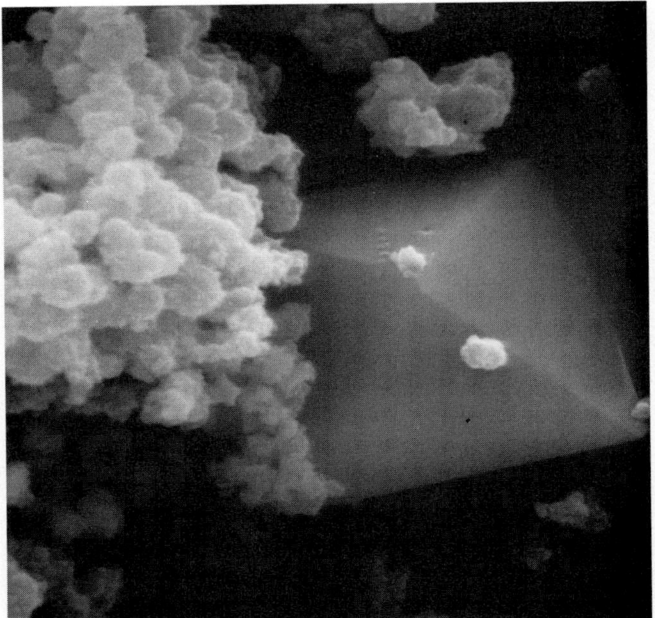

FIG. 7–34. Scanning electron micrograph of a calcium oxalate dihydrate crystal and numerous amorphous calcium phosphate crystals in the urine of a 3-year-old male Lhasa apso. The dog had calcium oxalate urocystoliths. (Magnification, 7920X.) (From Osborne CA, et al.: Identification and interpretation of crystalluria in domestic animals: A light and electron microscopic study. *Vet Med.* 1990; 85:18-37.)

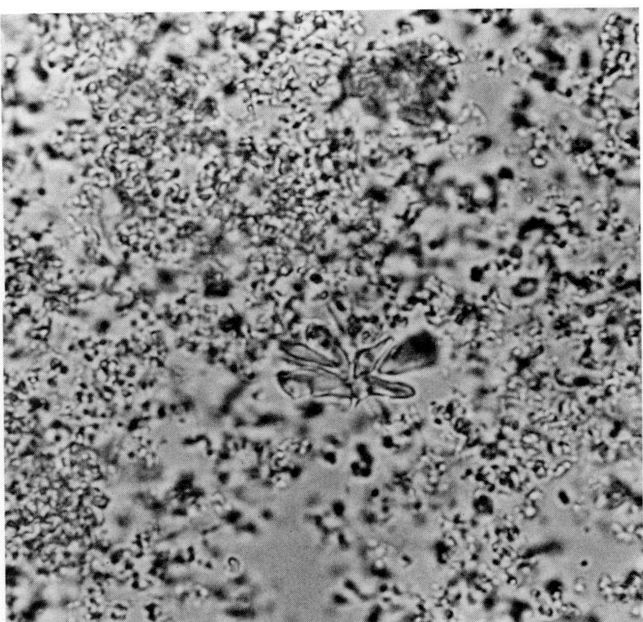

FIG. 7–35. Photomicrograph of canine urine sediment containing primarily amorphous calcium phosphate crystals. A small group of crystalline calcium phosphates are in the center of the illustration. Unstained. (Magnification, 160X.)

(1). Habit

(a). Calcium oxalate dihydrate crystals (weddellite) typically are colorless and have a characteristic octahedral or envelope shape. By light microscopy, they resemble small or large squares with corners that are connected by intersecting diagonal lines. Calcium oxalate crystals have been observed in acidic, neutral, and alkaline urine samples.

(b). Calcium oxalate monohydrate crystals (whewellite) vary in size and may have a spindle, oval (hempseed), or dumbbell shape. Calcium oxalate monohydrate crystals with hippuric acid-like morphologic findings have also been observed in dogs, especially those with ethylene glycol toxicity. They are soluble in hydrochloric acid but insoluble in acetic acid. They may occur in combination with calcium oxalate dihydrate and other types of crystals.

(2). Interpretation

(a). Calcium oxalate dihydrate crystals may occur in apparently normal

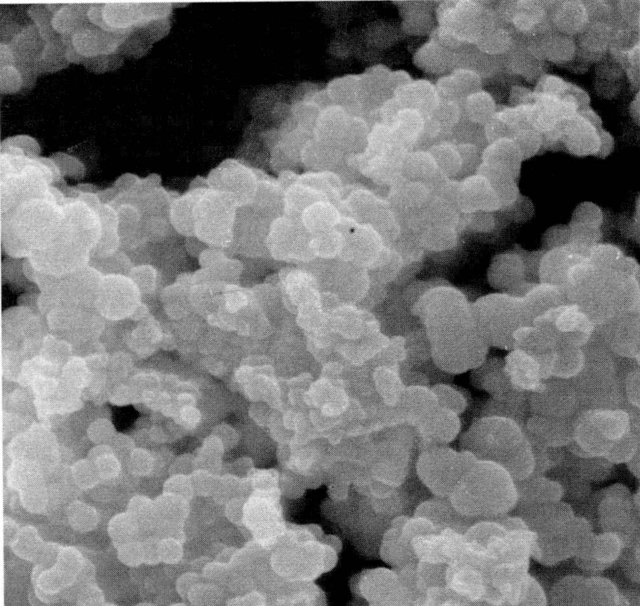

FIG. 7–36. Scanning electron micrograph of amorphous calcium phosphate crystals in the urine sediment of a 5-year-old male castrated Shih Tzu. (Magnification, 5760X.) (From Osborne CA, et al.: Identification and interpretation of crystalluria in domestic animals: A light and electron microscopic study. *Vet Med.* 1990; 85:18-37.)

dogs and cats and in dogs and cats with uroliths primarily composed of calcium oxalate. Although they may be observed in dogs intoxicated with ethylene glycol, they are less common than calcium oxalate monohydrate crystals (ethylene glycol toxicity may also occur without crystalluria).

(b). Calcium oxalate monohydrate crystals may occur alone or in combination with calcium oxalate dihydrate or other types of crystals. Large quantities of calcium oxalate monohydrate (or dihydrate) crystals in fresh urine should prompt consideration of hypercalciuric or hyperoxaluric disorders (such as ethylene glycol toxicity), especially if they occur in aggregates or grow to a large size.[35]

g. Calcium phosphate. (Figs. 7–34 through 7–37)

(1). Habit.

(a). There are many different types of calcium phosphate crystals. They appear to be variously described as amorphous phosphates and calcium phosphates.

(b). With the exception of brushite, calcium phosphate crystals tend to form in alkaline urine.

(c). By light microscopy, amorphous phosphates resemble amorphous urate. However, amorphous phosphates typically form in alkaline urine and are soluble in acetic acid. In contrast, amorphous urates often have a yellow granular appearance and are insoluble in acetic acid, but are soluble in alkali and at 60°C.

(d). Scanning electron micrographs of amorphous phosphates found in human urine revealed that they usually have a spheric habit, but may assume doughnut or cast forms. We have only recognized the spheric habit of calcium phosphate in dogs. Calcium phosphates may also form long, thin, colorless prisms, sometimes with one pointed end. These crystals may aggregate into rosettes or appear as needles. Calcium phosphate may also precipitate as elongated, lath-shaped brushite crystals in acidic urine.

(2). Interpretation.

(a). Care must be used in interpretation of amorphous crystals detected by light microscopy because they form

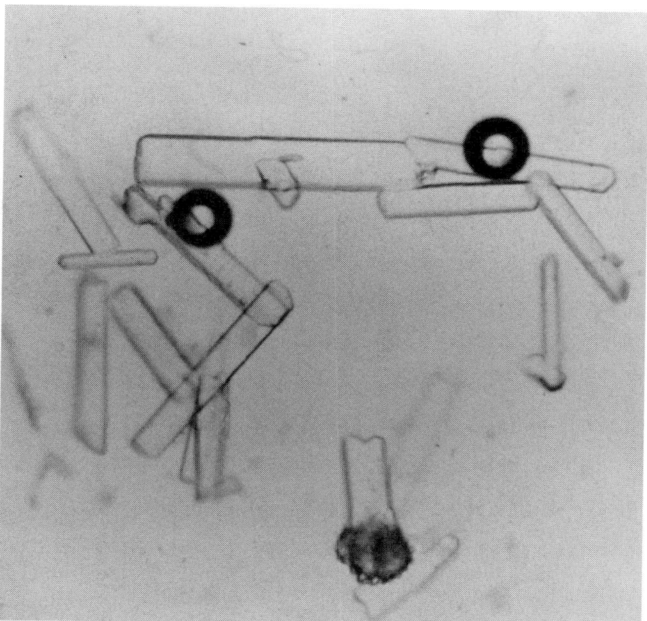

FIG. 7–37. Photomicrograph of urine sediment obtained from a 3-year-old male miniature schnauzer illustrates crystalline calcium phosphate crystals (brushite). The dog had urocystoliths composed of 85% calcium oxalate dihydrate and 15% calcium oxalate monohydrate. Unstained. (Magnification, 160X.) (From Osborne CA, et al.: Identification and interpretation of crystalluria in domestic animals: A light and electron microscopic study. *Vet Med.* 1990; 85:18-37.)

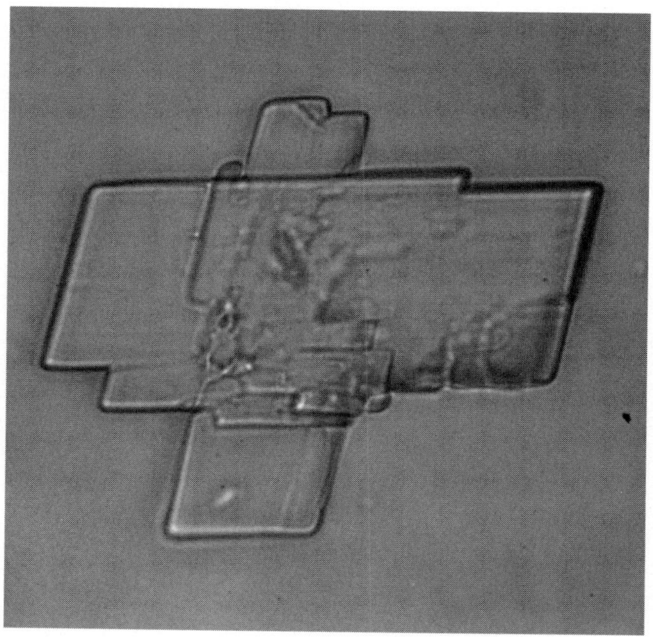

FIG. 7–38. Photomicrograph of canine urine illustrates typical cholesterol crystals. Unstained. (Magnification, 100X.)

from a variety of crystals, including calcium phosphate, ammonium urate, and xanthine.

(b). In our experience, many crystals presumed to be composed of calcium phosphate have been observed in apparently normal dogs, dogs with persistently alkaline urine, and dogs with calcium phosphate uroliths composed of a mixture of calcium phosphate and calcium oxalate. A few calcium phosphate crystals may occur in association with infection-induced struvite crystalluria.

h. Cholesterol (Fig. 7–38)

(1). Habit

(a). Cholesterol crystals typically appear as large, flat, rectangular plates with a characteristic notch in a corner.

(b). By light microscopy, they are colorless and transparent; by polarized light microscopy, a variety of brilliant colors typically are observed.

(2). Interpretation.

(a). In man, cholesterol crystals have been reported to be associated with excessive tissue destruction, the nephrotic syndrome, and chyluria.

(b). Veterinary experience with them has been too limited to formulate meaningful generalities. However, they have been observed in apparently normal dogs.

i. Cystine (Figs. 7–39 through 7–41)

(1). Habit.

(a). Cystine crystals are colorless and have a characteristic hexagonal (benzene ring) shape with equal or unequal sides. They may appear singly but commonly aggregate in layers. Their detection may be aided by reduced light intensity because they are thin.

(b). Cystine crystals most commonly form in concentrated acidic urine. Formation of markedly alkaline urine as a consequence of infection or contamination with urease-producing microbes may cause cystine crystals to dissolve.

(c). Addition of glacial acetic acid followed by refrigeration and centrifugation may enhance detection of typical crystals in alkaline urine samples. Cystine crystals are insoluble in acetic acid, alcohol, acetone, ether, and boiling water. They are soluble in ammonia and hydrochloric acid.

(2). Interpretation.

(a). Cystine crystalluria is not a normal phenomenon.

(b). Cystine uroliths may develop in

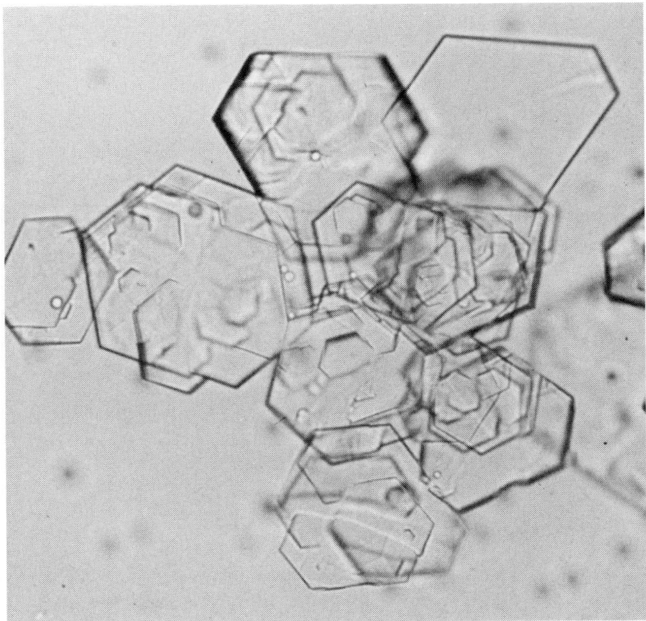

FIG. 7–39. Photomicrograph of urine sediment of a 9-month-old female Scottish terrier contains cystine crystals. Unstained. (Magnification, 40X.)

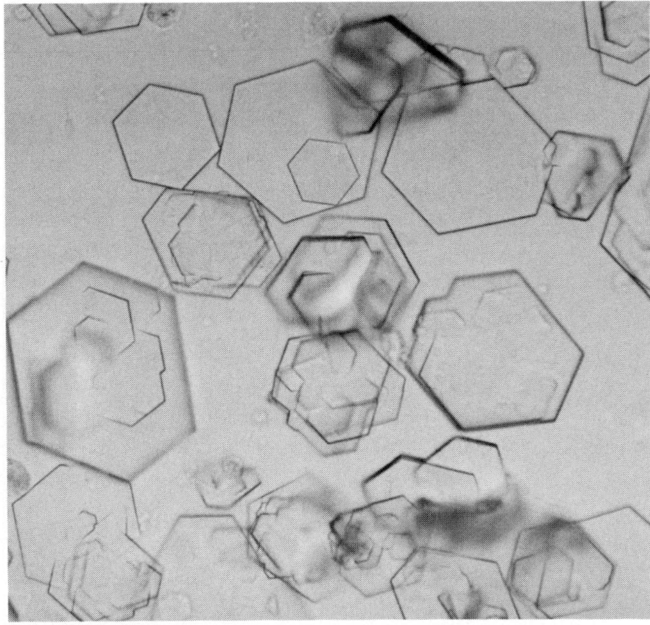

FIG. 7–40. Photomicrograph of cystine crystals formed in urine collected from a 22-month-old male Newfoundland dog. The dog had multiple cystine urocystoliths. (Magnification, 100X.)

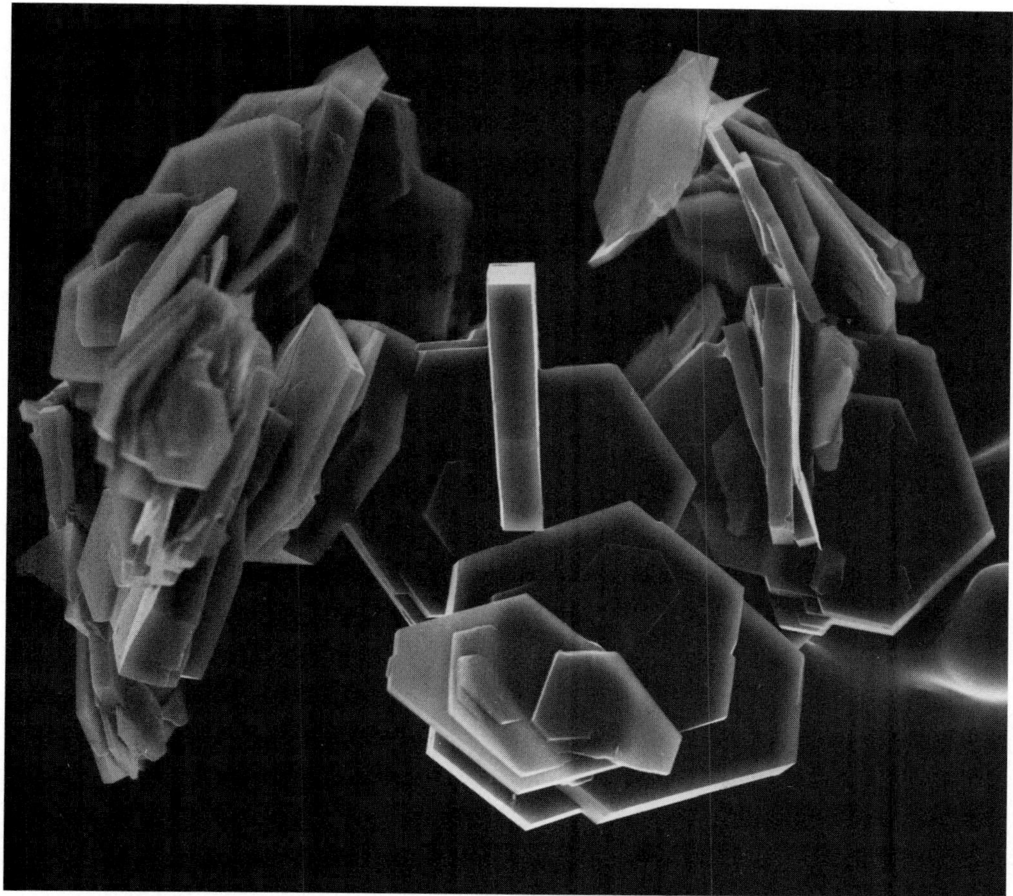

FIG. 7–41. Scanning electron micrograph of the cystine crystals obtained from the dog described in Figure 7–40. Notice the difference in size and thickness of the crystals and their tendency to adhere to each other in layers. (Magnification, 720X.)

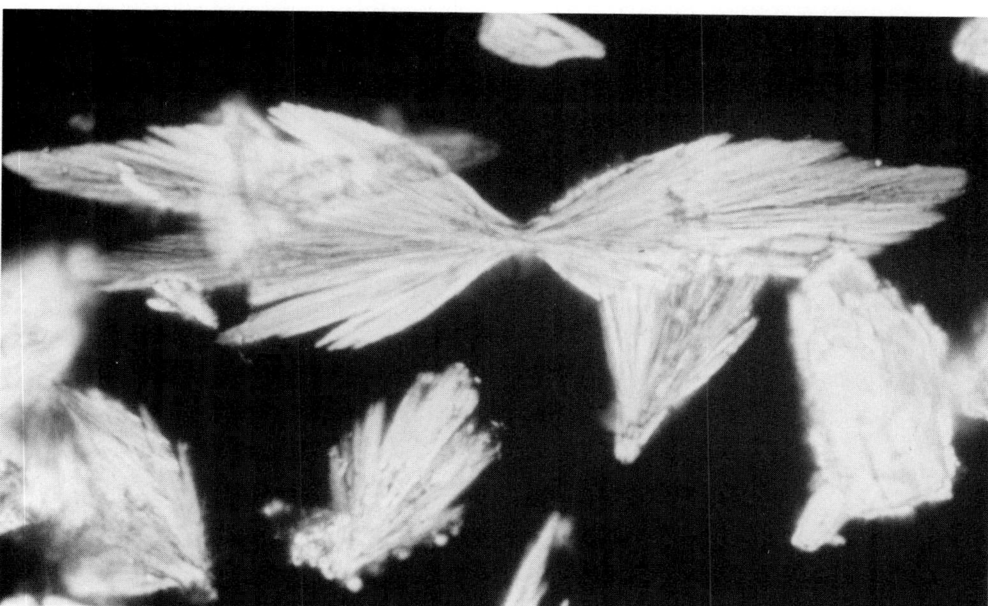

FIG. 7–42. Photomicrograph of sulfa crystals in the urine sediment of an adult male dog given sulfadiazine - trimethoprim orally. Unstained polarized light microscopy. (Magnification, 40X.)

dogs and cats with the metabolic disorder of cystinuria; however, not all patients with cystinuria develop cystine uroliths. (See following review of magnesium ammonium phosphate and uric acid crystalluria for details about differentiation of cystine crystals from struvite or uric acid crystals.)

j. Drug-associated crystalluria[73] (Fig. 7–42)
   (1). Various drugs excreted in urine may form crystals.
   (2). Perhaps the most familiar drug-associated crystalluria in dogs and cats is that occurring with sulfonamide administration. Sulfonamide drugs may precipitate in urine in characteristic sheaves of clear or brownish needles, usually with eccentric binding. They may also appear as amorphous crystals or spheroids with radial striations. A positive lignin test result supports a diagnosis of sulfonamide crystalluria. Compound uroliths containing varying quantities of sulfonamides have been observed in dogs and cats.
   (3). Other forms of drug-associated crystalluria have only been documented in man. Radiopaque contrast agents, such as Hypaque (Winthrop) and Renografin (Squibb), may precipitate in acidic urine as pleomorphic needles occurring singly or in sheaves. Primidone may precipitate as hexagonal plates resembling calcium oxalate monohydrate. Ciprofloxacin may precipitate in alkaline urine as sheaves with eccentric binding.

k. Hippuric acid.
   (1). Hippuric acid crystals are colorless, elongated structures of variable size. They typically have six sides that are connected by rounded corners.
   (2). They have attracted renewed interest in veterinary medicine because of their apparent association with ethylene glycol toxicity in dogs and cats.[52] However, in recent studies of dogs and cats with ethylene glycol poisoning, urine crystals presumed to be hippuric acid based on light microscopy were found to be composed of calcium oxalate monohydrate by x-ray diffraction.[35]

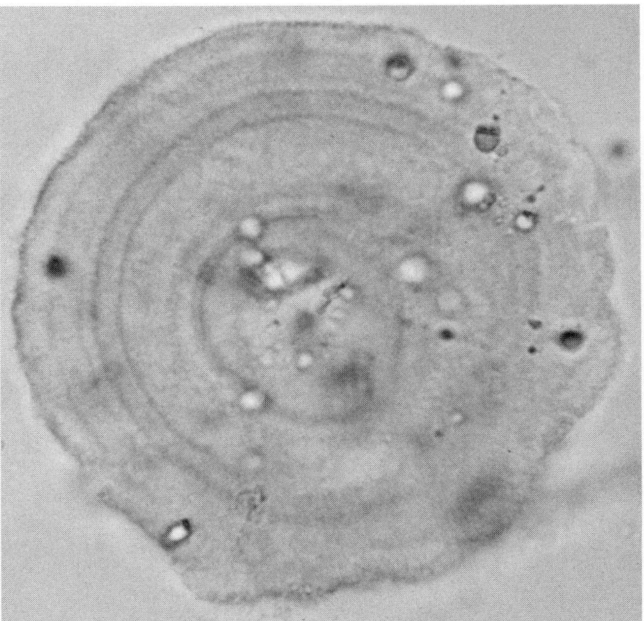

FIG. 7–43. Photomicrograph of crystals with morphologic characteristics similar to those of leucine. The crystals formed in the urine of an 11-year-old male mixed-breed dog. (Magnification, 160X.) (From Osborne CA, et al.: Identification and interpretation of crystalluria in domestic animals: A light and electron microscopic study. *Vet Med.* 1990; 85:18-37.)

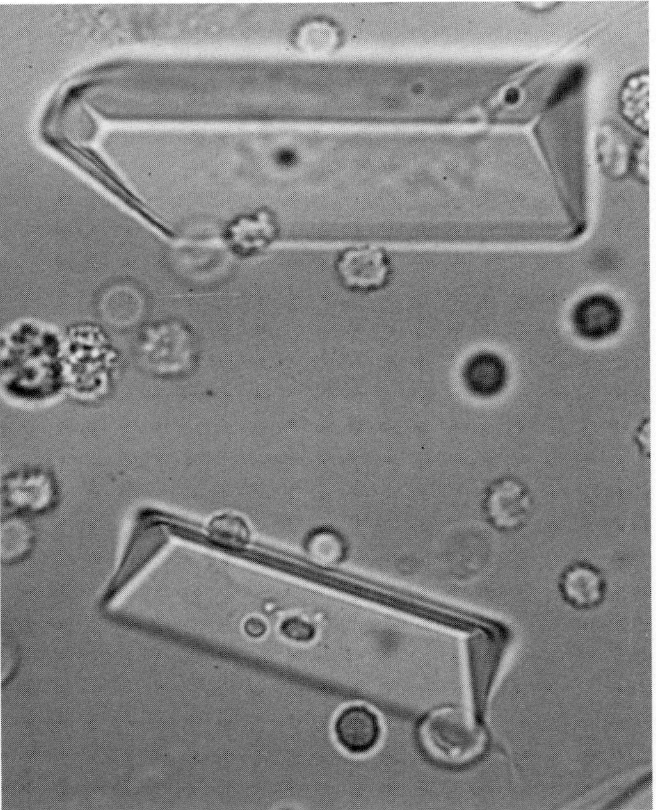

FIG. 7–44. Canine urine sediment containing magnesium ammonium phosphate crystals surrounded by crenated red cells, an occasional white cell, and occasional spermatozoa. Unstained. (Magnification, 100X.) (From Osborne CA, et al.: Identification and interpretation of crystalluria in domestic animals: A light and electron microscopic study. *Vet Med.* 1990; 85:18-37.)

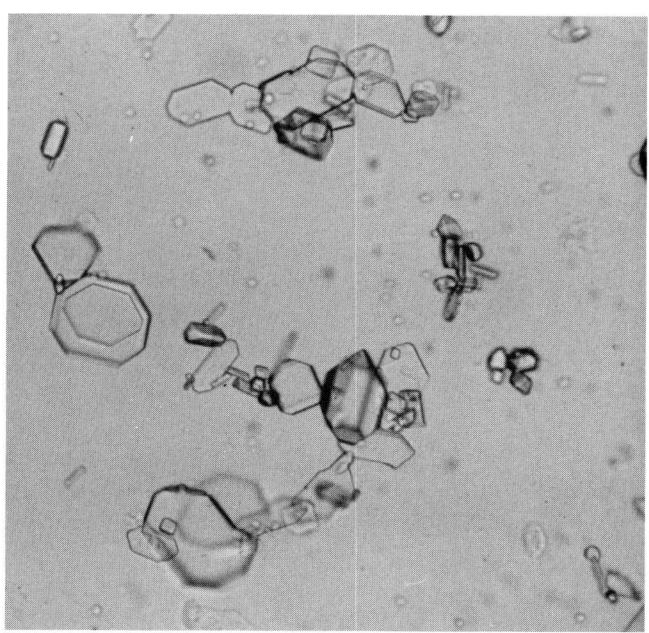

FIG. 7–45. Photomicrograph of magnesium ammonium phosphate crystals in urine sediment of a 2-year-old castrated male domestic short-haired cat. Unstained. (Magnification, 40X.) (From Osborne CA, et al.: Identification and interpretation of crystalluria in domestic animals: A light and electron microscopic study. *Vet Med.* 1990; 85:18-37.)

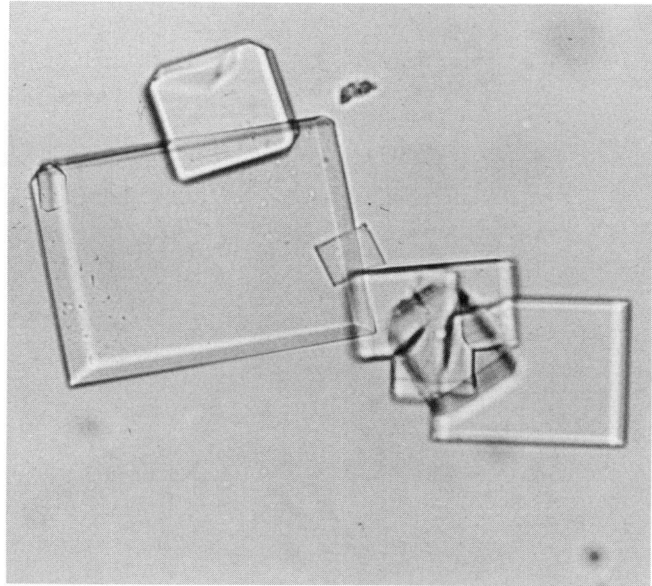

FIG. 7–46. Photomicrograph of urine sediment obtained from an adult male domestic short-haired cat contains magnesium ammonium phosphate crystals. Unstained. (Magnification, 40X.)

(3). True hippuric acid crystals are apparently rare in dogs and cats and therefore are of unknown significance.

l. Leucine (Fig. 7–43)

(1). Leucine crystals typically appear as large yellow or brown spheroids with radial concentric laminations. However, such spheroids may not be pure leucine because reports have revealed that pure leucine forms crystals that resemble hexagonal plates.

(2). In human beings, leucine crystals are indicative of severe liver disease. The significance of leucine crystals in dogs has not been well documented.

m. Magnesium ammonium phosphate (Figs. 7–44 through 7–46)

(1). Habit.

(a). Magnesium ammonium phosphate (struvite) crystals typically appear as colorless, orthorhombic (having three unequal axes intersecting at right angles), coffin-like prisms. They often have three to six or more sides and often have oblique ends. Six- to eight-sided struvite crystals in cats are sometimes mistaken for cystine crystals. Unlike cystine, however, they occur in association with other forms of struvite and readily dissolve following acidification with dilute acetic acid.

(b). On occasion, struvite crystals aggregate into fern-like structures. The sharp outlines of struvite crystals characteristically observed in fresh urine may become feather-like or motheaten as they dissolve.

(2). Interpretation.

(a). Struvite crystals commonly occur in dogs and occasionally in cats in association with free ammonia produced by microbial urease-induced hydrolysis of urea.

(b). Struvite crystals commonly occur in cats and occasionally in dogs in the absence of detectable urease. In this instance, the ammonium component of struvite presumably is generated by renal tubules.

(c). In our experience, struvite crystals may be observed in dogs and cats that:

(1′). Are apparently normal.

(2′). Have infection-induced struvite uroliths.

(3′). Have sterile struvite uroliths.

(4′). Have nonstruvite uroliths.

(5′). Have uroliths of mixed composition (e.g., a nucleus com-

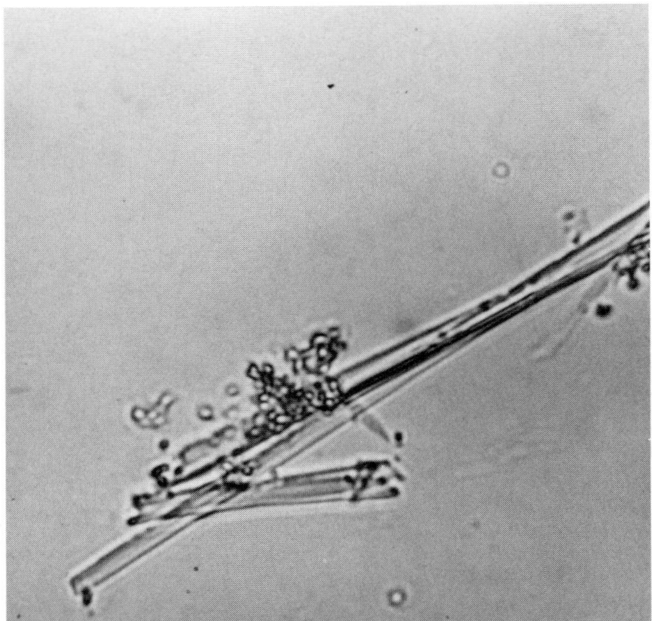

FIG. 7–47. Photomicrograph of canine urine sediment contains crystals with morphologic characteristics similar to those of tyrosine and calcium sulfate crystals. Unstained. (Magnification, 160X.) (From Osborne CA, et al.: Identification and interpretation of crystalluria in domestic animals: A light and electron microscopic study. *Vet Med.* 1990; 85:18-37.)

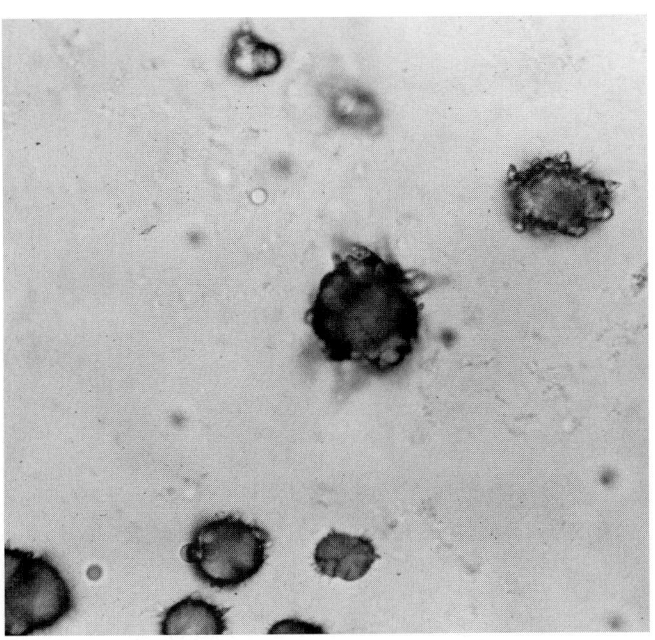

FIG. 7–49. Photomicrograph of canine urine sediment contains thorn-apple form of ammonium acid urate crystals. Unstained. (Magnification, 100X.) (From Osborne CA, et al.: Identification and interpretation of crystalluria in domestic animals: A light and electron microscopic study. *Vet Med.* 1990; 85:18-37.)

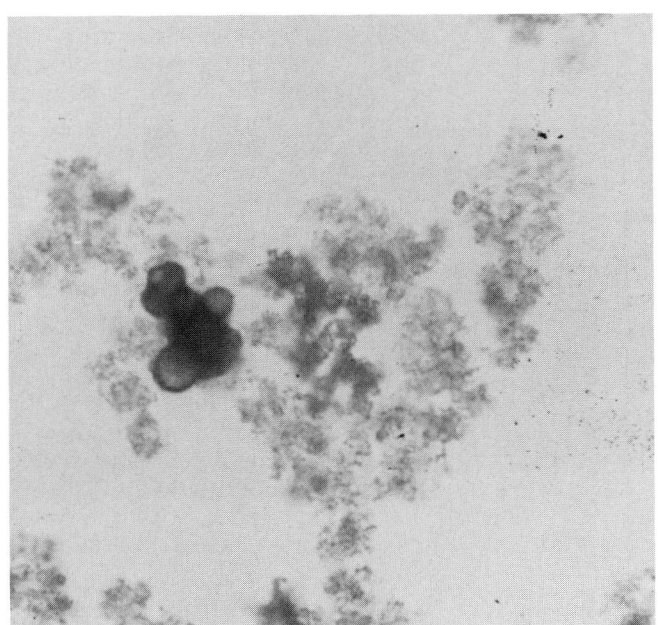

FIG. 7–48. Photomicrograph of ammonium urate crystals in urine sediment of a 1-year-old Persian with a portal vascular anomaly. Unstained. (Magnification, 128X.) (From Osborne CA, et al.: Identification and interpretation of crystalluria in domestic animals: A light and electron microscopic study. *Vet Med.* 1990; 85:18-37.)

posed of calcium oxalate and a shell composed of struvite).

(6′). Have urinary tract disease without uroliths.

n. Tyrosine (Fig. 7–47)
   (1). Tyrosine crystals appear as fine, highly refractile, colorless or yellow needles aggregated in sheaves or clusters.
   (2). In man, they have been reported to occur in association with severe liver disease. However, they have not been a common finding with canine or feline liver disorders.

o. Urates: Ammonium, sodium, and amorphous urate. (Figs. 7–48 through 7–50).
   (1). Habit.
      (a). Ammonium urate (also called ammonium biruate) crystals are commonly observed in slightly acidic, neutral, and alkaline urine. They are usually brown or yellow-brown and may form spherulites or spheric bodies with long irregular protrusions (so-called thorn-apple form).
      (b). Sodium, potassium, magnesium, and calcium urate salts may precipitate in amorphous form in acidic urine (so-called amorphous urates). They may resemble amorphous phosphates, but dissolve in an alka-

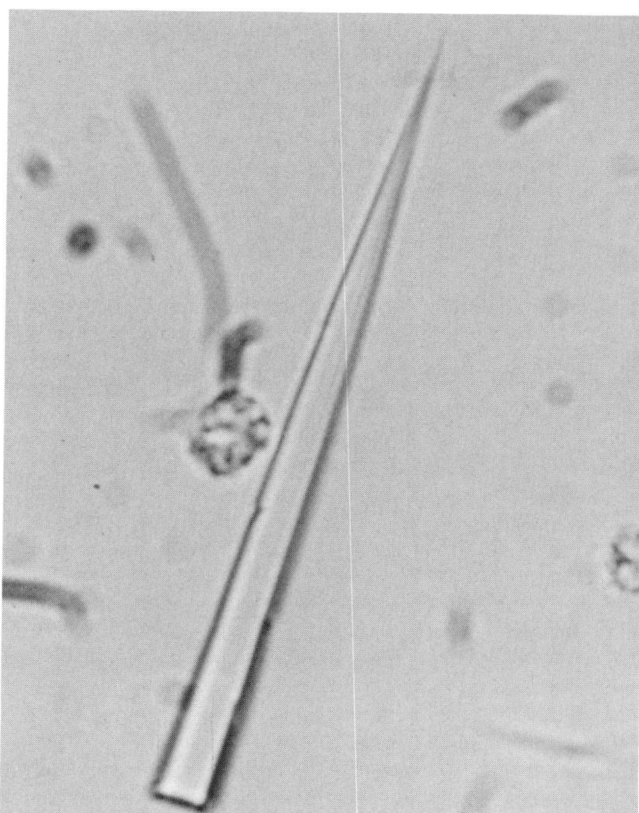

FIG. 7–50. Photomicrograph of a sodium urate crystal in the urine sediment of a 3-year-old male English bulldog. (Magnification, 250X.) (From Osborne CA, et al.: Identification and interpretation of crystalluria in domestic animals: A light and electron microscopic study. *Vet Med.* 1990; 85:18-37.)

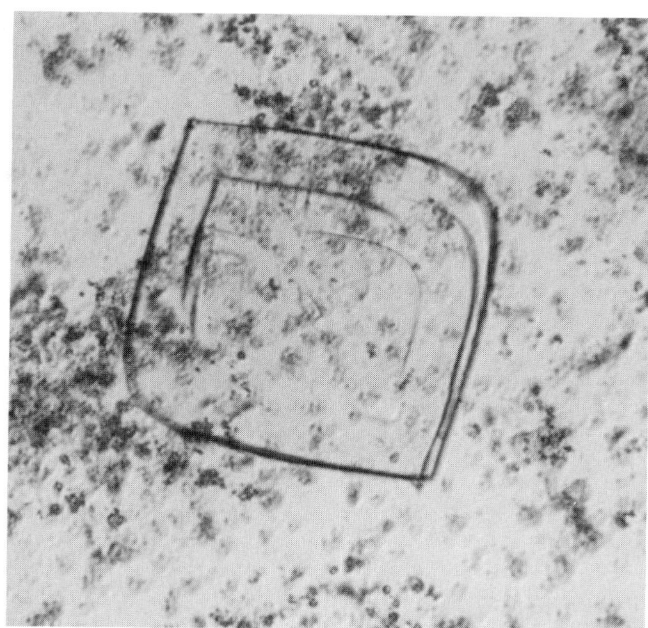

FIG. 7–51. Photomicrograph of urine sediment obtained from an adult male dalmatian contains a uric acid crystal. Unstained. (Magnification, 25X.)

line envirment. As the amorphous crystals grow, they develop a characteristic yellow or yellow-brown color. Sodium urate may also precipitate as colorless or yellowish needles or as slender prisms occurring in sheaves or clusters.

(c). Ammonium urate and amorphous urate crystals are insoluble in acetic acid. However, addition of 10% acetic acid to urine sediment containing these crystals often results in the appearance of uric acid and sometimes sodium urate crystals. (See the following section, "Uric Acid," for details.) Addition of acetic acid to amorphous phosphate crystals results in their rapid dissolution, whereas they persist in alkaline urine sediment.

(2). Interpretation

(a). Ammonium urate and amorphous urate may occur in apparently normal dogs and cats, but they are not common.

(b). They are frequently observed in dogs with portal vascular anomalies with or without concomitant ammonium urate uroliths.

(c). They are also commonly detected in dalmatians and English bulldogs. They may also be observed in dogs and cats with ammonium urate uroliths caused by disorders other than portal vascular anomalies.

p. Uric acid. (Fig. 7–51)

(1). Habit.

(a). Uric acid crystals are often yellow or yellow-brown and may occur in a variety of shapes. The most characteristic forms are diamond or rhombic plates, which may contain concentric rings.

(b). They may also appear as rosettes composed of aggregates of many uric acid crystals.

(c). Occasionally uric acid crystals form rhomboid plates with one or more paired protrusions from their sides.

(d). Less commonly they appear as six-sided crystals resembling cystine. However, the six-sided crystals occur in association with typical diamond-shape or rhomboid forms.

(e). Uric acid crystals are soluble in sodium hydroxide, but are insoluble

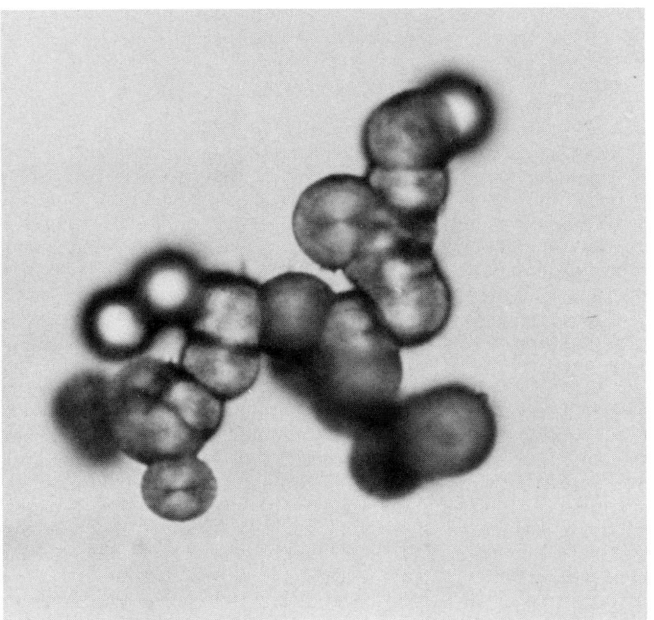

FIG. 7–52. Photomicrograph of xanthine crystals in the urine sediment of an adult female beagle given allopurinol orally. Compare to Figure 7–48. Unstained. (Magnification, 40X.)

in alcohol, hydrochloric acid, and acetic acid.

(2). Interpretation

(a). Although common in human beings, naturally occurring uric acid crystalluria is uncommon in dogs and cats. When detected, the crystals have the same significance as that described for ammonium and amorphous urates.

(b). Uric acid crystals readily form following the addition of 10% acetic acid to canine or feline urine sediment that contains amorphous urate or ammonium urate crystals. Sodium urate crystals may also appear. Exposure to acetic acid for approximately 20 to 30 minutes is often required before the uric acid crystals become visible. They may grow large if preserved overnight in a covered Petri dish humidified with a sponge soaked in water.

q. Xanthine (Fig. 7–52)

(1). Xanthine may precipitate in amorphous form in acidic urine, especially in dogs or

TABLE 7–11
NORMAL FINDINGS—FRESH CANINE AND FELINE URINE

Component	Adult Dog	Adult Cat
Color	Yellow	Yellow
Turbidity	Clear	Clear
Specific Gravity		
Minimum	1.001	1.001
Maximum	1.065+	1.080+
Typical Range	1.015-1.045	1.035-1.060
Volume (mL/kg body wt/d)	±20 to 40*	±15 to 30*
Osmolality		
Minimum	50	50
Maximum	±2400	±3000
Typical Range	500-1200	?
pH	4.5-8.5	4.5-8.5
Glucose	Negative	Negative
Ketones	Negative	Negative
Bilirubin	Trace to 1+†	Negative
Occult Blood	Negative	Negative
Protein	Trace†	Trace
RBC (per high-power field)	0-5 (?)	0-5 (?)
WBC (per high-power field)	0-5 (?)	0-5 (?)
Casts (per low-power field)	Occasional Hyaline	Occasional Hyaline
Epithelial cells (per high-power field)	Occasional	Occasional
Fat Droplets (per high-power field)	Uncommon	Common
Bacteria (per high-power field)	Negative	Negative
Crystals (per high-power field)	Variable	Variable

*Guesstimates only.
†In highly concentrated urine.

cats given allopurinol. Amorphous xanthine crystals resemble amorphous urate crystals.

(2). Detection of xanthine crystals suggests administration of excessive dosages of allopurinol in context of the amount of purine precursors in the diet.[5]

(3). In human beings, xanthine crystalluria has been reported to occur in association with hereditary xanthinuria. We have encountered xanthinuria and xanthine uroliths in cats.

REFERENCES

1. Adams LG, Polzin DJ, Osborne CA, O'Brien TD. Correlation of urine protein/creatinine ratio and twenty-four-hour urinary protein excretion in normal cats and cats with surgically induced chronic renal failure. *J Vet Intern Med.* 1992; 6:36-40.
2. Adams LG, Polzin DJ, Osborne CA, O'Brien TD. Effects of dietary protein restriction in clinically normal cats and cats with surgically induced chronic renal failure. *Am J Vet Res.* 1993; 54:1643-1662.
3. Allen TA, Jones RL, Purvance J: Microbiologic evaluation of canine urine: Direct microscopic examination and preservation of specimen quality for culture. *J Am Vet Med Assoc.* 1987; 190:1289-1291.
4. Barlough JE, Osborne CA, Stevens JB. Canine and feline urinalysis: Value of macroscopic and microscopic examination. *J Am Vet Med Assoc.* 1981; 178:61-63.
5. Bartges JW, Osborne CA, Felice LJ. Canine xanthine uroliths: Risk factor management. In: Kirk RW, Bonagura, JD, eds. *Current Veterinary Therapy.* XI Philadelphia, Pa: WB Saunders Co. 1992: 900-905.
6. Berggard I. Plasma proteins in normal human urine. In: Manuel Y, Revillard JP, Betuel H, eds. *Proteins in Normal and Pathological Urine.* Karger: Basel; 1970: 7–19.
7. Biewenga WJ, Gruys E, Hendricks HJ. Urinary protein loss in the dog. Nephrological study of 29 dogs without signs of renal disease. *Res Vet Sci.* 1982; 33:336-374.
8. Bovee KC. Urine osmolality as a definitive indicator of renal concentrating ability. *J Am Vet Med Assoc.* 1969; 155:30-35.
9. Bovee KC, Joyce T, Blazer-Yost B, et al. Characterization of renal defects in dogs with a syndrome similar to the Fanconi syndrome in man. *J Am Vet Med Assoc.* 1979; 174:1094-1099.
10. Bradley M, Schumann GB, Ward PCJ. Examination of urine. In: Henry JB, ed. *Clinical Diagnosis and Management by Laboratory Methods. I.* 17th ed. Philadelphia, Pa: WB Saunders; 1979: 559-634.
11. Breitschwerdt EB, Woody BJ, Zerbe CA, et al. Monoclonal grammopathy associated with naturally occurring canine ehrlichiosis. *J Vet Int Med.* 1987; 1:2-9.
12. Brown SA, Rakich PM, Barsanti JA, et al. Fanconi syndrome and acute renal failure associated with gentamicin therapy in a dog. *J Am Anim Hosp Assoc.* 1986; 22:635.
13. Center SA, Smith JF. Ocular lesions in a dog with serum hyperviscosity secondary to an IgA myeloma. *J Am Vet Med Assoc.* 1982; 181:811-813.
14. Center SA, Wilkinson E, Smith CA, et al. 24-hour urine protein/creatinine ratio in dogs with protein-losing nephropathies. *J Am Vet Med Assoc.* 1985; 187:820-823.
15. Chew DJ. Urinalysis. In: Bovee KC, ed. *Canine Nephrology.* Media, Pa: Harwall Publishing Co; 1984.
16. Chow FHC, Taton BS, Lewis LD, Hamar DW. Effect of dietary ammonium chloride, dl-methionine, sodium phosphate and ascorbic acid on urinary pH and electrolyte concentrations of male cats. *Feline Practice.* 1978; 8:29-34.
17. Cialla AP, Newsome B, Kaster J. Reagent strip method for specific gravity. An evaluation. *Lab Med.* 1985; 16:38-40.
18. Coye RD, Niehoff R, Rammer M, et al. Proteinuria associated with experimentally produced abscesses and fever in dogs. *Arch Pathol* 1959; 68:126-133.
19. Crawford MA. The urinary system. In: Hoskins JD, ed. *Veterinary Pediatrics.* Philadelphia, Pa: WB Saunders Co; 1990: 271-292.
20. Deen WM, Satvat B. Determinants of the glomerular filtration of proteins. *Am J Physiol.* 1981; 241:F162-F170.
21. Dennis VW, Robinson RR. Proteinuria. In: Seldin DW, Giebisch G, eds. *The Kidney: Physiology and Pathophysiology.* New York, NY: Raven Press; 1985:1805-1816.
22. DeSchepper J. Degradation of haemoglobin to bilirubin in the kidney of the dog. *Tijelschr Diergeneeskol.* 1974; 99:699-707.
23. DiBartola SP, Chew DJ, Jacobs G. Quantitative urinalysis including 24-hour protein excretion in the dog. *J Am Anim Hosp Assoc.* 1980; 16:537–546.
24. Dirks JH, Clapp JR, Berliner RW. The protein concentrations in the proximal tubule of the dog. *J Clin Invest.* 1964; 43:916-921.
25. Dooley MP, Pineda MH, Hopper JG, Hsu WH. *Retrograde Flow of Semen Caused by Electroejaculation in the Domestic Cat.* Urbana, Il: 10th International Congress on Animal & Artificial Insemination; June 10-14, 1981; 363.
26. Easley JR, Breitschwerdt EB. Glucosuria associated with renal tubular dysfunction in three basenji dogs. *J Am Vet Med Assoc.* 1976; 168:938-943.
27. Edelmann CM Jr, Barnett HL, Troupkov V. Renal concentrating mechanism in newborn infants. Effect of dietary protein and water content, role of urea, and responsiveness to antidiuretic hormone. *J Clin Invest.* 1960; 39:1062-1069.
28. Fairbanks VF, Klee GG. Biochemical aspects of haematology. In: Tietz NW, ed. *Textbook of Clinical Chemistry.* Philadelphia, Pa: WB Saunders Co; 1986: 1495-1588.
29. Fairley KF, Birch DF. A simple method for identifying glomerular bleeding. *Kidney Int.* 1982; 21:105-108.
30. Feeney DA, Osborne CA, Jessen CR. Effects of radiographic contrast media on the results of urinalysis. *J Am Vet Med Assoc.* 1980; 176:1378-1781.
31. Feeney DA, Walter PA, Johnston GR. The effect of radiopaque contrast media on the urinalysis. In: Kirk RW, ed. *Current Veterinary Therapy.* Vol. 9. Philadelphia, Pa: WB Saunders Co; 1986: 1115-1117.
32. Feldman EC, Nelson RW. *Canine and Feline Endocrinology and Reproduction.* Philadelphia, Pa: WB Saunders Co; 1987.
33. Ferguson JM, Renton JP. Observation on the presence of spermatozoa in canine urine. *J Small Anim Pract.* 1988; 29:691-694.
34. Finco DR. Kidney function. In: Kaneko JJ, ed. *Clinical Biochemistry of Domestic Animals.* 4th ed. New York, NY: Academic Press; 1989: 496-542.
35. Foit FF, et al. X-ray powder diffraction and microscopic analysis of crystalluria in dogs with ethylene glycol toxicity. *Am J Vet Res.* 1985; 46:2404-2408.
36. Free EL, Rupe CO, Metzler I. Studies with a new colorimetric method for proteinuria. *Clin Chem.* 1957; 3:716.
37. Gadeholt H. Quantitative examination of urinary sediment with special regard to sources of error. *Br Med.* 1964; 1:1547.
38. Giger U, Harvey JW. Hemolysis caused by phosphofructokinase deficiency in English springer spaniels. *J Am Vet Med Assoc.* 1987; 191:453-459.
39. Glover JF, Wallach J. Positive dipstick test for albumin when other renal function tests are normal. *J Am Vet Med Assoc.* 1973; 223:928.
40. Grauer GF, Thomas CB, Eicker SW, et al. Estimation of quantitative proteinuria in the dog using the urine protein-to-

creatinine ratio from a random voided sample. *Am J Vet Res.* 1985; 46:2216-2119.

41. Guignard P. Renal function in the newborn infant. *Pediatr Clin North Am.* 1982; 29:777-790.
42. Haber MH, Lindner LE. The surface ultrastructure of urinary casts. *Am J Clin Pathol.* 1977; 68:547-552.
43. Hall CW, Chung-Park M, Vacca CV, et al. The renal handling of beta 2-microglobulin in the dog. *Kidney Int.* 1982; 22:156-161.
44. Hardy RM, Osborne CA. Water deprivation test in the dog: Maximal normal values. *J Am Vet Med Assoc.* 1979; 174:479-484.
45. Harvey DG, Hou CM. The use of paper electrophoresis for routine identification of urinary proteins in the dog. *J Small Anim Pract.* 1966; 7:431-440.
46. Hayman JM, Shumway NP, Dunke P, et al. Experimental hyposthenuria. *J Clin Invest.* 1939; 18:195-211.
47. Horster M, Valtin H. Postnatal development of renal function. Micropuncture and clearance studies in the dog. *J Clin Invest.* 1971; 50:779-795.
48. Hoskins JD, Turnwald GH, Kearney MT, et al. Quantitative urinalysis in kittens from four to thirty weeks after birth. *Am J Vet Res.* 1991; 52:1295-1299.
49. Hoyer JR, Seiler MW. Pathophysiology of Tamm-Horsfall protein. *Kidney Int.* 1979; 16:279-289.
50. Jenkins RD, Fenn JP, Matsen JM. Review of urine microscopy for bacteria. *JAMA.* 1986; 255:3397-3404.
51. Klausner JS, Osborne CA, Stevens JB. Screening tests for the detection of significant bacteriuria. In: Kirk RW, ed. *Current Veterinary Therapy.* Vol 7. Philadelphia, Pa: WB Saunders Co; 1980:1154-1157.
52. Kramer JW, Bistline D, Sheridan P, et al. Identification of hippuric acid crystals in the urine of ethylene glycol-intoxicated dogs and cats. *J Am Vet Med Assoc.* 1984; 184:584.
53. Kruth SA, Cowgill LD. Renal glucose transport in the cat. In: *ACVIM Proceedings.* Washington DC; 1982:78.
54. Lambert PP, Gassee JP, Askenasi R. Physiologic basis of protein excretion. In: Manuel Y, Revillard JP, Betuel S, eds. *Proteins in Normal and Pathological Urine.* Basel: S Karger; 1970:67-82.
55. Lees GE, Hardy RM, Stevens JB, Osborne CA. Clinical implications of feline bilirubinuria. *J Am Anim Hosp Assoc.* 1981; 20:765-771.
56. Lees GE, Osborne CA, Stevens JB. Antibacterial properties of urine: Studies of feline urine specific gravity, osmolality, and pH. *J Am Anim Hosp Assoc.* 1979; 15:135-141.
57. Lewis LD, Morris ML, Hand MS. *Small Animal Clinical Nutrition, III.* Topeka, Kan: Mark Morris Associates; 1987.
58. Lindner LE, Haber MH. Hyaline casts in the urine: Mechanism of formation and morphologic transformations. *Am J Clin Pathol.* 1983; 80:347-352.
59. Lulich JP, Osborne CA. Interpretation of urine protein-creatinine ratios in dogs with glomerular and nonglomerular disorders. *Compendium of Continuing Education* 1990; 12:59-72.
60. Lulich JP, Osborne CA. Fungal urinary tract infections. In: Kirk RW, Bonagura JD, eds. *Current Veterinary Therapy, XI.* Philadelphia, Pa: WB Saunders Co; 1992:914-919.
61. Lulich JP, Osborne CA, O'Brien TD, Polzin DJ. Feline renal failure: Questions, answers, questions. *Comp Cont Educ.* 1992; 14:127-152.
62. Matus RE, Leifer CE, Gordon BR, et al. Plasmapheresis and chemotherapy of hyperviscosity syndrome associated with monoclonal gammopathy in the dog. *J Am Vet Med Assoc.* 1983; 183:215-218.
63. Matus RE, Leifer CE, MacEwen EG, et al. Prognostic factors for multiple myeloma in the dog. *J Am Vet Med Assoc.* 1986; 188:1288-1292.
64. McCaw DL, Knapp DW, Hewett JE. Effect of collection time and exercise restriction on the prediction of urine protein excretion using urine protein/creatinine ratio in dogs. *Am J Vet Res.* 1985; 46:1665-1669.
65. McKenzie JK, McQueen EG. Immunofluorescent localization of Tamm-Horsfall mucoprotein in human kidney. *J Clin Pathol.* 1969; 22:334.
66. McQueen EG. The nature of urinary casts. *J Clin Pathol.* 1962; 15:367-373.
67. McQueen EG, Engel GB. Factors determining the aggregation of urinary protein. *J Clin Pathol.* 1966; 19:392-396.
68. Miller C, Fish MB, Danelski TF. IgA multiple myeloma with multisystem manifestations in the dog: A case report. *J Am Anim Hosp Assoc.* 1982; 18:53-56.
69. Mori H, Yamasshita H, Nakanishi C, et al. *J Am Anim Hosp Assoc.* Proteinuria induced by transplantable rat pituitary tumor MLT SAS. *Lab Invest.* 1986; 54:636-644.
70. Nahata MC, Shimp L, Lampman T, Mcleod DC. Effect of ascorbic acid on urine pH in man. *Am J Hosp Pharm.* 1977; 34:1234-1237.
71. Nelson DA, Davey FR. Erythrocyte disorders. In: Henry JB, ed. *Clinical Diagnosis and Management by Laboratory Methods.* Philadelphia, Pa: WB Saunders Co; 1984:652-703.
72. Osborne CA, Davis LS, Sanna J, et al. Identification and interpretation of crystalluria in domestic animals: A light and scanning electron microscopic study. *Vet Med.* 1990; 85:18-37.
73. Osborne CA, O'Brien TD, Ghobrial HK, et al. Crystalluria: Observations, interpretations, and misinterpretations. *Vet Clin North Am.* 1986; 16:45-65.
74. Osborne CA, Stevens JB. Clinical significance of proteinuria. In: *Proceedings of the 45th Annual Meeting of the American Animal Hospital Association.* Salt Lake City, Ut: 1978:527-543.
75. Osborne CA, Stevens JB. *Handbook of Canine and Feline Urinalysis.* St. Louis, Mo: Ralston Purina Co; 1981.
76. Osborne CA, Stevens JB, Lees GE, et al. Clinical significance of bilirubinuria. *Comp Cont Educ.* 1980; 2:897-902.
77. Osborne CA, Stevens JB, Rakich P, Ogden B. Clinical significance of glucosuria. *Minn Vet.* 1980; 20:16-25.
78. Papper S. *Clinical Nephrology.* 2nd ed. Boston, Mass: Little, Brown and Co; 1980.
79. Pesce AJ. Methods used for analysis of proteins in urine. *Nephron.* 1974; 13:93-104.
80. Pesce AJ, First MR. *Proteinuria: An Integrated Review.* New York, NY: Marcel Dekker Inc.; 1979.
81. Pollak VE, Arbel C. The distribution of Tamm-Horsfall mucoprotein (Uromucoid) in the human nephron. *Nephron.* 1969; 6:667.
82. Poortman JR. Post exercise proteinuria in humans. *JAMA.* 1985; 253:236-240.
83. Porter P. Comparative study of the macromolecular components excreted in urine of dog and man. *J Comp Pathol.* 1964; 74:108-118.
84. Rahill WH, Subramanian S. Use of fetal animals to investigate renal development. *Lab Anim.* 1973; 23:92-96.
85. Ross LA, Finco DR. Relationship of selected renal function tests to glomerular filtration rate and renal blood flow in cats. *Am J Vet Res.* 1981; 42:1704-1710.
86. Rutecki GJ, Goldsmith C, Schreiner GE. Characterization of proteins in urinary casts: Fluorescent antibody identification of Tamm-Horsfall mucoprotein in matrix and serum proteins in granules. *N Engl J Med.* 1979; 284:1049-1052.
87. Schenk EA, Schwartz RH, Lewis RA. Tamm-Horsfall mucoprotein. I—Localization in the kidney. *Lab Invest.* 1971; 25:92-95.
88. Schull RM, Osborne CA, Barrett RE, et al. Serum hyperviscosity syndrome associated with IgA multiple myeloma in two dogs. *J Am Anim Hosp Assoc.* 1978; 14:58-70.

89. Searey GP, Tasker JB, Miller DB. Animal model: Pyruvate kinase deficiency in dogs. *Am J Pathol.* 1979; 94:689-692.
90. Shull RM, Hayden DW, Johnston GR. Urogenital blastomycosis in a dog. *J Am Vet Med Assoc.* 1977; 171:730-735.
91. Sternheimer R. A supravital cytodiagnostic stain for urinary sediments. *JAMA.* 1975; 231:826-832.
92. Terry R, Hawkins DR, Church EH, et al. Proteinuria related to hyperproteinemia in dogs following plasma given parenterally. *J Exp Med.* 1948; 87:561-573.
93. Thal SM, DeBellis CC, Iverson SA, Schumana GB. Comparison of dysmorphic erythrocytes with other urinary sediment parameters of renal bleeding. *Am J Clin Pathol.* 1986; 86:784-787.
94. Torrance AG, Fulton RB. Zinc-induced hemolytic anemia in a dog. *J Am Vet Med Assoc.* 1987; 191:443-444.
95. Vail DM, Allen TA, Weiser G. Applicability of leukocyte esterase test strip in detection of canine pyuria. *J Am Vet Med Assoc.* 1986; 189:1451-1453.
96. Vernier RL, Papermaster BW, Olness K, et al. Morphologic studies of the mechanism of proteinuria. *Am J Dis Child.* 1960; 100:476-478.
97. Weening JJ, VanGuildener C, Daha MR, et al. The pathophysiology of protein-overload proteinuria. *Am J Pathol.* 1987; 129:64-73.
98. White JV, Oliver NB, Reimana K, et al. Use of protein-to-creatinine ratio in a single urine specimen for quantitative estimation of canine proteinuria. *J Am Vet Med Assoc.* 1984; 185:882-883.
99. Worden AN, Waterhouse CE, Sellwood EHB. Studies of the composition of normal cat urine. *J Small Anim Pract.* 1960; 1:11-29.
100. Zwelling LA, Balow JE. Hypersthenuria in high dose carbenicillin therapy. *Ann Intern Med.* 1978; 89:225-226.

CHAPTER 

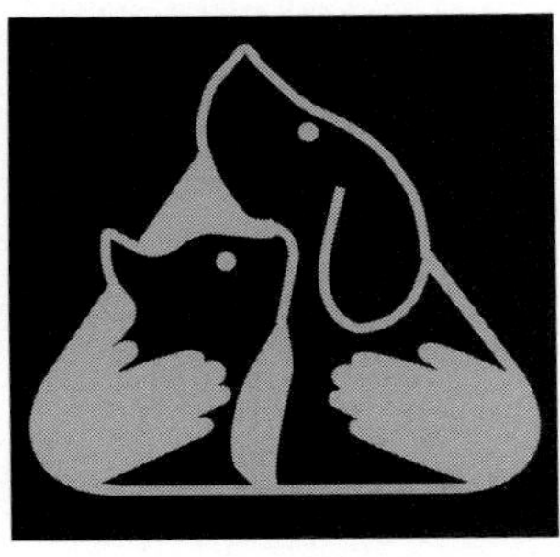

Diagnostic Urine Culture

CARL A. OSBORNE
GEORGE E. LEES

I. OVERVIEW

A. Urine culture is the goldstandard for diagnosis of urinary tract infections. Diagnosis of bacterial urinary tract infections solely on the basis of clinical signs usually results in overdiagnosis. Failure to perform urine cultures or failure to correctly interpret the results of urine cultures may lead not only to diagnostic errors, but to therapeutic failures as well.

B. Under some circumstances, therapy may be initiated without knowledge of urine culture results. (See Chapter 40, Bacterial Infections of the Canine And Feline Urinary Tract, Empirical Choice of Antimicrobial Agents.)

1. However, if cultures are to be performed, urine should be collected for culture before antibacterial therapy is initiated.
2. If antimicrobial therapy has already been instituted, it should be discontinued for approximately 3 to 5 days prior to urine culture to minimize the inhibition of in vivo and in vitro bacterial growth.

C. Because urine may be a good culture medium at room temperature (bacterial counts may double every 20 to 45 minutes), it should be cultured within 30 minutes from the time of collection if significant results are to be consistently obtained.[2] Multiplication or destruction of bacteria may be detected within an hour of collection.

1. If for any reason prompt culture is not possible, the samples should be immediately refrigerated following collection. Refrigerated samples may be stored for as many as 6 hours without significant additional growth of bacteria.[11] However, fastidious organisms may be killed in the urine environment if storage time is prolonged.
2. Alternatively, commercially manufactured collection tubes containing preservatives (B-D Urine C & S Transport Kit), combined with refrigeration, may be used to preserve specimens for as long as 72 hours.[1]

II. QUALITATIVE URINE CULTURE

A. Qualitative urine culture includes isolation and identification of bacteria in urine. It does not include determination of bacterial numbers.

B. Although urine contained in the urinary bladder is normally sterile, urine that passes through the urethra and genital tract may become contaminated with resident bacteria normally present in these locations (Table 8–1).

1. Gram-positive bacteria appear to be especially common inhabitants of the canine urethra.
2. The significance of bacteria in midstream (first portion of stream not included) urine samples, or in those obtained by manual compression of the bladder, is often difficult to interpret because such bacteria may represent pathogens or contaminants.

TABLE 8–1
BACTERIA DETECTED IN THE UROGENITAL TRACT OF NORMAL MALE AND FEMALE DOGS

Genus	Distal Urethra Males	Prepuce	Vagina
Acinetobacter	−	+	+
Bacteroides	−	−	+
Bacillus	−	+	+
Citrobacter	−	−	+
Corynebacterium	+	+	+
Enterococcus	−	−	+
Enterobacter	−	−	+
Escherichia	+	+	+
Flavobacterium	+	+	+
Haemophilus	+	+	+
Klebsiella	+	+	+
Micrococcus	−	−	+
Moraxella	−	+	+
Mycoplasma	+	+	+
Neisseria	−	−	+
Pasteurella	−	+	+
Proteus	−	+	+
Pseudomonas	−	−	+
Staphylococcus	+	+	+
Streptococcus	+	+	+
Ureaplasma	+	+	+

Key: + = presence; − = absence.

3. Even catheterized samples may be contaminated as the catheter passes through the lower genital tract and urethral lumen. For this reason, urine culture techniques should include estimation of the numbers of bacteria present in each milliliter of urine (quantitative culture) in addition to identification of bacterial organisms (qualitative culture).

C. Although qualitative culture is theoretically satisfactory when urine samples are obtained by cystocentesis, an element of doubt may exist concerning minor contamination via skin bacteria or urine transfer during the procedure. For this reason, quantitative urine culture also is recommended for samples collected by cystocentesis.

D. Several factors should be considered when interpreting the significance of qualitative bacterial culture of urine (Table 8–2).

1. Isolation of a single species is of special interest because contamination is more likely to be associated with multiple species.
2. Approximately 75% of the urinary tract infections in dogs are caused by a single species of pathogen, 18% are caused by 2 species, and 6% are caused by 3 species.[10]

TABLE 8–2
FACTORS INFLUENCING INTERPRETATION OF QUALITATIVE BACTERIAL CULTURE OF URINE

Method of collection.
Time lapse between collection and culture.
Method of preservation if not cultured within 30 minutes.
Whether pure or mixed culture.
Magnitude of inflammatory response (if any) detected by urinalysis.
Detection of bacteria in uncontaminated fresh unspun urine.

III. QUANTITATIVE URINE CULTURE

A. Significant bacteriuria.

1. Quantitative urine culture includes determination of the number of bacteria (colony forming units) per unit volume in addition to isolation and identification of bacteria. It is the preferred method of diagnostic culture for urine samples obtained by any collection method..
2. The concept of significant bacteriuria was introduced to aid differentiation between harmless bacterial contaminants of urine and pathogenic organisms causing infectious disease of the urinary system. This concept is based on the observation that a high bacterial count in a properly collected and cultured urine sample indicates the probability of urinary tract infection.
   a. In human beings, urine bacterial counts in excess of 100,000 organisms of a single species per milliliter of urine are considered to be significant.[7]
   b. Isolation of 10,000 to 100,000 bacteria of a single species per milliliter in catheterized or midstream urine samples is interpreted as suspected bacterial infection. Urine from patients with suspected bacteriuria should be cultured a second time. If the same organism is isolated at a similar or higher concentration, the presence of bacterial infection is confirmed because reproducible results would not be expected as a result of contamination.
   c. The presence of fewer than 10,000 bacteria of a single species per milliliter in midstream or catheterized urine samples usually represents contaminants.
3. Although controlled experiments with statistical analyses have not been performed, clinical studies of quantitative urine culture performed at the University Veterinary Hospital, University of Minnesota, and elsewhere[3,4] utilizing the calibrated-loop technique for quantitative culture have revealed that noncatheterized midstream urine samples and catheterized urine samples obtained from dogs with clinical, laboratory, and

TABLE 8–3
INTERPRETATION OF QUANTITATIVE URINE CULTURES IN DOGS AND CATS*

	Significant		Suspicious		Contaminant	
Collection Method	**Dog**	**Cat**	**Dog**	**Cat**	**Dog**	**Cat**
Cystocentesis	≥1,000†	≥1,000	100–1,000	100–1,000	≤100	≤100
Catheterization	≥10,000	≥1,000	1,000–10,000	100–1,000	≤1,000	≤100
Voluntary voiding	≥100,000‡	≥10,000	10,000–90,000	1,000–10,000	≤10,000	≤1,000
Manual compression	≥100,000‡	≥10,000	10,000–90,000	1,000–10,000	≤10,000	≤1,000

*The data represent generalities. On occasion, bacterial urinary tract infections may be detected in dogs and cats with smaller numbers of organisms (i.e., false-negative results).

†Numbers represent colony forming units of bacteria per milliliter of urine.

‡Caution: Contamination of midstream samples may result in colony counts of 10,000/mL or greater in some dogs and cats (i.e., false-positive results). Therefore, they should not be used for routine diagnostic culture of urine from dogs or cats.

radiographic evidence of urinary tract infection usually contained more than 100,000 bacteria per milliliter.

a. Although urine obtained from most dogs without urinary tract infections was either sterile or contained fewer than 10,000 bacteria per milliliter of urine (Table 8–3), counts of 100,000 bacteria per milliliter occurred with sufficient frequency to deem this form of urine collection unsatisfactory for routine diagnostic bacterial culture. Of note is that bacterial contamination of voided and catheterized samples is more likely to occur in female than in male dogs and cats.[6]

b. The lower limit of numbers of organisms that indicates significant bacteriuria in feline urine cultures has not been determined. However, it may be less than the limits in human beings and dogs because feline urine appears to be less conducive to bacterial growth than does urine of dogs or human beings (Table 8–3). In addition, other factors may influence results of quantitative culture of urine for bacteria (Table 8–4).

4. In general, cystocentesis should be used to collect urine samples for qualitative and quantitative bacterial culture.

5. If dysuria and pollakiuria prevent collection of urine by cystocentesis, urine for culture may need to be collected during voiding or by catheterization.

   a. In these situations, the external genitalia of males and females must be rinsed with an appropriate cleansing solution before urine is obtained.

   b. The hair surrounding the vulva of some long-haired female dogs may have to be clipped.

   c. Only sterilized catheters and collection containers should be used, and the containers should have tight-fitting lids. Sterile containers may be obtained by sterilizing paper cups in ethylene oxide gas, or they may be purchased from commercial manufacturers.

   d. If the results of quantitative urine culture of noncatheterized midstream or catheterized urine samples are equivocal following serial cultures, collection of urine by cystocentesis should be again considered.

6. The presence of even small numbers of bacteria in urine aseptically collected by cystocentesis indicates urinary tract infection. However, false-positive results may occur if the needle penetrates a loop of intestine during cystocentesis or if the sample is contaminated during transfer to culture media.

7. A diagnosis of bacterial prostatitis should be based on isolation of significant numbers of bacteria from prostate secretions and/or tissue.

   a. Significant prostatic bacteria is defined as greater than 100,000 bacteria per milliliter

TABLE 8–4
FACTORS THAT MAY INFLUENCE THE NUMBER OF BACTERIAL COLONY FORMING UNITS OBTAINED BY QUANTITATIVE URINE CULTURE

1. Species (dog, cat, other)
2. Collection method
3. Time lapse between collection and culture of urine
4. Method of preservation (if any)
5. Variables related to ability of bacteria to grow in vitro
6. Frequency of micturition
7. Magnitude of diuresis (if any)
8. Site(s) of bacterial infection
9. Administration of antimicrobial agents prior to bacterial culture

TABLE 8–5
IN VITRO CULTURE CHARACTERISTICS OF SOME BACTERIA THAT COMMONLY CAUSE URINARY TRACT INFECTIONS*

Pathogen	Gram Stain	Appearance on Blood Agar	Appearance on MacConkey Agar
Escherichia coli	Negative rods	Smooth gray colonies; may be hemolytic	Pink-red colonies (usually lactose positive)
Enterobacter spp	Negative rods	Smooth gray-white colonies	Pink-red colonies (lactose positive)
Enterococcus spp	Positive cocci	Smooth white colonies; ± partial hemolysis	No growth
Klebsiella spp	Negative rods	Mucoid gray-white colonies	Pink-red mucoid colonies (usually lactose positive)
Proteus mirabilis	Negative rods	Usually swarm	Colorless to tan (transparent) colonies (lactose negative)
Pseudomonas spp	Negative rods	Gray to green colonies; fruity or ammoniacal odor; often hemolytic	Colorless to greenish-tan (transparent) colonies (lactose negative)
Staphylococcus spp	Positive cocci	Small white or yellow colonies; often hemolytic	No growth
Streptococcus spp	Positive cocci	Small, often tiny pinpoint colonies; partial hemolysis or complete hemolysis	No growth

*Adapted from Biberstein EL. *Cal Vet.* 1977;31:10-17; and Ling GE. *J Am Vet Med Assoc.* 1984;185:1162-1164.

isolated from properly collected samples (postprostatic massage, prostatic portion of an ejaculate, or needle aspirate of prostate tissue), and an associated inflammatory response.

b. Fewer bacteria must be interpreted in conjunction with clinical signs and microscopic evaluation of ejaculates.

B. Techniques.

1. The most accurate results from quantitative bacterial culture of urine are obtained by dilution pour-plate methods. Unfortunately, this method is relatively time-consuming and, therefore, has not been adopted as a routine procedure by most veterinarians.
2. A less time-consuming technique involves the use of calibrated bacteriologic loops (available from Scientific Products, McGraw Park, Illinois) or microliter mechanical pipettes[5] that deliver exactly 0.01 or 0.001 ml of urine to culture plates.
   a. To facilitate qualitative and quantitative culture, urine is streaked over the surface of both blood agar and MacConkey agar by conventional methods.
   b. Blood agar supports growth of most aerobic organisms encountered in patients with urinary tract infections. MacConkey agar provides information that aids in identification of bacteria and prevents "swarming" of *Proteus* microbes (Table 8–5).
3. Although pour-plate and loop-dilution techniques provide accurate results, they have several disadvantages.
   a. Transport of urine specimens to a commercial microbiology laboratory results in an increase in time between urine collection and culture and therefore adds a potential source of erroneous results.
   b. Delay in obtaining results from a commercial laboratory may delay initiation of appropriate therapy.
   c. In addition, the cost of laboratory-performed quantitative urine cultures may be significant, especially when serial cultures from the same patient are required.
4. Many veterinarians do not perform urine cultures because of the time and expertise required to specifically identify bacteria. However, all individuals can recognize the fact that growth does not occur on culture plates. Therefore, we recommend that veterinarians culture urine on microbiologic plates utilizing calibrated loops.
   a. If no growth occurs after incubation for 18 to 30 hours, or if only small numbers of bacteria grow (contaminants), further efforts to identify bacterial species are unwarranted.
   b. If significant numbers of bacteria (colony forming units) are isolated, the microbiologic plates can be sent to commercial laboratories for species identifcation and antimicrobial susceptibility tests. Alternatively, bacteria from se-

lected colonies of the microbiologic plate could be collected on a swab and sent to commercial laboratories in transport media.

5. As an alternative, commercially manufactured screening culture kits designed to obtain quantitative bacterial counts may be utilized.[8,9]

REFERENCES

1. Allen TA, Jones RL, Purvance J. Microbiologic evaluation of canine urine: Direct microscopic examination and preservation of specimen quality for culture. *J Am Vet Med Assoc.* 1987;190: 1289-1291.
2. Asscher AW. Urine as a medium for bacterial growth. *Lancet.* 1966;2:1037-1041.
3. Barsanti JA, Blue J, Edmunds J. Urinary tract infection due to indwelling bladder catheters in dogs and cats. *J Am Vet Med Assoc.* 1985;187:384-388.
4. Chew DJ, Bartola SP. Diagnosis and pathophysiology of renal disease. In: Ettinger SJ, ed. *Textbook of Veterinary Internal Medicine.* Vol. 2. 3rd ed. Philadelphia, Pa: W.B. Saunders Co; 1989:1893-1961.
5. Chew DJ, Kowalski JA. Urinary tract infections. In: Bojrab MJ, ed. *Pathophysiology in Small Animal Surgery.* Philadelphia, Pa: Lea & Febiger; 1981.
6. Comer KM, Ling GV. Results of urinalysis and bacterial culture of canine urine obtained by antepubic cystocentesis, catheterization, and midstream voided methods. *J Am Vet Med Assoc.* 1981;179:891-895.
7. Kass EM. The role of asymptomatic bacteriuria in the pathogenesis of pyelonephritis. In: Quinn EL, Kass EM, eds. *Biology of Pyelonephritis.* Boston, Mass: Little Brown and Co; 1960.
8. Klausner JS, Osborne CA, Stevens JB. Screening tests for the detection of significant bacteriuria. In: Kirk RW, ed. *Current Veterinary Therapy,* Vol. 7. Philadelphia, Pa: W.B. Saunders Co; 1980.
9. Klausner JS, Osborne CA, Stevens JB. Clinical evaluation of commercial reagent strips for detection of significant bacteriuria in dogs and cats. *Am J Vet Res.* 1976;37:714-722.
10. Ling CV. Therapeutic strategies involving antimicrobial treatment of the canine urinary tract. *J Am Vet Med Assoc.* 1984;185: 1162-1164.
11. Padilla J, Osborne CA, Ward GE. Effects of storage time and temperature on quantitative culture of canine urine. *J Am Vet Med Assoc.* 1981;178:1077-1081.

CHAPTER 9

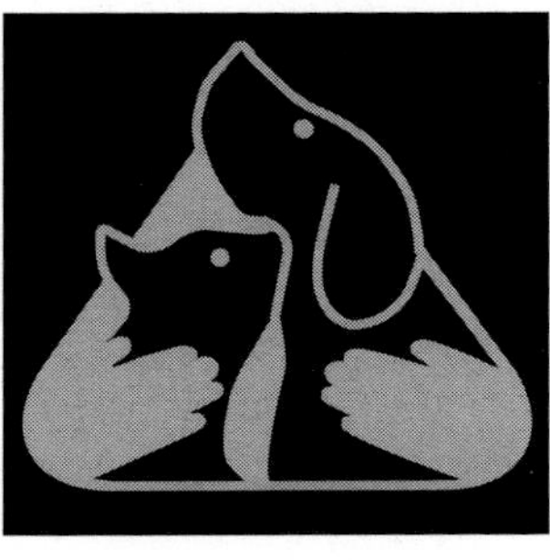

Urinary Protein Loss

DELMAR R. FINCO

I. INTRODUCTION

A. Definition of proteinuria.

1. Protein is present in urine from normal animals, but in quantities considerably less than those in animals with certain diseases.
2. Protein in the urine of normal dogs and cats is derived from filtered proteins not reabsorbed by the proximal tubule, Tamm-Horsfall proteins from nephron segments distal to the descending limb of the loop of Henle, and secretory globulins from the urinary tract.[6]
3. In this chapter, proteinuria refers to amounts of protein in the urine that are greater than normal.

B. Anatomic basis of proteinuria. Protein may appear in urine in association with prerenal, renal, and postrenal factors. These types of proteinuria must be distinguished from one another to avoid errors in diagnosis.

1. Prerenal proteinuria refers to protein loss from the blood into urine by normal kidneys as a consequence of either:
   a. Presence of abnormal, small-molecular-weight proteins in blood, allowing traversing of the normal filtration barrier. (Proteinuria associated with myeloma, hemoglobinuria, and myoglobinuria are examples.)
   b. Transient proteinuria caused by increased intraglomerular capillary pressure, which forces smaller-molecular-weight proteins normally present in the blood through the glomerular filtration barrier. (Proteinuria associated with venous stasis or with exercise is reported in humans, for example.)
2. Renal proteinuria is caused by disease of renal tissue.
   a. Glomerular proteinuria results from changes in the glomerular filtration barrier that allow normally restrained blood proteins to leak into Bowman's space. Because albumin has a molecular weight that is marginal for reflection (see Chapter 2, Applied Physiology of the Kidney), glomerular proteinuria is predominantly albumin.
   b. Tubular proteinuria results from lack of reabsorption of filtered protein by proximal tubule cells.
      (1). Small-molecular-weight globulins routinely pass through glomerular capillary walls and enter the proximal tubule, where they are reabsorbed by pinocytosis by proximal tubule cells.
      (2). If the proximal tubule cells lose capacity for this reabsorption, proteinuria ensues.
3. Postrenal proteinuria is caused by addition of protein to the urine at an anatomic site distal to the kidneys, usually by hemorrhage, inflammation, or both.

C. Protein concentration versus protein content.

1. Urine concentration of protein is the amount of protein per unit volume of urine.

2. Urine content of protein is the product of urine volume × urine protein concentration.
3. Measuring the concentration of protein in urine may not accurately reflect daily protein loss (i.e., the magnitude of proteinuria) because of fluctuations in urine volume with time in the same patient and because of interpatient differences in urine volume.
4. Knowing urine content of protein is superior to knowing concentration because the volume of urine being produced is considered.
   a. Usually, timed urine specimens are required for meaningful determinations of urine protein content; 24-hour specimens avoid potential errors associated with circadian rhythms in protein loss.
   b. In theory, determination of the urine protein/creatinine ratio (U-P/C) in a sample of urine circumvents the labor of 24-hour collections and provides information superior to protein concentration measurements. (See Section IIIB of this chapter.)

II. VARIATION BETWEEN METHODS FOR MEASURING URINE PROTEIN CONCENTRATION

A. Semiquantitative methods—urine protein concentration.

1. Urine dipsticks
   a. Detection of proteinuria with a urine dipstick depends on a color change in tetrabromphenol blue in the presence of protein. The color change is more sensitive to the presence of albumin than to globulins.
   b. Alkaline pH gives a false-positive reaction.
   c. Quaternary ammonium compounds give a false-negative reaction.
   d. Dipstick methods for determining urine protein concentration are notorious for false-positive reactions in small animals. Although dipsticks may be used as a screening test, they never should be relied on for a definitive diagnosis of proteinuria.
2. Sulfosalicylic acid, nitric acid tests.
   a. Both methods depend on acid precipitation of protein; the combination of urine and acid causes turbidity.
   b. These tests are probably more reliable than urine dipsticks.
   c. False-positive reactions may be observed in urine containing iodide radiocontrast media, penicillin, cephaloridine, and sulfisoxazole.

B. Quantitative methods—urine protein concentration.

1. Several colorimetric methods that are used for protein measurements in biochemistry are used for urine protein determination.
2. Each method has advantages, disadvantages, and limitations. Different methods may give considerably different results, because of different chemical bases for measuring protein.

III. URINE PROTEIN CONTENT

A. Twenty-four hour urine collections.

1. Method.
   a. A metabolism cage usually is required to avoid loss of urine.
   b. The dog or cat should be acclimated to the metabolism cage for at least 24 hours prior to initiating collections.
   c. The urinary bladder must be emptied prior to and at the conclusion of each 24-hour period, whether by voluntary voiding, catheterization, or manually expressing urine. Complete emptying of the urinary bladder before and after each 24-hour collection period is imperative.
   d. During 24-hour collections, a urinary preservative should be used to prevent microbial catabolism of urine protein (see Chapter 5, Techniques of Urine Collection and Preservation, IX., A.).
   e. Serial 24-hour collections are desirable to demonstrate repeatability of results.
2. Advantages.
   a. The 24-hour collection is the traditional and best-accepted method of determining urine protein content.
   b. Other data, such as endogenous creatinine clearance, also can be obtained if serum creatinine is measured.
3. Disadvantages.
   a. Expense of a metabolism cage.
   b. Twenty-four hour urine collections are cumbersome, time-consuming, and place the patient at risk for urinary tract infection if urinary catheterization is performed multiple times.
4. Considerable variation in normal values exists in reports from different laboratories (Table 9–1).

B. Urine protein/creatinine ratios (U-P/C).

1. Theoretic basis.
   a. Renal proteinuria occurs by two mechanisms:
      (1). An increase in porosity of the glomerular filtration barrier to plasma proteins exceeding the capacity of proximal tubule cells to reabsorb the proteins. This type of defect can cause mild to severe proteinuria.
      (2). Normal passage of lower-molecular-weight proteins (<70,000 daltons) through the normal filtration barrier, but faulty tubular reabsorption of the proteins. This type of defect causes only mild to moderate proteinuria.
   b. The rate of protein loss through a diseased filtration barrier depends on the type and degree of defect in the barrier and on glomerular filtration rate (GFR).
   c. The GFR in a normal animal and in animals with chronic renal failure remains fairly constant during a 24-hour period.

TABLE 9–1
TWENTY-FOUR HOUR URINARY PROTEIN EXCRETION BY CLINICALLY NORMAL DOGS

Author	Analytical method	No. dogs	Protein excretion (mg/kg/24 h) Mean	Range
Barsanti and Finco, 1979[3]	Coomassie blue	10	7.0	2.4–19.7
Barsanti and Finco, 1979[3]	Ponceau S	10*	3.8	0.8–15.1
Biewenga, et al., 1982[4]	Ponceau S	29	6.6	2.7–23.2
White, et al., 1984[16]	Ponceau S	8	4.8	1.9–11.1
McCaw, et al., 1985[14]	Coomassie blue	14	7.7	1.8–22.4
Grauer, et al., 1985[10]	Coomassie blue	16	2.3	0.6–5.1
Center, et al., 1985[5]	Turbidometric	19	2.5	0.2–7.7

*Same dogs as Barsanti, Coomassie blue method.

(1). In humans, some reports of diurnal variation in GFR exist.
(2). Comprehensive measurements in dogs and cats are lacking, but available data suggest that massive diurnal variations are unlikely.

d. Creatinine is excreted by the kidneys exclusively by glomerular filtration in cats,[8] and almost exclusively by glomerular filtration in dogs.[9] Thus, creatinine is a valid marker of GFR in these species.
e. Patients in stable renal failure excrete nearly the same amount of creatinine in their urine as do normal dogs, and nearly the same amount on a day-to-day basis.
f. Relating quantity of protein excreted to a urine component such as creatinine excretion eliminates variability associated with variable 24-hour urine volume.[7]
g. For U-P/C, the method routinely used for creatinine analysis (Jaffe method) is not specific for creatinine. Fortunately, in contrast to plasma, dog urine contains only a small percentage of noncreatinine chromogens.[7]

2. Performing U-P/C measurements.
   a. A urine sample is obtained and analyzed for creatinine and protein concentration. Values for both are expressed as mg/dL.
   b. The protein value divided by the creatinine value gives the unitless U-P/C.
3. Factors influencing U-P/C.
   a. Time of day. Initial studies done on "spot" samples of urine collected between 10 AM and 2 PM indicated excellent correlation between U-P/C and values for 24-hour collections.[17] Subsequent studies revealed excellent correlations with samples taken randomly throughout the day,[10] as well as day versus night.[15]
   b. Method of urine collection.
      (1). Overall, significant differences in protein concentration were not found in urine samples collected by voiding (midstream), cystocentesis, or catheterization.[3]
      (2). However, in both dogs[3] and cats,[16] voided urine from males had a higher protein concentration than that from females. Because cystocentesis samples did not differ in dogs, researchers concluded that the higher values in males resulted from lower tract addition of protein.
   c. Diet.
      (1). Dietary protein intake significantly affected U-P/C in both normal cats and cats with reduced renal mass.[1]
      (2). In dogs, one study failed to find an effect of a particular diet on U-P/C.[12]
      (3). Dietary protein may increase creatinine clearance; a proportionate increase in proteinuria would cause no change in U-P/C, whereas a disproportionate change in proteinuria compared with creatinine clearance could alter U-P/C.
   d. Hemorrhage.
      (1). Leakage of plasma proteins is expected when urinary tract hemorrhage occurs. An in vitro study employing addition of whole blood to urine indicated that U-P/C values were increased by blood addition.[2]
      (2). Entry of blood into hypotonic urine may result in hemolysis, thereby contributing hemoglobin, as well as plasma proteins, and increasing urine protein concentration.
   e. Inflammation. Cystotomy and experimentally induced urinary tract infection increased U-P/C in dogs, but the magnitude of the increase was not highly correlated with numbers of red blood cells or white blood cells found in the urine.[2]
   f. Exercise.

(1). In humans, strenuous exercise can cause transient proteinuria.

(2). Studies of hospitalized versus outpatient dogs have been done, but no meaningful conclusions could be drawn about the role of exercise because different dogs were used for the caged versus outpatient groups.[15]

(3). Effects of swimming and treadmill running were evaluated in normal beagle dogs. Swimming caused a small increase in proteinuria, but running had no effect on proteinuria.[14] Although dogs studied did not have impressive exertional proteinuria, effects of graded levels of exercise and possible dog and cat breed differences in degree of exertional proteinuria remain to be evaluated.

4. Determining abnormal U-P/C values.
   a. Values for U-P/C from normal dogs and cats have varied between laboratories, most likely because of the method used for urine protein analysis.
   b. The considerable increase in U-P/C observed with pathologic states means that interlaboratory variation in values may be masked by biologic difference in U-P/C between normal and abnormal levels of proteinuria.
   c. In dogs, the following guidelines should be used for interpretation of U-P/C values[14]:

      0-.3 = normal
      .3-1 = questionable
      >1 = abnormal

   d. Fewer studies have been done in cats.[1,7] A value of less than 0.7 on a voided urine sample was suggested as the lower limit of normal for adults.[1] In kittens from 4 to 30 weeks of age, maximum U-P/C was 0.34 ± 0.18.[11]
5. Interpreting U-P/C values.
   a. U-P/C values must be interpreted in the context of other information.
   b. Abnormal values can be expected with hematuria or urinary tract inflammation (pyuria), whether renal or postrenal. If inflammation or hemorrhage is causing the increased U-P/C, the U-P/C ratio should decrease into the normal range when the hemorrhage or inflammation is resolved.
   c. An elevated U-P/C ratio in the absence of urinary tract inflammation or hematuria suggests prerenal or renal proteinuria.
   d. With renal proteinuria, glomerular diseases generally have higher U-P/C ratios than do tubular causes of proteinuria. However, the magnitude of U-P/C with primary glomerular disease depends on its severity. Subcategorization of primary glomerular diseases based on U-P/C alone is probably unreliable, but the highest ratios have been reported with renal amyloidosis.[5]
6. Use of U-P/C to compute 24-hour protein loss.
   a. Based on regression equations devised by statistical comparison of 24-hour protein excretion and U-P/C ratios, one can compute one value, knowing the other.
   b. Whether such computations add usable information is questionable because:

(1). Computations add no diagnostic or prognostic information. Time comparisons of serial U-P/C are just as meaningful as time comparisons of serial 24-hour collections.

(2). Although a good correlation between U-P/C and 24-hour values has been reported in dogs and cats, individual values for 24-hour excretion may differ markedly from actual 24-hour excretion because of scatter of points along the regression line.

REFERENCES

1. Adams LG, Polzin DJ, Osborne CA, O'Brien TD. Correlation of urine protein/creatinine ratio and twenty-four-hour urinary protein excretion in normal cats and cats with surgically induced chronic renal failure. *J Vet Intern Med.* 1992;6:36-40.
2. Bagley RS, et al. The effect of experimental cystitis and iatrogenic blood contamination on the urine protein/creatinine ratio in the dog. *J Vet Intern Med.* 1991;5:66-70.
3. Barsanti JA, Finco DR. Protein concentration in urine of normal dogs. *Am J Vet Res.* 1979;40:1583-1588.
4. Biewenga WJ, Gruys E, Hendricks HJ. Urinary protein loss in the dog: nephrological study of 29 dogs without signs of renal disease. *Res Vet Sci.* 1982;33:366-374.
5. Center SA, et al. 24-hour urine protein/creatinine ratio in dogs with protein-losing nephropathies. *J Am Vet Med Assoc.* 1985;187: 820-824.
6. DiBartola SP, Chew DJ, Jacobs G. Quantitative urinalysis including 24-hour protein excretion in the dog. *J Am Anim Hosp Assoc.* 1980;16:537-546.
7. Finco DR. Kidney Function. In: Kaneko JJ, ed. *Clinical Biochemistry of Domestic Animals.* Orlando, Fla: Academic Press; 1989.
8. Finco DR, Barsanti JA. Mechanism of urinary excretion of creatinine by the cat. *Am J Vet Res.* 1982;43:2207-2209.
9. Finco DR, Brown SA, Crowell WA, Barsanti JA. Exogenous creatinine clearance as a measure of glomerular filtration rate in dogs with reduced renal mass. *Am J Vet Res.* 1991;52:1029-1032.
10. Grauer GF, Thomas CB, Eicker SW. Estimation of quantitative proteinuria in the dog, using the urine protein-to-creatinine ratio from a random, voided sample. *Am J Vet Res.* 1985;46:2116-2119.
11. Hoskins JD, et al. Quantitative urinalysis in kittens from four to thirty weeks from birth. *Am J Vet Res.* 1991;52:1295-1299.
12. Jergens AE, McCaw DL, Hewett JE. Effects of collection time and food consumption on the urine protein/creatinine ratio in the dog. *Am J Vet Res.* 1987;48:1106-1109.
13. Joles JA, Sanders M, Velthuizen JM, et al. Proteinuria in intact and splenectomized dogs after running and swimming. *Int J Sports Med.* 1984;5:311-316.
14. Lulich JP, Osborne CA. Interpretation of urine protein-creatinine ratios in dogs with glomerular and nonglomerular disorders. *Compendium.* 1990;12:59-73.

15. McCaw DL, Knapp DW, Hewett JE. Effect of collection time and exercise restriction on the prediction of urine protein excretion, using urine protein/creatinine ratio in dogs. *Am J Vet Res.* 1985;46:1665-1669.
16. Monroe WE, Davenport DJ, Saunders GK. Twenty-four-hour urinary protein loss in healthy cats and the urinary protein-creatinine ratio as an estimate. *Am J Vet Res.* 1989;50:1906-1909.
17. White JV, Olivier NB, Reimann K, Johnson C. Use of protein-to-creatinine ratio in a single urine specimen for quantitative estimation of canine proteinuria. *J Am Vet Med Assoc.* 1984;185:882-885.

CHAPTER 10

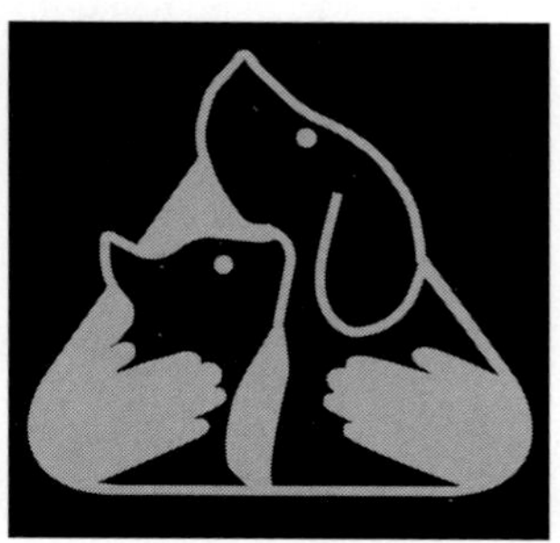

Evaluation of Renal Functions

DELMAR R. FINCO

I. INTRODUCTION

A. Motives for evaluation of renal function.

1. Motives for evaluation of renal function may vary, and the choice of renal function test employed may vary with the motives.
2. One motive is to determine if a clinical sign, or group of signs, is caused by renal dysfunction. Such signs include:
   a. Those attributable to uremia.
   b. Generalized edema.
   c. Polyuria.
3. Another motive is to assess renal function in a patient requiring major surgery to detect occult renal dysfunction and manage it properly.
4. A third motive is to monitor changes in renal function following implementation of some therapy.
5. The tests used may vary, depending on the information sought.

B. Errors in evaluation of renal function.

1. One type of error encountered is the conclusion that renal dysfunction does not exist, when it actually does.
   a. This type of error usually occurs when an insensitive test of renal function is used.
   b. A normal blood, serum, or plasma urea nitrogen concentration (BUN) or a normal plasma or serum creatinine concentration (SC) level could lead to this type of error because renal function must be reduced by 75% or more before BUN or SC increases above normal ranges.
2. The other type of error encountered is the conclusion that renal dysfunction exists, when it actually does not.
   a. This type of test error can occur with tests of any sensitivity and usually is the result of faulty technique or faulty interpretation.
   b. A BUN determination in the postprandial period following a high-protein meal may result in a slightly elevated value, even in the animal with normal renal function.[8,36]
   c. Failure to concentrate urine with water deprivation can be misinterpreted as an indication of generalized renal failure when the problem actually has a nonrenal cause.
   d. Prerenal and postrenal causes of azotemia may represent transient impairment of renal function, but could be erroneously interpreted as indicative of primary renal failure.
   e. Proteinuria of lower tract origin could erroneously be attributed to renal damage.
3. A knowledge of the basis for various renal function tests and of the strengths and weaknesses of each minimizes the occurrence of these errors.

C. Functional abnormalities without renal structural abnormalities.

1. Few renal function tests distinguish between function and structure.

2. Contraindications are the same as those for the abrupt test.
3. Procedure.
   a. An initial measurement of 24-hour water intake is made.
   b. The volume of water given daily is reduced by an amount equal to 2% of the body weight of the patient. For example, a 20-kg dog drinking 2.5 L per day would have water intake decreased on day 1 to 2.1 L.

$$2.5 - (0.02 \times 20 = 0.4 \text{ L}) = 2.1 \text{ L}$$

   c. On subsequent days, the same decrement (0.4 L) would be applied, so that, on day 2, 1.7 L of water would be given.
   d. Monitoring the patient's condition and response to deprivation should be conducted as for the abrupt water deprivation test.

E. Vasopressin (Pitressin) tests.

1. Indications.
   a. These tests may be used when water deprivation is risky.
   b. They also are indicated to confirm the presence of diabetes insipidus when water deprivation does not cause urine concentration.
2. Contraindications. The effects of vasopressin on smooth muscle should be considered in its usage.
3. Available forms of vasopressin.
   a. Aqueous vasopressin is available for injection, but has a short biologic half-life ($t\frac{1}{2}$).
   b. A synthetic analog of vasopressin (deamino D-arginine vasopressin, or DDAVP) is available for humans as an injectable agent and nasal spray. This compound has a $t\frac{1}{2}$ much longer than that of natural vasopressin.
   c. A repositol form of vasopressin (Pitressin Tannate in oil) is no longer commercially available.

F. DDAVP concentration test. Empiric usage suggests the following guidelines for a DDAVP urine concentration test in dogs.

1. Water need not be withheld prior to the test, but overnight fasting is preferable.
2. Regardless of the size of the dog, 10 µg of DDAVP is injected intravenously.
3. Urine is obtained for specific gravity or osmolality determinations at 1, 2, 4, 6, 12, and 24 hours.

G. Aqueous vasopressin (Pitressin) test.

1. Urine concentration tests using aqueous vasopressin have been advocated.
2. These tests have no advantage over the DDAVP test.
3. The aqueous vasopressin test has disadvantages, including:
   a. The short $t\frac{1}{2}$ of aqueous vasopressin requires its constant infusion.
   b. The shorter period used for evaluation of concentration does not allow re-establishment of the medullary osmotic gradient during the test.

H. Interpretation of urine concentration tests.

1. The same results would be anticipated whether exogenous administration of vasopressin or water deprivation were employed, but some studies in dogs indicate that urine concentration is greater after water deprivation.[37]
2. Studies on normal beagle dogs indicated that 16 hours or more of water deprivation resulted in urine specific gravity readings of 1.058 ± 0.008.[1]
3. In another study, urine specific gravity in 20 dogs was 1.062 ± 0.007 and osmolality was 2289 ± 251 mOsm/kg after a mean of 39.3 hours of water deprivation that resulted in 4 to 16% weight loss.[19]
4. In cats fed commercial dry food, abrupt water deprivation to achieve a 5 to 8% weight loss resulted in urine specific gravity readings of 1.064 ± 0.015 and urine osmolality readings of 2196 ± 533 mOsm/kg.[29]
5. Problems in use of data from normal animals abruptly deprived of water are:
   a. Pre-existing polyuria affects medullary interstitial osmotic gradients, and thus urine concentrations have not been considered.
   b. Protein content of the diet affects concentrating ability, and protein intake may vary between patients.
6. Because of these factors, the subsequent guidelines for interpretation of urine concentration tests should be considered as arbitrary.
7. Interpretations—dogs.
   a. With the abrupt water deprivation test, specific gravity readings of 1.040 and greater are considered evidence of normal concentrating ability.
   b. Readings of between 1.030 and 1.040 are considered questionable and worthy of further investigation.
   c. Readings of less than 1.030 are considered abnormal.
8. Interpretations—cats.
   a. At present, values from cats are interpreted using the same guidelines as in dogs.
   b. The ability of azotemic cats to concentrate urine suggests that standards for urine concentration should be higher.

IV. CLEARANCE METHODS FOR EVALUATING RENAL FUNCTION

A. Introduction.

1. See Chapter 2, Applied Physiology of the Kidney, for a review of renal clearance.
   a. To perform clearance measurements, plasma concentration of the material must be known so that the amount of substance to which the kidneys are exposed is known.
   b. The amount of the material excreted in the urine per unit time also must be known.

c. Clearance is calculated as:

$$C(\text{mL/min}) = \frac{U_c(\text{mg/mL}) \times U_v(\text{mL/min})}{P_c(\text{mg/mL})}$$

C = clearance
U_c = urine concentration of material
U_v = urine volume per unit time
P_c = plasma concentration of material

2. Clearance determinations have the advantage of being much more sensitive than BUN, SC, or urine concentration tests.
3. They have the disadvantage of being laborious to perform.
4. For clinical application, endogenous creatinine clearance or exogenous creatinine clearance can be readily determined in the dog; 24-hour endogenous creatinine clearance can be done in the cat, but reliable results are difficult to obtain unless catheterization is employed to completely empty the bladder.

B. Endogenous creatinine clearance—Jaffe method of creatinine analysis.

1. Because plasma creatinine concentration is relatively constant during each 24-hour period, a single SC determination and a timed urine collection are all that are required for determining endogenous creatinine clearance.
2. Both 24-hour[3] and 20-minute tests[10] have been used.
3. The 24-hour test.
   a. Advantages.
      (1). Short-term variations in renal function are less likely to cause spurious results.
      (2). Impeccable emptying of the urinary bladder at the beginning and end of the test is important, but less critical than with the short-term tests.
   b. Disadvantages.
      (1). A metabolism cage and overnight hospitalization are usually required.
      (2). Collection of urine by owner is usually not reliable.
   c. Procedure.
      (1). Water should be available *ad libitum* prior to and during the procedure, and food may be given.
      (2). The bladder is catheterized and completely emptied, as subsequently described for the short-term test. The exact time is noted.
      (3). All urine voided in the next 24 hours is collected. Urine should be refrigerated soon after it is voided to avoid metabolism of creatinine by bacteria. Alternatively, a urine preservative, such as thymol or hydrochloric acid, should be added to the urine collection container.
      (4). At 24 hours, a blood sample is obtained for SC measurement. The bladder is catheterized, and all urine collected is added to that already voided. The exact time is noted.
      (5). The volume of urine is measured in a graduated cylinder. Syringes are not reliable for measurement of volume.
      (6). The urine is mixed well, and a portion is used for creatinine analysis.
      (7). Endogenous creatinine clearance is calculated from the data obtained. Clearance usually is expressed as mL/min per kilogram of body weight.
4. The short-term test.
   a. Advantages.
      (1). The test is completed in about 30 minutes.
      (2). A metabolism cage is not required.
   b. Disadvantages.
      (1). Factors potentially altering creatinine clearance (excitement, apprehension) may lead to spurious results if the patient is not calm during the procedures.
      (2). Experience must be acquired in emptying and rinsing the urinary bladder before reliable results can be obtained. The short period of collection makes precise urine collection a critical factor.
   c. Procedure.
      (1). Water must be available *ad libitum* prior to the test. An overnight fast should be employed.
      (2). A urinary catheter is passed and left in place for the duration of the procedure. Placement of a retention catheter, such as a Foley catheter, facilitates the procedure.
      (3). Urine is gently aspirated from the bladder with a 20-ml syringe. A glass syringe is preferable to a plastic syringe because the glass is more sensitive to digital manipulations. Too forceful an aspiration may draw bladder mucosa into the catheter openings, causing trauma and preventing proper emptying of the bladder.
      (4). When the bladder is apparently empty, a syringeful of air is injected.
         (a). If it is entirely aspirated with no more than 1 or 2 ml of urine, the bladder has been adequately emptied.
         (b). If all the air cannot be aspirated, or if a large volume of urine accompanies the air, collection was not complete. Gentle compression of the bladder through the abdominal wall may facilitate retrieval of bladder contents. If not, movement or twisting of the catheter may help. Injecting more air may help by moving the tip of the catheter away from the bladder wall.
      (5). When emptied of urine and air, the blad-

der must be rinsed with sterile saline or sterile water.

(a). After injection of 5 to 20 ml (depending on patient size), all or nearly all of the solution should be retrieved. Succeeding rinses should recover any fluid injected but not retrieved during a previous rinse.

(b). At least three rinses with sterile saline should be performed, and they should be done quickly so that newly formed urine does not accumulate in the bladder. If the bladder has been emptied properly, the last rinse will not be colored with urine. The exact time of the completion of aspiration of the last rinse is recorded to the nearest 15 seconds; this point is the beginning of the clearance period.

(c). All urine and rinse removed prior to the beginning of the clearance period are discarded. All urine and rinses subsequently collected are saved. During the clearance period, urine may be kept in the urinary bladder by use of a three-way valve on the end of the catheter, or the urine may be allowed to drip into an appropriate container, such as a graduated cylinder.

(d). At about 20 minutes after the beginning of the clearance period, the bladder is emptied of all urine, and at least 2 rinses with sterile saline are performed quickly. Indications of the adequacy of bladder rinsing are the same as those given previously. The exact time of completion of the last rinse is recorded, and all rinses are added to the urine collected.

(e). A blood sample is obtained for analysis of SC.

(f). The volume of the combination of urine and final rinses is recorded, the combination is thoroughly mixed, and a sample is submitted for creatinine analysis.

(g). From the results, clearance is calculated and expressed as ml/min per kilogram of body weight.

(h). The reliability of the determination can be improved by extending the procedure to two clearance periods. The end of the first collection becomes the start of the second. The second collection is concluded in the same manner as the first. A single blood sample for SC suffices for both clearance periods.

d. Interpretation of results.

(1). Endogenous creatinine clearance measures GFR only under two conditions.

(a). When tubular secretion of creatinine is absent or is quantitatively negligible.

(b). When noncreatinine chromogens make up a negligible percentage of the value for SC.

(2). Tubular secretion of creatinine does not occur in female dogs or cats. The contribution of tubular secretion of creatinine by male dogs is negligible in the absence of urinary obstruction.

(3). The Jaffe method of creatinine analysis measures not only creatinine, but noncreatinine chromagens as well. Noncreatinine chromogens exist in variable quantities in blood, but do not appear in urine.[2]

(a). Some manufacturers of semiautomated analyzers claim that their kinetic methods of creatinine analysis measure only creatinine in plasma, but this claim is questionable.[17,34]

(b). The only way to determine if endogenous creatinine clearance is actually measuring GFR is to determine endogenous creatinine clearance and inulin clearance simultaneously, and then to compare the results.

(4). When the Jaffe method for creatinine analysis is used, endogenous creatinine clearance should not be referred to as a measure of GFR, nor should normal values for GFR be used for interpreting endogenous creatinine clearance data from a patient.

(5). Laboratory-to-laboratory differences in values for endogenous creatinine clearance dictate that each user determine his or her own normal values by performing clearance procedures in normal animals.

(6). Differing values—24-hour versus 20-minute clearance tests

(a). Some studies suggest that 24-hour endogenous creatinine clearance values are lower, on a mL/min basis, than are 20-minute values.[12]

(b). Yet, a laboratory has reported that 24-hour endogenous creatinine clearance values were higher than short-term clearance values in anesthetized dogs.[3]

(c). Factors that could result in different clearance values for short-term and 24-hour tests include diurnal variation in creatinine excretion, the effects of food ingestion on GFR, and changes in state of hydration.

(d). Until proved otherwise, normal values for 24-hour endogenous creatinine clearance and 20-minute clearance should not be used interchangeably.

(7). Endogenous creatinine clearance values, when compared to reliable values from normal animals, provide a relatively sensitive indication of renal function, even though numeric values are different from GFR.

C. Endogenous creatinine clearance—PAP creatinine method of creatinine analysis.

1. Recently, a new method of analyzing plasma and urine was developed that is reported to be specific for creatinine.
2. Studies indicate that the endogenous technique with PAP creatinine analysis is a valid measure of GFR when used for short-term clearance measurements in dogs (Fig. 10–4)[16] and probably is valid for 24-hour urine collections in dogs.
3. Studies in cats have not been reported.

D. Exogenous creatinine clearance determination.

1. Advantages. Exogenous creatinine clearance measures GFR accurately in both normal dogs and cats and in dogs and cats with renal failure.[15,34]
   a. Reliable measurement of GFR occurs because plasma creatinine levels are elevated by injection of creatinine.
   b. This reduces the error of noncreatinine chromogens (Jaffe method) to a negligible amount by dilution.
2. Disadvantage. Additional blood analyses are required to document the actual SC values, and creatinine must be injected to elevate plasma concentrations.
3. Procedure follows for determination of exogenous creatinine clearance after subcutaneous injection of creatinine.[17] Subcutaneous injection of creatinine elevates plasma creatinine concentration and results in a sufficiently constant plasma creatinine level to obtain accurate clearance measurements.
   a. Creatinine (Sigma Chem Co, St Louis, MO, product no. C-4255) is dissolved in distilled water (25 mg/mL) and sterilized by autoclaving.
   b. Creatinine is injected subcutaneously at a dose of 100 mg per kilogram of body weight for dogs less than 20 kg, and of 75 mg per kilogram of body weight for dogs more than 20 kg. Subsequent references to time are related to injection of creatinine at zero time.
   c. Immediately after injection, a stomach tube is passed, and a volume of water equal to 3% of body weight is given. For example, a 15-kg dog receives 15 kg × 0.03 = 0.45 kg = 450 mL.
   d. The procedure is planned so that the dog has a urinary catheter in place at 35 minutes after zero time.
   e. At 40 minutes, the bladder should be thoroughly rinsed as indicated for the 20-minute endogenous creatinine clearance procedure; the exact time of completion of the rinse is recorded.
   f. A blood sample is obtained for SC measurement immediately after the bladder rinse is completed.
   g. A precisely timed urine collection of about 20 minutes is made with appropriate rinses as indicated for endogenous creatinine clearance, and a blood sample is obtained for SC immediately upon conclusion of the rinse.
   h. For greater reliability, a second clearance period should be performed, using the end of the first period as the beginning of the second. A blood sample at the end of the second collection is required for SC measurement.
   i. For calculation of clearance, the mean of SC values at the beginning and at the end of each clearance period is calculated and used for the denominator of the clearance equation.
4. Normal values. Clearance of 4.09 ± 0.52 mL/min per kilogram of body weight was obtained in 10 normal dogs (5 of each sex).[17]

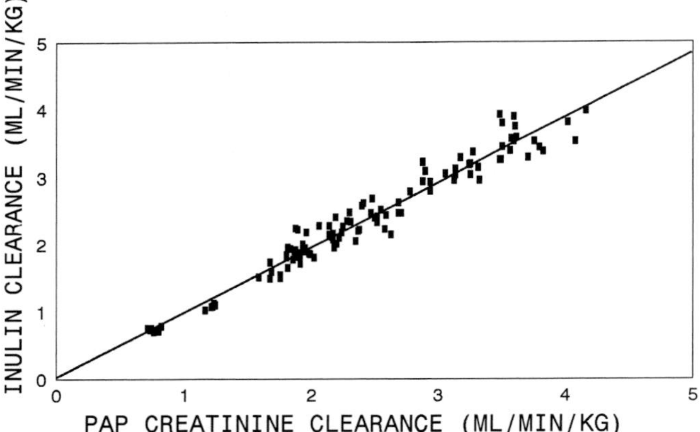

FIG. 10–4. Comparison indicating an excellent correlation between GFR (determined by inulin clearance) and endogenous creatinine clearance when the PAP creatinine method was used for creatinine measurement. In contrast, analysis of creatinine by the Jaffe method yields spuriously low values for GFR. (From Finco DR, Tabaru H, Brown SA, Barsanti JA. Endogenous creatinine clearance measurement of glomerular filtration rate in dogs. *Am J Vet Res.* 1993;54:1575-1578.)

E. Importance of hydration state when performing clearance procedures.

1. Studies in dogs indicate that change in hydration status markedly influences GFR values (Table 10–1).[34] Subclinically detectable dehydration could affect GFR values.
2. Animals should never have water restricted prior to clearance procedures.

3. Voluntary intake of water may be inadequate under certain circumstances, such as hospitalization.
4. To avoid errors associated with inadequate hydration, short-term clearance procedures should be preceded by water loading, as described for the exogenous creatinine clearance test. The water loading procedure
   a. Corrects any subclinical degree of dehydration that exists.
   b. Increases urine flow rates, making urine collection procedures more accurate.

V. SINGLE INJECTION-PLASMA DECAY TECHNIQUES

A. Rationale. For any substance excreted exclusively by the kidneys and not metabolized by the body, the rate of its disappearance from the plasma should be related to renal function.

B. Advantage. When disappearance of the test substance from the plasma is used as a measure of renal function, the need for collection of urine is obviated.

C. Disadvantages.

1. Plasma decay does not reflect renal function alone.
   a. Following intravenous injection, early decreases in plasma concentration represent mixing in the blood, as well as renal excretion.
   b. Few test substances are restricted to the blood. Plasma decay also is a reflection of equilibration between plasma and the interstitial or even the intracellular compartment.
   c. Inappropriate sampling times may result in spurious values for GFR when pharmacokinetic analyses of plasma decay curves are conducted.
2. Test substances that are logical choices for use are not analyzed by commercial laboratories.

D. Several substances have been advocated for use. These include:

1. Sodium sulfanilate.
2. Phenolsulfonphthalein (PSP).
3. Sodium para-aminohippurate.
4. ^{14}C-inulin.
5. Sodium iothalamate and sodium iodohippurate.
6. Iohexol.

E. Methods of data analysis.

1. After intravenous injection of test substance, serial samples of blood are procured for analysis.
2. Kinetic modeling of plasma decay curves may give numeric values for renal function.
3. Alternatively, a $t\frac{1}{2}$ may be computed.
   a. After mixing, many compounds have a decrease in plasma concentration that is linear when the $\log_{10}$ of plasma concentration is plotted against time.
   b. The time required for plasma concentration of test substance to be halved is referred to as the $t\frac{1}{2}$.
   c. This value is expected to be prolonged if renal function is decreased.
   d. The test is performed on normal animals to establish reference values for $t\frac{1}{2}$.
4. Of the compounds previously listed, sodium sulfanilate has been used most often.
   a. The technique for performing the analysis and normal values for $t\frac{1}{2}$ has been published for dogs[5] and for cats.[29]
   b. The test in dogs was sufficiently sensitive to detect acute unilateral nephrectomy.
   c. In cats, the test correlated fairly well with GFR (−0.70); this was superior to the correlation of GFR with plasma PSP decay (0.37).[29]

F. Some conclusions drawn about results from single-injection methods are questionable.

1. Because factors other than renal function influence the plasma decay curve, decay curves should be validated by simultaneous measurement of GFR or RPF by clearance procedures.
2. Some single-injection methods have been described as measures of GFR in cats[9] and dogs[27] without validation.
3. Subsequent studies in other laboratories indicated that the single-injection procedure in cats was poorly correlated with GFR.[28]

VI. QUANTITATIVE RENAL SCINTIGRAPHY

A. Description.

1. Renal scintigraphy is a technique of evaluating renal function in one or both kidneys by injecting an appropriate gamma-emitting compound and monitoring its accumulation in the kidneys with a gamma-detector.
2. The compound ^{99m}Tc-diethylenetriamenipenta-acetic acid is often used because it is excreted by the kidney only by glomerular filtration.

TABLE 10–1
EFFECTS OF DEHYDRATION, EUHYDRATION, AND FLUID ADMINISTRATION ON GFR IN CLINICALLY NORMAL DOGS

Clearance Procedure	Hydration State	Clearance (mL/min/kg)*†
	Water gavage	4.14 +/– 0.20
Exogenous creatinine	Baseline	3.64 +/– 0.10
	Dehydration	2.78 +/– 0.06
	Water gavage	2.94 +/– 0.12
Endogenous creatinine	Baseline	2.66 +/– 0.14
	Dehydration	2.15 +/– 0.09

*Mean +/– SEM

†Notice that GFR values change markedly with state of hydration, dictating that hydration state be standardized when making GFR measurements.

(From Tabaru H, Finco DR, Brown SA, Cooper T. Influence of hydration state on renal functions of dogs. *Am J Vet Res.* 1993;54:1758-1764.)

B. Advantages.

1. It provides a quick, noninvasive method of determining renal function. With appropriate development of the technique, it allows determination of GFR and RPF.[7,21,23,35]
2. Differences in function of right and left kidneys can be measured.
3. With some uses, renal size can be determined.
4. Urinary catheterization is not required.

C. Disadvantages.

1. Equipment needed is available only at universities or major referral centers.
2. Radiation exposure occurs, and isotope disposal is required.

VII. SPECIFIC RENAL FUNCTIONS

A. Previously, this chapter emphasized that nephron damage localized to a specific anatomic site usually causes generalized renal dysfunctions, including alteration of GFR. This generalization is the basis for advocating GFR, or tests that estimate GFR, as indices of renal functions. However, exceptions to this rule exist.

1. Genetic or acquired defects that have a specific biochemical effect may cause renal dysfunctions that are local. For example:
   a. Renal glycosuria is a rare disease in which the only renal defect is in glucose reabsorption by the proximal tubule.
   b. Fanconi syndrome in basenji dogs initially causes defects localized to the proximal tubule, although many functions at this site are abnormal.
2. Acutely after some forms of renal tubular damage, renal dysfunction may be more readily detectable by tests of tubular function than by GFR measurement.

B. Fractional excretion (FE) of materials.

1. FE refers to the fraction of filtered material that escapes reabsorption and thus appears in urine.
2. Renal tubular reabsorption of many materials is carefully modified to achieve body balance.
   a. The amount of each electrolyte filtered per unit time is the product of GFR and plasma concentration of the electrolyte. (This ignores plasma protein binding, which is negligible for sodium and potassium, minor for phosphorus and magnesium, and significant for calcium.)
   b. The amount filtered, but not reabsorbed, by the tubules appears in urine and can be measured there.
3. Classic methods for measurement of FE of electrolytes entail measurement of GFR and plasma concentration of the substance in question so that the amount of electrolyte filtered (filtered load) can be determined. Urinary excretion of the substance also is measured. FE is expressed as:

$$FE = \frac{\text{urinary excretion (amount/min)}}{\text{filtered load (amount/min)}}$$

4. A simpler "spot" method employed for determination of FE requires only single samples of blood and urine.
   a. The plasma/urine ratio of creatinine represents the concentration of creatinine in urine brought about by reabsorption of filtrate as urine traverses the tubule. The plasma/urine ratio of material represents the effect of net tubular reabsorption of water and electrolyte. By accounting for water reabsorption with creatinine measurements, the fraction of material reabsorbed can be determined. With this method, FE is expressed as:

$$FE = \frac{\text{plasma creatinine conc./urine creatinine conc.}}{\text{plasma material conc./urine material conc.}}$$

5. For the classic and "spot" methods for measuring FE to give the same values, certain requirements for the "spot" method must be fulfilled.[12,14] These are:
   a. Plasma creatinine measurements must be specific; noncreatinine chromogen measurement falsely elevates FE values.
   b. Plasma concentration of the material being studied must be constant during the period of time that urine accumulated in the bladder.
   c. The stimulus for renal tubular reabsorption or excretion of the material in question must have been constant while the urine procured was formed.
6. This FE method often is used for electrolytes. Diurnal rhythms exist for excretion of some electrolytes, and eating may have effects that are even greater than diurnal variations. The error of noncreatinine chromogens was reviewed in Section IV, B of this chapter.
7. Direct comparisons of classic and "spot" methods for FE have not been made for the dog and cat to determine the validity of the "spot" methods.
8. Until results of such comparisons are available, "spot" FE values must be interpreted with caution.
9. The following are tentative guidelines for conducting "spot" FE determinations, based on the theoretic concerns previously listed.
   a. The animal should be fasted beginning at 5 p.m., but should have ready access to water.
   b. The bladder should be emptied 15 hours later (8 a.m.); 3 hours should be allowed to elapse for new urine to form.
   c. Urine and blood can then be obtained for "spot" clearance determinations.
10. Interpretation of result.
    a. FE values of most electrolytes depend on their

dietary intake and intestinal absorption. For electrolytes restricted predominantly to the extracellular compartment (sodium, chloride), the 15-hour fast should minimize effects of diet. For electrolytes that are predominantly intracellular (potassium, phosphorus, magnesium), there is no assurance that FE values will not be influenced by diet, using the above guidelines. The only alternative would be to feed the patient a standard diet for several days before the determination.

b. The FE values can reflect normal renal tubular function in response to an abnormal external hormonal stimulus. For example, with primary hyperparathyroidism, FE for phosphorus is increased, although tubular function is normal.

c. The FE values can reflect compensatory homeostatic responses. For example, when functional renal mass is reduced, FE is increased for all electrolytes for which the kidney has homeostatic responsibility. (See Chapter 16, Pathophysiology of Renal Failure and Uremia.)

d. The FE values can reflect tubular dysfunctions. For example, FE values for all electrolytes and amino acids are increased in Fanconi syndrome because of transport defects in the proximal tubules.

11. Normal values should be determined by each user. When standardization of procedures occurs, universal normal values should be applicable.

C. Glucosuria, aminoaciduria.

1. Urine test strips give semiquantitative estimates of the amount of glucose in urine. (See Chapter 7, A Clinician's Analysis of Urinalysis.) To distinguish overflow glucosuria from a renal tubular reabsorptive defect, one must document urine glucose excretion during a period when blood glucose concentration remains constant. A potential error with measurement of blood and urine glucose concentrations on random samples occurs when glucosuria is a temporary event associated with a transient hyperglycemia. The hyperglycemia may be resolved at the time blood is obtained, but the urine produced during hyperglycemia may still be in the bladder. The following procedure circumvents this potential source of error.

   a. Place a urinary catheter in the bladder and empty the bladder completely. Rinse the bladder once with saline. Leave the catheter in place.
   b. Obtain a blood sample for glucose determination.
   c. Wait 10 minutes, and collect newly formed urine.
   d. Obtain a second blood sample.
   e. Analyze blood and urine samples for glucose.
   f. If urine glucose tests positive when normoglycemia exists, a renal tubular defect for glucose absorption exists or a false-positive urine glucose test exists. (See Chapter 7, A Clinician's Analysis of Urinalysis, for a review of false-positive tests.)

2. Quantitative assessment of a glucose reabsorptive defect.

   a. If glucosuria is known to occur during normoglycemia, the classic tubular maximum test for glucose reabsorption can be applied to measure the amount of glucose being reabsorbed.
   b. This measurement can be done by performing an exogenous creatinine clearance as previously described and analyzing blood and urine samples for glucose as well as creatinine.
   c. The tubular reabsorption of glucose is then calculated as follows:

$$\text{Filtered load of glucose} = \text{GFR} \times \text{plasma glucose concentration}$$

$$\text{Urine glucose excretion} = \text{Urine volume} \times \text{urine glucose concentration}$$

$$\text{Tubular reabsorption} = \text{filtered load} - \text{urine glucose excretion}$$

   d. Tubular reabsorption, when divided by GFR, standardizes the value for animals of different sizes. Normal values for maximum tubular glucose reabsorptive for the dog are 325 mg/dL filtrate.[11]

3. Aminoaciduria is not routinely evaluated and is likely to go undetected if some other clue to its existence is not present.

   a. Aminoacidurias may be specific biochemical defects of the transport mechanisms in the proximal tubule cell membranes. Such aminoacidurias are selective for those amino acids normally transported by that mechanism and occur at normal plasma amino acid concentrations.
   b. Aminoacidurias may occur because plasma amino acid concentrations exceed proximal tubule capacity to reabsorb them. Such aminoacidurias are generalized, representing the amino acids with increased plasma concentrations.

4. Measurement of amino acids in urine is beyond the scope of most clinical laboratory services. However, clinical laboratories can usually refer the clinician to the appropriate laboratory or can submit samples to such a laboratory. For differentiation of tubular defects from overflow aminoaci-

duria, plasma amino acid levels also must be known.

D. Urinary acidification.

1. Defects in renal acid-base homeostasis accompany renal failure and can lead to acid-base imbalances. (See Chapter 16, Pathophysiology of Renal Failure and Uremia.)
2. In contrast, renal tubular acidosis refers to seemingly rare cases that have normal or near normal GFR, but defects in acid-base homeostasis.
3. In man, types and subtypes of renal tubular acidosis are described.[25]
   a. Proximal tubular acidosis refers to defects in bicarbonate reabsorption at this site.
   b. Distal tubule acidosis refers to defects in hydrogen ion secretion in the distal tubule and collecting duct. This deficit may be caused by defective proton pumping or by backleak of protons once they are pumped.
4. In man, several tests have been recommended for distinguishing these types of renal tubular acidosis. Opinion is divided on the merits and limitations of the tests, and no single approach to testing has gained favor.
5. Too little is known about renal tubular acidosis in dogs or cats to provide definitive testing procedures. The following recommendations are tentative and subject to revision as more is learned.
   a. Proximal tubular acidosis should be considered a possibility when hypobicarbonatemia exists and when other evidence of proximal tubular function (increased FE of potassium, phosphorus, glucosuria, i.e., Fanconi syndrome) exists. Because distal tubule function may be normal, urine pH may be low (< 6.0).
   b. Distal tubular acidosis should be considered when an acidotic patient has a urine pH greater than 6.0 and renal function is otherwise normal.
6. However, the preceding recommendations refer to complete defects. When distal renal tubular acidosis is incomplete, urine pH values may be inappropriately high, with slight or equivocal decreases in plasma bicarbonate concentration. An ammonium chloride tolerance test has been described for the dog to aid in diagnosis of distal renal tubular acidosis under these conditions. This test is conducted as follows.[26]
   a. Administer ammonium chloride (as a solution to avoid vomiting) at a dose of 0.2 g per kilogram of body weight.
   b. Empty the bladder, and determine urine pH hourly for at least 6 hours.
   c. In 9 normal dogs, urine pH was reduced to 5.74 ± 0.19 at 5 hours after treatment. Failure to reduce urine pH to 6.0 or less supports the diagnosis of distal renal tubular acidosis.

E. Urinary enzymes.

1. Although not quantitative tests, enzyme assays have proved valuable for detecting organ dysfunctions.
2. Enzymes from damaged cells of many organs often are released into serum and are measured to aid in diagnosis of organ dysfunctions.
3. Unfortunately, no reliable serum enzyme assay has been discovered to detect renal damage.
4. This failure has led to the examination of urine for enzyme activity, with the rationale that enzymes from damaged kidneys may leak into urine rather than blood.
5. Several enzymes from two anatomic sites have been examined.
   a. Brush border enzymes
   b. Lysosomal enzymes
6. Unfortunately, urinary enzyme determinations have been fraught with problems.
   a. Enzyme inhibitors and enzyme accelerators have been found to interfere with assays.
   b. Clearcut results, with a definite advantage of enzyme assays over other methods of detection of renal damage, have not been obtained.
7. At present, urine enzyme assays have not reached a degree of reliability that justifies their routine clinical usage.

F. β_2-microglobulin clearance.

1. This compound is a protein with a molecular weight of 11,800.
2. It is a light chain component of class 1 major histocompatability antigens, which are normally shed into the blood.[30]
3. Because of the light chain's low molecular weight, it normally passes through the glomerular filter and is reabsorbed by the proximal tubule.
4. In humans, β_2-microglobulin clearance has been advocated for detection of diminished proximal tubular reabsorption.
5. However, many factors complicate analysis of urine for this compound.[30]
6. Data validating β_2-microglobulin clearance as a reliable test of tubular function in the dog have not been provided.

REFERENCES

1. Balazc T, Sekella R, Pauls, JF. Renal concentration test in beagle dogs. *Lab Anim Sci.* 1971;31:546-548.
2. Balint P, Visy M. "True creatinine" and "pseudocreatinine" in blood plasma of the dog. *Acta Physiol Acad Sci Hung.* 1965;28: 265-272.
3. Bovee KC, Joyce, T. Clinical evaluation of glomerular function: 24-hour creatinine clearance in dogs. *J Am Vet Med Assoc.* 1979;174:488-492.
4. Boylan, JW, Asshauer E. Depletion and restoration of the medullary osmotic gradient in the dog kidney. *Pflugers Arch.* 1962;176:99-216.
5. Carlson GP, Kaneko JJ. Simultaneous estimation of renal function in dogs, using sulfanilate and sodium iodohippurate ^{131}I. *J Am Vet Med Assoc.* 1971;158:1229-1234.

6. Coburn JW, Gonick HC, Rubini ME, Kleeman CR. Studies of experimental renal failure in the dog. I. Effect of 5/6 nephrectomy on concentrating and diluting capacity of residual nephrons. *J Clin Invest.* 1965;44:603-614.
7. Cowgill LD, Hornof WJ. Assessment of individual kidney function by quantitative renal scintigraphy. In: *Current* Kirk RW, ed. *Veterinary Therapy. IX.* Philadelphia, Pa: WB Saunders Co.; 1986.
8. Epstein ME, Barsanti JA, Finco DR, Cowgill LM. Postprandial changes in plasma urea nitrogen and plasma creatinine concentrations in dogs fed commercial diets. *J Am Anim Hosp Assoc.* 1984;20:779-782.
9. Fettman MJ, et al. Single-injection method for evaluation of renal function with ^{14}C-inulin and ^{3}H-tetraethyl ammonium bromide. *Am J Vet Res.* 1985;46:482-485.
10. Finco DR. Simultaneous determination of phenolsulfonphthalein excretion and endogenous creatinine clearance in the normal dog. *J Am Vet Med Assoc.* 1971;159:995-1003.
11. Finco DR. Familial renal disease in Norwegian elkhound dogs: Physiologic and biochemical examinations. *Am J Vet Res.* 1976; 37:87-91.
12. Finco DR. Renal functions. In: Kaneko JJ, ed. *Clinical Biochemistry of Domestic Animals.* New York, NY: Academic Press; 1988.
13. Finco DR, Barsanti JA. Mechanism of urinary excretion of creatinine by the cat. *Am J Vet Res.* 1982;43:2207-2209.
14. Finco DR, Brown SA, Barsanti JA. Solute fractional excretion rates. In: Kirk RW, Bonagura, JD, eds. *Current Veterinary Therapy. XI.* Philadelphia, Pa: WB Saunders Co; 1992.
15. Finco DR, Brown SA, Crowell WA, Barsanti JA. Exogenous creatinine clearance as a measure of glomerular filtration rate in dogs with reduced renal mass. *Am J Vet Res.* 1991;52:1029-1032.
16. Finco DR, Tabaru H, Brown SA, Barsanti JA. Endogenous creatinine clearance measurement of glomerular filtration rate in dogs. *Am J Vet Res.* 1993;54:1575-1578.
17. Finco DR, Coulter DB, Barsanti, JA. Simple, accurate method for clinical estimation of glomerular filtration rate. *Am J Vet Res.* 1981;42:1874-1877.
18. Finco DR, Duncan JR. Evaluation of blood urea nitrogen and serum creatinine concentrations as indicators of renal dysfunction: a study of 111 cases and a review of related literature. *J Am Vet Med Assoc.* 1976;168:593-601.
19. Hardy RM, Osborne CA. Water deprivation test in the dog: maximum normal values. *Am J Vet Res.* 1979;174:479-483.
20. Hayman JM, Shumuby NP, Dumke P, Miller M. Experimental hyposthenuria. *J Clin Invest.* 1939;18:195-212.
21. Itkin RJ, Krawiec DR, Twardock AR, Gelberg HB. Non-invasive determination of canine renal plasma flow. *Proceedings 10th Annual Veterinary Medical Forum.* 1992;802.
22. Jones JD, Burnett PC. Implications of creatinine and gut flora in the uremic syndrome: Induction of "creatinase" in colon contents of the rat by dietary creatinine. *Clin Chem.* 1972; 18:280-284.
23. Kraweic DR, et al. Evaluation of ^{99m}Tc-diethylenetriaminepentaacetic acid nuclear imaging for quantitative determination of the glomerular filtration rate of dogs. *Am J Vet Res.* 1986;147: 2175-2179.
24. Mitch WE, Collier VU, Walser M. Creatinine metabolism in chronic renal failure. *Clin Sci.* 1980;58:327-335.
25. Pohlman T, Hruska KA, Menon M. Renal tubular acidosis. *J Urol.* 1984;132:431-436.
26. Polzin DJ, Osborne CA. Detection and management of canine renal tubular acidosis. *Proceedings 5th Annual Veterinary Medical Forum.* Madison, Wis: Omnipress; 1985:4-67–4-69.
27. Powers TE, Powers JD, Garg RC. Study of the double isotope single injection method for estimating renal function in purebred beagle dogs. *Am J Vet Res.* 1977;38:1933-1936.
28. Rogers KS, et al. Comparison of four methods of estimating glomerular filtration rate in cats. *Am J Vet Res.* 1991;52:961-964.
29. Ross LA, Finco DR. Relationship of selected clinical renal function tests to glomerular filtration rate and renal blood flow in cats. *Am J Vet Res.* 1981;42:1704-1710.
30. Schardin GH, Statius van Eps LW. β_2-microglobulin: Its significance in the evaluation of renal function. *Kidney Int.* 1987;32: 635-641.
31. Schloerb PR. Total body water distribution of creatinine and urea in nephrectomized dogs. *Am J Physiol.* 1960;199:661-665.
32. Shannon JA. Glomerular filtration and urea excretion in relation to urine flow in the dog. *Am J Physiol.* 1936;117:206-218.
33. Swanson RE, Hakim AA. Stop-flow of creatinine excretion in the dog. *Am J Physiol.* 1962;203:980-984.
34. Tabaru H, Finco DR, Brown SA, Cooper, T. Influence of hydration state on renal functions of dogs. *Am J Vet Res.* 1993;54:1758-1764.
35. Uribe D, Krawiec, DR, Twardock, AR, Gelberg, HB. Quantitative renal scintigraphic determination of glomerular filtration rate in cats with normal and abnormal kidney function, using ^{99m}Tc-diethylenetriaminepentaacetic acid. *Am J Vet Res.* 1992;53:1101-1107.
36. Watson AD, Church DB, Fairburn AJ. Postprandial changes in plasma urea and creatinine concentrations in dogs. *Am J Vet Res.* 1981;42:1878-1880.
37. West CD, Traeger J, Kaplan, SA. A comparison of the relative effectiveness of hydropenia and of Pitressin in producing a concentrated urine. *J Clin Invest.* 1955;34:887-898.

CHAPTER 11

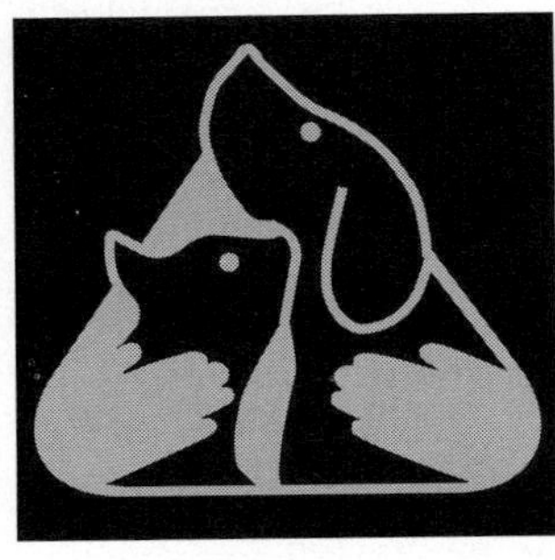

Diagnostic Imaging of the Urinary Tract

GARY R. JOHNSTON
PATRICIA A. WALTER
DANIEL A. FEENEY

I. ROLE OF IMAGING IN ASSESSMENT OF THE UROGENITAL SYSTEM

Urogenital imaging is performed to define organ structure and thereby confirm or refute a relationship between that organ or body system and clinical signs (Fig. 11–1).[1-3] Once the disease is localized, the extent of local or regional involvement of the organ or body system must be determined prior to formulating a treatment plan (Fig. 11–2). Prognoses, the likelihood that the disease, if treated, will be reversible, progressive, or static, also must be determined (Fig. 11–3). Once treatment is initiated, follow-up imaging can aid in assessing its effectiveness (Fig. 11–4). Imaging may also aid in determining whether a disease is congenital or acquired, and thus help to determine potential genetic ramifications should the animal be used for breeding (Fig. 11–3).[4]

II. RADIOGRAPHIC ASSESSMENT OF THE KIDNEYS

A. Role of radiographic imaging in kidney disease.

1. Radiographic imaging may allow assessment of whether a relationship exists between the upper urinary tract disease and clinical signs. For example, radiographic imaging would be used to confirm a relationship between upper urinary tract disease and idiopathic hematuria, or to confirm that a mass palpated during physical examination is originating in or invading the kidneys (Figs. 11–2 and 11–3).
2. Radiographic imaging may facilitate identification of congenital or heritable renal disease. Because laboratory and clinical signs of renal disease can be nonspecific for congenital/inherited renal disease versus acquired renal disease, renal imaging can link a small or irregularly marginated kidney in a high-risk breed to the diagnosis of congenital or inherited renal disease (Fig. 11–3).[4,5]
3. Radiographic versus ultrasonographic techniques.
   a. Advantages of radiography. Radiographic imaging of the kidneys has several advantages relevant to overall patient assessment. First, a qualitative assessment of renal function may be obtained by excretory urography.[6,7] In addition, a quantitative relationship between body size (length of the 2nd lumbar vertebral body) and kidney length facilitates identification of small and large kidneys.[1,6,8-10] Finally, excretory urography may provide insights into the pathophysiology of renal disease by way of characteristic nephrographic fading patterns (Figs. 11–5 and 11–6).[11] The relative rates of nephrographic opacification and fading provide subjective insight about renal blood flow, glomerular filtration rate, and the status of the renal outflow tract.
   b. Advantages of ultrasonography. Ultrasono-

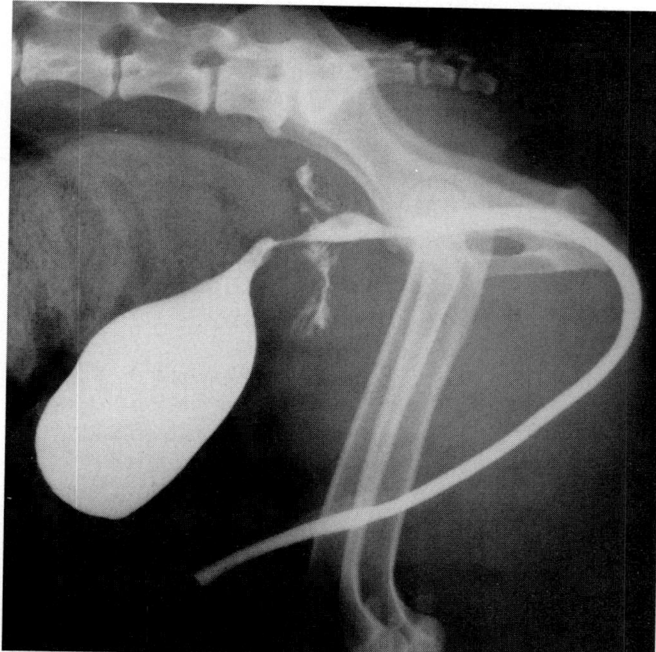

FIG. 11–1. Lateral abdominal view of a dog illustrates retrograde urethrocystography. Prominent narrowing and distortion of the cranial portion of the intraprostatic urethra are apparent. The location of the urethra indicates that the prostate gland is prominently enlarged. Note the massive accumulation of stool in the colon secondary to the prostomegaly. The diagnosis was prostatic carcinoma with urethral invasion.

graphic imaging techniques also provide strengths relative to the assessment of kidney disease. Although the information obtained by ultrasonography is not functional and is exclusively morphologic, this technique does not require use of ionizing radiation or systemically administered iodinated contrast media. In addition, ultrasonographic imaging does not depend on renal function, as does excretory urography.

B. Survey radiography.

1. Preparation for abdominal radiography. Routine preparation for abdominal radiography includes withholding food for 24 hours (except in emergency cases and diabetic patients).[1,8] Water should not be withheld, even prior to excretory urography. Tepid cleansing enemas are strongly suggested both the night before and approximately 2 hours before abdominal radiography to eliminate feces from the colon. Sedation should be necessary only for uncooperative patients and should be avoided when medically contraindicated. As part of the general abdominal radiography sequence, two orthogonal views are strongly recommended. Right lateral and ventrodorsal views are preferred for routine urinary tract imaging.
2. Practicality of survey radiography. Survey radiography has many practical aspects. The most prominent of these is definition of the radiographic characteristics of the kidneys, including size, shape, location, number, and density (Fig. 11–7).[1-3,9,10,12] In addition, survey radiographs can be of assistance in staging an abdominal mass relative to the kidneys and regional retroperitoneal vessels.
3. Shortcomings of survey radiography. Survey radiographic imaging has several disadvantages. First, it cannot be used to define the kidneys if retroperitoneal fat is lacking or if retroperitoneal fluid is present (Fig. 11–8A). Similarly, survey radiography cannot be used to characterize renal function. Survey radiography is of little value for diseases of the renal pelvis and ureters except to identify radiopaque materials, such as renoliths or dystrophic mineralization. Finally, survey radiography cannot differentiate between focal masses, diffuse infiltrates, or parenchymal cavitations, such as cysts or abscesses.

C. Excretory urography.

1. Definition(s). The excretory urogram is defined as sequential radiographic imaging that includes the opacification of the kidneys, renal pelves and

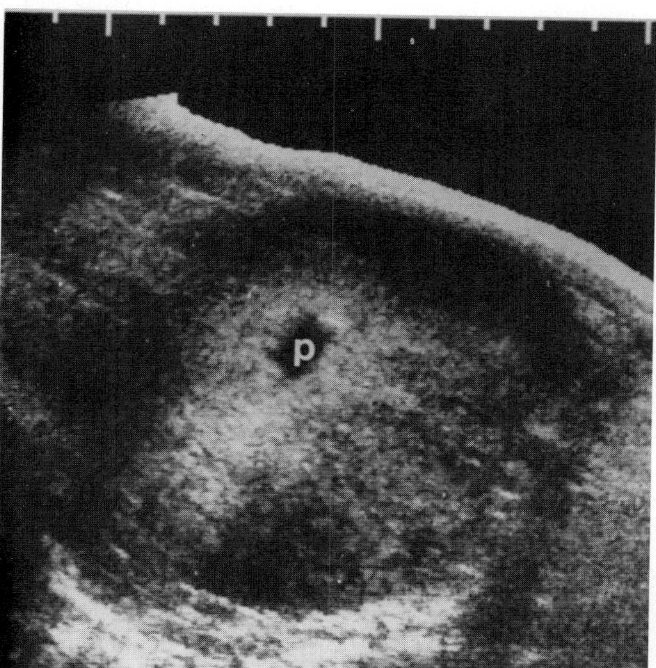

FIG. 11–2. Sagittal sonogram of a canine kidney with adenocarcinoma. Most of the renal architecture has been distorted by the invasive neoplastic echogenic mass, except for the renal pelvis (p). Reprinted with permission from Walter PA, Feeney DA, Johnston GR, O'Leary TP. Ultrasonographic evaluation of renal parenchymal diseases in the dog: 32 cases (1981-1986). *J Am Vet Med Assoc.* 1987;191:999.

recesses, and the ureters following the intravenous administration of iodinated contrast medium. The term "nephrogram" refers to opacification of the renal parenchyma, which results primarily from the concentration of contrast medium in the renal tubules. Vascular opacity contributes to renal opacification during the very early nephrogram phase, however. "Pyelogram" is a term that encompasses opacification of the renal collecting system, including the renal pelvic recesses and ureters.

2. Clinical considerations and contraindications. Several factors should be considered as part of the decision process leading to the use of excretory urography. First, we strongly recommend use of a short-term intravenous catheter.[1,8] Because excretory urography requires the intravascular administration of iodinated contrast medium, a small risk exists of a systemic contrast medium reaction, which could range from transient hypotension to anaphylactic shock.[13] In addition, some degree of renal function is needed to excrete a sufficient quantity of contrast medium to be detectable.[11] If renal function is severely compromised, one must either increase the dosage of contrast medium to allow for satisfactory opacification or consider an alternative imaging technique. Intravascular administration of contrast medium should be preceded by several considerations. First, these agents should not be administered to patients who are anuric, oliguric, or dehydrated.[1,11,14] In addition, systemic contrast medium can transiently affect renal function, thereby possibly influencing patient status and influencing analysis of renal function over the short term.[11,13] Finally, contrast medium can affect a series of clinical laboratory serum and urine analyses, which have been defined elsewhere.[15] Prior to performing the excretory urogram on a patient that is uncooperative, one must also consider the advantages and disadvantages of sedation.
3. Techniques of excretory urography. The technique of excretory urography is relatively straightforward.[1,8] Preparation for general abdominal radiography was defined in Section IIB of this chapter. Survey radiographs prior to intravenous administration of the contrast medium are mandatory. We recommend administration of contrast

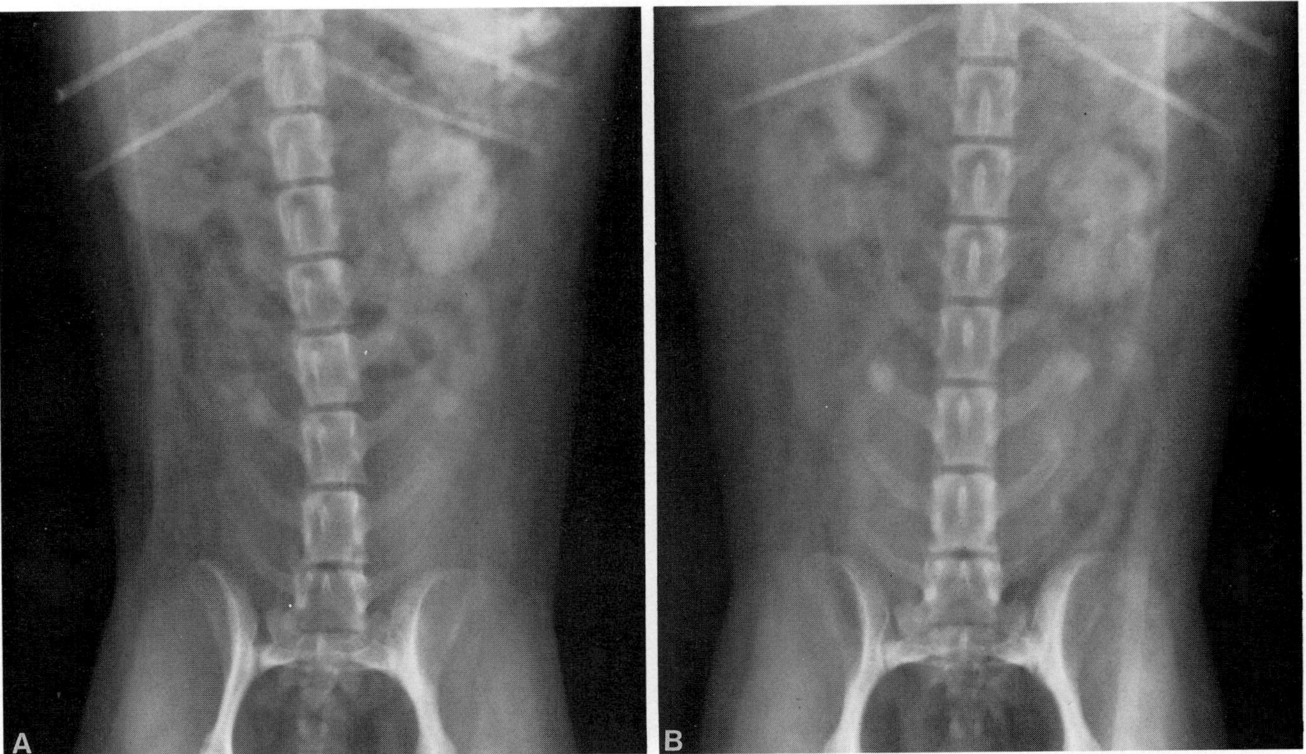

FIG. 11–3. Ventrodorsal views made at 10 seconds **(A)** and 5 minutes **(B)** after intravenous contrast medium injection into a 1-year-old Shih Tzu dog. The kidneys are small, nephrographic opacity is poor, and pyelographic opacity is barely discernible. The morphologic diagnosis was familial renal disease of the Shih Tzu. Reprinted with permission from Feeney DA, Johnston GR. The kidneys and ureters. In: Thrall DE, ed. *Textbook of Veterinary Diagnostic Radiology.* Philadelphia, Pa: WB Saunders Co; 1986.

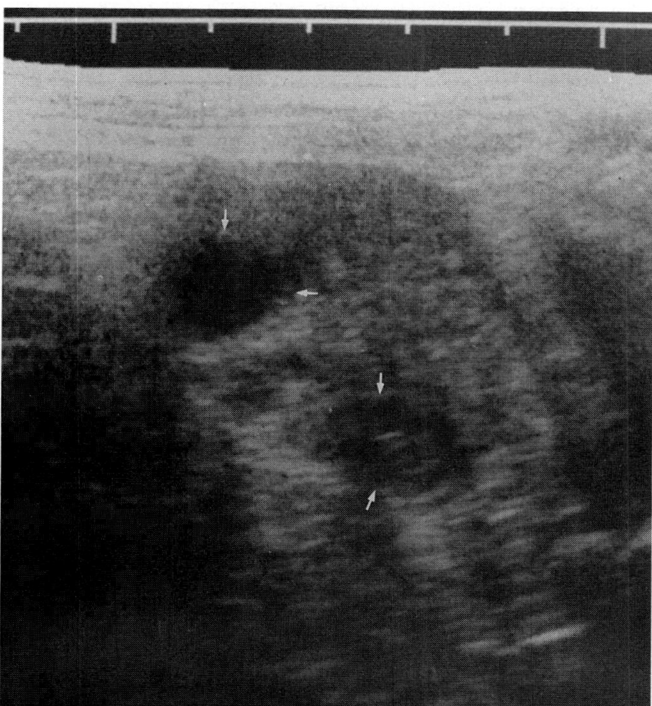

FIG. 11–4. Sagittal static ultrasonogram of a dog illustrates a lobulated outline of the prostate gland, which also contains 2 hypoechoic irregularly marginated cavitating lesions 2 cm in diameter (arrows) with some distant enhancement. Laparotomy revealed that these lesions were prostatic abscesses. Reprinted with permission from Feeney DA, et al. Canine prostatic disease: Comparison of ultrasonographic appearance with morphologic and microbiologic findings. *J Am Vet Med Assoc.* 1987;190:1027.

medium via a preplaced intravenous catheter, so that if a contrast medium reaction were to occur, catheter access to a vein would be available. The contrast medium should be given as a rapid intravenous (bolus) dose of approximately 400 mg of iodine per pound of body weight. We routinely use sodium-based ionic contrast medium. If the animal has a history of reaction to contrast media, a nonionic contrast medium should be considered. The filming sequence should include a ventrodorsal view at 5 to 15 seconds postinjection, followed by postinjection ventrodorsal views at 5, 20, and 40 minutes. Lateral views should be made at least 5 minutes postinjection, but are optional thereafter. Oblique views, as for ectopic ureters, are best performed at about the time 5-minute views are made. Abdominal compression is not suggested because of its effects on glomerular filtration rate and inconsistency associated with its use.[16]

4. Expectations of excretory urography. General expectations of excretory urography include:
   a. Further definition and clarification of survey radiographic findings.[1,14] Excretory urograms can be used to characterize the severity and distribution of focal, multifocal, or diffuse renal disease (Fig. 11–9). In addition, excretory urograms can be used to categorize opacification patterns of the nephrogram, which may aid in identifying probable differential pathophysiologic mechanisms of disease (Table 11–1, Fig. 11–6). It can also be used to locate a functional kidney (such as a pelvic kidney) not identified by survey radiography. Excretory urograms can also be used to characterize the relationship between renal masses and the renal pelvis and ureter (Fig. 11–10). The early nephrogram (almost nonselective angiogram) phase of excretory urograms can be used to characterize the relationship between renal masses and regional renal vessels, particularly the caudal vena cava and aorta. Also, excretory urograms may aid in differentiating focal cranial polar masses of the kidneys from adrenal masses (Fig. 11–11).
   b. Qualitatively assess overall and relative renal function. By use of a standardized technique, a subjective but useful qualitative assessment of renal function can be achieved using excretory urography.[6,7] The normal nephrographic opacification sequence is maximal opacity 5 to 20 seconds after bolus intravenous administration of the contrast medium, followed by progressive nephrographic fading until the opacity of the kidney parenchyma is no different from that seen on survey radiographs (Fig. 11–5). In addition, one can assess the relative opacity of both nephrogram and pyelogram phases, the degree of distention of pyelographic components (Fig. 11–6), the efficiency of ureteral peristalsis, and whether the ureters are intact (Fig. 11–8B).
   c. Gain insight into type of renal disorder by studying opacification patterns of the nephrogram. Variations from the generally expected nephrographic pattern of opacification and fading sequence provide insight into the pathophysiologic characteristics of renal disease (Table 11–2).[1,11,14] These sequences can be used to characterize the relationship of the disorder to systemic factors affecting renal blood flow, primary tubular or glomerular disorders, generalized renal deterioration, and extrarenal obstruction. An example is shown in Figure 11–6, wherein a poorly opacified, very slowly fading nephrogram is seen in an animal with renal disease caused by excessive dosages of aminoglycoside antibiotic.
   d. Identify and characterize the shape, function, and relative distention of the renal pelvis, pelvic recesses, and ureters (measure, if necessary). Assessment of renal and ureteral dimensions permits identification of, and differentiation among, numerous diseases affecting the

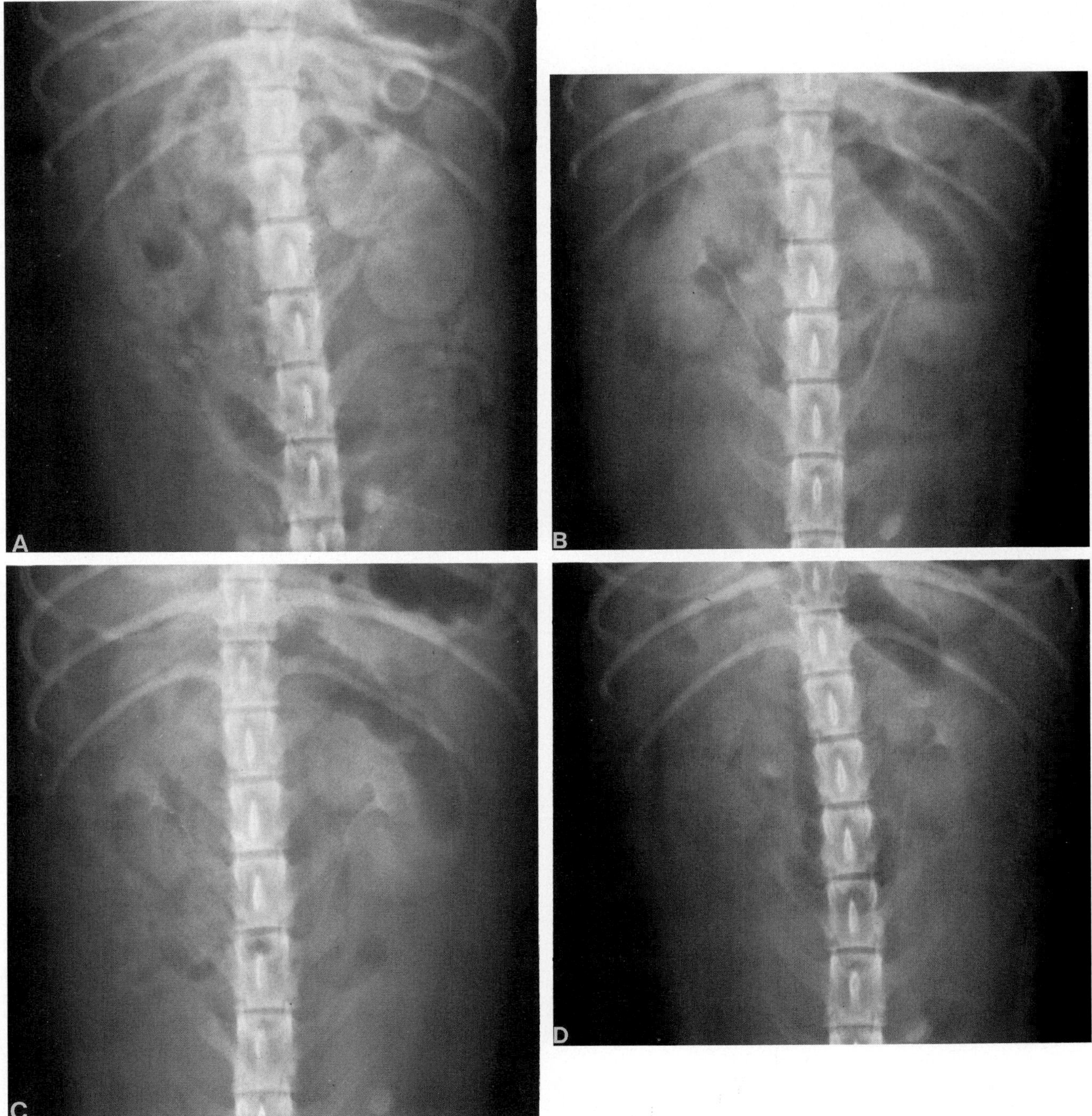

FIG. 11–5. Ventrodorsal views of the abdomen made 10 seconds (**A** and **E**), 5 minutes (**B** and **F**), 20 minutes (**C** and **G**), and 40 minutes (**D** and **H**) following intravenous administration of contrast medium into a normal dog (**A** through **D**).

renal collecting system (Table 11–3). These include hydronephrosis/hydroureter (Figs. 11–12 and 11–13),[1,14,17] acute and chronic pyelonephritis (Fig. 11–13),[1,3,14,18] intraluminal filling defects, including calculi, blood clots, and tumors (Fig. 11–12),[1,3,14,19,20] and distortion resulting from renal pelvic or renal parenchymal neoplasms and scarring (Fig. 11–10).[1,2,14]

5. Shortcomings of excretory urography. Excretory urograms have several shortcomings. In addition to those defined in Section IIC of this chapter, the following caveats should be considered when

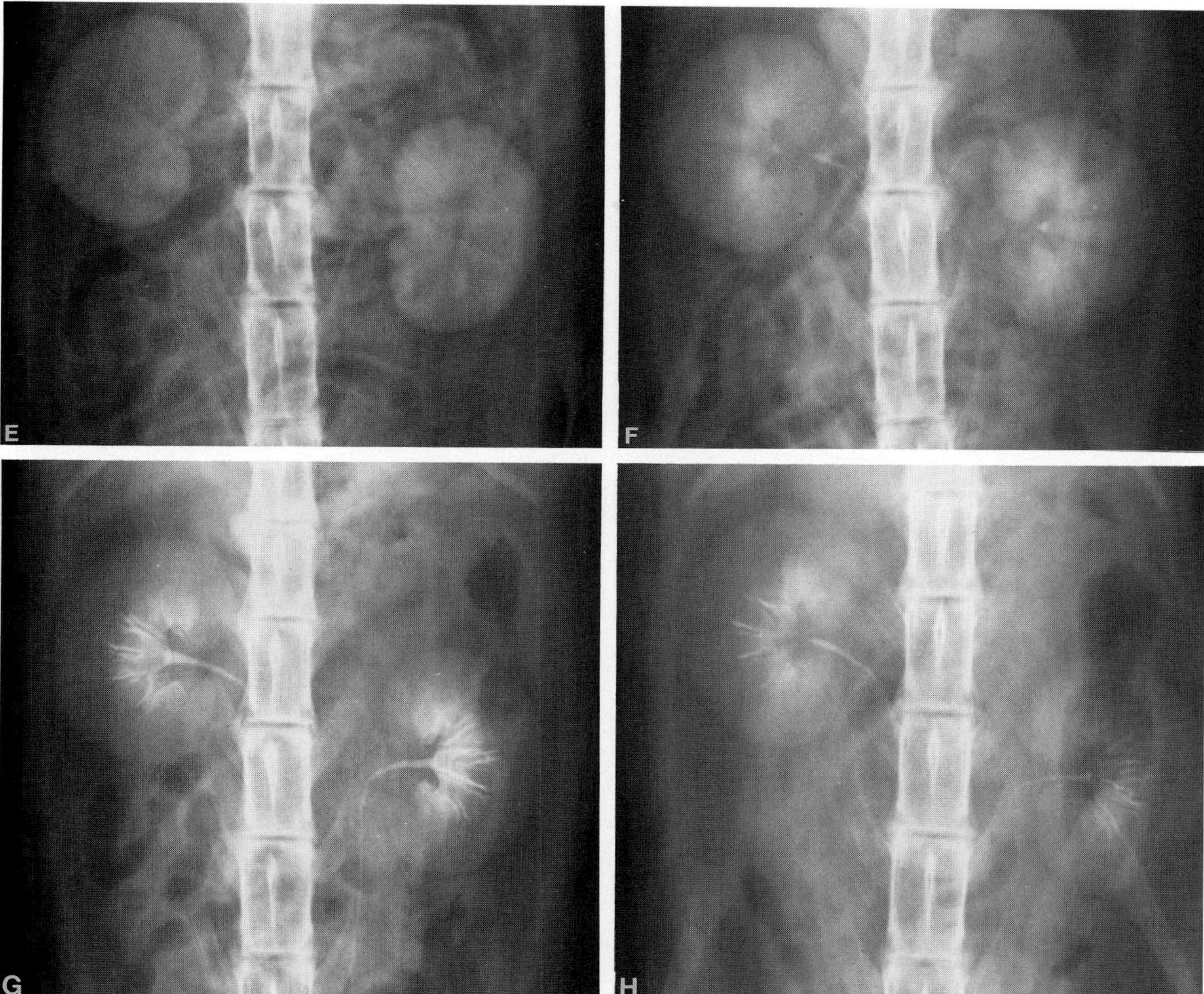

FIG. 11–5, cont'd. A normal cat (**E** through **H**).

performing and interpreting excretory urograms. First, if renal function is poor, the study probably will be nondiagnostic, particularly with standard dosages of contrast medium. Although associated with increased risk, doubling the dosage of contrast medium may yield sufficient diagnostic information to justify the risk of performing the procedure with this higher dosage. Small parenchymal lesions may be masked if the higher dosage results in an opaque nephrogram that causes scattered multifocal lesions to be missed. The appearance of the nephrogram may be delayed because of subacute pelvic or ureteral obstruction. This delay could lead to the misinterpretation of poor renal function, which would erroneously indicate an irreversible situation that is, in fact, reversible. One should remember the possibility of systemic contrast medium reaction both in the interpretation of the nephrographic fading pattern as well as in patient management after injection of the contrast medium.

III. ULTRASONOGRAPHIC ASSESSMENT OF THE KIDNEYS

A. **Role of ultrasonographic imaging of the kidney.** Ultrasonography is a noninvasive method that is complementary to traditional survey and contrast radiography.[21-26] The role of ultrasonography is to determine: 1) if the kidney/contralateral kidney is abnormal; 2) what area is affected and to what extent; 3) tissue composition (solid/cystic); and 4) presence of metastases. Laboratory tests and survey radiographs are recommended for routine screening. Survey abdominal radiographs may reveal the first indication that the kidney has an abnormal

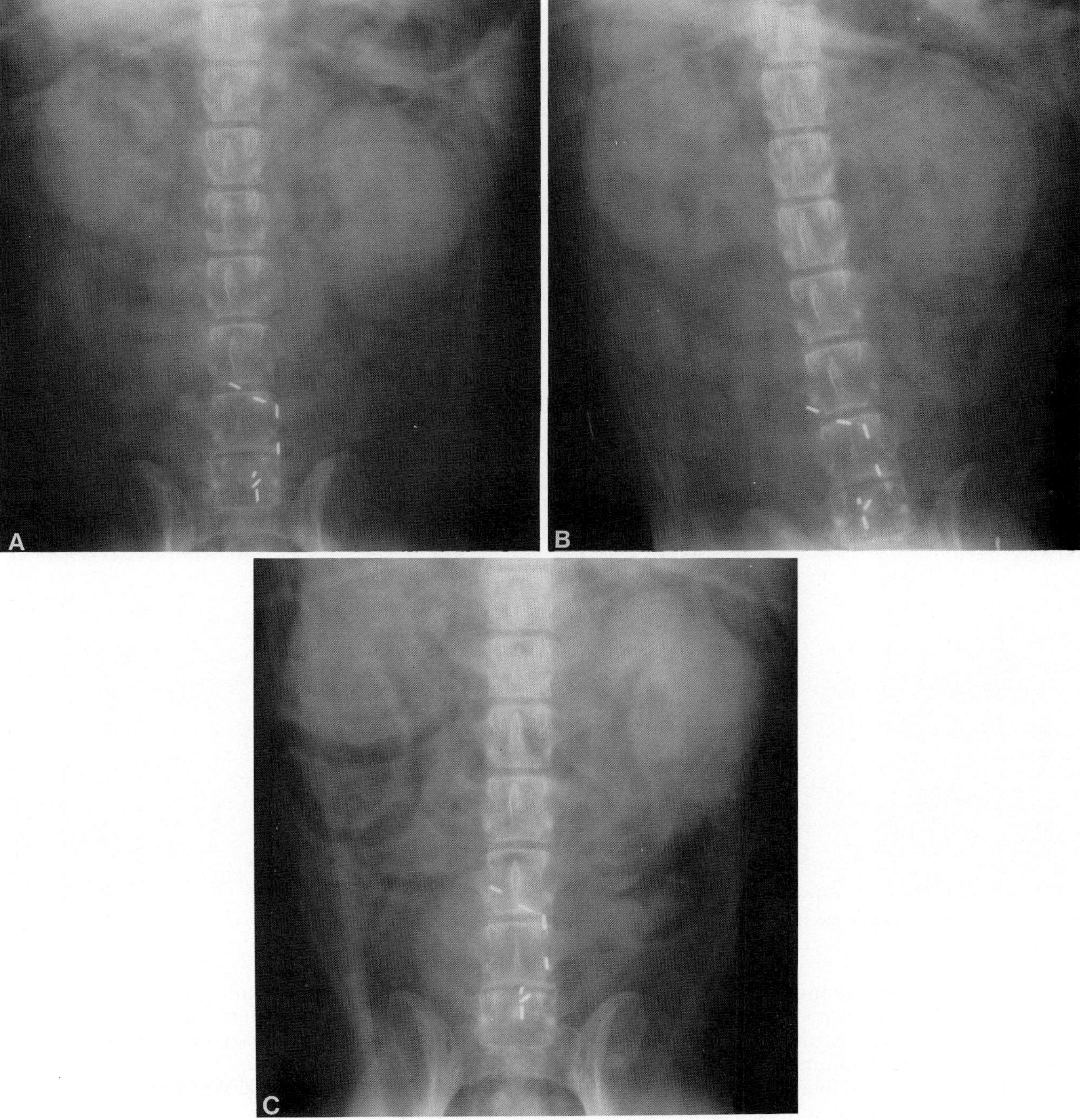

FIG. 11–6. Ventrodorsal views of a standard-dose excretory urogram made 10 seconds **(A)**, 5 minutes **(B)**, 20 minutes **(C)**,

shape or size or that a palpable mass is retroperitoneal. The examination should attempt to image kidneys, adrenal glands, regional vessels (aorta, vena cava), liver, spleen, urinary bladder and prostate gland or ovary, peritoneal surfaces, and regional lymph nodes. Ultrasonographic patterns are not always specific. However, the ability to distinguish solid from fluid-containing lesions and to assess the distribution of disease allows one to formulate differential considerations and management alternatives.

B. Indications for kidney sonography. Renal ultrasonography, one step in the evaluation of animals

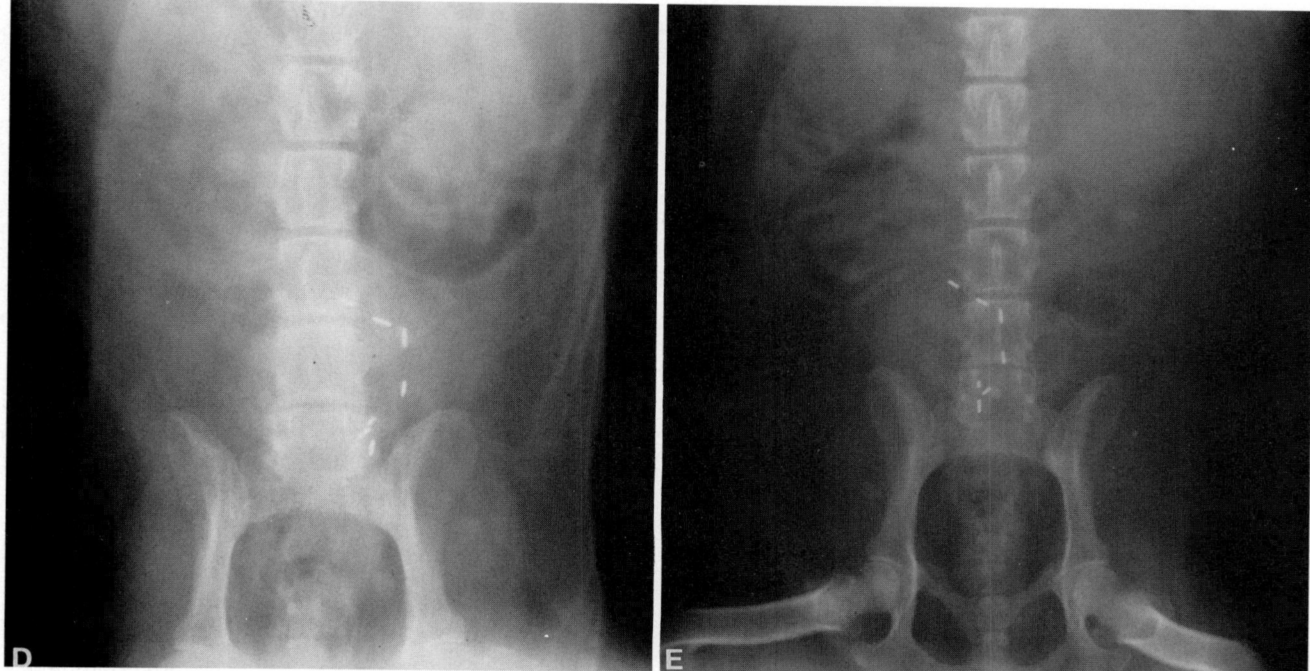

FIG. 11–6, cont'd. and 40 minutes **(D)** following intravenous administration of contrast medium. Note the poorly opacified but slowly fading nephrogram with negligible pyelographic opacification. This finding is typical of polyuric renal failure. This animal had renal failure induced by an aminoglycoside antibiotic. For perspective, the survey radiograph taken prior to administration of contrast medium is included **(E)**.

with clinical signs of renal disease, is generally performed after physical examination and acquisition of minimum data base, but before initiation of more invasive procedures (biopsy, surgery). Indications for sonography are: 1) abnormal laboratory findings indicative of urinary tract disease; 2) abnormal kidney size, contour, or renal mass on palpation; 3) poor intra-abdominal contrast (emaciation/effusion) that prevents visualization of kidneys on survey radiographs; 4) abnormal kidney shape, size, or opacity detected on survey radiographs or excretory urogram; and 5) nonvisualized kidney on survey radiographs or nonfunctional kidney on excretory urogram.

C. **Advantages of ultrasonography compared to uroradiography.** Primary advantages of sonography over conventional radiographic procedures are: 1) noninvasive, rapid, and cost-effective procedure; 2) assessment of intrarenal abnormalities not seen on survey radiographs (renal parenchyma and renal sinus); 3) alleviates use of contrast medium (safe for young and debilitated patients); 4) safe for patient and sonographer (no ionizing radiation); 5) effective when renal function is impaired (nondiagnostic excretory urogram); 6) allows determination of disease extent within the kidney, the contralateral kidney, and in the perirenal area; 7) guided biopsy facilitates visualization of tissue sampling; and 8) allows serial evaluation of structural change in response to surgical or medical therapy.

D. **Limitations of ultrasonography compared to uroradiography.** Limitations of sonography are: 1) inability to image kidneys through overlying bony structures, air-filled viscus, "free" intraperitoneal air, and barium sulfate suspension used for gastrointestinal series (water-soluble iodinated contrast media do not affect sound transmission); 2) does not facilitate quantitative or qualitative assessment of kidney function (except Doppler technique); 3) not a good screening method—best used when directed toward a specific problem identified by palpation, abdominal radiographs, or laboratory tests; 4) does not provide specific morphologic diagnosis, although many ultrasonographic patterns are quite specific; 5) user dependent—requires technical and interpretative skill and experience; and 6) in general, less effective than excretory urography for detection of subtle renal pelvic and ureteral abnormalities.

E. **Technique of renal ultrasonography.** Quality diagnostic images require adequate transducer contact, good depth penetration, image detail, and images of reference organs. For kidney scanning, the patient is restrained in dorsal recumbency with the head to the left of the sonographer. Sedation is rarely needed. A 7.5-MHz transducer provides optimal resolution for cats, whereas a 7.5- or a 5.0-MHz transducer is recommended for dogs. A full urinary bladder serves as control to adjust gain settings. Usually the patient's hair must be clipped around the margin of the costal arch, including the ventral flank and extending caudally to the pelvic brim. A coupling medium (gel) is applied between the transducer and the skin of the patient to displace air and to facilitate sound transmission. Air within the alimentary tract may prevent sound transmission. Withholding food minimizes this problem. Enemas should not be given to patients prior to sonography because they introduce air into the colon and lower small intestine. Varied positioning is often needed to move air-containing viscera away from the sonographic window. The kidneys, especially in cats, are extremely mobile. Transducer pressure on the abdominal wall and normal breathing patterns can affect the position of the kidneys. The appearance of the kidney is influenced by the plane in which the sound beam traverses the organ. Cranial and caudal curved borders of the kidneys are difficult to detect because of the absence of a perpendicular reflector.[21,23,27] True sagittal and transverse scans are important because measurements may be inaccurate if the beam slices the kidney at an obtuse angle. Sonographic measurements are smaller than actual *in vivo* measurements and magnified estimates made from radiographs with fixed focal film distance.[24,28] The right kidney lies in the renal impression of the liver. In dorsal recumbency, the cranial pole of the right kidney lies within the costal arch. The right kidney is traversed on its ventral surface by the ascending colon and descending duodenum. This topography makes scanning the right kidney more difficult because the sound beam may not be perpendicular to the longitudinal axis of the kidney, and if gas is within the bowel, it will reflect sound and prevent transmission to and from the kidney. The left kidney lies adjacent to the spleen, and this combination provides an excellent window. The comparatively caudal position of the left kidney makes it consistently easier to image. At least two orthogonal images are recommended to evaluate the kidneys (sagittal plane image showing an axial double hyperechoic bar pattern formed by the end-on renal pelvic recesses and a transverse plane image through the middle of the hilus.[29-31] Echogenicity of intrarenal

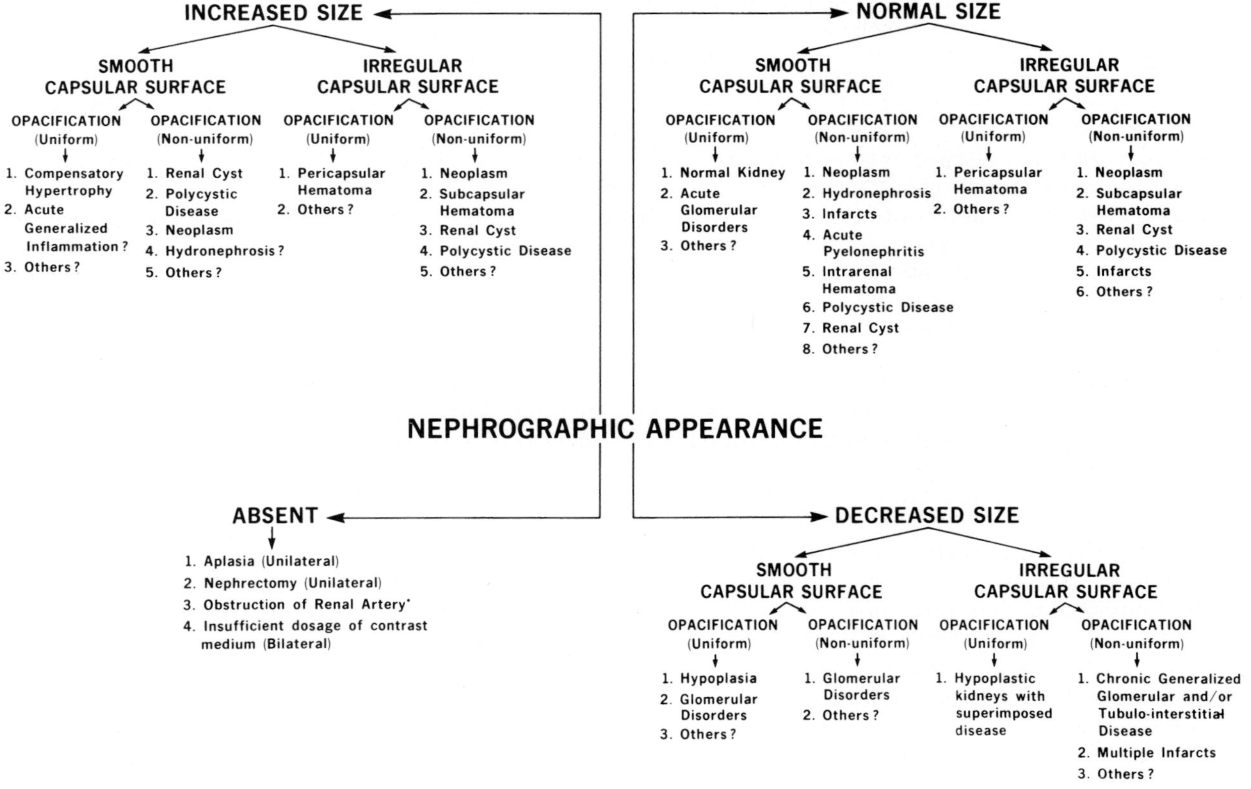

FIG. 11–7. Algorithm for interpretation of nephrograms produced by intravenous injection of radiographic contrast medium. Note: Bilateral obstruction of renal arteries (no. 3 under "Absent" heading) would result in death within a few days. Reprinted with permission from Feeney DA, Barber DL, Osborne CA. Advances in canine excretory urography. In: *30th Gaines Veterinary Symposium*. White Plains, NY: Gaines Dog Research Center; 1981:8-22.

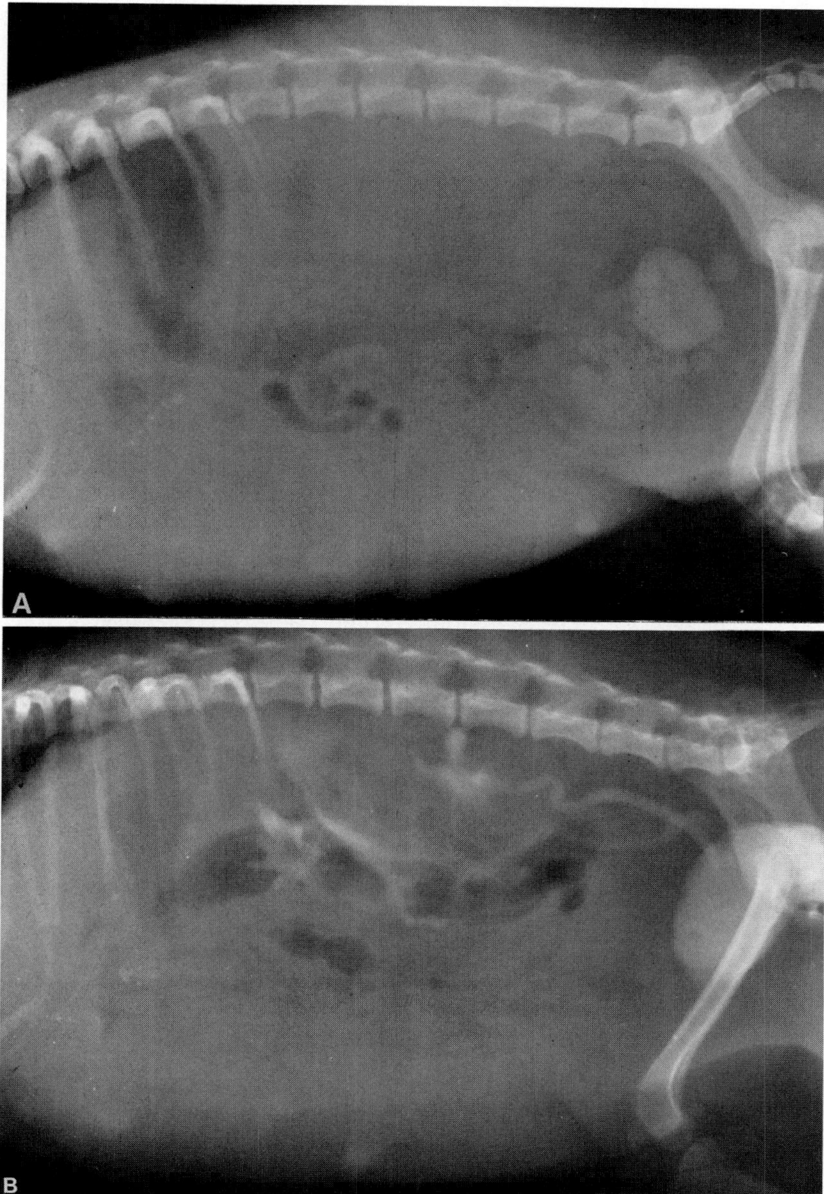

FIG. 11–8. Lateral views of a dog exposed before **(A)** and 30 minutes following **(B)** intravenous injection of contrast medium. Multiple urocystoliths are present. In **A,** note the lack of retroperitoneal contrast and the limited visualization of the kidneys. In **B,** note the spillage of contrast medium into the retroperitoneal space consistent with rupture of the right ureter. Reprinted with permission from Feeney DA, Johnston GR. The kidneys and ureters. In: Thrall DE, ed. *Textbook of Veterinary Diagnostic Radiology.* Philadelphia, Pa: WB Saunders Co; 1986.

structures should be compared, as should the echogenicity of one kidney with that of the contralateral kidney. The image of the liver or spleen may be used as an extrarenal control.

F. **Ultrasound-guided kidney biopsy.** Percutaneous ultrasound-guided punch biopsy or fine-needle aspiration allows visualization of the biopsy site, localization of lesions for sampling, accurate placement of the biopsy instrument, verification of tissue aspiration, and early detection of postbiopsy hemorrhage.[32] Renal biopsy may be especially useful in assessing diseases that are sonographically similar in appearance (e.g., immune-mediated glomerulopathies, amyloidosis, nephrocalcinosis, acute tubular necrosis). Preparation includes a coagulation profile and sedation or general anesthesia to minimize respiratory

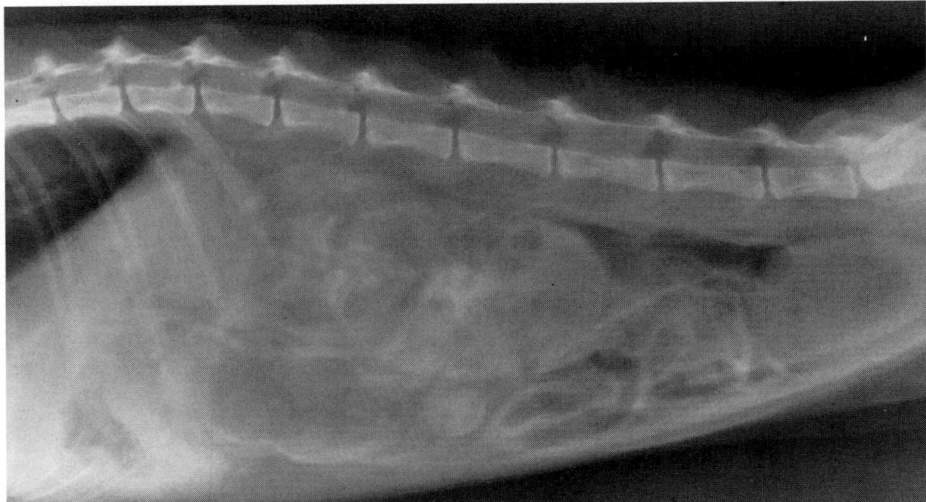

FIG. 11–9. Lateral view of the abdomen of a cat made approximately 5 minutes after intravenous contrast medium administration. Kidneys are enlarged, and nephrographic opacification is variable in a random patchy appearance. The morphologic diagnosis was feline polycystic renal disease. Reprinted with permission from Feeney DA, Johnston GR. The kidneys and ureters. In: Thrall DE, ed. *Textbook of Veterinary Diagnostic Radiology.* Philadelphia, Pa: WB Saunders Co; 1986.

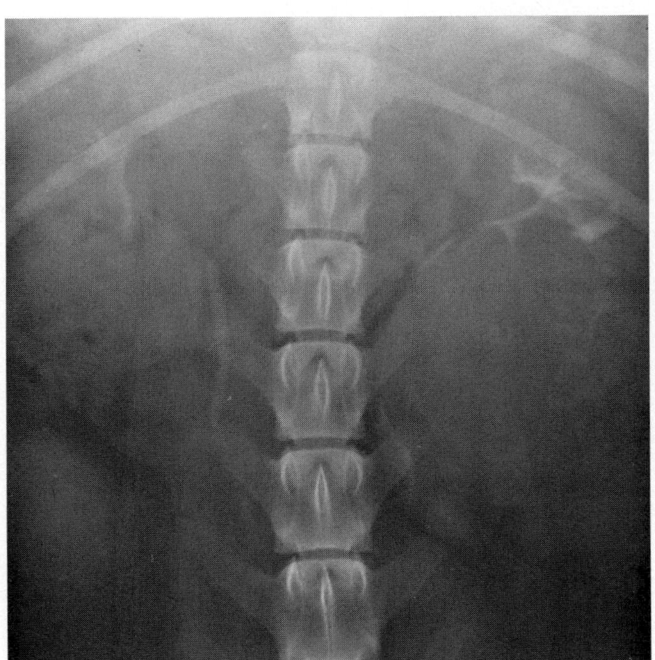

FIG. 11–10. Ventrodorsal view of the abdomen of a dog made about 5 minutes following intravenous injection of contrast medium. Note the distortion of the caudal aspect of the left renal pelvis and ureter, as well as the mass distorting the caudal pole of the left kidney. The morphologic diagnosis was renal adenocarcinoma. Reprinted with permission from Feeney DA, Johnston GR. The kidneys and ureters. In: Thrall DE, ed. *Textbook of Veterinary Diagnostic Radiology.* Philadelphia, Pa: WB Saunders Co; 1986.

rate and movement during the procedure. The animal is placed in right lateral recumbency (left kidney more accessible), the paralumbar region is clipped up to the costal arch, and the most desirable site for biopsy is located. Surgical preparation of the skin and application of sterile acoustic coupling gel minimize risk of contamination. A biopsy guide attached to the transducer can be used to direct the biopsy needle within the scanning image so that the procedure can be observed.

G. **Normal sonographic anatomy of the kidney.** Renal echogenicity is described relative to adjacent tissues and organs or in light of known normal relative tissue brightness (diaphragm > renal sinus > spleen > liver > renal cortex > medulla).[25] A marked distinction exists between the echogenic cortex and the almost anechoic medullary papillae. The renal cortex of cats appears brighter than the renal cortex of dogs because of higher fat content in the cat.[33] High-intensity echoes seen at the peripheral margin of the kidney, at the corticomedullary interface, and in the renal sinus are produced by reflective fibrous or fat interfaces in the capsule, renal pelvis and pelvic recesses, and vasculature. A hyperechoic ring at the corticomedullary junction in cats may be the result of microscopic mineralization.[33] The normal renal pelvis and ureter are not observed in dogs or cats, even during diuresis.[27,30,31,34] The normal sagittal sonographic patterns seen in the kidney of the dog and cat are: 1) mediad—renal sinus (renal pelvis and peripelvic fat and vessels) surrounded by the cortex and capsule; 2) midline—the pelvic recesses subdivide the medullary papilla surrounded by the cortex and

TABLE 11–1
STRUCTURAL NEPHROGRAPHIC OPACIFICATION PATTERNS ASSOCIATED WITH CERTAIN RENAL DISEASES*

Opacification Pattern	Renal Disease
Uniform	Normal Compensatory hypertrophy Acute glomerular or tubulo-interstitial disease Perirenal pseudocysts Hypoplasia Other(?)
Focal, nonuniform	Neoplasm Hematuria Cysts Single infarct Hydronephrosis Abscess Other(?)
Multifocal, nonuniform	Polycystic disease Multiple infarcts Acute pyelonephritis Chronic generalized glomerular or tubulo-interstitial disease Feline infectious peritonitis Infiltrative neoplasia Other(?)
Nonopacification	Aplasia/agenesis† Renal artery obstruction† Nephrectomy or nonfunctional renal parenchyma† Insufficient or extravascular contrast medium injection Other(?)

*Best identification on radiographs exposed 5 to 20 seconds or 5 minutes after contrast medium injection. Do not overinterpret corticomedullary separation on early postinjection radiographs.

†Only unilateral conditions compatible with life.

(Reprinted with permission from Feeney DA, Johnston GR. The kidneys and ureters. In: Thrall DE, ed. *Textbook of Veterinary Diagnostic Radiology.* Philadelphia, Pa: WB Saunders Co; 1986.)

capsule (Fig. 11–14); and 3) lateral—cortex and capsule only. The hyperechoic area of the renal sinus is best observed in the sagittal plane. A mildly dilated renal pelvis may be difficult to distinguish in this plane because of superimposed hilar structures. A transverse scan through the midkidney is most reliable to detect renal pelvic and ureteral dilatation because it distinguishes the outflow tract from the renal parenchyma. In normal kidneys, transverse scans typically reveal a bright crescent-shaped structure ("C" sign of the renal crest) surrounding the hypoechoic renal crest.[27,35]

H. Abnormal ultrasonographic patterns. Parenchymal diseases can be classified according to their distribution (Table 11–4). Diseases in which architecture is maintained are usually bilateral and lack a specific pattern, such as glomerulonephritis, nephrosclerosis, and tubular necrosis (e.g., ethylene glycol toxicosis).[35-39] These diseases are more likely to be hyperechoic than normal in appearance. As the disease progresses, scarring increases, demarcation between cortex and medulla decreases, and the kidney may shrink and become diffusely hyperechoic.[36] In diseases that disrupt normal architecture (e.g., cysts, hematomas, neoplasia, abscesses, and calculi), ultrasonography may aid in localizing a mass, determining its composition (fluid/solid), and defining the extent of disease.

1. Sonographic patterns of parenchyma diseases of dogs.
   a. Benign kidney masses. Solitary uncomplicated cysts, although rare in dogs, are easily distinguished from solid tissue or organizing lesions on the basis of a smooth well-defined inner wall, absence of internal echoes and septae, and distant enhancement.[22,23,26,34-37,40,41] The major differential diagnosis is a cystic tumor. Accuracy in identifying masses is greatest with

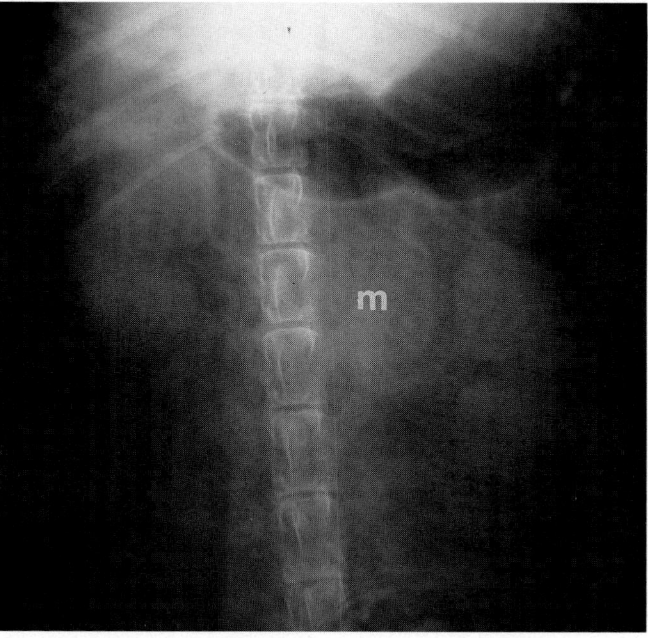

FIG. 11–11. Ventrodorsal view made 20 minutes after intravenous contrast medium administration. Note the distinct separation between the mass (m) in the left midhemiabdomen immediately adjacent to the 2nd lumbar vertebra and the left kidney. In addition to having an adrenal mass, which was confirmed to be a functional adenocarcinoma, this dog experienced contrast-medium-induced renal failure, which explains the lack of a pyelographic phase. Reprinted with permission from Feeney DA, Barber DL, Osborne CA. Advances in canine excretory urography. *Proceedings from the 30th Annual Gaines Veterinary Symposium.* White Plains, NY; 1981.

TABLE 11–2
NEPHROGRAPHIC OPACIFICATION PATTERNS ASSOCIATED WITH CERTAIN RENAL DISEASES

A	Good initial opacification followed by progressively decreasing opacity: Normal
B	Fair to good initial opacification followed by progressively increasing opacity: Systemic hypotension caused by radiocontrast agents Acute renal obstruction (including precipitated Tamm-Horsfall mucoprotein in renal tubules) Contrast-medium-induced renal failure Others
C	Fair to good initial opacification followed by persistent opacity: Acute renal tubular necrosis Contrast-medium-induced renal failure Systemic hypotension caused by radiocontrast agents Others
D	Poor initial opacification followed by progressively decreased opacity: Primary polyuric renal failure Inadequate contrast medium dosage Others
E	Poor initial opacification followed by progressively increased opacity: Acute extrarenal obstruction Systemic hypotension existing prior to contrast medium administration Renal ischemia (arterial or venous) Others
F	Poor initial opacification followed by persistent opacity: Primary glomerular dysfunction (chronic) Severe generalized renal disease

(Reprinted with permission from Feeney DA, Barber DL, Osborne CA. The functional aspects of the nephrogram in excretory urography: A review. *Vet Radiol.* 1982;23:42.)

lesions 2 cm or greater in diameter.[36] When cysts are identified in one kidney, the contralateral kidney and the liver should be examined. Infected or hemorrhagic cysts, abscesses, hematomas, or necrosis are likely to be hypoechoic with some distant enhancement,[37] but because of cellularity and fibrous components, echogenicity is variable and usually increases with time.[21,36] Size, shape, discrete margination, and minimal disruption distinguish a less aggressive benign lesion from aggressive neoplasia. Infarcts are usually hypoechoic, cause some contour deformity if they bulge from the surface, and become progressively hyperechoic as scar tissue develops.[42]

b. Diffuse tubulo-interstitial disease. Similar sonographic appearances are observed in diseases of unrelated causes (e.g., glomerulopathies, nephrocalcinosis, amyloidosis, acute tubular necrosis, granulomatous infiltrate, end-stage fibrosis) (Fig. 11–15).[25,26,29,38,41-43] The kidneys are most often hyperechoic, although some may appear normal.

c. Renal neoplasia. The more infiltrative, expansile, and disruptive a mass is, the more likely it is to be neoplastic. Most tumors are diffuse with a complex echogenicity or are multifocal and hyperechoic (Fig. 11–2).[26,29,34,44] Accuracy in distinguishing neoplastic disease is greatest for diffuse solid masses larger than 5 cm. Focal solid lesions smaller than 5 cm, especially those containing low-intensity echoes, are more difficult to distinguish from small nonneoplastic masses or fluid collections. The echogenicity of neoplasms suggests the homogeneity of the cellular type and varies with the amount of associated vascularity and hemorrhage or necrosis.[41,44,45] Sparsely vascular nonscirrhous tumors, such as lymphosarcomas, are usually

TABLE 11–3
PYELOGRAPHIC APPEARANCE OF SOME COMMON DISEASES OF THE KIDNEY

I. PYELONEPHRITIS
   A. Acute
      1. Pelvic Dilation
      2. Proximal Ureteral Dilation
      3. Absent or Incomplete Filling of Diverticula
   B. Chronic
      1. +/– Pelvic Dilation with Irregular Borders
      2. Proximal Ureteral Dilation
      3. Short-blunt Diverticula
II. HYDRONEPHROSIS
   A. Pelvic Dilation
   B. Dilation of Pelvic Diverticula (Note: Diverticula may not be distinguishable if pelvic dilation is severe)
   C. Ureteral Dilation
III. NEOPLASIA
   A. Of Renal Parenchyma
      1. Distortion or Deviation of Renal Pelvis, with +/– Dilation
      2. Distortion of Dilation of Pelvic Diverticula
   B. Of Renal Pelvis
      1. Distortion or Dilation of Renal Pelvis
      2. Filling Defects in Renal Pelvis
IV. UROLITHS
   A. Filling Defects in Renal Pelvis
   B. Uroliths Usually Radiolucent Compared to Contrast Medium
   C. May Be Changes as Seen in Pyelonephritis
   D. +/– Pelvic Dilation

(From Feeney DA, Barber DL, Osborne CA. Advances in canine excretory urography. *Proceedings from the 30th Annual Gaines Veterinary Symposium.* White Plains, NY; 1981.)

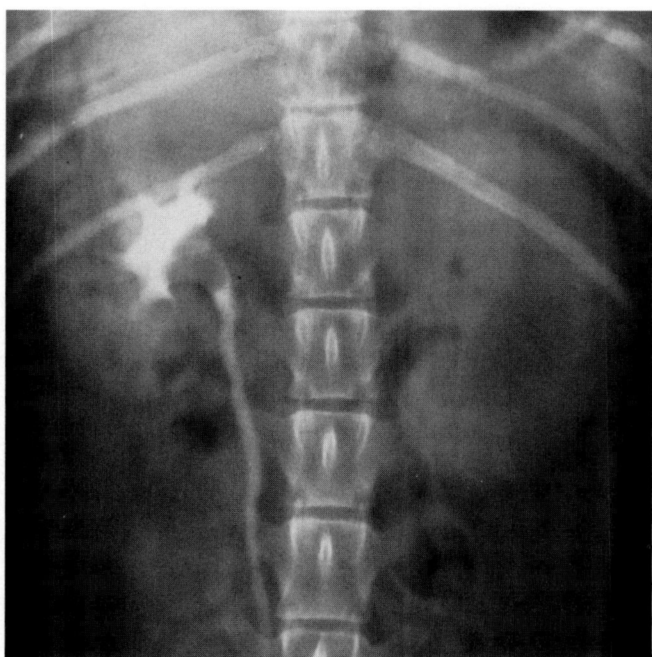

FIG. 11–12. Ventrodorsal view of the abdomen of a dog made approximately 5 minutes after intravenous contrast medium administration. The right renal pelvis is dilated, and a radiolucent filling defect is at the right ureteropelvic junction. Pyelographic opacification of the left upper urinary tract is not apparent, but a perihilar loss of nephrographic opacity suggests a dilated renal pelvis filled with nonopacified urine or possibly a mass. On survey radiographs, a calcific density was seen in the region of the right ureteropelvic junction and in the left proximal ureter. Radiographic diagnosis, which was surgically confirmed, was nonobstructive hydronephrosis of the right renal pelvis secondary to ureteropelvic calculus and obstructive hydronephrosis of the left kidney secondary to proximal left ureteral calculus. Reprinted with permission from Feeney DA, Barber DL, Osborne CA. Advances in canine excretory urography. *Proceedings from the 30th Annual Gaines Veterinary Symposium.* White Plains, NY; 1981.

hypoechoic. Vascular tumors without hemorrhage or necrosis are more echogenic. Adenocarcinomas, which tend to be extremely disruptive and expansile, are poorly demarcated, usually have a heterogeneic echo pattern, and are so invasive that little or no recognizable kidney structure is retained (Fig. 11–2).[36,41,44,45]

2. Sonographic patterns of parenchymal diseases in cats. Most diseases in cats have a multifocal/diffuse distribution.[5,41] Pattern specificity and interpretative confidence are greatest with focal or multifocal lesions 1 cm or greater in diameter.
   a. Benign kidney masses. Pattern specificity in feline polycystic disease makes sonographic diagnosis very accurate (Fig. 11–16).[5,41] Multifocal, sonolucent cysts have variable size (usually > 1 cm), smooth internal walls, and prominent distant enhancement. The hyperechoic renal sinus echo is usually preserved. Hepatic cysts may also be seen. Infected cysts are rare. Cysts smaller than 1 cm in diameter are often poorly separated from each other. The many reflecting interfaces typically produce a homogeneously hyperechoic kidney.
   b. Diffuse tubulo-interstitial disease. Diffuse parenchymal diseases in cats are most often hyperechoic, but pattern specificity is not apparent. Hyperechogenicity is associated with granulomatous infiltration in feline infectious peritonitis, glomerulointerstitial nephropathies, renal tubular necrosis, nephrocalcinosis, and amyloidosis.[38,41]
   c. Renal neoplasia. Focal renal neoplasms are unusual in cats. Most renal neoplasms affecting cats are diffuse lymphosarcomas, which appear as multifocal hypoechoic nodules with very-

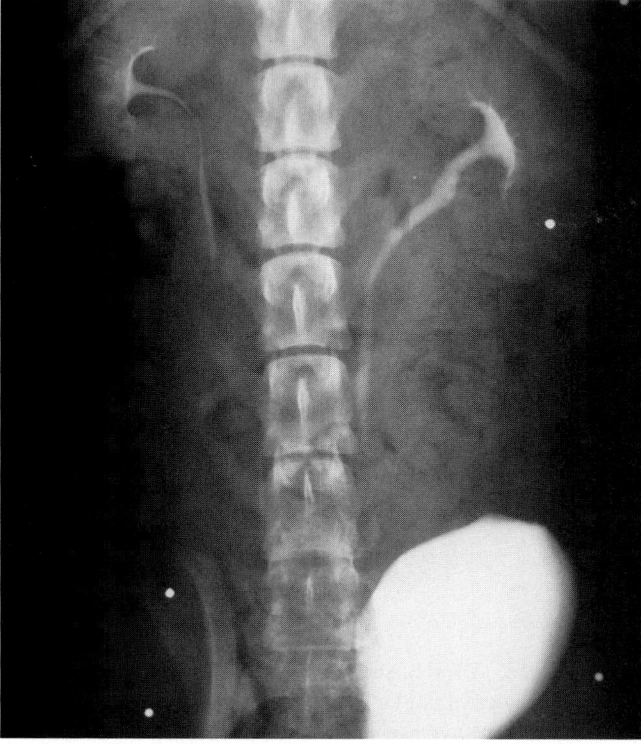

FIG. 11–13. Ventrodorsal radiograph of the abdomen of a dog made 40 minutes following intravenous contrast medium administration. This animal had induced pyelonephritis of the left kidney of about 10 days' duration. Note dilation of the left renal pelvis and proximal ureter with slight widening but prominent shortening and blunting of the left renal pelvic recesses. This appearance is characteristic of induced and naturally occurring pyelonephritis. Reprinted with permission from Feeney DA, Barber DL, Osborne CA. Advances in canine excretory urography. *Proceedings from the 30th Annual Gaines Veterinary Symposium.* White Plains, NY; 1981.

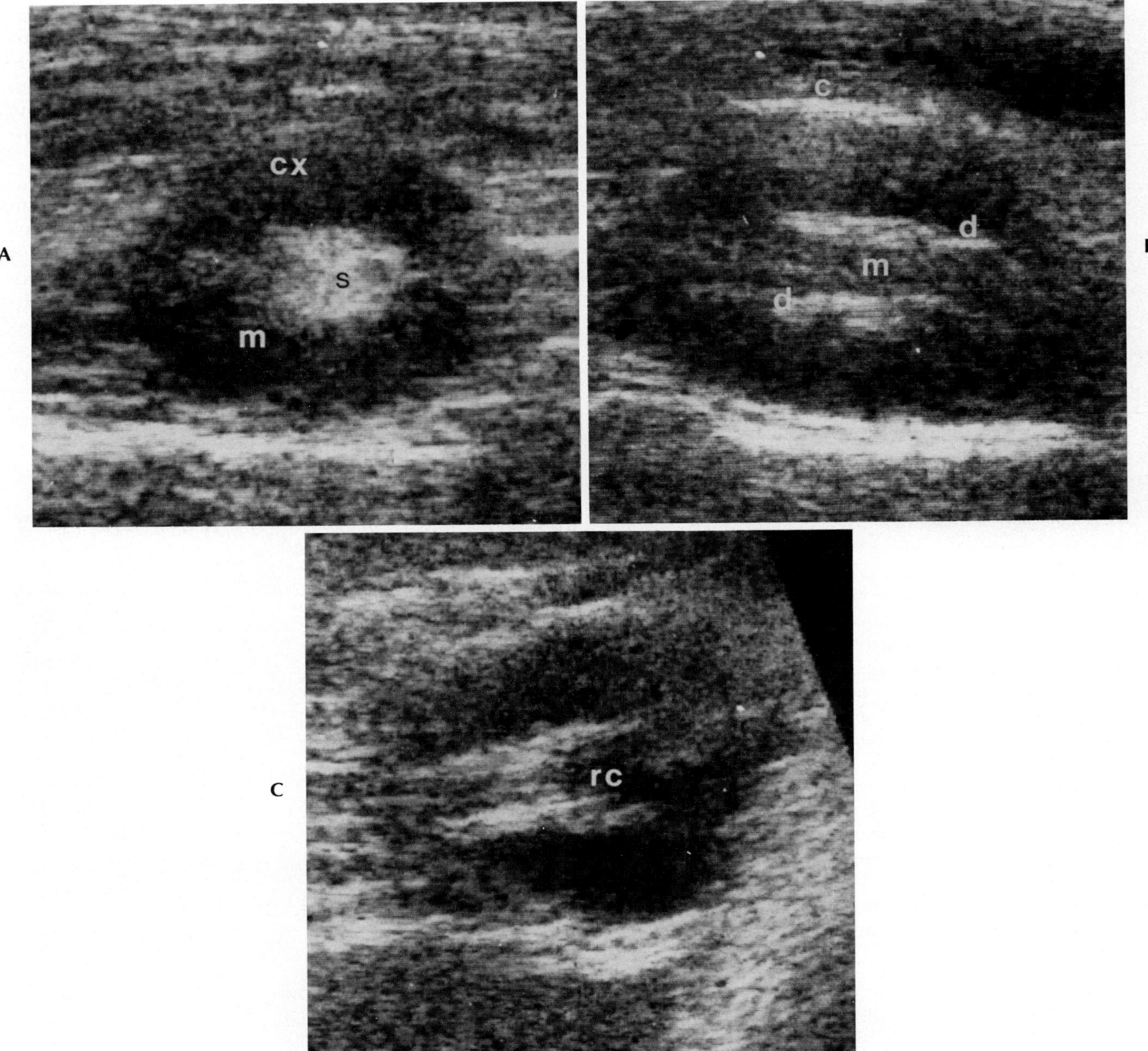

FIG. 11–14. A and **B,** Sagittal ultrasound images of normal cat kidney. **C,** Transverse ultrasound image of normal cat kidney. s = renal sinus; d = pelvic recesses; rc = renal crest c = capsule; cx = cortex; m = medulla. Reprinted with permission from Walter PA, et al. Renal ultrasonography in healthy cats. *Am J Vet Res.* 1987;48:600.

low-intensity echoes and minimal distant enhancement.[41] Diffuse hyperechogenicity is less frequently observed.[35,41] Architectural destruction is rare. Lack of a well-defined far wall and poor distant enhancement allow differentiation of lymphomatous nodules from cysts.[23]

3. Diseases of the renal pelvis and ureter in dogs and cats. Renal pelvic and ureteral diseases appear as fluid dilations (with or without calculi) or as space-occupying masses (Table 11–5). Mild renal pelvic dilation is seen as an anechoic fluid outline of the C-shaped outflow tract, which is often continuous with the ureter.[34,37] Fluid buildup expands the pelvis and separates the tightly opposed hyperechoic urothelium of the outflow region. Eventually, the sonolucent pelvic recesses become wider and flatter.

a. Inflammation of the kidney pelvis. For patients with uncomplicated pyelonephritis, sonography is not an adequate diagnostic substitute for excretory urography. Many cats and dogs with pyelonephritis have a normal hyperechoic renal sinus echo without evidence of dilation. Varying degrees of pelvic dilation (< 1 cm), some low-level echoes within the distended pelvic cavity, and mild separation without distortion of renal pelvic recesses are associated with inflammation (Fig. 11–17).[34] A hyperechoic halo around the periphery of a mildly dilated renal pelvis is likely the product of echoes from inflamed and edematous tissue.

b. Hydronephrosis. Sonographic diagnosis of hydronephrosis is accurate.[26,35,37] Absence of the pelvic sinus echo, anechoic dilation of the pelvic cavity with distant enhancement, and flattening of the pelvic recesses are hallmarks of hydronephrosis.[26,35,37] With moderate dilation, sonolucent outpouchings of the pelvic recesses extend peripherally from the central pelvic cavity to create a scalloped margin. Severe hydronephrosis is characterized by absence of this scalloping and by parenchymal atrophy (Fig. 11–18).[37] Hydronephrosis caused by distal obstruction usually affects the renal pelvis and recesses symmetrically, whereas asymmetric dilation suggests a ureteropelvic mass, especially if distant enhancement is reduced or absent when dilation of the lumen is significant. Fine low-level echoes or a debris fluid level within a dilated renal pelvis indicate cellular debris from infection or blood and must not be confused with electronic artifact.[34,46]

c. Renal pelvic masses. Renal pelvic masses are generally identified as low echogenic solid tissue expansion or fluid dilations. Most renal pelvic tumors create noticeable renal pelvic dilation that resembles hydronephrosis.[41,44] Transitional cell carcinomas are solid masses that separate the central renal sinus echo and are often demarcated from the renal parenchyma by an echogenic rim of sinus fat.[44] Transitional cell carcinomas are expansile, with renal pelvic fluid distention and compressed and distorted renal pelvic architecture. They often are associated with hydronephrosis because of secondary outflow tract obstruction. They may be anechoic, hypoechoic, or similar in echogenicity to renal parenchyma, but are hypoechoic to the normal renal sinus.[44] Squamous metaplasia and mineralization, if present, may be confused with calculi.[45] Lymphoma of the renal pelvis produces a centrally expansile, sound-attenuating mass with low-intensity internal echoes that causes renal pelvic dilation and minimal distant enhancement (Fig. 11–19).[45]

d. Renal pelvic calculi. Ultrasonography provides a sensitive method to detect radiopaque and nonradiopaque calculi.[26] Mineralized structures produce strong echo reflections/reverberations and characteristic shadowing (Fig. 11–20).[20,22,37] Localization of renal parenchymal mineralization depends on size/extent (> 3 mm)[23] of the beam angle and resolution. Iden-

TABLE 11–4
SONOGRAPHIC PATTERNS OF PARENCHYMAL KIDNEY DISEASE

	Echotexture*				
Distribution	**Anechoic**	**Hypoechoic**	**Normal**	**Hyperechoic**	**Complex**
Multifocal or Diffuse	Macrocysts†	Macrocysts† Abscesses Lymphosarcoma Mastocytoma	Glomerulointerstitial disease Renal tubular necrosis	Microcysts† Glomerulointerstitial disease Lymphosarcoma Renal tubular necrosis End-stage kidney Nephrocalcinosis Feline infectious peritonitis Amyloidosis	Carcinoma Sarcoma
Focal	Macrocysts†	Lymphosarcoma	Sarcoma Papilloma Adenoma	Sarcoma Nephroblastoma Hematoma	Carcinoma

*Compared to available normal intrarenal parenchyma, contralateral kidney, liver, or spleen.
†Nonneoplastic disease characterized by focal or multifocal accumulations of fluid within the renal parenchyma typified by feline polycystic renal disease.

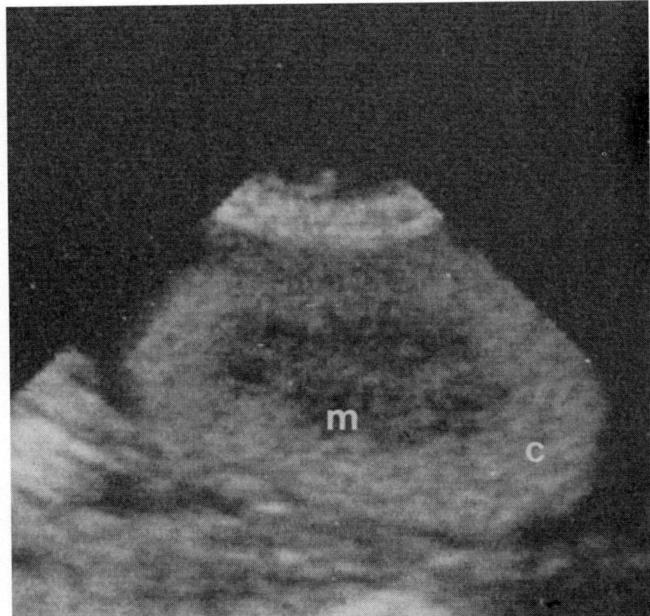

FIG. 11–15. Sagittal sonogram of a kidney in a dog with acute renal tubular necrosis caused by ethylene glycol toxicosis. The hyperechoic cortex (c) is clearly demarcated from the medulla (m). Reprinted with permission from Walter PA, Feeney DA, Johnston GR, O'Leary TP. Ultrasonographic evaluation of renal parenchymal diseases in the dog: 32 cases (1981-1986). *J Am Vet Med Assoc.* 1987;191:999.

tification of concomitant fluid dilation and subjective assessment of remaining potentially functional renal parenchyma are advantages of ultrasonography.[23]

IV. RADIOGRAPHIC ASSESSMENT OF THE URINARY BLADDER

A. Role of survey radiography in assessment of urinary bladder disorders. Survey abdominal radiographs are indicated prior to any contrast study of the lower urinary tract to detect concurrent renal, ureteral, or urethral diseases. Abnormal radiographic findings encountered on survey abdominal radiographs include alterations in size, shape, location, and radiographic density.

1. Structure
   a. Size. The size of the urinary bladder is variable and depends on the volume of urine in the bladder lumen. Urethral obstruction, neurogenic bladders, or normal distended urinary bladders all result in the appearance of an enlarged urinary bladder on survey radiographs.[2,3]
   b. Shape. The shape of the urinary bladder depends on the degree of distention; it may be round or oval in dogs and "teardrop" shaped in cats.[2,3] The shape of the urinary bladder is best defined by contrast cystography or urethrocystography when the bladder is maximally distended. Other abnormal shapes of the urinary bladder encountered on survey radiographs may be related to bladder urachal diverticula or adjacent caudal abdominal or pelvic diseases.
   c. Location. The location of the urinary bladder is influenced by the degree of urinary bladder

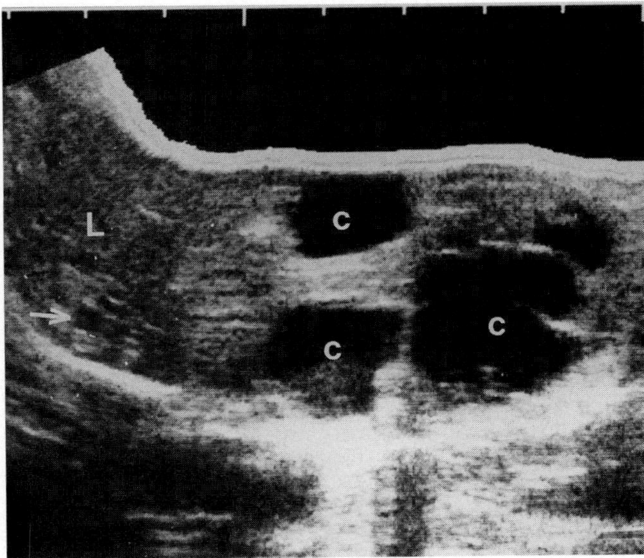

FIG. 11–16. Sagittal sonogram of a kidney in a cat with polycystic renal disease. Multiple anechoic cavitations with distant enhancement are seen (C). Cysts (arrow) are also seen in the liver (L). Reprinted with permission from Walter PA, Johnston GR, Feeney DA, O'Brien TD. Applications of ultrasonography in the diagnosis of parenchymal kidney disease in cats: 24 cases (1981-1986). *J Am Vet Med Assoc.* 1988;192:92.

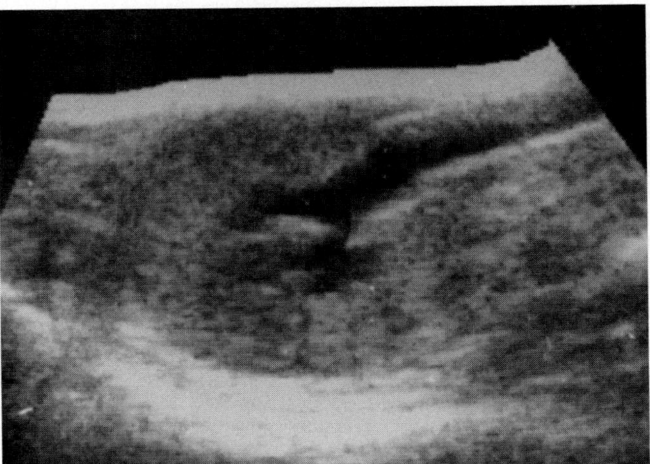

FIG. 11–17. Transverse sonogram of a kidney in a cat with pyelonephritis. Dilatation of the renal pelvis and echogenic material within the pelvic lumen are minimal.

TABLE 11–5
SONOGRAPHIC PATTERN OF RENAL PELVIC AND URETERAL DISEASE

	Echotexture				
Distribution	**Anechoic Cavitating**	**Hypoechoic Cavitating**	**Normal**	**Hypoechoic**	**Hyperechoic**
Renal Pelvis					
Focal	Pyelonephritis Hydronephrosis	Pyelonephritis Hydronephrosis	Pyelonephritis		Calculus*
Diffuse	Hydronephrosis Transitional cell carcinoma	Hydronephrosis		Lymphosarcoma	
Ureter					
Focal					Calculus*
Diffuse	Hydroureter				

*Distant shadowing identified.

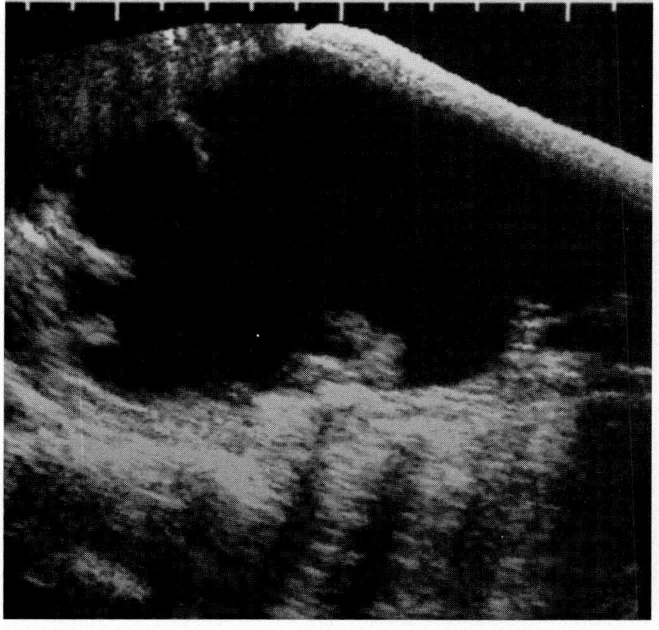

FIG. 11–18. Sagittal sonogram of a kidney in a dog with severe hydronephrosis. The anechoic renal pelvic cavity has a smooth contour and far enhancement is prominent. Loss of renal pelvic recesses and medullary papilla with a thin cortical shell suggests parenchymal atrophy.

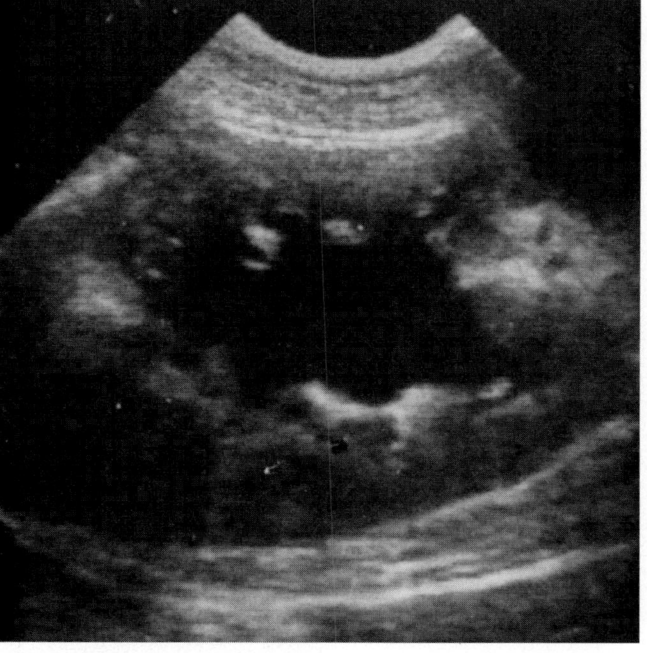

FIG. 11–19. Sagittal sonogram of a kidney in a dog with infiltrative lymphosarcoma of the renal pelvis. The mass is nearly anechoic. In comparison to the degree of renal pelvic dilatation, the distant enhancement is minimal, thereby allowing one to distinguish easily the mass effect from hydronephrosis.

distention.[2,3] In dogs, the urinary bladder may be totally or partially within the bony pelvis, depending on the degree of its distention.[47] In cats, the urinary bladder is normally in an intra-abdominal location, regardless of the degree of its distention.[47] Abdominal, inguinal, and perineal hernias may result in an abnormal location of the urinary bladder. Caudal abdominal masses caused by prostatic diseases, neoplastic cryptorchid testicles, sublumbar lymphadenopathy, and tumors of the bony pelvis can also result in abnormal locations of the urinary bladder detected by survey radiographs.

d. Radiographic opacity. Radiopacities or radiolucencies associated with the urinary bladder silhouette may be detected by survey radiography. The most common radiopacities are uroliths. Uroliths may be solitary or multiple and vary in size and shape (Fig. 11–8A). Radiographic characteristics of uroliths are influenced by their mineral composition and size. Dystrophic calcification of the urinary bladder identified by survey radiography has been reported in association with inflammatory polypoid cystitis and neoplastic disease.[48] Radiolucent structures associated with the urinary tract that may be detected by survey radiography include air bubbles within the urinary bladder lumen caused by catheterization or cystocentesis. Emphysematous cystitis (gas within the bladder wall and/or lumen) may be detected by survey radiography. This abnormality may be caused by traumatic catheterization or infectious inflammatory diseases, such as *Escherichia coli* or *Clostridium perfringens*, in patients with Cushing's disease or diabetes mellitus (Fig. 11–21).[2,3] Gas within the bladder wall in patients with emphysematous cystitis typically appears as radiolucent linear and coalescent lines associated with the peripheral silhouette of the urinary bladder.

2. Limitations. The main limitation of survey radiography is its inability to detect intramural and intraluminal soft tissue diseases.

B. Role of urocystography in assessment of urinary bladder disease.

1. Overview. Contrast evaluation of the urinary bladder (urocystography) is a simple, inexpensive, minimal-risk procedure. Patient preparation and pharmacologic restraint are the same as those described for abdominal radiography and excretory urography.
2. Clinical indications and contraindications.
   a. The indications for contrast urocystography include signs of lower urinary tract disease (e.g., hematuria, dysuria, pollakiuria), caudally located abdominal masses, radiopacities or radiolucencies associated with the urinary bladder detected by survey radiography, abnormal shape of the urinary bladder silhouette, and inability to visualize the urinary bladder on survey radiographs.[2,3]

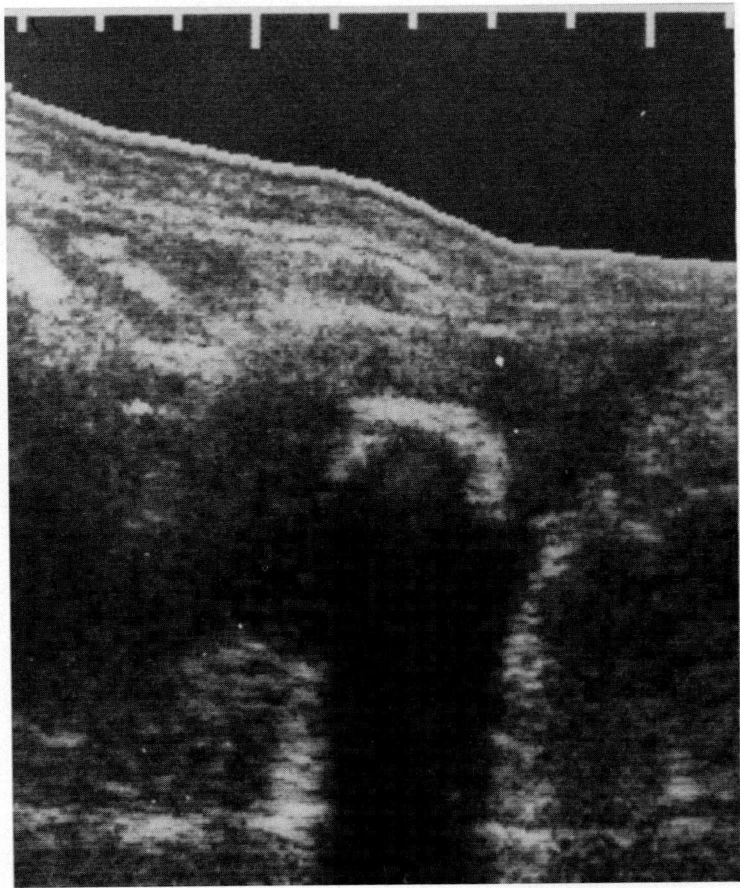

FIG. 11–20. Sagittal sonogram of a kidney in a dog with an intrapelvic calculus. The hyperechogenic stone produces strong reflections and shadowing.

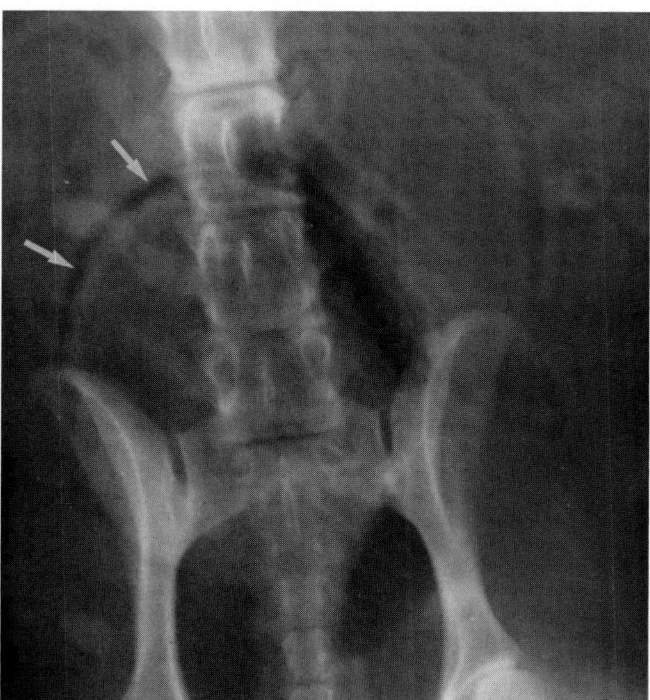

FIG. 11–21. Survey ventrodorsal radiograph of an 8-year-old female poodle with diabetes mellitus. The arrows indicate gas within the bladder wall, which is typical of emphysematous cystitis. Reprinted with permission from Johnston GR, Feeney DA, Osborne CA. Radiographic findings in urinary tract infection. *Vet Clin North Am.* 1979;9:749.

b. Contraindications for urocystography include patients with prior adverse reactions to positive contrast agents or anesthetic drugs. Frank hematuria is not a contraindication for contrast urocystography.

3. Techniques of urocystography.
   a. Overview. Three techniques of urocystography can be utilized to evaluate the urinary bladder: pneumocystography, double contrast cystography, and positive contrast cystography.[2] Pneumocystography, which involves use of a negative contrast agent infused through a urethral catheter to distend the urinary bladder, is simple, inexpensive, and quickly performed. However, pneumocystography provides poor mucosal detail and does not reveal small intraluminal filling defects. In patients with frank hematuria, air should be used cautiously to prevent the potential for fatal vascular embolization. Double contrast cystography incorporates use of positive and negative contrast agents. The volume of positive contrast medium used in double contrast cystography is small when compared to the volume of negative contrast agent used. The purpose of the positive contrast agent is to coat the dependent mucosal surface of the bladder and to outline filling defects in the dependent "puddle" of positive contrast medium. Double contrast cystography is more sensitive than pneumocystography or positive contrast cystography in detecting mucosal lesions, mural lesions, and free luminal or attached filling defects. Positive contrast cystography incorporates use of dilute iodinated contrast agent for distention of the urinary bladder. Positive contrast cystography has no advantages over pneumocystography or double contrast cystography for evaluation of mucosal or mural lesions or filling defects. It is best suited for patients with suspected bladder tears and/or rupture. It is more expensive because of the larger volume of positive contrast agents required compared to those used with the other techniques. Positive contrast cystography is the initial step in retrograde or antegrade urethrocystography, whereby the urinary bladder is maximally distended prior to urethral opacification to ensure the maximum distention of the urethra. Only the technique of double contrast cystography is described here.
   b. Technique and normal examples. The technique of double contrast cystography requires prior catheterization of the urinary bladder for removal of residual urine. The bladder should be maximally distended with air as determined by digital palpation (Fig. 11–22). A small volume of an undiluted iodinated contrast medium should then be injected through the catheter lumen into the bladder lumen. The thickness of the urinary bladder wall should be uniform throughout, and the dependent contrast puddle should show a smooth contour where it contacts the bladder wall, with no free luminal or attached filling defects.
   c. Complications. The most common complication associated with cystography is macroscopic hematuria following maximum distention of the urinary bladder.[48] Catheter-induced trauma to the urethra or bladder may be induced if stiff catheters are used. Damage to the urethral or urinary bladder mucosa may predispose the urinary tract to iatrogenic infection. Leakage of contrast medium into the walls of the urinary bladder may be encountered with maximum distention of the urinary bladder, but does not necessitate surgical intervention.[2,3,48,49] Mural leakage of contrast medium cannot be predicted prior to cystography and should not be considered synonymous with urinary bladder rupture. Unlike mural leakage of contrast medium, rupture of the urinary bladder is associated with extravasation of contrast medium into the peritoneal cavity and the loss of the bladder silhouette.

4. Abnormal contrast patterns
   a. Mucosal lesions. Mucosal lesions may be caused by artifacts or diseases, including infectious inflammatory, noninfectious inflammatory, or neoplastic disease (Fig. 11–23).[2,3] Focal, multifocal, or diffuse mucosal irregularities caused by inadequate urinary bladder distention cannot be differentiated from mucosal irregularities caused by disease. Mucosal diseases are best detected by double contrast or positive contrast cystography. Mucosal erosions or ulcerations are characterized radiographically by adherence of positive contrast medium to the mucosal surface, and are best detected by double contrast cystography (Fig. 11–23).
   b. Mural lesions. Mural lesions may be associated with mucosal lesions. They may be caused by artifacts or diseases and can be focal or diffuse in their distribution (Fig. 11–23).[2,3,49] Focal or diffuse mural thickening caused by inadequate urinary bladder distention is an artifact. Disease-related mural lesions may be focal, multifocal, or diffuse, and may be caused by infectious inflammatory, noninfectious inflammatory, or neoplastic diseases (Figs. 11–23 and 11–24). The most common radiographic manifestation of noninfectious and infectious inflammatory cystitis in dogs and cats is cranioventral bladder wall thickening viewed on lateral projections of cystograms (Fig. 11–23A). However, cranioventral bladder wall thickening (or focal mural thickening anywhere in the bladder) can also be associated with neoplastic disease or inadequate urinary bladder distention (Fig. 11–23B). Diffuse bladder wall thickening may be identified in dogs and cats with acute or chronic bladder disease caused by inflammatory or neoplastic disease (Fig. 11–24). Hemorrhage and edema of the bladder wall secondary to acute urethral obstruction in dogs and cats can also result in diffuse bladder wall thickening (Fig. 11–24A). However, diffuse bladder wall thickening caused by chronic cystitis is typically associated with diminished distensibility of the urinary bladder (Fig. 11–24B).
   c. Filling defects. Free intraluminal or attached filling defects of the urinary bladder are frequently encountered during cystography.[2,3,49]
      (1). Free intraluminal filling defects in the dog and cat include air bubbles (Fig. 11–22A), blood clots, matrix plugs (Figs. 11–24A and 11–25B), and uroliths (Figs. 11–25 and

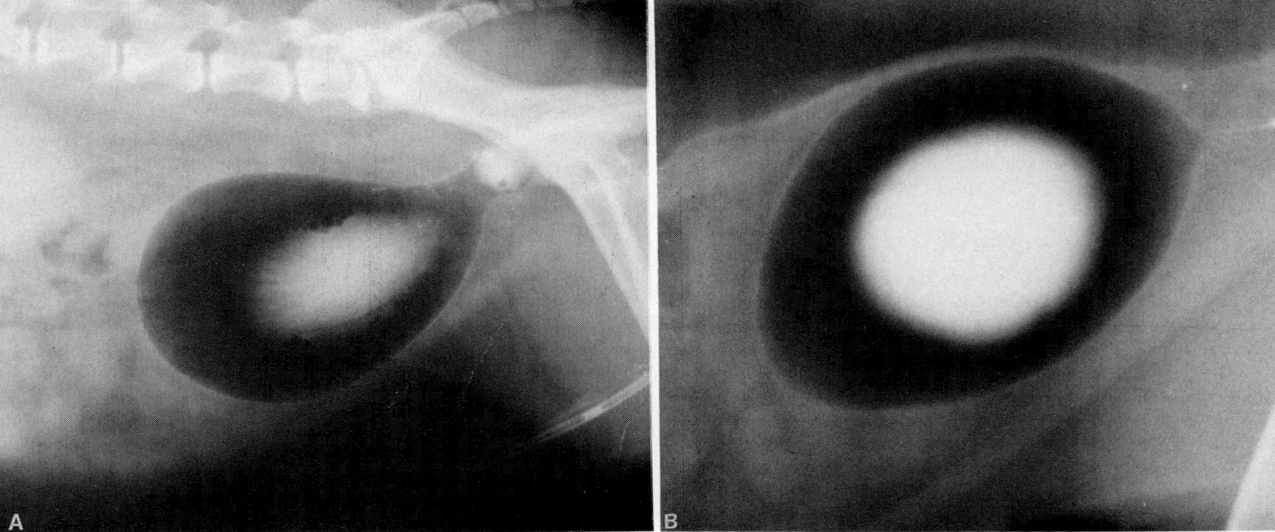

FIG. 11–22. Lateral views of normal double contrast cystograms from a 12-year-old miniature schnauzer **(A)** and a 14-year-old spayed domestic shorthair cat **(B).** The positive contrast medium in the double contrast cystogram on the dependent side should have a smooth interface with the mucosa of the urinary bladder. The thickness of the urinary bladder wall should be uniform if the urinary bladder is adequately distended. Radiolucent filling defects at the periphery of the contrast puddle in **A** are the result of air bubbles of variable size. Figure 11–22A reprinted with permission from Johnston GR, Feeney DA, Osborne CA. Radiographic findings in urinary tract infection. *Vet Clin North Am.* 1979;9:749. Figure 11–22B reprinted with permission from Johnston GR, Feeney DA, Osborne CA. Urethrography and cystography in cats. Part I. Techniques, normal radiographic anatomy, and artifacts. *Comp Cont Educ.* 1982;4:823.

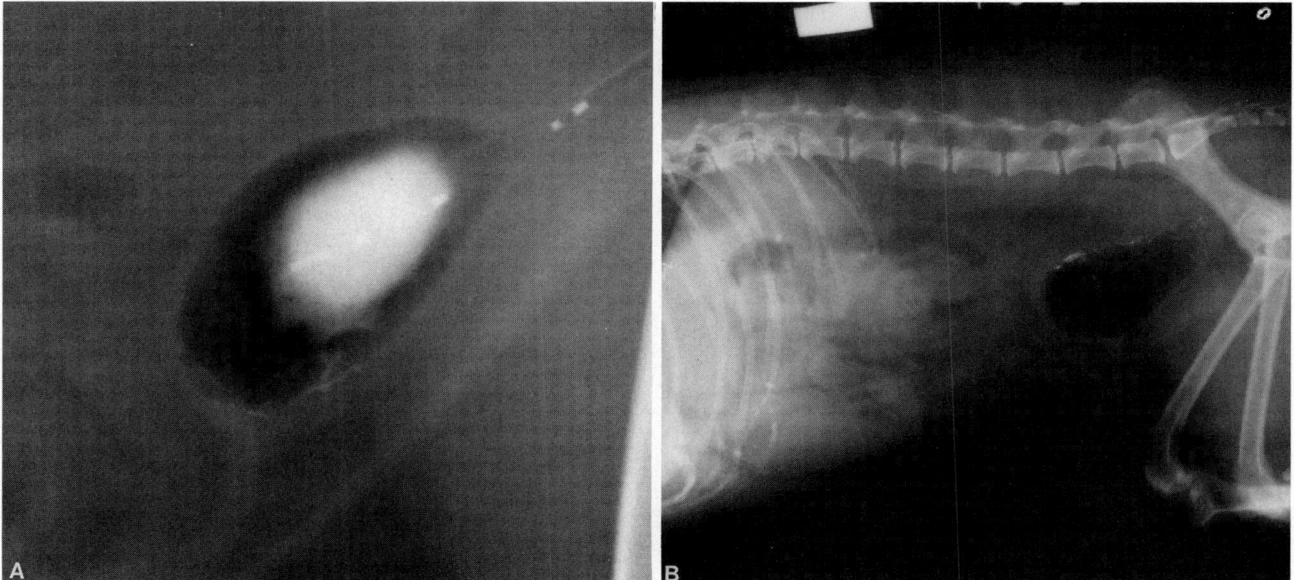

FIG. 11–23. A, Mucosal irregularity, contrast coating of the urinary bladder wall, and focal cranioventral bladder wall thickening are encountered on a lateral radiograph of a double contrast cystogram from an 8-year-old spayed female Siamese cat with hematuria and dysuria of 1 week's duration. Mucosal irregularity of the urinary bladder is frequently encountered in dogs and cats with acute or chronic lower urinary tract disease secondary to neoplastic or inflammatory disorders. **B,** Contrast coating of the bladder mucosa and focal thickening of the bladder wall and urethra encountered during double contrast cystography performed on an 8-year-old female miniature poodle with hematuria and dysuria secondary to a transitional cell carcinoma. Figure 11–23A reprinted with permission from Johnston GR, Feeney DA, Osborne CA. Urethrography and cystography in cats. Part II. Abnormal radiographic anatomy and complications. *Comp Cont Educ.* 1982;4:931. Figure 11–23B reprinted with permission from Johnston GR, Feeney DA. Radiographic evaluation of the urinary tract in dogs and cats. *Contemp Issues Small Anim Pract (Nephrol Urol).* 1986;4:203.

11–26). The differential radiographic characteristics of free intraluminal and attached filling defects encountered during cystography are included in Table 11–6.

(2). Intraluminal filling defects attached to the bladder wall may also be detected by cystography. Attached filling defects may be caused by blood clots and uroliths (Figs. 11–26 and 11–27A). Polypoid lesions attached to the mucosal surface may be neoplastic or nonneoplastic. Nonneoplastic attached filling defects include submucosal hematomas (Fig. 11–27B), blood clots (Fig. 11–27A), abscesses, and granulomas. Attached neoplastic filling defects may have a prominent intraluminal component called a polyp (Fig. 11–28). However, polypoid lesions are not pathognomonic for neoplastic disease. Both inflammatory (Fig. 11–28A) and neoplastic (Fig. 11–28B) diseases can have a polypoid component. The differential radiographic features of inflammatory polypoid cystitis and neoplastic polypoid lesions encountered during cystography are described in Table 11–7.[2,3,49] A definitive morphologic diagnosis of polypoid defects requires light microscopic examination of exfoliated cells or biopsy samples.

d. Extraluminal compression. Extraluminal compression of the urinary bladder of dogs and cats may be congenital or acquired.[2,3,49] Prostatic cysts, uterine stump granulomas, vaginal tumors, and congenital persistent uterus masculinus may cause urinary bladder displacement and compression. Cystography, ultrasonography, excretory urography, vaginography, and/or barium enemas may be required to further define and localize the disease. Mass lesions may compress the bladder neck or urethral junction and cause outflow obstruction. Extraluminal compression of the trigone of the urinary bladder may cause partial obstruction to the ureters and result in hydroureter or hydronephrosis. Inflammatory diseases that compress and displace the urinary bladder may invade the bladder and/or urethral wall.

e. Diverticula. Diverticula of the urinary bladder may be congenital or acquired (Fig. 11–29). Persistent urachal diverticula are a predisposing cause of bacterial urinary tract infections.[2,3,49] Urachal diverticula vary in appearance; they may be conical or rounded structures best defined by positive contrast cystography or urethrocystography.[2,3]

f. Vesicoureteral reflux. Vesicoureteral reflux may be detected during cystography or urethrocystography when positive and/or negative contrast agents reflux and partially or totally fill the ureteral lumen from the bladder trigone to the renal pelvis. Vesicoureteral reflux may be a normal event in young dogs because the vesicoureteral junction is not yet totally developed (Fig. 11–30A).[50] Vesicoureteral reflux may be influenced by the degree of urinary bladder distention, patient positioning, and degree of sedation (Fig. 11–30B).[51]

V. ULTRASONOGRAPHIC ASSESSMENT OF THE URINARY BLADDER

A. Indications for sonography of the urinary bladder. The indications for ultrasonographic assessment of the urinary bladder include difficulty in obtaining contrast radiographic studies because the urinary bladder is difficult to catheterize, as part of a complete abdominal ultrasound protocol, or for serial assessment of known bladder disease to help to evaluate response to medical management.

B. Advantages of urinary bladder sonography versus uroradiography. Major advantages include: 1) can obtain complementary information to uroradiography—can differentiate type of intraluminal material or filling defects seen with cystography, such as calculi, blood clots, or masses; 2) can be performed without sedation and catheterization if the bladder is adequately distended, thus avoiding complications; 3) provides a sonographic window to sublumbar lymph nodes; 4) uses no ionizing radiation; 5) is an examination that is relatively easy and quick to perform; 6) allows guided biopsy or aspira-

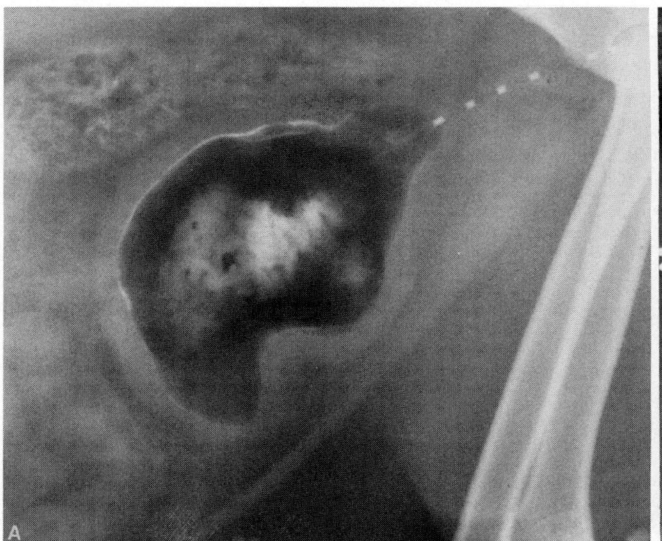

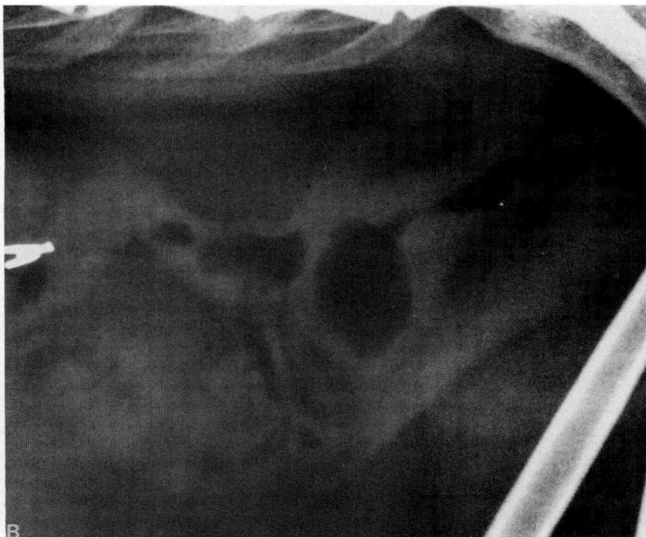

FIG. 11–24. Diffuse mural thickening may be caused by acute or chronic inflammatory bladder disease or neoplasia. **A,** Diffuse mural thickening, contrast coating of the bladder mucosa, and multiple free luminal blood clots, mucous plugs, and/or uroliths with an associated bladder wall invagination are present on a double contrast cystogram from a 3-year-old neutered male domestic shorthair cat 4 days following relief for urethral obstruction. A catheterized urine sample was positive for *Proteus mirabilis.* A chronic, necrotic, transmural cystitis was diagnosed at necropsy. **B,** A lateral radiograph from a pneumocystogram on an adult neutered male domestic shorthair cat with chronic hematuria and dysuria. Diffuse bladder wall thickening and nondistensibility were secondary to chronic inflammatory cystitis. Multifocal to diffuse bladder wall thickening can be secondary to neoplastic or inflammatory bladder disease. Figure 11–24A reprinted with permission from Johnston GR, Feeney DA, Osborne CA. Urethrography and cystography in cats. Part II. Abnormal radiographic anatomy and complications. *Comp Cont Educ.* 1982;4:931. Figure 11–24B reprinted with permission from Johnston GR, Feeney DA. Comparative organ imaging: Lower urinary tract. *Vet Radiol.* 1984;25:146.

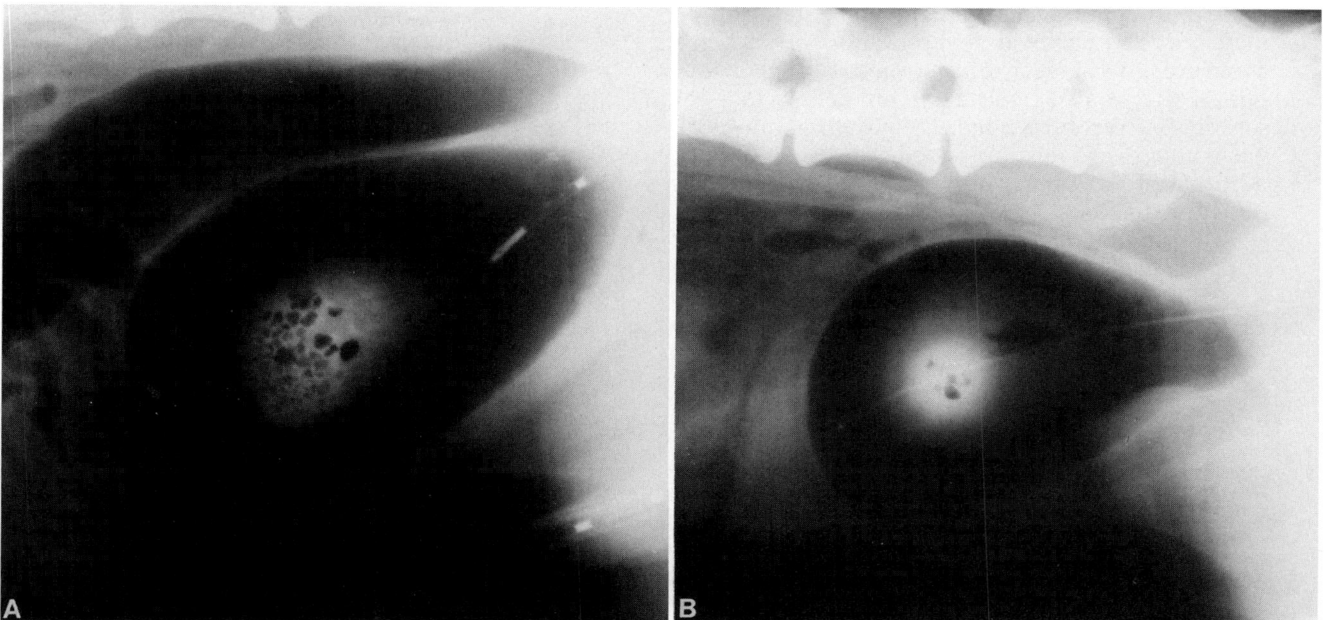

FIG. 11–25. A, Lateral view of a double contrast cystogram of a 6-year-old male Irish setter with multiple struvite uroliths. The uroliths appeared radiolucent when compared with the radiopaque contrast medium, but appeared radiopaque on survey radiographs. **B,** Lateral view of a double contrast cystogram of the dog described in **A** obtained several hours following a cystotomy to remove the uroliths. Six or more uroliths remain in the bladder lumen in addition to a large blood clot at the edge of the contrast puddle. The uroliths were not detected at the time of the cystotomy because they were located in the urethra. Reprinted with permission from Johnston GR, Feeney DA, Osborne CA. Radiographic findings in urinary tract infection. *Vet Clin North Am.* 1979;9:749.

tion to be performed; and 7) minimizes risk of air embolism.

C. **Limitations of sonography compared to uroradiography.** Sonography should be performed prior to cystography to avoid introduction of air, which may prevent sound transmission. Limitations include: 1) inaccuracy in identifying small objects (small uroliths) and in determining numbers of objects within the lumen—ability to differentiate objects as separated depends on transducer focal zone and resolution[20]; 2) ineffective in detecting bladder rupture; 3) less effective in determining the extent of disease; and 4) not effective in demonstrating urethral lesions.

D. **Normal ultrasonographic structure of the urinary bladder.** The bladder outline is round or pear-shaped, clearly marginated, and smooth. The bladder wall is thin and symmetric (Fig. 11–31). The muscular wall and mucosa cannot be distinguished. Normal ureters are usually not seen.[52] The echogenicity of the normal fluid-distended lumen is anechoic with prominent distant enhancement. Sediment that shifts in response to changing position of the animal may be a normal finding.[34]

E. **Technique of bladder sonography.** The bladder is easiest to identify and examine when it is distended with fluid. Because intraluminal air bubbles create ultrasonographic artifacts and prevent total visualization of the bladder, ultrasonography cannot be performed successfully following pneumocystography or double contrast cystography. It can be performed in conjunction with positive contrast cystography or excretory urography.[20,34] A cleansing enema is not recommended, but a 24-hour fast may be helpful to avoid gas and feces accumulation in the colon that may inhibit viewing or distort the contour of the bladder by pressure. The urinary bladder is most often scanned with the animal in dorsal recumbency. On occasion, the lateral recumbent position is used. If air bubbles are present, or if the animal resists restraint, the bladder may be scanned while the animal stands. Hair must be clipped from the area cranial to the pubic brim. The prepuce may be manipulated out of the viewing field. Gel is applied, and the transducer is placed on the ventral abdomen starting parallel to the long axis of the bladder. A 7.5- or 5.0-MHz frequency transducer is chosen to accommodate patient size. The bladder is located superficially. Information about the ventral bladder wall located in the near field of the transducer may be difficult to obtain. A tissue-equivalent stand-off pad may reduce near-field reverberation artifact.[52] To avoid creation of electronic noise within the bladder lumen that may be mistaken for debris, low-gain settings are recommended. Longitudinal and transverse images are recommended.

F. **Abnormal sonographic patterns in urinary bladder disease.**

1. Intraluminal material. Radiopaque and nonradiopaque calculi are typically hyperechoic and cause a sharply marginated shadow distal to the calculus because of marked sound attenuation by the stone (Fig. 11–20).[20,35,52] The accuracy of large calculus detection by ultrasonography is high. The ability to see shadowing is determined by the size of the stone and the frequency and focal zone of the transducer. The larger the calculus, the more distinctive and reliable the ultrasonographic findings. The echogenicity of blood clots depends on their fibrous tissue content. Blood clots are usually hypoechoic compared to the bladder wall (Fig. 11–32).[34] They are often irregular in shape, although this may not be easily determined by ultrasonography because of "edge fall-off" of the sound beam. As the clots become more organized, the intensity of reflected echoes increases. Some shadowing may occur, but it is not a consistent finding. Calculi and blood clots may be free floating or attached to the bladder wall. Changes in scanning direction or position of the animal are recommended to determine if these bodies are mobile, and to help to differentiate floating calculi from mural mineralization, and blood clots from mural masses. Unattached structures usually gravitate toward the most dependent area of the bladder, whereas the location of attached material remains unchanged despite a change in patient position. Attached blood clots are difficult to differentiate from intraluminal masses.[34] Gas bubbles within the bladder lumen inhibit sound transmission. Air migrates and coalesces in the most dorsal area of the bladder and produces reverberations and distant shadowing.[20]
2. Mural diseases. In acute cystitis, the echogenicity of the bladder wall is usually hypoechoic because of edema; typically a gradual zone of transition to normal tissue is evident.[53] Focal or diffuse thickening of the cranioventral bladder wall in response to chronic inflammation may be difficult to detect unless changes are dramatic.[34] Benign inflammatory polyps are identified as irregular, protruding, pedunculated, thickened areas of the bladder wall. The echogenicity of such wall masses is often similar to that of the bladder wall. Presence of sediment within the bladder lumen that changes location in response to altering the position of the animal may indicate urinary tract infection.[34,52] In contrast to other benign mass lesions, a congenital ureterocoele is usually elliptic, smoothly marginated, located within the wall, projecting into the lumen at the trigone, and fluid filled.[34,52] Neoplastic lesions are usually less echogenic than the normal bladder wall. They are viewed as complex focal masses that extend into the bladder lumen, diffuse infiltrative lesions which produce wall thickening with little protrusion, or large masses which obliterate the bladder lumen (Fig. 11–33).[53] Transition to normal tissue is usually abrupt in benign lesions and gradual in sessile malignant lesions. Accuracy of diagnosis depends on the size of the mass. Small masses of less than 0.3 cm, and those located in the trigone area, are difficult to detect.[53] Some masses may not be distinguished from wall thickening associated with bacterial cystitis until the masses become quite large. Causes of echogenic bladder masses include attached blood clot, granulomatous or polypoid cystitis, and neoplasia.[52] Ultrasonography is effective in identifying the site of a mass and in characterizing the mass as broad based or pedunculated. The openings of the ureters should be examined for invasion by masses or for evi-

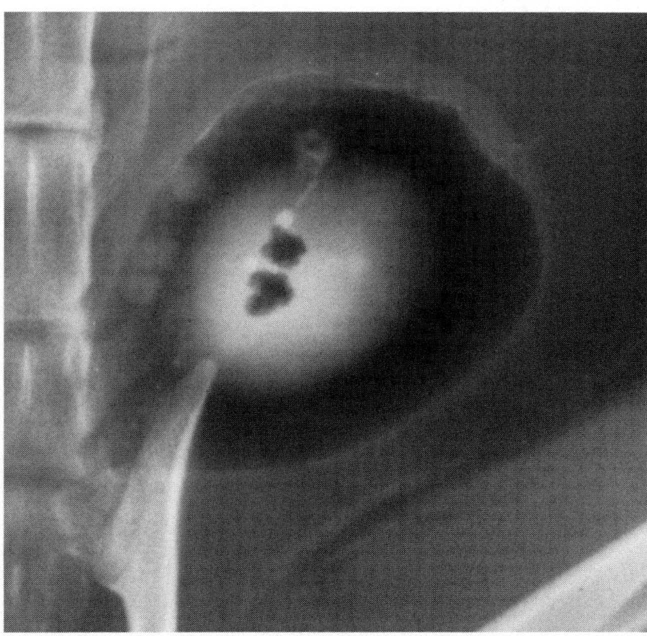

FIG. 11–26. Multiple urocystoliths detected by double contrast cystography of a 5-year-old neutered male domestic shorthair cat with dysuria and stranguria. Variations in the radiographic density of uroliths are related to their location in relationship to the positive or negative contrast medium. The uroliths that appear radiolucent are located in the dependent contrast puddle, whereas the radiopaque uroliths are attached to the bladder wall and are surrounded by air. Reprinted with permission from Johnston GR, Feeney DA, Osborne CA. Urethrography and cystography in cats. Part II. Abnormal radiographic anatomy and complications. *Comp Cont Educ.* 1982;4:931.

TABLE 11–6
DIFFERENTIAL RADIOGRAPHIC CHARACTERISTICS OF INTRALUMINAL FILLING DEFECTS OF THE URINARY BLADDER

Radiographic Criteria	Air Bubbles	Uroliths	Blood Clots
Size	Small to large Single, multiple, coalescent	Small to large Single or multiple	Small to large Single or multiple
Shape	Commonly round; if coalescing, ovoid or polyhedral	Spheroidal, ovoid, polygonal, pumpkin seed	Spheroidal, ovoid, polygonal, linear
Margination	Smooth and distinct	Smooth or irregular, distinct or indistinct	Indistinct and irregular
Location	Commonly at periphery of contrast puddle; if large and coalescing, anywhere	Center of contrast puddle or attached to bladder wall	Center of contrast puddle or attached to bladder wall
Density on survey radiography	Radiolucent	Water-dense (radiolucent) uroliths: nondetectable; Radiopaque uroliths: radiopaque or nondetectable (if small)	Nondetectable
Pneumocystography	Radiolucent	Water-dense uroliths: nondetectable or radiopaque (if attached) Radiopaque uroliths: radiopaque	Nondetectable or radiopaque (attached)
Double contrast cystography	Radiolucent	Water-dense uroliths: radiolucent or nondetectable	Nondetectable
Positive contrast urethrocystography	Radiolucent	Radiopaque uroliths: radiolucent or nondectable	

(With permission from Johnston GR, Feeney DA, Osborne CA. Urethrography and cystography in cats. Part II. Abnormal radiographic anatomy and complications. *Comp Cont Educ*. 1982;4:931.)

dence of hydroureter. These findings are especially important when surgery is being considered.

VI. RADIOGRAPHIC ASSESSMENT OF THE PROSTATE GLAND AND URETHRA

A. Role of radiographic imaging in prostatic disease and urethra.

1. Confirm/refute relationship between prostatic disease and clinical signs. The general categories of prostatic disease, as well as their diagnosis, prognosis, and therapeutic approach, have been defined elsewhere.[54,55] One of the most important aspects of radiographic imaging of the prostate gland is to help to determine if the clinical signs are related to morphologic prostatic abnormalities (Fig. 11–1).
2. Confirm/refute relationship between urethral disease and clinical signs. The clinical signs of lower urinary tract disease can be attributed to either urinary bladder and/or urethral disease. The site(s) of involvement must be identified so that appropriate management techniques can be implemented. In many cases, both cystography and urethrography are needed to identify all sites of involvement.
3. Radiographic techniques versus ultrasonographic techniques for assessment of the prostate gland.
   a. Advantages of radiography. Radiographic techniques facilitate determination of the size of the prostate gland by allowing comparison between the body size (as defined by the pubic-promontory distance) and the prostate gland dimensions.[56] Radiographic techniques allow similar comparisons between the relative diameters of the membranous and prostatic portions of the urethra (Fig. 11–34).[57,58] Survey radiographs are relatively sensitive for detection of parenchymal mineralization of the prostate gland, which is associated with prostatic carcinomas (Fig. 11–35).[56] Urethrocystographic techniques can also be used to delineate the degree of communication between the prostatic portion of the urethra and intraprostatic cavities (Fig. 11–36).[56,59]
   b. Advantages of ultrasonography. Ultrasonographic techniques do not require use of iodinated contrast medium or ionizing radiation. This technique is sensitive in detecting scarring, cavitation, and infiltration of soft tissues.

B. Survey radiography.

1. Preparation for abdominal radiography. Preparation for general abdominal radiography has been defined in Section IIB of this chapter.

2. Practicality of survey radiography for assessment of prostatic disease. As with the upper urinary tract, the practicality of survey radiography lies in its ability to define such characteristics as size, shape, location, and opacities of the prostate gland.[2,56,60-62] In addition, survey radiography is of value in staging abdominal masses in proximity to the prostate gland and in assessing caudal abdominal and pelvic organs, as well as the regional osseous and vascular structures.[56] This information helps to determine whether the prostate gland is the primary cause of clinical signs or is secondarily affected by other regional organs, particularly the colon and rectum (Fig. 11–1). By considering a combination of the external shape, size, and opacity of the prostate, probable causes of prostatic disease can be determined.[56,60-62]
3. Practicality of survey radiography for assessment of urethral disease. Because periurethral tissues and the urethra have the same density, the urethra can rarely be identified on survey radiographs. An exception is in obese female dogs and cats with sufficient urinary bladder distention to cause cranial displacement of the bladder so that the cranial portion of the urethra can be identified at its origin from the bladder neck. Iodinated contrast agents are required to assess the urethral lumen.

The most common abnormalities of the urethra detected by survey radiography are radiopaque uroliths. The most common site of urethroliths in male dogs is the area of the os penis (Fig. 11–37A). In male cats, the most common site of uroliths and urethral plugs is the narrowed portion of the penile urethra (Fig. 11–37B).

Urethral obstruction is less common in female dogs and cats than in male dogs and cats, but may occur anywhere along the length of the urethra, especially the bladder neck and adjacent to the external urethral orifice. The diameter of the female urethral lumen is smallest at the external urethral orifice. Radiolucent densities in the region of the urethra are uncommonly observed on survey radiographs. Subcutaneous cellulitis caused by gas-producing bacteria secondary to

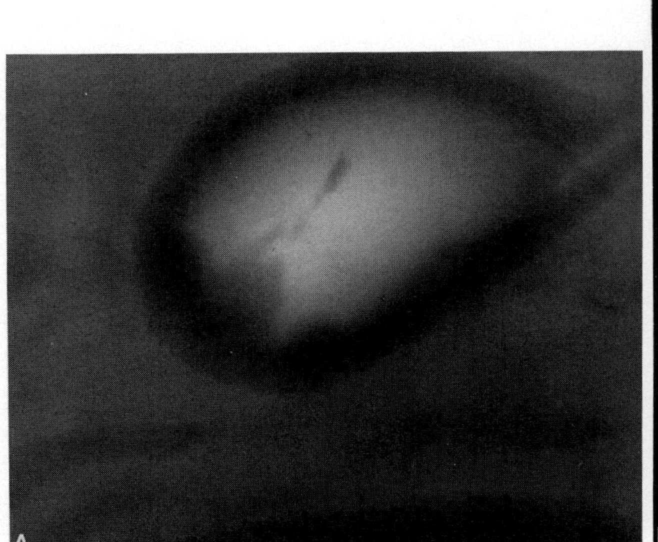

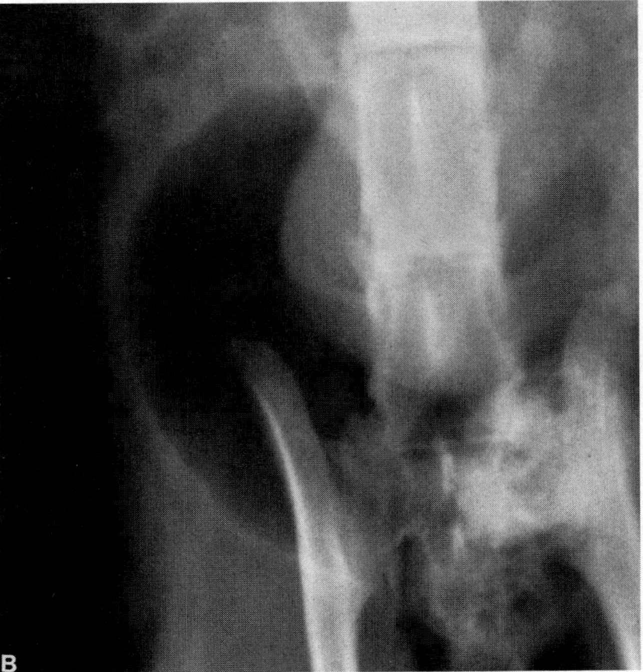

FIG. 11–27. A, Attached intraluminal filling defects encountered during double contrast cystography in a 4-year-old neutered male cat with intermittent hematuria of approximately 2 years' duration. Failure to identify the filling defects by survey radiography or pneumocystography indicates that they are composed of soft tissue. Potential causes include attached blood clots, attached polypoid lesions, or matrix uroliths. The filling defects subsequently were identified as attached blood clots. **B,** Ventrodorsal pneumocystogram from an 18-month-old neutered male Persian cat with lower urinary tract disease. Light microscopy of the large soft tissue mass revealed that it was a submucosal hematoma. Note the sharp transition between the normal and abnormal bladder wall. Reprinted with permission from Johnston GR, Feeney DA, Osborne CA. Urethrography and cystography in cats. Part II. Abnormal radiographic anatomy and complications. *Comp Cont Educ.* 1982;4:931.

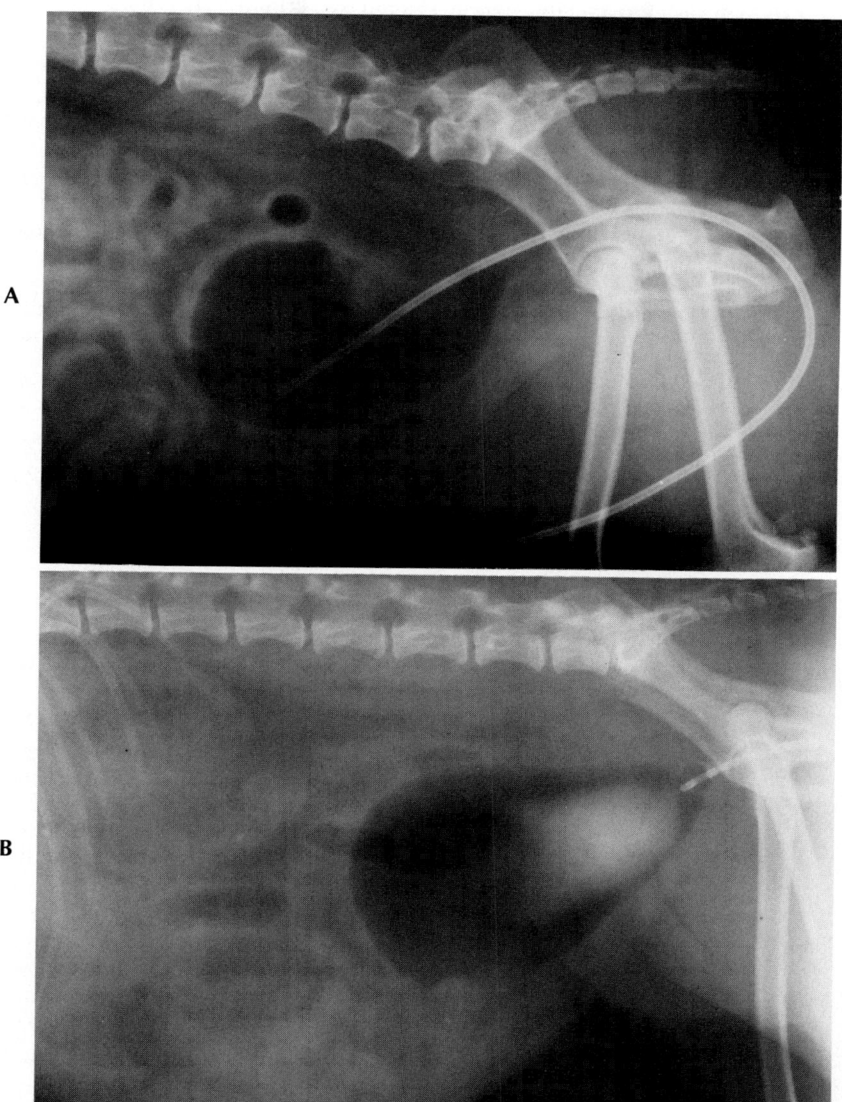

FIG. 11–28. A, Lateral view of a pneumocystogram of an 11–year-old West Highland white terrier with lower urinary tract disease. The attached filling defect was identified by catheter biopsy as a transitional cell carcinoma. Note the broad zone (shoulder) of transition between the normal and abnormal bladder wall. **B,** A lateral radiograph of a double contrast cystogram from an 8-year-old female mixed-breed dog with urinary tract infection. An attached filling defect on the cranioventral aspect of the bladder wall is identified. Microscopic examination of a surgical biopsy revealed that it was an inflammatory polyp. Note the minimal bladder wall thickening adjacent to the mass suggestive of a benign lesion. Figure 11–28A reprinted with permission from Johnston GR, Feeney DA, Osborne CA. Radiographic findings in urinary tract infection. *Vet Clin North Am.* 1979;9:749. Figure 11–28B reprinted with permission from Johnston GR, Feeney DA. Radiographic evaluation of the urinary tract in dogs and cats. *Contemp Issues Small Anim Pract (Nephrol Urol).* 1986;4:203.

TABLE 11–7
DIFFERENTIATION OF ATTACHED INTRALUMINAL FILLING DEFECTS OF THE URINARY BLADDER

Radiographic Criteria	Inflammatory Polyp	Neoplastic Polyp
Size	Small to large	Small to large
Number	Single or multiple	Single or multiple
Shape	Often symmetric, occasionally non-symmetric	Often symmetric, occasionally non-symmetric
Transition from normal to abnormal	Often sharp and distinct	Often gradual and distinct
Thickening of adjoining bladder wall	+ to ++	+ to ++++
Location	Anywhere	Anywhere
Intraluminal component	Prominent intraluminal filling defect with minimal mural component	Prominent intraluminal filling defect with or without minimal mural component
Density	Soft tissue (fluid)	Soft tissue (fluid) is uncommonly calcified

(With permission from Johnston GG, Feeney DA, Osborne CA. Radiographic findings in urinary tract infection. *Vet Clin North Am (Small Anim Pract).* 1979;9:749.)
+ = mild.
++ = moderate.
++++ = marked.

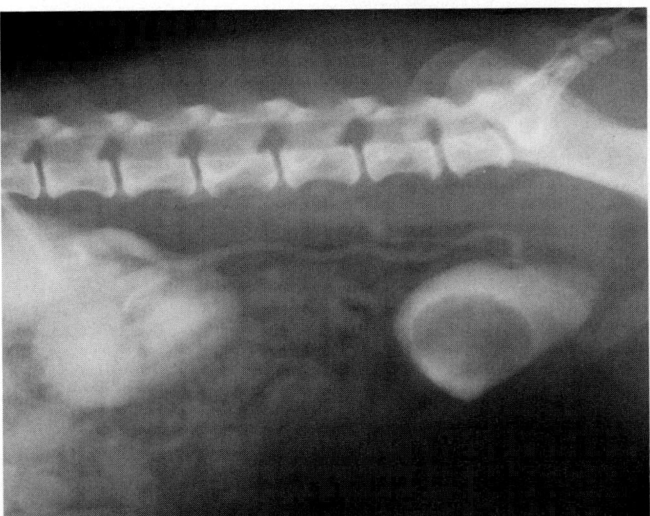

FIG. 11–29. Lateral view of an excretory urogram of a 4-year-old miniature schnauzer with a diverticulum of the cranioventral bladder wall, urinary tract infection, and a large struvite urocystourolith. The proximal lumen of the right ureter is dilated as a result of ascending pyelonephritis. Reprinted with permission from Johnston GR, Feeney DA, Osborne CA. Radiographic findings in urinary tract infection. *Vet Clin North Am.* 1979;9:749.

urethral rupture, periurethral abscesses, cutaneous lacerations, air injected with subcutaneous fluids, and subcutaneous emphysema secondary to trauma may produce radiolucent densities in the region of the urethra. Contrast urethrocystography is required to confirm urethral involvement.

4. Limitations of survey radiography in assessment of prostatic and urethral disease. Survey radiography for evaluation of the prostate gland is of limited value when peritoneal fat is lacking or peritoneal fluid is present.[56] Similarly, survey radiography is of little value for assessment of diseases of the prostatic urethra unless it has a density (usually radiopaque) different from that of glandular soft tissue. Survey radiographic techniques do not permit differentiation between focal or multifocal masses and diffuse infiltrates. In addition, they cannot be used to differentiate prostatic cavities caused by cysts from those caused by abscesses.[56]

C. Urethrocystography.

1. Overview. The term "urethrocystography" is defined as the simultaneous opacification of the urethra and urinary bladder. "Urethrocystography" also has been used as a synonym for retrograde contrast urethrocystography to imply that the urethra is opacified prior to opacification of the urinary bladder. "Cystourethrography" sometimes is used to imply that the urinary bladder is opacified prior to opacification of the urethra. Proper visualization of the urethra requires maximum distention of the urinary bladder. In practice, both the retrograde and antegrade techniques require prior distention of the urinary bladder with dilute contrast medium before the urethra is opacified. From a radiologist's point of view, the terms are interchangeable.

Pneumourethrocystography and double contrast urethrocystography are *not* recommended for

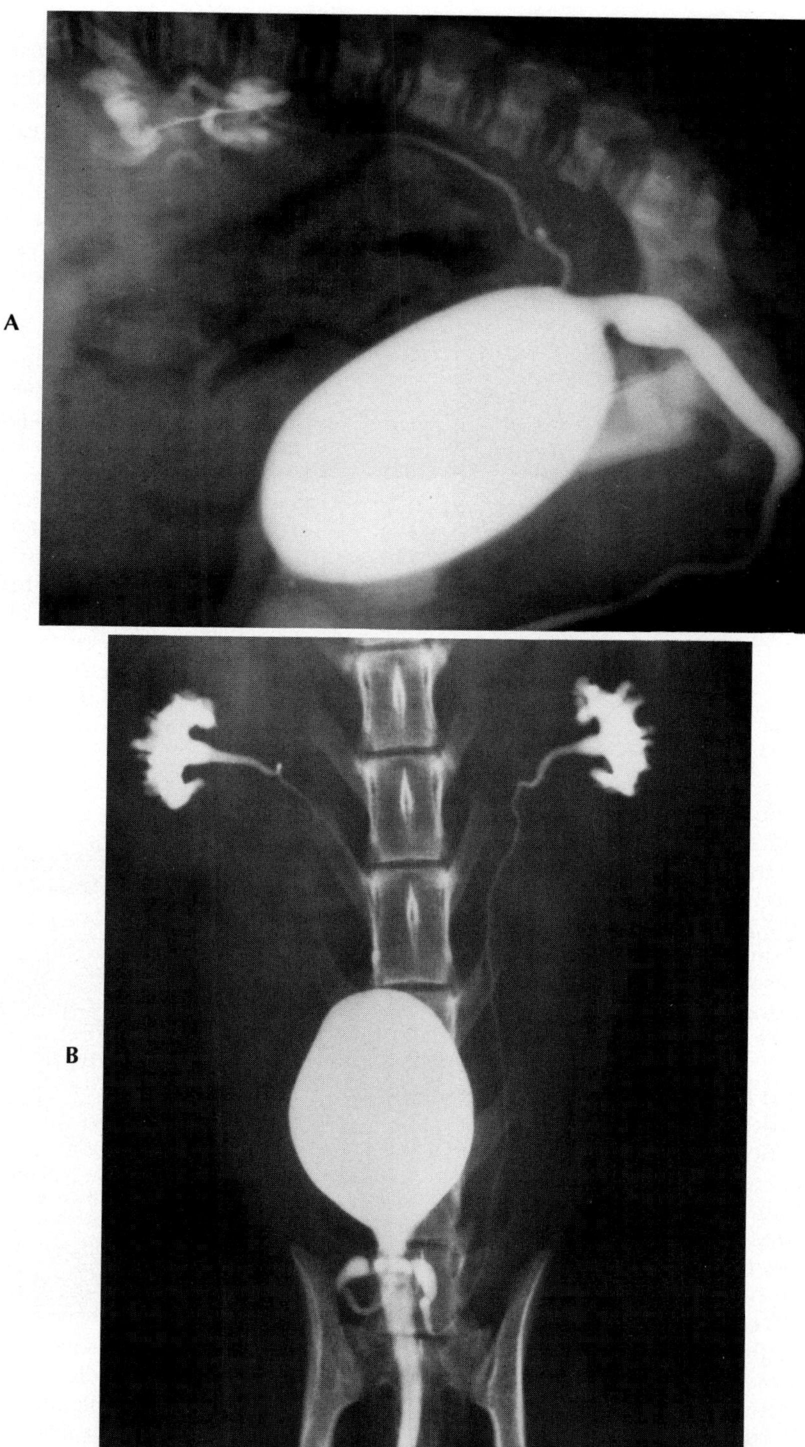

FIG. 11–30. A, Lateral view of a positive contrast retrograde urethrocystogram of a normal 8-week-old male beagle. Note vesicoureteral reflux associated with filling of the ureteral and renal pelvic lumens. **B,** Bilateral vesicoureteral reflux encountered during positive contrast retrograde urethrocystography in a 6-year-old male domestic shorthair cat with intermittent hematuria of several months' duration. A perineal urethrostomy had been performed 3 months previously. Overdistention of the bladder and urethra during general anesthesia may have predisposed the cat to the vesicoureteral reflux. Figure 11–30A reprinted with permission from Johnston GR, Feeney DA, Osborne CA. Radiographic findings in urinary tract infection. *Vet Clin North Am.* 1979;9:749. Figure 11–30B reprinted with permission from Johnston GR, Feeney DA, Osborne CA. Urethrography and cystography in cats. Part II. Abnormal radiographic anatomy and complications. *Comp Cont Educ.* 1982;4:931.

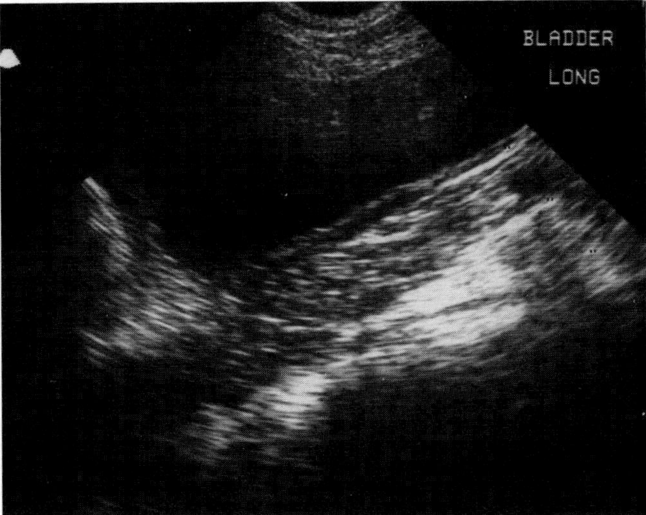

FIG. 11–31. Normal long axis (sagittal) sonogram of the urinary bladder of a 12-year-old neutered male golden retriever. The urinary bladder appears as an anechoic fluid-filled structure with a thin wall.

assessment of the prostate gland and urethra because these techniques do not improve the degree of contrast obtained by positive contrast urethrocystography. In patients with suspected urethral lacerations or tears, air should be avoided because of the potential for fatal vascular embolization. If aqueous iodinated contrast agents enter the subepithelial vascular plexus via urethral tears, fatal embolization would not be likely because these agents are approved for intravascular use.

2. Clinical considerations and contraindications. Before performing urethrographic techniques, consider the following. Some degree of sedation is usually required, except for depressed patients that do not object to catheterization.[20,48,51,63-65] Potential complications of urethral catheterization are described in Section B2c. Vesicoureteral reflux may occur as a result of distention of the urinary bladder. The net effect may be that infectious agents previously confined to the urethra or bladder now can gain access to the kidneys. The risk of iatrogenic overdistention of the bladder lumen that may result in rupture is always present. Radiopaque contrast requires the contrast medium may affect the results of urinalyses.[15]

   Urethrocystography is primarily indicated to localize and further characterize signs of lower urinary tract disease, including palpable periurethral masses, resistance to urethral catheterization, and blood dripping from the prepuce or vulva.

   Contraindications for urethrocystography are few, except in patients with a history of previous reactions to aqueous iodinated contrast agents.

3. Limitations. Periurethral diseases that do not communicate with the urethral lumen or that do not displace and/or compress the urethral lumen cannot be detected by contrast urethrocystography. Such abnormalities merit further investigation by ultrasonography. Contrast urethrocystography provides little information about urethral function.

   From an interpretative standpoint, three significant limitations of prostatic urethrocystography can be overcome by ultrasonography. First, urethrocystography does not permit differentiation of a prostatic mass caused by a neoplasm from a prostatic mass caused by a cyst or abscess if the mass does not communicate with the urethra.[56] Second, at times, relatively large lesions of the prostatic parenchyma do not create detectable changes in the prostatic urethra (Fig. 11–1). Third, urethral prostatic reflux of contrast medium is a subjective and nonspecific finding.[56,62,66]

4. Technique(s) of urethrography designed to evaluate the canine prostatic urethra and other urethral regions in male and female dogs and cats:

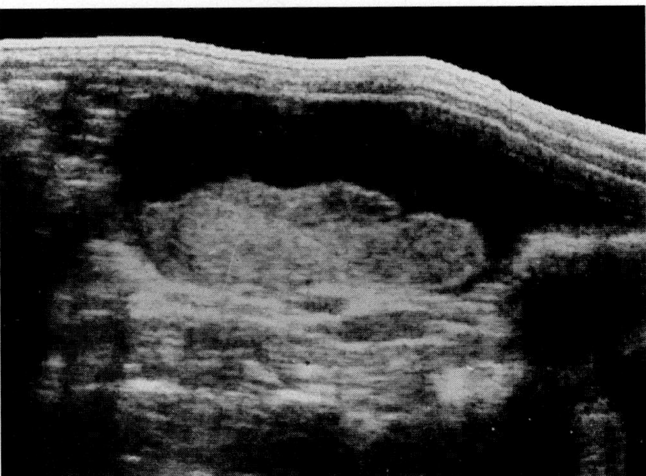

FIG. 11–32. Static B-mode sonogram of a 6-month-old male American Eskimo dog with idiopathic hematuria of the urinary bladder obtained with a 7.5-MHz transducer. The survey abdominal radiographs were unremarkable. The shape, size, and internal architecture, combined with the absence of acoustic shadowing caused by the filling defect, excludes the possibility of a nonradiopaque urolith. The transmission of sound waves deep to the filling defect is well defined. The filling defect was found to be a large blood clot. Reprinted with permission from Johnston GR, Walter PA, Feeney DA. Radiographic and ultrasonographic features of uroliths and other urinary tract filling defects. *Vet Clin North Am (Small Anim Pract).* 1986;16:261.

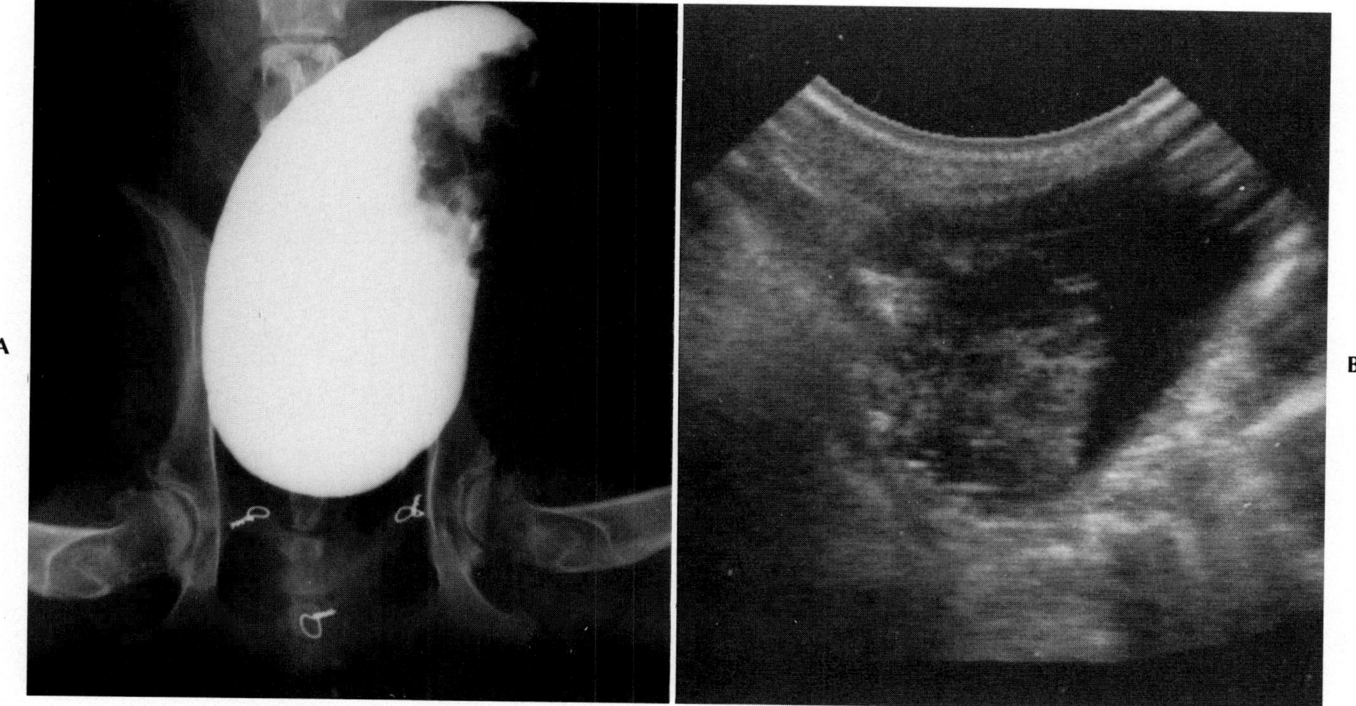

FIG. 11–33. A, Positive contrast cystogram in a dog with a transitional cell carcinoma of the bladder wall. **B,** Ultrasound of the urinary bladder reveals a mucosal mass extending into the bladder lumen.

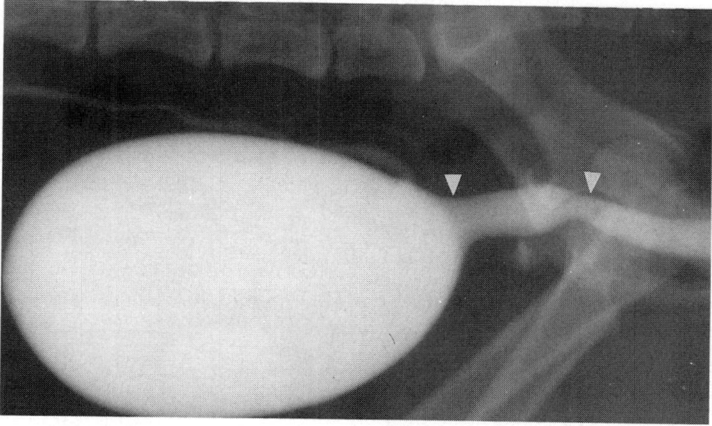

FIG. 11–34. Lateral view of a distention retrograde urethrocystogram of a normal male dog. Note that the prostatic portion of the urethra (between arrowheads) is larger than the intrapelvic membranous or penile portions of the urethra. Iatrogenic vesicoureteral reflux and a small amount of urethroprostatic reflux are apparent.

a. General abdominal preparation. The general preparation for abdominal radiography was defined in Section IIB of this chapter.

b. Types/protocols for urethrography. Urethrocystographic techniques and their interpretation have been extensively described.[2,57,65,67]

(1). Retrograde urethrography utilized to help to evaluate the prostate gland. The technique of retrograde urethrography consists of retrograde infusion of 5 to 20 mL of standard urographic contrast medium that has been diluted 1:3 with sterile water. Exposures are made during injection; lateral and ventrodorsal-oblique projections may be made to gain an orthogonal perspective of urethral lesions. Ventrodorsal-oblique views also limit superimposition of the prostatic urethra on the penile urethra, as seen in standard ventrodorsal views. This procedure permits assessment of patency of the urethral lumen and assessment of urethral lesions.

(2). Distention retrograde urethrocystography. This procedure involves retrograde infusion of a sufficient volume of diluted contrast medium (1:3 with sterile water) through a balloon-tipped catheter (No. 4-7 French Swan-Ganz) to palpably distend the urinary bladder. An additional 5 to 20 mL of less diluted contrast medium is then infused to distend the distal urethra. As with regular urethrography, lateral and ventrodorsal-oblique exposures are made during each injection. This technique allows assessment of the fully distended prostatic urethra. One can then determine if any external compression of the urethral lumen has occurred. Likewise, the technique facilitates urethroprostatic reflux, and thus allows the pattern of reflux to be characterized. Caution must be used not to overdistend the bladder lumen. This technique of urethrography is recommended in male and female dogs for evaluation of the entire urethra. An example of the normal distention retrograde urethrocystogram for evaluation of the prostate urethra in the male canine is seen in Figure 11–34.

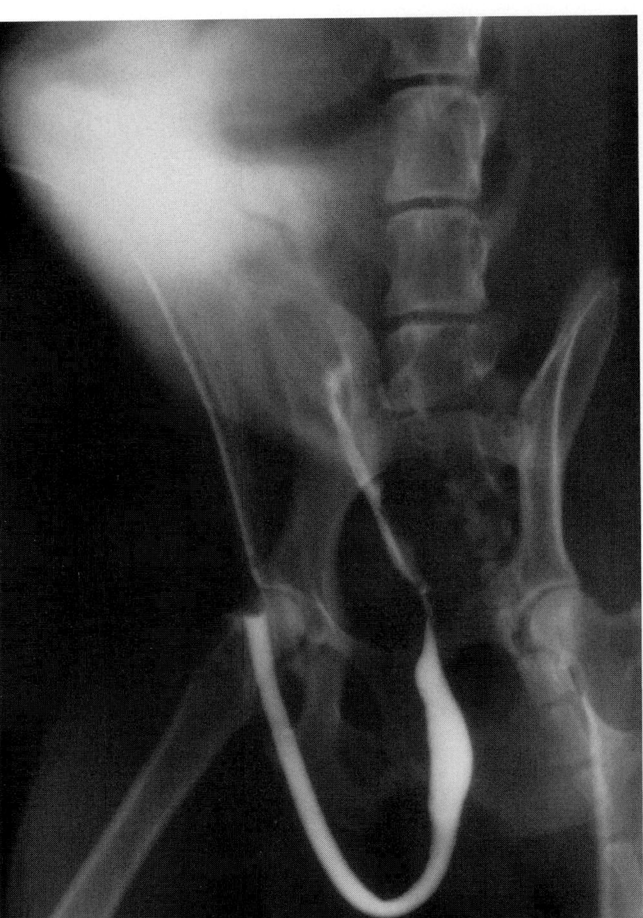

FIG. 11–36. Ventrodorsal-oblique view of the lower urinary tract of a dog during distention retrograde urethrocystography. Note lack of distention in the prostatic portion of the urethra and dilation of the membranous portion of the urethra. An extraluminal deviation of the caudal prostatic portion of the urethra is also evident. Changes are consistent with an intraprostatic extraurethral mass. Final diagnosis was prostatic abscess. Reprinted with permission from Feeney DA, et al. Canine prostatic disease: Comparison of radiographic appearance with morphologic and microbiologic findings. *J Am Vet Med Assoc.* 1987;190:1018.

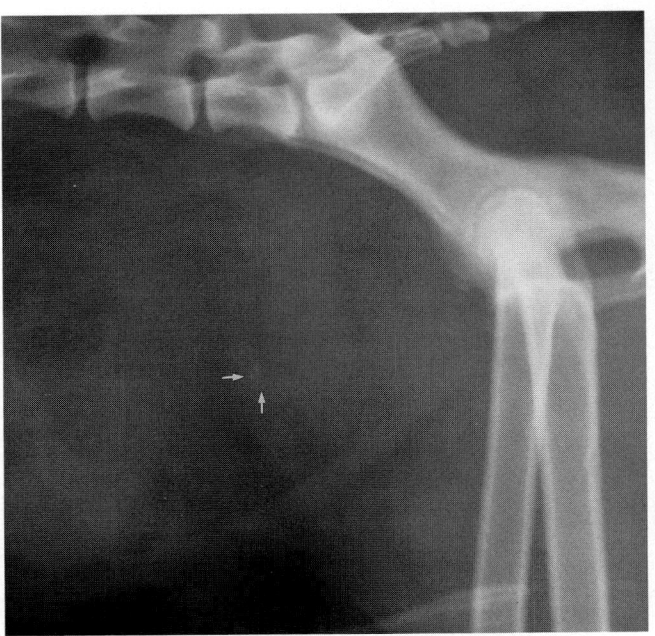

FIG. 11–35. Lateral survey radiograph of the abdomen of a dog in which caudal abdominal contrast is poor. The outline of the prostate gland cannot be clearly defined, but small foci of mineral density (arrowheads) are seen in what is presumed to be an enlarged prostate gland. Final morphologic diagnosis was schirrous prostatic adenocarcinoma. Reprinted with permission from Feeney DA, et al. Canine prostatic disease: Comparison of radiographic appearance with morphologic and microbiologic findings. *J Am Vet Med Assoc.* 1987;190:1018.

The male canine urethra is anatomically divided into three regions: prostatic,

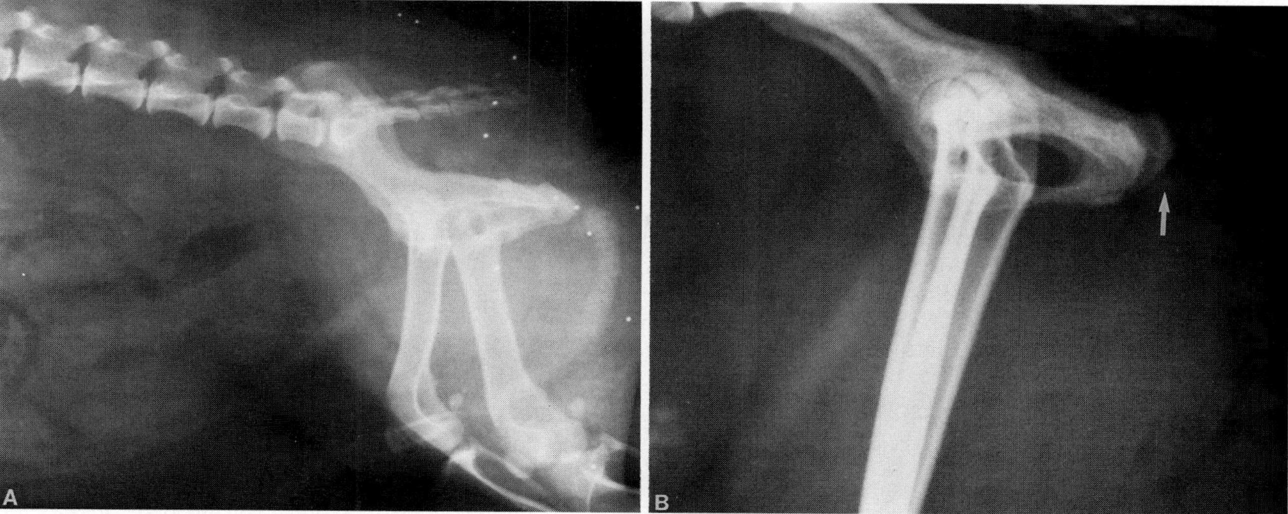

FIG. 11–37. A, Lateral survey abdominal radiograph of a male dog with multiple urethral calculi in the penile urethra extending from the ischial arch to the os penis. Although the penile urethra is the most common site of urethral obstruction in male dogs, other sites of obstruction throughout the length of the urethra may be involved. **B,** Lateral survey abdominal radiograph of the male cat described in Figure 11–26. Note the multiple urocystoliths and the solitary urethral urolith in the penile (arrow) urethra. Figure 11–37A reprinted with permission from Johnston GR, Walter PA, Feeney DA. Radiographic and ultrasonographic features of uroliths and other urinary tract filling defects. *Vet Clin North Am (Small Anim Pract).* 1986;16:261. Figure 11–37B reprinted with permission from Johnston GR, Feeney DA. Localization of feline urethral obstruction. *Vet Clin North Am.* 1984;14:555.

membranous, and penile (Fig. 11–38). The prostatic urethra is spindle shaped; its junctions between the bladder neck and the membranous urethra have a diameter narrower than that of the midprostatic urethra, which has the largest diameter of any region of the urethra. A filling defect in the dorsal wall of the prostatic urethra that is encountered on the ventrodorsal or ventrodorsal-oblique radiographic projection is caused by caliculus seminalis, the site of termination of the vas deferens (Fig. 11–38). When the prostatic urethra is maximally distended, the mucosal surface should be smooth. The membranous urethra connects the distal prostatic urethra to the penile urethra. The membranous urethra is more variable in diameter than is the penile or prostatic urethra. The causes for variable diameters of the membranous urethra include inadequate urinary bladder distention, peristaltic contractions of the smooth muscle in the wall of the membranous urethra, or spasms of the skeletal muscle (urethralis muscle) in the wall of the membranous urethra. These peristaltic contractions or muscle spasms must not be misinterpreted as strictures. If questions arise concerning the differentiation between a stricture and a peristaltic contraction or spasm, the procedure should be repeated, and the second set of radiographs should be compared to the original radiographs to determine if the abnormality in question is persistent. When the technique is properly performed, the penile urethra usually has a uniform diameter. However, variations in penile urethral diameter may be observed if the radiographic exposure is made after the injection of contrast medium. A variation in penile urethral diameter caused by muscular contraction in the wall of the urethra may occur adjacent to the site of balloon inflation. Focal and regional variations in penile urethral diameter may occur secondary to luminal or mural disease, but these variations must be differentiated from urethral peristaltic contractions or spasms.

The urethra of female dogs and cats is not divided into separate anatomic regions as in male dogs and cats; it is considered as one anatomic region (Figs. 11–39 and 11–40). Normal variations in urethral diameter of males and females are commonly encountered; they depend on the degree of urinary bladder distention. When the bladder is maximally distended, the entire length of the urethra has a uniform diameter from the bladder neck to the inflated balloon, except for the normally widened prostatic portion. When variations in urethral diameter are encountered, serial incremental injections of contrast medium followed by the radiographic exposure occurring toward the end of injection help to maximally distend the urethral lumen.

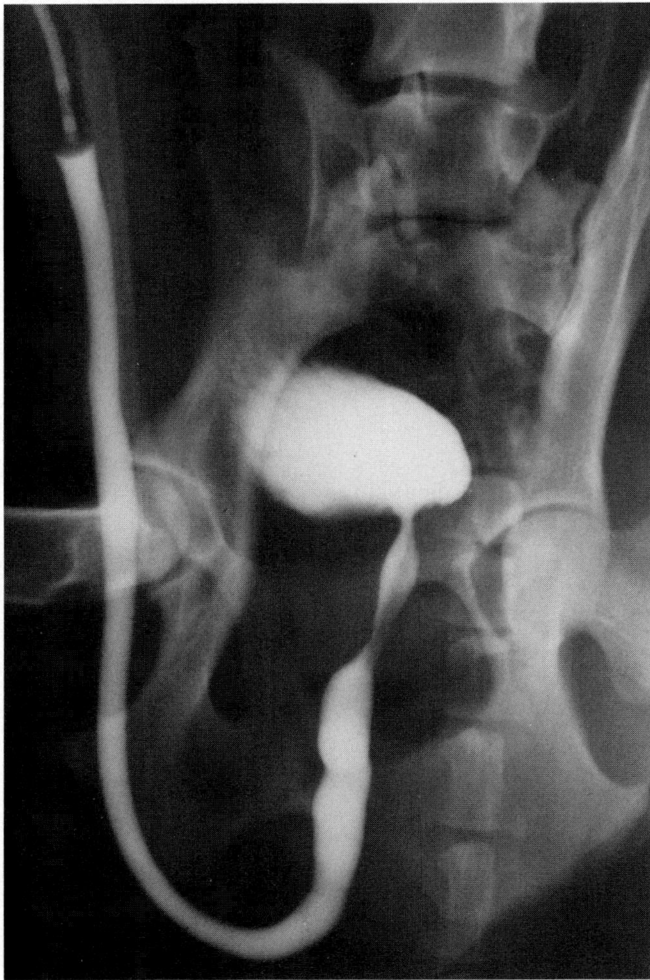

FIG. 11–38. Normal male canine retrograde urethrocystogram. The filling defect in the prostatic portion of the urethra is the caliculus seminalis, the site of termination of the vas deferens. The membranous urethra extends from the caudal portion of the prostatic urethra to the ischial arch and is variable in diameter. The penile urethra extends from the ischial arch to the external urethral orifice and usually has a uniform diameter. Reprinted with permission from Johnston GR, Feeney DA, Osborne CA. Radiographic findings in urinary tract infection. *Vet Clin North Am* 1979;9:749.

(3). Voiding cystourethrography. The voiding cystourethrogram has limited use in assessment of the prostatic portion of the urethra and the prostate gland. However, the antegrade technique of urethrocystography is recommended for male and female cats, for patients that are difficult to catheterize, and for patients at high risk for iatrogenic urinary tract infection. Antegrade urethrocystography is more "physiologic" than the retrograde technique. It may demonstrate vesicoureteral reflux and congenital or acquired urinary bladder or urethral diseases because the technique ensures maximum intravesical pressure during "voiding." The technique of antegrade urethrocystography is technically more difficult than retrograde urethrocystography because of the need for light general anesthesia and gradual bladder distention with contrast medium until reflex detrusor contraction is stimulated. The urinary bladder can be filled with contrast material either by intravenous excretory urography or by filling the bladder lumen via a urethral catheter or cystocentesis following removal of urine. Following distention of the urinary bladder with contrast medium, external pressure is applied with a wooden spoon or shielded hands to increase intravesical pressure sufficiently to induce spontaneous voiding. If voiding can be induced, the status of the prostatic urethra may be evaluated, although the distention retrograde urethrocystography technique consistently provides better distention of the prostatic urethra. Vesicoureteral reflux associated with this technique is also common. The normal male feline urethra is illustrated in Figure 11–41. Although the urethra of the male cat is divided into five anatomic regions (preprostatic, prostatic, postprostatic, membranous, and penile), these regions cannot be sharply demarcated by contrast radiography. When the urinary bladder is maximally distended prior to the retrograde injection of contrast medium, the segment of urethra that extends from the bladder neck to the ischial arch usually has a uniform diameter. The lumen of penile urethra gradually narrows from its largest diameter at the ischial arch to its smallest diameter at the urethral orifice. The radiographic appearance of the urethra of the female cat is similar to that of the urethra of female dogs; both normally have a uniform diameter along the entire length of the urethra. Urethral flexures caused by the

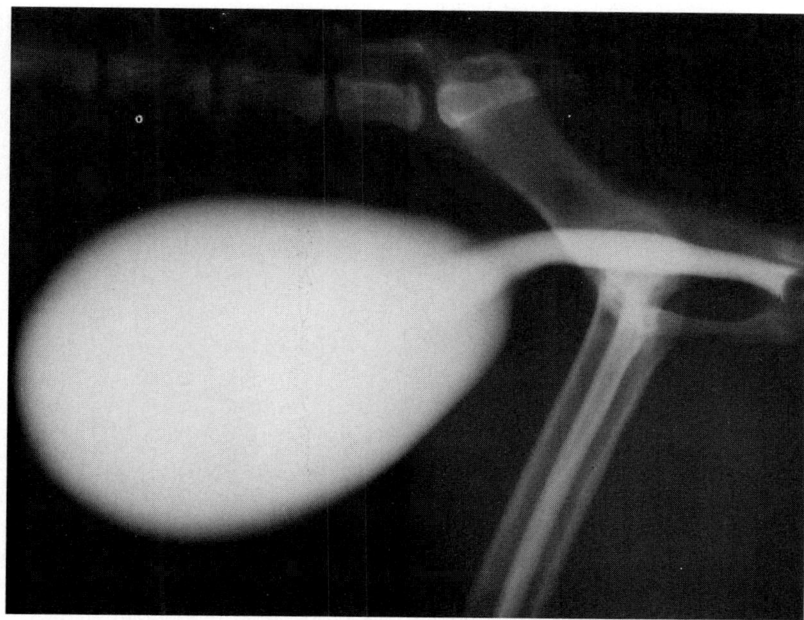

FIG. 11–39. Normal female canine retrograde urethrocystogram. When the bladder is maximally distended, the urethral diameter is uniform throughout its length from the bladder neck to the inflated balloon. Reprinted with permission from Johnston GR, Feeney DA, Osborne CA. Radiographic findings in urinary tract infection. *Vet Clin North Am.* 1979;9:749.

caudal displacement of the urinary bladder may be encountered in cats and can be differentiated from periurethral masses by obtaining a series of radiographic exposures during antegrade urethrocystography.

c. Expectations of urethrography.
   (1). Assess relationship between the prostate gland, urethra, periurethral or periprostatic masses, and caudal abdominal organs/vessels and clinical signs. Opacification of the urethra may help one to further characterize abnormalities of the prostate gland. In fact, contrast urethrography may assist in localizing the position of the prostate gland in patients with nonprostatic caudal abdominal masses that distort normal anatomic relationships.
   (2). Ensure maximum distention of the urethral lumen. One of the objectives of urethrocystography is to characterize the distensibility of the urethral lumen. Maximum distention of the urethra during urethrocystography can be ensured if the urinary bladder is maximally distended prior to opacification of the urethral lumen. Maximum distention of the urinary bladder results in maximal intravesical hydrostatic pressure, which promotes maximum distention of proximal portions of the urethral lumen.

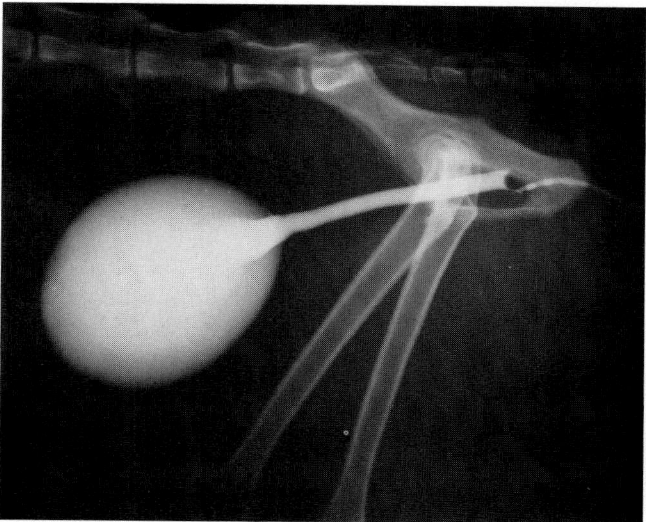

FIG. 11–40. Normal female feline antegrade urethrocystogram. When the bladder is maximally distended, the urethral diameter is uniform throughout its length from the bladder neck to the inflated balloon. Reprinted with permission from Johnston GR, Feeney DA, Osborne CA. Radiographic findings in urinary tract infection. *Vet Clin North Am.* 1979;9:749.

   (3). Differentiate prostate gland from urinary bladder. At times, one cannot determine by survey radiography whether a somewhat ovoid, caudoventral abdominal mass

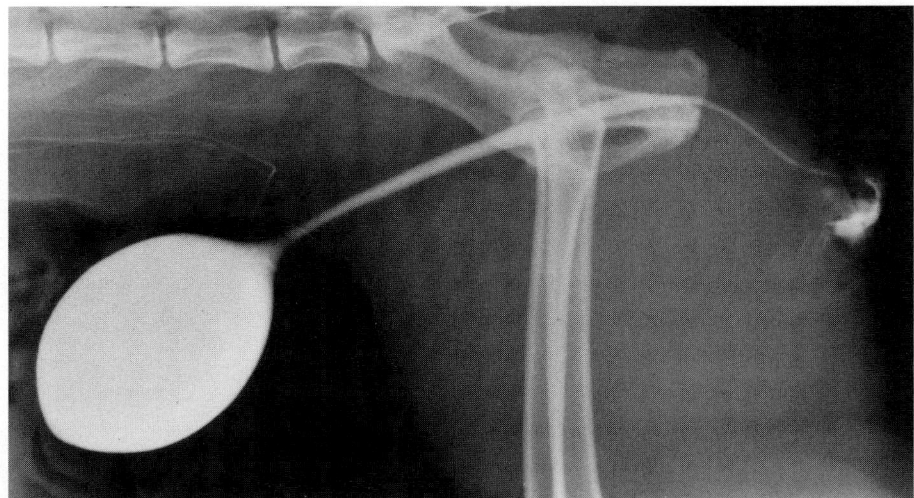

FIG. 11–41. Normal male feline antegrade urethrocystogram performed by external bladder compression with a wooden spoon. The five anatomic regions of the urethra cannot be individually identified. The portion of the urethra that extends from the bladder neck to the ischial arch should have a uniform diameter. The penile urethra gradually narrows from its largest diameter at the ischial arch to its smallest diameter at the urethral orifice. When the bladder is maximally distended, the urethral diameter is uniform throughout its length from the bladder neck to the inflated balloon. Reprinted with permission from Johnston GR, Feeney DA, Osborne CA. Urethrography and cystography in cats. Part I. Techniques, normal radiographic anatomy, and artifacts. *Comp Cont Educ.* 1982;4:823.

is actually the prostate gland or the urinary bladder. A turgid urinary bladder may be difficult to differentiate from prostomegaly by abdominal palpation. In this situation, retrograde urethrography allows one to differentiate the urinary bladder from the prostate gland.

(4). Assess effect of confirmed prostate gland on regional pelvic organs, particularly the colon and rectum. Although survey radiography usually allows one to determine the effects of prostate gland disease on regional pelvic organs, urethrographic techniques may allow further characterization of this relationship. For example, if the urethra is not distorted by prostatic disease, the underlying prostate lesion is probably a diffuse process rather than a focal mass (Fig. 11–1).

(5). Determine structure of prostatic portion of the urethra as indirect indicator of prostatic parenchymal disease. The anatomic structure of the prostatic urethra may be used as an indirect indicator of prostatic and bladder trigonal disease associated with clinical signs, particularly dysuria. The architecture of the prostatic parenchyma surrounding the prostatic portion of the urethra may indicate whether the underlying disease is diffuse or focal. In general, the canine prostatic urethra courses directly through the prostate gland and is evenly surrounded by parenchyma (Fig. 11–34). By comparison, deviations of the prostatic urethra or asymmetry of surrounding prostate tissue suggests a prostatic mass (Fig. 11–36). A combination of urethral distention characteristics, mucosal surface characteristics, and architecture of periurethral tissue can be used to characterize prostatic diseases as follows[2,56]:

(a). Smooth mucosal surface, uniform distention (larger than membranous part—distention technique), periurethral symmetry = normal (Fig. 11–34).

(b). Smooth mucosal surface, nonuniform distention, lack of periurethral symmetry = Prostatic mass (tumor, cyst, or abscess) (Fig. 11–36).

(c). Undulant mucosal surface, relatively uniform distention, periurethral symmetry = Chronic inflammation.

(d). Jagged mucosal surface, nonuniform distention, +/– periurethral symmetry = Neoplasia (Fig. 11–1).

(6). Characterize urethroprostatic reflux as an indirect index of normal and abnormal prostatic parenchyma. Urethroprostatic reflux is a common finding in dogs with normal and abnormal prostate glands as assessed by routine urethrography and, to a lesser degree, by most canine studies involving distention retrograde urethrocystography.[59,66] Therefore, detection of urethroprostatic reflux, particularly by standard urethrographic techniques, is of limited value in detecting and characterizing prostatic disease.[59,66] However, because the information about the character of urethroprostatic reflux is interpreted in light of general urethral structure, some generalities may be useful[56]:

(a). Minimal "fine" ≤ 1.0 urethral diameter penetration = Normal, particularly if a distention technique is used (Fig. 11–34).

(b). Moderate, noncoalescent ≥ 1.0 urethral diameter penetration = Abnormal, but nonspecific.

(c). Moderate to severe, smooth coalescent (pooling) ≥ 1.0 urethral diameter penetration = Cysts, abscesses, and possibly neoplasia (Fig. 11–36).

(d). Moderate to severe, jagged coalescent (pooling) ≥ 1.0 urethral diameter penetration = Neoplasia and possibly cysts or abscess.

(7). Assess abnormal contrast patterns.

(a). Overview. The goals of contrast urethrocystography are: 1) to help to localize the patient's disease; 2) to characterize its distribution; and 3) to characterize urethral involvement. From a pathophysiologic viewpoint, urethral diseases may be divided into categories similar to those described for bladder disease. They include mucosal defects, mural defects, intraluminal filling defects, communicating defects, and extraluminal abnormalities. Because different urethral diseases may be associated with one or more of these patterns, they are nonspecific.

(b). Mucosal patterns. Mucosal patterns may be focal or multifocal in distribution and may have a mural component (Fig. 11–42). Mucosal patterns are diagnostically nonspecific because they may originate from traumatic, infectious inflammatory, noninfectious inflammatory, or neoplastic diseases. Therefore, the significance of mucosal disease should be interpreted in light of the history, physical findings, urinalysis, urine culture, and other appropriate clinical laboratory data. Mucosal and mural lesions may exist concurrently as a manifestation of the same underlying

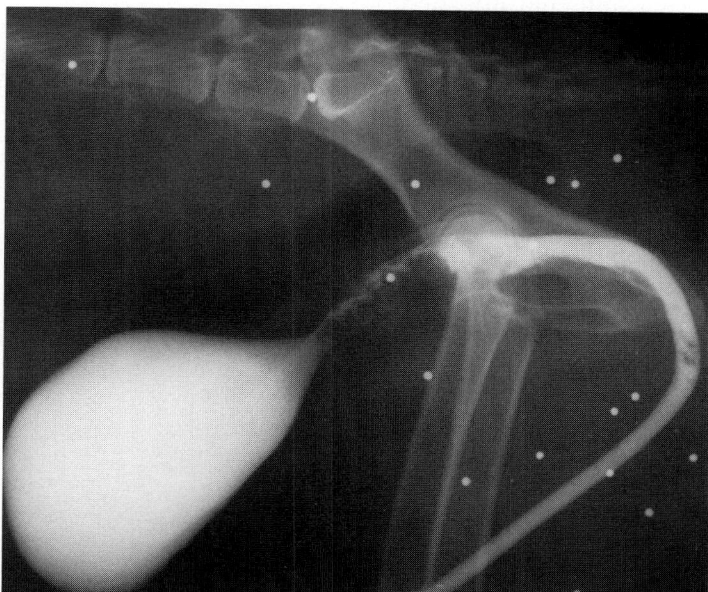

FIG. 11–42. Lateral radiograph of a positive contrast retrograde urethrocystogram from a neutered dog with a transitional cell carcinoma of the prostatic urethra. Note the ventral displacement of the descending colon caused by the sublumbar lymphadenopathy. The lumen of the prostatic urethra is characterized by a lack of distensibility and mucosal irregularity. Reprinted with permission from Johnston GR, Feeney DA, River B, Walter PA. Diagnostic imaging of the male canine reproductive organs. *Vet Clin North Am.* 1991;21:553.

disease. Frequently, mucosal disease can be differentiated from a combined mucosal and mural disease by evaluation of the distensibility of the urethral lumen. If a maximally distended urinary bladder is associated with a nondistensible urethral lumen with mucosal irregularity, an inflammatory or neoplastic infiltrate should be considered (Figs. 11–1 and 11–42). Focal mucosal irregularities may be associated with urethroliths, or catheter-induced urethral trauma of male dogs in the area of the ischial arch at the junction of the penile and membranous urethra. Multifocal to diffuse mucosal patterns may be encountered secondary to prolonged use of indwelling urethral catheters.

(c). Mural patterns. Mural diseases of the urethra are typically associated with mucosal irregularities. Nondistensibility of the urethral lumen is a reflection of a transmural disease, but is nonspecific and may indicate chronic inflammatory or neoplastic infiltrates (Fig. 11–42). Acute transmural hemorrhage and edema of the male feline penile urethra secondary to urethral obstruction are characterized by the narrowing of the urethral lumen (Fig. 11–43). Focal nondistensible regions may be encountered anywhere along the urethra and may be associated with congenital or acquired strictures. These focal areas of luminal narrowing should be evaluated carefully in relationship to urinary bladder distention. Normal peristaltic contractions of the urethral smooth muscle, and muscular spasms secondary to catheter trauma, may result in focal luminal narrowings that resemble strictures (Fig. 11–44). Serial exposures during urethrocystography may help to differentiate intermittent narrowing of the urethral lumen caused by muscular spasms from permanent luminal narrowing caused by strictures.

(d). Filling defects. Filling defects can occur anywhere in the excretory pathway and may be attached to the mucosa or free in the lumen. Free luminal filling defects are more common. Common urethral filling defects detected by radiography include uroliths, blood clots, air bubbles, and matrix-crystalline plugs (Figs. 11–43 through 11–45). The differential radiographic characteristics of urethral filling defects are summarized in Table 11–8.[2,3]

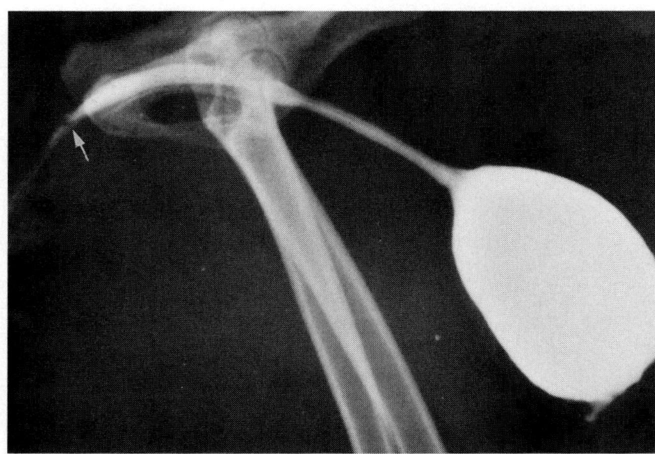

FIG. 11–43. Lateral view of an antegrade urethrocystogram from the cat described in Figure 11–26. Note the urachal diverticulum located in the cranioventral portion of the bladder, and the urethral calculus in the penile urethra (arrow). The urethral lumen is enlarged in the area of the urolith. Reprinted with permission from Johnston GR, Feeney DA, Osborne CA. Urethrography and cystography in cats. Part II. Abnormal radiographic anatomy and complications. *Comp Cont Educ.* 1982;4:931.

(1′). Free luminal. Uroliths typically are free in the urethral lumen, but occasionally are attached. In male dogs, they are commonly located in the penile urethra behind or within the os penis (Fig. 11–45). However, uroliths may also be located in the prostatic or membranous urethra (Fig. 11–46). In male cats, uroliths are most commonly located in the penile urethra (Fig. 11–43). However, the detection of a urolith in the penile urethra by catheterization does not exclude the possibility of uroliths elsewhere within the urethra. They can only be identified by urethrocystography (Fig. 11–46). Urethral uroliths in female dogs and cats may be found anywhere along its length, with a predilection for the bladder neck and just proximal to the external urethral orifice. These uroliths may be identified

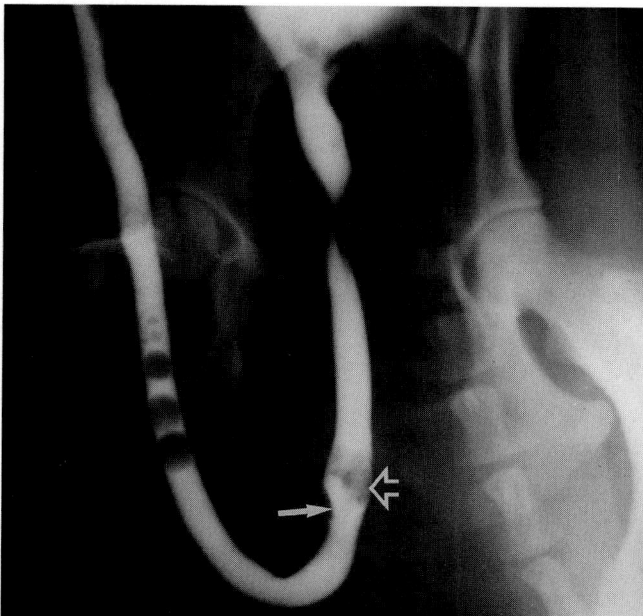

FIG. 11–44. Ventrodorsal-oblique radiograph of a positive contrast retrograde urethrocystogram of a 12-year-old male beagle with chronic hematuria and dysuria. Three large and several small air bubbles conforming to the lumen of the penile urethra are present. The irregular filling defect at the ischial arch is a blood clot (open arrow). The narrowed distal penile urethral lumen adjacent to the balloon catheter is caused by urethral spasm or peristaltic contraction. Mucosal irregularity at the junction of the membranous and penile urethra (white arrow) was caused by catheter trauma. Reprinted with permission from Johnston GR, Feeney DA, Osborne CA. Radiographic findings in urinary tract infection. *Vet Clin North Am.* 1979;9:749.

by vaginoscopic examination if they are lodged at the external urethral orifice. If the ventrodorsal and lateral survey abdominal radiographs do not include the caudal abdomen and pelvis, these uroliths may be missed on survey radiographs.

(2′). Attached. Attached urethral filling defects are encountered less commonly than are free luminal filling defects. The most common cause of attached filling defects is uroliths attached to the urethra following inflammation secondary to partial urethral obstruction. Other disorders that may be associated with attached filling defects include blood clots, urethral tumors, and iatrogenic and traumatic inflammatory lesions.

(e). Communicating patterns. Extravasation of control media beyond the urethra may be caused by congenital or acquired disorders, including urethrovaginal and urethrorectal fistulas (Fig. 11–47), trauma, or urethral obstruction (Fig. 11–45). The most common location of extravasation of contrast media in male dogs is in the region of the os penis (Fig. 11–45). Urethroprostatic reflux may be encountered in patients with prostatic disease and is described under Section VIC in this chapter.

VII. ULTRASONOGRAPHIC ASSESSMENT OF THE PROSTATE GLAND

A. Role of ultrasonographic imaging in prostatic disease. Use of ultrasonographic techniques to evaluate the prostate gland requires understanding of general ultrasonography and of ultrasonographic patterns of disease.[7,22,25,54,68-73]

1. Information gained complementary to that from survey radiographic and contrast urethrographic

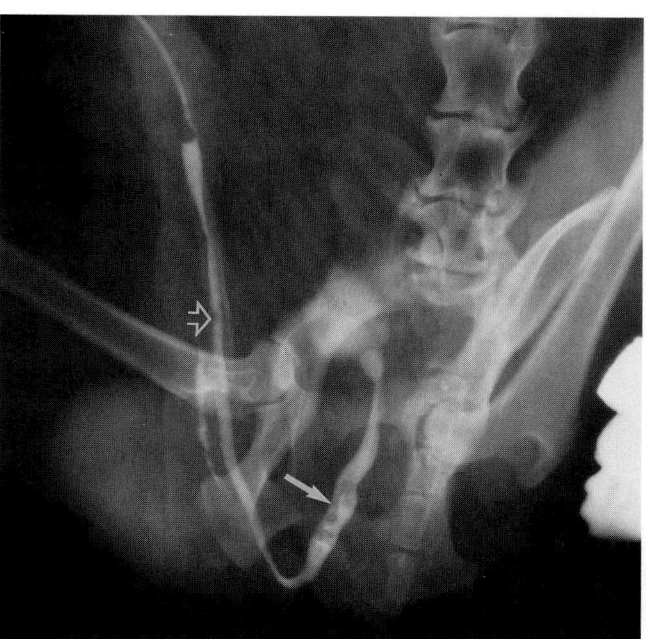

FIG. 11–45. Positive contrast retrograde urethrocystogram of a 6-year-old male Irish setter with lower urinary tract disease. Note a solitary urethral calculus in the penile urethra (open arrow), periurethral escape of contrast medium, periurethral soft tissue gas, multiple filling defects, including air bubbles, and a blood clot (arrowhead) in the membranous urethra. Reprinted with permission from Johnston GR, Feeney DA. Radiographic evaluation of the urinary tract in dogs and cats. *Contemp Issues Small Anim Pract (Nephrol Urol).* 1986;4:203.

TABLE 11–8
DIFFERENTIAL RADIOGRAPHIC CHARACTERISTICS OF INTRALUMINAL FILLING DEFECTS OF THE URETHRA ENCOUNTERED DURING POSITIVE CONTRAST URETHROCYSTOGRAPHY

Radiographic Criteria	Air Bubbles	Uroliths	Blood Clots
Size	Small, about 5-10 mm	Small, about 5-10 mm	Small
Number	Single, multiple, or coalescent	Single or multiple	Single or multiple
Shape	Round if smaller than urethral lumen; oval or polyhedral if coalescent	Spheroid, ovoid, polygonal, or pumpkin seed	Spheroid, ovoid, polygonal, or linear
Margination	Smooth and distinct	Smooth and irregular, commonly distinct	Irregular and indistinct
Location	Anywhere	Commonly in membranous urethra (ischeal arch) or penile urethra (os penis); may be attached or combined within a blood clot	Anywhere
Relationship to urethral lumen	Always conform to shape of urethra lumen	May cause focal distention if larger than urethral lumen; will conform to urethral lumen if small	Conform to shape of urethral lumen
Radiographic density	Radiolucent	Radiolucent	Radiolucent

(Reprinted with permission from Johnston GR, Feeney DA. Radiographic evaluation of the urinary tract in dogs and cats. *Contemp Issues Small Anim Pract (Nephrol/Urol).* 1986;4:203.)

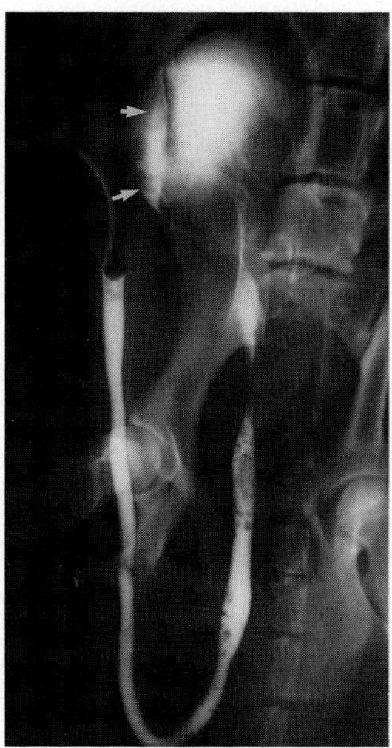

FIG. 11–46. Ventrodorsal-oblique radiograph of a positive contrast retrograde urethrocystogram of a 7-year-old male golden retriever. Many struvite uroliths are present in the lumen of the membranous and penile urethra. A blood clot attached to the bladder wall (arrows) was identified during surgery. Reprinted with permission from Johnston GR, Feeney DA, Osborne CA. Radiographic findings in urinary tract infection. *Vet Clin North Am.* 1979;9:749.

procedures. Information obtained from prostatic ultrasonography often complements information obtained from radiographic techniques.[71] Ultrasonography is especially useful in characterizing masses, cystic lesions, and infiltrates in the prostatic parenchyma. Ultrasonography overcomes many of the shortcomings of survey and contrast radiography. Ultrasonography of the prostate gland is not hampered by poor abdominal contrast or regional fluid.[54,70-73] Even though urethrograms are unremarkable, prominent intraprostatic masses may be identified by ultrasonographic techniques (Fig. 11–1).[71,72] Prostatic ultrasonography facilitates characterization of different types of intraprostatic masses, and also facilitates differentiation of paraprostatic and intraprostatic cysts from diffuse infiltrative prostatic masses and prostatic abscesses.[54,56,70-72] The overall prostatic architecture can be assessed and often clarified using ultrasonography (Figs. 11–4 and 11–36).[54,71,72] In addition, periprostatic structure and nonprostatic regional masses may be characterized by sonographic techniques.[54,71,72]

Urethrographic techniques facilitate assessment of the mucosa for evidence of inflammation and may also facilitate differentiation of infectious disorders from neoplastic processes (Fig. 11–36).[71,72] Urethrographic techniques may be required to localize and characterize strictures or leaks that cannot be detected by ultrasonographic

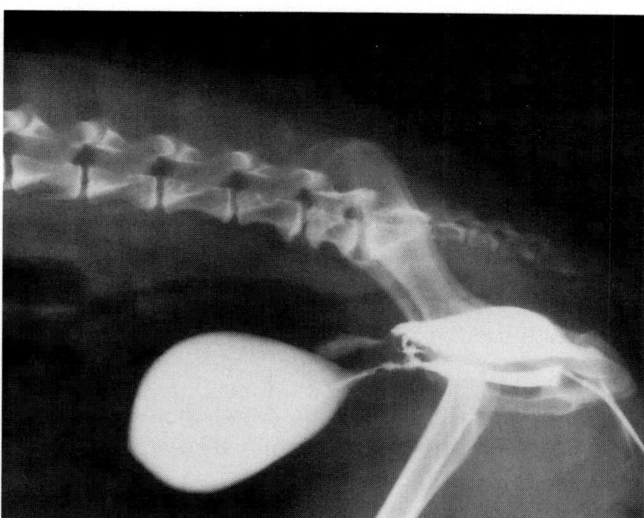

FIG. 11–47. Lateral radiograph of a positive contrast retrograde urethrocystogram of a 10-year-old female English setter with chronic hematuria and dysuria. Mucosal irregularity, nondistensibility of the proximal urethra, and a urethrovaginal fistula were caused by a transitional cell carcinoma of the proximal urethra. Reprinted with permission from Johnston GR, Feeney DA. Radiographic evaluation of the urinary tract in dogs and cats. *Contemp Issues Small Anim Pract (Nephrol Urol).* 1986;4:203.

techniques. Urethrocystographic techniques complement ultrasonography inasmuch as they help to detect communications between the prostatic portion of the urethra and sonographically identifiable intraprostatic cavities (Figs. 11–4) and 11–36). This information may facilitate diagnoses, particularly if the sonographic findings do not permit differentiation of cysts from abscesses.

2. Ultrasonographic images are often easier to interpret in light of survey and contrast radiographic findings. Radiographic findings facilitate evaluation of the architecture of the urethra and the relationship of the size of the prostate gland to the size of the dog (as assessed by pubic-promontory distance comparisons).[56] Ultrasonographic images provide information on the size and internal architecture of the prostate gland, the relationship of these to the prostatic portion of the urethra, and the effects on the colon.
3. Dimensions obtained by ultrasonography must be standardized against pubic-promontory distance derived radiographically to compensate for body size. Assessment of the dimensions of the prostate gland, although seemingly easy from a subjective standpoint, can be confused by misconceptions. The location of the prostate gland in the caudal portion of the abdomen may not be caused only by prostatomegaly. It has been observed in male dogs during the postsexual peak group wherein the prostate gland migrates out of the pelvic cavity into the caudal abdomen. This normal event should not be overinterpreted as prostatomegaly. In general, as many as 95% of normal dogs have prostate glands with dimensions less than 70% of the pubic-promontory distance.[56]
4. Summary. Urethrographic techniques provide information about the prostatic urethral lumen, whereas ultrasonographic techniques provide information about the prostate parenchyma.

B. Technical considerations for prostatic ultrasonography.

1. Little preparation is required for abdominal sonography. Enemas are undesirable because they tend to induce large bowel and small bowel gas accumulations that make ultrasound scanning more difficult. However, if ultrasonographic and radiographic techniques are to be performed in the same time frame, enema-induced gas causes less problems for the ultrasonographic interpretation than stool does for the radiographic interpretation. In this situation, enemas are recommended. Prior to ultrasonography, hair located up to 8 cm along either lateral side of the prepuce should be removed from the tip of the prepuce caudal to the pubic bone. This clipping is primarily to the prepubic window.
2. Prepubic window. The prepubic window is one of two sonographic approaches to the prostate gland. The other approach is the endorectal window. Advantages and disadvantages are associated with each technique. The prepubic window is best performed with the bladder lumen distended. We typically perform distention retrograde urethrocystograms first, immediately followed by prostatic ultrasonograms.
   a. Advantages. The advantage of this approach to the prostate is its ability to be performed with general real-time sector scanners, thus eliminating the need for specialized equipment designed for endorectal use. In addition, adequate images of the prostate gland can be obtained from most dogs that are "predisposed" by age to prostatic disease, because at that time of their life, the prostate gland has migrated into the caudal abdomen out of the pelvic canal. With the prepubic technique, both sagittal and transverse oblique planes can be made. In addition, the urinary bladder and retroperitoneal lymph nodes can be surveyed more easily with the prepubic technique than with the endorectal technique.
   b. Shortcomings. The main disadvantage of the prepubic technique of ultrasonography is inability to see clearly echoes from the capsule of the prostate gland. This situation limits one's ability to stage cranial and caudal prostatic masses relative to the capsule, which is germane in surgical decisions. The pubis can interfere with visualization of portions or all of

the prostate gland, particularly in young dogs.

3. Endorectal window. Small linear array scanners used for pregnancy detection in the horse can be used as endorectal scanners in medium- and large-breed dogs with little difficulty.
   a. Advantages. The primary advantage of the endorectal technique in dogs is good visualization of the prostatic capsule. In addition, other than maintaining coupling to the colon and rectal mucosa, adjacent organs do not tend to interfere with prostate gland visualization as they do with the prepubic technique. The entire prostate gland can be seen using the endorectal technique. Finally, the near field of view is improved because, with less tissue intervening between the scanner and the prostatic parenchyma, high frequency endorectal scanners may be used.
   b. Shortcomings. The shortcomings of the endorectal window procedure are basically related to technique. First, the imaging is limited to the sagittal plane with equine-oriented intrarectal linear array scanners; imaging is limited to transverse planes with most of the intrarectal or transvaginal sector scanners designed for use in human beings. In addition, patient tolerance to endorectal scans may be less than that with the prepubic scans. In our experience, sedation has rarely been required to perform prepubic prostatic ultrasonograms on the average dog. In contrast, any type of retrograde catheterization or invasion of a body orifice may necessitate more frequent use of sedation.

C. Applications of ultrasonographic techniques to prostatic disease.

1. Classification of prostatic disease relevant to ultrasonographic imaging. In an attempt to correlate imaging findings with pathologic findings, eight classifications of prostatic disease relevant to ultrasonographic and radiographic imaging were developed.[71] They are: 1) normal (Fig. 11–48); 2) noncavitating, nonbacterial/nonmycotic (basically benign hypertrophy/hyperplasia); 3) cavitating, noninfectious/nonmycotic (hyperplastic cysts or inclusion cysts); 4) noncavitating, bacterial/mycotic (nonabscessing prostatitis); 5) cavitating, bacterial/mycotic (prostatic abscess) (Fig. 11–4); 6) nonprostatic origin neoplasia (usually transitional cell carcinoma); 7) prostatic origin neoplasia (prostatic carcinoma) (Fig. 11–49); 8) and paraprostatic disease (usually paraprostatic cysts) (Fig. 11–50).
2. Characterize prostatic parenchymal and regional architecture. Detectable changes include an increase or decrease in size; the absence, presence, and number of intraparenchymal cavitations; the absence, presence, and distribution of echogenic reactions, usually secondary to scirrhous reactions caused by neoplasia or inflammation; and combinations of these possibilities.[70-73] Consider the four usual sonographic appearances of common prostatic diseases:
   1. Uniform prostatic echotexture (? acute in-

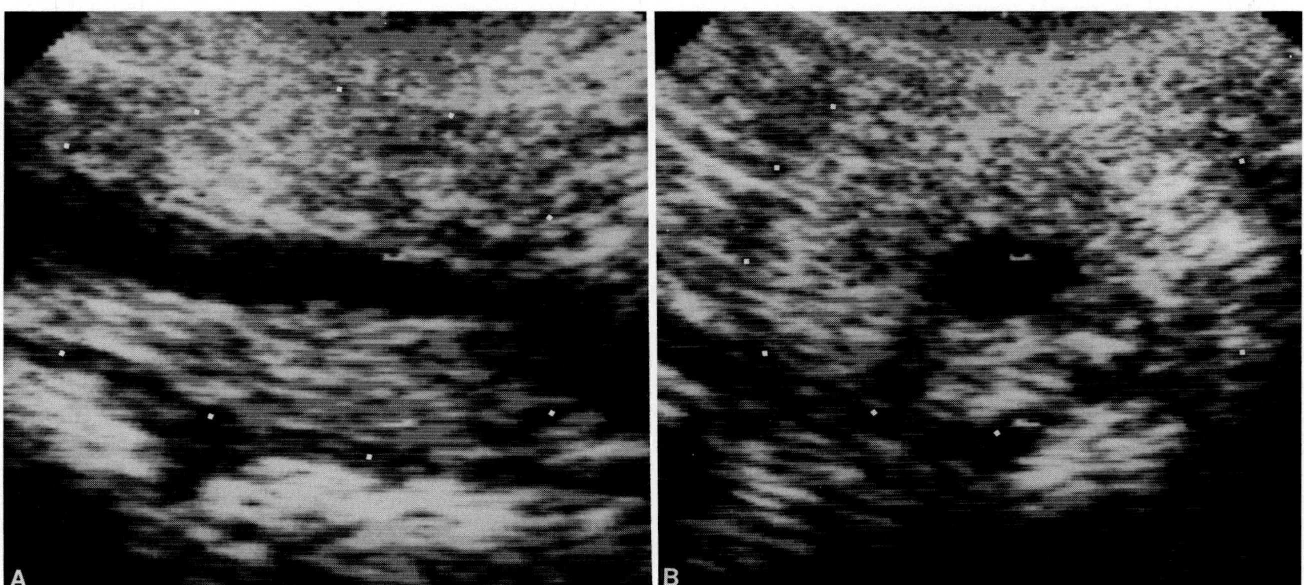

FIG. 11–48. Sagittal **(A)** and transverse **(B)** real-time ultrasonograms of a normal prostate gland. Notice the lack of definition of the capsule (outlined by dots) because this image was made via a prepubic window. The prostatic portion of the urethra is dilated because the image was made following distention retrograde urethrocystography.

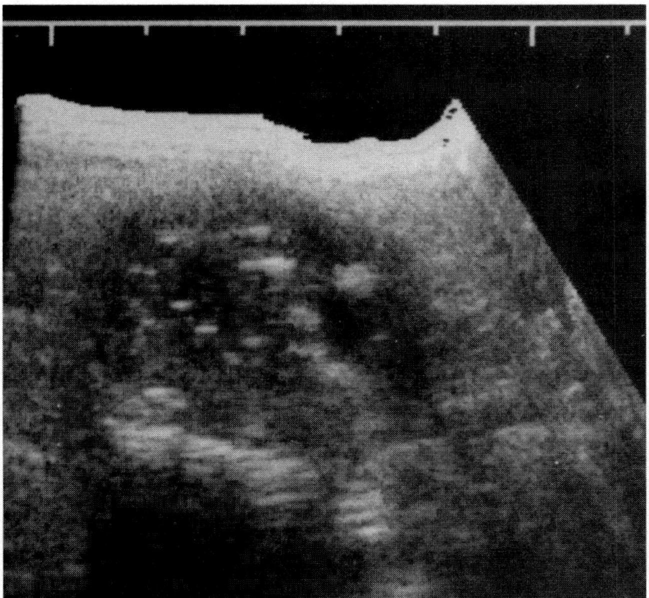

FIG. 11–49. Transverse static ultrasonogram of a canine prostate gland. Note the nonuniform echotexture with multiple hyperechoic foci and mixed background echotexture. The final diagnosis was prostatic carcinoma.

fection < normal < hypertrophy/hyperplasia or ? chronic infection).

2. Mixed echotexture (combination of focally increased and focally normal to decreased echogenicity) (probably neoplasia) (Fig. 11–49).
3. Focal to multifocal cavitations (> 1.5 cm in 1 dimension) (either cyst or abscess, ? cavitating tumor) (Fig. 11–4).
4. Differentiate solid from cavitating (far/distant enhancement) masses (e.g., distinguishing neoplasms from cysts or abscesses) (Fig. 11–50).

Prostatic sonography is highly useful in the staging of prostatic diseases, particularly neoplasms.[70-73] Prostatic ultrasonography is also useful in differentiating bladder from prostatic masses (primarily on the basis of their distribution). In addition, ultrasonography can be used to determine the relationship between caudal peritoneal and retroperitoneal masses and the prostate gland. Sonographic techniques facilitate staging disease relative to the prostatic portion of the urethra because distortion or enlargement of the hilar echo (central echo complex in the prostate gland resulting from the prostatic urethra and confluence of glandular tubules) is suggestive of urethral-related disease. Depending on the frequency characteristics of the equipment and the echogenicity of the surrounding prostate, this hilar echo complex may not be seen; thus, its absence is of no prognostic relevance. An advantage of prostatic imaging is its ability to determine the relationship of prostatic parenchymal masses to the prostatic portion of the urethra (Figs. 11–51 and 11–52).

D. Shortcomings of ultrasonography in the evaluation of prostatic disease. Unlike radiographic techniques, which can readily differentiate mineral from gas accumulations (depending on the resolving and contrast capabilities of the film-screen combination), ultrasonographic shadowing can be observed beyond both mineral and gas accumulations. This characteristic limits the utility of ultrasonography in finding prognostically relevant mineralization often associated with carcinoma.[56,71] Similarly, although parenchymal cavitations are relatively easy to identify with ultrasonography, one cannot confidently differentiate small- to medium-sized uncomplicated cysts from similar-sized abscesses based on the luminal and wall characteristics alone.[71] Therefore, cytologic and microbiologic procedures must be used on prostatic samples to facilitate this differentiation. Ultrasonography also has poor sensitivity for detecting and/or differentiating disease

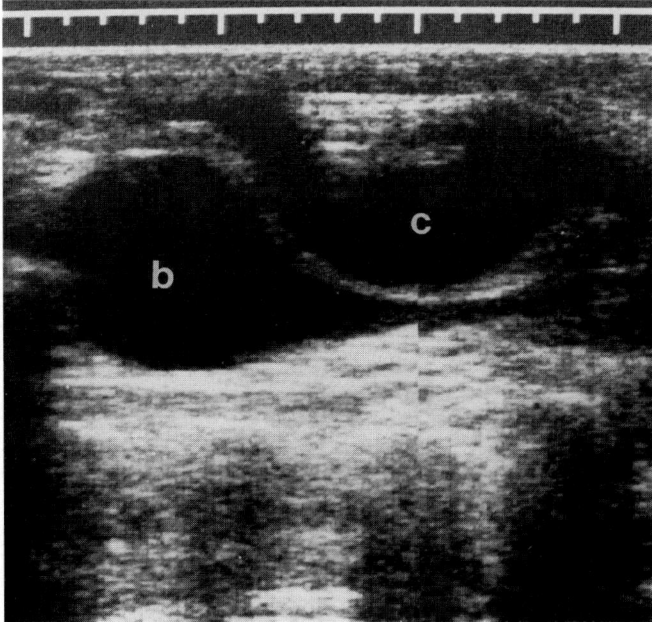

FIG. 11–50. Sagittal matched linear array real-time ultrasonogram of the bladder and prostate region of a dog. Note the two separate fluid-filled structures (the more cranial of which is the bladder [b]) leading into the prostatic portion of the urethra. The more caudal and ventral of the two fluid-filled structures (c) is a paraprostatic cyst that contained an echogenic mass in a nondependent portion. The final diagnosis was paraprostatic cyst associated with an undifferentiated carcinoma. Reprinted with permission from Feeney DA, et al. Canine prostatic disease: Comparison of ultrasonographic appearance with morphologic and microbiologic findings. *J Am Vet Med Assoc.* 1987;190:1027.

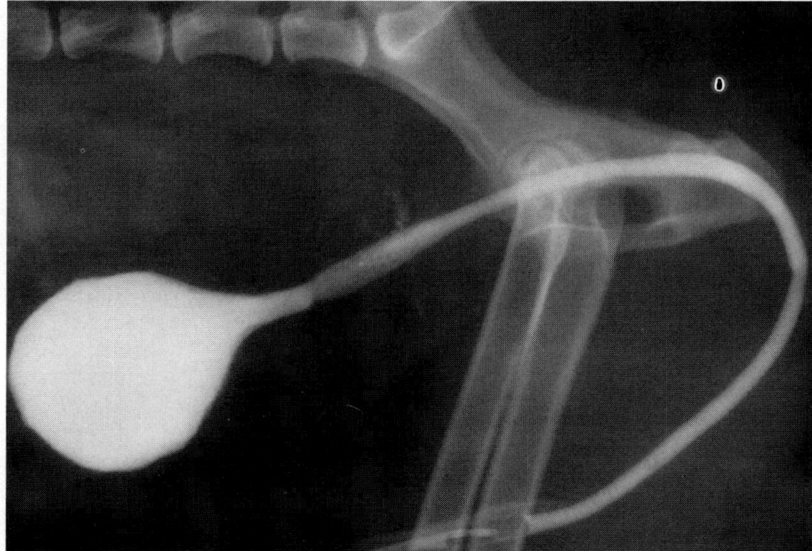

FIG. 11–51. Lateral view of the lower urinary tract a dog exposed during distention retrograde urethrocystography. Note the cranial displacement of the urinary bladder but lack of narrowing or distortion of the prostatic urethra. Urethral prostatic reflux is minimal. The final diagnosis was prostatic carcinoma without urethral invasion. Compare with Figure 11–52.

limited specifically to the urethral wall or the urethral lumen because of the unpredictability of the hilar echo complex.

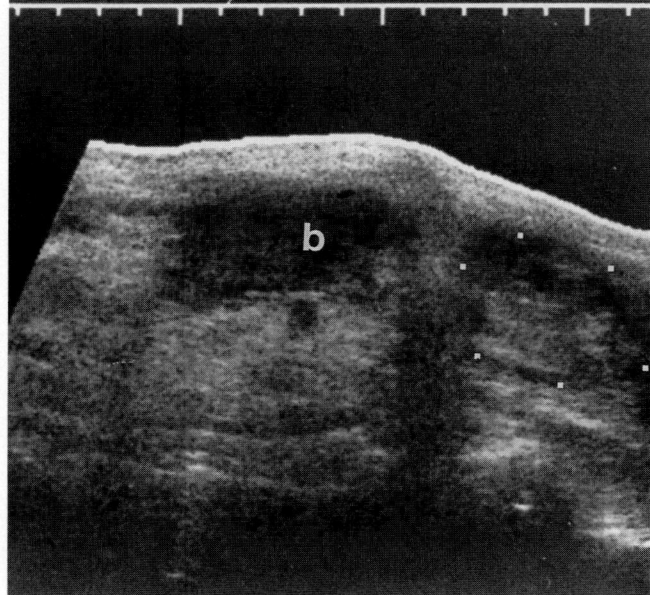

FIG. 11–52. Sagittal static ultrasonogram of the bladder (b) and prostate region (outlined by dots) of a dog in which amorphous echogenic material can be seen in the bladder. A mixture of normal and focally increased echotexture is apparent in the prostate gland. The final diagnosis was prostatic carcinoma; the material in the bladder was blood clots.

REFERENCES

1. Feeney DA, Johnston GR. The kidneys and ureters. In: Thrall DE, ed. *Textbook of Veterinary Diagnostic Radiology.* Philadelphia, Pa: WB Saunders Co; 1986.
2. Johnston GR, Feeney DA. Radiographic evaluation of the urinary tract in dogs and cats. *Contemp Issues Small Anim Pract.* 1986;4:203.
3. Johnston GR, Feeney DA, Osborne CA. Radiographic findings in urinary tract infection. *Vet Clin North Am (Small Anim Pract).* 1979;9:749.
4. Davenport DJ, DiBartola SP, Chew DJ. Familial renal disease in the dog and cat. *Contemp Issues Small Anim Pract.* 1986;4:137.
5. Lulich JP, Osborne CA, Walter PA, O'Brien TD. Feline idiopathic polycystic kidney disease. *Comp Cont Educ.* 1988;10:1030.
6. Feeney DA, et al. Normal canine excretory urogram: Effects of dose, time and individual dog variation. *Am J Vet Res.* 1979;40:1596.
7. Thrall DE, Finco DR. Canine excretory urography: Is quality a function of BUN? *J Am Anim Hosp Assoc.* 1976;12:446.
8. Feeney DA, Johnston GR, Osborne CA, Barber DL. The excretory urogram: Part 1. Techniques, normal radiographic appearance and misinterpretation. *Comp Cont Educ.* 1982;4:233.
9. Barrett RB, Kneller SK. Feline kidney measuration. *Acta Radiol (Diagn).* 1972;319:279.
10. Finco DR, et al. Radiographic estimation of kidney size in the dog. *J Am Vet Med Assoc.* 1971;159:995.
11. Feeney DA, Barber DL, Osborne CA. The functional aspects of the nephrogram in excretory urography: A review. *Vet Radiol.* 1982;23:42.

12. Kneller SK. Role of the excretory urogram in the diagnosis of renal and ureteral disease. *Vet Clin North Am (Small Anim Pract).* 1974;10:139.
13. Walter PA, Feeney DA, Johnston GR. Diagnosis and treatment of adverse reactions to radiopaque contrast agents. In: Kirk RW, ed. *Current Veterinary Therapy. IX.* Philadelphia, Pa: WB Saunders Co; 1985.
14. Feeney DA, Johnston GR, Osborne CA, Barber DL. The excretory urogram: Part 2. Interpretation of abnormal findings. *Comp Cont Educ.* 1982;4:321.
15. Feeney DA, Walter PA, Johnston GR. The effect of radiographic contrast media on the urinalysis. In: Kirk RW, ed. *Current Veterinary Therapy. IX.* Philadelphia, Pa: WB Saunders Co; 1985.
16. Olin TB, Rees DO. Renal function at urography with compression. *Acta Radiol [Diagn].* 1973;14:613.
17. Chambers JN, Selcer BA, Barsanti JH. Recovery from hydroureter and hydronephrosis after ureteral anastomosis in a dog. *J Am Vet Med Assoc.* 1987;191:1589.
18. Barber DL, Finco DR. Radiographic findings in induced bacterial pyelonephritis in dogs. *J Am Vet Med Assoc.* 1979;175:1183.
19. DiBartola SP, Myer CW, Boudrieau RJ, DeHoff WD. Chronic hematuria associated with renal pelvic blood clots in two dogs. *J Am Vet Med Assoc.* 1983;183:1102.
20. Johnston GR, Walter PA, Feeney DA. Radiographic and ultrasonographic features of uroliths and other urinary tract filling defects. *Vet Clin North Am (Small Anim Pract).* 1986;16:261.
21. Park RD, et al. B-mode gray-scale ultrasound: Imaging artifacts and interpretation principles. *Vet Radiol.* 1981;22:204.
22. Rantanen NW, Ewing RL. Principles of ultrasound applications in animals. *Vet Radiol.* 1981;22:196.
23. Feeney DA, Johnston GR, Walter PA. Ultrasonography of the kidney and prostate gland: Has gray-scale ultrasonography replaced contrast radiography? *Probl Vet Med.* 1991;3:619.
24. Christensen EE, Curry TS, Dowdey JE. *An Introduction to the Physics of Diagnostic Radiology.* 2nd ed. Philadelphia, Pa: Lea & Febiger; 1978.
25. Feeney DA, Johnston GR, Walter PA. Abdominal ultrasonography—1989: General interpretation and masses. *Semin Vet Med Surg.* 1989;4:77.
26. Konde LJ, et al. Comparison of radiography and ultrasonography in the evaluation of renal lesions in the dog. *J Am Vet Med Assoc.* 1986;188:1420.
27. Walter PA, et al. Feline renal ultrasonography: Quantitative analyses of imaged anatomy. *Am J Vet Res.* 1987;48:596.
28. Nyland TG, et al. Ultrasonic determination of kidney volume in the dog. *Vet Radiol.* 1989;30:174.
29. Walter PA, et al. Renal ultrasonography in healthy cats. *Am J Vet Res.* 1987;48:600.
30. Wood AKW, McCarthy PH. Ultrasonographic-anatomic correlation and imaging protocol for the normal canine kidney. *Am J Vet Res.* 1990;51:103.
31. Konde LJ, et al. Ultrasonographic anatomy of the normal canine kidney. *Vet Radiol.* 1984;25:173.
32. Poster RB, Jones DB, Spirt BA. Percutaneous pediatric renal biopsy: Use of the biopsy gun. *Radiology.* 1990;176:725.
33. Yeager AE, Anderson WI. Study of association between histologic features and echogenicity of architecturally normal cat kidneys. *Am J Vet Res.* 1989;50:860.
34. Barr FJ. *Diagnostic Ultrasound in the Dog and Cat.* Oxford: Blackwell Scientific Publications; 1990.
35. Cartee RE, Selcer BA, Patton CS. Ultrasonographic diagnosis of renal disease in small animals. *J Am Vet Med Assoc.* 1980;176:426.
36. Rosenfield A, Taylor F, Jaffe C. Clinical applications of ultrasound tissue characterization. *Radiol Clin North Am.* 1980;18:31.
37. Konde LJ. Renal sonography. *Semin Vet Med Surg.* 1989;4:32.
38. Adams WH, Toal RL, Breider MA. Ultrasonographic findings in dogs and cats with oxalate nephrosis attributed to ethylene glycol intoxication: 15 cases (1984-1988). *J Am Vet Med Assoc.* 1991;199:492.
39. Feeney DA, Johnston GR, Walter PA, Herring DS. Diagnostic ultrasonography: Veterinary medical applications. *Ultrasound Annu.* 1985;299.
40. Konde LJ. Sonography of the kidneys. *Vet Clin North Am.* 1985;15:1149.
41. Walter PA, Johnston GR, Feeney DA, O'Brien TD. Applications of ultrasonography in the diagnosis of parenchymal kidney disease in cats: 24 cases (1981-1986). *J Am Vet Med Assoc.* 1988;192:92.
42. Biller DS, Schenkman DI, Bortnowski H. Ultrasonographic appearance of renal infarcts in a dog. *J Am Anim Hosp Assoc.* 1991;27:370.
43. Konde LJ, et al. Sonographic appearance of renal neoplasia in the dog. *Vet Radiol.* 1985;26:74.
44. Barr FJ, et al. Hypercalcemic nephropathy in three dogs: Sonographic appearance. *Vet Radiol.* 1989;30:169.
45. Walter PA, Feeney DA, Johnston GR, O'Leary TP. Ultrasonographic evaluation of renal parenchymal diseases in the dog: 32 cases (1981-1986). *J Am Vet Med Assoc.* 1987;191:999.
46. Goldstein A, Madrazzo B. Slice-thickness artifacts in gray-scale ultrasound. *J Clin Ultrasound.* 1981;9:365.
47. Johnston GR, Osborne CA, Jessen CR, Feeney DA. Effects of urinary bladder distention on location of the urinary bladder and urethra of healthy dogs and cats. *Am J Vet Res.* 1986;47:404.
48. Johnston GR, et al. Complications of bladder distention during retrograde urethrography. *Am J Vet Res.* 1983;44:1248.
49. Johnston GR, Feeney DA. Comparative organ imaging: Lower urinary tract. *Vet Radiol.* 1984;25:146.
50. Christie BA. Vesicoureteral reflux in dogs. *J Am Vet Med Assoc.* 1973;162:772.
51. Feeney DA, Johnston GR, Osborne CA, Tomlinson MJ. Maximum-distention retrograde urethrocystography in healthy male dogs: Occurrence of vesicoureteral reflux. *Am J Vet Res.* 1984;45:953.
52. Biller DA, et al. Diagnostic ultrasound of the urinary bladder. *J Am Anim Hosp Assoc.* 1990;26:397.
53. Leveille R, et al. Sonographic investigation of transitional cell carcinoma of the urinary bladder in small animals. *Vet Radiol Ultrasound.* 1992;33:103.
54. Olson PN, Wrigley RH, Thrall MA, Husted PW. Disorders of the canine prostate gland: Pathogenesis, diagnosis, and medical therapy. *Compend Cont Educ Pract Vet (Small Anim).* 1987; 9:613.
55. O'Shea JD. Studies on the canine prostate gland. *J Comp Pathol.* 1962;72:321.
56. Feeney DA, et al. Canine prostatic disease: Comparison of radiographic appearance with morphologic and microbiologic findings. *J Am Vet Med Assoc.* 1987;190:1018.
57. Feeney DA, Johnston GR, Osborne CA, Tomlinson MJ. Dimensions of the prostatic and membranous urethra in normal male dogs during maximum distention retrograde urethrocystography. *Vet Radiol.* 1984;5:249.
58. Johnston GR, et al. Effects of intravesical hydrostatic pressure and volume on the distensibility of the canine prostatic portion of the urethra. *Am J Vet Res.* 1985;46:748.
59. Feeney DA, Johnston GR, Osborne CA, Tomlinson MJ. Maximum-distention retrograde urethrocystography in healthy male dogs: Occurrence and radiographic appearance of urethroprostatic reflux. *Am J Vet Res.* 1984;45:948.

60. Hornbuckle WE, et al. Prostatic disease in the dog. *Cornell Vet.* 1978;68(suppl 7):284.
61. Stone EA, Thrall DE, Barber DL. Radiographic interpretation of prostatic disease in the dog. *J Am Anim Hosp Assoc.* 1978; 14:115.
62. Thrall DE. Radiographic aspects of prostatic disease in the dog. *Compend Cont Educ Pract Vet.* 1981;3:718.
63. Barsanti JA, Crowell WA, Losonsky JM, Talkington FD. Complications of bladder distention during retrograde urethrography. *Am J Vet Res.* 1981;42:812.
64. Feeney DA, Osborne CA, Johnston GR. Vesicoureteral reflux induced by manual compression of the urinary bladder in dogs and cats. *J Am Vet Med Assoc.* 1983;182:795.
65. Mahaffey MB, Barber DL, Barsanti JA, Crowell WA. Simultaneous double-contrast cystography and cystometry in dogs. *Vet Radiol.* 1984;25:254.
66. Ackerman N. Prostatic reflux during positive contrast retrograde urethrography in the dog. *Vet Radiol.* 1983;24:251.
67. Park RD. Radiographic contrast studies of the lower urinary tract. *Vet Clin North Am (Small Anim Pract).* 1974;4:863.
68. Feeney DA, Fletcher TF, Hardy RM. *Atlas of Correlative Imaging Anatomy of the Normal Dog: Ultrasound & Computed Tomography.* Philadelphia, Pa: WB Saunders Co; 1991.
69. Nyland TG, et al. Gray-scale ultrasonography of the canine abdomen. *Vet Radiol.* 1981;22:220.
70. Cartee RE, Rowles T. Transabdominal sonographic evaluation of the canine prostate. *Vet Radiol.* 1983;24:156.
71. Feeney DA, et al. Canine prostatic disease: Comparison of ultrasonographic appearance with morphologic and microbiologic findings. *J Am Vet Med Assoc.* 1987;190:1027.
72. Feeney DA, Johnston GR, Klausner JS, Bell FW. Canine prostatic ultrasonography-1989. *Semin Vet Med Surg.* 1989;4:44.
73. Stowater JL, Lamb CR. Ultrasonographic features of paraprostatic cysts in nine dogs. *Vet Radiol.* 1989;30:232.

CHAPTER 12

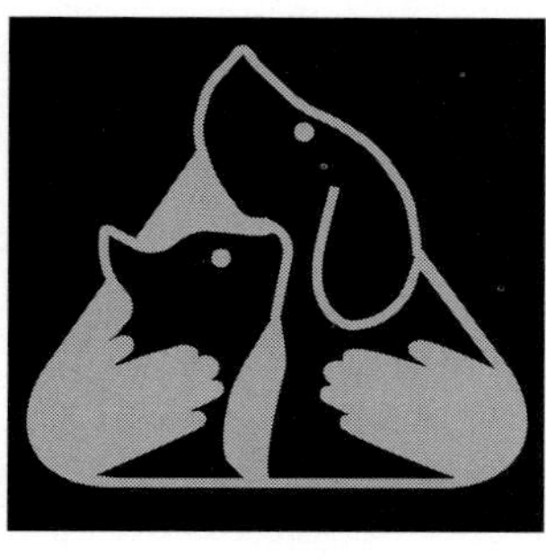

Canine and Feline Renal Biopsy

JOSEPH W. BARTGES
CARL A. OSBORNE

I. THERE ARE MANY INDICATIONS FOR BIOPSY OR FINE-NEEDLE ASPIRATION OF THE KIDNEY

A. Renal biopsy has evolved as an indispensable method of clinical evaluation of patients with primary renal failure because knowledge of morphologic alterations in the kidneys often provides a rapid assessment of the potential reversibility or irreversibility of the underlying disease process (Table 12–1; Figs. 12–1 to 12–4).[1-5]

1. To formulate effective therapy and establish a meaningful prognosis, one must differentiate renal failure caused by potentially reversible renal disease from renal failure caused by progressive irreversible renal disease.
   a. Detection of generalized renal diseases that are potentially reversible is justification for a guarded to favorable prognosis and vigorous employment of specific therapeutic techniques.
   b. Detection of generalized irreversible renal diseases may not warrant the same degree of effort and expense in treatment, and may be justification for establishing a guarded to poor prognosis.
   c. The reversibility or irreversibility of renal failure depends on the underlying cause.
   d. The distinction between potentially reversible and irreversible renal failure on the basis of clinical findings and laboratory data is often difficult because such findings are usually not sufficiently specific to establish a diagnosis other than the magnitude and duration of renal dysfunction.
   e. The clinical signs of uremia may vary from patient to patient, depending on the nature, severity, duration, and rate of progression of the underlying disease and on the presence or absence of predisposing or unrelated diseases.
2. Renal biopsy is indicated to confirm, support, or eliminate diagnostic probabilities formulated on the basis of the history, physical examination, radiographic or ultrasonographic evaluation, and laboratory data.
3. Renal function tests do not provide reliable evidence of the duration of the underlying renal disease or the likelihood of recovery from the renal disease.[6,7]
4. When renal biopsy permits establishment of a specific diagnosis, knowledge of the underlying cause of renal disease facilitates formulation of specific therapy and enhances the likelihood of accurately forecasting the probable future course of the disease process.
5. When the histologic changes do not indicate a specific diagnosis, the character and distribution of the lesions often allow one to determine whether the disease process is likely to undergo partial or

TABLE 12–1
ADVANTAGES AND DISADVANTAGES OF PERCUTANEOUS NEEDLE BIOPSY OF THE KIDNEY

Advantages	Disadvantages
Relatively noninvasive	Small tissue sample
Rapid technique	Sample may not be representative of generalized process
Good for patients who cannot be anesthetized	May not be possible to obtain a diagnostic sample of a focal disease process
Costly equipment is not necessary	Postbiopsy complications, such as hemorrhage, cannot be readily controlled

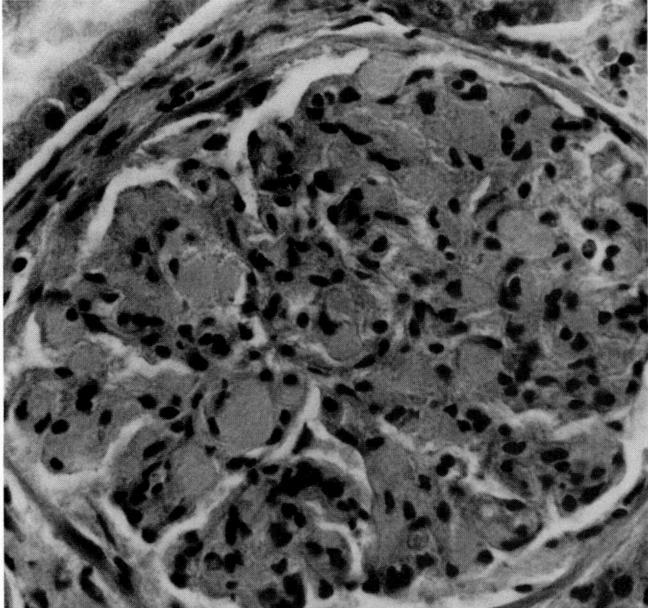

FIG. 12–1. Photomicrograph of a renal biopsy sample obtained from a 9-year-old male basset hound with oliguric renal failure of acute onset. All glomeruli contained in the biopsy sample contained massive quantities of amyloid and were similar in appearance to this glomerulus. This finding, associated with the presence of oliguric renal failure, indicated the irreversibility and progressive nature of the renal disease, and suggested the improbability of clinical recovery from renal failure. The dog died of renal failure 5 days after admittance to the hospital, despite intensive therapy to control renal failure. H & E stain. (Magnification, 1000×.)

complete resolution, remain static, or become progressive and irreversible.[8]

6. Serial biopsies of the kidney can be used to monitor therapeutic efficacy or progression of the renal disease.

B. Fine-needle aspiration biopsy of the kidney may provide useful information concerning the underlying disease process.

1. The primary advantage of fine-needle aspiration biopsy is technical ease and reduction in the incidence and severity of postbiopsy complications.
2. Fewer postbiopsy complications are associated with small-gauge aspiration biopsy needles.
3. The reduction in tissue trauma associated with fine-needle aspiration minimizes the admixture of peripheral blood with the aspirated sample.
4. The use of stylets to prevent contamination of biopsy material with cells from the skin is usually unnecessary when small-gauge needles are used.
5. Fine-needle aspiration is indicated when one suspects that a diagnosis may be established by microscopic examination of a few cells or of fluid obtained from the lesion.[9-16]
6. Fine-needle aspiration may be used as a screening diagnostic procedure.
7. A technique described for collection of well-

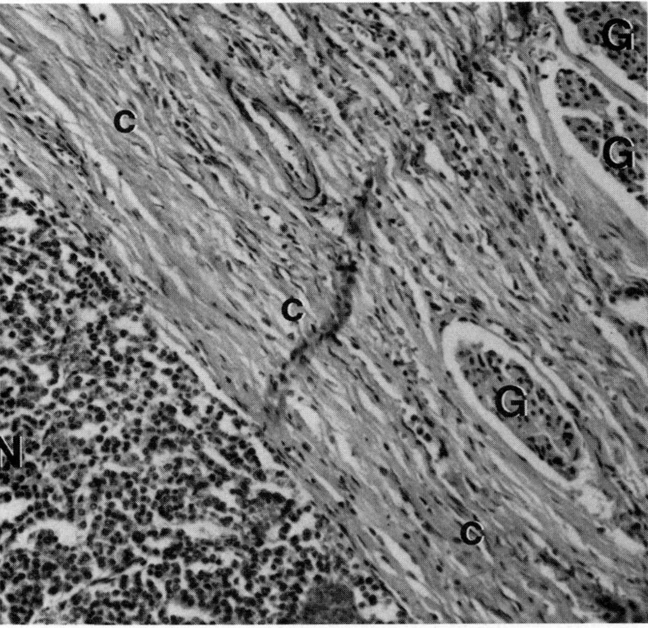

FIG. 12–2. Photomicrograph of a renal biopsy sample obtained from a 5-year-old female German shepherd dog. The only abnormalities noted by the owner were persistent hematuria and mild anorexia. Abdominal palpation revealed enlarged and asymmetric kidneys. Evaluation of survey radiographs of the thorax revealed findings consistent with metastatic neoplasia. Laboratory evaluation of renal functional capacity revealed no abnormalities. A diagnosis of renal cell carcinoma was established on the basis of microscopic examination of this sample. N = neoplastic tissue; C = compressed renal parenchyma adjacent to neoplastic tissue; G = compressed glomeruli. Hematoxylin and eosin stain. (Magnification, 400×.)

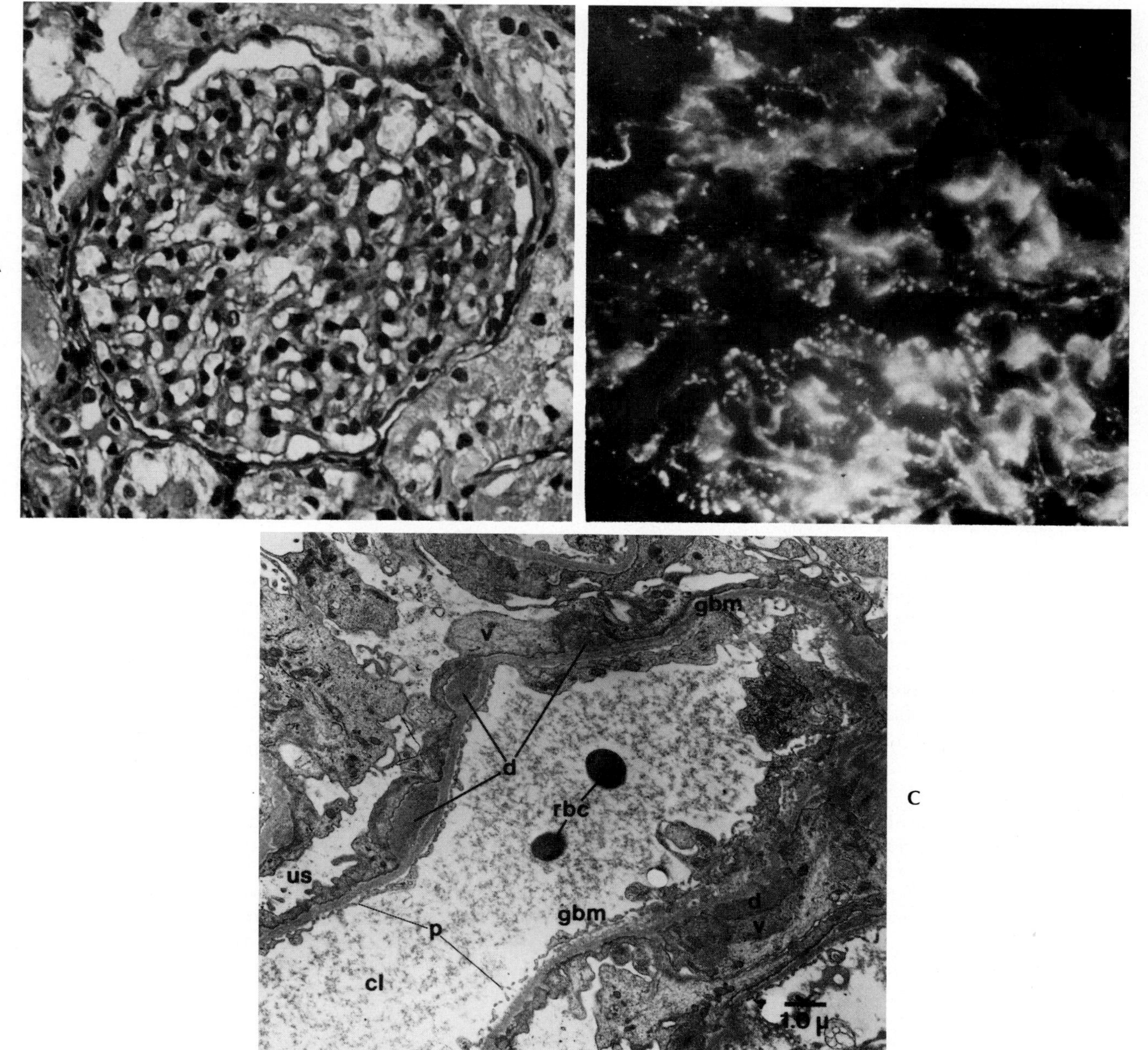

FIG. 12–3. A, Kidney biopsy sample obtained from a 2-year-old male German shepherd with the nephrotic syndrome evaluated by light microscopy. Generalized thickening of glomerular basement membranes and hypercellularity are evident. PAS stain. 2-μm section. (Magnification, 100×.) **B,** Kidney biopsy obtained from the same dog evaluated by immunofluorescent microscopy. Following staining with fluorescence labeled antiserum against canine immunoglobulin G (IgG), a diffuse pattern of interrupted glomerular immune deposits was detected in capillary walls and mesangium. (Magnification, 160×.) **C,** Kidney biopsy sample obtained from the same dog evaluated by transmission electron microscopy. Numerous electron-dense deposits (d), presumably immune complexes, are present in the subepithelial zone of the capillary wall adjacent to the glomerular basement membrane (gbm). Foot processes of visceral epithelial cells (v) are swollen. cl = capillary lumen; rbc = fragments of erythrocytes; p = pores in capillary endothelial cytoplasm; us = urinary space.

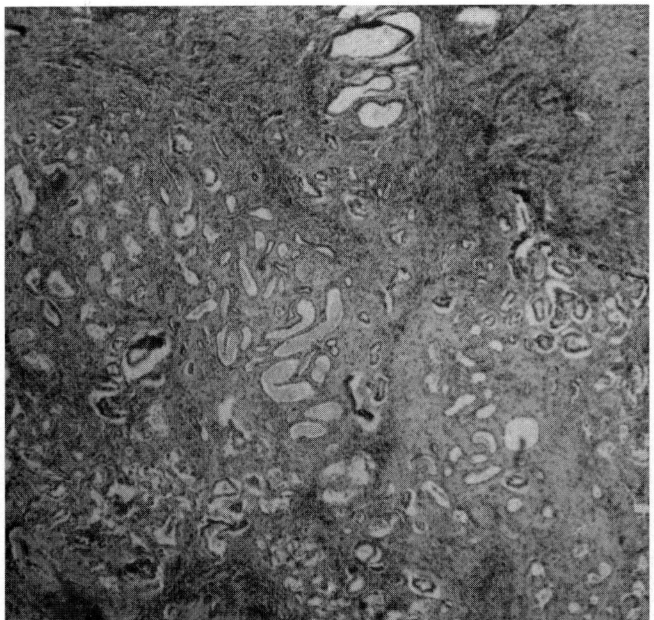

FIG. 12–4. Photomicrograph of a renal biopsy sample obtained from an 11½-year-old male mixed-breed dog with chronic renal failure. Microscopic examination of the biopsy sample revealed end-stage kidney disease of undetermined cause. Varying degrees of tubular atrophy and dilatation, interstitial mononuclear infiltration, calcification of basement membranes, and interstitial fibrosis are superimposed on compensatory hypertrophy and hyperplasia of a few viable nephrons. These changes indicate that the disease process is irreversible and, in all probability, progressive. Hematoxylin and eosin stain. (Magnification, 150×.)

preserved glomeruli from humans by fine-needle aspiration may be used in the diagnosis of glomerular diseases.[17,18]

8. Fine-needle aspiration is most popularly used as a means of detecting highly cellular neoplasms.[4,19-28]
9. If the results of microscopic examination of material obtained by fine-needle aspiration do not provide a specific diagnosis, other biopsy techniques that yield a larger quantity of tissue should be utilized.[29-31]
10. Fine-needle aspiration may be used to obtain culture material from some kidneys suspected of having infectious processes.[32-37]

II. CONTRAINDICATIONS AND DISADVANTAGES OF BIOPSY OR FINE-NEEDLE ASPIRATION OF THE KIDNEY ARE RELATIVELY FEW (TABLES 12–1 AND 12–2)

A. Excessive hemorrhage is one of the most serious potential complications following renal biopsy; therefore, patients with a hemorrhagic tendency should not be biopsied.[3,8,38-41]

1. Because uremia may induce changes in coagulation factor content and activity and in platelet number and function,[42] preliminary laboratory evaluation should include determination of packed cell volume, platelet numbers, activated clotting time, and, if necessary, other tests of hemostasis (such as activated partial thromboplastin time and prothrombin time).
2. Abnormalities in hemostasis should be corrected before biopsy is attempted.
3. If a hemorrhagic tendency cannot be corrected, biopsy of the kidney should not be performed.
4. The presence of hypertension has been associated with an increased incidence of hemorrhage and arteriovenous fistula formation in humans.[43-46]

B. Percutaneous biopsy of the kidney should not be attempted in patients with forced, violent, or unpredictable abdominal or thoracic movements.[47]

1. The kidneys are extremely difficult to localize under such circumstances.
2. Violent contraction of abdominal muscles or sudden unexpected movement of the rib cage while the biopsy needle is in the renal parenchyma may result in severe hemorrhage if the renal parenchyma and capsule are lacerated.

C. The rate of postbiopsy complications often occurs in inverse proportion to the experience of the individual performing the procedure.

1. Many biopsy techniques are not procedures that can be studied in a book the night before and attempted for the first time the following morning.
2. Prior to attempting biopsy techniques in patients, persons unfamiliar with the use of biopsy needles and techniques might gain experience by obtaining samples from animals at the time of euthanasia or from cadavers.
3. Careful attention to procedural detail is essential if adequate biopsy specimens are to be consistently obtained without serious risk to the patient.

D. Depending on the technique used, biopsy of the kidneys may substantially contribute to renal damage (Figs. 12–5 and 12–6).[48,49]

1. Varying degrees of ischemic damage and infarction, which occur secondary to vascular damage

TABLE 12–2
POTENTIAL CONTRAINDICATIONS TO NEEDLE BIOPSY OF THE KIDNEY

Uncontrollable bleeding disorders
Solitary kidney
Uncontrollable hypertension
Unilateral renal masses suspected of being neoplastic that may metastasize
Pyonephrosis
Renal abscess
Hydronephrosis
Small "end-stage" kidneys

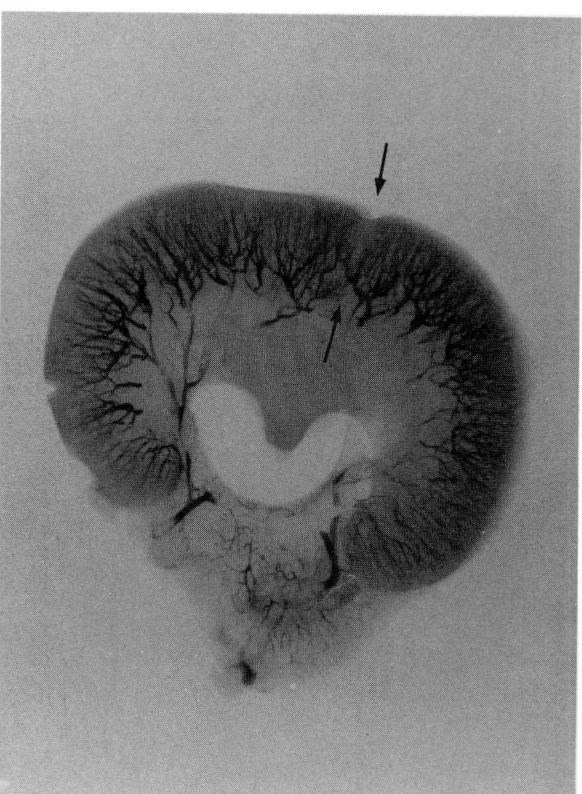

FIG. 12–5. Contrast angiogram of a section of a canine kidney biopsied 42 days previously. Damage to small renal cortical vessels resulted in a linear zone of vascular nonperfusion confined to the renal cortex (arrows).

induced with biopsy needles or scalpels, comprise a significantly greater portion of renal damage than that confined to biopsy tracts.[38,48-50]

2. The severity of damage caused by needle biopsy of the kidney depends on the size and number of renal vessels damaged.

E. A damaged needle is an absolute contraindication to needle biopsy because it may preclude procurement of an adequate sample and because repeated but futile attempts to obtain a biopsy sample increase the risk of postbiopsy complications.

F. Although nonobstructive pyelonephritis is considered by some to be a contraindication to renal biopsy,[51,52] clinical experience has revealed that renal biopsies may be performed in patients with this disorder without substantial risk of dissemination of the infectious process.

G. Although biopsy of the kidneys affected with hydronephrosis, pyonephrosis, or renal abscesses should not be performed with conventional biopsy instruments (Fig. 12–7), a fine-gauge needle and syringe may be used to aspirate a sample of fluid from such lesions for cytologic evaluation and bacterial culture.

H. A solitary functioning kidney may be considered as a relative contraindication for biopsy; however, if proper technique is used, biopsy of a solitary functioning kidney may be performed.[53]

I. Some diagnosticians consider severe uremia to be a contraindication to biopsy.

1. Uremic patients are poor anesthetic risks; in addition, coagulation defects may be associated with uremia.[42]
2. Extensive experience with renal biopsy in uremic dogs and cats indicates that they tolerate carefully administered and monitored anesthesia.
3. In one study, complication rates were not different between uremic and nonuremic human patients.[54]

J. Special consideration must be given to the anuric patient because bleeding after the biopsy may lead to clot formation in the renal pelvis and outflow obstruction.

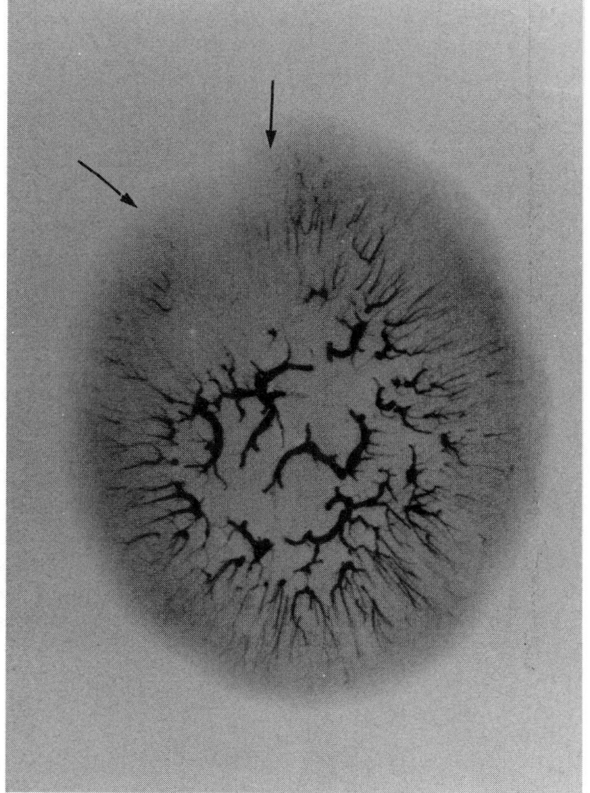

FIG. 12–6. Contrast angiogram of a section of a canine kidney biopsied 35 days previously. A large area of nonperfusion caused by needle-induced damage to larger renal vessels (arrows) is present above the biopsy tract. The biopsy tract could not be identified radiographically.

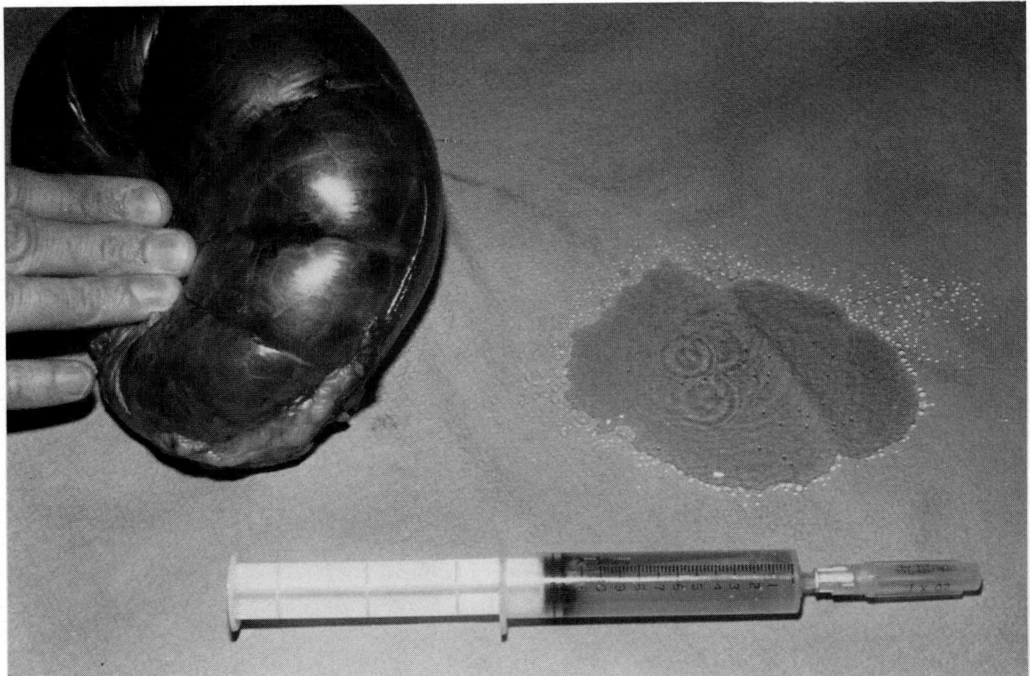

FIG. 12–7. Hydronephrotic kidney from an adult dog. Hydronephrosis was caused by outflow obstruction secondary to an ectopic ureter. Following aspiration of hydronephrotic fluid from the dilated renal pelvis, digital pressure applied to the kidney resulted in perirenal extravasation of substantial quantities of urine.

K. Animals that are prone to clot formation (such as those with antithrombin III deficiency associated with glomerulopathy) should be managed appropriately to minimize clot formation and obstruction. (See Section XIII of this chapter.)

L. Renal size is an important parameter when performing percutaneous biopsy.

1. Small contracted kidneys are more likely to bleed after biopsy because of increased likelihood of damaging large renal vessels.
2. Biopsy of patients with bilateral contracted kidneys is not likely to contribute to prognosis or treatment.

M. An objection often raised against needle biopsy is that it may induce metastases of malignant neoplasms by destroying natural barriers against neoplastic growth.

1. Neoplastic cell grafting along the biopsy tract induced by withdrawal of the needle from the neoplasm is a potential complication.
2. Experimental studies and empiric clinical observations suggest that this complication is infrequent.
3. Palpation and surgical extirpation probably impose equal or greater risk of neoplastic dissemination than that associated with needle biopsy.

N. Contraindications for fine-needle aspiration of the kidney are fewer than those for biopsy.

1. Although damage to the kidney by fine-needle aspiration is minimal, hemorrhage may occur, especially when the patient has a hemorrhagic tendency.
2. Evaluation of the morphologic character of a group of cells always provides information, but does not always provide a diagnosis.
   a. Because a small-gauge needle is used, relatively few cells may be aspirated and interpretation of microscopic findings may be exceedingly difficult.
   b. Fine-needle aspiration samples are of no value in evaluating diseases in which structural appearance and relationship are essential prerequisites to characterization of the lesions.
   c. Although a definitive diagnosis may be established on the basis of positive findings, tentative diagnoses cannot always be excluded on the basis of negative findings.
3. Considerable experience in the field of cytology is required.

III. FAMILIARITY WITH THE APPLIED ANATOMY OF THE KIDNEY AND ADJACENT STRUCTURES IS A PREREQUISITE TO RENAL BIOPSY (FIG. 12–8)[55,56]

A. Because the kidneys are identical pairs, either the right or the left kidney may be biopsied in patients with generalized renal disease.

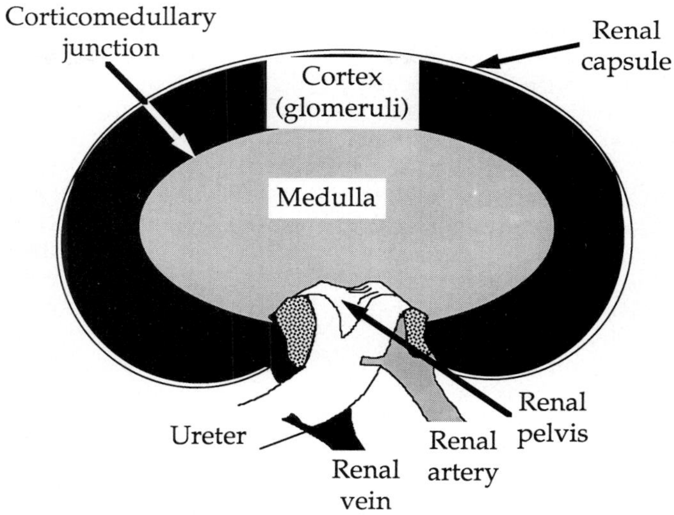

FIG. 12–8. Schematic illustration of applied renal anatomy.

1. The kidneys are retroperitoneal in position; they are covered with peritoneum on their ventral surface facing the abdominal cavity.
2. Each kidney has a cranial and caudal pole, a concave medial (hilar) and convex lateral border, and a dorsal and ventral surface.
3. The hilus is an indentation in the medial border through which the renal vessels, lymphatics, nerves, and the ureter enter and/or leave the organ.
4. The kidneys lie in the lumbar area to the right and left of the median plane.
5. A fibrous capsule covers the kidney; the firmness of the renal capsule can often be detected when a biopsy needle is introduced into the renal parenchyma.
6. The kidney parenchyma is divided into an outer dark-colored cortex and an inner light-colored medulla (Fig. 12–8).
   a. The cortex contains glomeruli and convoluted tubules.
   b. The medulla contains collecting tubules that unite to form papillary ducts, the foramina of which are visible on the medullary surface that faces the renal pelvis.
   c. Arcuate arteries are located at the junction of the medulla and cortex.

B. The kidneys of the dog are bean shaped and have a dark brownish-red or bluish-red color.

1. The position of the right kidney is as follows: the cranial pole lies at the level of the 12th or 13th rib in the renal impression of the liver; the caudal pole is opposite the 2nd or 3rd lumbar vertebra; it contacts the caudal vena cava medially; it is related to the abdominal wall laterally; and it is related ventrally to the descending duodenum and pancreas.

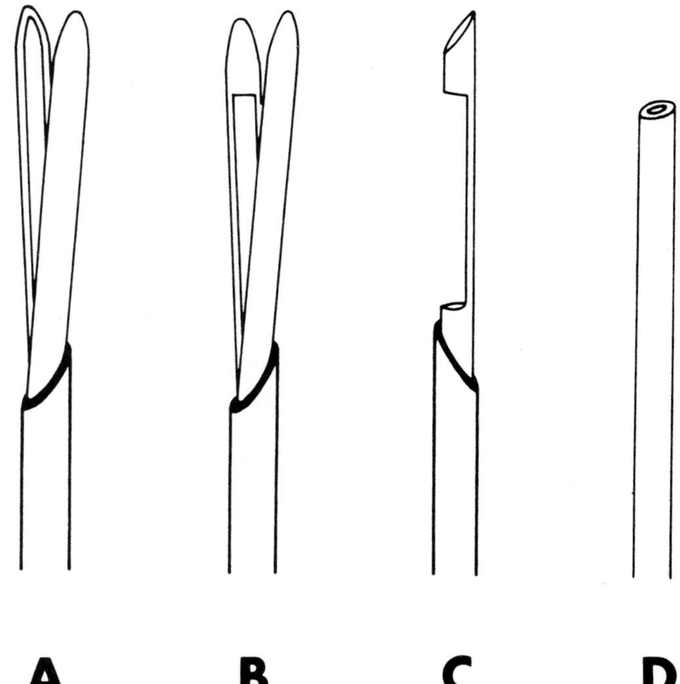

FIG. 12–9. Comparison of cutting portions of different biopsy needles. **A,** Unmodified Vim-Silverman biopsy needle with unsealed cutting prong tips. **B,** Franklin modified Vim-Silverman biopsy needle with sealed cutting prong tips. **C,** Tru-cut biopsy needle with specimen notch. **D,** Menghini aspiration biopsy needle.

2. The left kidney is less firmly fixed in position than is the right and has the following position: it contacts cranially the left lobe of the pancreas and stomach, when the stomach is distended; it is

related laterally to the spleen and abdominal wall; and it is related ventromedially to the descending colon.

3. Both kidneys may be palpated through the abdominal wall, although the right kidney is often difficult to palpate because of its more cranial position.
4. In dogs with generalized renal disease involving both kidneys, the right kidney is usually chosen for percutaneous biopsy or fine-needle aspiration because its anatomic position is more constant than that of the left kidney; however, the left kidney is often chosen for ultrasound-guided biopsy.
5. Unlike in some species, glomeruli are not within a wide peripheral zone of the outer cortical surface of the kidneys of dogs.

C. The anatomy of the kidneys of the cat is similar to that of the kidneys of the dog.

1. They are on the average 38 to 44 mm long, 27 to 31 mm wide, and 20 to 25 mm thick.
2. The kidneys of the cat lie more caudal in position than do those of the dog and are easily palpated.
   a. The right kidney lies ventral to the 1st to 4th lumbar transverse processes.
   b. The left kidney lies ventral to the 2nd to 5th transverse processes.
3. Because both can be localized and immobilized easily, either may be biopsied or aspirated with a needle.
4. The kidneys have subcapsular veins that make the cat more vulnerable to subcapsular and perirenal hemorrhage.[49]

IV. EQUIPMENT NEEDED FOR BIOPSY OR FINE-NEEDLE ASPIRATION OF THE KIDNEY MAY BE CLASSIFIED AS PUNCH BIOPSY NEEDLES, WIDE-BORE ASPIRATION NEEDLES, OR FINE-BORE ASPIRATION NEEDLES

A. Punch biopsy needles are designed to penetrate the kidney and to cut a core of tissue.

1. The Vim-Silverman biopsy needle was one of the first punch biopsy needles developed (Fig. 12–9).
   a. Vim-Silverman biopsy needles are 14-gauge punch biopsy needles and are available in lengths of 6 and 8.5 cm.
   b. Because the base of the tissue sample is not cut by the outer cannula, it must be removed by tearing the tissue sample from the kidney; therefore, the Vim-Silverman biopsy needle should not be used for biopsy of the kidney.
2. The Franklin modified Vim-Silverman biopsy needle (Becton, Dickenson, and Co., Rutherford, NJ, and V. Mueller Co., Chicago, IL) is a punch biopsy instrument similar to the Vim-Silverman biopsy needle; however, it is designed to completely isolate a plug of tissue (Figs. 12–9 and 12–10).
   a. The needle has three components: an outer beveled cutting cannula, a stylet with a matched point, and an inner cannula (cutting prongs) with a sample notch; Becton, Dickenson models also have a stylet for the cutting prongs.
   b. The Franklin modification consists of metal plugs (V. Mueller) or metal inserts (Becton, Dickenson) that seal the tips of the specimen notch on the inner cutting prongs; this modification allows the base of the biopsy specimen to be cut from the surrounding tissue.
   c. It is available in 3 lengths (8.5, 11.25, and 15 cm), the shortest of which is most satisfactory for use in dogs and cats.
   d. The Franklin modified Vim-Silverman biopsy needle may be used as follows (Fig. 12–10):
      (1). Place the biopsy needle with stylet against the renal capsule.
      (2). Remove the stylet from the outer cannula, and insert the cutting prongs; if the cutting prongs can be placed to their full depth without meeting resistance, the outer cannula is not in contact with the renal capsule.
      (3). Rapidly thrust the cutting prongs into the renal parenchyma; if the cutting prongs are advanced too slowly, the kidney will be moved a variable distance away from the biopsy instrument and the size of the biopsy sample will be reduced.
      (4). Grasp the hub of the cutting prongs with an index finger and thumb, and firmly hold them in this exact position.
      (5). Without changing the spatial relationship of the cutting prongs, advance the outer cannula over the blades; the outer cannula should be advanced just beyond the landmark in the shaft of the cutting prongs.
      (6). Care must be used so that countertraction is not applied on the cutting prongs while the outer cannula is being advanced into the kidney; if countertraction results in movement of the cutting prongs out of the kidney, the length of the biopsy specimen will be reduced or a biopsy specimen will not be obtained.[57]
      (7). Continuous altering rotation of the outer cannula 10° clockwise and then 10° counterclockwise as it is being advanced over the cutting prongs helps to prevent overpenetration of the outer cannula into the renal parenchyma.
      (8). Following movement of the outer cannula over the blades of the cutting prongs, the cutting prongs should be withdrawn back into the outer cannula for a short distance, and both should be removed as a single unit.
   e. The design of the Franklin modified Vim-Silverman biopsy needle does not allow one to

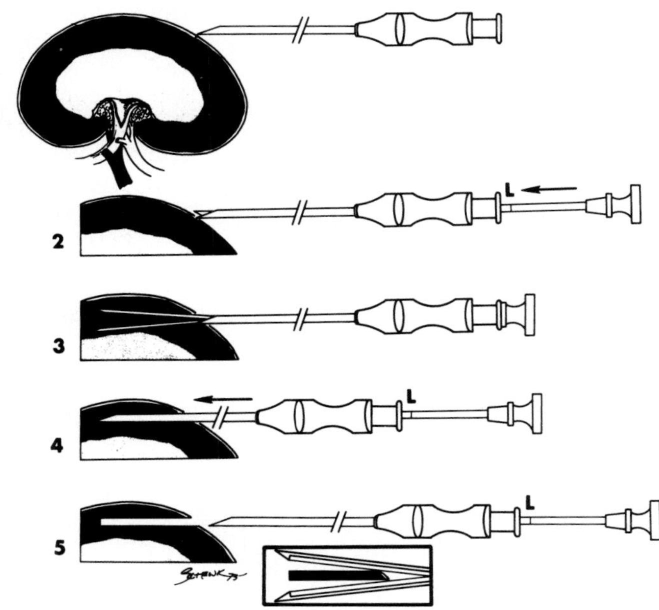

FIG. 12–10. Schematic illustration of mechanism of action of the Franklin modified Vim-Silverman biopsy needle.
1. The tip of the outer cannula with stylet is in contact with the renal capsule.
2. The stylet has been removed and replaced with cutting prongs.
3. The cutting prongs have been thrust into the kidney. The resistance imparted by the renal parenchyma has forced the blades of the cutting prongs to spread apart.
4. The outer cannula has been advanced over the cutting prongs, forcing them into apposition. The outer cannula has been advanced just beyond the landmark (L) filed in the shaft of the cutting prongs.
5. The outer cannula and cutting prongs containing a biopsy sample (insert) have been removed from the kidney.

determine the exact point at which the tips of the inner obturator have been covered by the outer cannula.

(1). Faulty technique may result in reduction of the quality and quantity of the biopsy sample or in overpenetration of the needle into the renal parenchyma.
   (a). If the outer cannula has not been advanced for a sufficient distance, an abnormally short biopsy sample or no biopsy sample will be obtained.
   (b). Overpenetration of the outer cannula serves no useful purpose and causes unnecessary damage to the renal parenchyma.[58]
   (c). Damage is not confined to the biopsy tract; its distribution is related to the size and number of renal vessels damaged.[48]

(2). To modify the Franklin modified Vim-Silverman biopsy needle so that one can determine the exact point at which the outer cannula covers the tips of the inner cutting prongs, one should scratch a mark into the surface of the upper portion of the shaft of the cutting prongs.
   (a). The exact location on the shaft of the inner cutting prongs at which the landmark should be placed can be determined by advancing the cutting prongs through the lumen of the outer cannula until the tips of the blades are just visible at the sharp end of the outer cannula.[59]
   (b). This modification does not physically limit the range of movement of the cutting prongs, and careful attention to procedural detail is still needed; however, it can be adapted to any conventional Franklin modified Vim-Silverman biopsy needle without use of special equipment or materials.

3. The Metcoff pediatric modification of the Franklin modified Vim-Silverman biopsy needle is a miniature replica of the Franklin modified Vim-Silverman biopsy needle.

a. The needle has four components: an outer beveled cutting cannula, a stylet with a matched point, an inner cannula (cutting prongs) with a sample notch, and a stylet for the cutting prongs.
b. Because portions of the needle are made of aluminum, it is lighter than the Franklin modified Vim-Silverman biopsy needle.
c. It is available in different gauges (14 and 15) and lengths (4, 5.5, and 7 cm).
d. The length of projection of the blades of the cutting prongs beyond the outer cannula (1, 1.3, and 2.2 cm) is shorter than that of the standard Franklin modified Vim-Silverman biopsy needle.
e. The Metcoff pediatric modification of the Franklin modified Vim-Silverman biopsy needle may be used for small dogs, cats, or patients with abnormally small kidneys.
f. The technique is similar to that for the Vim-Silverman biopsy needle.

4. The Tru-cut biopsy needle (Baxter Laboratories, Morton Grove, Illinois) is a 14-gauge punch biopsy needle (Figs. 12–9 and 12–11).
   a. The needle consists of an inner obturator specimen rod, with a cutting point and a trough (located behind the point to accommodate the tissue sample), enclosed in an outer protective cannula, which also has a cutting end; they are joined together by interlocking plastic handles.
   b. Tru-cut needles range in length from 10 cm (human pediatric size) to 15 cm.
      (1). The length of the Tru-cut biopsy needle may cause excessive damage from over-penetration of the kidney, especially in cats; therefore, the needle can be modified by shortening the length of the obturator tip (Fig. 12–12).[60]
         (a). The solid obturator tip is reduced by means of a rotary disc sander and is sharpened on an oil stone.
         (b). The original direction of the point is retained.
         (c). A hole is drilled through both sides of the T-shaped plastic handle at a position where only half of the specimen notch is exposed with the obturator extended.
         (d). A blunted 16-gauge hypodermic needle is then inserted between the 2 holes and is bent at a right angle to act as a barrier to further travel of the plastic-covered end of the obturator.
      (2). Tru-cut biopsy needles are less expensive, but much less durable, than the stainless steel and aluminum biopsy needles.
   c. The Tru-cut biopsy needle may be used as illustrated in (Fig. 12–13):
   d. They may be resterilized with ethylene oxide gas, but not by autoclaving because of the plastic components.

5. Automated punch biopsy needles are available.
   a. Some biopsy needles require the inner stylet with the sample notch to be advanced manu-

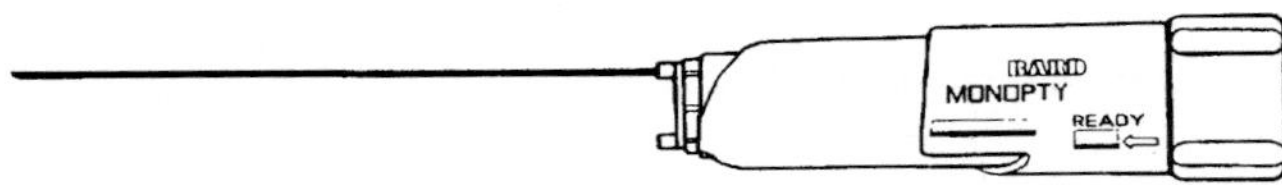

FIG. 12–11. Tru-cut disposable biopsy needle: R = plastic portion of inner obturator specimen rod; O = plastic portion of outer cannula; M = metal portion of outer cannula; S = magnified drawing (insert) of specimen notch in inner obturator specimen rod.

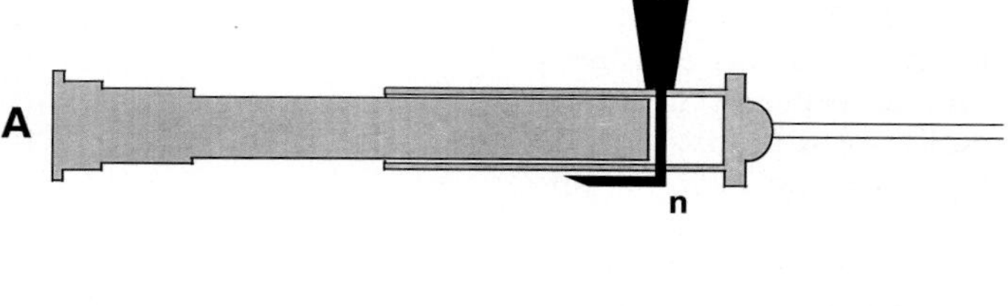

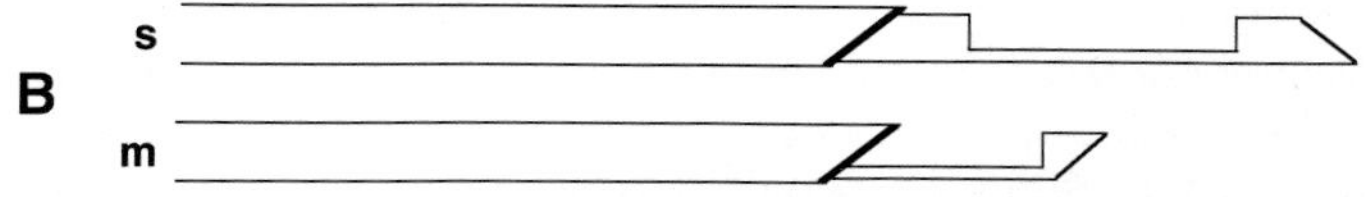

FIG. 12–12. Schematic illustration of Tru-cut biopsy needle modified for use in cats or dogs with small kidneys. **A,** Placement of 16-gauge hypodermic needle (n) into the outer plastic handle as a barrier to reduce the distance that the inner obturator specimen rod and thus the specimen notch extend past the outer cannula. **B,** Tip of inner obturator specimen rod modified to reduce its length. s = standard Tru-cut biopsy needle; m = modified Tru-cut biopsy needle.

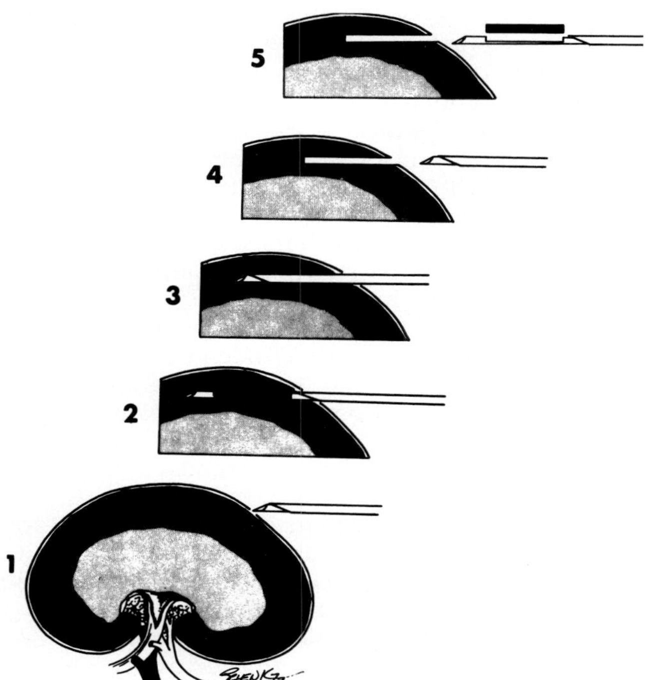

FIG. 12–13. Schematic illustration of procedure and mechanism of action of Tru-cut biopsy needle: 1. The tips of the outer cannula and inner obturator specimen rod are in contact with the renal capsule; 2. the inner obturator specimen rod has been thrust into the renal cortex; 3. the outer cannula has been advanced over the specimen notch in the stationary inner obturator specimen rod; 4. the biopsy needle containing a biopsy specimen has been removed from the kidney; 5. the outer cannula has been pulled back to expose the specimen notch containing a biopsy sample.

ally into the kidney; then a spring-loaded device activated by a trigger automatically advances the outer cannula over the stylet obtaining a core of tissue.

(1). The Roth biopsy needle (Cook Canada, Inc., Markham, Ontario, Canada) is available in 14 and 18 gauges and has been used for ultrasound-guided renal biopsy in humans.[61]

(2). The Cook biopsy gun (Cook, Bloomington, Indiana) is composed of a disposable biopsy needle and a reusable handle.[62]

(3). The Klear Kut biopsy gun (The Perry Group, St. Louis, Missouri) is available in 14 and 18 gauges.[62]

b. Some biopsy needles use a spring-loaded device that automatically advances the inner stylet with the sample notch and the outer cannula in rapid succession to obtain a core of tissue.

(1). We recommend the ASAP biopsy needle (Medi-tech, Watertown, MA), which is a single unit with a 17-mm Tru-cut needle-type specimen notch (Fig. 12–14).

(a). It is available as a single unit in the following sizes: 15-gauge and 15-cm length; 18-gauge and 10-, 15-, or 21-cm length; and 20-gauge and 15-cm length.

(1′). The biopsy needle is cocked for firing and is inserted through the abdominal wall until it contacts the renal capsule.

(2′). The spring-loaded trigger is pulled to obtain the biopsy.

(b). It is also available with a detachable handle and inner stylet with a length of 15 cm and 18 and 20 gauges for obtaining multiple specimens without removing the entire needle from the patient.

(1′). The outer cannula is inserted through the skin into the abdominal cavity until it contacts the renal capsule.

(2′). The inner stylet, which is attached to the handle, is inserted through the cannula and the biopsy is taken.

(3′). The inner stylet with biopsy sample may then be removed, the biopsy sample harvested, and the stylet replaced into the outer cannula to obtain another sample.

(2). The Monopty biopsy needle (Bard, Covington, Georgia) is a single unit and is available with 11- or 22-mm specimen notches, 18 or 20 gauges, and lengths of 10, 16, or 20 cm (Fig. 12–15).

(3). The Biopty biopsy instrument (Bard, Covington, Georgia) is composed of 2 separate parts, the cannula and the obturator, with a length of 16 cm and specimen notch of 9 or 17 mm, mounted in an automatic firing device (Biopty, Radioplast AB, Uppsala, Sweden).[63-65]

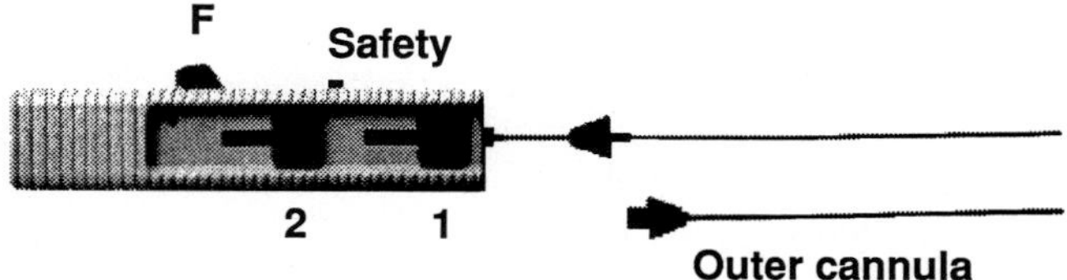

FIG. 12–14. ASAP biopsy needle. 1 = thumb tab that locks the outer stylet; 2 = thumb tab that locks the inner cannula with the specimen notch; F = firing trigger, which advances the inner cannula and the outer stylet in sequence to obtain a biopsy sample. The outer stylet is detachable, thereby permitting multiple biopsies to be obtained with one insertion of the biopsy cannula through the abdominal wall.

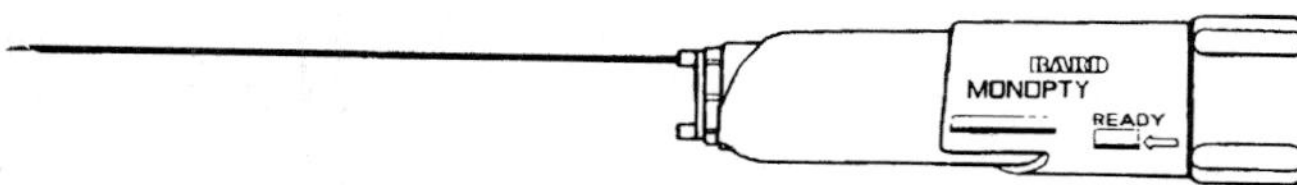

FIG. 12–15. Schematic illustration of the Monopty biopsy needle.

(a). The sample notch of the 18-gauge minicore needle obtains a sample with a volume that is 1/10 of the volume of the sample obtained by the Tru-cut biopsy needle.[63]

(b). The cost of the Biopty automatic firing device is approximately $2000; the biopsy needles are purchased separately and can be reused.

B. Wide-bore aspiration biopsy needles are available for sampling of vascular parenchymatous organs, such as the kidney.

1. The Menghini biopsy needle was designed to obtain biopsies of the liver, but it can also be used to obtain renal biopsy samples (Fig. 12–9).
   a. The apparatus consists of five parts:
      (1). A thin-walled needle with a beveled tip that is sharpened around the edge.
      (2). A sharp pointed trocar used to pierce the skin.
      (3). A biopsy stop (curved pin) to eliminate loss in handling and damage to the specimen by preventing the biopsy sample from being drawn into the cannula or syringe.
      (4). A fitted obturator for securing the biopsy stop in position.
      (5). An adjustable needle stop to control the depth of penetration.
   b. Menghini biopsy needles are available in gauges of 14 to 19 and in lengths of 4, 7, and 12 cm.
   c. The needle has a smooth outer leading edge with an inner convex edge designed to remove a core of tissue with minimal hemorrhage; however, the base of the sample is not cut from the surrounding tissue.
   d. The advantage of this needle is that less manipulation is required while the needle is within the kidney, making it easier to use and less likely to lacerate renal tissue.
   e. This needle has been used successfully in human patients with renal failure.[66]
   f. To use the Menghini biopsy needle, the operator advances the needle through the skin into the abdominal cavity with the trocar in place.
      (1). Once within the abdominal cavity, the trocar is removed and the biopsy stop is inserted.
      (2). The needle, with its special locking syringe filled with several milliliters of normal saline, is advanced down but not into the renal cortex.
      (3). One milliliter of saline is flushed from the syringe to clear the needle of debris.
      (4). The plunger is drawn back and locked, creating a vacuum within the syringe.
      (5). With a rapid in-and-out motion, the needle is advanced into the kidney and completely withdrawn.
      (6). The biopsy stop prevents aspiration of the sample into the syringe.
   g. A modified Menghini biopsy needle, the Klatskin needle, is available in gauges ranging from 15 to 19 and lengths of 5.6 and 10 cm.
2. The Jamshidi soft tissue aspiration biopsy needle (Kormed, Inc., St. Paul, Minnesota) procures a biopsy specimen in a manner similar to that of the Menghini biopsy needle.
   a. It is available in gauges from 15 through 19 and in lengths of 7, 10, and 15 cm.
   b. A specially prepared renal biopsy tray may be obtained from the manufacturer.
   c. The needle may be reused several times following sterilization with ethylene oxide.
   d. The needle has a uniform external and internal tubular configuration, except for the tapered distal portion.
   e. The interior diameter of the distal portion of the needle is tapered radically toward the cutting tip to prevent compression of the sample and occlusion of the needle lumen.
   f. Once the needle has penetrated the kidney parenchyma, suction is applied to the needle to draw a core of tissue into the needle shaft; the tissue is pinched off by the tapered end of the needle.
   g. The needle can be purchased with a syringe containing a notched plunger that can be rotated to lock the syringe in a vacuum position.
   h. A probe-like blocking device permanently attached to the syringe prevents the biopsy specimen from entering the syringe and aids in expelling the specimen from the needle.
   i. A needle guard can be broken off at predetermined levels to ensure the proper depth penetration of the kidney.

C. Fine-bore aspiration needles are used to obtain samples of body fluids or exudates or to obtain cell aspirates from organs, tissues, or lesions, such as tumors or inflammatory sites.

1. Fine-needle aspiration biopsy is defined as the removal of fluid, cells, or small bits of tissue from the body with a needle by means of negative pressure.
2. Hypodermic needles may be used for fine-needle aspiration biopsy of the kidney.
   a. Hypodermic needles of 22 to 25 gauge and lengths of 2.5 to 5 cm may be used to aspirate the kidney.

b. Hypodermic needles may also be used to aspirate fluid from cystic structures within or surrounding the kidneys; however, if the fluid is of high viscosity, a larger-gauge needle may be necessary.

3. Needles used for collection of cerebrospinal fluid or injection of topical anesthetics epidurally may be used for fine-needle aspiration biopsy of the kidney.
   a. Spinal needles are available in gauge sizes ranging from 18 through 25 and in lengths of 2.5, 3.75, 5, 6.25, 7.5, 8.75, 10, 11.25, 12.5, 15, 17.5, 20, 22.5, and 25 cm.
   b. The point on the spinal needles may be beveled 22, 30, 45, or 90°.
   c. Spinal needles are usually equipped with a stylet to aid in penetration of the body wall and perirenal tissue.
   d. The hub slot and cap guide of a spinal needle are aligned with the point of the needle to facilitate ease of orientation.
4. The Franseen fine-needle aspiration biopsy instrument is designed specifically for fine-needle aspiration biopsy of the liver, kidney, or other soft tissue structures.
   a. It consists of a 10-mL metal and glass syringe, a metal needle guide and finger ring, and fine-gauge needles (14, 16, 18, 20, and 22 gauge) of varying lengths (3.75, 11, 15, and 20 cm).
   b. The Franseen needle has a three-sided sharp point with cutting edges.
   c. The Franseen instrument allows puncture and aspiration with one hand, while the other hand is free to localize and immobilize the tissue or organ being biopsied.
   d. Although helpful, the metal and glass syringe, the needle guide, and the finger ring are not essential for the use of the fine-gauge needles.
   e. An adequate sample may be contained entirely within the lumen of the needle and not be visible in the syringe barrel.
5. Other fine-needle aspiration biopsy needles are available.
   a. The Turner biopsy needle (Cook, Bloomington, Indiana) has a sharp 45° beveled cannula.
      (1). It is available in gauges of 16, 18, and 20, and in lengths of 10 and 15 cm.
      (2). It is also available with an echogenic tip for ultrasound-guided biopsy.
   b. The Chiba biopsy needle (Cook, Bloomington, Indiana) has a short bevel.
      (1). The Chiba biopsy needle is available as a 22 or 23 gauge and in lengths of 15 and 20 cm.
      (2). It is also available with an echogenic tip.
   c. A thin "skinny core" biopsy needle, the Madayag biopsy needle, is available; however, compared to larger-diameter biopsy needles, such as the Tru-cut or Menghini, recovery of tissue with the Madayag biopsy needle is lower.[67]

D. Core biopsy and aspiration biopsy needles must be maintained in excellent condition if good renal biopsy specimens are to be consistently obtained.

1. All moveable parts should be examined prior to each use to ensure that they fit properly and slide with minimal resistance.
2. If excessive drag between components of biopsy instruments occurs, one may have difficulty determining when the cutting prongs (Franklin modified Vim-Silverman needle) or obturator specimen rod (Tru-cut needle) encounter renal tissue.
3. The cutting parts of all components must be sharp.
4. Biopsy needles often become dull after being used for 5 to 10 biopsies; therefore, they should be sharpened or disposed of if the blades become dull.
5. Needles used to obtain aspiration samples must be sharp; if the tip becomes dull, one should dispose of the needle.

V. PRIOR TO BIOPSY, THE PATIENT SHOULD BE EVALUATED TO DETERMINE RISKS AND BENEFITS OF PERFORMING THE PROCEDURE (TABLE 12–3)

A. In general, patients should be fasted for at least 8 hours prior to renal biopsy to reduce the likelihood of vomiting and bronchial aspiration that may occur with administration of anesthetics, sedatives, or tranquilizers.

B. Abnormalities in fluid and electrolyte balance should be corrected by parenteral fluid therapy prior to, during, and following biopsy.

C. Because hemorrhage is a major complication associated with biopsy, abnormalities in hemostasis should be corrected before biopsy is attempted.

D. Fine-needle aspiration of the kidney may be performed without sedation, tranquilization, or anesthesia; however, fine-needle aspiration should not be attempted in patients that are uncooperative or without adequate localization of the kidney.

VI. BIOPSY OF THE KIDNEY MAY BE PERFORMED WITH THE AID OF GENERAL ANESTHESIA, OR WITH SEDATION AND LOCAL ANESTHESIA; IN SOME PATIENTS, FINE-NEEDLE ASPIRATION OF THE KIDNEY MAY BE PERFORMED WITHOUT SEDATION OR GENERAL ANESTHESIA, BUT LOCAL ANESTHESIA MAY BE REQUIRED TO CONTROL PAIN AT THE POINT OF ENTRY OF THE NEEDLE THROUGH THE ABDOMINAL WALL

A. General anesthesia using inhalant anesthetics is preferred when biopsy of the kidney is performed utilizing the keyhole technique, laparoscopy, or laparotomy.

TABLE 12–3
PREBIOPSY EVALUATION

History and physical examination
- History of bleeding disorders?
- History of renal disease?

Laboratory evaluation
- Complete blood cell count and platelet count.
- Activated clotting time or complete testing of the coagulation system, including activated partial thromboplastin time, prothrombin time, thrombin time, fibrinogen concentration.
- Serum concentrations of urea nitrogen and creatinine.
- Serum concentrations of sodium, potassium, and total carbon dioxide.
- Urinalysis, including a quantitative urine culture with antimicrobic susceptibility or minimum inhibitory concentration.
- Urine protein/creatinine ratio or 24-hr urinary protein excretion if animal is proteinuric.
- Antithrombin III determination if proteinuric.
- Radiography, including intravenous urography and possibly ultrasonography to assess kidney size, function, presence of focal or diffuse disease, and ureteral obstruction.
- Arterial blood pressure.
- Other tests when indicated, such as immune panel, hepatic enzyme activities and function, arterial blood gases.

Discussion of benefits and risks with owner.

Appropriate preparation for biopsy, including withholding food for at least 8 hr prior to procedure, intravenous fluid therapy if indicated, and antibiotic therapy if indicated.

1. Inhalant anesthetics are preferred over most intravenous anesthetics in patients with renal failure because variables associated with drug metabolism and renal excretion are minimized.
2. Inhalant anesthetics permit rapid change in depth of anesthesia and allow rapid recovery following withdrawal.
3. Because medium- and short-acting barbiturate anesthetics are inactivated primarily by the liver, they may be used for induction; however, they are associated with systemic hypotension.
4. Other injectable drugs, such as opioids, benzodiazepines, or propofol, may be administered for induction of general anesthesia.

B. Injectable anesthetics or sedatives may be administered for quick procedures, such as blind or ultrasound-guided kidney biopsy, or for fine-needle aspiration of the kidney.

1. Opioids may provide satisfactory restraint and analgesia for most dogs.
2. Propofol provides short-term restraint; because it has little analgesic properties, it should be combined with an opioid.
3. Benzodiazepines may be combined with other injectable drugs to promote muscle relaxation and sedation.
4. In animals without renal failure, a tranquilizer (such as acepromazine) may be administered in combination with an opioid; however, profound systemic hypotension may occur.
5. Ketamine hydrochloride should be used with great caution in animals with renal failure because the drug is primarily excreted in active form in urine.

C. If the patient is severely depressed, local or regional techniques of anesthesia should be considered.[2]

1. Local anesthesia using lidocaine hydrochloride may suffice for profoundly depressed patients.
2. Local anesthesia may be combined with opioids, barbiturates, propofol, or tranquilizers for quick biopsy or aspiration procedures.
3. The greatest disadvantage to local and regional techniques of anesthesia prior to renal biopsy is that frequently the peritoneum is incompletely anesthesized.
   a. Penetration of the peritoneum is associated with forceful and unpredictable abdominal and thoracic movements caused by pain.
   b. Sudden movements seriously impair localization and immobilization of the kidney.

VII. BIOPSY OF THE KIDNEY MAY BE PERFORMED PERCUTANEOUSLY OR BY DIRECT VISUALIZATION VIA LAPAROSCOPY OR LAPAROTOMY; FINE-NEEDLE ASPIRATION BIOPSY OF THE KIDNEY IS USUALLY PERFORMED PERCUTANEOUSLY

A. Percutaneous biopsy of the kidney can be performed either with or without noninvasive means of visualization of the kidney.

1. The kidney may be biopsied percutaneously without image guidance.[8]
   a. Blind percutaneous biopsy of the kidney is easily accomplished when the kidney can be immobilized by abdominal palpation.
   b. Blind percutaneous biopsy of the kidney is technically easier to perform in cats because the kidneys are mobile and easily palpated.[2]
      (1). Surgically prepare the skin over the biopsy site and induce general or local anesthesia.
      (2). Localize and immobilize the kidney to be biopsied by digital palpation per abdomen.
      (3). Make a small skin incision over the biopsy site to facilitate entry of the biopsy needle.
      (4). Advance the biopsy needle through the incision and into the peritoneal cavity.
      (5). Position the tip of the needle against the renal capsule.
      (6). Direct the long axis of the needle away from the renal artery, vein, and renal

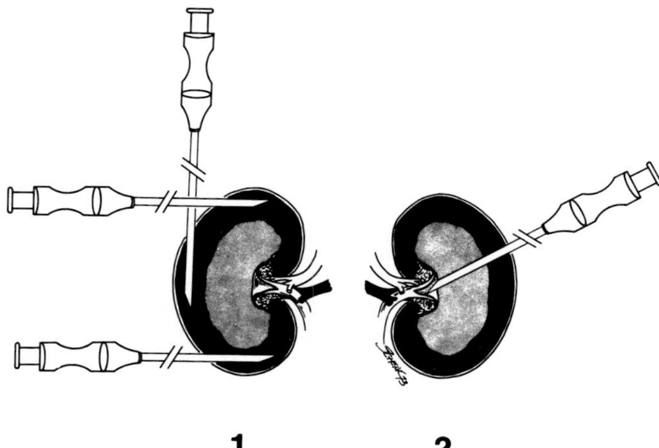

FIG. 12–16. Drawing depicting pathways of biopsy needle in the kidney. **1,** Several different pathways that may be used because they avoid the renal pelvis, renal artery, and renal vein. **2,** Biopsy needle incorrectly aimed and thrust into the renal pelvis.

pelvis to avoid damage to these vital structures (Fig. 12–16).

(7). Do not overpenetrate beyond the renal capsule; the quantity of renal cortex in the biopsy specimen will be inadequate if overpenetration occurs.

(8). Biopsy the kidney utilizing specific techniques designed for the needle being used.

(9). After the biopsy specimen is obtained, withdraw the biopsy needle.

c. Penetration of large thin-walled cysts or of markedly dilated renal pelves caused by obstructive uropathy may result in extravasation of fluid into the peritoneal cavity.

2. The keyhole technique may facilitate biopsy of kidneys that are not palpable, or may be used when image guidance is not available (Fig. 12–17).[2,8,58,68]
   a. In dogs, the right kidney is usually biopsied because its anatomic position is more constant than that of the left kidney.
   b. Although the left kidney may be more difficult to immobilize, it can usually be biopsied.
   c. The area over the kidney to be biopsied is surgically prepared, and general or local anesthesia is induced.

(1). With the patient in lateral recumbency, and with the animal's vertebrae facing the surgeon, an oblique paralumbar skin incision large enough to accommodate an index finger is made over the caudal pole of the kidney.

(a). The incision should be made just caudal to the last rib and just below the ventral border of the lumbar muscles.

(b). The long axis of the incision should be approximately equidistant between the last rib and the ventral border of the lumbar muscles.

(c). Care should be exercised so that the incision is placed in the correct location.

(d). If the incision is placed too far caudally or ventrally, the kidney may be impossible to palpate.

(e). If the incision is placed too far dorsally, dissection through a large quantity of vascular muscle tissue will be necessary.

(f). If the incision is placed too far cranially, the intercostal artery may be inadvertently transected.

(2). Bluntly dissect the underlying subcutaneous tissue, muscle, and peritoneum with sharp pointed tissue scissors.

(3). The intercostal artery located just caudal to the rib should be avoided.

(4). Insert an index finger through the incision and into the peritoneal cavity; palpate the kidney(s) and surrounding tissues.

(5). The size, shape, position, contour, and consistency of the kidneys should be evaluated.

(6). Make a separate incision in the body wall adjacent to the keyhole incision large enough to accommodate the biopsy needle.

(7). Guide the biopsy needle into the peritoneal cavity and then to the kidney with the index finger.

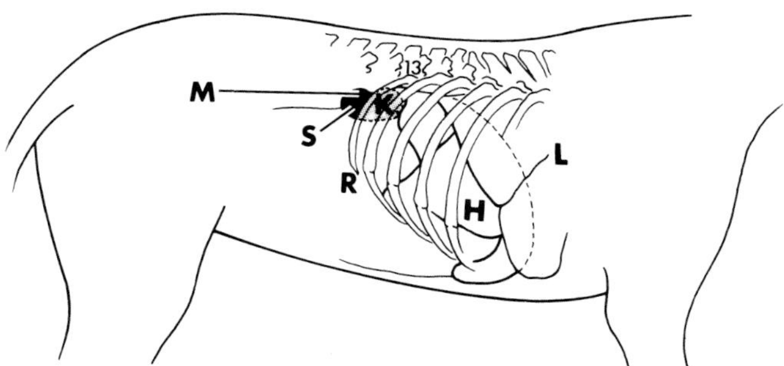

FIG. 12–17. Schematic drawing of landmarks for the keyhole technique of percutaneous renal biopsy. S = incision line in paralumbar fossa, which is equidistant between the caudal border of the 13th rib (R) and ventral border of the lumbar muscles (M). K = right kidney; H = liver; L = lungs.

(8). Immobilize the kidney by displacing it with the index finger against the body wall or other adjacent structures.

(9). Position the needle so that the exact route the cutting prongs will follow as they are thrust into the kidney can be predetermined.

(a). Direct the long axis of the needle away from the renal artery, vein, and renal pelvis to avoid damage to these vital structures (Fig. 12–16).

(b). Try to position the needle in such a way that the cutting prongs do not pass through the capsule twice.

(c). The tip of the needle should be in contact with the renal capsule.

(d). Do not overpenetrate beyond the renal capsule; the quantity of renal cortex in the biopsy specimen may be inadequate if overpenetration occurs.

(10). Biopsy the kidney utilizing specific techniques designed for the needle being used.

(11). After the biopsy specimen is obtained, withdraw the biopsy needle.

(12). While the needle is being withdrawn from the kidney, place the index finger adjacent to the shaft of the biopsy needle where it penetrated the kidney. Apply digital pressure over the biopsy site for several minutes; clotting may take from 3 to 8 minutes.[2]

(13). Prior to closure of the surgical wound in the abdominal wall, examine the operative area for the presence of excessive hemorrhage.

(a). In the event that uncontrollable hemorrhage continues, oxidized regenerated cellulose (Surgicel, Johnson & Johnson, New Brunswick, NJ) may be placed on the renal capsule over the biopsy site.

(b). If necessary, the keyhole incision should be lengthened to evaluate the renal biopsy site.

d. With the keyhole biopsy technique, one must occasionally displace the kidney for a considerable distance from its anatomic location to facilitate proper surgical exposure; however, doing so may compress the renal vein, resulting in congestion of peritubular and glomerular capillaries and erythrocytes in tubular lumens and Bowman's space.[57]

3. Biopsy of the kidney may be performed using ultrasound to help to guide the needle.[61,69-79]

a. Ultrasonography is an accurate, safe, and noninvasive method for depicting the kidneys.

(1). Ultrasonography can differentiate cystic versus solid lesions of the kidneys and is more sensitive than radiography in differentiating the internal characteristics of renal lesions.[80]

(2). The biopsy needle may be visualized and guided into the kidney.[61]

(3). Danger of radiation exposure to the patient or biopsy team is nonexistent.

(4). Postbiopsy ultrasonography may permit rapid detection of hemorrhage.

(5). Ultrasound-guided kidney biopsy may be performed using local anesthesia and sedation in animals that cannot tolerate general anesthesia.

b. The animal must be prepared for ultrasound-guided kidney biopsy.

(1). The hair over the ventral abdomen or the paracostal regions must be clipped, and sterile coupling gel is applied to the cleansed skin.

(2). The kidneys should be scanned in two planes, transversely and sagitally, to obtain information regarding their size, shape, position, internal structures, and determination of biopsy site(s).

(3). The left kidney is located by scanning approximately 2 cm caudal to the last rib (paralumbar fossa).

(4). The right kidney is located by scanning ventral to the costal arch of ribs 10 to 13 through the 11th or 12th intercostal space just ventral to the epaxial muscles.

(5). The renal cortex can be differentiated from the medulla because of its heterogeneity.

(a). The cortex produces more echoes because of the presence of glomeruli, tubules, and other cellular elements.

(b). The medulla is relatively anechoic.

c. A biopsy guide is attached to the transducer.

(1). Left and right biopsy guides with grooves that accommodate 14- to 22-gauge needles are available.

(2). Biopsy needles and guides should be sterilized prior to use.

(3). A sterile sleeve should be used to cover the transducer.

(4). Sterilized coupling gel is used to maintain contact between the transducer and the sleeve and also between the sleeved transducer and the skin.

d. Biopsy pathway guidelines that correspond to the needle pathway within the scanning plane of the kidney are electronically placed on the ultrasound screen, thereby allowing visualization of the needle as it passes into the intended biopsy site.

e. A stab incision is made through the skin with a scalpel blade to facilitate advancement of the needle through the body wall.
   (1). A second scan of the kidney is performed while the biopsy needle to be used is placed within the guide and passed through the abdominal wall.
   (2). The biopsy needle cannot be visualized until it contacts the capsule of the kidney.
   (3). During biopsy, the needle is seen as a bright image (echo) within the kidney parenchyma (Fig. 12–18).[81]

f. The kidney should be scanned after the procedure for evidence of postbiopsy hemorrhage and hematoma formation.

g. If substantial postbiopsy hemorrhage is suspected, its severity may be assessed by scanning the urinary bladder for hemorrhage and clot formation.[71]

4. Fluoroscopy may be used to help to guide the biopsy needle into the kidney.[82]
   a. A standard dose of intravenous contrast medium is given to visualize the kidneys.
   b. Once the kidneys are visualized, a radiopaque marker is placed on the patient's abdomen and is moved about until fluoroscopy shows that it is resting immediately over the intended site of biopsy.
   c. The biopsy needle is inserted at this point, and its progression toward the kidney is periodically checked with fluoroscopy.

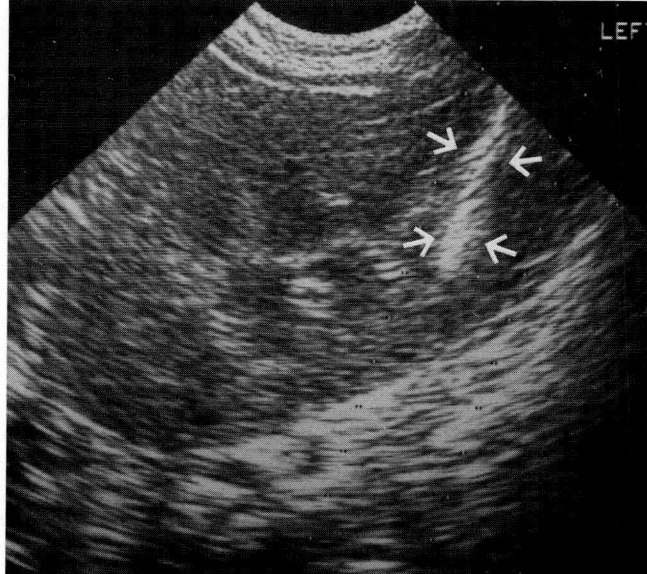

FIG. 12–18. Ultrasound image of right kidney of a beagle illustrates the tip of an ASAP biopsy needle in renal cortex (arrows).

   d. Once the needle is in contact with the renal capsule, the needle tip and the kidney appear to move in unison.
   e. The biopsy technique varies with the type of needle used.

5. Biopsy of the kidney may be accomplished using computerized tomography or magnetic resonance imaging; these techniques may be useful for biopsy of small lesions or for biopsy of lesions in multiple organs.[67,71]

6. Several studies to assess the effectiveness of renal biopsy utilizing different techniques have been reported.
   a. In one study of dogs, blind biopsy yielded adequate samples only when kidneys were pendulous and could easily be immobilized; otherwise, the keyhole technique was superior.[2]
   b. Similar results were observed in another study of dogs comparing the keyhole biopsy technique with the blind biopsy technique.[83]
   c. In one study of dogs, the standard keyhole technique yielded the highest percentage of adequate biopsy specimens; however, no statistical difference existed between specimens obtained by this technique and those obtained by modifications of this technique.[3]
   d. In a study of humans, diagnostic samples were obtained in 100% of the patients with an average of 3 to 4 passes using an ultrasound-guided Biopty instrument.[84]
   e. In another study of humans using ultrasound-guided Biopty instruments, 1.2-mm biopsy gun needles were superior to 0.9-mm biopsy gun needles (diagnostic accuracy was 69% for the 0.9-mm needle compared to 92% for the 1.2-mm needle); the difference was related to difficulties in guiding the 0.9-mm biopsy needle.[85]

B. Direct visualization of the kidney using laparoscopy or laparotomy may be considered for biopsy.

1. Laparoscopy, also known as peritoneoscopy or celioscopy, is a noninvasive technique that provides a view of the abdominal contents and peritoneal surfaces with a laparoscope; it is far less invasive than is celiotomy.[68,86,87]
   a. Only the intra-abdominal anatomy in the area of the laparoscopic entry point can be visualized; if the entry point is on the left, structures on the right side of the peritoneal cavity usually cannot be visualized.
   b. In addition to coagulopathies, contraindications for laparoscopy include: diaphragmatic hernia; cardiopulmonary dysfunction, which may be further impaired by distention of the abdominal cavity with air; massive ascites; and well-established adhesions formed between

the abdominal viscera and peritoneum resulting from previous surgeries or disease.[87]

c. For good visualization, the abdominal cavity is insufflated during laparoscopy.
   (1). Carbon dioxide or nitrous oxide is the gas of choice.
      (a). Carbon dioxide combines with water to form carbonic acid, which may be irritating to the peritoneum; therefore, more sedative or anesthesia may be needed with the use of carbon dioxide than with the use of nitrous oxide.
      (b). In the unusual situation when electrocoagulation is considered, carbon dioxide is the gas of choice because nitrous oxide supports combustion in mixtures with methane and hydrogen, which are gases that could come from the gastrointestinal tract.
   (2). Air should not be used because of the risk of embolization.
d. General or local anesthesia should be used to minimize discomfort to the patient and to provide adequate restraint for successful completion of the procedure.
e. Unless disease is present in the left kidney, entrance to the right side of the abdominal cavity and biopsy of the right kidney are usually preferred.
   (1). Because no large structures, such as a spleen, are on the right side, one is able to obtain an unobstructed view of the right kidney, as well as of other structures.
   (2). The technique for right-sided laparoscopy has been described.[68,86,87]
f. After entry into the abdominal cavity and prior to performing the kidney biopsy, abdominal structures should be visually evaluated.
g. Although some examiners prefer using a single-puncture technique whereby biopsy and surgical instruments are passed through the instrument channel of the operating laparoscope (celioscope), a double-puncture technique using an accessory trocar cannula unit is preferable.
   (1). For kidney biopsy, the second-puncture site should be in close proximity to the kidney.
   (2). The second-puncture site must be caudal to the diaphragm because pneumothorax from intraabdominal gas will develop if the diaphragm is penetrated.
h. Biopsies may be obtained from the kidney utilizing specific techniques mentioned in Section IV of this chapter.
i. If hemorrhage occurs following biopsy, the biopsy site may be compressed externally by pressing through the abdominal wall with a finger over the biopsy site.
j. After the completion of the procedure, the accessory trocar-cannula unit and the laparoscope are withdrawn from the abdominal cavity, the abdominal gas is removed, and the incision is closed.
k. Laparoscopic complications include air emboli, cardiac arrest, pneumothorax, damage to internal organs with the laparoscope or accessory trocar cannula, subcutaneous emphysema, and distention of a hollow organ with gas.[68,86]

2. Using an open surgical approach, biopsy of the kidney may be performed by taking a sample of tissue (core biopsy, wedge biopsy, partial nephrectomy) or by removing the entire kidney (total nephrectomy).[88-92]
   a. Prior to celiotomy, the number, size, and internal architecture of the kidneys should be determined.
   b. Total nephrectomy should be avoided unless absolutely necessary.
   c. At the time of celiotomy, a core of renal tissue may be obtained with a variety of different needle biopsy instruments.
   d. A wedge of tissue, 2- to 5-mm thick, can be removed for morphologic examination.[92]
      (1). The amount of biopsy-induced damage depends not only on the amount of tissue removed, but also on the number and size of renal end arteries that are transected.
      (2). The functional consequences of removal of this amount of tissue depend on the amount of function of the remaining nephrons.
   e. When excision biopsy is used as a form of treatment, partial or total nephrectomy may be indicated.[57,58,93-95]

C. Several novel techniques have been described for obtaining biopsies of the kidneys.

1. A technique of renal biopsy has been described using the transjugular route; it was designed for humans with clotting disorders in whom the percutaneous or open surgical route was contraindicated.[96]
   a. A transjugular liver biopsy needle, which is modified to prevent overpenetration into the renal parenchyma, is used (William Cook-Europe, Bjaeverskov, Denmark).
   b. Of 200 biopsies performed on 195 humans, transvenous renal biopsy yielded tissue in 88% of the attempts; the renal biopsy sample was diagnostically useful in 83% of these samples with an average of 10 ± 6 glomeruli per sample.
   c. Complications included nonsignificant perirenal hematoma formation (3%), clinically significant perirenal hematoma formation requir-

ing transfusions (1.5%), and macroscopic hematuria (7.5%).

2. A technique of transurethral renal punch biopsy in humans has also been described; the biopsy needle is advanced through the urethra, urinary bladder, and ureter, and into the renal pelvis.[97]

D. Aspiration of the kidney or renal pelvis may be performed using fine-bore needles.

1. Fine-needle aspiration (nephrocentesis) may be used to obtain culture material from kidneys suspected of having disease caused by infectious agents or to obtain dissociated cells from kidneys suspected of having highly cellular neoplasms.
   a. Fine-needle aspiration biopsies provide essentially no information concerning the structural architecture of normal and abnormal tissue; therefore, they are of no value in evaluating lesions in which structural appearance and relationship are essential prerequisites to characterization of the lesion.
   b. General anesthesia is usually not required to perform the procedure; local anesthesia, sedation, or tranquilization can be induced if the animal is uncooperative.
      (1). Localize and immobilize the kidney to be aspirated by digital palpation per abdomen.
      (2). Surgically prepare the skin over the aspiration site.
      (3). Advance a 22-gauge, 1½-inch needle attached to a 6-mL syringe through the abdominal wall and into the kidney cortex.
      (4). Apply negative pressure to the syringe to obtain an aspirate.
      (5). Release the negative pressure and withdraw the needle.
   c. If the results of microscopic examination of aspirated material do not provide information of significance in patients with clinical or laboratory evidence of renal disease or failure, a renal punch biopsy should be considered.
   d. In a study of four fine-needle aspiration biopsy needles, the Franseen needle produced the best yield.[98]
   e. Fine-needle aspiration cytology is commonly used for detection of renal transplantation rejection.[99]
   f. A fine-needle aspiration biopsy technique has been described for collection of well-preserved glomeruli; it may be used to aid in the diagnosis of glomerular diseases.[80]
2. Nephropyelocentesis is a technique designed to obtain urine from the renal pelvis percutaneously (Fig. 12–19).[100-102]
   a. Nephropyelocentesis may have clinical application in the management of upper urinary tract infection.[100,102]

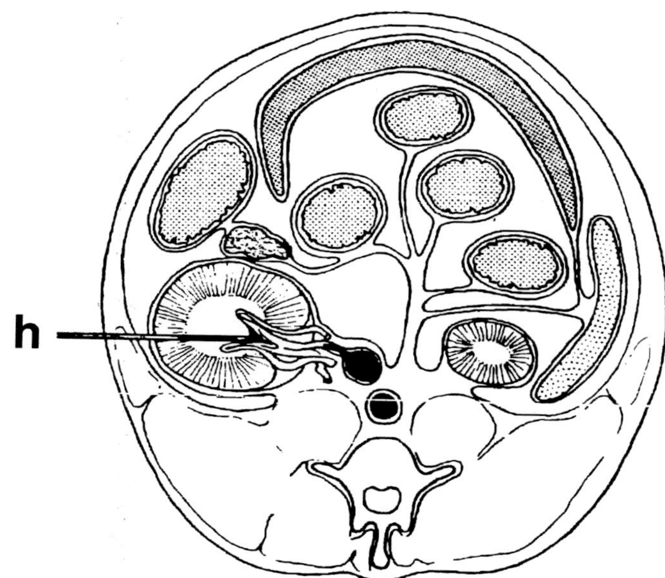

FIG. 12–19. Transverse section through the supine body of a dog at the level of the right renal pelvis illustrates the technique of nephropyelocentesis. h = hypodermic needle. (Reprinted with permission from Ling GV, et al. Percutaneous nephropyelocentesis and nephropyelostomy in the dog: A description of the technique. *Am J Vet Res.* 1979;40:1605.

   b. Patients should be anesthetized or heavily sedated and placed in dorsal recumbency.
      (1). The hair is clipped over the paralumbar fossa, and the skin is surgically prepared.
      (2). Fluoroscopy or ultrasonography may be used to guide the needle into the renal pelvis; if fluoroscopy is used, intravenously inject a standard dose of radiopaque contrast medium.
      (3). External compression of the caudal abdomen may be applied to partially obstruct outflow of urine, resulting in distention of the renal pelves.
      (4). Needles used in dogs may be 18 to 20 gauge in diameter and 7 to 15 cm in length; spinal needles, arterial needles, or hypodermic needles may be used.
      (5). The needle is introduced through the body wall until it contacts the lateral convex surface of the kidney.
      (6). With the aid of fluoroscopy or ultrasonography, the needle is positioned so that it is halfway between the cranial and caudal poles of the kidney; the needle is then advanced through the renal parenchyma into the renal pelvis, and urine is aspirated into a syringe.
   c. The urine sample obtained from the renal

TABLE 12–4
COMPLICATIONS OF RENAL BIOPSY

Hemorrhage
- Renal
  - Gross hematuria
  - Perinephric hematoma
  - Intrarenal hematoma
  - Retroperitoneal hematoma
  - Lacerated renal artery or vein
  - Laceration of ureter
  - Obstructon of renal pelvis or ureters with blood clots
- Nonrenal
  - Lacerated liver, spleen, or extrarenal artery or vein
  - Blood clots in urinary bladder

Inadequate biopsy
- Nonrenal tissue
  - Liver, pancreas, spleen, fat, muscle, bowel, adrenal gland, connective tissue, stomach
- Renal medulla
- No tissue

Perforation of hollow organ
- Bowel, gallbladder, lung, renal pelvis, or ureter

Infection
- Renal
- Perirenal
- Peritoneal
- Disseminated

Arteriovenous fistula
- Intrarenal
- Extrarenal

Miscellaneous
- Pain
- Ileus
- Fever
- Pancreatitis

pelvis may be cultured for infectious agents and/or examined microscopically.

VIII. FOLLOWING RENAL BIOPSY, PATIENTS SHOULD BE MONITORED (TABLE 12–4)

A. The most serious complication following renal biopsy of the dog and cat has been severe hemorrhage.[2,38]

1. Excessive hemorrhage almost always occurs as a result of faulty technique rather than as a result of the type of renal disease present.[38]
2. Unless postbiopsy hemorrhage is life threatening, a conservative course of therapy is usually indicated.
3. Perirenal hematomas have usually subsided without therapy, but blood transfusions have been given on occasion.[103-106]
4. In dogs and cats, whole blood transfusions control most serious bleeding problems in the event that they occur.
5. Most animals recover from perirenal hemorrhage without a blood transfusion if the packed cell volume does not decrease to less than 20%.[107]
6. In a study of 70 ultrasound-guided kidney biopsies, 5 patients had minor perirenal hemorrhage.[107]

B. Hematuria is a common finding following kidney biopsy.

1. Self-limiting microscopic hematuria usually occurs for 12 hours to 3 days in almost all patients following biopsy.[2,38,68]
2. Self-limiting gross hematuria has been observed in approximately 3% of dogs following renal biopsy.[2,68]
3. Uncommonly, blood clots that form in the renal pelvis may obstruct urine outflow and cause hydronephrosis.[2,38]
4. Hydronephrosis has been reported to occur in 4% of cases (Fig. 12–20).[38]
5. Parenteral administration of a sufficient quantity of lactated Ringer's solution to initiate a mild diuresis prior, during, or immediately following renal biopsy is usually effective in preventing the formation of blood clots in the excretory pathway.[8]

C. Excessive manipulation of the biopsied kidney should be avoided for a short time following completion of the procedure so that the clot at the biopsy site is not disturbed.

D. Depending on the technique used, biopsy of the kidneys may substantially contribute to renal damage (Figs. 12–5 and 12–6).[48,49]

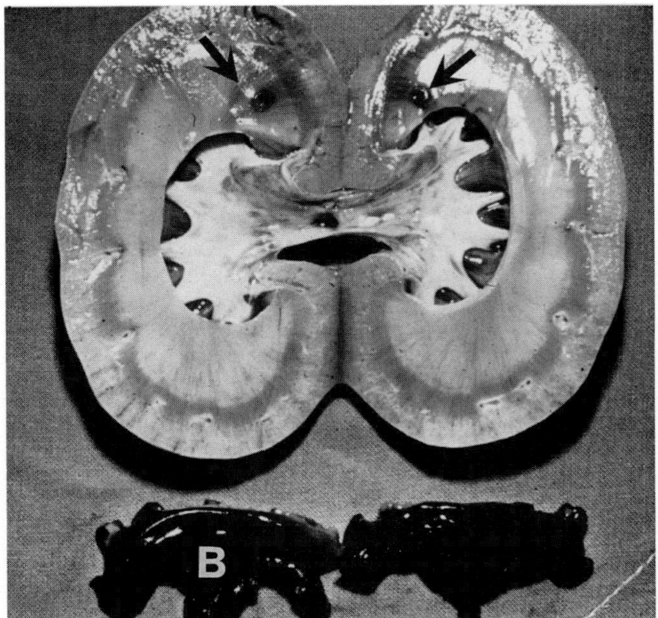

FIG. 12–20. Obstructing blood clot (B) removed from the dilated renal pelvis of a 7.5-year-old mixed-breed dog. A renal punch biopsy was obtained 8 days previously. The biopsy tract is visible in the renal medulla (arrows). Light microscopy of the kidney revealed chronic membranous glomerulonephritis.

1. Varying degrees of ischemic damage and infarction, which occur secondary to vascular damage induced with biopsy needles or scalpels, comprise a significantly greater portion of renal damage than that confined to biopsy tracts.[38,48-50]
2. The severity of damage caused by needle biopsy of the kidney depends on the size and number of renal vessels damaged.

E. Antibiotics are not essential if aseptic technique is maintained.

1. Antibiotics may be administered to debilitated patients or animals with infectious processes of the kidneys.
2. If the patient is in renal failure, antibiotics that are potentially nephrotoxic should be avoided.

F. Because of the small size of the needle, fine-needle aspiration of the kidney is usually not associated with serious complications.

1. Damage to the renal parenchyma is usually minimal; however, hemorrhage may be severe if laceration of an arcuate artery or of a renal artery or vein occurs.
2. Extravasation of urine into adjacent structures may occur through large thin-walled cystic structures or severely hydronephrotic kidneys; it may also occur if the renal pelvis or ureter is damaged by the needle (Fig. 12–7).

IX. EVALUATION OF RENAL BIOPSY SPECIMENS OR ASPIRATION SAMPLES IS INFLUENCED BY THEIR HANDLING, PROCESSING, AND STAINING[108]

A. Following removal of the biopsy specimen from the patient, great care must be used to prevent damage to the sample.

1. Biopsy samples should reach the fixative in the shortest time possible to inactive autolytic enzymes.
   a. The tissue must be handled delicately to avoid crushing or tearing portions of the specimen.
   b. Forceps should never be used to handle core biopsy specimens.
   c. If tissue cores obtained by needle biopsy are cut into smaller pieces to enhance fixation, they must be cut with a sharp blade using a slicing, rather than a crushing, motion.
   d. An adequate core biopsy sample should contain glomeruli that can be recognized with a small dissecting microscope or hand lens as tiny reddish structures of less than 1 mm in diameter.
   e. Two or three core biopsy samples should be obtained for light microscopy, immunofluorescence microscopy, and possibly transmission or scanning electron microscopy.
   f. If only one large core of tissue is available, it may be gently bisected longitudinally.
      (1). One half can be processed for light microscopy.
      (2). The second fragment is transected vertically, one half being used for immunofluorescence microscopy and one half for electron microscopy.
   g. Specimens obtained by wedge biopsy, partial nephrectomy, or total nephrectomy should be sectioned with a sharp blade and processed for light microscopy, fluorescence microscopy, and/or electron microscopy.
   h. If bacterial infection is suspected, a portion of the biopsy sample may be placed in culture medium; however, do not place the sample in the fixative first because the fixative rapidly sterilizes the sample.
2. After obtaining biopsy samples, the tissue must be placed in a fixative to prevent autolysis.
   a. Fixation is a process whereby a given cellular structure or activity is preserved or stabilized, often at the expense of other structures, for subsequent viewing with a microscope.
      (1). Fixatives prevent autolysis by inactivating enzymes.
      (2). Fixatives facilitate sectioning of tissues by hardening them.
      (3). Fixatives enhance staining by acting as a mordant.
      (4). Fixatives stabilize structural components in as near in vivo conditions as possible.
   b. Fixation is most commonly achieved by immersing the tissue in a solution of chemicals, but it may be accomplished by physical means, such as heat denaturation, freezing, or air drying.
      (1). Frequently used fixatives for light microscopy include 10% neutral buffered formalin, Zenker-formol, paraformaldehyde, and Bouin's solution.
         (a). Ten percent neutral buffered formalin preserves tissues indefinitely.
            (1′). It is prepared by adding 9 volumes of tap water or phosphate-buffered water to 1 volume of commercial formalin (40% w/v), and adding 10 g of calcium carbonate or bicarbonate to each gallon.
            (2′). A formalin fixation time of 2 to 4 hours has been recommended as ideal for the preparation of thin sections from renal punch biopsy sections.
            (3′). If thin sections are desired, a long fixation time should be avoided as it may cause the specimen to become brittle and may prevent satisfactory preparation of thin sections.
            (4′). A punch needle biopsy sample requires a minimum of 1 hour fixation.

(5′). For samples of larger size, formalin fixation is usually achieved within 24 hours.

(b). Paraformaldehyde may be used for both light microscopy and electron microscopy.

(2). Biopsy samples for immunofluorescence should be "snap frozen" in liquid nitrogen or fixed in Michel's solution.

(a). For snap freezing, isopentane chilled to approximately −70°C should be used.

(1′). Biopsy samples are laid flat on a saline-soaked sponge, placed in a tightly sealed container of isopentane, and immersed in liquid nitrogen.

(2′). After the tissue has been properly snap frozen, it may be stored at −70°C.

(3′). Storage for periods exceeding 4 to 6 weeks may result in desiccation, rendering the tissue uninterpretable.[108]

(4′). Snap freezing should never be used as a method of fixation for light or electron microscopy because the formation of intracellular ice crystals disrupts cell structure.

(b). Biopsy samples fixed in Michel's solution do not need to be frozen.

(1′). Michel's solution contains ammonium sulfate, N-ethyl maleimide, and magnesium sulfate in citrate buffer.

(2′). The fixative may be prepared by dissolving 55 g of ammonium sulfate in 100 mL of buffer.

(3′). The buffer is prepared by adding 2.5 mL of 1 mol/L potassium citrate buffer (pH 7), 5 mL of 1 mol/L magnesium sulfate, and 5 mL of 0.1 mol/L N-ethyl maleimide to 87.5 mL of distilled water.

(3). Three percent phosphate-buffered glutaraldehyde is a widely used fixative for electron microscopy.

(a). It is prepared from a stock solution of 25% glutaraldehyde.

(b). The diluted solution has a shelf life of no more than 2 months.

(c). At room temperature, 3% glutaraldehyde deteriorates within a few hours.

(d). Samples stored in glutaraldehyde may be refrigerated, but should not be frozen.

(4). Carson's fixative (4% formaldehyde and 1% glutaraldehyde) is an alternative fixative that is available commercially.

(5). Fixatives containing glutaraldehyde are not appropriate for light microscopy unless the free aldehyde groups are blocked; otherwise, the staining patterns are altered and the tissue becomes brittle and difficult to cut.

3. For light microscopy, samples should be sectioned into 2- to 3-μm slices; for electron microscopy, samples should be sectioned into 30- to 60-nm slices.

a. Although a tissue thickness of 0.4 to 6 μm has been recommended, thin sections of 0.4 to 3 μm are preferable because they facilitate evaluation of the number of the cells and the degree of cellularity of glomeruli.[57]

b. A technique has been described in which biopsy samples fixed in formalin and embedded in epoxy resin may be sectioned at 0.4 μm with an ultramicrotome.[109]

4. Many stains are available for examination of renal tissue by light microscopy.

a. Hematoxylin and eosin is a commonly used stain (Figs. 12–1, 12–2, and 12–4).

(1). Hematoxylin is basic and imparts a blue to purple color to acidic cell components, such as chromatin, and some secretory products.

(2). Eosin is acidic and imparts a pink to red color to basic cell components, such as cytoplasm, and many extracellular products.

(3). This general-purpose stain is used for general assessment of all components of renal parenchyma.

(4). It is less useful for detection of more subtle changes in glomeruli, especially those involving glomerular capillary walls.

b. Carbohydrates and carbohydrate-protein complexes may be stained with periodic acid-Schiff (Fig. 12–3A).

(1). The reaction involves oxidation of alpha-amino acids and/or 1,2-glycol groups to aldehydes by periodic acid.

(2). The tissue is then exposed to Schiff reagent, which has basic fuschin decolorized from its original red-violet by addition of sulfurous acid.

(3). Reaction with the Schiff reagent forms a complex that restores the magenta color.

(4). Periodic acid-Schiff accentuates glomerular capillary basement membranes, mesangial matrix, and the brush border of proximal tubular epithelial cells.

c. Methenamine silver stain is most useful for samples fixed in Bouin's solution.[110]

(1). Like periodic acid-Schiff, methenamine

silver stains glomerular capillary basement membranes, tubular basement membranes, and mesangial matrix.

(2). The stain has received widespread use in recognition of so-called "spikes" on the outer surface of thickened glomerular basement membranes sometimes seen during some stages of membranous glomerulonephropathy.

(3). Hematoxylin and eosin are commonly used as counter stains.

(4). A combination of methenamine silver, periodic acid-Schiff, and hematoxylin and eosin is especially useful for photomicrography.

d. Congo red is useful for detection of amyloid.

(1). Large quantities of amyloid can usually be detected with hematoxylin and eosin; however, smaller quantities can be detected with Congo red stain evaluated with light microscopy or polarizing light microscopy.

(2). When small quantities of amyloid are present, a thick section (6 to 8 μm) is preferable to provide sufficient dye binding for visualization with polarizing microscopy.

e. Other stains may be used to visualize specific components of the biopsy section.

(1). Von Kossa's silver nitrate stain is used for calcium.

(2). Van Gieson's stain is useful to visualize connective tissue.

(3). Masson's trichrome stain is useful to visualize collagen and subepithelial deposits.

5. For immunofluorescence microscopy, the tissue is cut in a cryostat at a temperature between −20 and −25°C.[108]

a. The sections should not exceed 6 μm; ideally they should be 3 to 4 μm in thickness.

b. The tissue sections are placed on glass slides, which are fixed for 5 to 10 minutes in acetone, dried at room temperature, washed in buffered saline, and covered for 30 minutes with a drop of fluorescein-labeled antiserum in a moist chamber that is light shielded.

c. Antibodies are used as a cytochemical reagent to carry a fluorescent dye that is visible in the ultraviolet range of light (Fig. 12–3B).

d. After several washes with buffer, the slides are mounted using buffered glycerol.

e. Fading of the fluorescence during storage can be delayed by adding phenylenediamine to the mounting medium.

6. For electron microscopy, the tissue is allowed to fix for a minimum of 2 hours and then is rinsed in buffer, postfixed in 1% osmic tetroxide, dehydrated, and embedded.[108]

a. Samples for transmission electron microscopy are fixed with glutaraldehyde, embedded in plastic, and cut in 30- to 60-nm sections to allow electron beam passage (Fig. 12–3C).

(1). Heavy metal stains (osmic acid, lead, uranium) are used to stain cell and extracellular components.

(2). When sections are too thin, insufficient scatter results; when sections are too thick, excessive electron absorption results.

b. Samples for scanning electron microscopy are processed in a manner similar to that described for transmission electron microscopy.

B. Samples obtained by fine-needle aspiration biopsy may be evaluated cytologically; portions may be cultured if a bacterial infection is suspected.

1. Following aspiration of renal tissue, the fine-gauge needle is removed from the hub of the syringe and approximately 1 mL of air is withdrawn into the syringe.
2. The needle is then placed on the syringe, and the contents of the hub of the needle are expelled onto one or more glass microscope slides.
3. After making a smear, slides are allowed to air dry prior to staining.
4. Cytologic preparations may be stained with a modified Wright's stain, new methylene blue, or Gram's stain.
5. Modification of fine-needle aspiration technique may yield preserved glomeruli.[17]

a. An aliquot of renal cortical material obtained by fine-needle aspiration is suspended in 1640 RPMI (Roswell Park Memorial Institute) solution supplemented with albumin and heparin.

b. The mixture is centrifuged in gelatin-coated plastic tubes for 10 minutes at 1000 rpm.

c. Following centrifugation, the supernatant is removed and the cellular pellet is entrapped in plasma clot produced by addition of plasma and thrombin to the sediment.

d. The resulting specimen is wrapped in absorbent paper (absorbent lens cleaning paper, Clay Adams Division of Beckton & Dickenson, Co., Parsippany, New Jersey) and fixed in glutaraldehyde for 1 hour.

e. Following fixation, the specimen may be processed for routine light microscopy and for special staining, as well as for polarizing microscopy and electron microscopy.

f. Using this technique, 25 or 30 fine-needle aspiration specimens in 1 study[17] contained glomeruli and occasional tubular fragments surrounded by fibrin and erythrocytes.

g. The average number of glomeruli per sample was 5.6 ± 2.6.

h. Light microscopy revealed that the structural

integrity of glomerular tufts was well preserved in 23 of 25 specimens; Bowman's capsule was preserved in approximately 30% of the specimens.

6. Samples obtained by fine-needle aspiration of cystic structures or nephropyelocentesis may be cultured for bacteria or fungi.

X. SERIAL PUNCH NEEDLE BIOPSIES OR WIDE-BORE OR FINE-BORE NEEDLE ASPIRATION BIOPSIES MAY BE OBTAINED FROM KIDNEYS

A. The use of repeat biopsies of the kidney with semiquantitative comparisons may give a dynamic view of the evolution of renal changes, especially that which occurs with inflammatory diseases.[111]

B. When serial biopsies are to be obtained from the same kidney at different intervals of time, the samples should not be obtained from the same area of the kidney.

1. If they are obtained from the same region, there is a high degree of probability that they will contain lesions induced by previous biopsies.[112]
2. Unsuspected discovery of iatrogenic lesions caused by previous needle biopsies might lead to erroneous conclusions about the disease being evaluated.
3. Serial biopsy samples obtained from opposite poles of the same kidney are unlikely to contain iatrogenic lesions.

C. Serial biopsy samples can be performed safely in cats and dogs if appropriate caution is used to avoid damage to major renal vessels.[50,112]

REFERENCES

1. Knecht CD, Reynolds HA. Needle punch biopsy procedures for obtaining specimens of liver, kidney and lymph nodes of dogs. *J Am Anim Hosp Assoc.* 1967;3:163.
2. Osborne CA. Clinical evaluation of needle biopsy of the kidney and its complications in the dog and cat. *J Am Vet Med Assoc.* 1971;158:1213.
3. Wise LA, Allen TA, Cartwright M. Comparison of renal biopsy techniques in dogs. *J Am Vet Med Assoc.* 1989;195:935.
4. Haubek A, Lundorf E, Lauridsen KN. Diagnostic strategy in renal mass lesions. *Scand J Urol Nephrol.* 1991;137 (suppl):35.
5. Montie JE. The incidental renal mass. Management alternatives. *Urol Clin North Am.* 1991;18:427.
6. Shirai T, et al. Correlation between renal functions and renal pathohistology. *Fukuoka Shika Daigaku Gakkai Zasshi.* 1987;14:205.
7. Waltzer WC, et al. Value of percutaneous core needle biopsy in the differential diagnosis of renal transplant dysfunction. *J Urol.* 1987;137:1117.
8. Osborne CA, Stevens JB, Perman V. Kidney biopsy. *Vet Clin North Am.* 1974;4:351.
9. Almirall J, et al. Aspiration cytology in the diagnosis of renal transplant rejection. *Med Clin (Barc).* 1991;97:410.
10. Amis E Jr., Cronan JJ, Pfister RC. Needle puncture of cystic renal masses: A survey of the Society of Uroradiology. *AJR.* 1987;148:297.
11. Capodicasa G, et al. Sequential fine needle aspiration biopsy in glomerulonephritis. *Int J Pediatr Nephrol.* 1986;7:3.
12. Danovitch GM, et al. Evaluation of fine-needle aspiration biopsy in the diagnosis of renal transplant dysfunction [published erratum appears in *Am J Kidney Dis.* March 1991; 17(suppl 3):362]. *Am J Kidney Dis.* 1991;17:206.
13. Egidi F, Stucchi L, Montagnino G. The role of fine needle aspiration biopsy in clinical transplantation. *Transplant Proc.* 1989;21:3576.
14. Hayry P, von-Willebrand E. Use of fine needle aspiration biopsy in differential diagnosis between nephrotoxicity and rejection. *Contrib Nephrol.* 1986;51:147.
15. Hayry PJ. Fine-needle aspiration biopsy in renal transplantation [clinical conference]. *Kidney Int.* 1989;36:130.
16. Jorgensen KA, et al. Fine needle aspiration biopsy during and after OKT3. *Transplant Proc.* 1989;21:3594.
17. Yussim A, et al. Use of modified fine needle aspiration for study of glomerular pathology in human kidneys. *Kidney Int.* 1990; 37:812.
18. Miller S, Belitsky P, Gupta R. Kidney glomeruli collected by fine needle aspiration biopsy. *Transplant Proc.* 1989;21:3614.
19. Akhtar M, et al. Fine-needle aspiration biopsy diagnosis of malignant rhabdoid tumor of the kidney. *Diagn Cytopathol.* 1991;7:36.
20. Clark SP, Kung IT, Tang SK. Fine-needle aspiration of cystic nephroma (multilocular cyst of the kidney). *Diagn Cytopathol.* 1992;8:349.
21. Cristallini EG, Paganelli C, Bolis GB. Role of fine-needle aspiration biopsy in the assessment of renal masses. *Diagn Cytopathol.* 1991;7:32.
22. Dey P, et al. Fine needle aspiration cytology of mesoblastic nephroma. A case report. *Acta Cytol.* 1992;36:404.
23. Leiman G. Audit of fine needle aspiration cytology of 120 renal lesions. *Cytopathology.* 1990;1:65.
24. Smith SA, Gharib H, Goellner JR. Fine-needle aspiration. Usefulness for diagnosis and management of metastatic carcinoma to the thyroid. *Arch Intern Med.* 1987;147:311.
25. Unger P, et al. Fine needle aspiration of a renal cell carcinoma with eosinophilic globules. A case report. *Acta Cytol.* 1993;37:201.
26. Valkov I, Bojikin B. Fine-needle aspiration biopsy of abdominal and retroperitoneal tumors in infants and children. *Diagn Cytopathol.* 1987;3:129.
27. Weaver MG, al-Kaisi N, Abdul-Karim FW. Fine-needle aspiration cytology of a renal cell adenocarcinoma with massive intracellular hemosiderin accumulation. *Diagn Cytopathol.* 1991;7:147.
28. Yazdi HM. Genitourinary cytology. *Clin Lab Med.* 1991;11:369.
29. Hughes DA, et al. Can incremental scoring of fine-needle aspirates predict histopathologic renal allograft rejection? *Transplant Proc.* 1988;20:690.
30. Lebron R, et al. Correlation between simultaneous fine needle aspiration biopsy and core biopsy in renal transplants. *Transplant Proc.* 1991;23:1762.
31. Reinholt FP, et al. Fine-needle aspiration cytology and conventional histology in 200 renal allografts. *Transplantation.* 1990; 49:910.
32. Surachno S, van-Oers MH, Wilmink JM. Early diagnosis of bacterial infection of renal allografts by fine needle aspiration biopsy [letter]. *Lancet.* 1986;1:686.
33. Lang EK. Renal cyst puncture studies. *Urol Clin North Am.* 1987;14:91.
34. Hernandez JA, et al. A novel use of fine-needle aspiration biopsy: Documentation of acute pyelonephritis of the transplanted kidney. *Transplant Proc.* 1988;20:632.

35. Horsburgh T, et al. Cell culture of fine-needle aspirates and Tru-cut biopsies. *Transplant Proc.* 1988;20:679.
36. Palmer BF, et al. Documentation of fungal pyelonephritis of the renal allograft by fine needle aspiration cytology. *Transplant Proc.* 1989;21:3598.
37. Palmer B, et al. Diagnosis of acute bacterial pyelonephritis of the renal allograft by fine-needle aspiration cytology. *Transplantation.* 1989;48:152.
38. Jeraj K, Osborne CA, Stevens JB. Evaluation of renal biopsy in 197 dogs and cats. *J Am Vet Med Assoc.* 1982;181:367.
39. Jamal Q, Jafarey NA, Naqvi AJ. A review of 1508 percutaneous renal biopsies. *J Pak Med Assoc.* 1988;38:272.
40. Dykes EH, et al. Risks and benefits of percutaneous biopsy and primary chemotherapy in advanced Wilms' tumour. *J Pediatr Surg.* 1991;26:610.
41. Alon U, Pery M. Percutaneous kidney needle biopsy in children is less traumatic than in adults. *Nephron.* 1988;50:57.
42. Harris CL, Krawiec DR. The pathophysiology of uremic bleeding. *Compend Contin Educ Pract Vet.* 1990;12:1294.
43. Carvajal HF, et al. Percutaneous renal biopsy in children—An analysis of complications in 890 consecutive biopsies. *Tex Rep Biol Med.* 1971;29:253.
44. Diaz-Buxo JA, Donadio JV. Complications of percutaneous renal biopsy: An analysis of 1,000 consecutive biopsies. *Clin Nephrol.* 1975;4:223.
45. O'Brien DP, et al. Renal arteriovenous fistulas. *Surg Gynecol Obstet.* 1974;139:739.
46. Harvey JM, et al. Renal biopsy findings in hypertensive patients with proteinuria. *Lancet.* 1992;340:1435.
47. Nadel L, Baumgartner BR, Bernardino ME. Percutaneous renal biopsies: Accuracy, safety, and indications. *Urol Radiol.* 1986;8:67.
48. Osborne CA, Low DG, Jessen CR. Renal parenchymal response to needle biopsy. *Invest Urol.* 1972;9:463.
49. Nash AS, et al. Renal biopsy in the normal cat: An examination of the effects of a single needle biopsy. *Res Vet Sci.* 1983;34:347.
50. Nash AS, et al. Renal biopsy in the normal cat: Examination of the effects of repeated needle biopsy. *Res Vet Sci.* 1986;40:112.
51. Kark RM, et al. An analysis of five hundred percutaneous renal biopsies. *Arch Intern Med.* 1958;101:439.
52. Samellas W. Death due to septicemia following percutaneous needle biopsy of the kidney. *J Urol.* 1964;91:317.
53. Schow DA, Vinson RK, Morrisseau PM. Percutaneous renal biopsy of the solitary kidney: A contraindication? *J Urol.* 1992;147:1235.
54. Mertz JHO, Lang E, Klingerman JJ. Percutaneous renal biopsy utilizing cinefluoroscopic monitoring. *J Urol.* 1966;95:618.
55. Nickel R, Schummer A, Seiferle E. The Viscera of the Domestic Mammals. 2nd Ed., New York, NY: Springer-Verlag; 1979:282.
56. Evans HE, Christensen GC: The urogential system. In: Evans HE, ed. *Miller's Anatomy of the Dog.* 3rd ed. Philadelphia, Pa: WB Saunders Co.; 1993:494.
57. Osborne CA, Low DG. Size, adequacy, and artifacts of canine renal biopsy samples. *Am J Vet Res.* 1971;32:1865.
58. Osborne CA. Experimental and clinical evaluation of needle biopsy of the kidney and its complications in the dog. Ph. D. Thesis. University of Minnesota. 1970.
59. Osborne CA. Modified Franklin-Silverman biopsy needle. *J Urol.* 1972;107:358.
60. Nash AS. Renal biopsy in the normal cat: Development of a modified disposable biopsy needle. *Res Vet Sci.* 1986;40:246.
61. Wiseman DA, et al. Percutaneous renal biopsy utilizing real time, ultrasonic guidance and a semiautomated biopsy device. *Kidney Int.* 1990;39:347.
62. Hopper KD, et al. Efficacy of automated biopsy gun versus conventional biopsy needles in the pygmy pig. *Radiology.* 1990;176:671.
63. Belitsky P, Gupta R. Minicore needle biopsy of kidney transplants: A safer sampling method. *J Urol.* 1990;144:310.
64. Elvin A, et al. Biopsy of the pancreas with a biopsy gun. *Radiology.* 1990;176:677.
65. Poster RB, Jones DB, Spirt BA. Percutaneous pediatric renal biopsy: Use of the biopsy gun. *Radiology.* 1990;176:725.
66. McEnery PT. Use of a modified Menghini needle for renal biopsy. *J Urol.* 1971;106:810.
67. Haaga JR, et al. Clinical comparison of small- and large-caliber cutting needles for biopsy. *Radiology.* 1983;146:665.
68. Grauer GF, Twedt DC, Mero KN. Evaluation of laparoscopy for obtaining renal biopsy specimens from dogs and cats. *J Am Vet Med Assoc.* 1983;183:677.
69. Hager DA, Nyland TG, Fisher P. Ultrasound-guided biopsy of the canine liver, kidney, and prostate. *Vet Radiol.* 1985;26:82.
70. Smith S. Ultrasound-guided biopsy. *Semin Vet Med Surg (Small Anim).* 1989;4:95.
71. Finn-Bodner ST, Hathcock JT. Image-guided percutaneous needle biopsy: Ultrasound, computed tomography, and magnetic resonance imaging. *Semin Vet Med Surg (Small Anim).* 1993;8:258.
72. Bogin-Iu N, et al. Clinical use of echotomography with target aspiration biopsy and urgent cytological examination. *Klin Med (Mosk).* 1990;68:94.
73. Buonocore E, Skipper TR. Steerable real-time sonographically guided needle biopsy. *Am J Radiol.* 1981;136:387.
74. Civardi G, et al. Echographically guided, percutaneous, fine-needle puncture in the diagnosis of renal masses suspected of malignancy. *Recenti Prog Med.* 1986;77:420.
75. Desrentes M, et al. Renal needle biopsy under echography. Apropos of 413 examinations. *Dakar Med.* 1990;35:114.
76. Goldberg BB, et al. Real-time aspiration-biopsy transducer. *Clin Ultrasound.* 1980;8:107.
77. Jakobeit C. Ultrasound-controlled puncture procedures: Free-hand puncture versus transducer biopsy puncture. 5 years' experience. *Ultraschall Med.* 1986;7:290.
78. Landolt-Weber U, Fattori S, Pedio G. The value of fine-needle biopsy under ultrasonic control in the diagnosis of kidney tumors. *Schweiz Rundsch Med Prax.* 1989;78:66.
79. Tiwari SC, et al. Ultrasound guided kidney biopsy. *J Assoc Physicians India.* 1988;36:327.
80. Konde LJ, et al. Comparison of radiography and ultrasonography in the evaluation of renal lesions in the dog. *J Am Vet Med Assoc.* 1986;188:1420.
81. Otto R, Dyhle R. Guided puncture under real-time sonographic control. *Radiology.* 1980;134:784.
82. Almkuist RD, Buckalew VMJ. Techniques in renal biopsy. *Urol Clin North Am.* 1979;6:503.
83. Srinivasan SR, et al. Evaluation of different renal biopsy techniques in canine. *Indian Vet J.* 1992;69:449.
84. Tartini A, Hood V, Rimmer J. Use of the Biopty instrument in percutaneous needle biopsy of the native kidney. *J Am Soc Nephrol.* 1990;1:219.
85. Elvin A, et al. Ultrasound-guided biopsies of neuroendocrine metastases. Comparison of 0.9 and 1.2 mm biopsy-gun needle biopsies. *Acta Radiol.* 1993;34:474.
86. Patterson JM. Laparoscopy in small animal medicine. In: Kirk RW, ed. *Current Veterinary Therapy. VII.* Philadelphia, Pa: WB Saunders Co; 1980:969.
87. Jones BD. Laparoscopy. *Vet Clin North Am (Small Anim Pract).* 1990;20:1243.

88. Caywood DD, Lipowitz AJ. *Atlas of General Small Animal Surgery.* St. Louis, Mo: C. V. Mosby Co; 1989:226.
89. Stone EA, Barsanti JA. *Urologic Surgery of the Dog and Cat.* Philadelphia, Pa: Lea & Febiger; 1992:100.
90. Gourley IM, Gregory CR. *Atlas of Small Animal Surgery.* New York, NY: Gower Medical Publishing; 1992:19.
91. Smith MM, Waldron DR. *Approaches for General Surgery of the Dog and Cat.* Philadelphia, Pa: WB Saunders Co; 1993:232.
92. Christie BA, Bjorling DE. Kidneys. In Slatter D, ed. *Textbook of Small Animal Surgery.* 2nd ed. Philadelphia, Pa: WB Saunders Co; 1993:1428.
93. Murphy JJ, Best R. The healing of renal wounds. 1. Partial nephrectomy. *J Urol.* 1957;78:504.
94. Williams DF. A new technique of partial nephrectomy. *J Urol.* 1967;97:955.
95. Kim SK. New techniques of partial nephrectomy. *J Urol.* 1969;102:165.
96. Mal F, et al. The diagnostic yield of transjugular renal biopsy. Experience in 200 cases. *Kidney Int.* 1992;41:445.
97. Leal JJ. A new technique for renal biopsy: The transurethral approach. *J Urol.* 1993;149:1061.
98. Dahnert WF, et al. Fine-needle aspiration biopsy of abdominal lesions: Diagnostic yield for different needle tip configurations. *Radiology.* 1992;185:263.
99. Gray DW, et al. A prospective, randomized, blind comparison of three biopsy techniques in the management of patients after renal transplantation. *Transplantation.* 1992;53:1226.
100. Ling GV, et al. Percutaneous nephropyelocentesis and nephropyelostomy in the dog: A description of the technique. *Am J Vet Res.* 1979;40:1605.
101. Ackerman N, Ling GV, Ruby AL. Percutaneous nephropyelocentesis and antegrade ureterography: A fluoroscopically assisted diagnostic technic in canine urology. *Vet Radiol.* 1980;21:117.
102. Ling GV, et al. Chronic urinary tract infection in dogs: Induction by inoculation with bacteria via percutaneous nephropyelostomy. *Am J Vet Res.* 1987;48:794.
103. Ackerman GL, Lipsmeyer EA. Prolonged hematuria after renal biopsy. *J Urol.* 1967;97:790.
104. Karafin L, Kendall AR, Fleisher DS. Urologic complications in percutaneous renal biopsy in children. *J Urol.* 1970;103:332.
105. Lee DA, et al. Late complications of percutaneous renal biopsy. *J Urol.* 1967;97:793.
106. Stern L, Langford C, Crossman BJ. Extravasation of urine. *Am J Dis Child.* 1970;119:88.
107. Leveille R, et al. Complications after ultrasound-guided biopsy of abdominal structures in dogs and cats: 246 cases (1984-1991). *J Am Vet Med Assoc.* 203:413, 1993.
108. Striker LJ, Olson JL, Striker GE. *The Renal Biopsy.* 2nd ed. Philadelphia, Pa: WB Saunders Co; 1990:282.
109. Eastham WN, Essex WB. Use of tissues embedded in epoxy resin for routine histological examination of renal biopsies. *J Clin Pathol.* 1969;22:99.
110. Bancroft JD, Stevens A. Histopathological stains and their diagnostic uses. New York, NY: Churchill Livingston; 1975.
111. Striker LJ. Modern renal biopsy interpretation: Can we predict glomerulosclerosis? *Semin Nephrol.* 1993;13:508.
112. Osborne CA, Low DG. Iatrogenic lesions in serial renal biopsy samples. *J Urol.* 1971;106:805.

CHAPTER 13

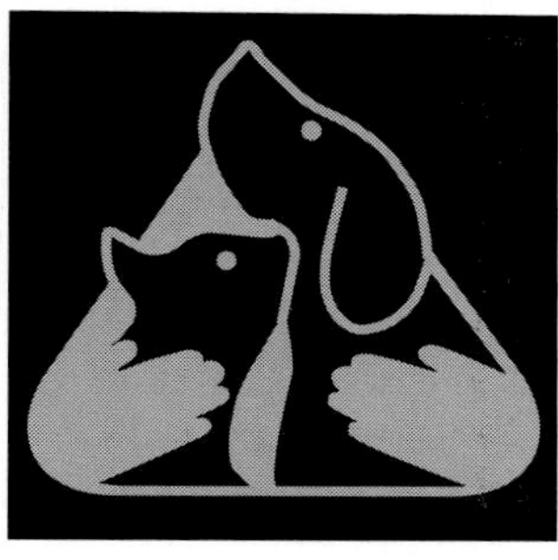

Endoscopy

DAVID F. SENIOR

I. INTRODUCTION

Cystoscopic techniques in human medicine allow many procedures to be performed without open surgery, and several procedures are more easily performed via cystoscope than by open surgery (e.g., prostatic resection and ureteral catheterization). Many of the same procedures used in human urologic practice can be performed cystoscopically in small animals, but several factors have prevented widespread application in veterinary medicine. Patients still must be anesthetized for cystoscopy, the equipment is expensive, open surgery meets with less resistance in veterinary medicine, and standard human cystoscopes are not readily suited for use in male dogs, small dogs, and all cats. Despite these limitations, cystoscopy is a useful adjunct to several urologic procedures in small animal veterinary medicine, and occasional cystoscopic procedures in small animals have been performed for many years.[2,3,7-9,13,25,26]

In veterinary patients, cystoscopy allows direct visualization of the epithelial surface of the bladder and urethra,[2,8,9,24,26] biopsy and photography of mucosal lesions,[2,8,24] ureteral catheterization for urine sampling and retrograde pyelography,[18] lithotripsy,[22] injection of polytetrafluoroethylene paste submucosally into the urethra to treat incontinence,[1] and resection of mucosal lesions. This chapter describes the equipment required and techniques used to perform cystoscopy in small animals, the cystoscopic appearance of the normal lower urinary tract, the cystoscopic appearance of several pathologic changes, and special procedures that may be performed via cystoscope.

II. INDICATIONS

The indications for cystoscopy in veterinary medicine include lower urinary tract inflammation of unknown cause, urolithiasis, recurrent urinary tract infection, urine retention, bladder or urethral masses, and urinary incontinence.

Several procedures have been described to examine the lower urinary tract of small animals endoscopically. Rigid telescopes provide the best visualization, and they can be introduced into the lower urinary tract through a standard urethral cystoscope or via a prepubic approach. Flexible endoscopes can be introduced into the urethra and bladder of large male dogs, but the fiberoptic image is less satisfactory. Also, a much wider range of instruments can be used through the rigid cystoscope than through a thin flexible fiberoptic endoscope.

III. RIGID CYSTOSCOPY

Rigid cystoscopes can be used to examine the bladder and urethra of female dogs and,

via a perineal urethrotomy, the bladder and proximal urethra of male dogs.[2,3,8,24]

A. Patient preparation and positioning.

1. Female dog.
   a. Under general anesthesia, the patient is positioned in dorsal recumbency with the hind end slightly beyond the end of the examination table. The hind legs may be lightly taped laterally and forward to stabilize the patient and to keep them out of the way, and a "V"-support in the lumbar region can be used to provide further stabilization. The dog is best situated on the end of the table that can be raised, because raising the table once the cystoscope is introduced allows easier examination.
   b. Hair around the vulva should be clipped, and the perivulva area is given a standard surgical scrub. A vaginal douche can be given prior to the surgical scrub if excessive vaginal discharge is noted; however, the indications for this procedure are not clear. A sterile drape is placed over the caudal half of the animal, thereby leaving the vulval area exposed.
2. Male dog.[3,25]
   a. Rigid cystoscopy in male dogs has only been reported in experimental studies, although the procedure could be used on such patients.[3,8,25] Access to the pelvic urethra is obtained through a perineal urethrotomy, which is left to heal after the completion of the procedure. Following urethrotomy, prolonged intermittent hemorrhage and transient hematuria may be minor problems, and subsequent stricture and creation of a permanent urethrostomy site are possible but unlikely.[3]
   b. Under general anesthesia, the patient is positioned in dorsal recumbency as described for the female dog. The perineal area is clipped and given a standard surgical scrub.
   c. A urethral catheter is introduced beyond the ischial arch, and a small incision is made in the skin and fascia overlying the palpable catheterized urethra in the mid-ischial region. The catheter is then withdrawn until the tip is felt just distal to the skin incision. Then, the urethra is distended by infusing saline through the catheter, and a needle is advanced obliquely through the skin incision into the lumen of the urethra. Saline flows from the needle when the urethral lumen is entered.
   d. A flexible guidewire (Amplatz Stiff Wire Guide, Cook Inc., Bloomington, Indiana 47402) is then advanced through the needle into the urethra and the bladder. With the guidewire in place, the needle is removed and taken off the wire. Fascial dilators (Amplatz Renal Dilator Set, Cook Inc., Bloomington, Indiana 47402) are introduced serially over the guidewire to dilate the urethrotomy from a diameter of 8 F to a diameter of 26 F.
   e. Finally, an Amplatz sheath is passed over the last dilator, the dilator is removed, and the cystoscope can be introduced into the bladder through the sheath. The diameter of the final dilator and Amplatz sheath is based on the size of the cystoscope to be used. Once the cystoscope is in place, the guidewire can be removed.

B. Equipment required.

1. Cystoscopic operating equipment for use in humans comes in two basic forms: the general-purpose diagnostic cystoscope sheath and the more dedicated resectoscope designed to remove prostatic and other tissue. The general-purpose cystoscope requires the following equipment (Fig. 13–1):
   a. Light-carrying cable
   b. Sheath
   c. Obturator
   d. Bridge (with or without Albarran deflector)
   e. Telescopes: 12 to 30° and 70 to 90°
   f. Light source (not shown)
2. To perform various procedures, the following instruments can be passed through the sheath:
   a. Biopsy and grasping forceps
   b. Electrocautery electrodes (various design)
   c. Stone baskets
   d. Electrohydraulic shock-wave lithotripsy cables
   e. Ultrasound sonotrodes
   f. Laser probes
   g. Ureteral catheters
3. Resectoscopes are specialized cystoscopes that are designed as complete units, with the telescope and electrocautery electrode arranged optimally for controlled endoscopic tissue resection. Resectoscopes were originally developed for transurethral prostatectomy in humans and are well suited for cystoscopic resection of bladder tumors in dogs.

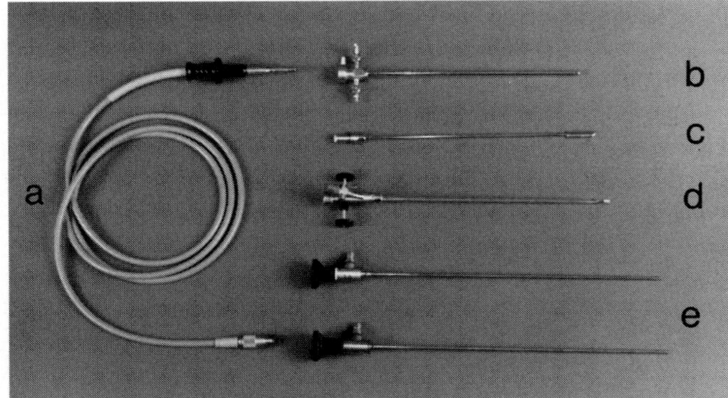

FIG. 13–1. Rigid cystoscopy equipment. a = light-carrying cable; b = cystoscope sheath; c = obturator; d = Albarran operating bridge; and e = telescopes.

IV. CHOOSING A CYSTOSCOPE

A. General-purpose cystoscope sheaths come in adult and pediatric lengths (approximately 12 cm versus approximately 23 cm, respectively). The outer diameter of adult-length cystoscope sheaths ranges from 17.5 to 26 F, whereas the pediatric diameter ranges from 12 to 15 F.

B. Selection of the most suitable cystoscope for a particular patient or operative procedure involves consideration of urethral diameter, urethral length, the size of the operating channel of the cystoscope sheath, and the instruments that will be required to perform the procedure.

1. The smallest cystoscope sheath through which all procedures can be performed is adult length, 23 F. This sheath can be passed comfortably into dogs of 25 kg body weight or more.
2. Sheath sizes as small as 17.5 F can accommodate all instruments except for a loop electrocautery electrode and a laser probe, although the biopsy and grasping forceps have smaller cups and obtain small, sometimes less adequate, tissue samples.
3. The 17.5 F sheath can be comfortably passed into dogs of 9 to 11 kg body weight or more.
4. Pediatric-length sheaths of 12 to 15 F diameter are suitable for dogs as small as 5.5 kg body weight, but the operating channels cannot accommodate substantial instruments.

V. INTRODUCTION OF THE CYSTOSCOPE

A. Once the patient is correctly positioned and prepared, the cystoscope sheath is introduced through the urethra into the bladder. The visualization of the urethral papilla and os in female dogs can be facilitated by drawing the ventral tip of the vulva caudoventrally while observing the vulva-vagina with a headlamp (Welch Allyn, Skaneateles Falls, New York 13158) and Killian nasal speculum (Henry Schein, Inc., Port Washington, New York 11050).[24] In female dogs for which the relative size of the cystoscope sheath suggests that introduction may be difficult, urethral dilation with balloon dilators (American Medical Systems, Minnetonka, Minnesota 55343) allows subsequent relatively atraumatic passage of the cystoscope (Fig. 13–2).[24] The well-lubricated balloon dilator should be introduced so that the balloon segment transverses the entire length of the urethra; the balloon is then inflated, and inflation is maintained for about 1 minute. The dilator is then deflated and removed, and the lubricated cystoscope sheath is introduced immediately. Extreme care should be taken when passing the cystoscope through the urethra to avoid urethral perforation.

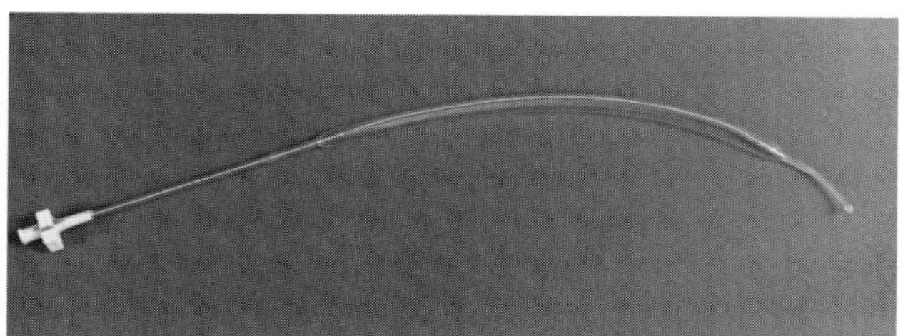

FIG. 13–2. Nephrostomy tract balloon dilator used for urethral dilation.

B. In most instances, the cystoscope sheath is introduced through the urethra with the obturator in place. The obturator tip matches the tip of the sheath and allows smooth and minimally traumatic introduction. Once the sheath is in place, the obturator is removed, the operating bridge and telescope are placed, the light cable and fluid lines are attached, and examination can begin. Sometimes urethral abnormalities, such as tumors or strictures, may result in difficult passage of the sheath and obturator. In these instances, the sheath, operating bridge, telescope, light lines, and fluid lines can be put together, and the lubricated cystoscope can be introduced fully assembled. Although introduction in this way may be a little more traumatic, this approach enables the operator to negotiate masses and strictures more easily under direct visualization.

VI. IRRIGATION SOLUTIONS

A. Repeated or continuous lavage with irrigation fluid is necessary to obtain a clear endoscopic view because bacteria, blood cells, crystals, lipid, mucus, and cellular debris otherwise cloud the image, making visualization difficult or impossible. Standard cystoscopes provide two taps connected to a single channel through which fluid can be intermittently instilled and evacuated. One tap is connected to an irrigation solution infusion set, whereas the other is connected to a drainage system. Both ingress and egress of fluid are driven by gravity flow and controlled by the taps mounted on the cystoscope sheath.

B. Resectoscopes are usually constructed to allow for continuous irrigation so that the operative procedure can continue uninterrupted by the need for fluid evacuation. The fluid enters via an inner sheath and is simultaneously sucked out through a separate outer channel.

C. The refractive index properties of all cystoscope lenses are designed to be used in a fluid medium. Irrigation allows distention of the bladder and urethra and washes away blood and debris. In several situations, the irrigation solution must have specific properties.[11] For electrocautery and cutting, the irrigant must be a non-electrolyte so that the current is not dissipated by the solution. Although sterile

water could be used, absorption into the vascular system can cause hemolysis; thus, the iso-osmotic nonelectrolyte solution 1.5% glycine (Travenol Lab, Inc., Atlanta, Georgia 30338), is most often used. For electrohydraulic shock-wave lithotripsy, 1/6 normal saline is used because more concentrated solutions tend to dissipate the current to such an extent that the required spark conformation is not achieved. For procedures not requiring electrical discharges, the best irrigants are physiologic solutions, such as normal saline. The integrity of biopsy specimens is preserved better by both 1.5% glycine and physiologic solutions than by more dilute solutions, such as 1/6 normal saline and sterile water.

VII. FLEXIBLE CYSTOSCOPY

A. Flexible fiberoptic endoscopes can be used to examine the lower urinary tract of both male and female dogs.[8] However, they are best confined to use in male dogs, because in females the image observed and the operating capability through a rigid cystoscope are so much better.

B. Patient preparation and positioning.

1. The male dog is placed in lateral recumbency with the upper hind limb raised.
2. After cleaning the penis with an appropriate irrigation solution, the bladder is catheterized, drained, rinsed several times with saline until the irrigation fluid is clear, and then partially distended.[2] The catheter is then withdrawn.

C. Equipment required.

1. A long (80-cm), fine (3.6-mm maximum diameter), flexible fiberoptic endoscope (PF25L 2.5 mm × 80 cm Ultrathin Bronchoscope, Olympus Corp., Lake Success, New York 11042) is required.
2. The most suitable are endoscopes originally intended for use in pediatric bronchoscopy.

D. Introduction of the flexible endoscope.

The endoscope is liberally lubricated and passed gently through the urethra into the bladder. The urethral diameter at the tip of the penis may be so narrow that initial passage of the endoscope is difficult. Dilation of the meatus can be achieved with a bougie or an Otis urethrotome knife (Olympus Corp., Lake Success, New York 11042) with the urethrotome blade removed.[8] After dilation, the well-lubricated endoscope can be introduced easily.

VIII. PREPUBIC PERCUTANEOUS CYSTOSCOPY

A. The length and diameter of the urethra often preclude urethral passage of endoscopic equipment; however, prepubic percutaneous cystoscopy allows endoscopic examination of the bladder of small dogs and cats of both sexes.[13]

B. Patient preparation and positioning.

1. Under general anesthesia, the patient is placed in dorsal recumbency, and the abdomen is shaved and given a surgical scrub.
2. The bladder is catheterized (via the urethra), emptied, rinsed several times, and then distended with saline.

C. Equipment required.

Needle endoscopes (2.7 to 5 mm outer diameter) suitable for arthroscopy or laparoscopy are used. An endoscopic trocar and cannula are used to introduce the needle endoscope into the bladder. Accessory equipment for performing biopsies includes an accessory instrument trocar and cannula and biopsy forceps.

D. Introduction of the prepubic percutaneous cystoscope.

1. A small skin incision is made ventrally over the distended bladder wall, and the trocar and cannula are advanced into the bladder through the abdominal wall in one motion.
2. Once the bladder lumen is entered, the trocar is replaced by the needle endoscope, and saline infusion is provided through the endoscopic irrigation port.
3. The urethral catheter is used for drainage of irrigation fluid to create a flow-through effect.
4. The accessory instruments for biopsy are introduced into the bladder through a separate trocar similarly placed in another part of the bladder.

E. Examination.

1. Once the cystoscope is introduced and assembled, the bladder should be flushed with irrigation fluid several times to obtain a clear view.
2. The bladder should be moderately distended at the time of examination so that lesions are not missed in mucosal folds of the contracted bladder wall.
3. The entire bladder wall should be examined systematically by successive advances and retractions of the cystoscope combined with partial rotation of the instrument. In this way, even small lesions are not missed.
4. Useful landmarks include air bubbles (Fig. 13–3A), the cranial pole, trigone with ureteral orifices (Fig. 13–3, B and C), neck of the bladder, (Fig. 13–3D) and proximal urethra (Fig. 13–3E). The ureteral orifices should be located and their positions noted.
5. The bladder neck and urethra are best examined by slowly withdrawing the cystoscope while irrigation fluid is instilled.

IX. CYSTOSCOPIC APPEARANCE OF THE LOWER URINARY TRACT

A. Normal appearance.

1. The mucosa of the contracted bladder has irregular mucosal folds, and the mucosal surface is wrinkled with a reddish hue (Fig. 13–4A).
2. When the bladder is distended, the mucosa is flat with a blanched appearance, and a fine submucosal vascular pattern is clearly visible (Fig. 13–4B).

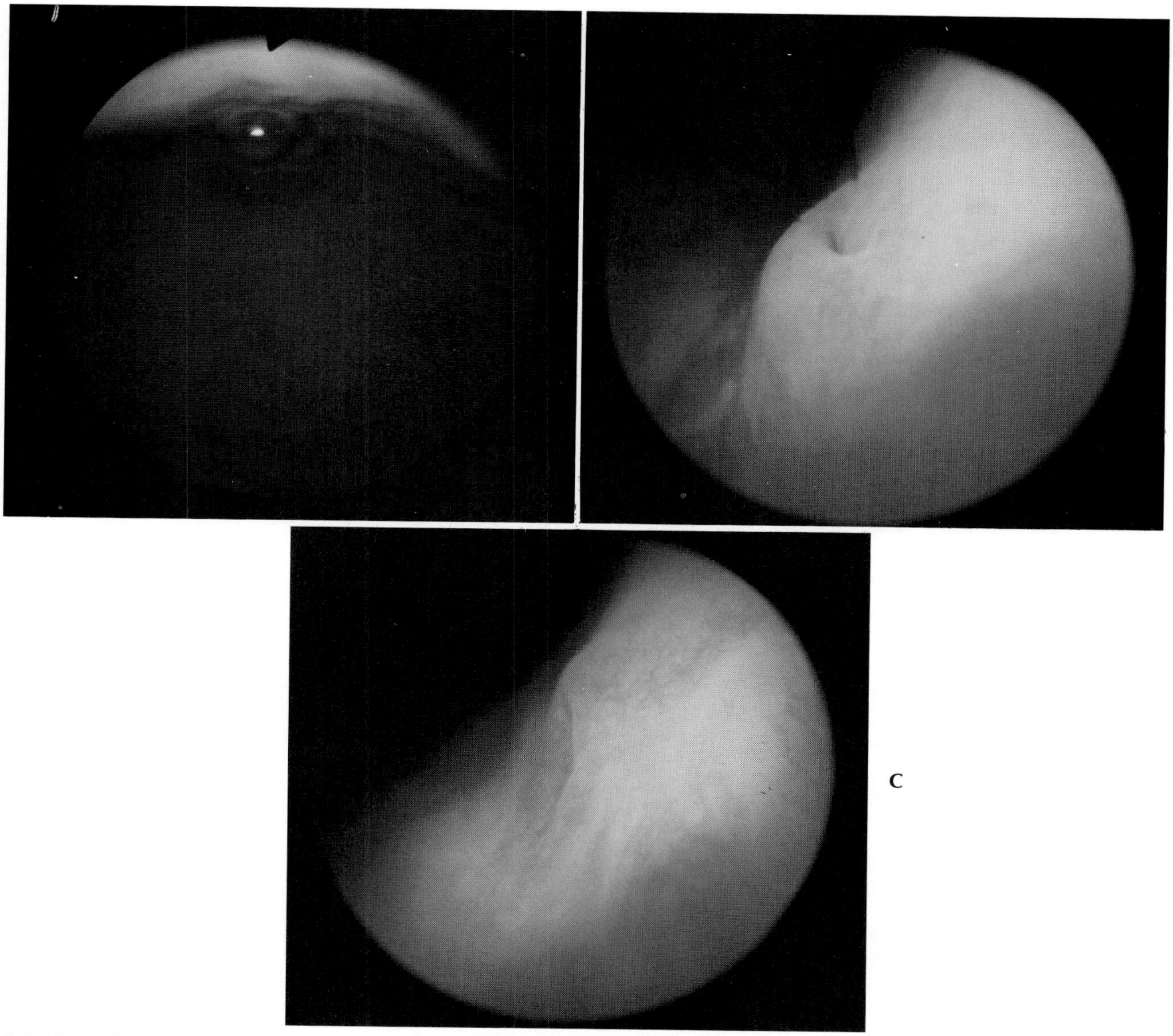

A

B

C

FIG. 13–3. Cystoscopic appearance of the normal bladder. **A,** Air bubbles collect at the ventrum of the bladder (dogs are placed in dorsal recumbency). **B,** Opening of the left ureter. **C,** Opening of the right ureter (the bladder is more distended, thus giving the opening a more flat, slit-like appearance).

3. The ureteral orifices are dorsal in the trigone area, although the location may vary in some animals with the trigone rotated away from dorsal midline.
4. The ureteral openings tend to face each other, and intermittent bursts of urine flow are evident several times a minute.
5. The urethral mucosa usually appears hyperemic and naturally contracts into longitudinal folds as the cystoscope is withdrawn.

B. Pathologic appearance.

1. Stones and crystals
   a. Stones are readily observed as solid brown-white structures (Fig. 13–5A). Blood clots can be observed adhering to the surface, and the bladder frequently has a hyperplastic cobblestone appearance, presumably the result of irritation from contact with the surface of the stone.
   b. Struvite crystals appear as small, white, sugar-like particles that tend to settle in dependent areas.
2. Polyps and tumors

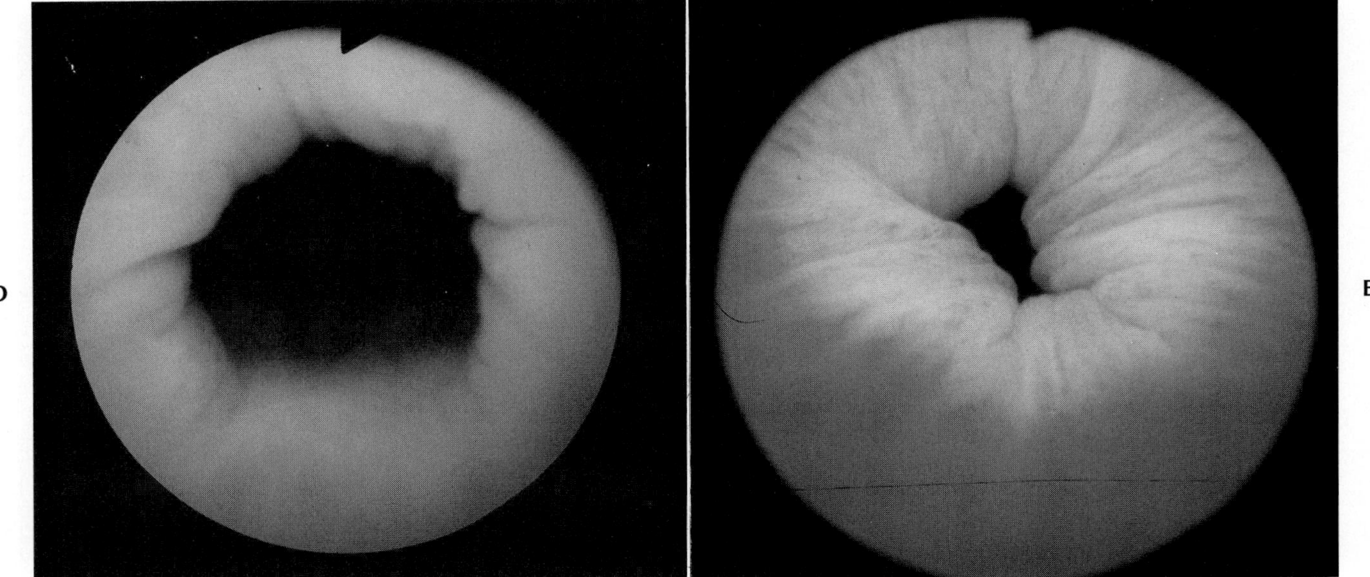

FIG. 13–3, cont'd. D, The neck of the bladder looking from the urethra toward the trigone area. **E,** The urethral mucosa (fluid is infused so that the urethral lumen tends to stay open).

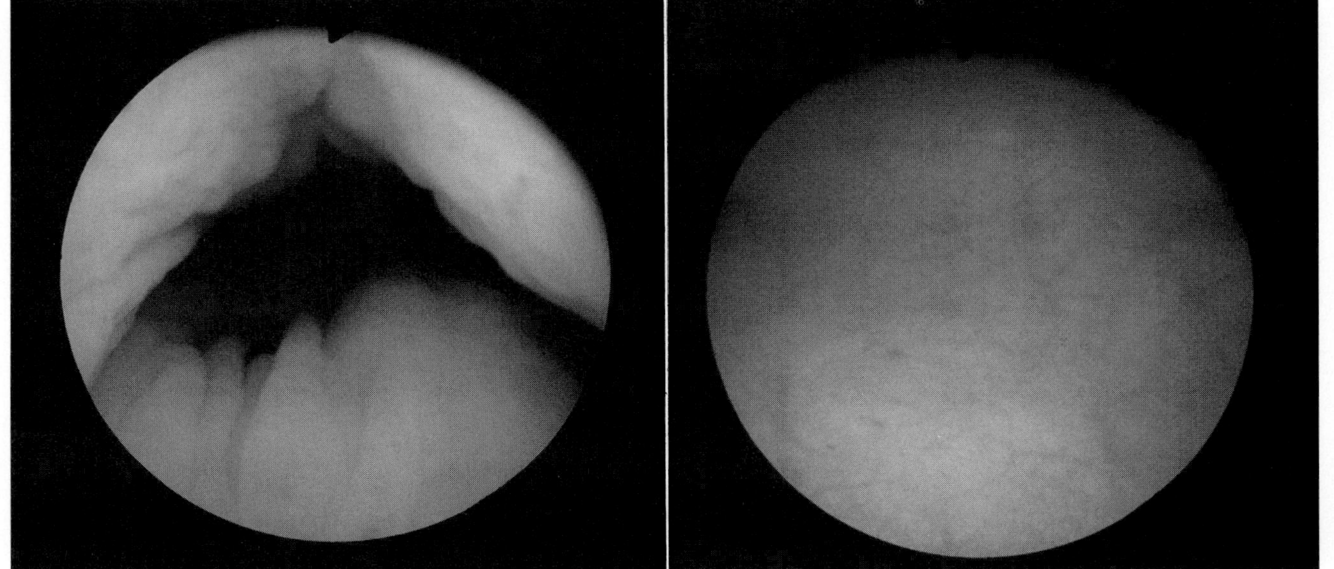

FIG. 13–4. The bladder mucosa. **A,** The bladder mucosa appears red-pink and thrown into folds when the bladder is contracted. **B,** The bladder mucosa appears blanched and submucosal vessels are visible when the bladder is distended.

a. Polypoid structures are easily identified and may be benign (Fig. 13–5B) or malignant (Figs. 13–5, C, D, E).
b. Malignant tumors tend to be larger with larger pedicle stalks or are sessile and exhibit more necrosis (Fig. 13–5C) than do inflammatory polyps.
c. Accurate differentiation between benign polyps and malignant tumors and between different types of malignant tumors (e.g., transi-

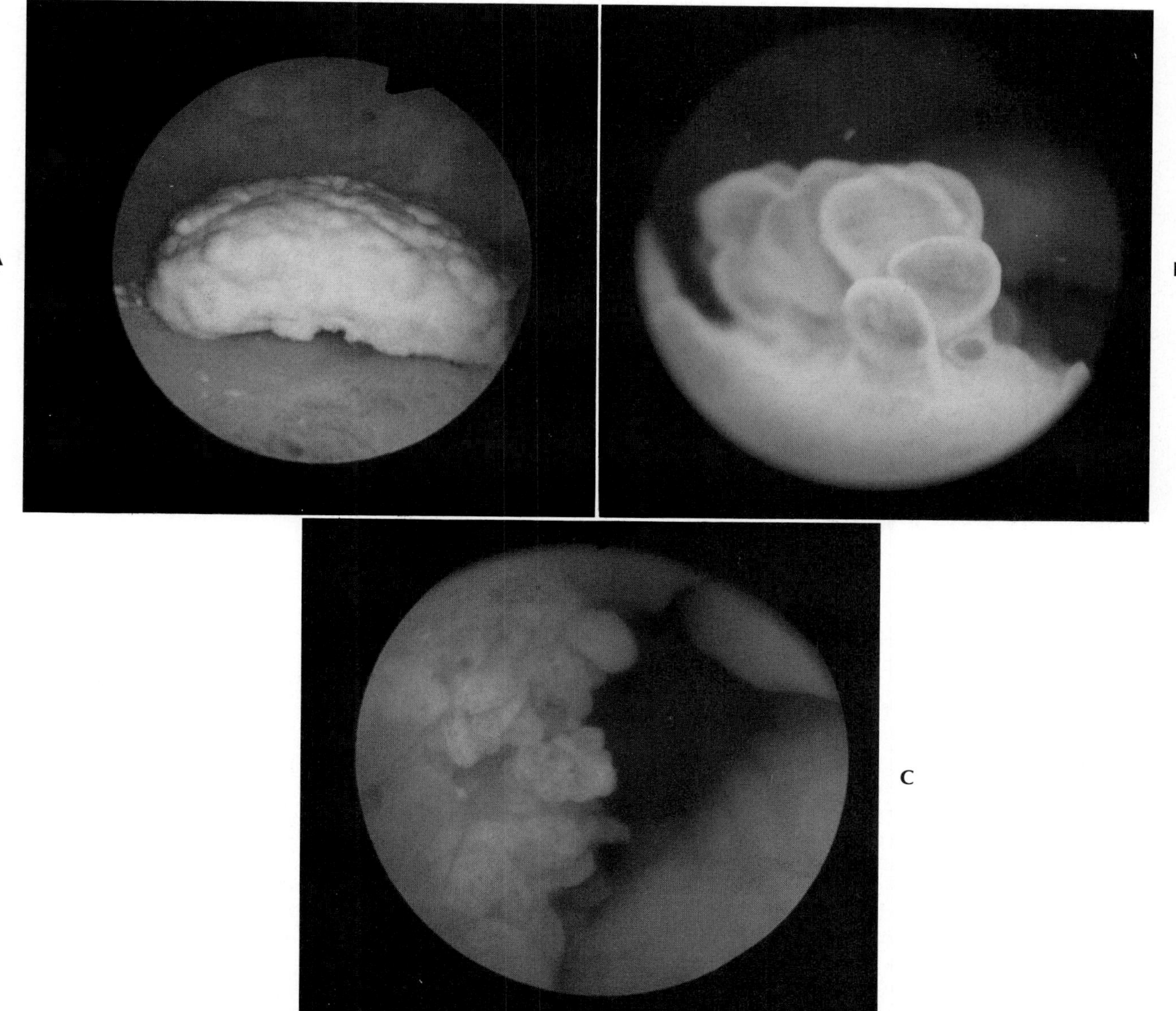

FIG. 13–5. Abnormalities seen via cystoscope. **A,** An infected struvite urolith. Notice the hyperplastic appearance of the bladder mucosa. **B,** Polypoid hyperplasia. **C,** Transitional cell carcinoma with areas of necrosis.

tional cell carcinoma versus adenocarcinoma) is not possible based on gross cystoscopic appearance.

3. Ectopic ureters
   a. The location of the final outlet of ectopic ureters is usually easy to establish via cystoscopy. In most instances, the ureter adopts a submucosal location where a normal ureteral orifice would have been, and then runs submucosally to the eventual opening some distance toward the bladder neck or in the urethra (Fig. 13–6A). The opening appears as a mucosal flap (Fig. 13–6B).
   b. Frequently the urethra has two small ridges running longitudinally distal from the ureteral opening for some of or almost the entire length of the urethra (Fig. 13–6C). These ridges could be vestigial remains of the wall of an even longer ectopic ureteral extension.
   c. The opening of the ectopic ureter can be identified much more easily if urine flow rate is high; thus, administration of diuretics prior to

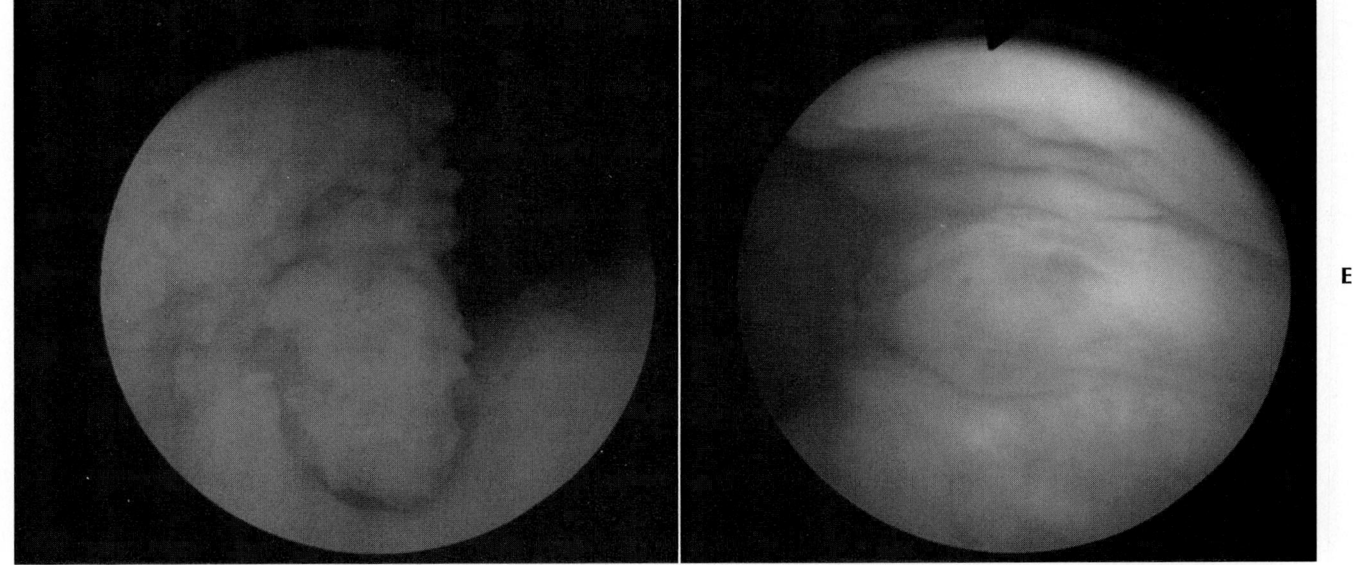

FIG. 13–5, cont'd. D, Transitional cell carcinoma. **E,** Transitional cell carcinoma.

cystoscopy can be helpful. If an excretory urogram is performed prior to cystoscopy, urine flow is usually sufficiently increased to allow easy identification of the ureteral opening.

X. CONTRAINDICATIONS AND PRECAUTIONS

A. Specific contraindications for cystoscopy have not been established in veterinary medicine. Urologists in human practice recommend that acute inflammatory processes, such as cystitis, prostatitis, and urethritis, be resolved before cystoscopy is attempted.[11]

B. Routine treatment with a broad-spectrum antimicrobial for 3 to 5 days following the cystoscopic procedure is probably advisable and is routinely employed in our clinic to prevent establishment of urinary tract infection secondary to trauma and introduction of pathogenic microorganisms.

XI. SPECIAL PROCEDURES

A. Biopsy.

1. Equipment Required
   a. Flexible biopsy forceps (Fig. 13–7A) and grasping forceps (Fig. 13–7B) of several sizes are available for obtaining tissue specimens via cystoscopy.
   b. There are limitations in the size of the biopsy instrument that can be passed through various sizes of cystoscope sheath. A 5 F biopsy forceps can be used through a 14 F or larger cystoscope sheath, a 7 F can be used through a 19.5 F or larger sheath, and a 10 F can be used through a 21 F or larger sheath.
   c. With smaller instruments, the tissue specimens are more likely to be inadequate for complete histologic assessment.
   d. Biopsy forceps should be maintained in good working order to prevent crush artifact as a result of tearing off rather than biting off pieces of tissue. The forceps should be lubricated on a regular basis and thoroughly cleaned and dried immediately after use to prevent corrosion of the hinge mechanism that operates the biopsy cups.
2. Technique. The biopsy forceps are advanced through the operating channel of the cystoscope sheath, and tissue samples are obtained under direct visualization.

B. Resection of polyps and tumors.

1. Tissue can be resected from the bladder by direct mechanical cutting with scissors, by electrocautery, and by laser.
2. Equipment
   a. Flexible scissors (Fig. 13–7C) are available for operating via cystoscopy. Because the smallest scissors size is 10 F, they are limited to use through a 21 F or larger cystoscope sheath.
   b. Electrocautery instruments (Figs. 13–7D, E, F, G) shaped as knives, probes, buttons, and loops are available. The smallest available size of all instruments but the loop electrode is 5 F, which can be passed through a 14 F or larger cystoscope sheath. The smallest loop electrode is 10 F and can be passed through a 21 F or larger sheath.
   c. The neodymium:YAG laser is well suited to tissue resection and coagulation via cystoscopy.[11] The laser emits light of 1060-μ wave-

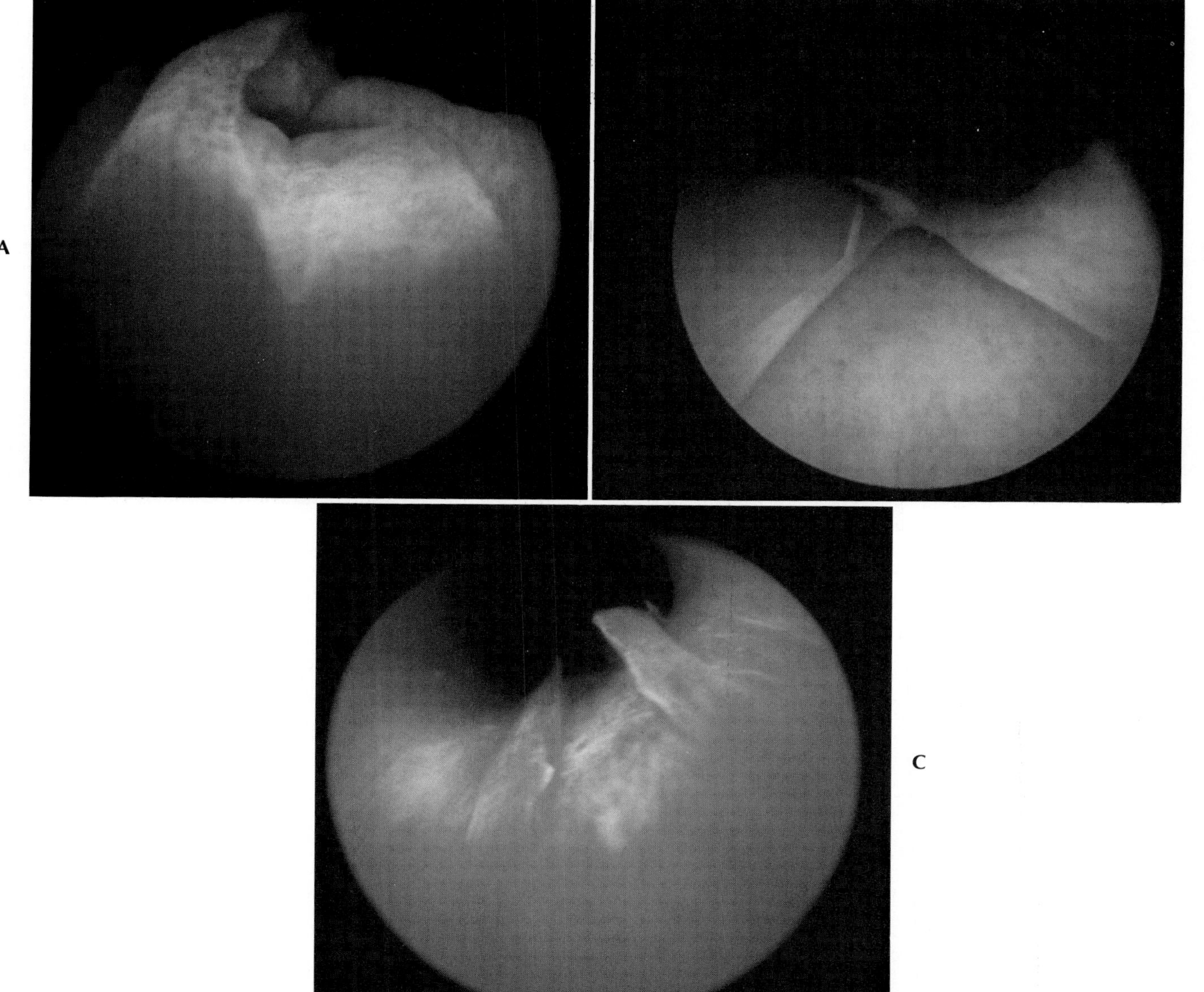

FIG. 13–6. Ectopic ureter. The ureteral opening is at an abnormal site in the bladder neck or urethral area **(A)** and appears as a tissue flap **(B).** Ridges exist along the urethra caudal to the ureteral opening **(C).**

length, which is easily transmitted by optical fibers, passes well through water, and can penetrate tissues to a depth of 4 to 5 mm. The laser light is capable of causing reproducible full-thickness bladder wall coagulation while maintaining bladder wall stability and integrity. Tissue sloughing occurs over a period of time following the procedure. Because the typical laser fiber sizes are 18 and 22 mm outer diameter, laser resection can be performed only through a 19 F or larger cystoscope sheath.

3. Technique
   a. Polypoid masses can be transected near the base. The base may then be lasered, or alternatively, the stalk may be cut and the base coagulated with cutting or resection electrocautery.
   b. Care should be taken to avoid bladder perforation or full-thickness destruction of the bladder wall with the laser.
   c. Nodular or sessile masses may be removed, but any suggestion that the neoplastic process in-

volves the muscularis layer should be a contraindication for total cystoscopic resection.

d. In the case of multiple tumors, those near the bubble should be resected first because accumulation of gas from previous resections occludes a good view of such tumors if they are not resected first.

e. Some experience is necessary when gauging the depth of laser tissue coagulation to avoid full-thickness bladder damage. Less chance of perforation is probable if the bladder is not fully distended because the bladder wall is thicker in the nondistended state.

C. Lithotripsy.

1. Mechanical litholapaxy
   a. Most mechanical devices useful for crushing and removing cystic uroliths in humans are too large or have an impractical shape for use in dogs and cats.
   b. Some of the specialized instruments could be used, but they are relatively expensive and not thought to have more utility than other medical or surgical approaches.
2. Electrohydraulic shock-wave lithotripsy (EHL)[27,28]
   a. EHL has been used on an experimental basis to remove bladder stones in dogs.[22] This system is capable of disintegrating hard uroliths.[11]
   b. Equipment required
      (1). A special spark generator and electrode system is required to deliver a series of shocks at the stone surface.
      (2). Each electrode lasts for about 15 to 50 seconds of operating time before wearing out (usually long enough to complete the disintegration of 1 stone).[6]
      (3). The EHL probes come in sizes 5, 7, and 9 F and can be used through 14, 19.5, and 21 F cystoscope sheaths, respectively(Fig. 13–7H).
      (4). The probes have a special tip that generates a spark between an axial and a cylindric electrode.
   c. Theoretic basis
      (1). When an electrical spark superheats water, a plasma bubble of superheated steam develops around the spark and generates a shock wave. When the spark stops, the plasma bubble collapses and another shock wave is produced. The spark generator develops DC pulses 50 or 100 times per second.
      (2). The successive high-pressure shock waves transmit sufficient energy to disrupt solid objects, such as uroliths.
   d. Technique
      (1). The procedure is performed while the bladder lumen contains a fluid medium, such as saline, to transmit hydraulic shock waves.
      (2). The electrode is advanced to within 1 mm of the urolith surface because the force of the shock wave varies inversely with the square of its distance from the spark.[17] Also, the electrode tip should be some distance from the end of the telescope because the shock waves can damage the telescope lens.
      (3). Using short 1- to 2-second bursts, the urolith is disintegrated (Fig. 13–8A). Larger fragments can be further broken up with successive shock waves (Fig. 13–8B).
      (4). Care should be taken to avoid applying the activated electrode directly on the bladder wall because severe mucosal and submucosal damage may lead to perforation.[6]
      (5). When the stone is sufficiently broken up, smaller fragments can be removed from the bladder with repeated in-and-out flushes through the cystoscope sheath using an Ellick evacuator (Richard Wolf Medical Instruments Corp., Rosemont, Illinois 60018). Larger fragments can be removed with a stone basket.

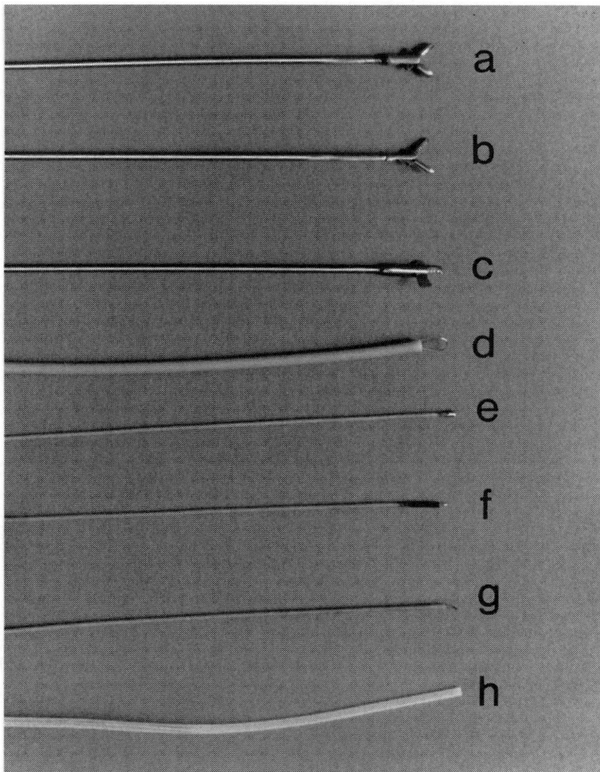

FIG. 13–7 Accessory instruments for cystoscopy include biopsy forceps **(a)**, grasping forceps **(b)**, scissors **(c)**, electrocautery instruments **(d, e, f, g)**, and electrohydraulic shock wave lithotriptor electrode **(h)**.

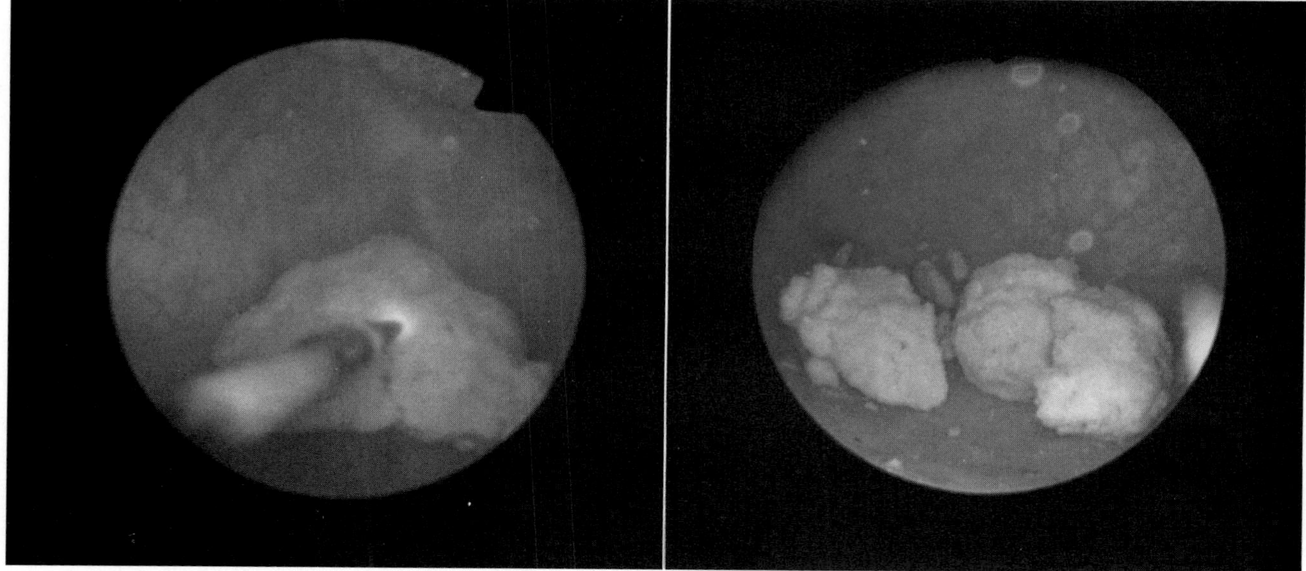

FIG. 13–8. A, Electrohydraulic shock wave lithotriptor electrode during activation **B,** The appearance of a urolith subsequent to fragmentation.

3. Ultrasonic lithotripsy[16,21]
   a. Use of ultrasonic lithotripsy has not been reported in veterinary medicine. Not all ultrasonic lithotriptors tested in my laboratory appeared capable of disintegrating dense struvite stones from dogs.
   b. Equipment required
      (1). Several companies manufacture cystoscopic equipment for ultrasonic removal of stones.
      (2). The smallest system available uses a 1.5-mm outer diameter sonotrode capable of being passed through an 11 F integrated sheath (Ultrasonic Lithotrite, Richard Wolf Medical Instruments Corp., Rosemont, Illinois 60018).
   c. Theoretic basis and technique
      (1). All ultrasonic lithotriptors utilize piezoceramic elements in a transducer to generate ultrasonic energy that is applied to a metal tip (sometimes jawed). The vibrations are usually 23 to 27 kHz.
      (2). The sonotrode is advanced into the bladder until it contacts the surface of the urolith. The tip of the probe is hollow. An irrigation system allows constant ingress of fluid into the bladder with subsequent egress out of the bladder via the lumen inside the hollow tip. Thus, as ultrasonic energy causes fragments to break away from the surface of the stone, they are suctioned out of the bladder, and the constant flow of irrigation fluid keeps the tip of the sonotrode cool.
      (3). One major advantage of ultrasonic lithotripsy is that tissue is not significantly damaged even when the mucosal surface is directly contacted with the activated probe tip.
      (4). The smallest ultrasonic lithotriptors available can be passed through an 11 F sheath; thus, the method is technically feasible in quite small dogs. Ultrasonic lithotriptors are rigid and cannot be used in a flexible endoscopy system.
      (5). At this time, the high cost of this equipment has precluded routine use of ultrasonic lithotripsy in dogs.

D. Ureteral catheterization.

1. Indications
   a. In humans, cystoscopic ureteral catheterization has been used for several purposes, including:
      (1). Localizing urinary tract infection
      (2). Performing retrograde pyelography
      (3). Diagnosing filling defects observed on intravenous pyelogram
      (4). Localizing stone in extracorporeal shockwave lithotripsy
      (5). Placing ureteral stents for drainage of obstructed kidneys
      (6). Removing ureteral stones with a stone basket
      (7). Performing brush biopsy of the renal pelvis
      (8). Performing differential clearance studies
      (9). Identifying ureters more readily during open surgery.[5,10,11,18,23]

b. We have found presurgical placement of a ureteral catheter into the ectopic ureter via cystoscopy useful in helping the surgeon to identify the exact location of the submucosal ureteral extension and in creating a new ureteral opening.

2. Equipment required. The most useful assemblies consist of a 70-cm 3 or 4 F whistle-tip ureteral catheter (Bard Urological Div., CR Bard, Inc., Murray Hill, New Jersey 07974) matched to a corresponding 145-cm long 0.018- or 0.021-inch J-tipped guidewire (Rosen Curved Safe-T-J Wire Guide, Cook Inc., Bloomington, Indiana 47402), respectively.[23]
3. Technique[23]
   a. The J-tipped guidewire is passed into the lumen of the whistle-tip catheter until the catheter and wire are tip-to-tip.
   b. The catheter-wire combination is inserted through the cystoscope and advanced about 1 to 2 cm into the ureteral orifice. At this point, resistance to further introduction is usually observed.
   c. The J-tipped guidewire is then advanced gently beyond the tip of the catheter into the ureter until resistance is met. Then the wire is held on tension while the catheter is advanced over the wire up toward the renal collection system.
   d. Sometimes the wire and then the catheter have to be advanced in turn several times before the catheter can be passed up to the renal pelvis without resistance.
   e. Once the catheter is in position, the J-tipped guidewire can be removed from the catheter.

E. Periurethral injection of polytetrafluorothylene paste.

1. Periurethral injection of polytetrafluoroethylene paste (Polytef Paste for Injection, Mentor, Norwell, Massachusetts 02061) via cystoscope in dogs has been used to treat urinary incontinence.[1] The paste adds bulk to the periurethral and urethral tissues, and with inflation of these tissues, compression of the urethral lumen results.[1,19] This procedure has given good to excellent results in humans for many years, is well tolerated, and has induced minimal complications.[19,20]
2. In dogs, the procedure was reserved for animals that did not respond to or could not tolerate medical treatment for urinary incontinence and in which the history, physical examination, and urodynamic findings suggested urethral incompetence.[1] The paste used contained 50% polytetrafluoroethylene and 50% polyethylene glycol.
3. In female dogs, the cystoscope was passed transurethrally to the site of injection, whereas in male dogs the cystoscope was passed via cystotomy or could be passed via urethrotomy.
4. Three Teflon deposits were injected into the urethral submucosa at 4, 8, and 12 o'clock positions, all approximately 1.5 cm caudal to the junction between the bladder neck and urethra.[1] Most dogs required injection of a total volume of 1.5 to 2 ml subdivided between all 3 sites. Upon completion of the procedure, the cystoscopic appearance indicated that the injection sites were nearly apposed to one another and the urethral lumen was almost occluded.[1]
5. In the series of 22 dogs treated with periurethral Teflon, urinary incontinence recurred in 14 dogs (64%), but was subsequently controlled by a second Teflon injection in 11 of 12 dogs (92%).[1] Several minor complications observed following the procedure included transient stranguria with or without hematuria (4 of 35 procedures) and temporary partial urethral obstruction in 1 dog. Histologic examination indicated cell-free Teflon surrounded by fibrous tissue in 2 dogs, but a granulomatous reaction developed in 1 dog.
6. Although tissue migration of Teflon was not observed in this study, previous studies in dogs revealed that periurethral and subureteric injection resulted in migration of Teflon particles to the pelvic lymph nodes, liver, spleen, kidneys, lung, and brain.[14,15] The recent development of glutaraldehyde cross-linked bovine collagen used in place of Teflon has promise because local tissue reaction and migration do not appear to be a problem.[4,12]

XII. PHOTOGRAPHY AND VIDEO IMAGING

A. For still photography, a suitable camera with a lens adaptor for attachment to the eyepiece of the cystoscope telescope is required. To obtain good still photographs and video imaging, all equipment must be of the highest quality. Telescopes and light-carrying cables capable of carrying maximum light should be used, and the light source should have a quartz-glass xenon arc-light bulb. The high-quality light sources are equipped with automatic systems for flash still photography.

B. When taking still photographs, some experience is necessary in framing and composing the field of view so that over- and underexposure of the subject are avoided. Because insufficient light is available to adequately illuminate a large depth of field view, photographs are usually limited to single subjects.

C. For video imaging, a camera attachment for the cystoscope telescope, a video monitor, and a video recorder are required. A very powerful light source is mandatory to obtain a good image. The video monitor can be used by the operator to perform procedures without direct visualization through the telescope eyepiece. All systems result in a loss in quality of the image compared to that seen directly through the telescope eyepiece, but in many procedures, the loss of quality is sufficiently minor to

make no difference in the ability to adequately perform the procedure. However, the initial examination of the urinary tract should be done using direct visualization so that small lesions and subtle changes are not missed.

When recording cystoscopic procedures, the VHS recorder should be set on high speed (SP) to record an image of the highest possible quality.

REFERENCES

1. Arnold S, et al. Treatment of urinary incontinence in dogs by endoscopic injection of Teflon. *J Am Vet Med Assoc.* 1989;195: 1369-1374.
2. Brearley MJ, Cooper JE. The diagnosis of bladder disease in dogs by cystoscopy. *J Small Anim Pract.* 1987;28:75-85.
3. Brearley MJ, Milroy EJD, Rickards D. A percutaneous approach for cystoscopy in male dogs. *Res Vet Sci.* 1988;44:380-382.
4. Canning DA, Peters CA, Gearhart JR, Jeffs RD. Local tissue response to glutaraldehyde cross-linked bovine collagen in the rabbit bladder. *J Urol.* 1988;139(pt 2):258A. Abstract.
5. Chaussy C, et al. First clinical experience with extracorporeally induced destruction of kidney stones by shock waves. *J Urol.* 1982;127:417-420.
6. Comisarow RH, Barkin M. Electrohydraulic cystolithopaxy. *Can J Surg.* 1979;22:525-526.
7. Cooper JE, Brearley MJ. Urothelial abnormalities in the canine bladder. *Vet Rec.* 1986;118:513-514.
8. Cooper JE, et al. Cystoscopic examination of male and female dogs. *Vet Rec.* 1984;115:571-574.
9. Ensor RD, Boyarsky S, Glenn JF. Cystoscopy and ureteral catheterization in the dog. *J Am Vet Med Assoc.* 1966;149:1067-1072.
10. Hunter PT, et al. Hawkins-Hunter retrograde transcutaneous nephrostomy: A new technique. *Urology.* 1983;22:583-587.
11. Lange PH. Diagnostic and therapeutic urologic instrumentation. In: Walsh PC, Gitter RF, Perlmutter AD, Stamey TA, eds. *Campbell's Urology.* Philadelphia, Pennsylvania: WB Saunders Co; 1986.
12. Leonard MP, et al. Local tissue reaction to the subureteral injection of glutaraldehyde cross-linked bovine collagen in humans. *J Urol.* 1990;143:1209-1212.
13. McCarthy TC, McDermaid SL. Prepubic percutaneous cystoscopy in the dog and cat. *J Am Anim Hosp Assoc.* 1986;22:213-219.
14. Malizia AA, et al. Migration and granulomatous reaction after periurethral injection of Polytef (Teflon). *JAMA.* 1984;251:3277-3281.
15. Malizia AA, et al. Migration and granulomatous reaction after intravesical/subureteric injection of Polytef. *J Urol.* 1987;137(pt 2):122A. Abstract.
16. Marberger M. Disintegration of renal and ureteral calculi with ultrasound. *Urol Clin North Am.* 1983;10:729-742.
17. Martin EC, Wolff M, Neff RA, Casarella WJ. Use of electrohydraulic lithotriptor in the biliary tree of dogs. *Radiology.* 1981; 139:215-217.
18. Newman RC, et al. ESWL—effect on canine renal and neurologic tissue. In: Gravenstein JS, Peter K, eds. *Extracorporeal Shock Wave Lithotripsy.* Stoneham, Massachusetts: Butterworth Publishing Co; 1986.
19. Politano VA. Periurethral polytetrafluoroethylene injection for urinary incontinence. *J Urol.* 1982;127:439-442.
20. Politano VA, Small MP, Harper JM. Periurethral Teflon injection for urinary incontinence. In: Transactions of the XVI Congres de la Societe Internatinale d'Urologie, Amsterdam: Diffusion Doin Editeurs, 1973;459.
21. Raney AM. Electrohydraulic cystolithotripsy. *Urology.* 1976;7: 379-381.
22. Senior DF. Electrohydraulic shock-wave lithotripsy in experimental canine struvite bladder stone disease. *Vet Surg.* 1984;13: 143-148.
23. Senior DF, Newman RC. Retrograde ureteral catheterization in female dogs. *J Am Anim Hosp Assoc.* 1986;22:831-834.
24. Senior DF, Sundstrom DA. Cystoscopy in female dogs. *Comp Contin Educ Pract Vet.* 1988;10:890-895.
25. Trindade JCS, Lantenschlager MFM, de Araujo CG. Endoscopic surgery: A new teaching method. *J Urol.* 1981;126:192.
26. Vermooten V. Cystoscopy in male and female dogs. *J Lab Clin Med.* 1930;15:650-657.
27. Watson BW. Urat-1: Instrument for crushing calculi in the urinary bladder by electrohydraulics. *Biomed Eng.* 1970;5:21-22.
28. Yutkin LA. *Electrohydraulic Effect.* Published Union of Soviet Socialist Republics, 1955. English translation US Dept of Commerce Office of Technical Services Dept, 62-14184, MCL, 1207/1-2.

CHAPTER 14

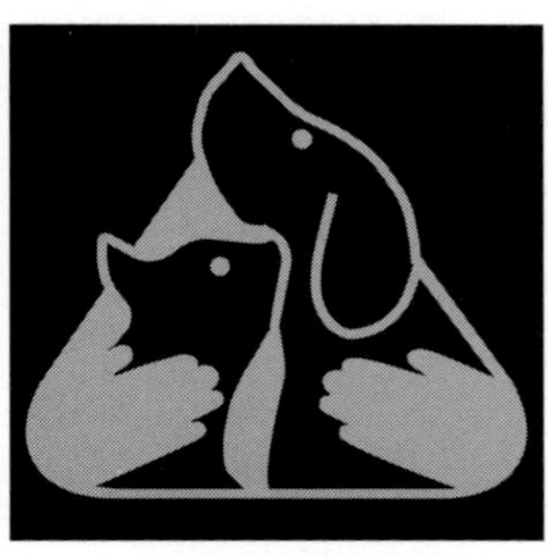

Tests of Lower Urinary Tract Function in Dogs and Cats

JEANNE A. BARSANTI

I. INDICATIONS FOR EVALUATING LOWER URINARY TRACT FUNCTION

A. Incontinence.

1. Incontinence is defined as the involuntary leakage of urine from the urethral orifice. (See Chapter 37, Disorders of Micturition, for a more complete review.) Incontinence must be distinguished from a urethral discharge caused by urethral disease in males or females, a urethral discharge caused by prostatic disease in males, a vaginal discharge in females, or a preputial discharge in males. This distinction is usually made by vaginal or preputial examination and by comparing fluid discharge with urine collected from the bladder by cystocentesis or catheterization.
2. Incontinence always indicates dysfunction of the lower urinary tract, which normally stores urine and evacuates it under voluntary control. This dysfunction may be primarily the result of abnormalities in neurologic pathways controlling micturition (neurogenic incontinence) or may be the result of anatomic or physiologic abnormalities in the bladder or urethra.
3. Neurogenic incontinence is often associated with other abnormalities on neurologic examination, such as paraplegia or a decreased perineal reflex. In such cases, the diagnostic plan entails the localization and identification of the neurologic lesion rather than the examination of the lower urinary tract per se. Extensive testing of lower urinary tract function usually is not performed in such cases unless the pattern of incontinence does not correlate with the localization of the neurologic lesion or unless the incontinence is being pursued to assist in localizing the neurologic lesion.
4. Electrodiagnostic tests of lower urinary tract function are indicated in cases of nonneurogenic incontinence.
   a. When less invasive tests have failed to indicate a cause for incontinence.
   b. When therapy for the most likely cause of the incontinence fails.
   c. When incontinence is associated with another cause of lower urinary tract dysfunction. The most common example is the presence of ectopic ureters, which are often associated with urethral incompetence.[30]
5. Most cases of incontinence can be diagnosed successfully and treated without electrodiagnostic tests if other approaches, such as history, physical examination, urinalysis, and radiography, are used appropriately. However, some cases cannot be diagnosed or treated effectively without urodynamic testing.[31] These cases may be referred to centers with electrodiagnostic testing equipment.

B. Inability to empty the bladder.

1. An animal that is unable to empty its bladder, but that has intact sensation from the bladder, attempts to void frequently and may strain (dys-

uria). On physical examination, the bladder is at least partially distended. Sometimes the animal is also incontinent.

2. The most common nonneurogenic cause of this problem is complete or partial obstruction to urine flow in the urethra or bladder neck. A complete obstruction may be excluded by passing a urethral catheter. Note, though, that some soft tissue lesions that prevent normal passage of urine allow retrograde passage of a urinary catheter. Detailed radiographic studies (including voiding and retrograde urethrograms, with the bladder both empty and distended) are necessary to exclude a partial obstruction. Ultrasonography may also be used to identify bladder neck and prostatic urethral lesions.
3. When no evidence of obstruction is found on these studies, urodynamic testing is warranted to evaluate detrusor function and to evaluate further the possibility of urethral obstruction or constriction.

C. Severe prostatic disease.

1. Marked prostatomegaly can adversely affect lower urinary tract function. Signs of lower urinary tract dysfunction may not be noted because of the severity of signs related to the prostate disease itself.[6] Once the disease is treated, especially if the disease is treated surgically by prostatectomy,[6,21] incontinence may become a major problem.
2. Results of pre-operative electrodiagnostic testing allow surgeons to more accurately advise an owner of the potential for postoperative problems with urination, including incontinence.

II. TESTS OF LOWER URINARY TRACT FUNCTION

A. History.

1. The patient's history is an important part of determining the cause of lower urinary tract dysfunction.
2. The precise nature of the problem must be determined. Is the animal dribbling fluid? If so, when, how often, and where? What is the nature of the fluid? Some owners confuse behavioral problems with urination, such as marking and submissive urination, with incontinence. At what age did the problem begin? Is it getting better or worse? Did neutering have any relationship to the onset of incontinence?
3. One must determine whether the animal ever urinates normally. When the animal initiates urination, does urination appear to be normal or does the animal strain? Is the volume of urine voided normal? When does incontinence occur in relation to urination?
4. One should establish whether the patient is receiving any drugs that may affect urinary tract function or that may cause polyuria. Polyuria with increased bladder volume may lead to incontinence in animals with marginal urethral competence or with decreased bladder capacity.
5. In addition to the questions specifically related to urination, a thorough general history should be obtained to detect any neurologic or systemic diseases that may be related to incontinence.

B. Physical examination/observation of micturition.

1. The physical examination is another important part of evaluation of lower urinary tract function. The bladder and urethra should be palpated in males and females, and the prostate gland should be palpated in male dogs even if the dog has been neutered (Fig. 14–1). (See Chapter 39, Diseases of the Prostate Gland.) Anal tone and the integrity of the perineal reflex can be evaluated during the rectal examination. Portions of the urethra in the male dog also can be palpated under the skin from the perineal region to the os penis. The urethral orifice can be observed in males by retracting the prepuce from over the penis and in females by vaginal examination.
2. The act of urination should be observed as an extension of the physical examination, and the bladder should be palpated prior to and after urination to determine whether the animal can empty the bladder (Fig. 14–2). If the bladder cannot be palpated well because the animal is tense or obese, catheterization of the bladder after the patient has urinated may be necessary to determine residual volume. Residual volume should be low. Less than 0.1 ml/kg residual volume was found in 10- to 30-kg male and female dogs in a study.[34] Alterna-

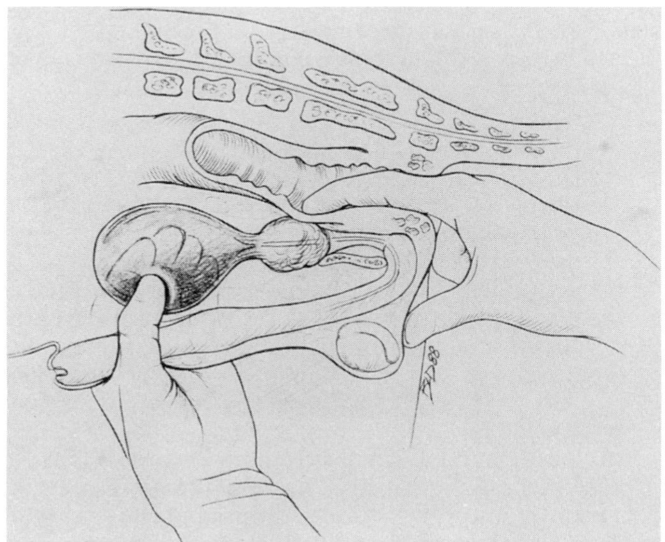

FIG. 14–1 Palpation of the prostate gland per rectum and the urinary bladder per abdomen in a male dog. The urethra also can be palpated per rectum in male and female dogs. Occasionally, depending on prostatic position, the prostate gland can be palpated per abdomen.

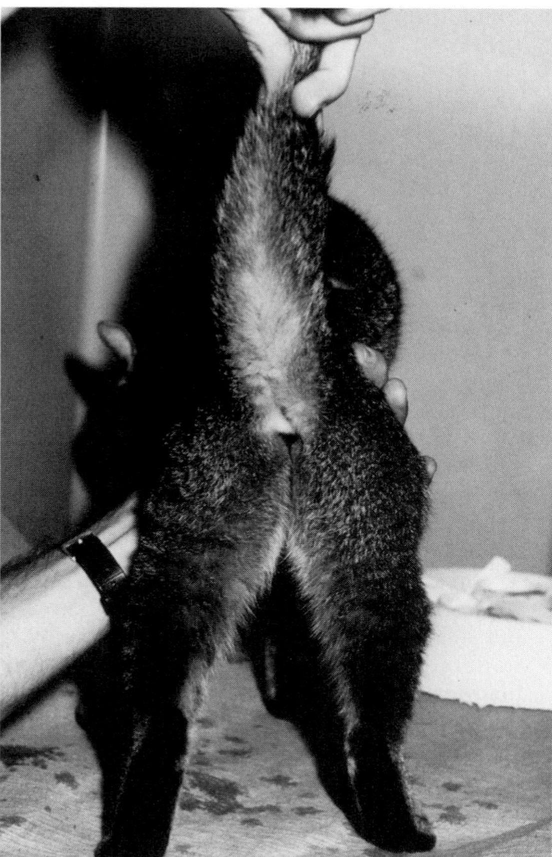

FIG. 14–2 Palpation of the caudal abdomen of a cat with urinary incontinence. The numerous small dark spots on the cage paper were urine that dripped from the vulva as the cat walked about. Palpation of the bladder when incontinence is occurring determines whether incontinence is associated with a full bladder (suggesting a problem in emptying the bladder) or with a small bladder (indicating a problem in ability to store urine).

tively, radiography or ultrasonography can be used to determine bladder size.

C. Urodynamic studies: an overview.

1. To understand urodynamics, one must understand the anatomy of the lower urinary tract and the normal physiology of the storage and emptying phases of micturition. (See Chapter 1, Applied Anatomy of the Urinary System with Clinicopathologic Correlation.)
2. Urodynamics can be used to evaluate bladder function (cystometry), urethral function (urethral profilometry), or both (uroflowmetry). In addition, electromyography can be combined with urodynamic techniques to evaluate associated muscle function, particularly of the urethra and anal sphincter.
3. These tests require specialized equipment and are not available in all referral centers.

III. URODYNAMIC TESTS

A. Cystometry.

1. Technique
   a. Cystometry is used to evaluate the ability of the bladder to relax and store appropriate urine volumes and to evaluate its ability to contract when full.[37] Cystometry is most useful to determine whether the bladder is capable of contracting and to determine whether bladder storage capacity is normal.
   b. Cystometry is usually performed with xylazine restraint. The usual dose is 2.2 mg/kg subcutaneously or intramuscularly,[28,37,38] but a dose of 1 mg/kg subcutaneously also has been reported.[8] Intravenous xylazine at 1.1 mg/kg can also be used. Xylazine has minimal effects on the detrusor reflex (approximately 85% of normal dogs sedated with xylazine have a detrusor reflex),[28,34,37] but provides sedation to reduce both movement artifact and incidence of voluntary inhibition of the detrusor reflex, both of which occur in unsedated animals.[28,38] Potential adverse effects of xylazine include nausea, vomiting, and periods of excitement characterized by twitching, snapping, and curling of the lips in dogs. Heart rate is also markedly reduced.[29] Atropine (0.04 to 0.06 mg/kg, subcutaneously) can be used to counteract the bradycardia[4,26,28]; however, atropine also potentiates xylazine-induced hypertension.[26] Although atropine does not significantly affect most of the components measured during cystometry,[4,28] atropine has been shown experimentally to decrease maximal contraction pressure, decrease the ability of the bladder to sustain a contraction, and decrease bladder emptying in dogs and cats. Dosage of atropine may be important, because higher doses are often used experimentally (0.05 to 0.4 mg/kg).[1,10,11,13,46] The effects of atropine have only been evaluated in normal animals. Effects in animals with abnormalities in the lower urinary tract may be different.[27] We do not routinely use atropine, and find clinically significant adverse reactions to xylazine to be infrequent. Drugs that reportedly alter or decrease the detrusor reflex (at least at the dosages studied) include acepromazine maleate, fentanyl-droperidol, ketamine, diazepam with ketamine, pentobarbital, methoxyflurane, and halothane.[28,37] Results with oxymorphone and low dosages of acepromazine have been inconsistent.[3,28,36]
   c. Before cystometry is performed, the bladder is catheterized and emptied. Retention catheters (Foley catheters) are usually used in female dogs and rubber urethral catheters are used in male dogs and cats.[28,37] Plastic tomcat catheters can also be used in cats. Size 8 or 10 F catheters

are usually used in dogs, and 3 or 5 F sizes are used in cats. The catheter should barely reach the bladder so that it does not kink. Kinking in the catheter causes artifacts in the recording. The catheter is connected to a device to record pressure, and either sterile fluid (usually saline) or carbon dioxide is infused by a nonpulsatile pump at a known rate (Fig. 14–3). The transducer used to detect the pressure should be at the same height as the bladder. A chart records the amount infused per unit time and the bladder pressure. The recording of changes in intravesicular pressure during filling and contraction of the urinary bladder is referred to as a cystometrogram (CMG). Cystometry has also been performed, at least in normal animals, by percutaneously placing a catheter(s) directly into the bladder for infusion and pressure recording.[34,36,44]

d. The rate of fluid infusion should be proportional to the size of the animal. The bladder should be allowed to distend gradually during at least 5 minutes. Rates used for small dogs and cats should be about 3 mL/min, whereas rates for large dogs can be as great as 100 mL/min. These rates still greatly exceed physiologic filling rates. (Urine production is estimated to be 0.02 to 0.04 mL/min/kg.) Intravesicular pressure should not be allowed to exceed 40 cm H_2O during filling.[28] Overdistention of the bladder can lead to transient hematuria.[3,4,28] If a detrusor reflex does not occur on the first recording, cystometry should be repeated once to ensure that the response of the animal is consistent.[28]

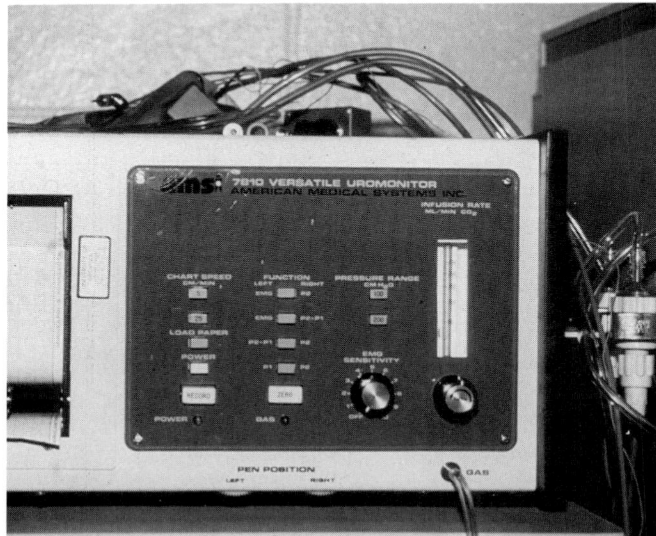

FIG. 14–3 Example of an instrument used to perform cystometry in dogs and cats. The instrument contains an internal carbon dioxide cartridge and has an adjustable infusion rate. The transducer on the right detects pressure in the bladder via a transurethral catheter. The pressure is recorded on the paper to the left. An electromyogram can be recorded by the same instrument.

e. Cystometry can be done at the same time as contrast radiography, with the advantages of direct correlation of anatomic with functional changes and of correct positioning of the urinary catheter.[32]

f. A potential adverse effect of cystometry is development of urinary tract infection, probably as a result of urinary tract manipulation.[7] Infection has been reported in approximately 12% of the animals tested.[28] A broad-spectrum antibiotic, such as ampicillin, may be administered on the day of cystometry in an attempt to prevent such infections.[4] Whether or not antibiotics are used, a urinalysis should be performed a few days after cystometry to be sure that infection did not result.

g. Potential sources of error in cystometry include failure to adequately calibrate the instruments, the presence of air bubbles in the recording catheters or transducers if fluid infusion is used, variation in the location of the catheter in the bladder or kinking of the catheter, injury to the bladder from the catheter, and variation in degree of sedation or the sedative used.

2. Normal Findings
   a. Normally, bladder pressure rises slowly during filling. When threshold volume and pressure are reached, the bladder contracts (detrusor reflex). During contraction, pressure rises rapidly and then falls as the fluid (or carbon dioxide) is expelled (Fig. 14–4).
   b. Values recorded are (Fig. 14–4)[37]:
      (1). T-I: intravesicular pressure at the beginning of the infusion.
      (2). T-II: the change in pressure from T-I to threshold pressure (or to T-III) in relation to the volume infused; a measure of bladder compliance.
      (3). T-III: a significant increase in pressure occurring after T-II and prior to the detrusor reflex; rarely noted in CMGs in dogs or cats.[28,37]
      (4). $T_{threshold}$ or T_{thresh}: intravesicular pressure at the onset of the detrusor reflex.
      (5). T_{max}: maximal intravesicular pressure during the detrusor reflex; this value is often not measured when retention (Foley) catheters are used because the gas cannot be expelled; when a retention catheter is used, the catheter for infusion should be disconnected when the detrusor contraction is sustained so the gas can be expelled.
      (6). TV: volume of fluid or gas infused to initiate a detrusor reflex; measure of blad-

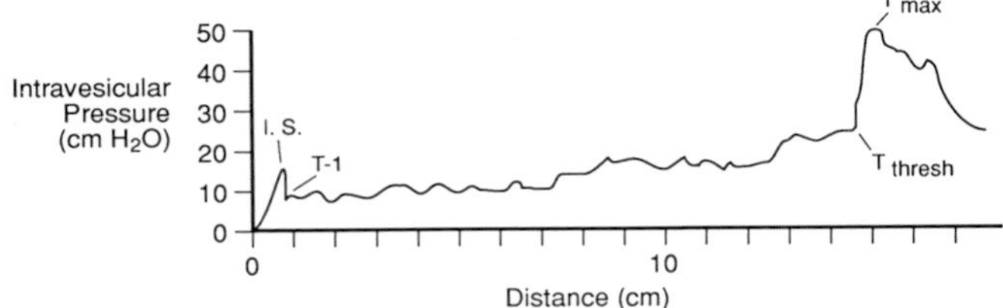

FIG. 14–4 Cystometrogram from a normal dog under xylazine restraint. The vertical axis records intravesicular pressure. The horizontal axis indicates intravesicular volume with knowledge of chart speed and infusion rate. The initial spike (I.S.) is an artifact of the gas filling the catheter. T-I is the intravesicular pressure at the beginning of the infusion. T-II measures the change in pressure in relation to volume of CO_2 infused. T-II is calculated by subtracting T-I from T_{thresh} and dividing by bladder volume. Note that there is little change in pressure as the bladder fills, but a rapid increase in pressure occurs as the bladder contracts. T_{thresh} is the pressure at the onset of the detrusor reflex. When the bladder contracts, the intravesicular pressure rises rapidly to a maximum (T_{max}) and then falls as the CO_2 is expelled. Bladder volume (TV) to initiate a detrusor reflex is determined by knowing the infusion rate (e.g., 50 ml/min) and the chart speed (e.g., 5 cm/min), counting the distance from T-I to T_{thresh} (e.g., 13.4 cm), and calculating the milliliters infused in 13.4 cm (e.g., 50 mL/min divided by 5 cm/min equals 10 mL/cm; therefore, 13.4 cm indicates 134 ml were infused).

der capacity. A direct correlation exists between body weight and bladder capacity.[3,37]

c. CMGs have been found to be reproducible when immediately repeated,[37] with the exception that normal animals that fail to have a detrusor reflex on the first recording occasionally have a contraction on a second trial.[28] CMGs also have been found to be reproducible on different days and with either intravenous or intramuscular xylazine.[36]

d. Normal Values (Table 14–1): Note that these values are based on relatively few animals of limited size variation and with different techniques.
   (1). Male cats: Some normal male cats had apparent detrusor hyperactivity (bladder contraction at low intravesicular volumes).
   (2). Normal male and female dogs: In general, results from male and female dogs have been similar.

3. Examples of Major Abnormalities
   a. Absence of a detrusor reflex
      (1). Absence of a detrusor reflex (Fig. 14–5) can be the result of voluntary inhibition, of an effect of the drug used for restraint, or of inability to contract. Whether the animal can void voluntarily should be assessed to help to distinguish voluntary

TABLE 14–1.
NORMAL VALUES REPORTED FOR CYSTOMETRY IN DOGS AND MALE CATS

Animals Studied (Reference No.)	T-I (cm H_2O)	T-II (cm H_2O/100 mL)	$T_{threshold}$ (cm H_2O)	Threshold Volume (mL)	Threshold Volume (mL/kg)	T_{max} (cm H_2O)
12 dogs, 9.5-25.9 kg* (4)	6 (S.D. 3)	26 (S.D. 16)	34 (S.D. 9)	130 (S.D. 73)	6.6 (S.D. 2.3)	40 (S.D. 7)
10 dogs, 20-30 kg* (28)	Not given	8 (S.D. 4.1)	22.9 (S.D. 8.5)	Not given	10.0 (S.D. 3.8)	Not given
23 dogs, 5-30 kg* (37,38)	9.7 (S.D. 4.3)	12.6 (S.D. 12.2)	24.4 (S.D. 10.0)	206.6 (S.D. 184.4)	Not given	77.6 (S.D. 33.8)
11 intact male cats, 2.5-6.0 kg† (44)	Not given	Not given	19.32 (S.D. 16.83)	24 (S.D. 24)	Not given	64.32 (S.D. 24.11)
6 male dogs, 13.1-27.5 kg‡ (34)	8.2 (S.D. 3.0)	Not given	31.2 (S.D. 11.1)	Not given	8.4 (S.D. 2.9)	62.0 (S.D. 15.2)
6 female dogs, 16.2-26.6 kg (34)	8.0 (S.D. 3.8)	Not given	27.7 (S.D. 11.1)	Not given	11.6 (S.D. 5.0)	37.6 (S.D. 8.1)

*Xylazine sedation with CO_2 infusion through a transurethral catheter.
†Xylazine sedation (0.1 mg/kg 1M) and ketamine (1 mg/kg 1M) restraint through a percutaneous intravesicular catheter with fluid infusion.
‡Xylazine restraint through a percutaneous intravesicular catheter with fluid infusion.
S.D. = standard deviation.

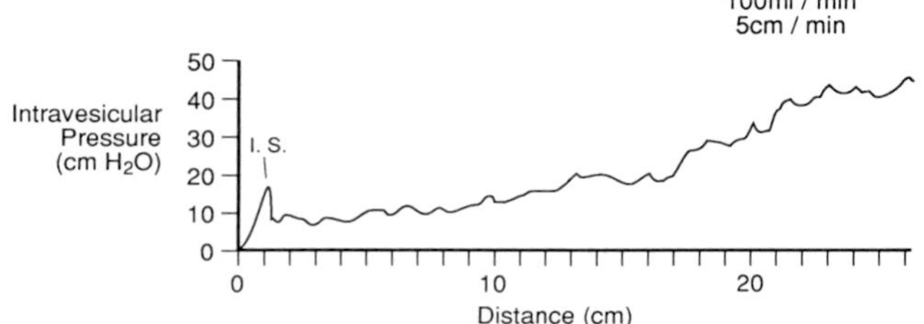

FIG. 14–5 An example of a cystometrogram showing absence of a detrusor reflex. A gradual rise in intravesicular pressure is shown. No sharp increase in pressure, indicative of a detrusor reflex, occurs. The infusion is stopped when bladder pressure exceeds 40 cm H_2O to avoid bladder injury from overdistention. I.S. = initial spike. Reprinted with permission from Barsanti, JA. *Small Animal Medical Diagnosis.* Philadelphia, PA: JB Lippincott Co; 1987:348.

inhibition and drug effects. Animals that voluntarily inhibit voiding may also become restless and attempt to move about when the bladder is full. If no detrusor reflex occurs on the first CMG, the CMG should be repeated because the reflex may not be inhibited on the second attempt.[28]

(2). Inability of the detrusor to contract can be the result of lack of innervation (as per a sacral spinal cord injury) or of detrusor muscle injury (as per chronic overdistention). Other findings on the neurologic examination or abnormalities on an electromyogram (EMG) of the perineal area can be used to help to distinguish these possibilities.

(3). Lack of a detrusor reflex on a CMG should not be used prognostically. Absence of the reflex does not mean that the reflex cannot be re-established.

b. Small bladder capacity/decreased compliance (Fig. 14–6)

(1). Reduced bladder capacity, decreased compliance, or rapid detrusor contraction (detrusor instability) can be caused by:[5,31]

(a). Changes in the bladder wall associated with inflammation, fibrosis, or neoplasia

(b). Decreased bladder size, either congenital or secondary to disease or cystectomy

(c). Neuropathy (detrusor hyperreflexia)

(d). Idiopathy. Detrusor instability secondary to prostatectomy for a prostatic abscess has also been reported.[6]

(2). Separation of these possibilities requires urinalysis, urine culture, and contrast radiography and/or ultrasonography. Only cystometry can confirm that detrusor hyperactivity (detrusor instability) exists.

(3). Too rapid a rate of filling can also result in erroneous diagnosis of decreased capacity and decreased compliance because the bladder cannot accommodate to rapid fluid infusions.[9] To exclude this possibility, cystometry should be repeated with a slower infusion rate.

c. Increased bladder capacity/increased bladder compliance

(1). These findings are often associated with decreased bladder contractility. However, some dogs with these findings have normal contractility.[34]

(2). If bladder contractility is normal, as indicated by a normal detrusor reflex, such abnormal findings related to capacity and compliance are usually not pursued.

(3). If bladder contractility is reduced, these findings may be the result of chronic overdistention. These findings do not reliably indicate prognosis for return of bladder function, as they may be reversed with appropriate therapy for overdistention.

B. Urethral pressure profilometry.

1. Technique

a. The function of the urethra can be evaluated by measuring pressure throughout the entire urethra at rest (a resting urethral pressure profile).[42,43] The urethral pressure profile measures the response of the urethral smooth and striated musculature and fibroelastic tissue. The profile is also affected by the diameter of the urethral lumen. The urethral pressure profile is used to determine whether intraurethral pressure is normal or reduced or whether areas of increased pressure, associated with partial urethral obstruction, are detectable.

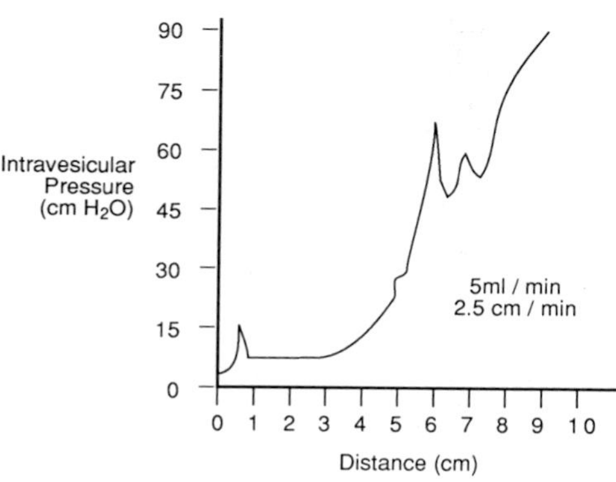

FIG. 14–6 A cystometrogram from a cat shows two detrusor reflexes that were not sustained followed by a strong sustained contraction. Note that the detrusor reflexes occurred at a small bladder volume, thus indicating detrusor instability.

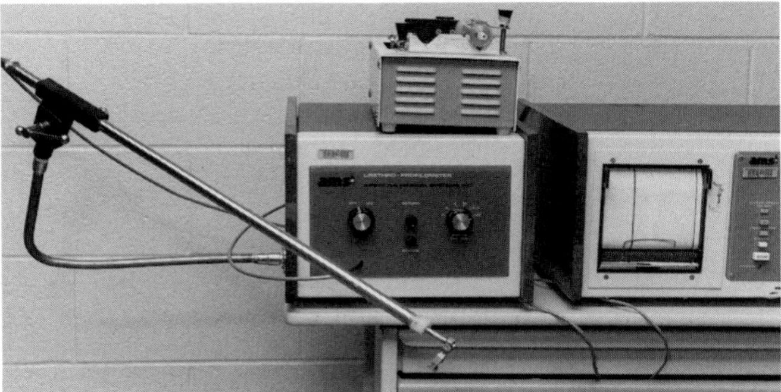

FIG. 14–7 Example of an instrument that can be used for urethral pressure profilometry in dogs and cats. A nonpulsatile pump (on the top of the instrument) is used to infuse sterile saline through a transurethral catheter at a known rate. Pressure is detected by connecting the catheter to a transducer, which transfers the result to the strip chart recorder. With this instrument, a robot arm withdraws the catheter at a preset speed. An EMG can be recorded at the same time by using the second channel on the chart.

b. The urethral pressure profile can be performed without sedation,[33,40,41] with xylazine restraint,[17,18,42,43] or with general anesthesia.[19] The dosages of xylazine used for profilometry are the same as those used for cystometry. Xylazine restraint results in lower urethral pressures and eliminates or attenuates the EMG response in dogs,[40] and lowers midurethral pressures in male cats.[33] General anesthesia also lowers resting urethral pressures.[19,24] Atropine has little effect on the urethral pressure profile in dogs.[2,4,14]

c. For urethral profilometry, the animal is usually placed in right lateral recumbency, although dorsal recumbency has been used in cats.[33,45] A urinary catheter is inserted into the bladder, the bladder is emptied, and the catheter is connected to a pressure transducer. The pressure transducer should be at the same height as the bladder and urethra (Fig. 14–7). Ordinary urinary catheters (8 F in dogs and 3 or 3.5 F in cats) with a single side hole are usually used, with the exception that the orientation of the side hole within the urethra will vary somewhat with each recording.[42] The catheter is infused with sterile fluid, such as saline, at a known, slow rate (2 mL/min has been recommended).[17,42] The catheter is withdrawn at a known, constant speed. Most normal values in dogs have been established at withdrawal rates of 5 or 6 cm/min.[40,42] Catheter withdrawal speeds of 6 versus 18 cm/min resulted in significant differences in maximal urethral closure pressure, but no differences in functional profile length.[19] During withdrawal, resting urethral pressure imposed against the fluid leaving the catheter is recorded. The resulting graph is called a urethral pressure profile. One alternative technique measures intravesicular pressure during urethral pressure measurement ("simultaneous" urethral pressure profilometry), but no diagnostic advantage was found with this technique in dogs.[24] Another technique uses a pressure transducer attached to the catheter to measure urethral pressure directly without fluid infusion.[19,22,25,33]

d. Potential sources of error or variation in urethral pressure profilometry include failure to calibrate the instrument adequately, the presence of air bubbles in the recording catheter/transducer system when fluid infusion is used, failure to empty the bladder prior to the test, injury to the urethra by the catheter, and type and degree of sedation. The type and size of catheter compared to patient size may also affect results.[23]

e. Urinary tract infections were uncommon in cats that underwent repetitive urethral pressure profilometry.[33] However, in dogs, urinary tract infection occurs with urodynamic testing (as with cystometry). Prophylactic treatment and a urinalysis and/or urine culture should be performed a few days after a urethral pressure profile to determine if infection was induced.

2. Normal Findings

a. The tracing begins with intravesicular pressure, which should be similar to T-I on the CMG. As the catheter enters the urethra, pressure rises. In female dogs, the pressure peaks at approximately the middle to the distal one third of the urethra and then declines to zero as the catheter exits the urethral orifice (Fig. 14–8).[4,19,24,40,42] In female cats, the maximal ure-

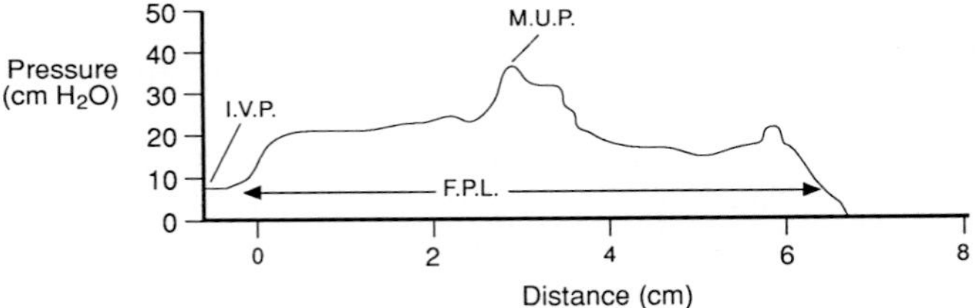

FIG. 14–8 Example of a urethral pressure profile using fluid infusion in a female dog under xylazine restraint. A similar curve is found in unsedated dogs, but pressures are higher. Pressure is recorded on the vertical axis and distance on the horizontal axis. The initial catheter position in the bladder records intravesicular pressure (I.V.P.). When the catheter is withdrawn from the bladder and enters the urethra, pressure begins to increase. Maximal urethral pressure (M.U.P.) is exerted in the midurethra in female dogs. Maximal urethral closure pressure (MUCP) is the difference between maximal urethral pressure and intravesicular pressure. F.P.L. indicates functional urethral (profile) length, the distance over which urethral pressure exceeds bladder pressure. Reprinted with permission from Barsanti JA. *Small Animal Medical Diagnosis.* Philadelphia, PA: JB Lippincott Co; 1987:350.

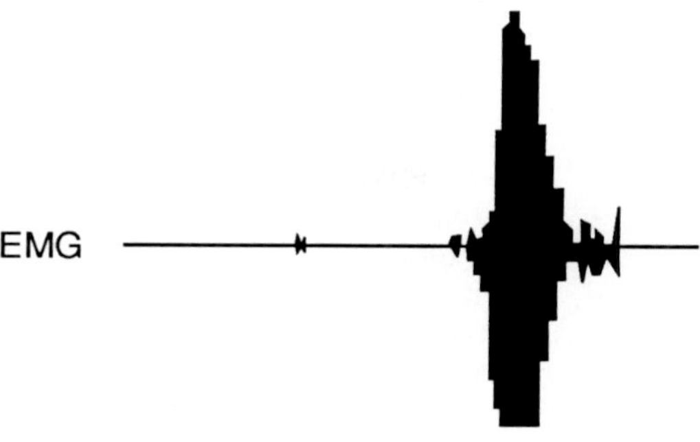

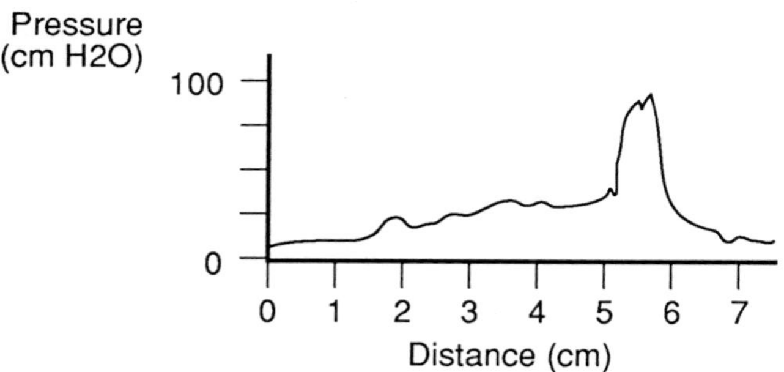

FIG. 14–9 Example of a urethral pressure profile using fluid infusion in a female cat sedated with xylazine. Also shown is an EMG from electrodes placed on the urethral catheter. Measurements made are similar to those in Figure 14–8. Reprinted with permission from Gregory CR, Willits NH. Electromyographic and urethral pressure evaluations: Assessment of urethral function in female and ovariohysterectomized female cats. *Am J Vet Res.* 1986;47:1472.

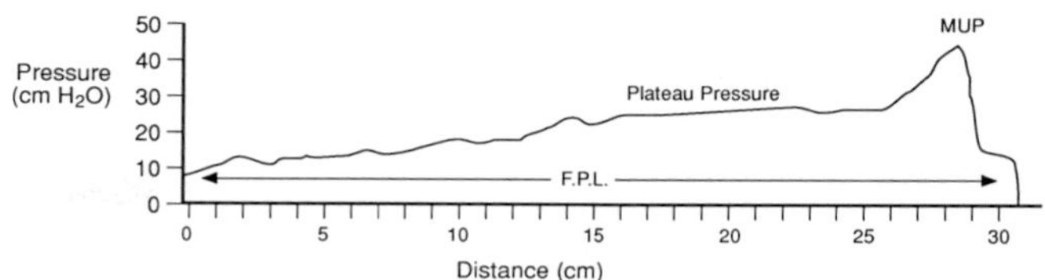

FIG. 14–10 Example of a urethral pressure profile using fluid infusion in a male dog under xylazine restraint. Note that a long pressure plateau is in the membranous urethra, with maximal pressure in this tracing in the distal urethra. MUP = maximal urethral pressure; F.P.L. = functional profile length.

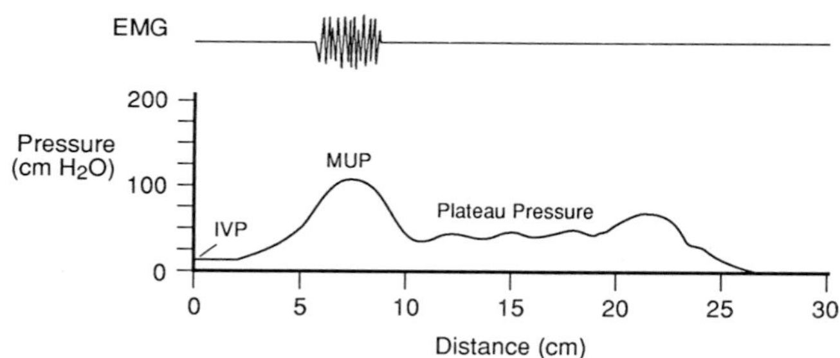

FIG. 14–11 Example of a urethral pressure profile using fluid infusion in an unsedated dog recorded with an EMG from electrodes placed on the urethral catheter. Note that maximal pressure and EMG activity occur in the proximal urethra with a prolonged plateau of pressure in the membranous urethra. Note that pressures are much higher than those in xylazine-restrained dogs (see Fig. 14–10). IVP = intravesicular pressure; MUP = maximal urethral pressure. Reprinted with permission from Basinger RR, et al. Urodynamic alterations after prostatectomy in dogs without clinical prostatic disease. *Vet Surg.* 1987;16:405.

thral pressure occurs in the distal one third of the urethra (Fig. 14–9).[18] In male dogs with xylazine restraint, the pressure reaches an initial plateau in the prostatic urethra, rises to reach another plateau in the membranous/penile urethra, rises to a maximum in the distal penile urethra, and declines to zero as the catheter exits the urethral orifice (Fig. 14–10).[4,40,42] The rise in the distal urethra could result from lack of urethral distensibility in the area of the os penis or from changes in engorgement of the bulbus glandis during catheter withdrawal. Because this rise might be an artifact of technique, pressure in the membranous urethra (plateau pressure) also should be examined. In nonsedated male dogs, the maximal urethral pressure occurs in the membranous urethra, just caudal to the prostate gland (Fig. 14–11)[40] where the highest concentration of striated muscle fibers is located.[12] In male cats, a marked increase in pressure occurs in the postprostatic urethra, and a further increase occurs in the penile urethra (Fig. 14–12).[16,17] These are areas of striated muscle in

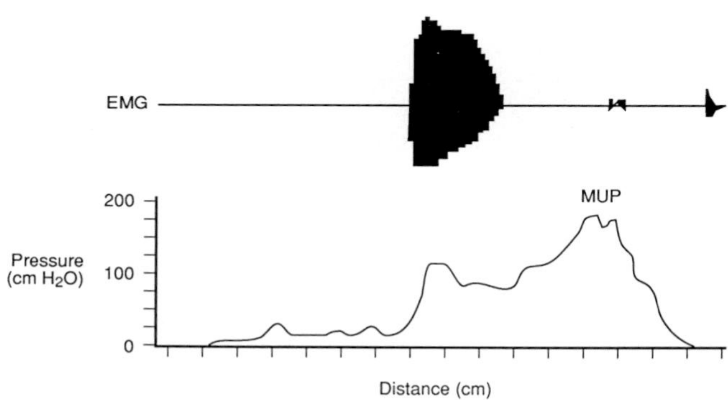

FIG. 14–12 Example of a urethral pressure profile using fluid infusion and an EMG from electrodes placed on the urethral catheter in a male cat sedated with xylazine. Note that variation has been reported in normal cats, with the maximal pressure (MUP) occurring in either the penile or the prostatic/postprostatic urethra. Reprinted with permission from Gregory CR, Willits NH. Electromyographic and urethral pressure evaluations: Assessment of urethral function in female and ovariohysterectomized female cats. *Am J Vet Res.* 1986;47:1472.

cats; in addition, the penile urethra is of small diameter, thereby leading to recording of increased pressure.

b. Values recorded
   (1). Maximum Urethral Pressure (MUP): the maximum pressure recorded.
   (2). Maximum Urethral Closing Pressure (MUCP): the difference between the maximal urethral pressure and the resting bladder pressure.
   (3). Plateau Pressure: pressure in the membranous urethra in male dogs.
   (4). Functional Profile Length (FPL): the length of the urethra along which urethral pressure exceeds bladder pressure; normally correlates well with anatomic length.
c. Normal values in female dogs are shown in Table 14–2.
d. Normal values in male dogs are shown in Table 14–3.
e. Normal values in cats are shown in Table 14-4. One study[33] reported lower values for intraurethral pressures. The authors attributed this

TABLE 14–2.
NORMAL VALUES REPORTED FOR URETHRAL PRESSURE PROFILOMETRY IN FEMALE DOGS

Number and Weight of Animals Studied (Reference No.)	Maximal Urethral Pressure (MUP) (cm H_2O)	Maximal Urethral Closure Pressure (MUCP) (cm H_2O)	Functional Profile Length (FPL) (cm)	Intravesicular Pressure (cm H_2O)
25, 17-37.5 kg* (24)	Not given	11.9 (2.5-40.5) range	6.8 (2.8-13.3) range	4.4 (2-10) range
20, 10-43.5 kg* (19)	Not given	7.81 (SEM 0.67)	7.2 (SEM 0.25)	Not given
7, 10-30 kg† (42)	37 (S.D. 17)	33 (S.D. 16)	7.2 (S.D. 1.9)	Not given
11, 20-30 kg† (40)	330 (SEM 4.54)	23 (SEM 4.54)	6.23 (SEM 0.98)	10.0 (SEM 0)
11, 20-30 kg‡ (40)	90.18 (SEM 4.48)	79.72 (SEM 4.61)	8.68 (SEM 0.57)	10.45 (SEM 0.43)
6, 18-22 kg† (4)	26 (S.D. 9)	18 (S.D. 5)	5.1 (S.D. 0.9)	Not given

*General anesthesia with catheter microtransducers.
†Xylazine with fluid infusion.
‡Unsedated with fluid infusion.
S.D. = standard deviation; SEM = standard error of the mean.

TABLE 14–3.
NORMAL VALUES REPORTED FOR URETHRAL PRESSURE PROFILOMETRY IN MALE DOGS

Number and Weight of Animals Studied (Reference No.)	Maximal Urethral Pressure (MUP) (cm H_2O)	Maximal Urethral Closure Pressure (MUCP) (cm H_2O)	Plateau Pressure (cm H_2O)	Functional Profile Length (cm)	Intravesicular Pressure (cm H_2O)
6, 10-30 kg* (42)	44 (S.D. 5.6)	38 (S.D. 5)	Not given	28.3 (S.D. 3.9)	Not given
13, 20-30 kg* (40)	52 (SEM 6)	42 (SEM 6)	26 (SEM 2)	19 (SEM 2)	11 (SEM 1)
6, 9.5-25.0 kg* (4)	37 (S.D. 17)	30 (S.D. 17)	Not given	23 (S.D. 5)	Not given
13, 20-30 kg† (40)	110 (SEM 11.5)	100 (SEM 12)	43 (SEM 4)	24 (SEM 1)	10 (SEM 0.5)

*Xylazine with fluid infusion.
†Unsedated with fluid infusion.
S.D. = standard deviation; SEM = standard error of the mean.

TABLE 14–4.
NORMAL VALUES REPORTED FOR URETHRAL PRESSURE PROFILOMETRY IN CATS

Number and Sex of Animals Studied (Reference No.)	Maximal Urethral Pressure (MUP) (cm H_2O)	Maximal Urethral Closure Pressure (MUCP) (cm H_2O)	Functional Profile Length (FPL) (cm)	Intravesicular Pressure (cm H_2O)
10 intact males* (34,33)	82.6 (S.D. 18.7)	Not given	Not given	Not given
10 intact males† (34,33)	53.4 (S.D. 25.7)	Not given	Not given	Not given
10 intact males† (17)	163.2 (S.D. 47.5)	161.6 (S.D. 47.1)	10.53 (S.D. 0.53)	Not given
10 neutered males‡ (20)	Not given	151 (S.D. 52)	Not given	5.4 (S.D. 3.8)
11 intact males§ (46)	Not done	93.1 (S.D. 13.29)	8.1 (S.D. 0.93)	Not done
10 intact females‡ (18)	76.6 (S.D. 26.7)	71.4 (S.D. 25)	4.4 (S.D. 1.5)	Not given
10 neutered females‡ (18)	81.3 (S.D. 31.7)	77.5 (S.D. 31.3)	5.78 (S.D. 0.9)	Not given

*Intermittent recordings, unsedated with catheter microtransducer.
†Intermittent recordings, xylazine restraint with catheter microtransducer. Note that the lower values in this study were attributed to a difference in technique (see text).
‡Continuous recordings xylazine restraint with fluid infusion. Note that in the female cats the intact cats were younger and smaller, perhaps explaining the difference in FPL.
§Continuous recordings, xylazine (0.1 mg/kg 1M) and ketamine (1 mg/kg 1M) with fluid infusion.
S.D. = standard deviation.

difference to technique. Instead of recording pressures constantly as the catheter was withdrawn, the catheter was moved and stopped at 1-cm intervals, at which time pressure was recorded. The authors stated that movement of the catheter caused a dramatic increase in urethral pressure, which was avoided by allowing time for the pressure to stabilize once catheter movement was stopped.

f. Urethral pressure profiles have been reproducible in normal dogs and cats, tested on the same or different days with or without xylazine sedation, as long as the profiles were repeated only a few times each day.[17,18,40,42,45] However, other studies in dogs and humans have shown inconsistent pressure measurements, with only functional profile length measurements being consistent.[15,22,25,47] The differences in reproducibility may be the result of differences in technique or differences in quantities and types of measurements made.

3. Examples of Major Abnormalities[43]
   a. Reduced urethral pressure suggests decreased ability of the urethra to maintain normal resting tone. One example is "spay" or "hormonally responsive" incontinence.[41] In this condition, the decrease in pressure occurs throughout the urethra (Fig. 14–13).[42] Lesions of the pudendal nerve (or cauda equina in the sacral spinal canal) or of the hypogastric nerve also result in reduced urethral pressure. Decreases in urethral pressure are greatest with pudendal lesions in the area of striated muscle (midurethra in female dogs and membranous urethra in male dogs) and are associated with EMG changes and other potential neurologic deficits.
   b. A focal area of increased urethral pressure suggests urethral obstruction caused by either an intraluminal mass or an extraluminal compression. This finding on the urethral pressure

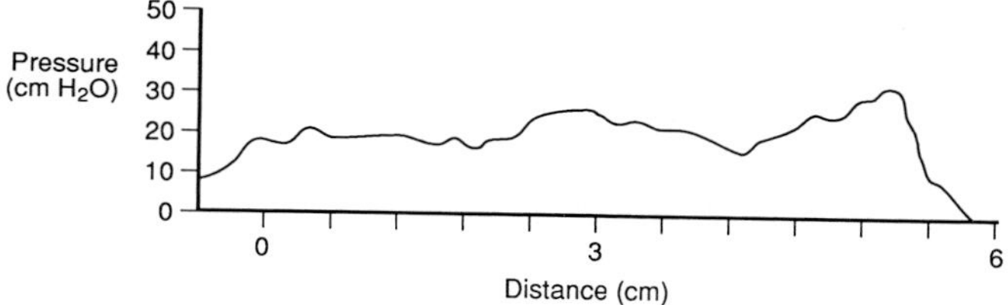

FIG. 14–13 A urethral pressure profile from a neutered female dog with "spay" incontinence under xylazine restraint. The normal increase in pressure in the midurethra is absent, and the pressure recording is flat as compared to normal (see Fig. 14–8). Reprinted with permission from Barsanti JA. *Small Animal Medical Diagnosis.* Philadelphia, PA: JB Lippincott Co; 1987:350.

profile should be correlated with radiographic contrast studies and/or endoscopy.

c. Decreased functional urethral length also suggests decreased urethral competence. Decrease in functional length may or may not be associated with decreased anatomic length, which can only be determined radiographically.

C. Uroflowmetry.

1. Technique

a. The contractile function of the bladder and the resistance of the urethra can be assessed by measuring fluid flow through the urethra (urethral flowmetry) during micturition.[34,35,44]

b. Cystometry and urethral pressure profilometry have been utilized in dogs and cats more frequently to date than has urethral flowmetry. Urethral flowmetry has mainly been performed in normal animals. Potential risks remain to be determined in animals with abnormal bladder walls.

c. Uroflowmetry is usually performed using xylazine in the same dosage as that used for cystometry.[34,36]

d. Uroflowmetry is performed by placing either one or two catheters percutaneously directly into the bladder under aseptic conditions. Placement of the percutaneous intravesicular catheter is facilitated when the bladder is initially filled with sterile saline through a urethral catheter. After placing the percutaneous catheters, the bladder is emptied and the transurethral catheter is removed. The percutaneous intravesicular catheter or catheters are used to infuse the bladder with sterile fluid (usually saline) and to record intravesicular pressure. In more sophisticated systems, an electromagnetic flow transducer is mounted on tubing connected to a funnel that is used to collect all fluid voided.

e. Intracystic pressure at which urination begins is recorded. With appropriate recording devices, flow rate of fluid out of the urethra can also be determined, as can bladder pressure at the time of maximal fluid flow through the urethra. The amount of fluid voided and the residual volume can be determined. A urethral resistance factor can be calculated.[35] Because the procedure includes continuous measurement of bladder pressure, all CMG measurements can also be made.

f. As with cystometry, hematuria and urinary tract infections can result from urinary tract manipulation. An infection rate of almost 20% was found in normal dogs.[36] Risk of infection was greater in female than in male dogs. A broad-spectrum antibiotic can be administered on the day of the study to try to reduce this infection rate. Whether antibiotics are administered or not, a urinalysis or urine culture should be performed a few days after the procedure to determine if the patient is free of infection.

g. Sources of error in uroflowmetry are similar to those in cystometry.

2. Normal Findings

a. The values recorded are the same as those for the CMG, with the additions of the intravesicular pressures during fluid flow through the urethra and fluid flow rate from the urethra.

b. In cats, significant variation in pressures has been noted in recordings taken in the same individual on different days,[44] thus indicating that caution must be used in interpreting changes in an individual case and in establishing normal values. More consistent results were found in dogs.[36]

c. Intravesicular pressures are recorded initially as in a CMG. Just after the detrusor reflex begins, fluid begins to flow from the urethra. Fluid flow continues as the detrusor reflex is sustained. The intravesicular pressure recording may show pulsations of varying magnitude and duration. As intravesicular pressure declines, fluid flow decreases fairly abruptly. Another contraction of the detrusor may occur at the end of fluid flow (after-contraction). Occasionally, in normal dogs a small amount of fluid leaks from the urethra prior to detrusor contraction.

d. Normal Values

(1). Male cats with ketamine/xylazine restraint[44]: intravesicular pressure at onset of urine flow is 44 cm H_2O (range 12 to 110 cm H_2O)

(2). Female dogs, 10 to 30 kg, with xylazine restraint[34]:

(a). intravesicular pressure at onset of urine flow: 39 cm H_2O (S.D. 14)

(b). urine flow at maximum intravesicular pressure: 12 mL/sec (S.D. 4)

(c). maximal urine flow: 15.5 ml/sec (S.D. 3.2)

(3). Male dogs, 10 to 30 kg, xylazine restraint[34]:

(a). intravesicular pressure at onset of urine flow: 50.5 cm H_2O (S.D. 13)

(b). urine flow at maximum intravesicular pressure: 6.7 mL/sec (S.D. 3)

(c). maximal urine flow: 9 mL/sec (S.D. 4)

3. Examples of Abnormalities[35]

a. Increased urethral resistance

(1). With increased urethral resistance, intravesicular pressure to initiate fluid flow is higher than normal and urine flow rate is reduced.

(2). The major diagnostic possibility for increased urethral resistance is urethral obstruction caused by an intraluminal mass or by extraluminal urethral compression.

(3). Another possibility for increased urethral resistance during voiding is detrusor-urethral dyssynergia (reflex dyssynergia). Uroflowmetry is the only electrodiagnostic test that can confirm this possibility when urethral obstruction has been excluded by contrast radiographic techniques and/or endoscopy. Only uroflowmetry can document that the urethra fails to relax during micturition. Urethral pressure profilometry measures urethral resistance only during bladder storage of urine and not during micturition, and is normal in reflex dyssynergia.[43]

b. Decreased urethral resistance

(1). Flow of fluid through the urethra during bladder filling, but prior to the detrusor reflex, suggests decreased resting urethral pressure, although this abnormal flow does occur occasionally in normal dogs. Maximal urine flow rates occur at lower than usual intravesicular pressure, leading to a decrease in the calculated urethral resistance.

(2). Decreased urethral competence, either congenital or related to neutering, is the most common reason for decreased urethral resistance.

D. Electromyography (EMG).

1. Technique

a. The purpose of the EMG is to record muscle activity. In relation to the lower urinary tract, the EMG has been used to evaluate muscle activity in the urethra.

b. The EMG can be recorded from a fine-wire electrode placed percutaneously into or near the striated muscle of the urethra[44,45] or in the anal sphincter, which is also innervated by the pudendal nerve.[39] In humans, however, EMG activity in the anal sphincter does not always correlate with urethral sphincter response.[9] Alternatively, a bipolar electrode can be mounted on the urethral catheter for pressure recordings from within the urethral lumen. Usually smaller urethral catheters (3.5 F in cats and 5 or 6 F in dogs) are used because of the added size of the electrodes.[17,18,40] Which of these techniques is best is controversial. Fine-wire electrodes placed percutaneously in the striated urethral sphincter record activity in that area of the urethra throughout the procedure, whereas intraurethral electrodes record activity in each area of the urethra as the catheter passes. The techniques require comparison in many clinical cases of known cause before any meaningful conclusions can be made.

c. Xylazine markedly attenuated the EMG response in dogs,[40] but xylazine sedation has been used without interference in cats.[17,18,44,45]

2. Normal Findings

a. Needle recordings from one area of the urethra in male cats show slight to moderate activity during bladder filling and minimal activity during bladder emptying. In some male cats, maximal activity occurs at the completion of the detrusor reflex and is associated with pulsatile elimination of small amounts of urine.[44] With intraurethral pressure recordings, maximal EMG activity occurs in the postprostatic urethra in male cats and in the distal urethra in female cats (Figs. 14–9 and 14–12).[16-18] The areas of maximal EMG activity correlate with areas of striated muscle.

b. When recorded from within the urethra during the urethral pressure profile, maximal EMG activity corresponds to the area of maximal urethral pressure in dogs (Fig. 14–11).[40] This finding corresponds to the areas with the largest amount of striated muscle that is innervated by the pudendal nerve.

3. Examples of Abnormalities

a. Sedative drugs, such as xylazine, can depress EMG activity at the dosages usually used for cystometry and urethral pressure profilometry in dogs.

b. To date, few EMG abnormalities associated with clinical cases of lower urinary tract dysfunction have been described in the literature.

(1). EMG activity was normal in dogs with primary urethral sphincter incompetence.[41]

(2). EMG activity was decreased in male dogs with severe prostatic disease.[6]

(3). Injury to the pudendal nerve or injury to the area of the spinal cord from which the nerve originates would most likely result in EMG changes.

(4). Disease or injury to the striated muscle itself would be expected to result in decreased or altered EMG activity.

REFERENCES

1. Abdel-Rahman M, Galeano C, Elhilali M. New approach to study of voiding cycle in cat. *Urology.* 1983;22:91.
2. Awad SA, Downie JW. Relative contributions of smooth and striated muscles to the canine urethral pressure profile. *Br J Urol.* 1976;48:347.
3. Barsanti JA, Mahaffey MB, Crowell WA, Barber DL. Cystometry in dogs using oxymorphone and acepromazine restraint. *Am J Vet Res.* 1984;45:2152.
4. Barsanti JA, Finco DR, Brown J. Effect of atropine on cystometry and urethral pressure profilometry in the dog. *Am J Vet Res.* 1988;49:112.
5. Basinger RR, et al. Urodynamic alterations after prostatectomy in dogs without clinical prostatic disease. *Vet Surg.* 1987;16:405.

6. Basinger RR, Rawlings CA, Barsanti JA, Oliver JE. Urodynamic alterations associated with clinical prostatic diseases and prostatic surgery. *J Am Anim Hosp Assoc.* 1989;25:385.
7. Biertuempfel PH, Ling GV, Ling GA. Urinary tract infection resulting from catheterization in healthy adult dogs. *J Am Vet Med Assoc.* 1981;178:989.
8. Biewenga WJ, de Vries HW, Stokhof AA, deBruyne JJ. Evaluation of the risk of xylazine sedation in cystometric studies in dogs. *Vet Anesth.* 1978;5:8.
9. Blaivas JG. A critical appraisal of specific diagnostic techniques. In: Krane RJ, Siroky MB, eds. *Clinical Neuro-Urology.* Boston, Mass: Little, Brown and Co; 1979.
10. Craggs MD, Stephenson JD. The effects of parasympathetic blocking agents on bladder electromyograms and function in conscious and anesthetized cats. *Neuropharmacology.* 1982;21:695.
11. Creed KE, Tulloch AGS. The effect of pelvic nerve stimulation and some drugs on the urethra and bladder of the dog. *Br J Urol.* 1978;50:398.
12. Cullen CW, Fletcher TF, Bradley WE. Histology of the canine urethra. II. Morphometry of the male pelvic urethra. *Anat Rec.* 1981;199:187.
13. Edvardsen P. Nervous control of the urinary bladder in cats. *Acta Physiol Scand.* 1968;72:183.
14. Ghoneim MA, Fretin JA, Gagnon DJ, Susset JG. The influence of vesical distension on urethral resistance to flow: The expulsion phase. *Br J Urol.* 1975;47:663.
15. Ghoneim MA, et al. Urethral pressure profile. Standardization of technique and study of reproducibility. *Urology.* 1975;5:632.
16. Gregory CR. Electromyographic and urethral pressure profilometry. *Vet Clin North Am.* 1984;14:567.
17. Gregory CR, et al. Electromyographic and urethral pressure profilometry: Assessment of urethral function before and after perineal urethrostomy in cats. *Am J Vet Res.* 1984;45:2062.
18. Gregory CR, Willits NH. Electromyographic and urethral pressure evaluations: Assessment of urethral function in female and ovariohysterectomized female cats. *Am J Vet Res.* 1986;47:1472.
19. Gregory SP, Holt PE, Parkinson TJ. Comparison of two catheter withdrawal speeds during simultaneous urethral pressure profilometry in anesthetized bitches. *Am J Vet Res.* 1992;53:355.
20. Griffin DW, Gregory CR, Kitchell RL. Preservation of striated-muscle urethral sphincter function with use of a surgical technique for perineal urethrostomy in cats. *J Am Vet Med Assoc.* 1989;194:1057.
21. Hardie EM, Barsanti JA, Rawlings CA. Complications of prostatic surgery. *J Am Anim Hosp Assoc.* 1984;20:50.
22. Holt PE. "Simultaneous" urethral pressure profilometry in the bitch: Methodology and reproducibility of the technique. *Res Vet Sci.* 1989;47:110.
23. Holt PE. Urethral pressure profilometry in the bitch—artifact or reality? In: *Proceedings of the 4th Symposium of the European Society of Veterinary Nephrology and Urology.* Giesen, West Germany; 1989.
24. Holt PE. Urethral pressure profile in the anaesthetised bitch: A comparison between double and single sensor recording. *Res Vet Sci.* 1989;47:346.
25. Holt PE. Simultaneous urethral pressure profilometry using microtip transducer catheters in the bitch: A comparison of catheter material. *J Small Anim Pract.* 1990;31:431.
26. Hsu WH, Lu ZX, Hembrough FB. Effect of xylazine on heart rate and arterial blood pressure in conscious dogs, as influenced by atropine, 4-aminopyridine, doxapram, and yohimbine. *J Am Vet Med Assoc.* 1985;186:153.
27. Jensen D. Pharmacological studies of the uninhibited neurogenic bladder. *Acta Neurol Scand.* 1981;64:175.
28. Johnson CA, et al. Effects of various sedatives on air cystometry in dogs. *Am J Vet Res.* 1988;49:1525.
29. Klide AM, Calderwood HW, Soma LR. Cardiopulmonary effects of xylazine in dogs. *Am J Vet Res.* 1975;36:931.
30. Lane IF, Lappin MR. Predictive value of urodynamic measurements in the management of ectopic ureters in the dog. *J Vet Intern Med.* 1992;6:119. Abstract.
31. Lappin MR, Barsanti JA. Urinary incontinence secondary to idiopathic detrusor instability: Cystometrographic diagnosis and pharmacologic management of two dogs and a cat. *J Am Vet Med Assoc.* 1987;191:1439.
32. Mahaffey MB, Barber DL, Barsanti JA, Crowell WA. Simultaneous double-contrast cystography and cystometry in dogs. *Vet Radiol.* 1984;25:254.
33. Mawby DI, et al. Pharmacologic relaxation of the urethra in male cats: A study of the effects of phenoxybenzamine, diazepam, nifedipine, and xylazine. *Can J Vet Res.* 1990;55:28.
34. Moreau PM, Lees GE, Gross DR. Simultaneous cystometry and uroflowmetry for evaluation of the caudal part of the urinary tract function in dogs: Reference values for healthy animals sedated with xylazine. *Am J Vet Res.* 1983;44:1774.
35. Moreau PM, Lees GE, Hobson HP. Simultaneous cystometry and uroflowmetry for evaluation of micturition in two dogs. *J Am Vet Med Assoc.* 1983;183:1084.
36. Moreau PM, Lees GE, Gross DR. Simultaneous cystometry and uroflowmetry (micturition study) for evaluation of the caudal part of the urinary tract in dogs: Studies of technique. *Am J Vet Res.* 1983;44:1769.
37. Oliver JE, Young WO. Air cystometry in dogs under xylazine-induced restraint. *Am J Vet Res.* 1973;34:1433.
38. Oliver JE, Young WO. Evaluation of pharmacologic agents for restraint in cystometry in the dog and cat. *Am J Vet Res.* 1973;34:665.
39. Oliver JE, Selcer RR. Neurogenic causes of abnormal micturition in the dog and cat. *Vet Clin North Am.* 1974;4:517.
40. Richter KP, Ling GV. Effects of xylazine on the urethral pressure profile of healthy dogs. *Am J Vet Res.* 1985;46:1881.
41. Richter KP, Ling GV. Clinical response and urethral pressure profile changes following phenylpropanolamine in dogs with primary sphincter incompetence. *J Am Vet Med Assoc.* 1985;187:605.
42. Rosin A, Rosin E, Oliver J. Canine urethral pressure profile. *Am J Vet Res.* 1980;41:1113.
43. Rosin AE, Barsanti JA. Diagnosis of urinary incontinence in dogs: Role of the urethral pressure profile. *J Am Vet Med Assoc.* 1981;178:814.
44. Sackman JE, Sims MH. Electromyographic evaluation of the external urethral sphincter during cystometry in male cats. *Am J Vet Res.* 1990;51:1237.
45. Sackman JE, Sims MH. Use of fine-wire electrodes for electromyographic evaluation of the external urethral sphincter during urethral pressure profilometry in male cats. *Am J Vet Res.* 1991;52:314.
46. Sjostrand SE, Sjogren C, Schmiterlow CG. Responses of the rabbit and cat urinary bladders in situ to drugs and to nerve stimulation. *Acta Pharmacol Toxicol.* 1972;31:241.
47. Toguri AG, Bee DE, Bunce H. Variability of water urethral closure pressure profiles. *J Urol.* 1980;124:407.

CHAPTER 15

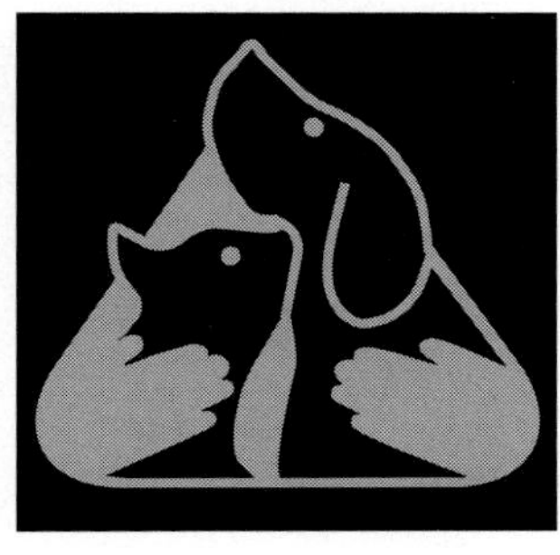

Catheter and Forceps Biopsy of the Urethra, Urinary Bladder, and Prostate Gland

CARL A. OSBORNE
JODY P. LULICH

I. INDICATIONS

A. Evaluation of the morphologic characteristics of various types of cells (e.g., transitional epithelium, red blood cell, white blood cell) found in urine sediment is of proven value in the investigation of inflammatory and neoplastic diseases of the urogenital system.

B. Evaluation of the morphologic characteristics of individual cells found in urine is often more difficult than examination of cytologic preparations obtained from most other body organs and systems. This difficulty is partly associated with the fact that cells present in urine are subjected to osmotic and pH levels that are markedly different from those in their normal environment. In addition, they may be exposed to toxic concentrations of enzymes and other metabolites excreted in urine. The problem may also be compounded by the fact that relatively few cells originating from the site of the lesion may be available for examination.

II. CATHETER BIOPSY OF THE URETHRA, URINARY BLADDER, AND PROSTATE GLAND

A. We have had varying degrees of success by using a flexible urinary catheter to obtain aspiration biopsy specimens from lesions in the bladder, urethra, and/or prostate gland of dogs. The procedure may also be used in cats and other animals. The advantage of the catheter biopsy technique over conventional exfoliative cytologic methods for urine sediment is the collection of a relatively large quantity of fresh cells from a specific site within the genitourinary tract in a fluid of similar composition to that of extracellular fluid. The major disadvantage of the technique is related to the fact that, although evaluation of the morphologic characteristics of a group of cells provides information, it does not always provide a diagnosis. Although a definitive diagnosis may be established on the basis of positive findings, tentative diagnoses cannot always be eliminated by exclusion on the basis of negative findings.

B. We have had the greatest success with this technique in confirming diagnosis of transitional cell carcinomas of the urethra and urinary bladder, thereby eliminating the need for diagnostic surgical procedures. It also has been of value in the evaluation of inflammatory and neoplastic lesions of the prostate gland. In addition to microscopic examination of the cell population, aspirated tissues may be cultured for microorganisms.

C. We recommend this technique as an adjunct to the clinical evaluation of diseases of the lower urinary tract and prostate gland. Because it is easy to perform, of minimal discomfort to the

patient, and inexpensive, the use of this procedure does not preclude further clinical investigations by radiography, punch biopsy, or exploratory surgery.

D. Materials.

1. A flexible urethral or ureteral catheter with openings (eyes) on the sides of the proximal end should be used. The size of the catheter, and thus of its openings, should be as large as is consistent with atraumatic passage through the urethra to maximize the quantity of the biopsy sample.
2. Once the sample is obtained, it must be rapidly fixed to minimize artifactual changes caused by autolysis. If chunks of tissue are obtained with the catheter, they should immediately be transferred to a bottle of 10% buffered formalin solution for processing by routine histologic techniques.
3. The liquid portion of the sample may be processed in a variety of ways. To insure proper handling of the specimen, we suggest consultation with the laboratory to which the sample is to be delivered before the sample is taken.
4. A few drops of the noncentrifuged sample may be placed on a microscopic slide, fixed by air drying, and stained with such stains as new methylene blue or Wright's stain. The same technique may be used for examination of sediment prepared from the sample (see the following).
5. Concentration of cellular material may be achieved by routine preparation of urine sediment (i.e., centrifugation at 1500 to 2000 rpm for 5 minutes). After removal of the supernatant, the sediment may be placed on several microscopic slides and fixed by air drying, proprietary cytologic fixatives, or Aqua-Net hair spray. A nucleopore filter may be used to concentrate cells in lieu of centrifugation.
6. A cell block for routine histologic sectioning may be prepared by adding 2 drops of plasma and 2 drops of thrombin to the sediment. The clot that forms should be fixed in 10% buffered formalin solution.

E. Technique.

1. Localize the site of the lesion in the urinary bladder, urethra, or prostate gland by palpation, catheterization, or radiography. Remove the urine from the bladder by catheterization. Insert the catheter through the urethra until the catheter openings are adjacent to the lesion. Correct positioning of the catheter may be facilitated by rectal or vaginal palpation or by radiography (using a radiopaque catheter).
2. Attach a 12-ml syringe containing 3 to 10 ml of an isotonic solution (i.e., physiologic saline solution or lactated Ringer's solution) to the catheter and inject all but 1 ml of the solution into the urinary tract. Create negative pressure in the system by pulling the syringe plunger outward. The objective of this maneuver is to aspirate a small portion of the mucosal surface of the urinary tract into the openings of the catheter (Fig. 15–1). With the syringe plunger pulled out, move the catheter a short distance forward and backward. The aspiration portion of the procedure should be rapidly performed to minimize admixture of peripheral blood elements with the biopsy sample.

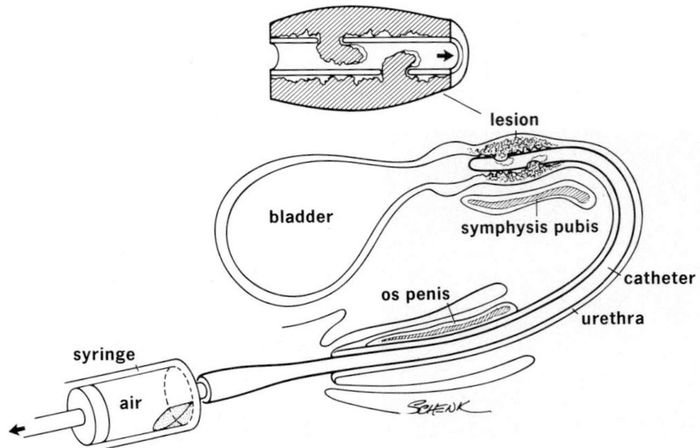

FIG. 15–1. Schematic illustration of catheter biopsy of a urethral lesion in a male dog. A portion of the lesion has been aspirated into the lumen of the urinary catheter as a result of negative pressure created with a syringe. If a significant quantity of lesion enters the lumen of the urethra (insert), a small plug of tissue may be harvested as the catheter is withdrawn. Reprinted with permission from Melhoff T, Osborne CA. Catheter biopsy of the urethra, urinary bladder, and prostate gland. In: Kirk RW, ed. *Current Veterinary Therapy.* Vol 6. Philadelphia, Pennsylvania: WB Saunders Co; 1977:1175.

3. The negative pressure created with the syringe should gradually be released by allowing the plunger to return to its normal resting position. This goal should be accomplished before withdrawing the catheter to prevent contamination of the biopsy sample with cells located between the lesion and the external urethral orifice.
4. If material from the prostate gland is desired, the yield and representativeness of the sample may be improved by massaging the prostate gland per rectum during the biopsy procedure.
5. The biopsy sample may be removed from the catheter by injecting the remaining portion of isotonic solution through its lumen and harvesting the mixture in a test tube or small vial. Chunks of tissue should be removed with a wooden applicator stick and placed in 10% buffered formalin solution. The remaining portion of the sample should be processed as described under the following section on materials.
6. Postoperative antibiotics are indicated because the integrity of the mucosal surface of the lower urinary tract is damaged by this procedure.

III. FORCEPS BIOPSY OF THE LOWER URINARY TRACT

A. Materials.

1. Flexible endoscope forceps (not the endoscope) are inserted into the urethra to obtain tissue samples (Fig. 15–2). Several types of grasping units on the end of the forceps are available. We have had the most experience using the standard fenestrated grasping unit.
2. Once the sample is obtained, it can be blotted and tissue impressions can be made on glass slides for immediate staining and microscopic evaluation. The sample is then placed into 10% buffered formalin prior to histologic processing.

B. Technique.

1. Identify the site for biopsy by palpation, catheterization, or radiography.
2. With the grasping unit closed, insert the endoscope forceps into the urethra.
3. Advance the forceps until the grasping unit is near the area to be biopsied. The tip of the grasping unit can be positioned by abdominal palpation, rectal palpation, fluoroscopy, or ultrasonography.
4. Open the grasping unit of the forceps and advance against the lesion.
5. Close the grasping unit. With the grasping unit closed, the endoscope forceps and tissue samples are retracted from the urinary tract.
6. The biopsy sample can be removed from the forceps by lifting the sample from the cup of the grasping unit with a 22- or 25-gauge needle.
7. In most cases, several samples can be obtained.
8. Postbiopsy antibiotics are indicated because the integrity of the mucosal surface of the lower urinary tract is damaged by this procedure.

C. Advantages.

1. Structurally intact samples can be obtained quickly.
2. Any section of the lower urinary tract is accessible for biopsy.

D. Limitations.

1. Specialized biopsy equipment is needed.
2. Patients may need to be sedated.
3. Sample processing delays sample evaluation.

IV. INTERPRETATION

A. Knowledge of the normal histologic and cytologic characteristics of the urinary tract is prerequisite to meaningful interpretation of biopsy samples. Although examination of cytologic preparations by the clinician should be performed, consultation with a competent pathologist, including confirmation of findings, is recommended.

B. A diagnosis of neoplasia following the examination of cytologic preparations is based on multiple criteria, including abnormal changes in individual cells and their nuclei and modification of cellular interrelationships. Undifferentiated malignant cells derived from transitional cell carcinomas can usually be identified, provided that such cells are contained in the biopsy sample. Recognition of benign or well-

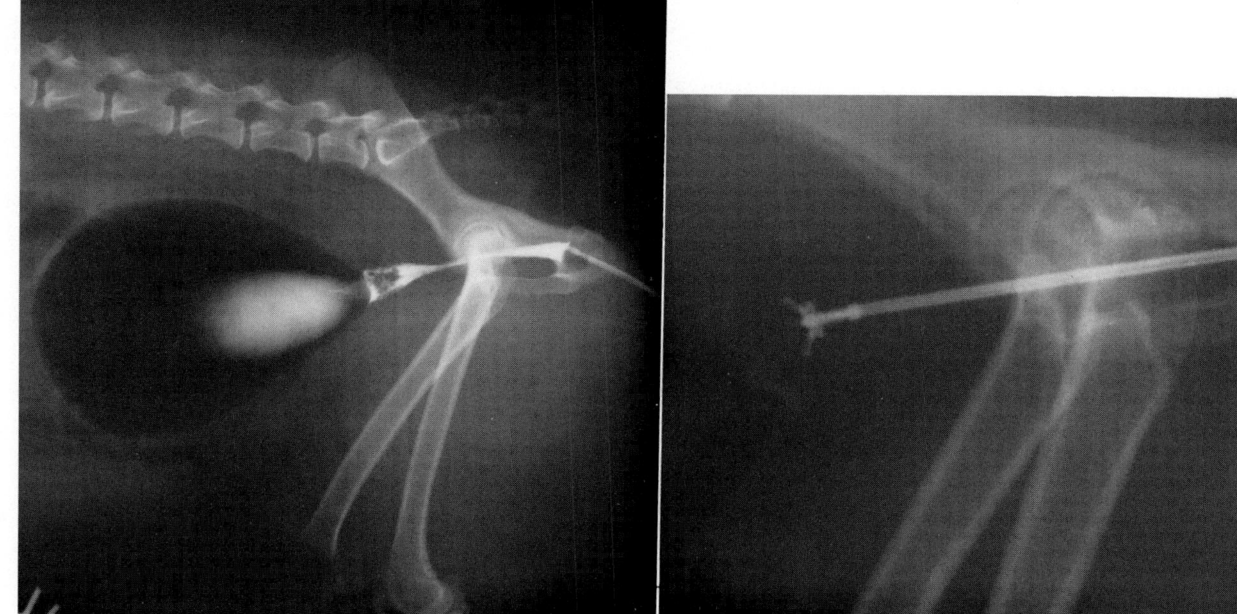

FIG. 15–2. A, Retrograde urethrogram of an 11-year-old American Eskimo dog with a proliferative mass in the neck of the urinary bladder. **B,** Endoscopy forceps were used to biopsy the mass after its position was localized with fluoroscopy.

differentiated malignant neoplasms on the basis of cytologic preparations may be difficult, however, because exfoliated cells may differ little from hyperplastic or even normal transitional epithelial cells.

C. Regardless of the type and degree of differentiation of the underlying tumor, secondary bacterial infection of neoplastic lesions may result in the collection of samples that are primarily composed of inflammatory cells and that contain relatively few neoplastic cells. Thus, a negative result does not exclude the presence of a neoplasm.

D. Because of difficulties that are sometimes encountered in evaluation of the significance of biopsy findings, the results should always be interpreted in association with other clinical, laboratory, and radiographic findings.

PART III

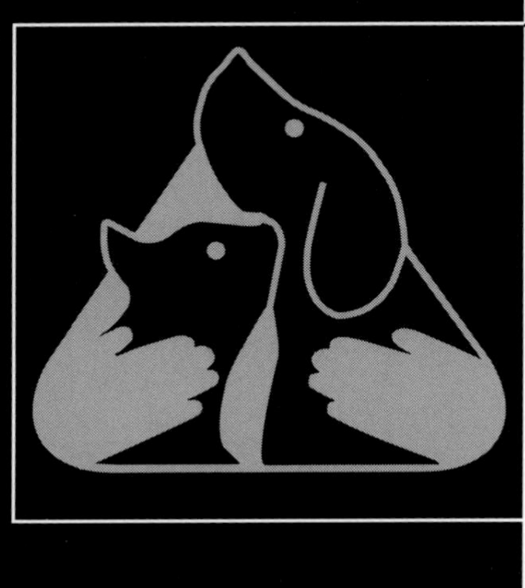

DISEASES OF THE KIDNEY

CHAPTER 16

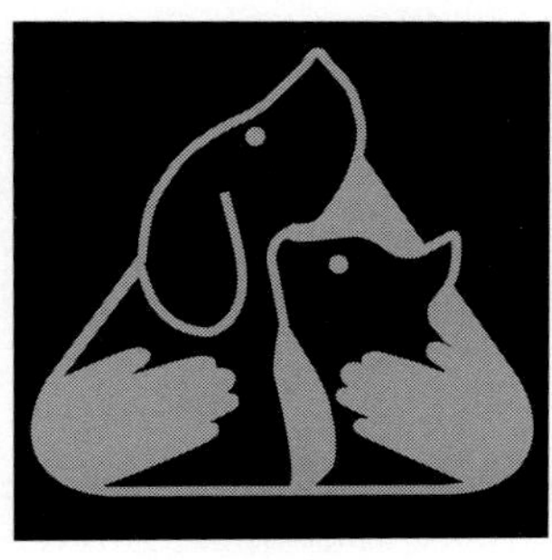

Pathophysiology of Renal Failure and Uremia

DAVID J. POLZIN
CARL A. OSBORNE

I. TERMS AND CONCEPTS

A. Azotemia.

1. Azotemia is an abnormal concentration of urea, creatinine, or other nonprotein nitrogenous substances in blood, plasma, or serum.
   a. Azotemia is a laboratory finding with fundamentally different causes.
   b. Since nonprotein nitrogenous compounds are endogenous substances, abnormally elevated concentrations in serum may be caused by an increased rate of production (by the liver for urea; by muscles for creatinine) or a decreased rate of loss (primarily by the kidneys).
   c. Because azotemia may be caused by factors that are not directly related to the urinary system, and by abnormalities of the lower urinary tract not directly related to the kidney, azotemia should not be used as a synonym for renal failure or uremia.
2. Azotemia may occur when renal structure and function are normal, when renal structure is normal but renal function is abnormal, and/or when renal structure and function are abnormal.
   a. Determination of the underlying cause(s) of azotemia has much clinical significance, since this information significantly influences prognosis and therapy.
   b. Failure to identify the cause may lead to formulation of ineffective or even contraindicated therapy.
3. Because azotemia by definition depends on accumulation of nonprotein nitrogenous substances produced by the body in blood, plasma, or serum, the underlying mechanisms must be related to an increased rate of production, a decreased rate of excretion, or both.
   a. Increased rates of production of urea and creatinine may cause a mild degree of azotemia.
   b. If the normal endogenous rates of production of urea and creatinine are constant, however, azotemia results from reduced glomerular filtration.
4. Glomerular filtration may be reduced owing to alterations in blood volume, blood pressure, colloidal osmotic pressure, the number of patent renal arteries and glomerular capillaries, the permeability of glomerular capillaries, renal interstitial pressure, or renal intratubular pressure.
   a. Glomerular filtration is dependent on prerenal components (blood volume, blood pressure, colloidal osmotic pressure), renal components (patency of renal arteries and glomerular capillaries, permeability of glomerular capillaries, renal interstitial pressure, renal intratubular pressure), and postrenal components (influence of patency of ureters, bladder, and urethra on intratubular pressure).
   b. Therefore, the cause(s) of reduction in glomerular filtration may be categorized as prerenal, renal, postrenal, or combinations of these factors.

c. Because of clinically significant differences in pathogenesis, prognosis, and treatment, causes of decreased glomerular filtration associated with azotemia always should be localized according to this classification.

d. The fact that different forms of azotemia commonly coexist must also be considered.

B. Uremia.

1. Uremia is defined as abnormal quantities of urine constituents in blood caused by primary generalized disease and the polysystemic toxic syndrome that results from abnormal renal function.
   a. When the structural and functional integrity of both kidneys has been compromised to such a degree that polysystemic signs of renal failure become manifest clinically, the relatively predictable symptom complex called uremia appears, regardless of underlying cause.
   b. In some instances, uremic crises may suddenly be precipitated by prerenal disorders (i.e., congestive heart failure, acute pancreatitis, hypoadrenocorticism) or, less commonly, by postrenal disorders (urethral obstruction, displacement of the urinary bladder into a perineal hernia, and so forth) in patients with previously compensated primary renal failure.
2. Uremia is characterized by multiple physiologic and metabolic alterations that result from renal failure.
   a. Primary renal failure may be caused by many disease processes that have in common impairment of at least three quarters of the nephrons of both kidneys.*
   b. Depending on the biologic behavior of the disease in question, primary renal failure may be reversible or irreversible, acute or chronic, and oliguric, nonoliguric, or polyuric.

C. Renal disease.

1. Because of the tremendous reserve capacity of the kidneys, the term renal disease should not be used interchangeably with uremia or renal failure unless it is described as generalized renal disease. Depending on the quantity of renal parenchyma affected and the severity and duration of lesions, renal disease(s) may or may not cause renal failure or uremia. The clinical relevance of the difference between renal disease and renal failure is emphasized by the fact that symptomatic and supportive therapy designed to correct fluid, electrolyte, acid-base, nutrient, and endocrine imbalances in patients with renal failure may not be appropriate for patients with renal disease without renal dysfunction.
2. The term renal disease appropriately describes:
   a. Renal conditions associated with dysfunction (some forms of nephrogenic diabetes insipidus) or biochemical abnormalities (cystinuria) without detectable morphologic alterations.
   b. Renal lesions (anomalies, infection, endogenous or exogenous toxins, obstruction to urine flow, neoplasms, and others) in one or both kidneys. Renal disease may affect glomeruli, tubules, interstitial tissue, and/or vessels. The disease may regress, persist, or advance.
3. The specific cause(s) of renal disease(s) may or may not be known; however, quantitative information about renal function (or dysfunction) is not defined by the term renal disease.

D. Renal failure.

1. Failure is defined as an inability to perform. The term renal failure is analogous to liver failure or heart failure in that a level of organ dysfunction—rather than a specific disease entity—is described.
   a. The kidneys perform multiple functions, including excretory, regulatory, and biosynthetic functions.
      (1). Renal excretory function entails the elimination of waste products of metabolism, toxins, and drugs.
      (2). Regulatory function refers to the role the kidneys play in maintaining fluid and electrolyte balance.
      (3). The biosynthetic functions of the kidneys include the formation of a variety of regulatory autacoids and hormones that have important local and systemic functions.
   b. The clinical and laboratory effects of chronic renal failure result from loss of these functions.
2. Renal failure implies that two thirds to three fourths or more of the functional capacity of both kidneys has been impaired. The term often is used to connote a less severe state of renal dysfunction that is not (yet) associated with polysystemic clinical manifestations (i.e., uremia).
   a. In dogs, loss of adequate ability to concentrate urine (a measure of regulatory function) caused by primary renal disease cannot be detected by evaluation of urine specific gravity or urine osmolality until the functional capacity of about two thirds of the nephrons of both kidneys has been surgically removed.
   b. Although the serum concentrations of both urea and creatinine vary inversely with glomerular filtration rate (GFR), primary renal azotemia (a measure of excretory function) and retention of other metabolites normally

*Abrupt reduction in nephron number and function by 75% or greater results in azotemic renal failure. However, compensatory hypertrophy develops in surviving nephrons, so that, several months after loss of 75% of nephrons, renal function will be reduced by only 50% or less from baseline levels. At this time azotemia would not be present, and some degree of urine-concentrating ability often is retained (typically to urine specific gravity values greater than 1.025 to 1.030 in dogs and 1.035 in cats). Thus, 75% reduction in nephron numbers is associated with renal failure only in the absence of compensatory hypertrophy. The clinical implication of this observation is that most dogs and cats with azotemic chronic renal failure have lost substantially more than 75% of their nephrons.

excreted by the kidneys usually are not recognized until the functional capacity of 70 to 75% of the nephrons is affected.

3. Renal function adequate for homeostasis does not require that all nephrons be functional. The concept that adequate renal function is not synonymous with total renal function is important in understanding the difference between renal disease and renal failure, in formulating meaningful prognoses, and in formulating specific, supportive, and symptomatic therapy.
4. Failure to perform all these functions is not an "all-or-none phenomenon," and graded loss of functions is accompanied by progressively advanced evidence of disease.
   a. Clinical signs of polysystemic disorders caused by abnormalities of water, electrolyte, acid-base, endocrine, and nutrient balance are not invariably present in patients with primary renal failure (i.e., not all patients with primary renal failure are uremic).
   b. This is related, at least in part, to the reserve capacity of the kidneys and the ability of unaffected nephrons to undergo compensatory hypertrophy and hyperplasia.
5. Although compensatory mechanisms of the body maintain a state of biochemical homeostasis despite significant renal dysfunction, a price is paid for loss of functional reserve capacity.
   a. Patients with presymptomatic primary renal failure have reduced capacity to respond to physiologic and pathologic stresses.
   b. As renal failure progresses, patients are forced to live in a narrowed state of physiologic activity. A uremic crisis may be suddenly precipitated by decreased intake of nutrients or water, development of concomitant but unrelated diseases, and/or inappropriate administration of certain drugs.

E. Polyuria, nonoliguria, oliguria, and anuria.

1. Polyuria is defined as formation and elimination of large quantities of urine. Depending on the body's need to conserve or eliminate water and solutes, polyuria may be normal (physiologic) or abnormal. The significance of polyuria, and the establishment of whether it is an obligatory or adaptive process, cannot be determined without information obtained from the medical history, physical examination, and laboratory evaluations.
2. Nonoliguria is most often used to describe certain patients with acute tubular necrosis. Nonoliguria means that urine output is greater than 0.5 ml/kg/h. The patient's urine output may be within the normal range or in the polyuric range. Although the patient is not technically oliguric, urine output may be fixed in that it does not appropriately increase in response to the administration of fluids.
3. Oliguria is defined as a decrease in the rate of formation or elimination of urine. It may be prerenal (physiologic), primary renal, or postrenal. Pathologic oliguria presumably exists if urine volume is too low to excrete metabolic waste products without concomitant alteration in body fluid composition and balance. In dogs, oliguria has been calculated to be urine production of less than approximately 0.5 mL/kg/h.[1]
   a. Prerenal (or physiologic) oliguria is a compensatory response by normal kidneys to conserve water in excess of solute to maintain or restore normal body fluid balance. It is associated with formation of a reduced volume of highly concentrated urine with a low sodium concentration. It may be associated with azotemia if there is a concomitant reduction in renal blood flow and glomerular filtration.
   b. Pathologic primary renal oliguria may occur in patients with acute or chronic renal failure. It generally indicates that renal injury is severe.
      (1). Oliguria may develop during the early phase of acute primary renal failure caused by acute tubular necrosis. In such patients, oliguria may persist for hours, days, or weeks. The specific gravity and osmolality of urine obtained from patients with acute oliguric renal failure reflect impaired tubular capacity to concentrate or dilute glomerular filtrate. If sufficient nephrons have been damaged, isosthenuria may occur.
      (2). Oliguria may occur in patients with chronic primary polyuric renal failure if some prerenal abnormality (such as dehydration or cardiac decompensation) develops. If the prerenal cause of reduced perfusion is removed, and if additional acute nephron damage has not occurred, polyuria will resume. Primary renal oliguria may also develop as a terminal event in patients with chronic, progressive, generalized renal disease.
   c. Oliguria may occur in association with diseases of the lower urinary tract that impair flow of urine through the excretory pathway.
4. Anuria indicates a lack of urine formation by the kidneys and failure to eliminate urine from the body. Although anuria could occur as a result of complete shutdown of renal function caused by lack of renal perfusion or primary renal failure, it is usually associated with urinary obstruction or rents in the lower urinary tract.
5. The significance of determining urine output is that the type and magnitude of excesses and deficits associated with fluid, electrolyte, acid-base, nutrient, and endocrine imbalances in patients with renal failure characterized by oliguria or anuria are different from those observed in patients with nonoliguria or polyuria.

a. Polyuric renal failure tends to be characterized by greater deficits caused by impaired tubular modification of glomerular filtrate. Biochemical trends associated with primary polyuric renal failure include deficits in water, sodium, chloride, bicarbonate, calcium, vitamins, erythropoietin, amino acids, and calories, and excesses in phosphates, sulfates, hydrogen ion, parathyroid hormone (PTH), and nitrogenous wastes. Although polyuric patients are usually normokalemic, they may become hypokalemic (especially cats) or, rarely, hyperkalemic.

b. Primary oliguric renal failure tends to be associated with greater excesses caused by profound reductions in renal blood flow and GFR. Biochemical trends associated with pathologic oliguria include excesses in water, potassium, hydrogen ion, sodium, chloride, phosphates, sulfates, and nitrogenous wastes, and deficits in calories, amino acids, and vitamins. Negative body water balance may result from gastrointestinal losses.

F. Chronic renal failure.

1. Chronic renal failure is defined as primary renal failure that has persisted for an extended period, usually months to years. Regardless of the cause(s) of nephron loss, chronic renal failure is characterized by irreversible renal structural lesions.
   a. After correcting reversible primary diseases and/or prerenal or postrenal components of renal dysfunction, further improvement in renal function should not be expected in patients with chronic renal failure, because compensatory and adaptive changes designed to sustain renal function have likely reached their maximum.
   b. Likewise, unless additional forms of renal injury occur, rapid deterioration of intrinsic renal function is also unusual.
2. In spite of the poor long-term prognosis, patients with chronic renal failure often survive for many months to years with a good quality of life. Although no treatment can correct existing irreversible renal lesions of chronic renal failure, the clinical and biochemical consequences of reduced renal function can be minimized by symptomatic and supportive therapy.

G. Acute renal failure.

1. Acute renal failure is defined as rapid onset of azotemia over hours to days (at most 2 weeks), or pathologic oliguria that could not have been present for more than a few days.[2] Rapid onset of azotemia or oliguria indicates rapid deterioration or loss of renal function. The rapid deterioration of renal function characteristic of acute renal failure contrasts with the indolent, inevitable progression of chronic renal failure over months to years. Implicit in the diagnosis of acute renal failure is the potential for reversibility and improved function owing to development of compensatory adaptations.
2. Acute renal failure most commonly results from the effects of renal ischemia or nephrotoxins, a syndrome known as acute tubular necrosis. However, other acute renal diseases (e.g., leptospirosis, hypercalcemic nephropathy, acute glomerulonephritis) may cause acute renal failure.

H. End-stage renal failure.

1. The term end-stage kidney implies the presence of renal diseases that are generalized, progressive, irreversible, and at an extremely advanced, or "end" stage of development.
   a. End-stage kidneys are one step beyond chronic generalized nephropathy, and the term applies to all cases in which the antecedent cause of renal destruction cannot be identified or localized to any particular portion of the nephron.
   b. In some cases, disease processes initially responsible for renal damage are no longer present or active in these kidneys.
2. The histopathologic appearance of such kidneys is consistently characterized by sclerotic glomeruli, abundant mononuclear tubulo-interstitial infiltrate, interstitial fibrosis, dilated tubules, and atrophic tubular epithelium that are superimposed on compensatory changes in remaining viable nephrons.

II. RENAL ADAPTATIONS TO THE LOSS OF NEPHRONS

A. Alterations in glomerular structure and function.

1. Reduction in renal mass is associated with an increase in glomerular size in dogs and cats (Fig. 16–1).[3,4]
   a. Hypertrophy of cellular and matrix constituents of glomeruli is at least partially responsible for the glomerular enlargement.
      (1). In young rats, prominent increases in glomerular endothelial, mesangial, and epithelial cells were observed following uninephrectomy.[5]
      (2). In a recent study, glomerular epithelial cells did not appear to increase in response to extensive renal ablation in older rats.[6] The authors speculated that epithelial cell injury may promote glomerulosclerosis in this model.
   b. A portion of the glomerular enlargement may also be caused by hemodynamically mediated increases in glomerular capillary volume.
   c. Although surviving glomeruli and nephrons become hypertrophic after ablation of renal tissue, new glomeruli and nephrons do not develop.
2. A progressive increase in whole kidney blood flow and GFR occurs within days to weeks following abrupt reduction in renal mass.[3]
   a. This observed increase in whole kidney renal

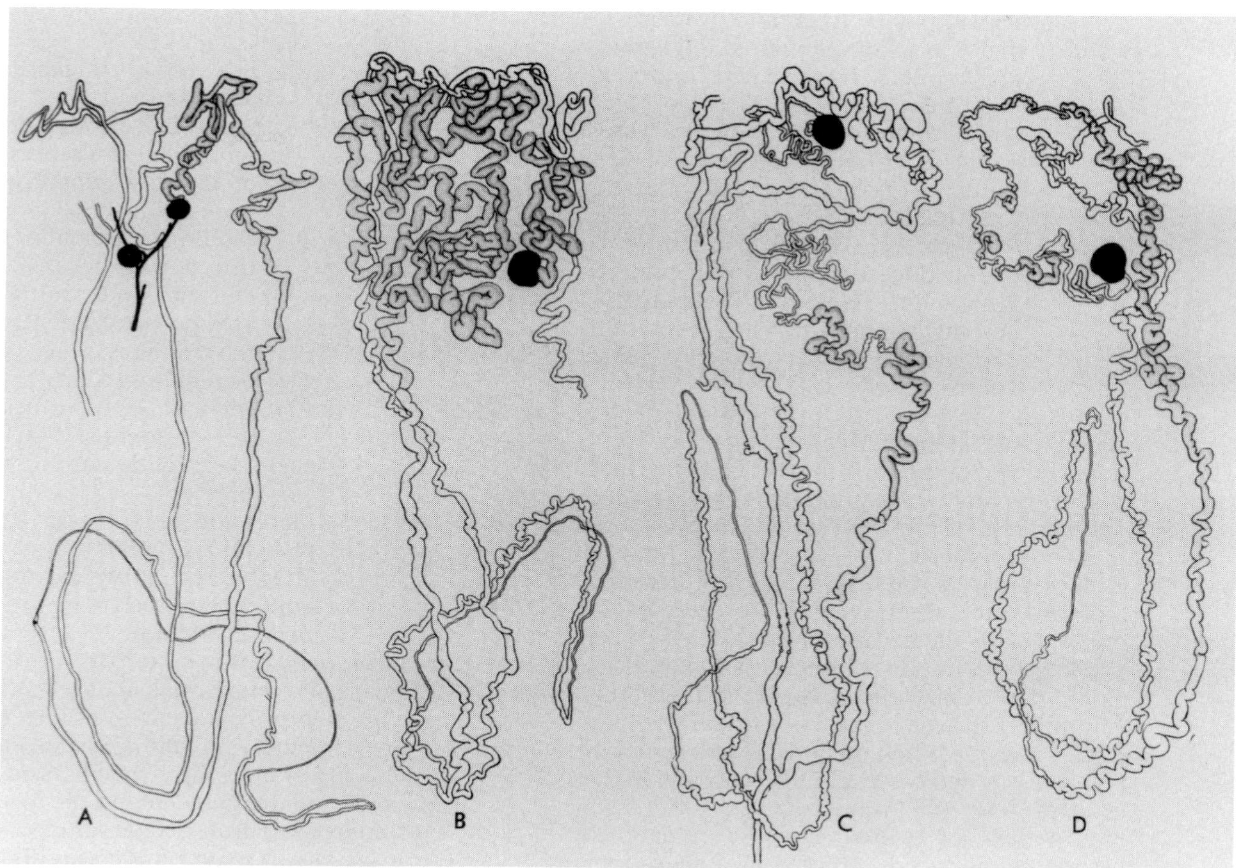

FIG. 16–1. Camera lucida drawing of nephrons isolated by microdissection from dog kidneys and stained vitally with trypan blue. In all nephrons, the dye is localized only in the proximal convoluted tubules. **A,** A normal dog kidney. **B, C, D,** Kidneys of dogs with compensated end-stage renal disease. **B,** The proximal convolution shows marked hypertrophy and hyperplasia and is filled with dye granules in a normal manner throughout its course. **C** and **D,** The proximal convolutions show atrophic dye-free stretches as well as hypertrophic dye-containing stretches. Reprinted with permission from Bloom F. *Pathology of the Dog and Cat. The Genitourinary System, With Clinical Considerations.* Evanston, Illinois: American Veterinary Publications; 1954.

function is attributable to increases in single-nephron GFR (SNGFR) and renal blood flow among surviving nephrons.[3,7]

b. Increased SNGFR is associated with an increase in glomerular capillary pressure or glomerular hypertension.[8]
   (1). In rats, glomerular hypertension has been causally linked to glomerular injury and progression of renal failure (Fig. 16–2).[9]
   (2). The magnitude of glomerular capillary hypertension observed in dogs with surgically reduced renal mass is similar to or greater than that observed in rats.[7]
   (3). Single-nephron adaptive changes observed in dogs are similar to those observed in rats, with two notable exceptions.[3,10]

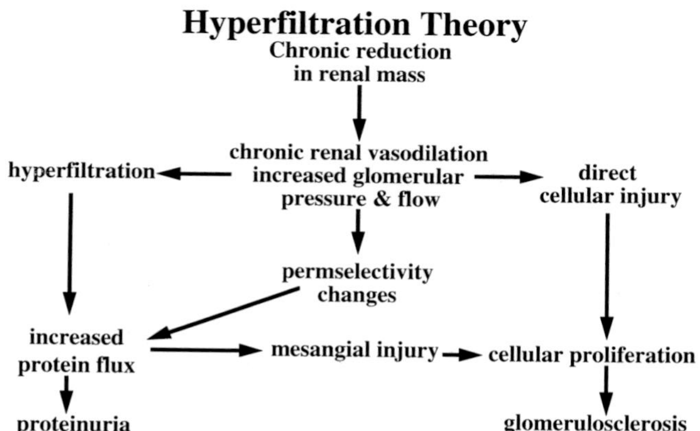

FIG. 16–2. Hemodynamic adaptations that follow reduction in nephrons have been proposed to promote glomerular injury. Enhanced proteinuria may also promote tubular injury.

(a). Transcapillary hydraulic pressure, a major factor incriminated in glomerular capillary hypertensive injury, is only marginally increased in dogs with a three-fourths reduction in renal mass, although it may be significantly increased with more extensive renal ablation.

(b). Systemic hypertension is less prominent in dogs than in rats with induced renal failure; however, systemic hypertension appears to be common in dogs with naturally occurring renal failure.

c. Adaptation in SNGFR is proportional to the extent of reduction in nephron quantity.

d. Changes in glomerular function and structure appear to parallel one another.[3]

3. Urinary protein excretion typically increases as renal mass is reduced.

a. In dogs and cats, the magnitude of proteinuria is often 1.5 to 2 times normal or greater, and is influenced by dietary protein intake.[4,11]

b. While proteinuria is considered a hallmark of glomerular injury and dysfunction, the observation that the magnitude of proteinuria may rapidly change when dietary protein intake is increased or decreased has led some researchers to propose that proteinuria in chronic renal failure may be related, at least in part, to hemodynamic and physiologic alterations rather than to glomerular lesions.[12,13]

(1). Disturbances in intraglomerular hemodynamics can induce proteinuria even in the absence of detectable structural abnormalities in the filtration barrier.[12]

(2). Dietary protein intake has been thought to influence proteinuria, at least in rats, by modifying intraglomerular capillary pressure. Protein restriction in rats has been shown to improve glomerular size permselectivity (the ability of the glomerular barrier to limit passage of proteins according to their size) by a mechanism independent of its protective effect on glomerular structure.[13]

(a). Dietary protein restriction may decrease proteinuria by reducing the proportion of glomerular filtrate permeating a non–size discriminatory shunt pathway.

(b). Acute and chronic effects of dietary protein intake on proteinuria may be different.

(1′). While acute increases in proteinuria associated with high-protein feeding may be of hemodynamic and physiologic origin, the magnitude of this proteinuria typically remains stable.

(2′). Progressive increases in proteinuria associated with long-term high-protein feeding are more likely to represent development of glomerular structural lesions.

(3′). Studies in our laboratory indicate that in dogs with induced chronic renal failure, onset of an increasing magnitude of proteinuria may precede a decline in renal function.

(4′). Increasing proteinuria is an adverse prognostic factor in humans with chronic renal failure.[14,15]

(c). Increasing angiotensin II promotes proteinuria by hemodynamic effects and by regulating sieving function and macromolecular processing of the mesangium.[16]

B. Alterations in tubular structure and function.

1. Structural and functional changes occurring in surviving nephrons appear to reflect a combination of a general hypertrophic response associated with hyperfiltration, and specific structural and functional adaptations required for increased nephron excretion of specific solutes.[3]

2. The mass of surviving renal tissue increases following loss of nephrons. Most of this increase in renal mass is caused by growth of proximal tubules; other nephron segments exhibit less growth.[3]

a. The increase in proximal tubular size is proportional to the extent of reduction in nephron quantity.

b. Enlargement of proximal nephrons is associated with increased proximal reabsorption of glomerular filtrate.

(1). The increase in proximal reabsorption approximates the increase in SNGFR, thus preserving glomerulotubular balance.

(2). Increased delivery of filtrate to the proximal tubules (owing to increased SNGFR) likely triggers increased proximal fluid reabsorption, which, in turn, stimulates proximal tubule hypertrophy.

(3). Some tubular functions are altered in proportion to changes in tubule mass, whereas others are not.

(a). Proximal glucose and amino acid reabsorption is altered in proportion to changes in tubule mass, presumably to facilitate conservation of these nutrients.

(b). Phosphate reabsorption is decreased per unit of tubule mass, facilitating the increase in fractional excretion of phosphate that occurs with constant dietary phosphate intake and declining renal function.

(c). Activities of proximal nephron enzymes required for ammoniagenesis increase, facilitating the capacity of surviving nephrons to excrete acid derived from the daily diet.

(d). Proximal sodium-hydrogen ion exchange is increased in excess of the need for proximal bicarbonate reabsorption. This change may be a general manifestation of tubule cell hypertrophy rather than an adaptive response.

3. Loop of Henle mass appears to increase minimally following reduction in nephron quantity, but fluid reabsorption in the thick ascending limb appears to increase in proportion to SNGFR.[3]
4. Functional and structural adaptations occur in distal tubules.[3]
   a. Distal nephron mass increases following loss of nephrons, but the magnitude of hypertrophy is less than that in the proximal nephron.
   b. Distal nephron potassium secretion increases as nephrons are lost to facilitate increased fractional potassium excretion necessary to prevent hyperkalemia.
      (1). The increase in potassium secretion is a function of a long-term increase in dietary potassium load per nephron.
      (2). Increased potassium secretion can be prevented by proportionally reducing potassium load per nephron; however, reducing potassium intake does not appear to prevent hypertrophy of the collecting ducts.

C. Mechanisms of compensatory adaptation.

1. Proposed mechanisms of renal growth and hypertrophy
   a. Although existence of a renotropic hormone responsible for promoting renal hypertrophy has been proposed, no such factor has been identified.[17] Further, the stimulus responsible for initiating renal compensatory hypertrophy (growth) has not been established.
      (1). Many compounds have been shown to promote renal growth.[3,17]
         (a). Substances known to promote renal growth include insulin-like growth factor I (IGF-I), epidermal growth factor (EGF), platelet-derived growth factor (PDGF), prostaglandin E_2 (PGE_2), hydrocortisone, thyroxine, arginine, vasopressin, and angiotensin.
         (b). None of these factors promotes exclusively renal hypertrophy.
      (2). Although the systemic circulation is a potential source of peptide growth factors, such as IGF-I and EGF, recent evidence suggests that these substances act in an autocrine or short-loop paracrine fashion rather than in an endocrine manner.[17]
      (3). Because kidney cells can produce substances that both promote and inhibit cell growth, growth of the renal epithelium may be subject to multiple influences, including local autocrine control. Compensatory hypertrophy may be mediated by altered sensitivity to these factors.[3,17]
   b. Renal hypertrophy has been proposed to reflect a tubular response to increased reabsorption of solutes, principally sodium, associated with increased GFR (so-called "work hypertrophy").[3]
      (1). In general, renal plasma flow (RPF), GFR, and renal mass tend to increase proportionally.
      (2). Initially, hypertrophy associated with feeding a high-protein diet (a recognized stimulus for hyperfiltration) was thought to result from the workload imposed by the necessity of excreting large quantities of urea. We now know that renal energy consumption is devoted predominantly to cation reabsorption rather than to urea excretion.
      (3). Indications that renal hypertrophy may precede hyperfiltration tend to argue against the "work hypothesis" as the primary stimulus for renal hypertrophy.[18]
      (4). Alternatively, renal hypertrophy may be the cause for hyperfiltration rather than a consequence of it.
         (a). Antidiuretic hormone (ADH)–mediated renal tubule hypertrophy and increased fluid reabsorption in the medullary thick ascending limb have been proposed to induce hyperfiltration secondarily.[3,19]
         (b). By increasing salt transport in the thick ascending limb, salt concentration at the macula densa is reduced, thus depressing tubuloglomerular feedback, and leading to increased GFR.
2. Proposed mechanisms responsible for glomerular hyperperfusion, hypertension, and hyperfiltration.
   a. Glomerular hemodynamics and filtration are influenced by an array of circulating and local mediators.[20]
      (1). Vasodilators and vasoconstrictors are necessary to allow the renal microcirculation to autoregulate and adapt to a wide variety of physiologic conditions.
      (2). The relative availability of vasodilators

and vasoconstrictors determines renal vascular resistance.

(3). Glomerular perfusion, glomerular capillary pressure, and glomerular filtration are controlled by modulating preglomerular arteriolar and postglomerular arteriolar resistances. Alterations in preglomerular and postglomerular arteriolar resistances often do not parallel one another.

b. The primary renal hemodynamic event following reduction in renal mass appears to be renal arteriolar vasodilation. Glomerular hypertension and hyperfiltration appear to be promoted by preferential dilation of preglomerular arterioles. Although presumably compensatory in origin, the precise factors responsible for initiating these hemodynamic events following reduction in renal mass have not been firmly established.

(1). Structural hypertrophy may alter arteriolar resistance and promote glomerular hypertension.[3]

(2). In the setting of systemic hypertension, glomerular hypertension has been proposed to result from impaired afferent arteriolar autoregulation.[3] That is, glomerular capillaries are not protected by autoregulation from increases in systemic pressure; however, glomerular hypertension may occur in absence of systemic hypertension, particularly in dogs.[7]

(3). A variety of vasoactive mediators has been found to influence the hemodynamic adaptations that occur in renal failure.

(a). The observation that chronic inhibition of angiotensin I–converting enzyme normalizes glomerular capillary pressure implicates increased angiotensin II activity in the genesis of glomerular hypertension.[21] Increased angiotensin II activity promotes intrarenal vasoconstriction, preferentially enhancing efferent arteriolar resistance. Thus, limiting angiotensin II production preferentially lowers efferent arteriolar resistance, which in turn reduces glomerular capillary pressure. In addition to influencing renal function, angiotensin II may also affect cellular hypertrophy.

(b). Several studies have indicated that renal vasodilation and hyperfiltration may be mediated partly by nitric oxide (NO) production.[20] Endothelium-derived relaxing factor/nitrous oxide (EDNO), a substance derived from L-arginine, is one of several vasoactive mediators produced by endothelial cells. NO appears to modulate renin release and the renal vascular effects of angiotensin II.[22–24] It acts as a physiologic antagonist of angiotensin II by affecting both glomeruli and renal tubules.[25] NO also modulates renal tubular function, participating in the renal adaptation to increased sodium intake by facilitating sodium excretion and allowing maintenance of normal blood pressure.[26] Recent data support a role for macula densa–derived NO in modifying glomerular capillary pressure via tubuloglomerular feedback in response to tubular fluid delivery and reabsorption.[27] In addition, NO has been proposed to be involved in the renal vasodilatory actions of IGF-I.

(c). Synthesis of vasodilator prostaglandins E_2 and I_2, and vasoconstrictor thromboxane A_2, is increased in glomeruli isolated from subtotally nephrectomized rats.[3] These prostanoids may influence glomerular hemodynamic function and glomerulotubular balance. Prostaglandin synthesis inhibition reduces RPF and GFR in rats with reduced renal mass; however, RPF and GFR were not affected by prostaglandin synthesis inhibitors in dogs with reduced renal mass.[28] These contrasting findings emphasize that there may be important species-related differences in pathophysiologic mechanisms.

D. Factors that influence renal compensatory adaptations.

1. Dietary protein intake is an important determinant of renal function and renal mass.
   a. Increasing dietary protein intake increases renal function and renal mass, whereas reducing protein intake limits renal function and mass.[11]
   b. However, dietary protein restriction does not prevent compensatory increases in renal function or renal mass.[3,29,30] The effects of dietary protein intake appear to be limited to modifying basal GFR and renal mass.
   c. Dietary protein intake and subtotal nephrectomy appear to have additive effects on renal function and hypertrophy.
2. Endocrine hormones influence renal function and growth.[3]
   a. Pituitary ablation reduces renal weight, but as with dietary protein restriction, compensatory renal hypertrophy is not impeded.
   b. Likewise, thyroidectomy and adrenalectomy reduce renal weight and GFR, but the renal

hypertrophic response to subtotal renal ablation is not limited.

c. Androgens increase kidney weight in female rats and mice, but androgens do not appear to enhance compensatory renal hypertrophy.

3. Age has a proven effect on the magnitude of compensatory renal hypertrophy.[3]
   a. Increases in renal mass and GFR are substantially greater in young animals as compared with older animals.
   b. Findings in experimental animals that have also been confirmed in humans indicate that the magnitude of compensatory renal adaptations following uninephrectomy is substantially greater for young patients than for adults.
   c. This age-related effect on organ growth following reduction in total organ mass is not limited to the kidneys.

E. The intact nephron hypothesis.

1. The intact nephron hypothesis, originally proposed by Bricker and colleagues, states that despite morphologic heterogeneity and wide variations in SNGFR among surviving nephrons, glomerular and tubular function remain as closely integrated in diseased kidneys as they do in normal kidneys.[31]
   a. Maintenance of body fluid homeostasis by diseased kidneys depends on the ability of a heterogeneous nephron population to control water and solute excretion.
   b. It is highly unlikely that physiologically appropriate handling of solutes and water by diseased kidneys represents a fortuitous combination of elevated solute excretion by some nephrons and reduced solute excretion by others.
   c. It is most plausible that surviving functional nephrons transport solute and water in proportion to their individual GFR values, i.e., glomerulotubular balance is maintained in diseased nephrons.
   d. It has been confirmed that glomerulotubular balance is maintained over a wide range of SNGFR values in both tubulo-interstitial and glomerular diseases.[3]
2. The balance between intake of water and nutrients and their excretion by the kidneys may be maintained without therapy during the earlier phases of renal failure by the same biologic control mechanisms operative in normal patients.
   a. To achieve these adaptations, each surviving nephron must accept a greater proportion of overall nephron function.
   b. As renal function declines, the excretory response of each surviving nephron must increase in inverse proportion to the number of surviving nephrons. This phenomenon, which has been termed the magnification phenomenon, represents further refinement of the intact nephron hypothesis.[32]

F. Compensatory adaptation and progressive renal injury.

1. Chronic renal failure is an inherently progressive disease.
   a. Progression of renal failure most likely results from continuing renal damage induced by whatever disease process is responsible for its onset.[33]
   b. Findings over the past 2 decades suggest that renal insufficiency may also progress to end-stage renal failure through mechanisms that are independent of the initiating insult.[34]
      (1). Surgical resection or infarction of approximately three quarters or more of the functional renal mass in rats resulted in a syndrome of progressive azotemia, proteinuria, arterial hypertension, and, eventually, death from uremia.[35] Progression occurs in this rodent model of renal failure despite the fact that remaining renal tissue is initially normal, albeit reduced in quantity.
      (2). Such findings have led to the hypothesis that reduction in nephrons beyond some critical threshold leads to failure of the remaining nephrons.[36]
      (3). Mechanisms responsible for spontaneous, self-perpetuation of chronic renal failure have not been fully elucidated but are thought to relate in part to adverse consequences of compensatory adaptations that follow reduction in nephrons (Fig. 16–3).[8,36]
         (a). Although these compensatory adaptations may be initially beneficial in facilitating fluid and solute homeostasis and enhancing waste excretion, they may eventually prove injurious to surviving nephrons.
         (b). Several lines of evidence suggest that hemodynamic and hypertrophic adaptations to the loss of nephrons may lead to glomerular injury that promotes spontaneous self-perpetuation of chronic renal failure.[36–38]
         (c). Other factors that may contribute to progressive renal injury include tubulo-interstitial injury, hyperlipidemia, and glomerular capillary thrombosis.
   c. Clinical impressions suggest that chronic renal failure is progressive in dogs and cats. However, few studies have been designed to confirm this impression in dogs; even less is known of the course of spontaneous chronic renal failure in cats.
      (1). In rats with induced chronic renal failure, and in some humans with spontaneous renal disease, renal function reportedly

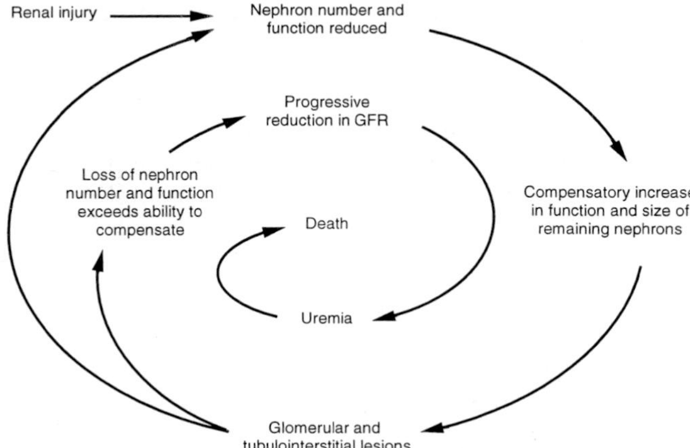

FIG. 16–3. An initial insult or injury to the kidney results in both structural and functional compensatory reactions by the remaining nephrons. Over time, these adaptations lead to further glomerular and tubulo-interstitial damage. Continued destruction initiates further compensation, promoting a self-perpetuating cycle of adaptation and injury. The compensatory changes maintain clinically stable disease until structural and functional damage exceeds a threshold, beyond which progression of renal function and clinical signs of uremia occur. Reprinted with permission from Churchill J, Polzin D, Osborne C, Adams L. The influence of dietary protein intake on progression of chronic renal failure. *Semin Vet Med Surg (Small Animal).* 1992;7:244-250.

declines in a predictable, and often linear, fashion.[8]

(2). Serial evaluation of renal function in dogs with induced or spontaneous renal failure has revealed more varied patterns, including stable, episodically declining, and linearly declining renal function.[39,40]

2. Glomerular hypertension and hyperfiltration, the hyperfiltration theory.
   a. The hyperfiltration theory proposes that compensatory intraglomerular hypertension, hyperperfusion, and hyperfiltration occur initially as adaptive responses to reduction in nephrons, but eventually lead to progressive proteinuria, glomerular sclerosis, and loss of functional nephrons (see Figs. 16–2, 16–3).
   b. This hypothesis is based on the observation that blunting these hemodynamic adaptations by feeding reduced-protein diets prevents development of proteinuria, glomerular sclerosis, and progressive renal dysfunction in subtotally nephrectomized rats.[35,36]
   c. The mechanism(s) by which increased glomerular pressure, increased perfusion, and increased filtration promote glomerular sclerosis and proteinuria are not fully understood, but they may involve, in part, hypertension-mediated endothelial injury, activation of platelets leading to intraglomerular thrombosis as a result of endothelial injury, release of platelet-derived growth promoters, and increased flux of plasma proteins through the mesangium owing to hyperfiltration.[35,36,41]
   d. Although hyperfiltration and glomerular capillary hypertension occur in subtotally nephrectomized dogs, a link between glomerular hyperfiltration and hypertension and a progressive decline in renal function has yet to be confirmed in this species.[33,42]
   e. High-protein feeding has been associated with increases in GFR and glomerular lesions in subtotally nephrectomized cats, but glomerular capillary pressures were not determined in this study. Renal function remained stable despite development of glomerular lesions.[4]
   f. Systemic hypertension may be an important risk factor promoting glomerular hypertension–induced glomerulopathy.
      (1). Reducing renal mass in rats typically results in systemic and glomerular hypertension, progressive glomerular injury, and loss of surviving nephrons.
      (2). Glomerular injury and nephron loss did not occur in rats that remained normotensive after subtotal nephrectomy.[43] Rats in this study had marked increases in SNGFR, but glomerular capillary pressures were only slightly increased. The researchers proposed that, in the absence of systemic hypertension, increases in glomerular capillary pressure may not be sufficient to initiate progressive glomerular injury and nephron loss.
      (3). Although subtotal nephrectomy also increases systemic blood pressure in dogs and cats, the increases are modest compared to changes typically observed in rats.
         (a). Relative resistance to development of systemic hypertension following subtotal nephrectomy may be one reason dogs and cats appear to be less susceptible to progressive renal injury in this model of renal failure.
         (b). Because systemic hypertension appears to be common in dogs and cats with spontaneous chronic renal failure,[44,45] studies on the progression of chronic renal failure utilizing the subtotal nephrectomy (remnant kidney) model should be interpreted with caution in these species.
3. Glomerular hypertrophy may be an important step preceding development of glomerular sclerosis and progression of chronic renal failure.[46,47]
   a. The observation that glomerular sclerosis may develop in rats with unilateral nephrectomy in the absence of glomerular hypertension sug-

gests that mechanisms other than hyperfiltration may contribute to progression of chronic renal failure.[48]

b. A striking correlation has been observed between hypertrophic glomeruli and development of glomerular sclerosis.
   (1). In addition, glomerular hypertrophy has been observed to precede onset of several clinical renal diseases in human beings, including diabetes mellitus, oligomeganephronia, and sickle cell disease.[47]
   (2). Dietary protein restriction has been proposed to minimize development of glomerular sclerosis and progression of chronic renal failure in subtotally nephrectomized rats by limiting renal and glomerular hypertrophy.[48]
c. The mechanisms by which glomerular hypertrophy promote glomerular injury have not been established.
   (1). "Growth promoters" acting on the glomerulus may enhance mesangial and epithelial cell proliferation and mesangial matrix production, leading to glomerular sclerosis and progressive nephron loss.
   (2). Glomerular hypertrophy may exacerbate glomerular injury by increasing glomerular capillary wall tension.
   (3). Failure of visceral epithelial cells to increase in quantity during glomerular hypertrophy may impair their ability to maintain normal permselectivity.[6]
d. Glomerular hypertrophy may act alone or in concert with hemodynamic factors to promote glomerular injury following loss of renal mass.[47] The effects of glomerular hypertrophy and glomerular hypertension appear to be additive.[3]

4. Although the emphasis of much of the research investigating the cause of progressive renal disease has focused on glomerular pathology, primary tubulo-interstitial injury also occurs with subtotal nephrectomy and may contribute to progression of renal failure.
   a. Tubular atrophy and dilation, interstitial fibrosis, and inflammatory interstitial infiltration are common following subtotal nephrectomy.[3,4,11]
   b. Tubulo-interstitial injury is often regarded as secondary to the glomerulopathy observed in surviving nephrons.[3]
      (1). Proteinuria is thought to result in tubule obstruction and dilation.
      (2). Glomerular sclerosis is thought to induce remnant nephron hypoproliferation and tubule atrophy.
   c. Tubulo-interstitial injury may occur by mechanisms independent of those that cause glomerulosclerosis and may promote progression of chronic renal failure. Altered phosphate metabolism, increased renal ammoniagenesis, hypokalemia, and cellular hypermetabolism have been implicated in the genesis of primary tubulo-interstitial injury.
   d. Limiting dietary intake of phosphorus limits tubulo-interstitial injury and progression of renal failure in subtotally nephrectomized rats.[49]
      (1). The adverse effect of dietary phosphorus, hyperphosphatemia, and hyperparathyroidism on progressive renal dysfunction has been hypothesized to result from precipitation of phosphorus salts within the renal parenchyma, stimulating renal interstitial inflammation and fibrosis.[50]
      (2). Dietary phosphorus restriction may prevent renal cell injury by limiting cellular calcium uptake.[51]
      (3). Dietary phosphate restriction has been shown to slow progression of chronic renal failure in studies of dogs.[42,52,53]
         (a). In these studies, a substantial increase in renal phosphorus content and a massive increase in renal calcium content were detected after 2 years of renal failure.[42] However, dietary phosphorus intake did not influence the concentrations of calcium or phosphorus in renal tissue. Nonetheless, dogs dying of uremia in these studies had greater renal mineralization and fibrosis than did the dogs that survived the study.
         (b). The mechanisms by which phosphorus restriction improved survival in these dogs is unclear, but the authors hypothesized a role for extrarenal mechanisms.
         (c). Phosphorus restriction has also been shown to limit renal mineralization in cats with induced chronic renal failure, but renal function remained unchanged in this study.[54]
   e. Increased renal ammoniagenesis and elevated intrarenal ammonia concentrations appear to promote renal tubulo-interstitial injury.[55,56]
      (1). Renal ammoniagenesis is increased with chronic metabolic acidosis, hypokalemia, subtotal renal ablation, a high-protein diet, diabetic nephropathy, and antioxidant (vitamin E or selenium) deficiency. All these states have been associated with induction or progression of renal failure in an experimental model or clinical disease state.[56]
      (2). High concentrations of ammonium in the renal interstitium are hypothesized to activate the third component of comple-

ment by the alternate pathway, initiating complement-mediated renal inflammation, which culminates in tubulo-interstitial injury.

(3). Increased ammoniagenesis and elevated intrarenal concentrations of ammonia may also contribute to progression by promoting renal hypertrophy.

(4). Prevention of metabolic acidosis by dietary supplementation with sodium bicarbonate prevented development of tubulo-interstitial lesions in rats with induced chronic renal failure.[57]

f. Chronic potassium depletion and hypokalemia have been linked to a form of tubulo-interstitial injury sometimes referred to as hypokalemic nephropathy.

(1). In rats and humans, affected kidneys are enlarged, proximal tubule cells become vacuolated, tubulo-interstitial inflammatory lesions develop, and urine-concentrating ability is lost; hypokalemic nephropathy can progress to end-stage renal disease if the potassium depletion is not corrected.

(2). Renal vasoconstriction associated with increased thromboxane and prostaglandin levels are thought to contribute to the pathogenesis of hypokalemic nephropathy. Furthermore, augmentation of renal ammoniagenesis predisposes to ammonium-mediated progression of renal damage, as previously described.

(3). A similar, although not identical, syndrome of hypokalemic nephropathy has been reported in cats.[58,59]

(a). A strong association between renal failure and hypokalemia has been reported in cats.[60] Feeding a high-protein diet with relatively low dietary potassium content seems to promote potassium depletion in cats; metabolic acidosis may exacerbate the condition.

(b). In a recent uncontrolled study, renal lesions characterized by lymphoplasmacytic interstitial infiltrates and interstitial fibrosis reportedly developed in five of nine healthy cats fed a low-potassium, high-protein diet.[59] Fewer cats in this study developed clinical and laboratory evidence of renal dysfunction.

g. Renal hypermetabolism characterized by increased renal oxygen consumption and superoxide radical production may expose renal tubule cells to increased risk of oxidant injury.[61,62]

5. Considerable evidence from rodent studies suggests a role for dietary lipids in modulating the progression of renal disease.[63–66]

a. The effects of lipids on the progression of chronic renal failure may be related to renal eicosanoid production and plasma lipid concentrations.

b. The specific composition of dietary lipids may influence systemic blood pressure, blood lipid composition, platelet aggregation, blood viscosity, the immune system, and fibrinolytic activity.[66]

c. Although conflicting data exist, researchers have hypothesized that accumulation of lipid macromolecules in the mesangium, especially cholesterol and cholesterol esters, may contribute to mesangial cell injury and may stimulate production of mesangial matrix, thus promoting glomerular sclerosis.[67,68]

(1). A close correlation appears to exist between the lipid status of the glomerulus and the presence or absence of macrophages.[69,70]

(2). Glomeruli with mesangial deposits of antibody or macromolecules release a lipid chemoattractant substance specific for monocytes. Macrophages, which comprise a major portion of atherosclerotic plaque in humans, may contribute to or modulate many of the following processes thought to contribute to progressive renal injury.

(a). Release of PDGF (a mesangial cell mitogen).

(b). Interleukin-1 (a mesangial cell activator).

(c). Cytokines that induce the leukocyte adhesion proteins on endothelial cells and membrane-bound procoagulant activity on endothelial cells.[69]

d. Systemic hypertension appears to enhance the adverse effects of hyperlipidemia on glomeruli.[38]

6. Glomerular capillary thrombosis, a prominent finding in rats following subtotal nephrectomy, is thought to contribute to glomerular sclerosis by direct occlusion of glomerular capillaries and by release of platelet-derived substances that aggravate glomerular injury.[3]

a. Microthrombi also occur in dogs following subtotal nephrectomy, although this lesion appears to be less prominent in dogs than in rats.[11]

b. Endothelial damage, presumably induced by glomerular hypertension or hypertrophy, may expose circulating plasma proteins and platelets to basement membrane constituents, precipitating intracapillary coagulation.

c. Anticoagulants and thromboxane synthesis inhibition limit development of glomerular sclerosis.[1,3]

(1). Heparin is particularly effective in limiting glomerular injury; however, in addition to its anticoagulant properties, heparin may: (1) ameliorate systemic hypertension, (2) limit proliferation of smooth muscle cells, and (3) abolish the effects of growth factors derived from mononuclear cells. Therefore, the effects of heparin on glomerular pathology and progression of renal failure may involve factors other than coagulation.

(2). Aspirin has been shown to prevent hyperfiltration and glomerular basement membrane thickening in rats with experimental diabetes mellitus. The mechanism of aspirin in this model is not known, but it may relate more to inhibition of prostaglandin synthesis than to anticoagulant properties of aspirin.

III. PATHOPHYSIOLOGY OF UREMIA

A. Overview of uremia and uremic toxins.

1. The onset and spectrum of clinical and biochemical events in patients with renal failure may vary depending on the nature, severity, duration, rate of progression of the underlying disease, presence of coexisting but unrelated disease(s), age and species of the patient, and administration of therapeutic agents. In most instances, uremia is the clinical state toward which all progressive, generalized renal diseases ultimately converge, and associated signs are more similar than dissimilar. The diverse clinical and laboratory findings characteristic of uremia emphasize its polysystemic nature (Table 16–1). Such diverse organ involvement implies that uremia must be associated with impairment of one or more fundamental cell functions.[71]

2. The clinical manifestations of uremia have been attributed, at least in part, to retention of uremic toxins. Searches for uremic toxins have thus far failed to identify any single toxin as the cause for uremic signs. The list of potential uremic toxins is extensive (Table 16–2), although a cause-and-effect relationship between these various compounds and manifestations of the uremic syndrome has not been established in most instances.

   a. Byproducts of endogenous and exogenous protein metabolism are an important source of uremic toxins.

      (1). The well-recognized association between clinical signs of uremia and dietary protein intake supports the hypothesis that products of protein metabolism act as uremic toxins.

         (a). Protein restriction reduces blood urea nitrogen concentrations and ameliorates clinical signs of uremia.

         (b). The magnitude of elevation of blood urea nitrogen concentrations is crudely related to the severity of clinical signs of uremia. Although urea fulfills criteria to be a uremic toxin, it appears to do so only in extremely high concentrations.[71] More likely, urea is a marker of the retention of other protein-derived uremic toxins. High levels of urea may exert feedback inhibition of urea production and channel waste nitrogen into more toxic compounds.

         (c). Studies on human dialysis patients have suggested that dialyzable substances with molecular weights of approximately 500 to 3000 daltons, called middle molecules, may contribute importantly to uremic signs. The significance of these substances and their chemical nature remains unclear.

TABLE 16–1.
FEATURES OF THE UREMIC SYNDROME

Gastrointestinal manifestations: anorexia, nausea, vomiting, gastritis and duodenitis, enterocolitis, uremic stomatitis and gingivitis, uriniferous breath, hyperamylasemia, hyperlipasemia
Neuromuscular manifestations: dullness, fatigue, drowsiness, lethargy, irritability, tremors, behavioral changes, dementia, seizures, stupor, coma, peripheral neuropathies
Musculoskeletal manifestations: gait imbalance, flaccid muscle weakness, myoclonus, renal osteodystrophy
Endocrinologic manifestations: secondary hyperparathyroidism, carbohydrate intolerance, hyperlipidemia, reproductive dysfunction
Cardiopulmonary manifestations: left ventricular hypertrophy, cardiomyopathy, pericarditis, pneumonitis, pleuritis
Hematopoietic manifestations: anemia, hemorrhagic diathesis, immune dysfunction (altered neutrophil and lymphocyte function)
Ophthalmic manifestations: scleral and conjunctival injection

TABLE 16–2.
A PARTIAL LIST OF POTENTIAL UREMIC TOXINS

Urea	Phenols	Indoles
Skatols	Hormones	Polyamines
Trace elements	Serum proteases	Pyradine derivatives
Guanidine compounds	β_2-Microglobulin	Aliphatic amines
Hippurate esters	"Middle molecules"	Aromatic amines

(d). In addition to nitrogenous wastes, protein metabolism also produces a variety of inorganic ions, such as sulfate, phosphate, and hydrogen, that may contribute to signs of uremia.

(2). Bacterial metabolism within the intestines also provides an additional source of protein-derived waste products.[71] If bacterial overgrowth occurs in the small intestines of patients with chronic renal failure, it will exacerbate this effect.

b. Uremia may also result from a variety of endocrine perturbations that occur in renal failure.

(1). The kidneys play a major role in production, modulation, and disposition of many hormones.

(2). Endocrine defects that may occur in chronic renal failure include[71]:

(a). Diminished renal production of erythropoietin and calcitriol.

(b). Adaptive hypersecretion of PTH in an attempt to re-establish calcium and phosphate balance.

(c). Decreased metabolic clearance of follicle-stimulating hormone (FSH), luteinizing hormone (LH), prolactin, growth hormone (GH), melanocyte-stimulating hormone (MSH), and gastrin.

(d). Blunting of feedback response causing increased secretion of LH, adrenocorticotropic hormone (ACTH), and prolactin.

(e). Defective tissue conversion of thyroxine (T_4) to tri-iodothyronine (T_3). Hypothermia is often observed in uremic patients.

(f). Decreased testosterone production.

(g). Diminished end-organ responsiveness to T_3, insulin, and PTH.

(h). Increased circulating somatomedin inhibitory factor.

(3). Although largely unproved in dogs and cats, elevated serum PTH caused by secondary hyperparathyroidism has been hypothesized to function as a "uremic toxin," promoting several important clinical consequences of uremia, including renal osteodystrophy, mental dullness and lethargy resulting from toxic effects of PTH on the brain, immunodeficiency as a consequence of deranged leukocyte function, impaired cardiac and skeletal muscle function resulting from impaired mitochondrial energy metabolism and myofiber mineralization, decreased appetite and energy metabolism resulting from inhibited insulin secretion, and progressive loss of renal function caused by nephrocalcinosis.[72] The toxicity of PTH appears to be mediated through enhanced entry of calcium into cells having plasma membrane receptors for PTH.[72] Excess PTH promotes too great a flux of calcium into these cells, thus activating enzymes that destroy phospholipids, proteins, and nucleic acids. These effects result in cell dysfunction and death.[73]

c. Abnormal metabolism of trace minerals may contribute to the uremic syndrome.[71,74]

(1). Serum vanadium levels may increase with chronic uremia. Oxidized vanadium can inhibit adenosine triphosphatases (ATPases), including sodium-potassium–dependent ATPases.

(2). Aluminum toxicity, associated with long-term, excessive intake of aluminum-containing phosphate-binding agents, may promote renal osteodystrophy, encephalopathy, and defective erythropoiesis.

(3). Zinc deficiency may promote abnormal taste, defective cell-mediated immunity, and reproductive dysfunction.

B. Metabolic disturbances in uremia.

1. Fluid balance

a. Among the earliest clinical manifestations of chronic renal failure is the onset of obligatory polyuria and compensatory polydipsia as a result of reduced urine-concentrating ability.

(1). Depending on the cause of nephron loss, some degree of urine-concentrating and urine-diluting capacity may be retained in early renal failure.[29,75,76]

(a). Renal disease that profoundly disturbs renal medullary architecture may cause disproportionate impairment of concentrating ability at any level of renal dysfunction.[3] Reduced urine-concentrating ability is more likely to develop during early stages of tubulo-interstitial renal diseases, such as pyelonephritis.

(b). In contrast, patients with primary glomerulopathies may retain substantial urine-concentrating capacity even after the onset of azotemia. However, glomerular and tubulo-interstitial diseases cannot be reliably differentiated on the basis of urine-concentrating ability because secondary tubulo-interstitial lesions and impairments in urine-concentrating ability commonly develop as glomerulopathies progress.

(c). Substantial urine-concentrating ability has been shown to persist in dogs and cats with mild to moderate chronic renal failure induced by subtotal nephrectomy.[29,75,76] This model of renal failure minimally alters renal medullary architecture and function. Guidelines defining adequate urine-concentrating ability for dogs and cats have been extrapolated largely from studies using this model of chronic renal failure.

(d). In more advanced renal failure, urine-concentrating and urine-diluting capacities are largely lost and isosthenuria (failure to alter urine osmolality from that of the plasma and glomerular filtrate) is common, regardless of the initiating renal disease.

(2). These signs appear to be recognized less often by cat owners, presumably because of the greater intrinsic concentrating ability of cats and the nature of their voiding habits.[77,78]

b. Reduction in urine-concentrating and urine-diluting capacity is multifactorial in origin.

(1). Renal disease may directly impair urine concentration and dilution by disrupting the renal medullary architecture and countercurrent multiplier system.

(2). Solute diuresis appears to be an important contributor to polyuria and loss of urine-concentrating and urine-diluting capacity in patients with substantial reduction of GRF (e.g., they are azotemic). With renal failure, solute diuresis occurs because the same quantity of solute must be excreted by fewer functioning nephrons. However, studies in dogs confirm that solute diuresis is not the sole factor responsible for altered concentrating and diluting capacity in renal failure.[79]

(a). Concentration of urine requires maintenance of hypertonicity of the medullary interstitium. Disrupting medullary architecture may limit urine concentration and dilution by impairing the ability to maintain hypertonicity of the medullary interstitium.

(b). Deranged countercurrent flow in medullary vasa recta may contribute to the inability to maintain medullary interstitial hypertonicity.

(3). Impaired renal responsiveness to ADH may occur in renal failure and contribute to decreased urine-concentrating ability.[3]

(a). Loss of renal responsiveness to ADH may result from an increase in distal renal tubule flow rate, which limits equilibration of tubular fluid with the hypertonic medullary interstitium.

(b). Additionally, ADH-stimulated adenyl cyclase activity and water permeability in the distal nephron may be impaired in uremia.

c. Free access to water and compensatory polydipsia prevent dehydration in polyuric renal failure.

(1). If fluid intake fails to keep pace with urinary fluid losses, dehydration will ensue because of the inability of the patient to conserve water appropriately by concentrating urine.

(2). Dehydration subsequent to inadequate fluid intake appears to be a common problem in cats with chronic renal failure. It is often manifested in part as constipation.

2. Serum and body sodium balance.

a. Normal sodium balance and extracellular fluid volume are maintained remarkably close to normal by patients with chronic renal failure. Homeostasis is maintained by increasing the fractional excretion of sodium in proportion to the decline in GFR.[3]

(1). For patients with reduced GFR to continue to completely excrete their daily sodium load, the quantity of filtered sodium that is reabsorbed by the tubules must decrease in proportion to the decrease in GFR.

(a). Studies indicate that, at least in rats, these adaptive changes in renal tubular sodium handling occur in the distal portions of the nephron.

(b). This finding is consistent with the concept that fine-tuning of sodium excretion occurs at distal nephron sites.

(2). Enhanced excretion of sodium in patients with renal failure has been linked to production of natriuretic factors.

(a). Fractions of serum and urine from animals with renal failure have been shown to induce natriuresis in normal rats.[3]

(b). The identity of this natriuretic factor(s) remains elusive. Atrial natriuretic peptide appears to be an important factor in contributing to maintenance of sodium balance by inhibiting sodium reabsorption at the distal nephron.[80] Other factors have also been implicated.

b. Although sodium balance is well maintained in renal failure, adaptation to changes in sodium intake may occur more slowly in patients with renal failure than in normal persons.[81]

(1). Renal conservation of sodium may require time for adaptation to occur. Although this theory has not been proved, abrupt reduction in sodium intake has been suggested to be a risk factor for acute decompensation in renal function in dogs with renal failure.[29]

(2). In a recent study, abrupt changes in sodium intake did not appear to adversely affect renal function in dogs with mild renal impairment[82]; however, dogs in the study were not in renal failure and timing of renal function studies in this report was such that reductions in GFR could have been missed.

3. Metabolic acidosis.
   a. Metabolic acidosis is characteristic of renal failure. In a retrospective case series of cats with renal failure, approximately 80% had metabolic acidosis based on decreased venous blood pH values and bicarbonate concentration.[78]
   b. Metabolic acidosis in renal failure results principally from the limited ability of failing kidneys to excrete hydrogen ions and regenerate bicarbonate.
      (1). Normal acid-base balance is maintained by a combination of tubular reabsorption of filtered bicarbonate and excretion of hydrogen ions with ammonia and urinary buffers, primarily HPO_4^{2-}(termed titratable acidity). Renal excretion of hydrogen ions effectively regenerates bicarbonate lost via the gastrointestinal or urinary tract or through respiratory buffering of metabolic acids.
      (2). As the quantity of functioning renal mass declines in chronic renal failure, hydrogen ion secretion is sustained largely by increasing the secretion of ammonium by surviving nephrons to buffer hydrogen ions; however, at some level of renal dysfunction, the capacity to further increase renal ammoniagenesis is lost and metabolic acidosis ensues. The fall in total ammonium excretion that occurs in advanced renal failure is assumed to result from the limited number of functioning nephrons. Decreased medullary recycling of ammonia resulting from structural renal damage may also contribute to impaired ammonium excretion.[83]
      (3). Feline kidneys may respond differently to metabolic acidosis. Acidosis fails to increase the rate of ammoniagenesis in cultured feline proximal tubular cells.[84] Whether cats are at increased risk for developing metabolic acidosis because of this limitation is unknown.
   c. In addition to renal modulation of acid-base balance, other factors also influence acidosis in renal failure.
      (1). Increased gastrointestinal acid excretion may be an important defense against uremic acidosis.[85]
      (2). The severity of metabolic acidosis in renal failure may be limited by the buffer action of skeletal calcium salts; however, recently, the long-standing belief that bone serves as an important buffer system in chronic metabolic acidosis has been challenged after a re-examination of the amount of buffer available in bone.[86]
      (3). Diet may be a major factor in the development of uremic acidosis.
         (a). The amino acid composition of the proteins, organic anions, and fixed ions and their solubility all influence the net effect of the diet on acid-base balance.
         (b). In addition to the effects of amino acid metabolism, gastrointestinal acid or alkali secretion and the complex interactions of nonabsorbable components influence the effects of diet on body pH.[87]
         (c). The effect of diet on acidosis may be complicated by the misuse of acidifying diets designed to minimize crystalluria, particularly in cats.
   d. Chronic metabolic acidosis may promote a variety of adverse clinical effects.
      (1). Long-term mineral acid feeding increased urinary calcium excretion and promoted progressive bone demineralization in dogs.[88] Chronic metabolic acidosis in cats can cause negative calcium balance and bone demineralization or negative potassium balance, which may in turn promote hypokalemia, renal disease, or taurine depletion.[89,90] Metabolic acidosis may lead to skeletal and calcium disturbances by promoting phosphaturia, hypophosphatemia, and cellular phosphate depletion, thus elevating serum 1,25-dihydroxycholecalciferol concentrations.[91] Whether chronic metabolic acidosis associated with naturally occurring chronic renal failure can have these same adverse effects in dogs and cats is unclear.
      (2). The combined effects of uremic inhibition of protein synthesis and accelerated proteolysis resulting from metabolic acidosis may promote negative nitrogen balance and protein malnutrition.[92]
         (a). Chronic acidosis may enhance protein catabolism to provide a source of nitrogen for hepatic glutamine synthesis, glutamine being the substrate for renal ammoniagenesis.[93]
         (b). Protein degradation is stimulated by metabolic acidosis, even in nonuremic states.[94] Altered branched-chain amino acid metabolism appears to be involved in this process.[95]

Chronic metabolic acidosis increases the activity of muscle branched-chain ketoacid dehydrogenase, the rate-limiting enzyme in branched-chain amino acid catabolism. This is important because branched-chain amino acids are rate limiting in protein synthesis and play a role in regulation of protein turnover. Alkalization therapy effectively reverses acidosis-associated protein breakdown. There is speculation that changes in intracellular pH accompanying acidosis may lead to alterations in gene transcription that increase the activity the cytosolic, ATP- and ubiquitin-dependent protein degradation pathways.[93,96]

(c). Severe chronic metabolic acidosis has the potential to induce a cycle of progressive protein malnutrition and metabolic acidosis. Excessive protein catabolism may lead to protein malnutrition, despite adequate dietary intake. This process may then accelerate breakdown of endogenous cationic and sulfur-containing amino acids, thus promoting further acidosis.

(d). Acidosis poses an additional risk for patients with chronic renal failure that consume a protein-restricted diet. When acid-base status is normal, adaptive reductions in skeletal muscle protein degradation protect patients that eat a low-protein diet from losses in lean body mass. In rats and humans, these adaptive responses are overridden even when mild acidosis is present.

(3). Metabolic acidosis has been associated with anorexia, lethargy, nausea, vomiting, muscle weakness, and weight loss.[83] Severe metabolic acidosis may also impair myocardial contractility and enhance venoconstriction, making the patient relatively susceptible to signs of fluid overload with intravenous fluid therapy.

4. Hyperphosphatemia and phosphate retention.
   a. Phosphorus is absorbed from the gastrointestinal tract and excreted primarily by the kidneys. Renal excretion of phosphorus reflects the net effect of glomerular filtration and tubular reabsorption. If dietary phosphorus intake remains constant, a decline in GFR will lead to phosphorus retention, and ultimately hyperphosphatemia.
   b. During the early stages of renal failure, serum phosphorus concentrations remain within the normal range because of a compensatory increase in phosphate excretion in surviving nephrons.
      (1). This adaptive phenomenon may be partly an effect of renal secondary hyperparathyroidism (see the following). An increased PTH level promotes renal excretion of phosphate by reducing the tubular transport maximum for phosphate reabsorption in the proximal tubule via the adenyl cyclase system.
      (2). However, fractional excretion of phosphorus has been shown to increase following partial renal ablation in thyroparathyroidectomized dogs and rats, indicating that this phenomenon is not dependent on PTH.[3,97] The mechanism of nonPTH-mediated phosphaturia has not been elucidated.
      (3). Loss of nephrons and PTH likely have separate and additive effects on phosphate excretion.[3] Although hyperparathyroidism is no longer regarded as being responsible for maintaining phosphate excretion in renal failure, excessive phosphate intake does promote hyperparathyroidism.
   c. When the GFR drops below about 20% of normal, renal adaptive effects have been maximized and hyperphosphatemia ensues. Thereafter, the serum phosphate concentration roughly parallels the serum urea nitrogen concentration, unless modified by therapy. Hyperphosphatemia caused by renal disease does not typically occur before the onset of azotemia.
   d. Hyperphosphatemia has been linked to many clinical consequences of chronic renal failure, including renal secondary hyperparathyroidism, reduced calcitriol level, soft tissue calcification, renal osteodystrophy, and hypocalcemia, but it does not typically induce clinical signs directly in uremic patients. Increases in serum PTH activities in dogs with chronic renal failure are usually related to the degree of hyperphosphatemia.[73]
5. Renal secondary hyperparathyroidism.
   a. Renal secondary hyperparathyroidism is multifactorial in origin.
      (1). Factors involved include hypocalcemia, phosphorus retention, calcitriol deficiency, and skeletal resistance to PTH.[98]
         (a). Hypocalcemia and calcitriol deficiency both directly stimulate PTH synthesis and secretion.
         (b). Phosphorus retention and calcitriol deficiency independently contribute to the decreased calcemic response to PTH.
         (c). Phosphorus retention decreases calcitriol production and promotes hypocalcemia.

(d). Phosphorus retention may directly stimulate PTH secretion.[99] Preliminary findings suggest that phosphorus may also directly stimulate PTH mRNA.[98]

(2). Dietary calcium and phosphorus, and the magnitude of renal dysfunction, appear to be important in determining which pathogenic factors are involved in the genesis of secondary hyperparathyroidism. The relative contributions of these pathogenic factors was recently studied in a model of graded renal failure in rats.[98]

(a). High dietary phosphate intake induced the most profound degree of hyperparathyroidism, regardless of the magnitude of renal dysfunction, probably because it inhibited all the counterregulatory factors that normally moderate severity of renal secondary hyperparathyroidism. Phosphorus-induced hyperparathyroidism in these rats could be attributed to a cumulative effect of phosphorus retention, calcitriol deficiency, decreased skeletal calcemic response to PTH, and hypocalcemia.

(b). High dietary calcium intake appeared to induce hyperparathyroidism principally by suppressing calcitriol production.

(c). Moderate dietary calcium and phosphorus intake induced hyperparathyroidism primarily by decreasing calcemic response to PTH. Although decreased calcemic response to PTH in renal failure has traditionally been attributed to phosphorus retention, calcitriol deficiency, and down-regulation of PTH receptors, findings in this study suggested that a factor intrinsic to uremia might have been responsible.

(d). Even at the same magnitude of renal dysfunction, the relative contributions of different pathogenic factors appeared to vary considerably.

(3). In most instances, relative or absolute deficiency of 1,25-dihydroxycholecalciferol (calcitriol) plays a pivotal role in development of renal secondary hyperparathyroidism.

(a). Calcitriol, the most active form of vitamin D, is formed by renal 1α-hydroxylation of 25-hydroxycholecalciferol. Renal 1α-hydroxylase activity and formation of calcitriol are promoted by PTH. In turn, calcitriol limits PTH synthesis by feedback inhibition.

(b). Early in the course of chronic renal failure, calcitriol production is limited by the inhibitory effects of phosphate retention on 1α-hydroxylase activity in renal tubular cells. Because calcitriol normally limits PTH synthesis, reduced calcitriol synthesis promotes renal secondary hyperparathyroidism.

(c). Initially, the resultant hyperparathyroidism promotes phosphaturia and increases 1α-hydroxylase activity, thus returning plasma phosphate concentration and calcitriol production toward normal. However, normalization of plasma phosphate concentration and calcitriol production occur at the expense of persistently elevated plasma PTH activity, a classic example of the trade-off hypothesis.*

(d). As renal failure progresses, loss of viable renal tubular cells ultimately limits renal calcitriol synthetic capacity, and calcitriol levels subsequently remain low.[101] Deficiency of calcitriol leads to skeletal resistance to the action of PTH and elevates the setpoint for calcium-induced suppression of PTH secretion. Skeletal resistance to PTH limits skeletal release of calcium, whereas elevating the setpoint for PTH secretion allows hyperparathyroidism to persist even when ionized calcium concentrations in plasma are normal or elevated.[72]

b. Chronic renal secondary hyperparathyroidism results in renal osteodystrophy (the general term for metabolic bone disorders characteristic of chronic renal failure) and soft tissue mineralization.

(1). Clinical signs of renal osteodystrophy are uncommon in dogs and cats with chronic renal failure.

(a). When they occur, such signs most often appear in immature patients, presumably because metabolically active growing bone is more susceptible to the adverse effects of hyperparathyroidism.

(b). For an unexplained reason, bones of

*The trade-off hypothesis states that the biologic price to be paid for maintaining external homeostasis for a given solute is one or more of the abnormalities of the uremia.[100] The biologic price to be paid for maintaining phosphate homeostasis is the diverse pathophysiologic consequences of renal secondary hyperparathyroidism. In this sense, PTH functions as a uremic toxin at markedly elevated concentrations.

the skull are most severely affected. They may become so demineralized that the teeth become moveable and the jaw can be bent or twisted without fracturing (so-called rubber jaw syndrome; Fig. 16–4). Marked proliferation of connective tissue associated with the maxilla may cause severe distortion of the face (Figs. 16–5 and 16–6).

(c). Pathologic fractures may occur, but are seemingly uncommon in dogs and cats with chronic renal failure. When they occur, they commonly affect the mandible.

(d). Other seemingly uncommon clinical manifestations of severe renal osteodystrophy include skeletal decalcification, cystic bone lesions, bone pain, and growth retardation.

(2). Soft tissue calcification, another complication of renal secondary hyperparathyroidism, is common in dogs and cats with advanced chronic renal failure (Fig. 16–7).[102] It appears most commonly to affect the lungs, kidneys, arteries, stomach, and myocardium.

c. Elevated PTH activity has been characterized as a "uremic toxin" that promotes several other important clinical consequences of uremia, including mental dullness and lethargy resulting from toxic effects of PTH on the brain, immunodeficiency as a consequence of deranged leukocyte function, impaired cardiac and skeletal muscle function resulting from impaired mitochondrial energy metabolism and myofiber mineralization, decreased appetite and energy metabolism resulting from inhibited insulin secretion, and progressive loss of renal function caused by nephrocalcinosis.[72]

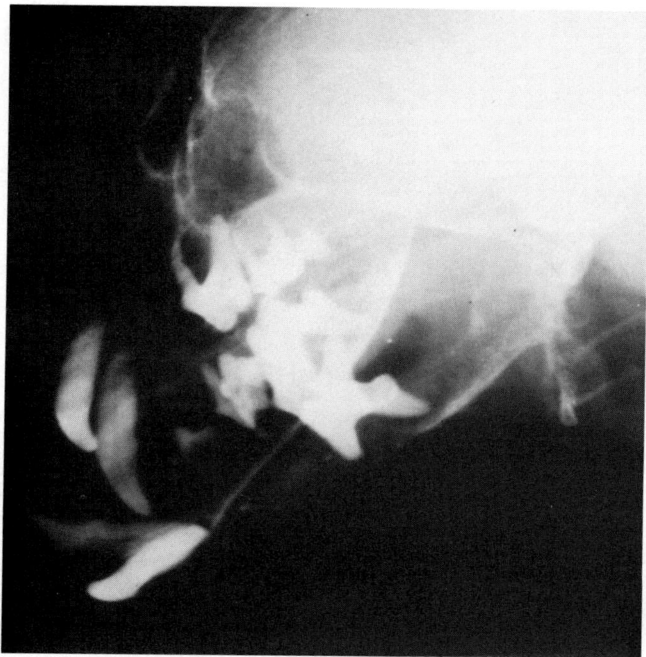

FIG. 16–5. Radiograph of the skull of a 5-year-old male mixed-breed dog with osteodystrophy secondary to chronic uremia. Marked proliferation of connective tissue was not observed.

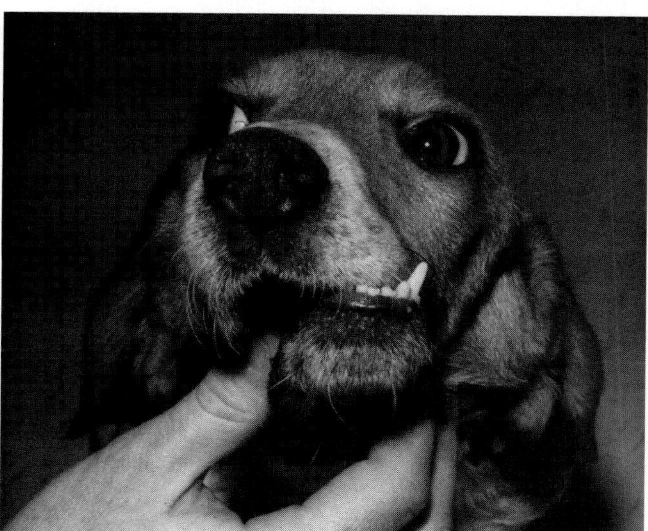

FIG. 16–4. A 2-year-old beagle dog with chronic renal failure. The maxilla has lost its rigidity owing to demineralization associated with renal osteodystrophy.

(1). Nagode and colleagues have reported that administration of calcitriol ameliorates some clinical signs, including anorexia, in uremic dogs.[103]

(2). The toxicity of PTH is likely mediated through enhanced entry of calcium into cells that have plasma membrane receptors for PTH.[72] In addition to PTH-mediated influx of calcium into cells, extrusion of calcium out of cells is decreased owing to reduced activity of the enzymes responsible for pumping calcium out of the cells. The combination of increased entry and decreased exit of calcium results in elevated intracellular calcium content.

(a). Available data are consistent with the notion that chronic renal failure is a state of cellular calcium toxicity, which underlies many of the associated metabolic and functional derangements.[104] Elevation in the basal levels of cytosolic calcium is, in large part, responsible for organ dysfunction associated with chronic renal failure.

(b). Preventing secondary hyperparathyroidism in chronic renal failure, or blocking the effect of PTH by a calcium channel blocker, results in normalization of intracellular calcium and restoration of cell function.

6. Serum and body potassium balance.

a. Although dogs are seemingly capable of maintaining potassium balance until more advanced stages of chronic renal failure, an association between polyuric renal failure and hypokalemia has been recognized in cats by several groups of investigators.[58–60,77,78] Hypokalemia is among the most common biochemical derangements observed in cats with renal failure. In a retrospective study of 132 cats with renal failure performed at the University of Minne-

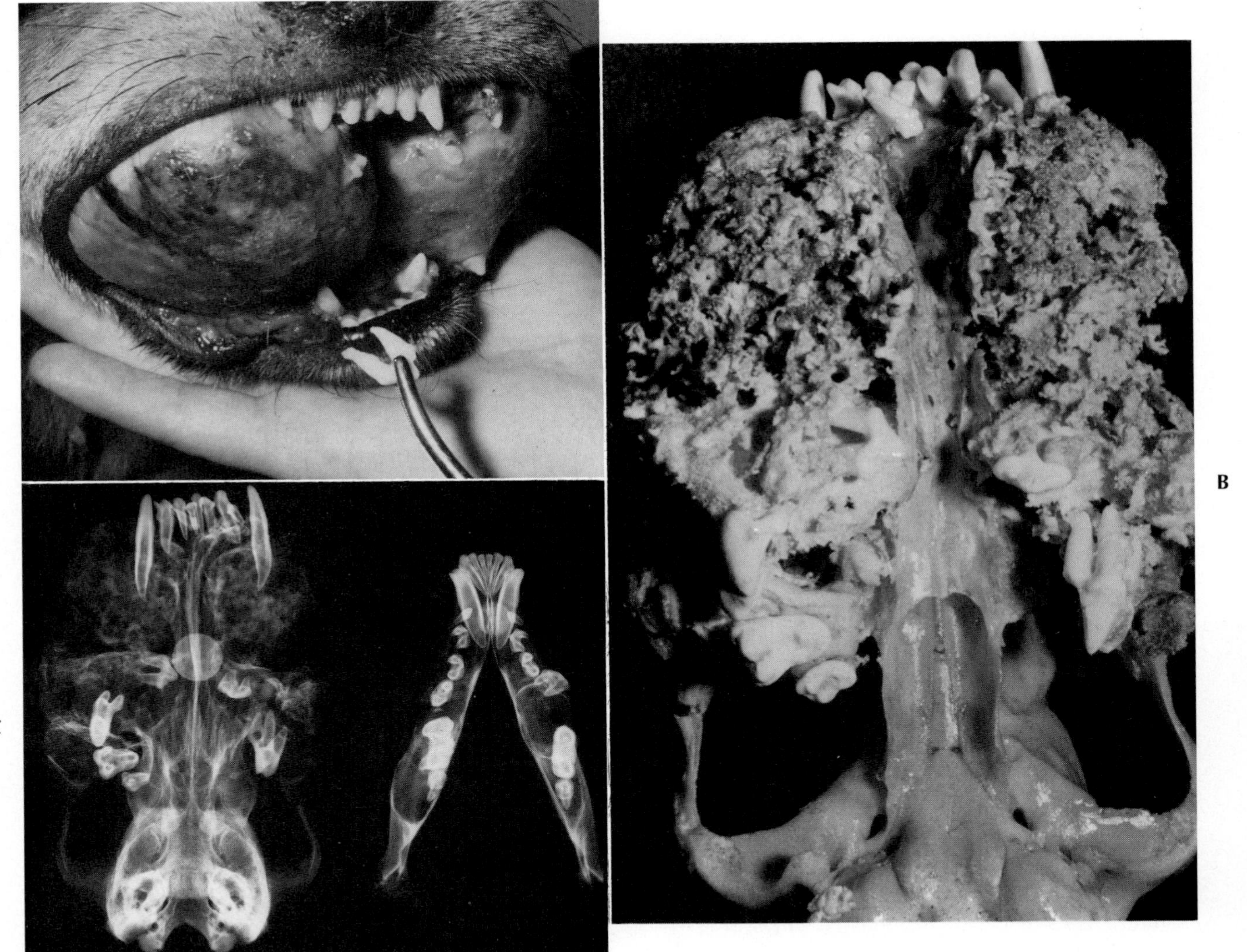

FIG. 16–6. A, Advanced fibrous osteodystrophy of the head of a 9-month-old male mixed-breed dog with chronic renal failure. The teeth are being extruded as a result of displacement by proliferation of fibrous connective tissue. Portions of the oral mucosa that were constantly exposed to air have been ulcerated. **B,** The proliferative nature of the maxillary lesions is shown in this photograph of the skull, which was taken after removal of the soft tissue by a colony of beetles. (Courtesy of Dr. Walter Mackey.) **C,** A radiograph of the skull reveals the extent of demineralization and fibro-cystic changes. The circular structure on the midline of the maxillary bones is the outline of a piece of plastic used to support the skull. (Courtesy of Dr. Carl Jessen.)

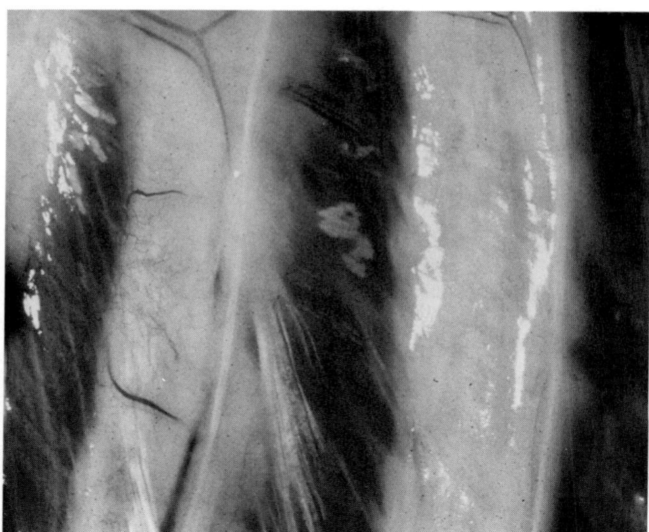

FIG. 16–7. Uremic calcification in the parietal pleura of a 13-year-old male Irish setter with chronic uremia.

sota, 19% were hypokalemic (serum potassium less than 3.5 mEq/L).[78] In a study of 74 cats with chronic renal disease at the Ohio State University, 29.7% had hypokalemia.[77] Because potassium is an intracellular anion, the extracellular potassium concentration does not necessarily reflect the total body potassium content.

b. Potassium is excreted primarily via renal secretion; small quantities are lost in feces and sweat.
   (1). Although large quantities of potassium appear in glomerular filtrate, essentially all is reabsorbed before it reaches the distal tubules. The majority of potassium appears in urine as a result of potassium secretion in the distal nephron.
   (2). Potassium excretion in the distal nephron segments is quite sensitive to tubular flow rates; diuresis promotes potassium secretion, whereas antidiuresis limits potassium secretion.
   (3). Distal potassium secretion is modulated by potassium reabsorption by the intercalated cells in the cortical and outer medullary collecting tubules.[83] With potassium depletion, net potassium absorption, rather than secretion, may occur in the distal nephron.

c. In patients with chronic renal failure, the residual nephrons maintain potassium balance by increasing fractional excretion of potassium in proportion to the decline in GFR by enhancing distal tubular secretion of potassium.[1] Gastrointestinal secretion of potassium (primarily in the colon) also appears to increase in chronic renal failure, and it may play an important role in modulating potassium balance in this setting.
   (1). Because of these adaptations, most dogs and cats with chronic renal failure are able to tolerate normal dietary potassium intake (about 0.6% dry matter) until renal dysfunction is severe.
   (2). The ability to excrete a potassium load rapidly may be impaired in chronic renal failure. Thus, transient hyperkalemia may follow ingestion of a potassium-rich meal.
   (3). Severe reductions in renal function, typically characterized by oliguria, may result in hyperkalemia. Although hyperkalemia is an important complication of chronic renal failure in humans, most dogs and cats successfully managed by conservative medical therapy have sufficient renal function that physiologically significant hyperkalemia is rare.

d. Potassium serves two major physiologic functions.
   (1). The ratio of intracellular and extracellular potassium concentrations is the major determinant of the resting membrane potential across cell membranes.
   (2). Potassium plays an important role in cell metabolism.[83]
      (a). Because of the impact of potassium on resting cell membrane potentials, potassium imbalance typically manifests clinically as neuromuscular dysfunction.
         (1′). Hypokalemia increases the magnitude of the resting potential (i.e., increases electronegativity), thus hyperpolarizing the cell membrane and making it less sensitive to exciting stimuli.
         (2′). The cardinal, and most dramatic, sign of hypokalemia, regardless of cause, is generalized muscle weakness. Muscle weakness and pain associated with hypokalemic polymyopathy may be recognized clinically as cervical ventroflexion and a stiff, stilted gait (Fig. 16–8).[77,105,106]
         (3′). Activity of serum creatinine kinase and other muscle enzymes may be elevated with hypokalemic polymyopathy. In severe instances, rhabdomyolysis may occur.
      (b). By influencing cell metabolism, potassium imbalances may disrupt a variety of cell functions.

(1′). Hypokalemia-impaired protein synthesis may promote weight loss and poor haircoat.[105]

(2′). Marked potassium depletion has also been linked to polyuria resulting from decreased renal responsiveness to ADH. This antagonism to ADH appears to result from interference with generation and action of cyclic adenosine monophosphate (AMP) and to impairment of the countercurrent mechanism.[83] Locally generated prostaglandins may mediate at least part of this effect.

e. Chronic potassium depletion impairs renal function in cats.[89]

(1). In many cats with chronic renal failure and hypokalemia, renal function improves following restoration of normokalemia by potassium supplementation. This suggests that hypokalemia may induce a reversible, functional decline in chronic renal failure.

(2). Inadequate dietary potassium intake has been linked to development of renal dysfunction in normal cats.

(a). Renal function was adversely affected in normal cats when an acidified, potassium restricted diet was fed.[89] Potassium depletion and acidosis appeared to have additive effects in impairing renal function in this study.

(b). In a recent uncontrolled study of the long-term effects of feeding a potassium-restricted, acidifying diet to cats, evidence of renal dysfunction developed in three of nine cats, and renal lesions consisting of lymphoplasmacytic interstitial nephritis and interstitial fibrosis were observed in five of the nine cats.[59]

f. The mechanisms involved in development of hypokalemia in cats with chronic renal failure remain unresolved.

(1). Although initially thought to result from excessive kaliuresis,[60] more recent studies suggest that hypokalemia in cats with chronic renal failure may not be caused by increased urinary potassium losses.[89,107]

(a). Twenty-four–hour urinary potassium excretion did not appear to increase in cats with experimentally induced chronic renal failure, even among those that developed hypokalemia.[107]

(b). Fractional excretion of potassium is increased in most cats with chronic renal failure, but this increase is at least partially adaptive rather than

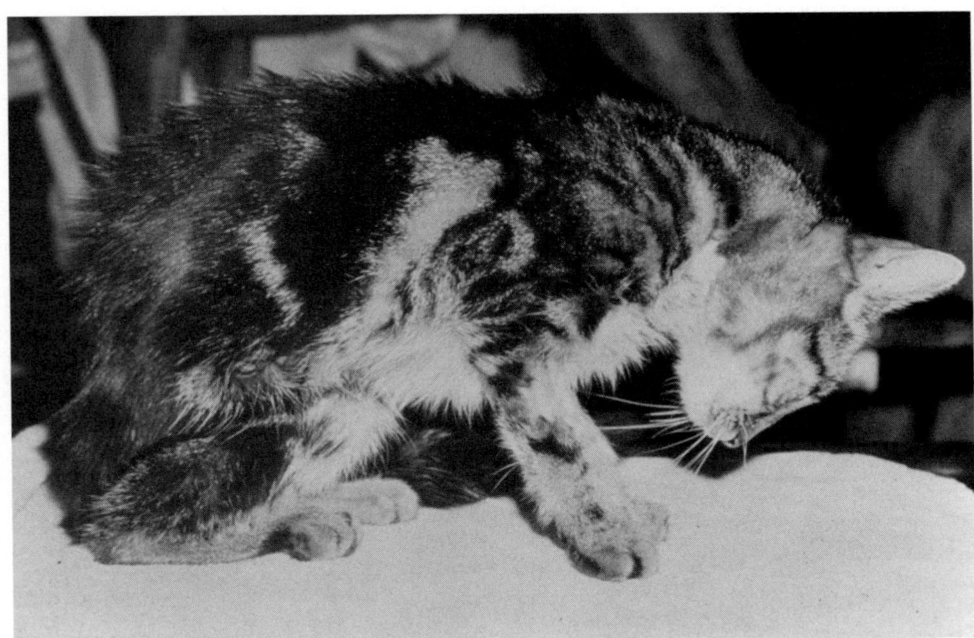

FIG. 16–8. A 1-year-old cat with typical signs of hypokalemic myopathy associated with chronic renal failure.

pathologic. Diagnosis of excessive or inappropriate kaliuresis should be based on measurement of 24-hour urine potassium excretion.

(2). Inadequate dietary potassium intake (it should be at least 0.6% dry matter for cats) appears to be an important factor in promoting hypokalemia in chronic renal failure.[89,105,107]

(a). Other dietary factors that appear to promote hypokalemia include diets that contain acidifying metabolites and those that contain reduced amounts of magnesium.[58,60,108,109]

(b). Dietary protein may also be a factor, because dietary potassium requirement increases as dietary protein content increases.[110]

(3). In normal cats fed an acidified, potassium-restricted diet, evidence suggests that potassium depletion may result from decreased gastrointestinal absorption and/or increased gastrointestinal excretion of potassium.[89]

(4). Hypokalemia may be a cause of chronic renal failure rather than simply a consequence of it.

(a). Hypokalemia promotes renal injury in rats by enhancing renal ammoniagenesis (see the previous section on acidosis for details).[111]

(b). As previously described, some evidence suggests that potassium-restricted diets may impair renal function or induce renal lesions in seemingly normal cats.[59]

(c). However, evidence also shows that renal impairment may be a risk factor for hypokalemia. Hypokalemia occurred in 4 of 7 cats with induced chronic renal failure fed a diet containing 0.3% potassium, whereas hypokalemia did not develop in 4 control cats fed the same diet.[76]

7. Abnormalities in insulin metabolism.

a. Abnormalities of insulin metabolism associated with uremia include hyperinsulinemia, mild hyperglycemia, peripheral resistance to insulin, deranged pancreatic islet cell responses to glucose loads, and spontaneous hypoglycemia.[74,112,113]

(1). Insulin levels are elevated in uremia, in part owing to reduced degradation of insulin by the kidneys and other tissues.[112]

(a). Insulin is readily cleared by glomerular filtration and reabsorbed by the renal tubules; however, renal clearance of insulin greatly exceeds GFR, suggesting that substantial insulin uptake and degradation occurs in peritubular epithelial and endothelial cell membranes.

(b). In humans, little change in metabolic clearance of insulin occurs until GFR declines below about 40% of normal. Below about 15 to 20% of normal GFR, renal insulin degradation declines precipitously. Impaired degradation of insulin in extrarenal tissues (liver, muscle) also occurs in uremia, apparently owing to the effects of undefined dialyzable uremic toxins.

(c). Insulin requirements of diabetic patients typically decline with renal failure.

(2). Carbohydrate (glucose) intolerance and mild hyperglycemia probably result from peripheral resistance to the action of insulin and impaired release of insulin from pancreatic islet cells.[112]

(a). Impaired cellular glucose uptake (insulin resistance) in uremia occurs principally in muscle cells.

(1′). Because insulin receptor quantity and affinity appear to be normal, uremia is thought to cause insulin resistance by affecting a postbinding event in insulin-mediated glucose metabolism.[71,112]

(2′). Uremic insulin resistance has been corrected by dialysis or by feeding a low-protein diet, suggesting uremic toxins are likely responsible for insulin resistance. Evidence suggests that the uremic toxins may be "middle molecules."

(b). Augmented insulin secretion maintains euglycemia despite insulin resistance, albeit at elevated circulating insulin levels. However, beta-cell insulin secretion may be impaired with chronic renal failure. When insulin secretion is impaired, mild hyperglycemia and carbohydrate intolerance result.

(1′). Renal secondary hyperparathyroidism impairs glucose-induced insulin secretion.[114]

(2′). Glucose-insulin signaling in pancreatic islet cells is deranged by increases in intracellular cytosolic calcium content.[115]

(3′). Calcitriol therapy ameliorates carbohydrate intolerance in uremia, either by suppressing hyperparathyroidism, correcting 1,25-dihydroxyvitamin D deficiency, or both.[116]

b. Abnormal insulin metabolism may contribute to several clinical abnormalities of uremia.[112]
   (1). Impaired insulin action on amino acid transport and metabolism and regulation of protein turnover may be responsible for the muscle-wasting characteristic of uremia.
   (2). Abnormal insulin metabolism may contribute to growth retardation commonly observed in children and growing animals affected by chronic renal failure.
   (3). Insulin resistance may promote hypertriglyceridemia.

c. Potassium-induced insulin secretion is also impaired in chronic renal failure.[114]
   (1). The mechanisms of this defect appear to be the same as those for carbohydrate intolerance of uremia, being mediated by hyperparathyroidism and cellular calcium overload.
   (2). The clinical impact of this metabolic derangement is that extrarenal disposal of potassium may be impaired in patients with chronic renal failure. In normal persons, ingestion of a large potassium load does not lead to hyperkalemia because mild diet-induced hyperkalemia stimulates insulin release, which in turn enhances intracellular translocation of potassium. Potassium then slowly leaches out of cells, to be gradually excreted by the kidneys.

8. Hyperamylasemia and hyperlipasemia.
   a. Serum amylase and lipase activity is commonly increased in dogs with chronic renal failure.[117]
      (1). In dogs with chronic renal failure, serum amylase activity reportedly increases approximately 2.5-fold over normal values, whereas serum lipase activity increases 2- to 4-fold.
      (2). Pancreatic enzyme activities are not consistently increased in patients with renal failure; amylase values are increased more frequently than those for lipase.
      (3). Marked increases in serum amylase and/or lipase activity rarely develop solely as a result of renal failure.
   b. The mechanisms underlying elevated amylase and lipase activity in renal failure are unclear.
      (1). Hyperamylasemia and hyperlipasemia of chronic renal failure were thought to result, at least in part, from reduced renal excretion or degradation of these enzymes.[117,118]
         (a). In dogs, the magnitude of enzyme elevation does not appear to correlate well with the severity of renal dysfunction.
         (b). Total serum amylase activity correlates significantly with GFR in humans; however, serum lipase activity did not correlate with GFR.[119]
      (2). More recent studies indicate that the kidneys are not an important route of amylase excretion in dogs.[120] Amylase apparently is not filtered by the glomerulus in dogs because formation of polymers or complexation of canine amylase and other serum proteins results in complexes too large to pass through the filter.[121]
      (3). Acute pancreatitis reportedly occurs in some human patients with chronic renal failure,[122] and renal failure has been hypothesized to promote or induce development of "uremic pancreatitis." A more recent study suggests that, although histologic evidence of pancreatic alterations is common in humans with chronic renal failure, these lesions are probably not the cause of hyperamylasemia.[123]
      (4). No evidence suggests that dogs and cats develop "uremic pancreatitis." In dogs with induced chronic renal failure whose serum amylase and lipase activity is increased, histopathologic examination of the pancreas failed to reveal evidence of inflammatory pancreatic lesions.[117]

9. Lipid abnormalities.
   a. Disturbances in lipoprotein transport are common in humans with chronic renal failure.[124] Recent findings suggest that dyslipoproteinemia in chronic renal failure is not always reflected in hyperlipidemia and thus may be more prevalent than was previously thought. Lipoprotein abnormalities are demonstrable over a wide spectrum of decreased renal function, becoming more pronounced as renal failure advances.
      (1). Defective triglyceride metabolism, the most important abnormality of lipid transport in chronic renal failure,[124] is commonly manifest as hypertriglyceridemia, usually of moderate degree.
      (2). Alterations in cholesterol metabolism appear to be largely a reflection of disturbed triglyceride metabolism. Plasma cholesterol concentrations are often within normal range, but may be elevated with more marked hypertriglyceridemia.[124]
   b. Hypertriglyceridemia results from decreased catabolism rather than increased production of lipoproteins.[124,125]
      (1). Plasma concentration of lipoproteins results from a balance between the rates of production and of catabolism. A substantial body of evidence indicated that, in renal failure, impaired transport and catabolism of triglyceride-rich lipoproteins

leads to accumulation of these lipoproteins at various stages of catabolism. Renal failure may be characterized by disturbed catabolism of chylomicron and accumulation of very–low-density (VLDL) and intermediate-density (IDL) lipoproteins, as well as by incompletely cleared remnant particles, whereas low-density lipoprotein (LDL) levels are diminished.[126] Some hypertriglyceridemic persons may also have elevated production of triglycerides.

(2). Decreased triglyceride catabolism and removal may result from decreased activity of lipolytic enzymes (lipoprotein lipase, hepatic triglyceride lipase, and lecithin cholesterol acyltransferase), altered lipoprotein substrates, and decreased receptor-mediated and non–receptor-mediated uptake of lipoproteins.

(a). Catabolism of triglyceride-rich lipoproteins is mediated mainly by lipoprotein lipase and hepatic triglyceride lipase.

(b). Mechanisms responsible for reduced lipoprotein lipase activity are not known, but they may involve insulin deficiency or resistance, hyperparathyroidism, and uremic inhibitors.[125,127]

(c). Uremic patients with hypertriglyceridemia incorporate fatty acids into adipose tissue more slowly than normal, which may also retard catabolism and elevate triglyceride levels.

c. Hypertriglyceridemias of renal failure appear to be influenced by diet. Protein content of the diet probably has little effect on lipid or apolipoprotein levels, but the carbohydrate or lipid composition of the diet may be important.

d. The major clinical implications of lipid disorders in humans with renal failure appear to be related to development of atherosclerotic vascular and cardiovascular diseases and progression of renal failure. However, the clinical significance and need for treatment of uremic dyslipoproteinemia remains unclear.[124–126]

C. Gastrointestinal manifestations.

1. Gastrointestinal complications, among the most common and prominent clinical effects of uremia, include stomatitis, gastroduodenitis, enterocolitis, and associated clinical signs of anorexia, nausea, vomiting, and diarrhea.

a. Severe chronic renal failure may result in uremic stomatitis characterized by oral ulcerations (particularly on the buccal mucosa and tongue), brownish discoloration of the dorsal surface of the tongue, necrosis and sloughing of the anterior portion of the tongue, and "uremic" breath (Fig. 16–9). The mucous membranes may also become dry (xerostomia). Degradation of urea to ammonia by bacterial urease may contribute to many of these signs. Poor oral hygiene and dental disease may exacerbate the onset and severity of uremic stomatitis, perhaps because of increased oral

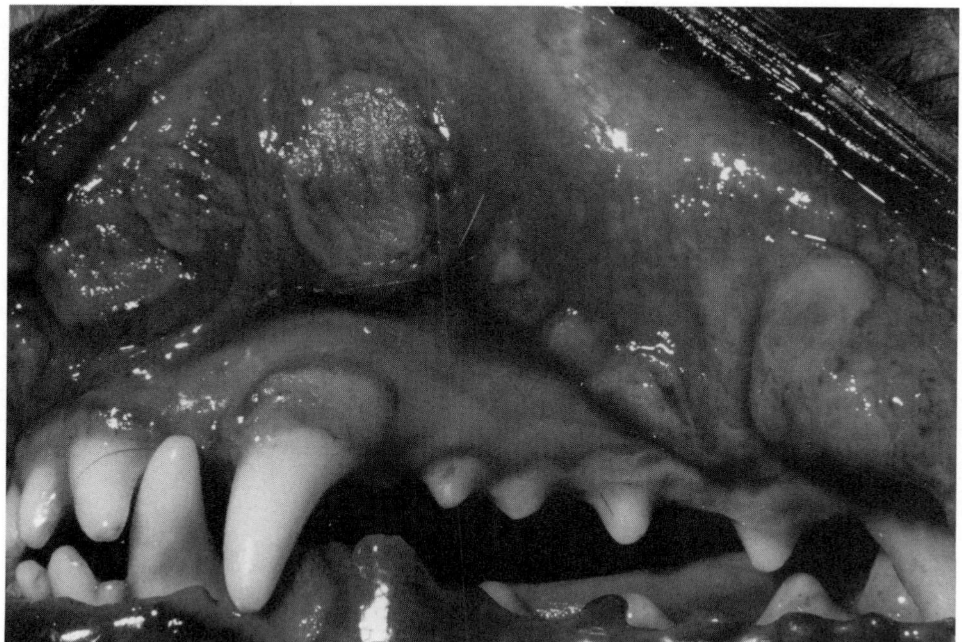

FIG. 16–9. Oral ulcers in a 1-year-old male beagle with advanced uremia.

bacterial flora. Tongue tip necrosis in uremia may result from fibrinoid necrosis and arteritis with focal ischemia, necrosis, and ulceration.[74]

b. Uremic gastropathy in dogs is characterized by glandular atrophy, edema of the lamina propria, mast call infiltration, fibroplasia, mineralization, and submucosal arteritis.[74]
   (1). Elevated gastrin levels have been implicated in development of uremic gastropathy in several species.
      (a). Gastrin stimulates receptors located on parietal cells in the stomach mucosa to produce and secrete hydrogen ions. The resultant gastric hyperacidity causes mucosal irritation, ulceration, and hemorrhage.
      (b). Back-diffusion of hydrochloric acid and pepsin into the stomach wall leads to hemorrhage, inflammation, and the release of histamine from mast cells. This cycle may be perpetuated as mast cell–derived histamine causes further stimulation of parietal cells to produce hydrogen ions.
      (c). The mechanism of hypergastrinemia is controversial.[128]
         (1′). Hypergastrinemia has traditionally been attributed to impaired renal degradation of this hormone, but more recent studies have discounted this mechanism as a major contributing factor.
         (2′). Hypergastrinemia likely results from gastrin hypersecretion. The cause of increased gastrin secretion has not been established, but one possible causative factor is an accumulation of aliphatic amines in gastric juice. Aliphatic amines, which are amino acid metabolites, are increased severalfold in the serum of uremic patients.[128]
      (d). Pentagastrin-stimulated acid output is greater in rats with induced renal failure than in normal rats.[129] Although the mechanism of increased pentagastrin-stimulated acid output remains obscure, preliminary findings suggest that the parietal cell mass may be increased in rats with renal failure.
      (e). The pathogenesis of gastric mucosal lesions in uremia has not been clearly shown to result from gastric hyperacidity. Various studies have found increased, normal, and decreased gastric acidity associated with uremia.[130,131] A possible mechanism for normal or decreased gastric acidity in uremia is neutralization of gastric acid by elevated concentrations of ammonium ion in gastric fluids. Increased gastric ammonium content results from the action of bacterial urease on gastric urea. In humans, *Helicobacter pylori* infection has been associated with increased gastric ammonia levels in uremia, although the presence of this bacterium does not correlate with clinical signs.[131,132]
   (2). Because uremic gastritis is not always characterized by gastric hyperacidity, renal failure has been suggested to interfere with the normal gastric mucosal barrier, increasing proton permeability and enhancing susceptibility to acid injury.[130]
      (a). Increased susceptibility to acid injury may be enhanced in uremia by reduced function of pre-epithelial, epithelial, and postepithelial elements of the gastric mucosa.
      (b). Studies in rats suggest that permeability of the gastric mucosa to acid may be increased in renal failure. Increased acid permeability may in part result from thinning of the gastric mucous gel layer. A decrease in gastric transmural potential difference, suggesting either increased mucosal ion permeability or altered ion secretion rates, may also participate. Impairment of epithelial tight junctions may also promote increased gastric mucosal susceptibility to acid permeability and injury.
      (c). Increased gastric mucosal blood flow provides a protective function by facilitating disposal of protons back-diffusing into the gastric mucosa. In rats, uremia is associated with increased basal gastric mucosal blood flow, mediated by locally produced endothelium-derived nitric oxide, which may minimize the effects of proton back-diffusion.[129,130] However, the hyperemic response to gastric barrier disruption may be limited in uremia, perhaps because increased basal mucosal blood flow limits the potential for additional vasodilation, thus increasing susceptibility to back-diffusion of acid.
   (3). Other factors implicated in the genesis of uremic gastropathy include psychologic stress related to illness, an increase in proton back-diffusion caused by high urea

levels, erosions caused by ammonia liberated by bacterial urease acting on urea, ischemia caused by vascular lesions, decreased concentration and turnover of gastric mucus, and biliary reflux caused by pyloric incompetence (which may be an indirect consequence of elevated gastrin levels).[74,132,133] Platelet functional defects may contribute to the hemorrhagic nature of uremic gastroduodenitis.

(4). Gastroduodenal hyperplastic or metaplastic changes are occasionally sufficient to cause obstruction in humans.[131] We have observed a few dogs with hyperplastic pyloric lesions causing obstruction. These dogs typically had metabolic alkalosis associated with gastric vomiting.

c. Vomiting is a frequent, but inconsistent, finding of uremia in dogs. Uremic cats appear to vomit less frequently than do uremic dogs. Although often an early manifestation of acute renal failure, vomiting may not occur until the later stages of chronic renal failure, particularly when systemic signs have been minimized by properly formulated symptomatic and supportive therapy. The severity of vomiting correlates variably with the magnitude of azotemia.

(1). Vomiting and nausea (with associated anorexia) are presumed to result from the effects of as yet unidentified uremic toxins on the medullary emetic chemoreceptor trigger zone. Uremic gastroenteritis may also contribute to nausea and vomiting. Altered taste sensation may also contribute to anorexia of uremia.[133]

(2). Hematemesis may occur in association with uremic gastric ulcerations. The hemorrhagic diathesis associated with uremia also contributes to hematemesis.

(3). Chronic renal failure appears to affect the function of the smooth muscle of the foregut, resulting in motility disorders that likely contribute to anorexia, nausea, and vomiting in chronic renal failure.[134]

(a). Motility disorders that have been recognized in uremic children include gastroesophageal reflux and altered gastric emptying half-times for milk and glucose.

(b). Gastric antral electrical control activity was abnormal with different types of gastric dysrhythmias in many of these children.

(c). All children with anorexia and vomiting had one or more disorder of foregut motility.

(d). Adults with renal failure may have normal or delayed gastric emptying times.[131]

d. Uremic enterocolitis, manifested as diarrhea, may occur in dogs and cats with severe uremia, but it is less common than uremic gastritis.

(1). Uremic enterocolitis may be hemorrhagic, as a consequence of colonic ulcerations and telangiectasias and the hemorrhagic diathesis of uremia.[131] A high colonic ammonia concentration may contribute to mucosal lesions owing to colonic bacterial degradation of urea. The incidence of gastrointestinal hemorrhage in uremic dogs and cats is unknown, in part because even considerable gastrointestinal hemorrhage may escape routine clinical detection.

(2). Small intestinal malfunction with impaired absorption of glucose, calcium, fat, and folate and increased intestinal loss of albumin have been reported in uremic humans[131]; however, jejunal structure and disaccharidase levels have variously been found to be normal and abnormal.

(3). Constipation is a relatively common complication of CRF, particularly in cats. It most often indicates dehydration, but can occur as a complication of intestinal phosphate binding agents or physical inactivity. Bowel perforation is a potential complication in severe cases.

D. Neurologic manifestations.

1. Clinical signs of cerebral cortical dysfunction in uremic dogs and cats (uremic encephalopathy) may include dullness, drowsiness, lethargy, restlessness, disorientation, tremors, gait imbalance, myoclonus, bizarre behavior, seizures, stupor, and coma. Anorexia, nausea, and vomiting may also be mediated by central nervous system disorders.

a. A progressive decline in appetite, alertness, and awareness occurs early in uremia. Patients initially appear depressed, fatigued, and apathetic. In some patients, stupor, coma, or seizures may develop acutely. Rarely, seizures may be the primary presenting complaint.[135] In one dog, electroencephalographic changes characterized by slowing of alpha activity with paroxysms of high-voltage spikes were observed. These changes have also been reported in uremic humans.

b. In patients with advanced chronic renal failure, clinical signs of neurologic dysfunction may be episodic and vary from day to day. Severity of signs may be related to the rate of onset of azotemia, with more rapid increases in azotemia inducing more severe clinical signs.

c. Many of these signs appear to be reversible with treatment.

2. The pathogenesis of the neurologic manifestation of uremia appears to be multifactorial.

a. Many of the neurologic signs of chronic renal

failure appear to result from the effects of uremic toxins.[133]

b. Elevated PTH levels may be a major factor in the development of "uremic encephalopathy." Increased brain calcium content and typical electroencephalographic changes may occur in uremic dogs.[74] Treatment of hyperparathyroidism may ameliorate some or all of the neurologic symptoms of uremic humans.[133]

c. Mineral and electrolyte disturbances in uremia may contribute to neurologic signs. For example, tremors, myoclonus, and tetany may develop secondary to hypocalcemia.

d. Arterial hypertension may also lead to neurologic signs in patients with otherwise well-controlled renal failure. Hypertensive encephalopathy associated with an acute severe increase in blood pressure and cerebrovascular hemorrhage has been described in humans, and is suspected to occur in hypertensive dogs and cats. Clinical signs are acute in onset and may include seizures, behavioral changes, dementia, isolated cranial nerve deficits, and death.[136]

e. Retention of drugs and toxins secondary to reduced renal function may promote encephalopathies. A frequently cited cause of encephalopathy in humans with chronic renal failure is aluminum intoxication associated with long-term administration of antacids containing aluminum. Although aluminum content in the brain may be increased in dogs with renal failure, the role of aluminum intoxication in the genesis of neurologic signs in dogs has not been studied.[74]

3. A peripheral neuropathy ("uremic neuropathy") reported to occur in uremic humans has been characterized as an insidious, distal, symmetric, mixed polyneuropathy that develops over an extended time in patients with GFR of less than 10% of normal.[74] Sensory components precede motor symptoms, which may include muscle atrophy, myoclonus, and transient paralysis. Decreased motor nerve conduction velocity is observed with this condition. Peripheral neuropathy is presumed to result from chronic, cumulative effects of uremic toxins. This condition has not been described in dogs or cats with spontaneous renal failure.

4. An autonomic neuropathy that affects both the sympathetic and the parasympathetic nervous system has been recognized in uremic humans. It appears to correlate with peripheral neuropathy and improves with dialysis therapy.[133] Relative end-organ resistance to norepinephrine may be a contributing factor.

E. Uremic myopathies.

1. Lethargy, fatigue, and muscle weakness are common in chronic renal failure and may be manifestations of a metabolic myopathy ("uremic myopathy").[137] Although skeletal muscle is probably widely affected by uremic myopathy, functional responses of different muscle groups may vary.[137]

2. The pathogenesis of uremic myopathy is likely multifactorial.

a. Aerobic and anaerobic energy production appears to be impaired by uremia.[138] Skeletal muscle metabolism is deranged in uremic humans, owing at least in part, to mitochondrial dysfunction.[139] Anemia contributes to, but does not fully explain, cellular energy dysfunction in uremia. Mitochondrial dysfunction may be a later manifestation of chronic renal failure.[140,141]

b. In humans with chronic renal failure, accumulation of a dialyzable uremic toxin derived from dietary protein promotes abnormalities in sarcolemmal ion flux, leading to reduced muscle membrane potential.[142]

c. Aluminum intoxication consequent to use of aluminum-containing phosphorus-binding agents may be associated with myopathy in renal failure patients.[143]

d. Malnutrition also probably contributes to uremic myopathy.[140]

F. Cardiovascular manifestations.

1. Cardiovascular manifestations of chronic renal failure in humans include systemic hypertension, increased cardiac index, impaired left ventricular function, and increased cardiac work. Echocardiographic findings include increased left ventricular cavity size, thickened left ventricular posterior wall, thickened left ventricular septal wall, decrease in normalized rigidity, impaired contractility, atrial enlargement, and atrial septal hypertrophy.[133]

a. Systemic hypertension is the most commonly recognized cardiovascular complication of chronic renal failure in dogs and cats.[44,45,144]

(1). Hypertension of renal failure appears to develop principally as a consequence of increased extracellular fluid volume and vasoconstriction caused by activity of the renin-angiotensin axis.[133] These effects may be aggravated by a reversible sympathetic activation, which appears to be mediated by an afferent signal arising in the failing kidneys.[145]

(2). Reports have revealed that most dogs and cats with chronic moderate to severe hypertension have evidence of left ventricular hypertrophy (LVH).[146] Low-grade mitral murmur and cardiomegaly are commonly observed in these patients. Vascular lesions typical of chronic systemic hypertension have also been reported in dogs.[44]

(3). The reader should consult Chapter 18, Primary Tubulo-Interstitial Diseases of the Kidney, for additional details on the pathophysiology and consequences of systemic hypertension in chronic renal failure.

b. The most common cardiac complication of chronic renal failure is development of LVH.[74,147]
   (1). LVH results from chronic flow and pressure overload. Flow overload may be attributable to salt and water overload and anemia. Pressure overload is related to increased systemic arterial pressure and alterations in physical properties of large arteries characterized by increased stiffness. Systolic function of the ventricle is reportedly preserved, but diastolic filling is impaired.
   (2). Congestive heart failure is unlikely to occur as a consequence of renal failure-induced LVH except in patients with preexisting cardiac disease.
   (3). Secondary hyperparathyroidism may affect myocardial contractility and hypertrophy.[148] Further, myocardial and coronary vascular mineralization may occur consequent to renal secondary hyperparathyroidism. Mineralization has been linked to death from arrhythmias and congestive heart failure in humans.[133]

c. Uremic pericarditis is a rare complication of renal failure. Its pathogenesis remains obscure. Suggested causative factors include a direct effect of dialyzable uremic toxins, overhydration, decreased plasma fibrinolytic activity, and immune-mediated mechanisms.[74,133]

d. "Uremic pneumonitis," characterized as noncardiogenic pulmonary edema, has been reported in dogs and humans with renal failure,[133,149] although in both species it appears to be rare.
   (1). Findings in affected dogs included radiographic evidence of diffuse pulmonary infiltrates (three of ten dogs) and severe dyspnea and cyanosis (four of ten dogs). Edema was subclinical in most dogs. Affected dogs had fibrin-rich alveolar fluid, variably thickened alveolar septae, engorged capillaries, and moderate amounts of mononuclear infiltrates.* Similar histopathologic findings are characteristic of uremic pneumonitis in humans.
   (2). Uremic humans reportedly have increased capillary permeability, which predisposes them to pulmonary edema. The observation that uremic patients are at increased risk of accumulating fluid in the pleural, pericardial, and peritoneal cavities suggests the possibility of a generalized increase in vascular permeability in uremia; however, other factors may also play a role.
   (3). Unrelated to uremic pneumonitis, dogs and cats with renal failure may have pulmonary mineralization. Pulmonary mineralization does not usually cause respiratory signs.

*Dogs were selected for study on the basis of these histopathologic findings, which were similar to findings reported in humans with uremic pneumonitis. During the study interval, 10 of 73 dogs with renal disease and pulmonary edema fit this classification.

G. Hematopoietic manifestations.

1. A progressive hypoproliferative anemia is the most obvious hematologic manifestation of chronic renal failure in dogs and cats. The pathophysiology and treatment of this condition is described in detail in Chapter 29, Medical Management of the Anemia of Chronic Renal Failure.
2. Uremia may also be characterized by a hemorrhagic tendency, which typically presents as bruising, gastrointestinal hemorrhage with hematemesis or melena, bleeding from the gums, or hemorrhage subsequent to venipuncture. Gastrointestinal hemorrhage can be an important route of blood loss leading to anemia and exacerbating azotemia and uremia.
   a. Hemorrhage in patients with renal failure results from decreased platelet function and abnormalities in the interaction of platelets and vessel walls.[150] Platelet production and clotting factors are generally normal in renal failure, except in patients with the nephrotic syndrome. Bleeding time has been advocated as the best screening test to assess the platelet-associated bleeding tendency characteristic of renal failure.[150]
   b. Evidence from humans and rats indicates that platelet dysfunction and hemorrhage in uremia may result from enhanced NO synthesis.[151]
      (1). Uremic plasma has been found to be a potent inducer of NO synthesis.
      (2). Administration of *N*-monomethyl-L-arginine, a competitive inhibitor of NO synthesis, completely normalizes bleeding time in uremic rats.
      (3). Nitric oxide interacts with primary hemostasis by:
         (a). Counteracting vessel injury–induced vasoconstriction.
         (b). Inhibiting platelet adhesion to damaged endothelium.
         (c). Interfering with the process of platelet-platelet interaction.
         (d). Activating soluble guanylate cyclase, thereby increasing platelet cyclic guanosine monophosphate (the NO second messenger).

H. Immune system manifestations.

1. Bacterial infection is an important complication and frequent cause of death in patients with renal failure.

2. Increased susceptibility to infection may result from impaired neutrophil function and deranged cell-mediated immunity.[74,133]
   a. Neutrophilic leukocytosis is commonly observed in patients with chronic renal failure; however, several tests of neutrophil function may be abnormal in uremic patients, including impaired neutrophil chemotaxis, adherence, and phagocytosis.
   b. Circulating B and T cells are often reduced in uremia; immunoglobulin levels are typically within normal limits. Lymphocyte function tests may be impaired in renal failure.

REFERENCES

1. Polzin DJ, Osborne CA, O'Brien TD. Diseases of the kidneys and ureters. In: Ettinger SJ (ed). *Textbook of Veterinary Internal Medicine.* Philadelphia, Pennsylvania: WB Saunders; 1989: 1963.
2. Brenner BM, Coe F, Rector FC. *Acute Renal Failure.* Philadelphia, Pennsylvania: WB Saunders; 1987:36.
3. Meyer T, Scholey J, Brenner B. Nephron adaptation to renal injury. In: Brenner B, Rector F (eds). *The Kidney.* Philadelphia, Pennsylvania: WB Saunders; 1991:1871.
4. Adams L, Polzin D, Osborne C, O'Brien T, Hostetter T. Influence of dietary protein-calorie intake on renal morphology and function in cats with 5/6 nephrectomy. *Lab Invest.* 1994;70: 347-357.
5. Olivetti G, Anversa P, Melissari M, Loud A. Morphometry of the renal corpuscle during postnatal growth and compensatory hypertrophy. *Kidney Int.* 1980;17:438.
6. Fries J, Sandstrom D, Meyer T, Rennke H. Glomerular cell hypertrophy and epithelial cell injury modulate progressive glomerulosclerosis in the rat. *Lab Invest.* 1989;60:205.
7. Brown SA, Finco DR, Crowell WA, Choat DC, Navar LG. Single-nephron adaptations to partial renal ablation in the dog. *Am J Physiol.* 1990;258:F495.
8. Churchill J, Polzin D, Osborne C, Adams L. The influence of dietary protein intake on progression of chronic renal failure. *Semin Vet Med Surg (Small Anim).* 1992;7:244.
9. Anderson S, et al. Antihypertensive therapy must control glomerular hypertension to limit glomerular injury. *J Hypertension.* 1986;4:S242.
10. Brown S. Glomerular hypertension. Proceedings of the Tenth Annual Veterinary Medical Forum. San Diego, California: American College of Veterinary Internal Medicine; 1992:560.
11. Polzin DJ, Leininger JR, Osborne CA, Jeraj K. Development of renal lesions in dogs after 11/12 reduction of renal mass: Influences of dietary protein intake. *Lab Invest.* 1988;58:172.
12. Kanwar Y, Liu Z, Kashihara N, and Wallner E. Current status of the structural and functional basis of glomerular filtration and proteinuria. *Semin Nephrol.* 1991;11:390.
13. Neugarten J, Kozin A, Gayner R, Schacht R, Baldwin D. Dietary protein restriction and glomerular permselectivity in nephrotoxic serum nephritis. *Kidney Int.* 1991;40:57.
14. Stenvinkel P, Alvestrand A, Bergstrom J. Factors influencing progression in patients with chronic renal failure. *J Intern Med.* 1989;226:183.
15. Wright J, Salzano S, Brown C, el Nahas A. Natural history of chronic renal failure: A reappraisal. *Nephrol Dial Transplant.* 1992;7:379.
16. Burns K, Homma T, Harris R. The intrarenal renin-angiotensin system. *Semin Nephrol.* 1993;13:13.
17. Fine L, Hammerman M, Abboud H. Evolving role of growth factors in the renal response to acute and chronic disease. *J Am Soc Nephrol.* 1992;2:1163.
18. Miskell C, Simpson D. Hyperplasia precedes increased glomerular filtration rate in rat remnant kidney. *Kidney Int.* 1990; 37:758.
19. Bouby N, Bachmann S, Bichet D, Bankir L. Effect of water intake on the progression of chronic renal failure in the 5/6 nephrectomized rat. *Am J Physiol.* 1990;258:F973.
20. King A, Troy J, Anderson S, Neuringer J, Gunning M. Nitric oxide: A potential mediator of amino acid–induced renal hyperemia and hyperfiltration. *J Am Soc Nephrol.* 1991; 1:1271.
21. Anderson S, Meyer T, Rennke H, Brenner B. Control of glomerular hypertension limits glomerular injury in rats with reduced renal mass. *J Clin Invest.* 1985;76:612.
22. Naess PA, Christensen G, Kirkeboen KA, Kiil F. Effect on renin release of inhibiting renal nitric oxide synthesis in anaesthetized dogs. *Acta Physiol Scand.* 1993;148:137.
23. Persson PB, Baumann JE, Ehmke H, Hackenthal E, Kirchheim HR, Nafz B. Endothelium-derived NO stimulates pressure-dependent renin release in conscious dogs. *Am J Physiol.* 1993;264:F943.
24. Manning R Jr, Hu L, Mizelle HL, Granger JP. Role of nitric oxide in long-term angiotensin II–induced renal vasoconstriction. *Hypertension.* 1993;21:949.
25. De-Nicola L, Blantz RC, Gabbai FB. Nitric oxide and angiotensin II. Glomerular and tubular interaction in the rat. *J Clin Invest.* 1992;89:1248.
26. Shultz PJ, Tolins JP. Adaptation to increased dietary salt intake in the rat. Role of endogenous nitric oxide. *J Clin Invest.* 1993;91:642.
27. Wilcox CS, Welch WJ, Murad F, et al. Nitric oxide synthase in macula densa regulates glomerular capillary pressure. *Proc Natl Acad Sci USA.* 1992;89:11993.
28. Altsheler P, Klahe S, Rosenbaum R, Slatopolsky E. Effects of inhibitors of prostaglandin synthesis on renal sodium excretion in normal dogs and dogs with decreased renal mass. *Am J Physiol.* 1978;235:F338.
29. Polzin DJ, Osborne CA, Hayden DW, Stevens JB. Influence of reduced protein diets on morbidity, mortality, and renal function in dogs with induced chronic renal failure. *Am J Vet Res.* 1984;45:506.
30. Brown SA, Finco DR, Crowell WA, Navar LG. Dietary protein intake and the glomerular adaptations to partial nephrectomy in dogs. *J Nutrition.* 1991;121:S125.
31. Bricker N. On the meaning of the intact nephron hypothesis. *Am J Med.* 1969;46:1.
32. Bricker N, Fine L, Kaplan M, Epstein M, Bourgoigne J, Light A. Magnification phenomenon in chronic renal disease. *N Engl J Med.* 1978;299:1287.
33. Brown S. Dietary protein restriction: Some unanswered questions. *Semin Vet Med Surg.* 1992;7:237.
34. Shimamura T, Morrison A. A progressive glomerulosclerosis occurring in partial five-sixth nephrectomized rats. *Am J Pathol.* 1975;79:95.
35. Hostetter T. The hyperfiltering glomerulus. *Med Clin North Am.* 1984;62:387.
36. Brenner BM, Meter TW, Hostetter TH. Dietary protein intake and the progressive nature of kidney disease: The role of hemodynamically mediated glomerular injury in the pathogenesis of progressive glomerular sclerosis in aging, renal ablation, and intrinsic renal disease. *N Engl J Med.* 1982;307: 652.
37. Ichikawa I, Ikoma M, Fogo A. Glomerular growth promoters,

the common key mediator for progressive glomerular sclerosis in chronic renal diseases. *Adv Nephrol Necker Hosp.* 1991; 20:127.

38. Keane WF, Kasiske BL, O'Donnell MP, Kim Y. Hypertension, hyperlipidemia, and renal damage. *Am J Kidney Dis.* 1993; 21:43.
39. Barsanti J, Finco D. Dietary management of chronic renal failure in dogs. *J Am Animal Hosp Assoc.* 1985;21:371.
40. Allen T, Jaenke R, Fettman M. A technique for estimating progression of chronic renal failure in the dog. *J Am Vet Med Assoc.* 1987;190:866.
41. Fujihara CK, Limongi DMZPRF, Graudenz MS, Zatz R. Pathogenesis of glomerular sclerosis in subtotally nephrectomized analbuminemic rats. *Am J Physiol.* 1991;261:F256.
42. Finco D, Brown S, Crowell W, Duncan R, Barsanti J, Bennett S. Effects of dietary phosphorus and protein in dogs with chronic renal failure. *Am J Vet Res.* 1992;53:2264.
43. Bidani AK, Mitchell KD, Schwartz MM, Navar LG, Lewis EJ. Absence of glomerular injury or nephron loss in a normotensive rat remnant kidney model. *Kidney Int.* 1990;38:28.
44. Cowgill L, Kallet A. Systemic hypertension. In: Kirk, R. ed. *Current Veterinary Therapy IX.* Philadelphia, Pennsylvania: WB Saunders; 1986;360.
45. Kobayashi D, Peterson M, Graves T, Lesser M, Nichols C. Hypertension in cats with chronic renal failure or hyperthyroidism. *J Vet Intern Med.* 1990;4:58.
46. Yoshiyuki Y, Fogo A, Ichikawa I. Glomerular hemodynamic changes vs hypertrophy in experimental glomerular sclerosis. *Kidney Int.* 1989;35:654.
47. Daniels B, Hostetter T. Adverse effects of growth in the glomerular microcirculation. *Am J Physiol.* 1990;27:F1409.
48. O'Donnell M, Kasiske B, Schmitz P, et al. High protein intake accelerates glomerulosclerosis independent of effects on glomerular hemodynamics. *Kidney Int.* 1990;37:1263.
49. Ibels L, Alfrey ALH, We H. Preservation of renal function in experimental renal disease by dietary restriction of phosphates. *N Engl J Med.* 1978;298:122.
50. Lau K. Phosphate excess and progressive renal failure: The precipitation-calcification hypothesis. *Kidney Int.* 1989;36:918.
51. Lumlertgul D, Burke T, Gillum D, et al. Phosphate depletion arrests progression of chronic renal failure independent of protein intake. *Kidney Int.* 1986;29:658.
52. Finco D, Brown S, Crowell W, Groves C, Duncan J, Barsanti J. Effects of phosphorus/calcium–restricted and phosphorus/calcium–replete 32% protein diets in dogs with chronic renal failure. *Am J Vet Res.* 1992;53:157.
53. Brown SA, Crowell WA, Barsanti JA, White JV, Finco DR. Beneficial effects of dietary mineral restriction in dogs with marked reduction of functional renal mass. *J Am Soc Nephrol.* 1991;1:1169.
54. Ross LA, Finco DR, Crowell WA. Effect of dietary phosphorus restriction on the kidneys of cats with reduced renal mass. *Am J Vet Res.* 1982;43:1023.
55. Nath K, Hostetter M, Hostetter T. Ammonia-complement interaction in the pathogenesis of progressive renal injury. *Kidney Int.* 1989;36:S-52.
56. Nath K, Hostetter M, Hostetter T. Increased ammoniagenesis as a determinant of progressive renal injury. *Am J Kidney Dis.* 1991;17:654.
57. Nath KA, Hostetter MK, Hostetter TH. Pathophysiology of chronic tubulo-interstitial disease in rats: Interactions of dietary acid load, ammonia, and complement component C3. *J Clin Invest.* 1985;76:667.
58. Dow S, Fettman M. Renal disease in cats: The potassium connection. In: Kirk R, Bonagura J. eds. *Current Veterinary Therapy XI.* Philadelphia, Pennsylvania: WB Saunders; 1992;820.
59. DiBartola S, Buffington C, Chew D, McLoughlin M, Sparks R. Development of chronic renal disease in cats fed a commercial diet. *J Am Vet Med Assoc.* 1993;202:744.
60. Dow SW, Fettman MJ, LeCouteur RA, Hamar DW. Potassium depletion in cats: Renal and dietary influences. *J Am Vet Med Assoc.* 1987;191:1569.
61. Harris D, Chan L, Schrier R. Remnant kidney hypermetabolism and progression of chronic renal failure. *Am J Physiol.* 1988; 254:F267-F276.
62. Schrier R, Harris D, Chan L, et al. Tubular hypermetabolism as a factor in the progression of chronic renal failure. *Am J Kidney Dis.* 1988;12:243.
63. Glomset J. Fish, fatty acids, and human health. *N Engl J Med.* 1985;312:1253.
64. Heifets M, David T, Tegtmeyer E, Klahr S. Exercise training ameliorates progressive renal disease in rats with subtotal nephrectomy. *Kidney Int.* 1987;32:815.
65. Scharschmidt L, Gibbons N, et al. Effects of dietary fish oil on renal insufficiency in rats with subtotal nephrectomy. *Kidney Int.* 1987;32:700.
66. Barcelli U, Pollak V. Is there a role for polyunsaturated fatty acids in the prevention of renal disease and renal failure? *Nephron.* 1985;41:209.
67. Moorehead J, El-Nahas M, et al. Lipid nephrotoxicity in chronic progressive glomerular and tubulo-interstitial disease. *Lancet.* 1982;ii:1309.
68. Rayner H, Ross-Gilbertson V, Walls J. The role of lipids in the pathogenesis of glomerulosclerosis in the rat following subtotal nephrectomy. *Eur J Clin Invest.* 1990;20:97.
69. Schreiner G. Pathways leading from glomerular injury to glomerulosclerosis. In: Gurland H, Morgan J, Wetzels E, eds. *Immunologic Perspectives in Chronic Renal Failure. Contributions in Nephrology.* Basel: Karger; 1990;86:1.
70. Kasiske BL, O'Donnell MP, Schmitz PG, Kim Y, Keane WF. Renal injury of diet-induced hypercholesterolemia in rats. *Kidney Int.* 1990;37:880.
71. May R, Kelly R, Mitch W. Pathophysiology of uremia. In: Brenner B, Rector F, eds. *The Kidney,* 4th ed. Philadelphia, Pennsylvania: WB Saunders; 1991.
72. Nagode L, Chew D, Steinmeyer C, Carothers M. Renal secondary hyperparathyroidism: Toxic aspects, mechanisms of development, and control by oral calcitriol treatment. 11th Annual Veterinary Medical Forum. Washington, DC: 1993;154.
73. Nagode L, Chew D. Nephrocalcinosis caused by hyperparathyroidism in progression of renal failure: Treatment with calcitriol. *Semin Vet Med Surg (Small Animal).* 1992;7:202.
74. Chew D, DiBartola S. Diagnosis and pathophysiology of renal disease. In: Ettinger S, ed. *Textbook of Veterinary Internal Medicine,* 3rd ed. Philadelphia, Pennsylvania: WB Saunders; 1989:1893.
75. Ross LA, Finco DR. Relationship of selected clinical renal function tests to glomerular filtration rate and renal blood flow in cats. *Am J Vet Res.* 1981;42:1704.
76. Adams L, Polzin D, Osborne C, O'Brien T. Effects of dietary protein restriction in clinically normal cats and cats with induced chronic renal failure. *Am J Vet Res.* 1993;54:1653.
77. DiBartola SP, Rutgers HC, Zack PM, Tarr MJ. Clinicopathologic findings associated with chronic renal disease in cats: 74 cases (1973–1984). *J Am Vet Med Assoc.* 1987;190:1196.
78. Lulich J, Osborne C, O'Brien T, Polzin D. Feline renal failure: Questions, answers, questions. *Comp Cont Educ Pract Vet.* 1992; 14:127.
79. Coburn J, Gonick H, Rubinin M, Kleeman C. Studies of

experimental renal failure in dogs: I. Effect of 5/6 nephrectomy on concentrating and diluting capacity of residual nephrons. *J Clin Invest.* 1965;44:603.

80. Ardaillou R, Dussaule J-C. Role of atrial natriuretic peptide in the control of sodium balance in chronic renal failure. *Nephron.* 1994;66:249.
81. Danovitch G, Bourgoigne J, Bricker N. Reversibility of the "salt losing" tendency of chronic renal failure. *N Engl J Med.* 1977; 296:14.
82. Greco D, Lees G, Dzendzel G, Komkov A, Carter A. Effect of dietary sodium intake on glomerular filtration rate in partially nephrectomized dogs. *Am J Vet Res.* 1994;55:152.
83. Rose BD. *Clinical Physiology of Acid-Base and Electrolyte Disorders.* 3rd ed. New York, New York: McGraw-Hill; 1989.
84. Lemieux GCL, Duplessis S, Berkofsky J. Metabolic characteristics of the cat kidney: Failure to adapt to metabolic acidosis. *Am J Physiol.* 1990;259:R277.
85. Giovannetti S, Cupisti A, Barsotti G. The metabolic acidosis of chronic renal failure: Pathophysiology and treatment. *Contrib Nephrol.* 1992;100:48.
86. Oh M. Irrelevance of bone buffering to acid-base homeostasis in chronic metabolic acidosis. *Nephron.* 1991;59:7.
87. Berlyne G, Adler A, Barth R, Burke D, Palant C. Perspectives in acid-base balance in advanced chronic renal failure. *Contrib Nephrol.* 1992;100:105.
88. Green J, Kleeman C. The role of bone in the regulation of systemic acid-base balance. *Contrib Nephrol.* 1991;91:61.
89. Dow SW, Fettman MJ, Smith KR, et al. Effects of dietary acidification and potassium depletion on acid-base balance, mineral metabolism and renal function in adult cats. *J Nutrition.* 1990;120:569.
90. Fettman M, Coble J, Hamar D, et al. Effect of dietary phosphoric acid supplementation on acid-base balance and mineral and bone metabolism in adult cats. *Am J Vet Res.* 1992;53:2125.
91. Krapf R, Vetsch R, Vetsch W, et al. Metabolic acidosis increases serum 1,25-(OH)2D concentration. *J Clin Invest.* 1992;90:2456.
92. Maniar S, Laouari D, Caldas A, Kleinknecht C. Protein synthesis and growth in uremic rats with and without chronic metabolic acidosis. *Mineral Electrolyte Metab.* 1992;18:250.
93. Mitch W, Jurkovitz C, England B. Mechanisms that cause protein and amino acid catabolism in uremia. *Am J Kidney Dis.* 1993;21:91.
94. May R, Kelly R, Mitch W. Mechanisms for defects in muscle protein metabolism in rats with chronic uremia: The influence of metabolic acidosis. *J Clin Invest.* 1987;79:1099.
95. May R, Kelly R, Mitch W. Metabolic acidosis accelerates whole body protein degredation and leucine oxidation by a glucocorticoid-dependent mechanism. *Mineral Electrolyte Metab.* 1992;18:245.
96. Greiber S, Mitch W. Catabolism in uremia: Metabolic acidosis and activation of specific pathways. *Contrib Nephrol.* 1992; 98:20.
97. Swenson R, Weisinger J, Ruggeri J. Evidence that parathyroid hormone is not required for phosphate homeostasis in renal failure. *Metabolism.* 1975;24:199.
98. Bover J, Rodriguez M, Trinidad P, et al. Factors in development of secondary hyperparathyroidism during graded renal failure in the rat. *Kidney Int.* 1994;45:953.
99. Lopez-Hilker S, Dusso A, Rapp N, Martin K, Slatopolski E. Phosphorus restriction reverses hyperparathyroidism in uremia independent of changes in calcium and calcitriol. *Am J Physiol.* 1990;259:F432.
100. Bricker N. On the pathogenesis of the uremic state: An exposition of the "trade-off" hypothesis. *N Engl J Med.* 1972; 286:1093.
101. Chew D, Nagode L. Calcitriol in treatment of chronic renal failure. In: Kirk R, Bonagura J, eds. *Current Veterinary Therapy XI.* Philadelphia, Pennsylvania: WB Saunders; 1992:857.
102. Barber DL, Rowland GN. Radiographically detectable soft tissue calcification in chronic renal failure. *Vet Radiol.* 1979;20: 117.
103. Nagode L, Chew D. The use of calcitriol in treatment of renal disease of the dog and cat. Purina Internationa Nutrition Symposium. Orlando, Florida: Ralston Purina Company; 1991:39.
104. Massry SG, Fadda GZ. Chronic renal failure is a state of cellular calcium toxicity. *Am J Kidney Dis.* 1993;21:81.
105. Dow SW, LeCouteur RA, Fettman MJ, Spurgeon TL. Potassium depletion in cats: Hypokalemic polymyopathy. *J Am Vet Med Assoc.* 1987;191:1563.
106. Grevel V, Opitz M, Stteb C, Skrodzki M. Myopathy due to potassium deficiency in eight cats and a dog. *Berl Munch Tierartzl Wochenschr.* 1993;106:20.
107. Adams LG, Polzin DJ, Osborne CA, O'Brien TD. Comparison of fractional excretion and twenty-four-hour urinary excretion of sodium and potassium in clinically normal cats and cats with induced chronic renal failure. *Am J Vet Res.* 1991;52:718.
108. Ching S, Fettman M, Hamar D, Nagode L, Smith K. The effect of chronic dietary acidification using ammonium chloride on acid-base and mineral metabolism in the adult cat. *J Nutrition.* 1989;119:902.
109. Whang R, Whang DD, Ryan MP. Refractory potassium repletion—a consequence of magnesium deficiency. *Arch Intern Med.* 1992;152:40.
110. Hills D, Morris J, Rogers Q. Potassium requirement of kittens as affected by dietary protein. *J Nutrition.* 1982;112:216.
111. Tolins JP, Hostetter MK, Hostetter TH. Hypokalemic nephropathy in the rat: Role of ammonia in chronic tubular injury. *J Clin Invest.* 1987;79:1447.
112. Mak RH, DeFronzo RA. Glucose and insulin metabolism in uremia. *Nephron.* 1992;61:377.
113. Cianciaruso B, Bellizzi V, Napoli R, Sacca L, Kopple JD. Hepatic uptake and release of glucose, lactate, and amino acids in acutely uremic dogs. *Metabolism.* 1991;40:261.
114. Fadda GZ, Thanakitcharu P, Comunale R, Lipson LG, Massry SG. Impaired potassium-induced insulin secretion in chronic renal failure. *Kidney Int.* 1991;40:413.
115. Fadda GZ, Massry SG. Impaired glucose-induced calcium signal in pancreatic islets in chronic renal failure. *Am J Nephrol.* 1991;11:475.
116. Turk S, Yeksan M, Tamer N, et al. Effect of 1,25-(OH)2D3 treatment on glucose intolerance in uraemia. *Nephrol Dial Transplant.* 1992;7:1207.
117. Polzin D, Osborne C, Stevens J, Hayden D. Serum amylase and lipase activities in dogs with chronic polyuric renal failure. *Am J Vet Res.* 1983;44:404.
118. Hudson E, Strombeck D. Effects of functional nephrectomy on the disappearance rates of canine serum amylase and lipase. *Am J Vet Res.* 1978;39:1316.
119. Buchman AL, Ament ME, Moukarzel A. Total serum amylase but not lipase correlates with measured glomerular filtration rate. *J Clin Gastroenterol.* 1993;16:204.
120. Jacobs R. Renal disposition of amylase, lipase, and lysozyme in the dog. *Vet Pathol.* 1988;25:443.
121. Jacobs R. Relationship of urinary amylase activity and proteinuria in the dog. *Vet Pathol.* 1989;26:349.
122. Rutsky E, et al. Acute pancreatitis in patients with end-stage renal disease without transplantation. *Arch Intern Med.* 1986; 146:1741.
123. Araki T, Ueda M, Ogawa K, Tsuji T. Histological pancreatitis in end-stage renal disease. *Int J Pancreatol.* 1992;12:263.

124. Attman P-O, Alaupovic P. Lipid abnormalities in chronic renal insufficiency. *Kidney Int.* 1991;39:S-16.

125. Attman PO, Samuelsson O, Alaupovic P. Lipoprotein metabolism and renal failure. *Am J Kidney Dis.* 1993;21:573.

126. Wanner C, Frommherz K, Horl WH. Hyperlipoproteinemia in chronic renal failure: Pathophysiological and therapeutic aspects. *Cardiology.* 1991;78:202.

127. Akmal M, Perkins S, Kasim SE, Oh HY, Smogorzewski M, Massry SG. Verapamil prevents chronic renal failure-induced abnormalities in lipid metabolism. *Am J Kidney Dis.* 1993; 22:158.

128. Lichtenberger LM, Gardner JW, Barreto JC, Dial EJ, Weinman EJ. Accumulation of aliphatic amines in gastric juice of acute renal failure patients. Possible cause of hypergastrinemia associated with uremia. *Dig Dis Sci.* 1993;38:1885.

129. Quintero E, Guth PH. Renal failure increases gastric mucosal blood flow and acid secretion in rats: Role of endothelium-derived nitric oxide. *Am J Physiol.* 1992;263:G75.

130. Quintero E, Kaunitz J, Nishizaki Y, De-Giorgio R, Sternini C, Guth PH. Uremia increases gastric mucosal permeability and acid back-diffusion injury in the rat. *Gastroenterology.* 1992;103: 1762.

131. Kang JY. The gastrointestinal tract in uremia. *Dig Dis Sci.* 1993;38:257.

132. Triebling AT, Korsten MA, Dlugosz JW, Paronetto F, Lieber CS. Severity of *Helicobacter*-induced gastric injury correlates with gastric juice ammonia. *Dig Dis Sci.* 1991;36:1089.

133. Lazarus J, Hakim R. Medical aspects of hemodialysis. In: Brenner B, Rector F, eds. *The Kidney.* Philadelphia, Pennsylvania: WB Saunders; 1991:2223.

134. Ravelli AM, Ledermann SE, Bisset WM, Trompeter RS, Barratt TM, Milla PJ. Foregut motor function in chronic renal failure. *Arch Dis Child.* 1992;67:1343.

135. Wolf A. Canine uremic encephalopathy. *J Am Animal Hosp Assoc.* 1980;16:735.

136. Littman M. Update: Treatment of hypertension in dogs and cats. In: Kirk R, Bonagura J, eds. *Current Veterinary Therapy XI.* Philadelphia, Pennsylvania: WB Saunders;1992:838.

137. Tarasuik A, Heimer D, Bark H. Effect of chronic renal failure on skeletal and diaphragmatic muscle contraction. *Am Rev Respir Dis.* 1992;146:1383.

138. Nishida A, Kubo K, Nihei H. Impaired muscle energy metabolism in uremia as monitored by 31P-NMR. *Nippon Jinzo Gakkai Shi.* 1991;33:65.

139. Thompson CH, Kemp GJ, Taylor DJ, Ledingham JG, Radda GK, Rajagopalan B. Effect of chronic uraemia on skeletal muscle metabolism in man. *Nephrol Dial Transplant.* 1993;8:218.

140. Clyne N, Esbjornsson M, Jansson E, Jogestrand T, Lins LE, Pehrsson SK. Effects of renal failure on skeletal muscle. *Nephron.* 1993;63:395.

141. Thompson CH, Kemp GJ, Green YS, Rix LK, Radda GK, Ledingham JG. Skeletal muscle metabolism in uremic rats: A 31P-magnetic resonance study. *Nephron.* 1993;63:330.

142. Cotton J, Knochel J. Correction of a uremic cellular injury with a protein-restricted, amino acid supplemented diet. *Am J Kidney Dis.* 1985;5:233.

143. Delmez JA, Slatopolsky E. Hyperphosphatemia—its consequences and treatment in patients with chronic renal disease. *Am J Kid Dis.* 1992;19:303.

144. Ross L. Hypertension and chronic renal failure. *Semin Vet Med Surg (Small Animals).* 1992;7:221.

145. Converse R Jr, Jacobsen TN, Toto RD, et al. Sympathetic overactivity in patients with chronic renal failure. *N Engl J Med.* 1992;327:1912.

146. Littman M. Chronic spontaneous systemic hypertension in dogs and cats. In: *Proceedings of the 8th Annual Veterinary Medical Forum.* Washington, DC: American College of Veterinary Internal Medicine; 1990;209.

147. London G, Marchais S, Guerin A, Metivier F, Pannier B. Cardiac hypertrophy and arterial alterations in end-stage renal disease: Hemodynamic factors. *Kidney Int.* 1993;43(Suppl) 41:S-42.

148. London G, De Vernejoul M-C, Fabiani F, et al. Secondary hyperparathyroidism and cardiac hypertrophy in hemodialysis patients. *Kidney Int.* 1987;32:900.

149. Moon M, Greenlee P, Burk R. Uremic pneumonitis-like syndrome in ten dogs. *J Am Animal Hosp Assoc.* 1986;22:687.

150. Eschbach J, Adamson J. Hematologic consequences of renal failure. In: Brenner B, Rector F, eds. *The Kidney,* Philadelphia, Pennsylvania: WB Saunders; 4th ed. 1991:2019.

151. Noris M, Benigni A, Boccardo P, et al. Enhanced nitric oxide synthesis in uremia: Implications for platelet dysfunction and dialysis hypotension. *Kidney Int.* 1993;44:445.

CHAPTER 17

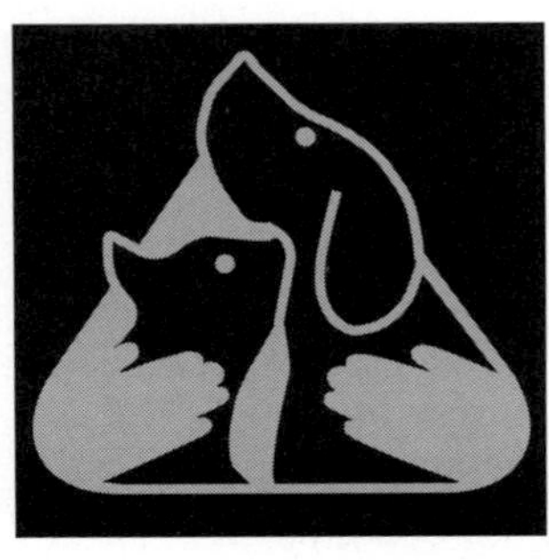

Primary Diseases of Glomeruli

SCOTT A. BROWN

I. AN APPRECIATION OF THE STRUCTURE AND FUNCTION OF THE GLOMERULUS IS A PREREQUISITE TO UNDERSTANDING GLOMERULAR DISEASES. (SEE CHAPTER 1, APPLIED ANATOMY OF THE URINARY SYSTEM WITH CLINICOPATHOLOGIC CORRELATION, AND CHAPTER 2, APPLIED PHYSIOLOGY OF THE KIDNEY.)

A. Proteinuria is the hallmark of glomerular disease. The glomerular filtration barrier, composed of endothelial cells, basement membrane, and foot processes of epithelial cells, presents both a size-selective and a charge-selective barrier to the passage of plasma proteins.

B. A disruption of the size-selective barrier results in proteinuria of variable magnitude and is usually associated with changes in glomerular structure visible by light microscopy.

C. A disruption of the charge-selective barrier results in proteinuria of variable magnitude and may be associated with biochemical changes in the glomerulus that are not detectable by light microscopy.

D. Frequently, glomerular disease disrupts both the size- and the charge-selective barriers to proteinuria.[19]

II. CHARACTERIZATION OF GLOMERULAR DISEASES

A. Introduction.

1. The term glomerular disease represents a diverse array of disorders of different pathogenic mechanisms, morphologic expressions, clinical courses, and responses to therapy.
2. Although the approach to these disorders in dogs and cats has traditionally emphasized a classification scheme based on light microscopic evaluation of renal tissue, there are other equally important considerations in the categorization of glomerular diseases (Table 17–1).

B. Glomerular diseases may be classified on the basis of whether they are primary or secondary to a systemic disorder.

1. Primary glomerular diseases are a diverse group of disorders in which the renal glomerulus is the sole or principal tissue involved. Using this terminology, primary glomerular diseases may be idiopathic or of known cause.
2. Secondary glomerular diseases occur in patients who have a primary disease that is extrarenal in origin. Causes of secondary glomerular diseases include drugs, infectious agents, multisystem diseases, biochemical disturbances, and heredofamilial diseases. Examples in dogs and cats include glomerular diseases observed in animals with diabetes mellitus, systemic lupus erythematosus, canine pyometra, dirofilariasis, feline leukemia virus infection, and hereditary glomerulopathies.

TABLE 17–1.
CHARACTERIZATION OF GLOMERULAR DISEASES IN DOGS AND CATS

Characteristic	Variations
Extrarenal involvement	Primary Secondary
Clinical signs	Proteinuria Edema, ascites, and/or hydrothorax (nephrotic syndrome) Polyuria, azotemia, and/or uremia
Clinical syndromes	Asymptomatic proteinuria Acute glomerulonephritis Rapidly progressive glomerulonephritis Chronic glomerulonephritis Nephrotic syndrome
Clinical course	Progressive Nonprogressive
Type of primary injury	Immune-mediated Non–immune-mediated
Light microscopic findings	Proliferative glomerulonephritis Membranoproliferative glomerulonephritis Minimal change disease Glomerulosclerosis Amyloidosis
Immunofluorescence findings	Class of immunoglobulin Location of deposits: subepithelial, subendothelial, or mesangial Linear versus granular immunoglobulin deposition Presence of complement or other antigens

For a review of secondary glomerular diseases, see Chapter 26, Renal Manifestations of Polysystemic Diseases. For a review of heredofamilial glomerular diseases, see Chapter 24, Congenital, Inherited, and Familial Renal Diseases.

3. This distinction between primary and secondary glomerular diseases is somewhat arbitrary. Some disorders classified as primary glomerular diseases may be associated with lesions in other tissues. Alternatively, animals with secondary glomerular disease may initially exhibit only renal involvement (e.g., systemic lupus erythematosus). Many dogs and cats considered to have a primary glomerular disease are likely to have a secondary disease and an undiagnosed extrarenal disorder.

C. Glomerular disease may be classified on the basis of clinical signs. The same clinical signs may be observed in animals with primary or secondary glomerular diseases.

1. Although a mild glomerular disease could be present without a detectable increase in urinary protein excretion, proteinuria is the hallmark of glomerular disease and is generally presumed to be present if an animal has a significant, generalized glomerular lesion. Proteinuria may represent the initial stage of other syndromes or may persist for months or years in some animals and may be observed in dogs with apparently normal glomerular morphology.[16,123] A relation between glomerular deposition of immunoglobulin A and proteinuria in these dogs has been suggested.[16]
2. Conversely, proteinuria is not diagnostic of glomerular disease, because lower tract sources of protein are common.
3. Some animals present with peripheral edema, ascites, and/or hydrothorax, manifestations of the nephrotic syndrome. This constellation of abnormalities associated with edema may include proteinuria, hypoalbuminemia, and hypercholesterolemia. In cats, membranous glomerulonephritis,[7,40,99,135] and, in dogs, membranous glomerulonephritis,[16,30,75,83,135] minimal change disease,[126] hereditary nephropathy,[77] and amyloidosis[44] may present as the nephrotic syndrome. The most common presenting complaint of dogs and cats with glomerular disease is the nephrotic syndrome; however, dogs and cats with the nephrotic syndrome exhibit only some of the classic signs and/or laboratory abnormalities at a single point in time.
4. Animals with a substantial reduction of glomerular filtration rate (GFR) may exhibit the typical clinical manifestations of polyuria and/or uremia. Although animals with nephrotic syndrome may survive many months or years,[7,30,99] the presence of azotemia or uremia appears to be a poor prognostic sign.[7,30]
5. In some animals, the nephrotic syndrome coexists with uremia (or azotemia).

D. Glomerular diseases may be classified on the basis of clinical syndromes, as in affected human beings.[57] These clinical syndromes are not specific for primary glomerular diseases, and the same classification system can be used for secondary glomerular diseases. To date, this system has not been routinely employed in dogs and cats, as morphologic classification systems have predominated in surveys of glomerular disease.

1. Asymptomatic proteinuria/hematuria is characterized by glomerular disease whose only clinical abnormality is mild proteinuria and/or hematuria in an animal that exhibits no evidence of other abnormalities. This may be identified on routine urinalysis of dogs or cats, and further testing (sequential urinalysis with or without renal biopsy) is necessary to determine if the lesion is a stable subclinical glomerulopathy, a resolving glo-

merular injury, or an early stage of a progressive glomerulopathy.

2. Acute glomerulonephritis, also referred to as acute nephritic syndrome, in humans is characterized by sudden onset and is frequently associated with an infectious agent. Features of the syndrome in humans include hematuria, proteinuria, reduced GFR, sodium and fluid retention, and systemic hypertension. In people it sometimes resolves spontaneously. Although the glomerulopathy of some infectious diseases, such as ehrlichiosis[33] or canine adenovirus infection,[133] may exhibit an acute phase, a syndrome in dogs and cats that closely resembles acute glomerulonephritis is rarely observed in people.
3. Rapidly progressive glomerulonephritis is characterized in humans by progressive loss of renal function, often leading to oliguria. Spontaneous recovery is rare. In dogs and cats, some glomerulopathies have a progressive course,[6,7,30,85,99,135] but most are insidious in onset and frequently exhibit an erratic (waxing and waning) clinical course.[7,30,99,101,103]
4. Chronic glomerulonephritis, also called chronic nephritic syndrome, is characterized in people by an insidious onset with hematuria, proteinuria, and systemic hypertension. The course is generally progressive over a variable period. This clinical syndrome represents a conglomeration of diseases of different pathogenesis, prognosis, and response to therapy. Terminally, the kidney is shrunken and involved with tubular atrophy, interstitial nephritis, and glomerular obliteration or sclerosis. As reviewed elsewhere,[103] chronic end-stage renal disease in dogs with a histologic diagnosis of chronic interstitial nephritis was once believed to represent end-stage chronic glomerulonephritis. Subsequently, investigators had attributed this disease to a primary tubulo-interstitial nephropathy, termed chronic interstitial nephritis. Recent evidence demonstrating a correlation between primary glomerular lesions and secondary tubulointerstitial lesions in dogs[83] has reopened this question. Some investigators have suggested that primary glomerular disease in dogs is more common than was previously thought.[88]
5. The nephrotic syndrome is characterized by proteinuria accompanied by varying degrees of hypoalbuminemia, hypercholesterolemia, systemic hypertension, and edema. Azotemia may be present or absent.
   a. Most reported cases of glomerular disease in dogs and cats fall in the category of nephrotic syndrome.
   b. Cases of the nephrotic syndrome may be subcategorized on the basis of morphologic appearance on renal biopsy (see the following).
   c. This syndrome is generally of insidious onset and the clinical course is erratic, with apparent remissions, often followed weeks or months later by exacerbation.
   d. Clinical indices of renal function, such as level of azotemia or proteinuria, may not accurately reflect the extent of morphologic injury.

E. Glomerular diseases may be classified on the basis of whether they are or are not progressive.

1. Successive increases in proteinuria and/or level of azotemia for three sequential determinations are suggestive of progressive disease.
2. Some glomerular diseases may be progressive at one point in time yet subsequently demonstrate clinical remission. This variable course is typical of canine and feline glomerulopathies,[6,7,30,99,101,103,135] making it difficult to interpret responses to therapy.

F. Glomerular diseases may be classified on the basis of the presence or absence of an immune-mediated mechanism of injury.

1. Two basic pathogenic mechanisms are described: immune complex disease and antiglomerular basement membrane disease.
   a. Immune complexes accumulate within the filtration barrier, producing glomerular injury as a result of a localized type III hypersensitivity reaction. Immune complexes may accumulate by trapping of circulating, preformed antigen-antibody complexes, or an antigen may bind to the glomerulus, serving as a "planted antigen."[62,87,127] On immunofluorescence microscopy, focal deposits of immunoglobulin and/or complement are visible as a "lumpy-bumpy" or granular pattern.
   b. Renal glomerular antigens may serve as the target of an antibody in antiglomerular basement membrane disease. On immunofluorescence microscopy, deposits of immunoglobulin and/or complement are arranged linearly along the glomerular basement membrane in a smooth pattern. This disease is uncommon in humans, though it has been produced experimentally in dogs[137] and documented in one horse,[8] it is believed to be rare in pet dogs and cats.
   c. Both types of immune-mediated glomerulopathy represent a localized type III hypersensitivity reaction. Renal injury is caused by involvement of resident glomerular cells and circulating leukocytes, platelets, complement, coagulation factors, and a variety of other mediators of inflammation.
2. Nonimmunologic causes of glomerular injury include a variety of hemodynamic changes, metabolic disorders, and drugs. (See Chapter 26, Renal Manifestations of Polysystemic Diseases.)
   a. Glomerular hypertension.[20,22,25]
   b. Systemic hypertension.[13]
   c. Glomerular hypertrophy and associated in-

creases in intrarenal concentrations of peptide growth factors.[22,25,89]

d. Hyperglycemia of diabetes mellitus.[22,121,130]
e. Hyperlipidemia.[82]
f. Intrarenal coagulation.[108]
g. Hyperphosphatemia and/or hyperparathyroidism.[23,50]
h. Glucocorticoids.[30,128]
i. Urinary tract infections, especially in animals receiving immunosuppressant therapy.[74]

3. Many primary glomerular diseases either are idiopathic or have a multifactorial cause. Frequently, both immunologic and nonimmunologic factors contribute to renal injury in affected animals, and identification of the primary cause may be difficult.

G. Glomerular diseases may be classified on the basis of findings of immunofluorescence microscopy. Findings include the class of immunoglobulin (Ig) present (generally IgG, IgM, or IgA), the location of the deposits (intramesangial versus subepithelial or subendothelial along the basement membrane), or pattern of deposition along the basement membrane (granular versus linear). Other antigens, such as components of the complement cascade (especially the third component) and fibrin-related antigens, may be demonstrable in some canine or feline glomerulopathies.

H. Light microscopic findings.

1. Surveys of glomerular diseases in dogs and cats have more often been divided, on the basis of changes in glomerular structure, into proliferative (mesangial) glomerulonephritis, membranous glomerulonephritis, membranoproliferative glomerulonephritis, minimal change disease, glomerulosclerosis, and amyloidosis. (See Chapter 20, Renal Amyloidosis.)
2. This morphologic classification system is most useful for chronic glomerular disease. A morphologic classification system, particularly one based on light microscopic examination, should not be used as the only criterion for classification of glomerular disease. As an example, although IgA nephropathy (Berger's disease in humans) may present in dogs with characteristics described later as membranoproliferative glomerulonephritis,[70] in humans it may produce glomerular lesions characterized as proliferative or as membranoproliferative glomerulonephritis.[57]
3. Establishing a morphologic diagnosis requires the integration of results of light, electron, and immunofluorescence microscopic examination of a renal biopsy specimen. (See Chapter 12, Canine and Feline Renal Biopsy.) Because most glomerular diseases are diffuse (i.e., they involve all glomeruli), needle biopsy of the renal cortex generally suffices to establish a diagnosis.
4. Though a morphologic classification system is central to clinical management of affected persons, its utility for veterinary glomerulopathies remains to be established. Unfortunately, renal biopsies are not always obtained from affected animals. The applicability of a morphologic classification system is further limited by the infrequent use of electron microscopy, immunofluorescence, and immunoserology in the examination of renal biopsy specimens of pet dogs and cats. Relying solely on light microscopic examination of renal tissue results in inaccuracies in diagnosis.
5. The World Health Organization (WHO) has proposed an alternate system for morphologic classification of glomerulonephritis that is commonly used to group human glomerulopathies. Though in this chapter I do not use the WHO system, it has been applied to proteinuria in dogs.[88]

III. MORPHOLOGIC CLASSIFICATION SYSTEM FOR GLOMERULAR DISEASE IN DOGS AND CATS

A. Introduction.

1. In humans, primary glomerular diseases are categorized on the basis of morphologic appearance under light, immunofluorescence, and electron microscopy.
2. For dogs and cats, light microscopic evaluation alone is often employed.
3. Although this classification system is reserved for primary glomerular disease of humans, similar morphologic changes occur in both primary and secondary glomerular diseases. Animals with secondary glomerular diseases (e.g., heredofamilial disease,[97] systemic lupus erythematosus,[67] or diabetes mellitus,[22,121,130]) can be placed within these morphologic categories. But, because a single disease may produce more than one morphologic type of glomerular disease,[132] the generally more useful approach categorizes secondary glomerular diseases on the basis of the causal mechanism. The goal of a categorization scheme is to establish a definable population of animals for which some generalities about pathogenesis, prognosis, and response to therapy can be made. Because each category is comprised of a population of animals with heterogeneous glomerular diseases of diverse pathogenic mechanisms, the utility of such generalities about the clinical management of patients is limited.
4. Although the utility of renal biopsy has been questioned by some,[45] a biopsy is required to establish morphologic type of glomerulopathy.[92,122] Guessing the type of glomerular lesion from clinical data has proved to be of limited utility in humans.
5. Classification of morphologic findings in animals with primary nephrotic syndrome. (In the following section, information on clinical findings and response to therapy in affected people is provided

for illustrative purposes. The magnitudes of variances in response to therapy between species and between individuals within a species are largely unknown.)

B. Minimal change disease.

1. Normal to mild increases in mesangial cellularity on light microscopic examination.
   a. Cases with more substantial mesangial proliferation may be indistinguishable from mesangioproliferative glomerulonephritis.
   b. Minimal change disease may be indistinguishable from early membranous nephropathy by light microscopy.
2. Abnormalities of epithelial foot processes are observable by electron microscopy.
3. Absence or paucity of glomerular immunoglobulin deposition on immunofluorescence microscopy.
4. Marked proteinuria.
5. Thromboembolism may complicate the clinical course.
6. Minimal change disease in humans.[57]
   a. Often affects young persons.
   b. Exhibits spontaneous remission in as many as 50% of affected people.
   c. Is usually steroid responsive. Nonresponsive cases may progress to glomerulosclerosis. Some patients are steroid dependent or require cytotoxic therapy (e.g., cyclophosphamide, chlorambucil, or azathioprine). Cyclosporine could be considered for steroid-unresponsive cases.
7. Minimal change nephropathy reported in a 4-year-old female collie.[126]
   a. The dog was azotemic, markedly proteinuric with hypoproteinemia and edema, and euthanized without treatment.
   b. Light microscopy revealed minimal glomerular changes.
   c. Immunofluorescence microscopy revealed deposits of IgM and complement C3.
   d. Ultrastructural studies revealed podocyte foot process loss.

C. Proliferative glomerulonephritis.

1. Differentiation between a mild increase in mesangial cellularity (as occasionally observed in minimal change disease) and clear-cut mesangial proliferation may be difficult.
2. Proliferative (mesangioproliferative) glomerulonephritis in humans.[57]
   a. As the disease progresses, sclerotic glomeruli may become more prominent.
   b. Frequently, IgM is detectable with immunofluorescence and the condition has been called IgM nephropathy.
   c. If IgA is present on immunofluorescence microscopy of human tissue, it is referred to as Berger's disease or IgA nephropathy.
   d. Progression to renal failure may be observed.
   e. Spontaneous remission can also occur.
   f. Approximately 50% of patients respond to steroids.
   g. Adjunctive cytotoxic therapy (e.g., cyclophosphamide, chlorambucil, or azathioprine) sometimes is required.
3. Proliferative glomerulonephritis in cats.
   a. Although most reported cases of glomerular diseases in cats are membranous, proliferative glomerulonephritis has been observed.
   b. One report of cats with viral feline infectious peritonitis documented 16 cases of proliferative glomerular disease.[71]
4. Proliferative glomerulonephritis in dogs (Table 17–2).
   a. Surveys of morphologic findings of glomerular disease in dogs have frequently identified cases of proliferative glomerulonephritis.[30,83,88,95,96,116]
   b. Although proteinuria is not usually marked, clinical signs compatible with the nephrotic syndrome may develop in some animals.[30]
5. IgA nephropathy.
   a. In humans, proliferative or membranoproliferative glomerulonephritis in which deposition of IgA and the complement C3 predominate is referred to as IgA nephropathy or Berger's disease.[10] Other diseases, such as Henoch-Schönlein purpura, also are characterized by mesangial IgA deposits, but patients affected with this disorder also frequently display arthralgia, abdominal pain, and nonthrombocytopenic purpura.
   b. One report documented three cases of IgA glomerulonephritis in three young, male dogs co-housed in a blood donor facility.[70] The light microscopic lesions were characterized as membranoproliferative.
   c. In proteinuric dogs, glomerular IgA deposition may be nonspecifically associated with the glomerular lesions.[16]
   d. In a report of 100 autopsied dogs,[91] 47% of dogs had IgA in glomeruli on immunofluorescence studies. Dogs with enteritis or hepatic disease had the highest prevalence of IgA deposition. IgG, IgM, and complement were often codeposited. Localization of immune complexes within the glomerulus does not necessarily equate with the presence of significant glomerular injury. Nonrenal diseases may directly cause glomerular deposition of immune complexes, especially IgA, in hepatic diseases.[46] Although glomerular lesions were identified in some dogs that exhibited IgA deposition, the relation between glomerular deposition of immunoglobulin and clinical renal disease is sometimes unclear.

D. Membranous glomerulonephritis (Fig. 17–1).

1. Diffuse thickening of capillary wall and subepithelial immune complex deposition are typical of this class.
2. Subcategorization is done on the basis of cause.
   a. The cause may be unknown.

TABLE 17–2.
PREVALENCE OF SELECTED CLINICAL CHARACTERISTICS IN DOGS WITH GLOMERULAR DISEASE

Investigator	Cases (No.)	Age Mean (range) (yr.)	Sex*	Morphologic Type	Prevalence (%)	Clinical Presentation	Prevalence (%)
Kurtz et al.[85]	8	7.3 (3–12)	4M/4F	MP	100	Edema/ascites	0
						Hypoalbuminemia	100
						Azotemia	100
Murray et al.[96]	42	7.7 (0.8–14.5)	24M/18F	M	12	†	
				P	74		
				MP	14		
DiBartola et al.[41]	21	6.5	†	M	33	Edema/ascites	14
				MP	19	Hypoalbuminemia	76
				AMY	29	Hypercholesterolemia	94
				ATR	19	Thromboembolism	29
Wright et al.[135]	5	4.5 (2–8.5)	4M/1F	M	100	Edema/ascites	80
						Azotemia	20
						Thromboembolism	60
Jeraj et al.[78]	4	6.3 (5–8)	4F	†		Hypoalbuminemia	100
						Hypercholesterolemia	100
						Azotemia	100
Jaenke et al.[75]	14	6.5 (1–14)	7M/7F	M	100††	Edema/ascites	43
						Azotemia	50
MacDougall et al.[88]	40	7.7	22M/18F	M	0	†	
				MP	20		
				P	33		
				AMY	29		
				SCL	17		
Center et al.[30]	41	7.4 (0.8–18)	23M/18F	M	29	Edema/ascites	15
				MP	34	Hypoalbuminemia	61
				P	37	Hypercholesterolemia	79
						Thromboembolism	29
						Azotemia	53

Key: MP, membranoproliferative glomerulonephritis; M, membranous glomerulonephritis; P, proliferative glomerulonephritis; AMY, glomerular amyloidosis; SCL, glomerulosclerosis.

*M, male or male castrate; F, female or spayed female.

†Data not provided or provided in a different format.

††These investigators also identified 7 cases of glomerulosclerosis, 12 cases of amyloidosis, and 11 cases with tubulo-interstitial disease or no renal lesions but reported data for the 14 membranous glomerulonephritis cases only.

b. The condition can be secondary to an underlying disease.
   (1). Infectious diseases (e.g., infection with feline leukemia virus[6,52,58] or feline infectious peritonitis virus[71]).
   (2). Metabolic diseases (e.g., diabetes mellitus).[22,121,130]
   (3). Drug-induced (morphologic glomerulopathy incompletely documented in clinical cases in veterinary medicine).[30,34,56]
   (4). Neoplasms.[4,40,52,58,99]
   (5). Systemic lupus erythematosus.[118,120]

3. This category is termed primary if no identifiable underlying disease is identified. Frequently, underlying disease may be present but not yet expressed.

4. Light microscopic findings include diffuse, uniform thickening of the capillary wall without cellular proliferation. Silver stains may reveal the presence of subepithelial spikes comprised of laminin that project toward the urinary space.[53]
5. Characteristic electron microscopic findings include subepithelial deposits (immune complexes) surrounded by spikes of basement membrane–like material (laminin).[53]
6. Characteristic immunofluorescence findings include IgG outlining all capillary loops in a granular or "lumpy-bumpy" pattern. In humans, early immunofluorescence findings may have a linear pattern, causing confusion with antiglomerular basement membrane disease.[57]
7. The genesis of the immune complexes is usually unknown. They may represent trapping of preformed circulating immune complexes or binding *in situ* of a circulating antibody to an antigen "planted" in the glomerulus by virtue of an affinity of the antigen for the glomerulus.[62,87,127] Antibodies may be directed against antigens within the glomerular basement membrane.[8,137]
8. Membranous nephropathy in humans.[57]
   a. Clinical course is indolent and progressive, with multiple remissions and exacerbations.
   b. Spontaneous remissions occur in about 25% of cases. The role of steroid therapy and/or cytotoxic agents is unknown.
9. Membranous nephropathy in cats (Table 17–3).
   a. It has been associated with infection with feline leukemia virus,[4,6,7,52] feline infectious peritonitis,[71] and systemic lupus erythematosus.[7,118] An association with neoplasms, especially lymphoid types, has also been noted.[4,52,58,99] (See Chapter 26, Renal Manifestations of Polysystemic Diseases.)
   b. Feline leukemia virus–induced nephropathy is an immune complex disease.[52,58,79,117] The death rate for affected animals with feline leukemia virus infection is as high as 30%.[52]
   c. Feline immunodeficiency virus has been associated with chronic renal disease in a survey of 15 affected elderly cats.[106] Because age-matched control data were not provided, cause and effect was not established by this study.
   d. Membranous nephropathy with a possible heredofamilial component has been reported in related cats on two occasions.[38,98] Immune complex deposition was apparently responsible for the nephropathy.
   e. Most cases of feline membranous glomerulonephritis are idiopathic (see Table 17–3).[85,96]
      (1). It affects young cats (mean age 3.3 years).
      (2). Males appear to be overrepresented.
      (3). It may present with nephrotic syndrome, azotemic renal failure, or both.
      (4). Most cats have nephrotic syndrome at presentation.
      (5). Prevalence of azotemia at presentation varies.
      (6). Cats with membranous glomerulonephritis frequently exhibit hypercholesterolemia, hypoalbuminemia, and anemia at presentation.
      (7). The clinical course is irregular and unpredictable and varies dramatically among individual cats. In general, the disease is progressive.[6,7,99,135] Azotemia at presentation is a poor prognostic sign. In nonazotemic cats, survival of several years with symptomatic therapy (diuretics or dietary therapy) is observed in as many as one third of affected cats.[7,99,135]
      (8). Although steroid responsiveness has been suggested,[48] the clinical course of this disease is erratic, with apparent remission noted in some animals. Consequently, effectiveness of treatment is difficult to judge from anecdotal reports. Other investigators have reported spontaneous remission in a dog with glomerular disease,[101] an association between glomerulonephritis and corticosteroid administration in dogs,[30] and lack of evidence of efficacy of corticosteroids in affected cats.[99] Consequently, corticosteroid therapy is controversial and has no clear rationale at this time.
10. Membranous nephropathy in dogs (see Table 17–2).

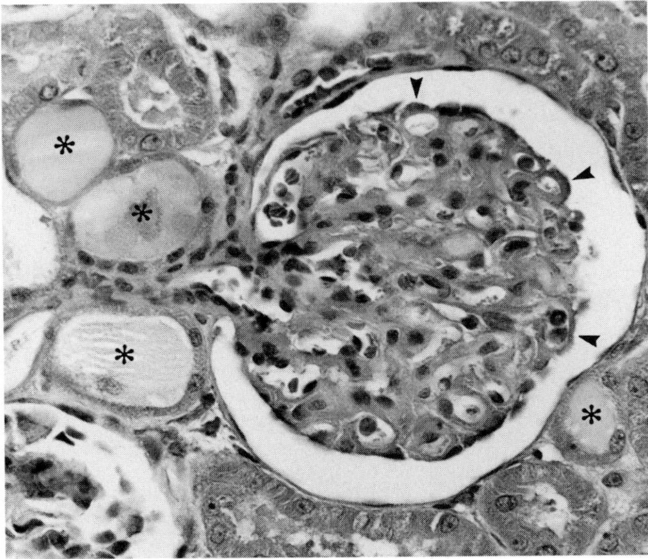

FIG. 17–1. Membranous glomerulonephritis in a cat infected with feline leukemia virus. Note the generalized increase in thickness of the capillary loops within the glomerulus (arrows). Intraluminal casts (asterisks) provide evidence of glomerular protein leak. (Courtesy of C.A. Brown.)

TABLE 17–3.
PREVALENCE OF SELECTED CLINICAL CHARACTERISTICS IN CATS WITH MEMBRANOUS NEPHROPATHY

Investigator	Subjects (No.)	Mean Age (Range) (yr.)	Sex*	Clinical Presentation	Prevalence (%)
Nash et al.[99]	13	4.0 (2.5–7)	13M	Edema/ascites	62
				Hypoalbuminemia	85
				Azotemia	54
				Hypercholesterolemia	85
				Anemia	85
Wright et al.[135]	11	3.3 (1–7)	8M/3F	Edema/ascites	91
Arthur et al.[7]	24	3.2 (2.5–6)	16M/8F	Edema/ascites	75
				Hypoalbuminemia	96
				Azotemia	67
				Hypercholesterolemia	77
				Anemia	63

*M, male or male castrate; F, female or spayed female.

a. The condition is reportedly associated with neoplasia.[96]
b. Most cases of canine membranous glomerulonephritis are idiopathic.[85,96]
c. A predisposition for massive proteinuria and development of clinical signs of nephrotic syndrome is reported.[15,17,103,136]
d. The clinical course is erratic; apparent remission is noted in some animals.[101]

E. Membranoproliferative glomerulonephritis (see Fig. 17–2).

1. Proliferation of glomerular mesangial cells with extension of mesangial cell cytoplasm into peripheral capillary loops produces a "railroad track" double-walled appearance of the capillary walls. This is sometimes incorrectly referred to as *split basement membrane.*
2. Membranoproliferative glomerulonephritis may be primary or secondary to a variety of diseases, such as systemic lupus erythematosus or a hereditary nephropathy. Familial glomerulonephritis of Doberman pinscher dogs is an example of membranoproliferative glomerulonephritis.[104,131] (See Chapter 24, Congenital, Inherited, and Familial Renal Diseases.)
3. Light microscopic findings include expansion of mesangial matrix, duplication of the wall of peripheral capillaries, and proliferation of mesangial cells.
4. Immunofluorescence findings frequently include immunoglobulin and complement deposition, particularly in "railroad tracks."
5. It has been observed in several surveys of canine glomerular diseases (see Table 17–2).

F. Glomerulosclerosis (Fig. 17–3).

1. Lesions typically exhibit a segmental increase in mesangial matrix and basement membrane.
2. Lesions may be more prominent in juxtamedullary glomeruli.

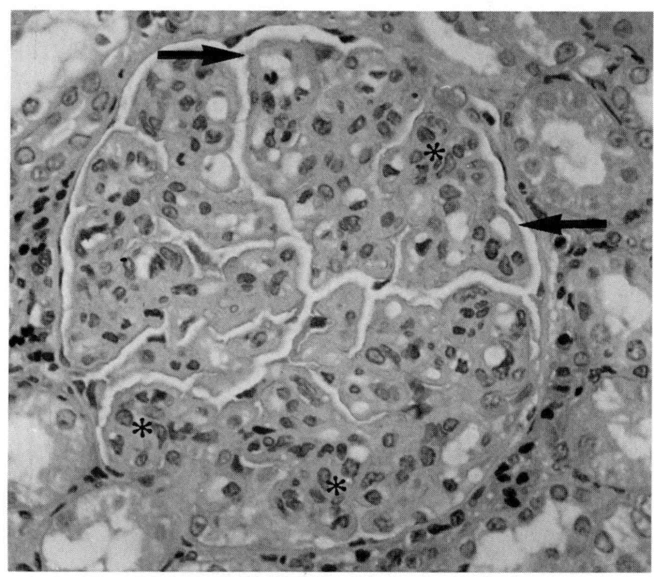

FIG. 17–2. Membranoproliferative glomerulonephritis in a Doberman pinscher dog. Note the increase in both cell numbers (asterisks) and thickness of the capillary loops within the glomerulus (arrows). (Courtesy of C.A. Brown.)

3. Segmental lesions may progress to global sclerosis within individual glomeruli.
4. The term glomerular tip lesion is used when it involves the tubular pole only.
5. Glomerulosclerosis in humans.[57]
   a. It may be superimposed on minimal change disease, proliferative glomerulonephritis, membranous glomerulonephritis, or any disease that causes a marked reduction in renal function.
   b. Some forms respond to steroids.
   c. It may be secondary to hemodynamic changes in glomeruli as a result of reduced renal function of any cause.

d. The long-term course is usually progressive, and glomerulosclerosis is an ominous finding.

6. Glomerulosclerosis in dogs and cats.
   a. It may be superimposed on other glomerular diseases or on renal disease of any type.
   b. It has been reported in dogs with heredofamilial disorders[84] and diabetes mellitus,[22,54,121,130] and following radiation exposure.[68,76,139]
   c. One theory proposes that glomerulosclerosis is the renal lesion of progressive renal disease in all animals.[20] Glomerulosclerosis is observed in dogs[23,107] and cats[2] with surgically reduced renal mass.

G. Miscellaneous glomerular diseases.

1. Idiopathic vascular disease in racing greyhounds.[28]
   a. This idiopathic disease is most frequently identified in racing greyhounds but has been identified in other breeds.
   b. It is characterized by slowly healing cutaneous ulcers, glomerular infarction, and necrosis.
   c. Intravascular coagulation with fibrinoid arteritis and thrombosis is the underlying morphologic lesion. This disease may represent an analog of hemolytic uremic syndrome in humans.
   d. Increased prevalence in greyhounds may be the result of a genetic predisposition or it may be related to management practices.
2. Glomerular lipidosis.[51]
   a. Focal deposition of lipid within mesangial cells typifies the lesion.
   b. The cause is unknown.
   c. Its significance is ill-understood; it may be an incidental finding in clinically normal animals.

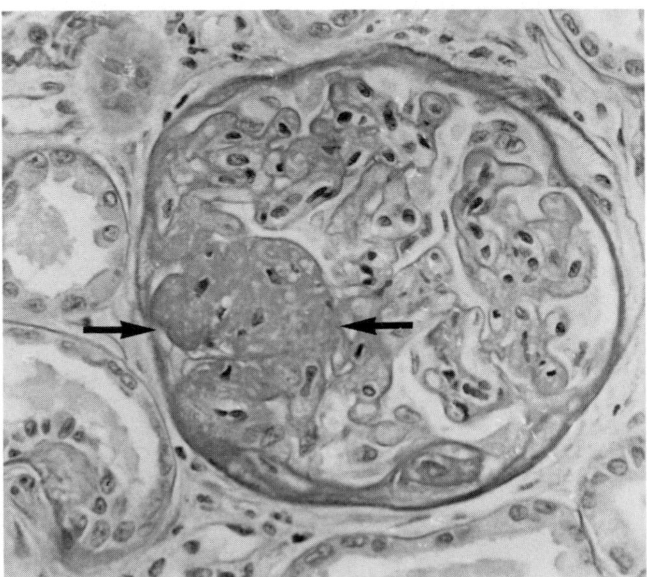

FIG. 17–3. Segmental glomerulosclerosis in a dog. Note the segmental increase in mesangial matrix within the glomerulus (arrows). (Courtesy of C.A. Brown.)

IV. CONSEQUENCES OF GLOMERULAR DISEASES

A. Proteinuria is the hallmark of glomerular disease.

1. See Chapter 9, Urinary Protein Loss, for a review of appropriate diagnostic methods.
2. Albumin, transferrin, immunoglobulin G, various apolipoproteins, and antithrombin III are prominent proteins lost. Many other proteins are also present in the urine in abnormally elevated amounts. Some are pathophysiologically significant.
3. Hypoalbuminemia, the most commonly identified consequence of proteinuria, is a consequence of renal loss exceeding hepatic production. A substantial portion of the albumin leaking through the glomerulus is absorbed, degraded into constituent amino acids by the proximal tubule epithelium, and returned to the blood. Dietary protein intake and other maneuvers may affect both synthesis and loss of albumin.
4. Although the permeability of the glomerular filtration barrier to albumin is the primary determinant of the extent of proteinuria, the magnitude of proteinuria is directly affected by the GFR, plasma concentration of albumin, and, in rats,[81] by dietary protein intake. If plasma albumin concentration falls, the filtered load of albumin falls, causing renal excretion to decrease. Thus, hypoalbuminemia contributes to achieving a balance between hepatic production and renal loss.
5. Edema, ascites, or hydrothorax occurs as a result of hypoalbuminemia, the consequent drop in plasma oncotic pressure, and fluid retention. Although the pathogenesis of the fluid retention in nephrotic syndrome is controversial, enhanced production of angiotensin II, antidiuretic hormone, and atrial natriuretic factor, as well as ill-understood intrarenal mechanisms, all appear to play a role.

B. Hyperlipidemia.

1. In clinical surveys of animals with glomerulopathies, hypercholesterolemia and hypertriglyceridemia are often observed (see Tables 17–2 and 17–3).
2. The distribution of canine and feline lipoproteins differs from that of people, with higher-density lipoproteins predominating.[39,69,90,111] Consequently, data pertaining to the pattern of changes in plasma lipoproteins in people with nephrotic syndrome may not apply to dogs and cats.
3. Hyperlipidemia has been attributed to an increase in hepatic production and reduced peripheral catabolism of lower-density lipoproteins. The inciting cause of these metabolic changes appears to be a reduction in plasma oncotic pressure and/or the loss of a regulatory protein in the urine.[11,55,138]

The degree of fasting hyperlipidemia is directly related to the extent of hypoalbuminemia.

4. Lipiduria may be observed as the presence of refractile lipid bodies in the urine sediment, but it is not diagnostic of lipidemia because lipids are normal components of feline urine.
5. Studies in humans and rats have demonstrated that hypercholesterolemia is a risk factor for a variety of vascular diseases, including progressive renal disease.[82] Although hypercholesterolemia might contribute to progressive loss of GFR in dogs and cats, effects are generally unknown. Preliminary results of one study indicate that hypercholesterolemia is associated with progressive renal disease in dogs, but a cause-and-effect relationship has not been established (personal observations).

C. The nephrotic syndrome is defined as marked proteinuria plus edema, hypoalbuminemia, and hypercholesterolemia.

1. The syndrome occurs as a consequence of marked glomerular proteinuria.
2. Although proteinuria is always present, expression of the other components of the nephrotic syndrome varies (see Tables 17–2 and 17–3).
3. A wide variety of primary and secondary glomerular diseases can cause the nephrotic syndrome.

D. Systemic hypertension.

1. A common complication in people affected with glomerular diseases is systemic hypertension.
2. It may contribute to the progressive loss of renal function.[14,54]
3. A prevalence of systemic hypertension of 80% was reported in dogs with glomerular disease or persistent proteinuria.[37]
4. Although a recent study demonstrated a beneficial effect of an angiotensin-converting enzyme inhibitor in uninephrectomized, diabetic beagles,[22,54] the consequences of systemic hypertension to cats and to nondiabetic dogs with glomerulopathy remain largely unknown.

E. Azotemia.

1. Azotemia occurs as the result of a decrement of GFR. This results in the contrasting combination of increased glomerular loss of plasma proteins coupled with reduced glomerular filtration of water and dissolved solutes (including nitrogenous wastes). The decrement in GFR has been attributed to the complete destruction of some nephrons and the loss of filtration surface area in many of the surviving glomeruli.
2. Azotemia (uremia) and the nephrotic syndrome may occur independently or in concert in animals with glomerular disease (see Tables 17–2 and 17–3).

F. A hypercoagulable state may be present.

1. The hypercoagulable state in dogs with nephrotic syndrome may lead to thromboses of pulmonary and systemic vessels (see Tables 17–2 and 17–3). Thrombotic disease is apparently rare in cats with glomerulopathy. The tendency for renal vein thrombosis in humans with nephrotic syndrome does not appear to be present in dogs and cats, though it has been reported in dogs with amyloidosis.[44,119]
2. Antithrombin III (heparin cofactor) is an α_2-globulin with a molecular weight of approximately 65,000. Antithrombin III inhibits the coagulation process but is lost in the urine of animals with glomerular disease.[65]
   a. Antithrombin III deficiency is associated with a hypercoagulable state in dogs and humans, apparently contributing to the genesis of vascular thromboses.
   b. The degree of proteinuria is loosely related to the extent of antithrombin III deficiency.
3. Hypoalbuminemia and/or hyperfibrinogenemia may enhance platelet aggregability, contributing further to a hypercoagulable state.[66]
4. The function of the anticoagulant factors protein S and protein C may also be diminished in similarly affected humans.[115]

G. Altered pharmacokinetics.

1. The volume of distribution of drugs may be increased in proteinuric patients,[110] potentially resulting in a subtherapeutic plasma concentration of a drug administered in standard dosages. This complicates drug dosing regimens, especially use of nephrotoxic agents or adjustment of dosage in an animal with concurrent azotemia and nephrotic syndrome.
2. Hypoalbuminemia limits drug binding sites, so protein-bound medications should be administered with this in mind.
3. Reductions of GFR and tubular secretory mass alter pharmacokinetics of drugs eliminated partially or solely by the kidneys.
4. See Chapter 30, Drug Therapy during Renal Disease and Renal Failure, for considerations related to drug therapy of patients with glomerular disease.

H. Other substances normally bound to proteins may also be lost in the urine of animals with nephrotic syndrome. These substances have received little attention in veterinary medicine.

1. Theoretically, urinary loss of iron could lead to microcytic, hypochromic anemia, or loss of zinc could interfere with wound healing or immune function.
2. Loss of calcitriol-binding globulin may interfere with metabolism of vitamin D, elevating plasma parathyroid hormone levels.[59]
3. Loss of thyroid-binding globulin may interfere with thyroid hormone metabolism.[49]
4. Loss of immunoglobulins may enhance susceptibility to bacterial infections, particularly in animals with virus-induced immunosuppression.

V. DIAGNOSIS OF GLOMERULAR DISEASES

A. Laboratory findings.

1. Proteinuria is the hallmark of glomerular disease.
   a. See Chapter 9, Urinary Protein Loss, for a review of methods for assessment of proteinuria.
   b. Proteinuria of glomerular origin is predominantly albumin.
   c. Proteinuria varies in magnitude, and in certain glomerular diseases or early in any glomerular disease, it may be mild or even below detectable limits, depending on the method of assessment.
   d. The extent of proteinuria may be poorly related to the degree of azotemia or to the morphologic evidence of glomerular injury.
2. Hematuria is a frequent finding in humans with glomerular diseases but has received little attention in affected dogs and cats.
   a. Either urinary tract hemorrhage or glomerular disease may cause hematuria and proteinuria. The cause of hematuria may be difficult to determine by urinalysis alone. Other clinical evidence (e.g., history of trauma, blood chemistry determinations, excretory urography, renal biopsy) may be required to identify the cause of proteinuria.
   b. In hypotonic urine, red blood cells may lyse, producing an artifactual elevation in urine protein content. In this case, proteinuria parallels the degree of hematuria, but generally is mild, and urine protein electrophoresis reveals protein molecules migrating in the β-globulin region (hemoglobin).
   c. In humans with glomerular disease, red blood cells that are fragmented, distorted, uneven in size, and pallid when examined by phase microscopy are referred to as dysmorphic and may indicate a glomerular origin.[47] Urinary red blood cells that are of small volume may also indicate a glomerular source.[60] These changes in red cell shape and size in humans with glomerular hematuria reflect the effects of red cell transit through the tubule and the osmotic stresses of this environment. Unfortunately, the predictive value of these observations has not been reported in dogs and cats.
3. Cylindruria is a consistent finding in affected dogs and cats. Casts may be hyaline, granular, cellular (red or white), waxy, or broad.
4. In some animals, urine-concentrating ability may be intact despite the presence of azotemia or renal origin.
   a. Urine-concentrating ability may be intact in cats with renal azotemia[113] that is caused by any type of renal disease.
   b. Glomerular disease should be suspected in proteinuric dogs with renal azotemia whose urine-concentrating ability is intact (urine specific gravity greater than 1.025).
5. Other laboratory tests.
   a. In humans with glomerular disease, a variety of serologic tests is routinely performed to subdivide and further characterize the glomerulopathy. These tests include an evaluation for antibodies directed against streptococcal enzymes in acute glomerulonephritis, antineutrophil cytoplasmic antibody (ANCA) in systemic vasculitides, antiglomerular basement membrane antibodies, antiDNA antibodies, rheumatoid factor, antiDNase B antibodies, and plasma concentrations of components of the complement system.
   b. In addition to routine hemogram, urinalysis, and urine protein quantification, and plasma biochemical panel, appropriate diagnostic evaluation in dogs or cats might include radiographic or ultrasonographic images and tests for feline leukemia virus, feline immunodeficiency, antinuclear antibodies, lupus erythematosus, cells, *Dirofilaria immitis* organisms, and systemic hypertension.

B. Renal biopsy.

1. Renal biopsy is generally the only definitive method for establishing a diagnosis of glomerular disease and classifying the disease.
2. Light microscopy is the most widely used tool for the morphologic classification of glomerulopathies. A commonly used classification system outlined previously (see Section III of this chapter) divides glomerular diseases into proliferative, membranoproliferative, membranous, amyloid, and sclerotic.
3. Electron microscopy frequently must be employed to differentiate between morphologic types when light microscopy by itself is not adequate. Although infrequently used in veterinary medicine, electron microscopy is routinely used to classify glomerulopathies in humans.
4. Immunofluorescence microscopy.
   a. Immunoglobulin deposition may be identified by fluorescent antibody examination of renal biopsy specimens. The presence of antibody deposition, the subclass of immunoglobulin, and the location of the antibody (subepithelial versus subendothelial) may be useful in establishing a diagnosis.
   b. The presence of antibody within the glomerulus does not confirm immune complex or antiglomerular basement membrane disease. Normally some trapping of immunoglobulin occurs within the glomerulus, and the amount is often enhanced in glomerulopathy of any cause. In particular, removal of IgA is slow and deposition of immune complexes is directly enhanced by some extrarenal diseases.[46]

c. The pattern of immunofluorescence is also important. In immune complex disease, a "lumpy-bumpy" or granular pattern of antibody deposition is noted. In antiglomerular basement membrane disease, a linear pattern of antibody deposition is evident; however, some animals with a linear pattern of immunofluorescence do not have antiglomerular basement membrane disease.[30] In veterinary medicine, a case of antiglomerular basement membrane disease has been characterized in a horse.[8] A definitive diagnosis of antiglomerular basement membrane disease requires the presence either of circulating antibodies directed against the glomerular basement membrane or of antibodies eluted from the glomerulus specifically directed against glomerular basement membrane antigens. In nearly all cases, antibody deposition in dogs and cats is believed to be the result of immune complex disease.

d. The presence of various other antigens within glomeruli may indicate the pathogenesis of the disease. Examples include the components of the complement system, fibrin-related antigens, and coagulation factors. With the exception of fluorescent antibody staining for complement, these tests are not routinely performed in veterinary medicine.

VI. GENERAL PRINCIPLES OF SPECIFIC THERAPY IN PRIMARY GLOMERULAR DISEASES

A. Knowledge of the type of glomerular disease is a prerequisite for the appropriate choice of specific therapy. For example, people with minimal change disease are generally steroid responsive, whereas those with acute post-streptococcal glomerulonephritis generally recover spontaneously and may actually be harmed by the use of corticosteroids.[57]

B. A variety of therapeutic maneuvers has been attempted in dogs and cats with glomerular diseases. Although the response to therapy may vary with the type of glomerular disease, available data are inadequate to draw firm conclusions about most glomerular diseases.

C. Some diseases or their clinical manifestations exhibit spontaneous remission,[101] which may be transient. In some cases, apparent clinical improvement is not reflected in improvement in renal morphology. In one case, edema resolved spontaneously but renal lesions persisted in serial biopsy examinations.[64]

D. Glomerulonephritis.

1. Agents aimed at modifying immune function could be considered when a renal specimen reveals severe morphologic changes, such as glomerular crescent formation, particularly when the clinical course is progressive. Unfortunately, no data in veterinary medicine is currently available upon which to base recommendations.
   a. Aggressive therapy that includes steroids and cytotoxic agents (cyclophosphamide or azathioprine), cyclosporin A, and/or plasmapharesis may be considered, particularly in animals that exhibit clear evidence of a progressive disease. Response of affected patients to cyclosporin A has been disappointing.[124]
   b. In some severe forms of human glomerular disease for which steroid therapy is indicated, the use of intravenous pulse therapy with methylprednisolone is of added benefit.[112]
   c. Prednisolone may enhance glomerular permeability to plasma proteins[129] and may slow immune complex removal from the glomeruli. High levels of endogenous or exogenous corticosteroids have been associated with exacerbation of renal disease.[30,128]
2. Thromboxane synthase inhibitors may lessen immune-mediated renal injury.
   a. Beneficial effects were demonstrated in two experimental models of immune complex glomerulonephritis.[63,87]
   b. Treatment of a whippet with spontaneous membranoproliferative glomerulonephritis reduced proteinuria and apparently led to resolution of edema and ascites but did not reduce glomerular histologic changes.[64]

E. Glomerulosclerosis.

1. As previously noted, this is generally believed to be a secondary lesion, and therapeutic maneuvers center on efforts to interrupt mechanisms that contribute to ongoing renal injury.
2. When systemic hypertension and azotemia are documented in an animal, appropriate use of antihypertensive therapy should be considered.
   a. See Chapter 19, Pathophysiology and Management of Systemic Hypertension Associated with Renal Dysfunction, for a review of the diagnosis and management of this disorder.
   b. Theoretic reasons exist for considering the appropriate use of an angiotensin-converting enzyme inhibitor and avoiding the use of a calcium channel antagonist in these patients.[5,22] (At this time, no data support the preferential use of one member of this class of therapeutic agents.)
3. For animals with glomerulosclerosis that also have documented diabetes mellitus and azotemia, an angiotensin-converting enzyme inhibitor may be considered. (At this time, no data support the preferential use of one member of this class of therapeutic agents.[54])
4. In patients with glomerular disease and uremia, dietary protein restriction should be employed, as necessary, to control the extent of clinical signs. See Chapter 22, Acute Renal Failure: Ischemia and

Chemical Nephrosis, Chapter 28, Conservative Medical Management of Chronic Renal Failure, Chapter 29, Medical Management of the Anemia of Chronic Renal Failure, and Chapter 31, Application of Peritoneal Dialysis and Hemodialysis in the Management of Renal Failure, for a review of the management of this and other manifestations of renal failure.

5. In patients with the nephrotic syndrome, dietary protein intake should be adjusted as necessary to control proteinuria and edema. (See Section VIII A of this chapter.)
6. On the basis of currently available evidence, indiscriminate use of antihypertensive therapy or dietary modification is not indicated for all patients with any form of renal disease.

F. See Chapter 20, Renal Amyloidosis.

VII. GENERAL PRINCIPLES OF THERAPY DIRECTED AT THE COMPLICATIONS OF PRIMARY GLOMERULAR DISEASES

A. Agents to reduce the magnitude of proteinuria.

1. Massive proteinuria may lead to protein malnutrition and fluid retention with associated edema, ascites, and/or hydrothorax.
2. Animals with marked proteinuria, hypoalbuminemia, and edema may benefit from maneuvers designed to limit proteinuria.
   a. Dietary protein intake directly affects both renal excretion and hepatic synthesis of protein.[81] In many animals, dietary protein restriction modifies plasma albumin concentration very little, since reductions in dietary protein intake may reduce both hepatic synthesis and renal excretion of protein, resulting in approximately equal opposing effects on plasma albumin concentration. The net effects, however, vary with the individual, and little is known about the net effects of dietary protein restriction on serum albumin concentration in dogs and cats with nephrotic syndrome. Dietary protein restriction, to approximately 2.0 to 3.0 g/kg body weight per day in dogs (commercial diets consisting of approximately 14 to 20% protein on a dry matter basis) and 4.0 g/kg body weight per day in cats (commercial diets consisting of approximately 28 to 32% protein on a dry matter basis), is appropriate for animals with nephrotic syndrome. Careful monitoring is required to determine the net effect of dietary therapy on serum albumin concentration.
   b. Antihypertensive medications may reduce proteinuria, through effects on systemic arterial pressure, glomerular hemodynamics, or glomerular permselectivity. Angiotensin-converting enzyme inhibitors and calcium channel antagonists have been evaluated in an experimental model of diabetic glomerulopathy in dogs.[22,54] Although both reduced the extent of proteinuria, the calcium channel antagonist promoted glomerulosclerosis. Angiotensin-converting enzyme inhibitors seem to be the agents of choice for diabetic animals. At this time, no data support the preferential use of one agent of this group of compounds. Administration of angiotensin-converting enzyme inhibitors may reduce proteinuria without affecting hepatic synthesis, regardless of protein intake. If so, a larger amount of dietary protein may be given to encourage hepatic synthesis.
   c. Nonsteroidal anti-inflammatory agents may reduce the extent of proteinuria.
      (1). Nonsteroidal anti-inflammatory agents may lower glomerular capillary pressure and the extent of proteinuria, possibly by reducing glomerular production of vasodilatory prostanoids believed to be responsible for afferent arteriolar dilation.[100]
      (2). Because of the gastrointestinal and renal toxicity of these compounds and their unproven efficacy in dogs and cats, they cannot be recommended for routine use at this time. Thromboxane synthase inhibitors may be a related therapeutic alternative, and, theoretically, they possess less potential for toxicity. Commercially available agents are not yet readily available.

B. Edema: Therapy consists of sequential use of the following measures:

1. Efforts designed to effect a positive balance of albumin. (See Section VIIIA of this chapter.)
2. Dietary sodium restriction; Reduce intake to 15 to 40 mg/kg per day by feeding a diet containing 0.1 to 0.4% sodium.
3. Diuretics.
   a. Thiazide or loop diuretics are acceptable.
   b. Potassium supplementation should be considered.
   c. Volume depletion associated with hypoalbuminemia, dietary sodium restriction, and aggressive diuretic therapy may result in weakness from systemic hypotension.

C. Hypercoagulable state.[65]

1. Pulmonary and systemic thromboses have been reported in a variety of glomerular diseases.
2. A deficiency of antithrombin III and hypoalbuminemia is causally associated with a hypercoagulable state in dogs and humans.
3. Efforts to effect a positive albumin balance should be instituted. (See Section VIIIA of this chapter.)
4. Dogs with less than 70% of normal antithrombin III activity should receive anticoagulant therapy (e.g., aspirin or heparin).[65] Heparin utilizes antithrombin III as a cofactor and enhances the turnover of antithrombin III. Consequently, animals with marked reduction of antithrombin III activity

may be less responsive to heparin than to other anticoagulant drugs.

D. Progressive renal dysfunction.

1. Therapy aimed at the primary inciting factor should receive consideration. Secondary therapy, such as dietary modification, may be appropriate.
2. Maneuvers designed to slow progression of renal disease from nonimmune factors include dietary phosphate restriction, dietary protein restriction, antihypertensive therapy, dietary alkalinization, modification of dietary fatty acid composition, and eradication of urinary tract infections.
   a. With the exception of dietary phosphate restriction in dogs and cats with reduced renal function,[24,50,114] angiotensin-converting enzyme inhibitors in dogs with diabetic nephropathy,[22,54] and combined dietary energy and protein restriction in cats with reduced renal function,[3] the efficacy of these maneuvers is generally unknown.
   b. Although dietary protein restriction is employed with a rationale of reducing the extent of glomerular hypertension,[20,26] no controlled studies of the effects of dietary protein restriction on glomerular hemodynamics have been published in dogs or cats with renal dysfunction: however, hyperaminoacidemia, as occurs after protein ingestion, elevates glomerular capillary pressure in normal dogs.[27]
   c. For animals that exhibit clear evidence of progression of renal disease, dietary protein restriction, to approximately 2.0 to 3.0 g/kg body weight per day in dogs (commercial diets consisting of approximately 14 to 20% protein on a dry matter basis) and 4.0 g/kg body weight per day in cats (commercial diets of approximately 28 to 32% protein on a dry matter basis), can be considered. Plasma creatinine and albumin concentration and the urine protein/creatinine ratio should be monitored sequentially. A consistent pattern of beneficial change in these parameters over the subsequent 3 to 6 months is justification for continuing dietary protein restriction; however, if the initial reduction in dietary protein intake is not effective, further reductions to less than 2.0 g/kg body weight per day should be considered in dogs. Restricting dietary protein intake limits renal excretion and hepatic synthesis of protein.[81] The net effect on albumin balance should be assessed in each animal by sequential measurement of serum albumin concentration. Very-low–protein diets should be used with caution, as they may produce hypoalbuminemia and elevations in liver enzymes.
   d. If dietary protein restriction for animals with progressive disease worsens hypoalbuminemia, other therapy designed to slow progression of renal disease should be considered. For example, angiotensin-converting enzyme inhibitors may lower glomerular capillary pressure and the extent of proteinuria, without adversely affecting hepatic synthesis of albumin.

E. In azotemic patients, therapy for secondary events common to the clinical course of renal disease may be required. (See Chapter 22, Acute Renal Failure: Ischemia and Chemical Nephrosis, Chapter 28, Conservative Medical Management of Chronic Renal Failure, Chapter 29, Medical Management of the Anemia of Chronic Renal Failure, and Chapter 31, Application of Peritoneal Dialysis and Hemodialysis in the Management of Renal Failure.) These include: (1) systemic hypertension, (2) hyperparathyroidism, (3) urinary tract infections, (4) anemia, (5) electrolyte and mineral imbalances, and (6) vomiting and other signs of uremia.

VIII. MONITORING THE ANIMAL FOR EVIDENCE OF RESPONSE TO THERAPY IS CRITICAL. DAY-TO-DAY VARIATIONS IN THE URINE PROTEIN/CREATININE RATIO OR SERUM ALBUMIN CONCENTRATION SHOULD NOT BE MISINTERPRETED AS EVIDENCE OF RESPONSE TO THERAPY. EACH PARAMETER SHOULD BE EVALUATED ON THREE OR MORE OCCASIONS BEFORE A DECISION IS MADE TO ALTER THERAPY. A TYPICAL PROTOCOL FOR EVALUATION OF RESPONSE TO THERAPEUTIC MANEUVERS IS OUTLINED AS FOLLOWS:

A. Establish baseline values for urine protein/creatinine ratio (at least 2 measurements separated by at least 2 days), serum albumin concentration, serum creatinine (SC), and blood urea nitrogen (BUN).

B. Administer therapy for a minimum of 4 weeks.

C. Re-evaluate response to therapy by re-evaluating the urine protein/creatinine ratio (at least 2 measurements separated by at least 2 days), serum albumin concentration, SC, and BUN.

D. Re-evaluate the animal in 1 month.

E. Consider changes in therapy after the second evaluation. In some animals, sequential renal biopsies should be considered to judge effectiveness of therapy or the need for continued therapy, a strategy routinely employed in affected humans.

IX. SECONDARY GLOMERULAR DISEASE IN DOGS AND CATS

A. In dogs, commonly identified secondary glomerulopathies include amyloidosis,[18,32,42–44] neoplasia,[9,30,41,75,88,94,96,116] infectious agents,[9,15,30,61,88,105,133] heartworm disease,[1,29,30,41,62] inflammatory diseases,[15,30,41] familial disorders,[12,21,31,35,42,72,73,77,80,84,93,102,104,109,125,131] systemic

and intrarenal hypertension,[22,54] radiation,[68,76,139] excess endogenous or exogenous steroids,[15,30] diabetes mellitus,[22,54,121] immune deficiency,[36] and drug therapy.[56,86,134]

B. In cats, glomerulopathies frequently are associated with viral infections and are usually manifested as membranous nephropathy. (See Section III E of this chapter.)

C. See Chapter 19, Pathophysiology and Management of Systemic Hypertension Associated with Renal Dysfunction, Chapter 20, Renal Amyloidosis, Chapter 24, Congenital, Inherited, and Familial Renal Diseases, and Chapter 26, Renal Manifestations of Polysystemic Diseases, for a review of these disorders.

REFERENCES

1. Abramowsky CR, Powers M, Aikawa M, Swinehart G. *Dirofilaria immitis:* 5. Immunopathology of filarial nephropathy in dogs. *Am J Pathol.* 1981;104:1.
2. Adams L, Polzin DJ, Osborne CA, O'Brien TD, Hostetter TH. Influence of dietary protein/calorie intake on renal morphology and function in cats with 5/6 nephrectomy. *Lab Invest.* 1994;70:347.
3. Adams LG, Polzin DJ, Osborne CA, O'Brien TD. Effects of dietary protein and calorie restriction in clinically normal cats and in cats with surgically induced chronic renal failure. *Am J Vet Res.* 1993;54:1653.
4. Anderson LA, Jarrett W. Membranous glomerulonephritis associated with leukaemia in cats. *Res Vet Sci.* 1971;12:179.
5. Anderson S, Meyer TW, Rennke HG, et al. Control of glomerular hypertension limits glomerular injury in rats with reduced renal mass. *J Clin Invest* 1985;76:612.
6. Arthur J, Lucke V, Newby T, Bourne F. An immunohistological study of feline glomerulonephritis using the peroxidase-antiperoxidase method. *Res Vet Sci.* 1984;37:12.
7. Arthur JE, Lucke VM, Newby TJ, Bourne FJ. The long-term prognosis of feline membranous glomerulonephritis. *J Am Anim Hosp Assoc.* 1986;22:731.
8. Banks KL, Henson JB. Immunologically mediated glomerulitis in horses. *Lab Invest.* 1972;26:708.
9. Benderitter T, Casanova P, Nashkidachvili L, Quilici M. Glomerulonephritis in dogs with canine leishmaniasis. *Trop Med Parasitol.* 1988;82:335.
10. Berger J. IgA glomerular deposits in renal disease. *Transplant Proc.* 1969;1:939.
11. Bernard D. Extrarenal complications of the nephrotic syndrome. *Kidney Int.* 1988;33:1184.
12. Bernard MA, Valli VE. Familial renal disease in Samoyed dogs. *Can Vet J.* 1977;18:181.
13. Bidani A, Mitchell K, Schwartz MM, Navar LG, Lewis EJ. Absence of glomerular injury or nephron loss in a normotensive rat remnant kidney model. *Kidney Int.* 1990;38:28.
14. Bidani AK, Schwartz MM, Lewis EJ. Renal autoregulation and vulnerability to hypertensive injury in remnant kidney. *Am J Physiol.* 1987;252:F1003.
15. Biewanga WJ. Proteinuria in the dog: A clinicopathological study in 51 proteinuric dogs. *Res Vet Sci.* 1986;41:257.
16. Biewanga WJ, Gruys E, Hendricks HJ. Urinary protein loss in the dog: nephrological study of 29 dogs without signs of renal disease. *Res Vet Sci.* 1982;33:366.
17. Bown P. Glomerulonephritis in the dog: A clinical review. *J Sm Anim Pract.* 1977;18:93.
18. Boyce J, DiBartola SP, Chew DJ, Gasper PW. Familial renal amyloidosis in Abyssinian cats. *Vet Pathol.* 1984;21:33.
19. Brenner B, Hostetter T, Humes H. Molecular basis of proteinuria of glomerular origin. *N Engl J Med.* 1978;298:826.
20. Brenner BM, Meyer TW, Hostetter TH. Dietary protein intake and the progressive nature of renal disease: The role of hemodynamically mediated glomerular injury in the pathogenesis of progressive glomerular sclerosis in aging, renal ablation, and intrinsic renal disease. *N Engl J Med.* 1982; 307:652.
21. Brown CA, Crowell WA, Brown SA, Barsanti JA, Finco DR. Suspected familial renal disease in chow chows. *J Am Vet Med Assoc.* 1990;196:1279.
22. Brown S, Walton C, Crawford P, Bakris G. Long-term effects of antihypertensive regimens on renal hemodynamics and proteinuria. *Kidney Int.* 1993;43:1210.
23. Brown SA, Crowell WA, Barsanti JA, White JV, Finco DR. Beneficial effects of dietary mineral restriction in dogs with marked reduction of functional renal mass. *J Am Soc Nephr.* 1991;1:1169.
24. Brown SA, Finco DR, Crowell WA, et al. Beneficial effect of moderate phosphate restriction in partially nephrectomized dogs on a low protein diet. *Kidney Int.* 1987;31:380.
25. Brown SA, Finco DR, Crowell WA, Choat DC, Navar LG. Single-nephron adaptations to partial renal ablation in the dog. *Am J Physiol.* 1990;258:F495.
26. Brown SA, Finco DR, Crowell WA, Navar LG. Dietary protein intake and the glomerular adaptations to partial nephrectomy in dogs. *J Nutrition.* 1991;121:S125.
27. Brown SA, Navar LG. Single-nephron responses to systemic administration of amino acids in dogs. *Am J Physiol.* 1990;259: F736.
28. Carpenter J, Andelman N, Moore F, King N. Idiopathic cutaneous and renal glomerular vasculopathy of greyhounds. *Vet Pathol.* 1988;25:401.
29. Casery HW, Splitter GA. Membranous glomerulonephritis in dogs infected with *Dirofilaria immitis. Vet Pathol.* 1975;12:111.
30. Center S, Smith C, Wilkinson E, Erb H, Lewis R. Clinicopathologic, renal immunofluorescent, and light microscopic features of glomerolonephritis in the dog: 41 cases (1975–1985). *J Am Vet Med Assoc.* 1987;190:81.
31. Chew DJ, DiBartola SP, Boyce JT, et al. Juvenile renal disease in Doberman pinscher dogs. *J Am Vet Med Assoc.* 1983;182:481.
32. Chew DJ, DiBartola SP, Boyce JT, Gasper PW. Renal amyloidosis in related Abyssinian cats. *J Am Vet Med Assoc.* 1982; 181:139.
33. Codner EC, Caceci T, Saunders GK, et al. Investigation of glomerular lesions in dogs with acute experimentally induced *Ehrlichia canis* infection. *Am J Vet Res.* 1992;53:2286.
34. Commens P. Experimental hydralazine disease and its similarity to disseminated lupus erythematosus. *J Lab Clin Med.* 1956;47:444.
35. Cook SM, Dean DF, Golden DL, Wilkinson JE, Means TL. Renal failure attributable to atrophic glomerulopathy in four related Rottweilers. *J Am Vet Med Assoc.* 1993;202:107.
36. Cork LC, Morris JM, Olson JL, Krakowka S, Swift AJ, Winkelstein. Membranoproliferative glomerulonephritis in dogs with a genetically determined deficiency of the third component of complement. *Clin Immunol Immunopathol.* 1991;60:455.
37. Cowgill LD, Kallet AJ. Recognition and management of hypertension in the dog. In: Kirk RW, eds. *Current Veterinary Therapy VIII.* Philadelphia, Pennsylvania: WB Saunders; 1983:1025.
38. Crowell W, Barsanti J. Membranous glomerulopathy in two feline siblings. *J Am Vet Med Assoc.* 1983;182:1244.
39. Demacker PNM, van Heijst PJ, Hak-Lemmers HLM, Stalenhof

AFH. A study of the lipid transport system in the cat, *Felix domesticus*. *Atherosclerosis*. 1987;66:113.

40. DiBartola S, Rutgers H, Zack P, Tarr M. Clinicopathologic findings associated with chronic renal disease in cats: 74 cases (1973–1984). *J Am Vet Med Assoc*. 1987;190:1196.
41. DiBartola S, Spaulding G, Chew D, Lewis R. Urinary protein excretion and immunopathologic findings in dogs with glomerular disease. *J Am Vet Med Assoc*. 1980;177:73.
42. DiBartola S, Tarr M, Webb D, Giger U. Familial renal amyloidosis in Chinese Shar Pei dogs. *J Am Vet Med Assoc*. 1990;197:483.
43. DiBartola SP, Tarr MJ, Benson MD. Tissue distribution of amyloid deposits in Abyssinian cats with familial amyloidosis. *J Comp Pathol*. 1986;96:387.
44. DiBartola SP, Tarr MJ, Webb DM, et al. Clinicopathological findings in dogs with renal amyloidosis: 59 cases (1976–1986). *J Am Vet Med Assoc*. 1989;195:358.
45. Donadio J. The limitations of renal biopsy. *Am J Kidney Dis*. 1982;1:249.
46. Emancipator SN, Gallo GR, Razaboni R, Lamm ME. Experimental cholestasis promotes the deposition of glomerular IgA immune complexes. *Am J Pathol*. 1983;113:19.
47. Fairley KF, Birch DF. Hematuria: A simple method for identifying glomerular bleeding. *Kidney Int*. 1982;21:105.
48. Farrow BRH, Huxtable CR, McGovern VJ. Membranous nephropathy and the nephrotic syndrome in the cats. *J Comp Pathol*. 1971;81:463.
49. Feinstein E, Kaptien E, Nicoloff J, Massry S. Thyroid function in patients with nephrotic syndrome and normal renal function. *Am J Nephrol*. 1982;2:70.
50. Finco DR, Brown SA, Crowell WA, Groves CA, Duncan JR, Barsanti JA. Effects of phosphorous/calcium-restricted and phosphorous/calcium-replete 32% protein diets in dogs with chronic renal failure. *Am J Vet Res*. 1992;53:157.
51. Fisher ER, Fisher B. Glomerular lipoidosis in the dog. *Am J Vet Res*. 1954;285:285.
52. Francis DP, Essex M, Jakowski RM, Cotter SM, Lerer TJ, Hardy WD. Increased risk for lymphoma and glomerulonephritis in a closed population of cats exposed to feline leukemia virus. *Am J Epidemiol*. 1980;111:337.
53. Fukatsu A, Matsuo S, Killen P, et al. The glomerular distribution of type IV collagen and laminin in human membranous glomerulonephritis. *Hum Pathol*. 1988;19:64.
54. Gaber L, Walton C, Brown S, Bakris G. Effects of antihypertensive agents on the morphologic progression of diabetic nephropathy in dogs. *Kidney Int*. 1994;46:161.
55. Garber D, Gottlieb B, March JB, Sparks C. Catabolism of very low–density lipoproteins in experimental nephrosis. *J Clin Invest*. 1984;74:1375.
56. Giger U, Werner LL, Millichamp NJ, et al. Sulfadiazine-induced allergy in six Doberman pinschers. *J Am Vet Med Assoc*. 1985; 186:479.
57. Glassock R, et al. Primary glomerular diseases. In: Brenner B, Rector F, eds. *The Kidney*. Philadelphia, Pennsylvania: WB Saunders; 1991:1182.
58. Glick AD, Horn RG, Holscher M. Characterization of feline glomerulonephritis associated with viral-induced hematopoietic neoplasms. *Am J Pathol*. 1978;92:321.
59. Goldstein D, Oda Y, Kurokawa K, Massry S. Blood levels of 25-hydroxy vitamin D in nephrotic syndrome. *Ann Intern Med*. 1977;87:664.
60. Goldwasser P, Antignani, Norbergs A, et al. Urinary red blood cell volume differentiates glomerular and non-glomerular hematuria. *Kidney Int*. 1988;33:191.
61. Grauer G. Renal lesions associated with *Borrelia burgdorferi* infection in a dog. *J Am Vet Med Assoc*. 1988;193:237.
62. Grauer G, Culham C, Dubielzig R, Longhofer S, Grieve R. Experimental *Dirofilaria immitis*–associated glomerulonephritis induced in part by in situ formation of glomerular capillary wall. *J Parasitol*. 1989;75:585.
63. Grauer G, Culman C, Dubielzig R, et al. Effects of a specific thromboxane synthetase on development of experimental *Dirofilaria immitis* immune complex glomerulonephritis in the dog. *J Vet Intern Med*. 1988;2:192.
64. Grauer GF, Frisbie DD, Snyder PS, Dubielzig RR, Panciera DL. Treatment of membranoproliferative glomerulonephritis and nephrotic syndrome in a dog with thromboxane synthetase inhibitor. *J Vet Intern Med*. 1992;6:77.
65. Green R, Kabel A. Hypercoagulable state in 3 dogs with nephrotic syndrome: Role of acquired antithrombin III deficiency. *J Am Vet Med Assoc*. 1982;181:914.
66. Green RA, Russo EA, Greene RT, Kabel AL. Hypoalbuminemia-related platelet hypersensitivity in two dogs with nephrotic syndrome. *J Am Vet Med Assoc*. 1985;186:485.
67. Grindem CB, Johnson KH. Systemic lupus erythematosus: Literature review and report of 42 new canine cases. *J Am Anim Hosp Assoc*. 1983;19:489.
68. Guttman PH, Andersen AC. Progressive intercapillary glomerulosclerosis in aging and irradiated beagles. *J Pathol*. 1968; 35:45.
69. Hahley RW, Weisgraber KH. Canine lipoproteins and atherosclerosis I. Isolation and characterization of plasma lipoproteins from control dogs. *Circ Res*. 1974;35:713.
70. Harris CH, Krawiec DR, Gelberg HB, Shapiro SZ. Canine IgA glomerulonephropathy. *Vet Immunol Immunopathol*. 1993;36:1.
71. Hayashi T, Ishida T, Fujiwara K. Glomerulonephritis associated with feline infectious peritonitis. *Jpn J Vet Sci*. 1982;44:909.
72. Hood JC, Robinson WF, Clark WT, et al. Proteinuria as an indicator of early renal disease in bull terriers with hereditary nephritis. *J Small Anim Pract*. 1991;32:241.
73. Hood JC, Robinson WF, Huxtable CR, Bradley JS, Sutherland RJ, Thomas MAB. Hereditary nephritis in the bull terrier: Evidence for inheritance by an autosomal dominant gene. *Vet Rec*. 1990;126:456.
74. Ihrke PJ, Norton AL, Ling GV, Stannard AA. Urinary tract infection associated with longterm corticosteroid administration in dogs with chronic skin diseases. *J Am Vet Med Assoc*. 1985;184:43.
75. Jaenke R, Allen T. Membranous nephropathy in the dog. *Vet Pathol*. 1986;23:718.
76. Jaenke R, Phemister R, Norrdin R. Progressive glomerulosclerosis and renal failure following perinatal gamma radiation in the beagle. *Lab Invest*. 1980;42:643.
77. Jansen B, Valli V, Thorner P, Baumal R, Lumsden J. Samoyed hereditary glomerulopathy: Serial clinical and laboratory studies. *Can J Vet Res*. 1987;51:387.
78. Jeraj K, Vernier R, Polzin D, et al. Idiopathic immune complex glomerulonephritis in dogs with multisystem involvement. *Am J Vet Res*. 1984;45:1699.
79. Jeraj KP, Hardy R, O'Leary TP, Vernier RL, Michael AF. Immune complex glomerulonephritis in a cat with renal lymphosarcoma. *Vet Pathol*. 1985;22:287.
80. Jones BR, Gething MA, Badcoe LM, Pauli JV, Davies E. Familial progressive nephropathy in young bull terriers. *N Z Vet J*. 1989;37:79.
81. Kaysen G, Jones H, Martin V, Hutchison F. A low-protein diet restricts albumin synthesis in nephrotic rats. *J Clin Invest*. 1989;83:1623.
82. Keane WF, Kasiske BL, O'Donnell MP. Hyperlipidemia and the progression of renal disease. *Am J Clin Nutr*. 1988;47:157.
83. Koeman JP, Biewanga WJ, Gruys E. Proteinuria in the dog: A

pathomorphological study of 51 proteinuric dogs. *Res Vet Sci.* 1987;43:367.

84. Koeman JP, Biewanga WJ, Gruys E. Proteinuria associated with glomerulosclerosis and glomerular collagen formation in three Newfoundland dog littermates. *Vet Pathol.* 1994;31:188.
85. Kurtz JM, et al. Naturally occurring canine glomerulonephritis. *Am J Pathol.* 1972;67:471.
86. Leifer CE, Page RL, Matus RE, Patnaik AK, MacEwen EG. Proliferative glomerulonephritis and chronic active hepatitis with cirrhosis associated with *Corynebacterium parvum* immunotherapy in a dog. *J Am Vet Med Assoc.* 1987;190:78.
87. Longhofer SL, Frisbie DD, Johnson HC, et al. Effects of thromboxane synthetase inhibition on immune complex glomerulonephritis. *Am J Vet Res.* 1991;52:480.
88. MacDougall DG, Cook T, Steward AP, Cattell V. Canine chronic renal disease: Prevalence and types of glomerulonephritis in the dog. *Kidney Int.* 1986;29:1144.
89. MacKay K, Striker LJ, Stauffer JW, Agodoa LY, Striker GE. Relationship of glomerular hypertrophy and sclerosis: Studies in SV 40 transgenic mice. *Kidney Int.* 1990;37:741.
90. Manning PJ, Corwin LA, Middleton CC. Familial hyperlipoproteinemia and thyroid dysfunction of beagles. *Exp Molec Pathol.* 1973;19:378.
91. Miyauchi Y, Nakayama H, Uchida K, Uetska K, Hasegawa A, Goto N. Glomerulopathy with IgA deposition in the dog. *J Vet Med Sci.* 1992;54:969.
92. Morel-Maroger L. The value of renal biopsy. *Am J Kid Dis.* 1982;1:244.
93. Morton LD, Sanecki RK, Gordon DE, Sopiarz RL, Bell JS, Sakas PS. Juvenile renal disease in miniature schnauzer dogs. *Vet Pathol.* 1990;27:455.
94. Muller-Peddinghaus R, Trautwein G. Spontaneous glomerulonephritis in dogs II. Correlation of glomerulonephritis with age, chronic interstitial nephritis and extrarenal lesions. *Vet Pathol.* 1977;14:121.
95. Muller-Peddinghaus R, Trautwein G. Spontaneous glomerulonephritis in dogs I. Classification and immunopathology. *Vet Pathol.* 1977;14:1.
96. Murray M, Wright N. A morphological study of canine glomerulonephritis. *Lab Invest.* 1974;30:213.
97. Nash A. Familial renal disease in dogs. *J Small Anim Pract.* 1989;30:178.
98. Nash A, Wright N. Membranous nephropathy in sibling cats. *Vet Rec.* 1983;113:180.
99. Nash A, Wright N, Spencer A, Thompson H, Fisher E. Membranous nephropathy in the cat: A clinical and pathological study. *Vet Rec.* 1979;105:71.
100. Nath KA, Chmielewski DH, Hostetter TH. Regulatory role of prostanoids in glomerular microcirculation of remnant nephrons. *Am J Physiol.* 1987;252:F829.
101. Osborne CA, Hammer RF, Resnick JS, Stevens JB, Yano BL, Vernier RL. Natural remission of nephrotic syndrome in a dog with immune-complex glomerular disease. *J Am Vet Med Assoc.* 1976;168:129.
102. Osborne CA, O'Brien T. Renal dysplasia in Lhasa Apso and Shih Tzu dogs. In: Kirk RW eds. *Current Veterinary Therapy VIII.* Philadelphia, Pennsylvania: WB Saunders; 1983:971.
103. Osborne CA, Vernier RL. Glomerulonephritis in the dog and cat: A comparative review. *J Am Anim Hosp Assoc.* 1973;9:101.
104. Picut C, Lewis R. Juvenile renal disease in the Doberman pinscher: Ultrastructural changes of the glomerular basement membrane. *Comp Pathol.* 1987;97:587.
105. Poli A, Abramo F, Mancianti F, Nigro M, Pieri S, Bionda A. Renal involvement in canine leishmaniasis. *Nephron.* 1991;57:444.
106. Poli A, Abramo F, Taccini E, et al. Renal involvement in feline immunodeficiency virus infection: A clinicopathological study. *Nephron.* 1993;64:282.
107. Polzin DL, Leininger JR, Osborne CA, Jeraj K. Development of renal lesions in dogs after 11/12 reduction of renal mass. *Lab Invest.* 1988;58:172.
108. Purkerson ML, Hoffstein PE, Klahr S. Pathogenesis of the glomerulopathy associated with renal infarction in rats. *Kidney Int.* 1976;9:407.
109. Reusche VT, Liehs M, Bren G. A new familial membranoproliferative glomerulonephritis in Bernese mountain dogs. *J Vet Intern Med.* 1992;6:120.
110. Riviere JE, Coppoc GL, Hinsman EJ, et al. Gentamicin pharmacokinetics changes in induced acute canine nephrotoxic glomerulonephritis. *Antimicrob Agents Chemother.* 1981;20:387.
111. Rogers WA, Donovan EF, Kociba GJ. Lipids and lipoproteins in normal dogs and in dogs with secondary hyperlipoproteinemia. *J Am Vet Med Assoc.* 1975;166:1092.
112. Rose G, et al. The treatment of severe glomerulopathies in children using high-dose intravenous methylprednisolone pulses. *Am J Kid Dis.* 1981;1:148.
113. Ross LA, Finco DR. Relationship of selected clinical renal function tests to glomerular filtration rate and renal blood flow in cats. *Am J Vet Res.* 1981;42:1704.
114. Ross LA, Finco DR, Crowell WA. Effect of dietary phosphorus restriction on the kidneys of cats with reduced renal mass. *Am J Vet Res.* 1982;43:1023.
115. Rostokev G, Parent T, Peck M, et al. Natural anticoagulase factors in adult nephrotic syndrome. *Clin Nephrol.* 1988;29:214.
116. Rouse B, Lewis R. Canine glomerulonephritis: Prevalence in dogs submitted at random for euthanasia. *Can J Comp Med.* 1975;39:365.
117. Saegusa S, Shimizu F, Nagase M, Hasegawa A. Concurrent feline immune-complex nephritis. *Arch Pathol Lab Med.* 1979;103:475.
118. Slauson D, Russell S, Schechter R. Naturally occurring immune complex glomerulonephritis in the cat. *J Pathol.* 1971;103:131.
119. Slauson DO, Griggle DH. Thrombosis complicating renal amyloidosis in dogs. *Vet Pathol.* 1971;8:352.
120. Slauson DO, Lewis RM. Comparative pathology of glomerulonephritis in animals. *Vet Pathol.* 1979;16:135.
121. Steffes MW, Buchwald H, Wigness BD, et al. Diabetic nephropathy in the uninephrectomized dog: Microscopic lesions after one year. *Kidney Int.* 1982;21:721.
122. Striker G. Controversy: The role of renal biopsy in modern medicine. *Am J Kid Dis.* 1982;1:241.
123. Stuart B, Phemister R, Thomassen R. Glomerular lesions associated with proteinuria in clinically healthy dogs. *Vet Pathol.* 1975;12:125.
124. Vaden SL, et al. Effects of cyclosporine A in dogs with glomerular disease. *J Vet Intern Med.* (in review, 1994).
125. Vilafranca M, Ferrer L. Juvenile nephropathy in Alaskan malamute littermates. *Vet Pathol.* 1994;31:375.
126. Vilafranca M, Wohlsein P, Leopold-Temmler B, Trautwein G. A canine nephropathy resembling minimal change nephrotic syndrome in man. *J Comp Pathol.* 1993;109:271.
127. Vogt A, Batsford S, Rodrigues-Iturbe B, Garcia R. Cationic antigens in poststreptococcal glomerulonephritis. *Clin Nephrol.* 1983;20:271.
128. Walser M, Ward L. Progression of chronic renal failure is related to glucocorticoid production. *Kidney Int.* 1988;34:859.
129. Wetzels J, Sluiter H, Hortsma A, et al. Prednisolone can increase glomerular permeability to proteins in nephrotic syndrome. *Kidney Int.* 1988;33:1169.
130. Whiteside C, Katz A, Cho C, Silverman M. Diabetic glomeru-

lopathy following unilateral nephrectomy in the dog. *Clin Invest Med.* 1990;13:279.

131. Wilcock B, Patterson J. Familial glomerulonephritis in Doberman pinscher dogs. *Can Vet J.* 1979;20:244.
132. Wilson CB. The renal response to immunologic injury. In: Brenner B, Rector, eds. *The Kidney.* Philadelphia, Pennsylvania: WB Saunders; 1991:1062.
133. Wright N, Cornwell H. Experimental canine adenovirus glomerulonephritis: Histological, immunofluorescence and ultrastructural features of the early glomerular changes. *Br J Exp Pathol.* 1983;64:312.
134. Wright N, Nash A. Experimental ampicillin glomerulonephropathy. *J Comp Pathol.* 1984;94:357.
135. Wright N, Path M, Nash A, Thompson H, Fisher E. Membranous nephropathy in the cat and dog. *Lab Invest.* 1981;45:269.
136. Wright NG, Nash AS. Glomerulonephritis in the dog and cat. *Irish Vet J.* 1983;37:4.
137. Wright NG, Thompson H, Cornwell HJC. Canine nephrotoxic glomerulonephritis: A combined light, immunofluorescent, and ultrastructural study. *Vet Pathol.* 1973;10:69.
138. Yedgar S, Eilam O, Shafrir E. Regulation of plasma lipid levels by plasma viscosity in nephrotic rats. *Am J Physiol.* 1985;248: E10.
139. Zook BC, Bradley JW, Rogers CC. Morphologic effects of fast neutrons or photons on the canine kidney. *Int J Radiol Oncol Biol Physiol.* 1992;23:821.

CHAPTER 18

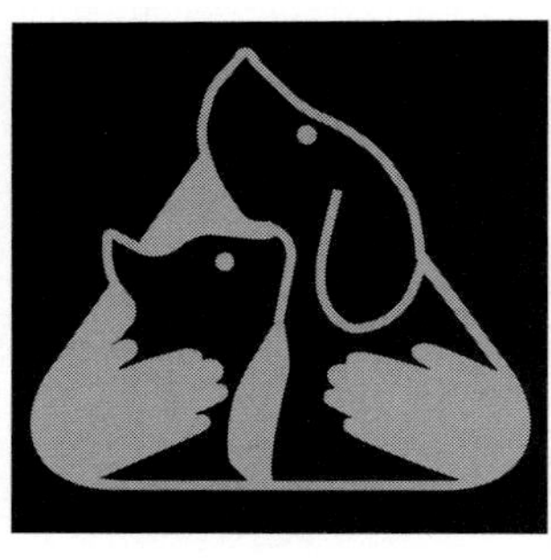

Primary Tubulo-Interstitial Diseases of the Kidney

DELMAR R. FINCO
CATHY A. BROWN

I. INTRODUCTION

A. Description.

1. Primary tubulo-interstitial diseases are characterized by a predominance of tubular and interstitial lesions compared to glomerular lesions.
2. Mononuclear cell (lymphocyte, plasma cell) infiltration, tubular atrophy, and interstitial and periglomerular fibrosis are common lesions (see Fig. 18–1). These lesions lead to occupation of less space by functional tubules, and thus interstitial volume or interstitial space is increased.

B. Clinical correlation.

1. Most dogs and cats with end-stage renal disease have lesions that pathologists categorize as predominantly tubulo-interstitial disease. Although glomerular lesions often are present, they usually appear less severe than the tubulo-interstitial lesions.
2. In advanced stages of kidney damage, determining the primary or initiating site of damage (glomerular versus tubulo-interstitial) is difficult if not impossible.
3. Many dogs and cats with chronic, end-stage renal disease have mild to moderate proteinuria, compared to the severe proteinuria observed with many forms of primary glomerular disease. This observation suggests (but does not prove) that the tubulo-interstitial lesions are primary.
4. Studies of naturally occurring renal diseases of humans indicate that, even when glomerular disease is primary, tubulo-interstitial lesions develop. Although unexplained, several studies of human glomerular disease indicate that the histologic character of the tubulointerstitium is better correlated with glomerular filtration rate (GFR) and with progression of renal failure than are glomerular lesions.[2,11,15]
5. Thus, reason dictates that the state of the tubulo-interstitium should be considered in the clinical management of renal diseases of the dog and cat.
6. Subsequently, several possible mechanisms for development of primary tubulo-interstitial disease will be described. Clinically, one should recognize that primary tubulo-interstitial nephritis represents an anatomic localization and a histologic description, but not a specific etiologic diagnosis.

II. ANATOMIC AND PHYSIOLOGIC STATE OF THE RENAL TUBULO-INTERSTITIUM

A. Morphologic characteristics of renal tubules are well described by anatomists (see Chapter 1, Applied Anatomy of the Urinary System with Clinicopathologic Correlation), but the nature of the renal interstitium and the dynamics of its function have received less attention. Certain aspects of structure-function

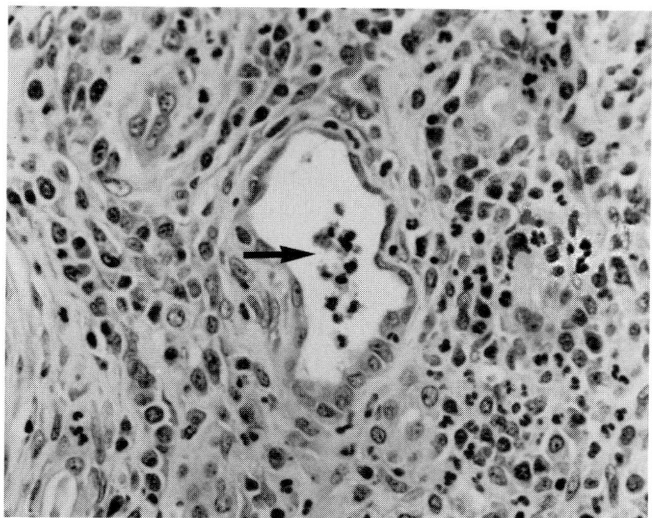

FIG. 18–1. Acute tubulo-interstitial nephritis in a dog with leptospirosis. Note the interstitial inflammatory cells and the neutrophils within dilated tubules (arrow).

relationships of the tubulo-interstitium are relevant to disease.

B. **Hemodynamics, transport functions.**
   1. High intraglomerular capillary pressure may place glomeruli at risk for pressure damage.
      a. A popular theory of progression of renal failure is based on glomerular capillary hypertension secondary to systemic hypertension or afferent arteriolar dilation.
      b. Primary tubulo-interstitial damage may impede peritubular capillary flow and thus increase intraglomerular pressure by such outflow impingement. Thus, glomerular injury may occur secondary to tubulo-interstitial disease.
   2. Renal tubules and the interstitium are not at jeopardy from high intravascular hydraulic forces because cortical peritubular capillaries and vasa recta are low-pressure vessels. However, the tubules depend on adequate flow of blood from the glomeruli via the efferent glomerular arterioles and the peritubular capillaries. Renal cortical blood flow rate is high, and thus delivery of blood components to the cortical tubules is high. This flow rate is coupled with high metabolic rate of tubular cells compared to glomerular cells, making tubular cells particularly vulnerable to ischemia and to nephrotoxic agents.
   3. Medullary blood flow via vasa recta is much slower than cortical flow. Consequently, the ascending limb of the loop of Henle, which is very active metabolically, is even more vulnerable to ischemia than is the cortex.
   4. Experimental chronic renal ischemia in rats results in marked tubulo-interstitial damage with good preservation of glomerular structure. Researchers have postulated that the ischemia alters the antigenic profile of tubular epithelium, thereby initiating a cell-mediated immune response.[13] (See Section IIIB of this chapter.)

C. **Renal interstitial space represents space between tubular and vascular structures.**
   1. Overall renal interstitial space normally occupies about 7% of renal volume, but percentage increases progressively from cortex to renal papilla.[1]
   2. Extracellular matrix in the interstitium is a hydrated gel composed of glycosaminoglycans.
   3. Enmeshed in the gel are fibers of collagen, fibronectin, and vitronectin. These are connected to tubule basement membrane constituents.
   4. Massive amounts of water and particles move through the interstitial space in the course of tubular modification of glomerular filtrate. Thus, processes impeding this traffic, such as inflammation and fibrosis, may interfere with tubular functions on a purely mechanical basis.

D. **Normal cells of the renal interstitium.**[1]
   1. Cell infiltration into renal interstitium occurs, but resident cells also may play a role in tubulo-interstitial nephritis.
   2. Two types of interstitial cortical cell types have been described.
      a. A fibroblast-like cell is most abundant.
      b. A lymphocyte-like cell also exists.
   3. Three types of interstitial medullary cells have been described in the inner stripe and inner zone.
      a. A lipid-laden fibroblast-like cell.
      b. A lymphocyte-like cell.
      c. A pericyte associated with the vasa recta.
   4. The function of renal interstitial cells is unclear.
      a. The fibroblast-like cells may secrete extracellular ground substances, such as collagen and reticular fibers, and possibly have a phagocytic activity.
      b. Medullary lipid-laden cells may play a role in regulation of systemic blood pressure. Phagocytic functions and structural support functions also have been postulated.
      c. The lymphocytic cells are postulated to be resident progeners for mononuclear cells that accumulate during tubulo-interstitial disease.

III. PATHOGENESIS OF TUBULO-INTERSTITIAL DAMAGE[2,6,10,11,17]

A. **Introduction.**
   1. Study of several models of renal disease has generated considerable information on the genesis of tubulo-interstitial damage.
   2. As with primary glomerular damage, most studies have been conducted in highly inbred strains of rats, and thus may or may not relate to naturally occurring diseases in other species. The following information on pathogenesis should be considered as attractive theory that remains to be proved or disproved in diseases of dogs or cats.
   3. Glomeruli, tubules, or interstitium may be the

initiating site of the process of development of tubulo-interstitial nephritis.

B. Glomerular injury may result in leakage of plasma elements that are noxious to tubule cells by a variety of mechanisms.

1. Glomerular leakage of protein is followed by increased proximal tubule protein endocytosis and degradation by lysosomal enzymes. Excessive or aberrant release of lysosomal enzymes could cause tubulo-interstitial damage.
2. Glomerular proteinuria may affect tubules via immune mechanisms. Plasma complement activation by glomerular processes or by brush border activation of the alternate complement cascade may result in tubule cell injury. Antigens can arrive at the apical surface of proximal tubule cells via glomerular leakage.
3. Glomerular leakage of transferrin may cause tubular injury secondary to transferrin release of iron. Glomerular leakage of red cells also may injure tubules via iron release. Iron can generate oxidants that may damage apical membranes or intracellular structures.
4. Glomerular damage may cause tubulo-interstitial disease via cytokines and growth factors that are generated in diseased glomeruli, but that move to the interstitial space via the glomerular mesangial stalk.

C. Tubular processes.

1. Immune-mediated disease of tubules may be incited by both humoral and cellular mechanisms. Potential but benign antigens presented to the apical membrane of tubule cells via proteinuria or to the basolateral membranes via paracellular channels may be "processed" by tubule cells into molecules inciting immune-mediated disease. Proteins leaked via glomerular lesions and engulfed by pinocytosis may be antigenic without tubular modification.
2. Tubular metabolism may be altered to cause cell injury. Generation of oxidants via "hypermetabolism" may lead to tubule cell injury. Increased ammonium generation, primarily from glutamine, also may cause renal tubule cell injury via complement activation.
3. Increased fluid flow rate through residual nephrons may have adverse consequences. Alterations in tubular wall tension associated with the increased fluid flow rate may cause structural, functional, and biochemical changes.
4. Production of autacoids, cytokines, and growth factors by tubule cells may have adverse effects by recruiting and activating circulating cells or by activating resident interstitial cells (see the following).

D. Interstitial processes.

1. The role of resident interstitial cells versus that of infiltrating cells in the development of tubulo-interstitial disease is not resolved.
2. Increase in mononuclear cells in the interstitium is often interpreted to support an immunologic basis of tubulo-interstitial injury.
3. Several experimental models of immunologically mediated tubulo-interstitial nephritis have been developed, usually in rats, guinea pigs, or rabbits.
4. Models include both antibody and cell-mediated mechanisms and both autologous and heterologous antigens.
5. Efforts have been made to diagnose immune-mediated renal diseases in dogs and cats, but emphasis has been placed on diseases of the glomeruli. (See Chapter 17, Primary Diseases of Glomeruli.)
6. Although not studied in dogs or cats, one intriguing humoral autologous model of tubulo-interstitial nephritis is associated with Tamm-Horsfall protein.
   a. This protein is apparently produced in the ascending limb of the loop of Henle and functions to maintain this segment of the nephron in a water-impermeable state.[4]
   b. In a variety of human tubulo-interstitial nephridites, 32% had periodic acid-Schiff (PAS)-positive deposits that were located identically to immunoreactive Tamm-Horsfall glycoprotein.[18]
   c. Rats immunized with Tamm-Horsfall proteins had *in situ* formation of immune complexes in the ascending limb of the loop of Henle and developed some interstitial lesions.[5]
   d. Immunized guinea pigs developed tubulo-interstitial nephritis, and transfer of spleen cells or lymphocytes of affected guinea pigs to non-immunized guinea pigs caused renal lesions in the nonimmunized animals as well.
7. Fibrosis.[8]
   a. Multiple pathways for induction of fibrosis are known to exist in tissues other than the kidney; the same mechanisms may operate in the kidney.
   b. Fibroblast growth and collagen production can be modulated by several cytokines produced by immune cells.
      (1). Transforming growth factor beta.
      (2). Interleukin-2.
      (3). Platelet-derived growth factor.

IV. CAUSES OF TUBULO-INTERSTITIAL DISEASES

A. Infectious agents.

1. Leptospirosis.
   a. Leptospirosis may be associated with an acute tubulo-interstitial nephritis in dogs (Fig. 18–1).
   b. Common serotypes described include *Leptospira icterohaemorrhagiae* and *L. canicola*, but *L. pomona* and *L. grippotyphosa* also have been incriminated.[12]
   c. Although acute or subacute interstitial nephritis is known to occur with leptospirosis, several

observations suggest that leptospirosis is not a common cause of chronic tubulo-interstitial nephritis.

(1). Chronic tubulo-interstitial nephritis is commonly observed in geographic areas where leptospirosis is not detectable clinically, immunochemically, or serologically.[7]

(2). Dogs that made a clinical recovery from experimental infection with leptospires had no residual renal effects. Azotemia resolved, GFR returned to normal, and histologic lesions of the kidneys were absent for periods of as long as 4 years after acute infection.[9]

d. Leptospirosis is uncommon in cats.

2. Several other multisystem infectious agents are known to cause tubulo-interstitial nephritis, including canine hepatitis virus.[16] However, lesions are not reported to be sufficiently severe to cause clinical signs of renal failure. (See Chapter 26, Renal Manifestations of Polysystemic Diseases.)

3. Pyelonephritis.
   a. Historically, the terms tubulo-interstitial nephritis and pyelonephritis once were used synonymously, and the cause was assumed to be bacterial infection of the urinary tract.
   b. At present, both pyelonephritis and tubulo-interstitial nephritis are histologic diagnoses, and pathologists differ in their opinions regarding use of the terms synonymously.
   c. Cortical contraction (Fig. 18–2) and typical histologic lesions have been produced in dogs with experimentally induced bacterial nephritis, thus indicating that bacterial infection can cause tubulo-interstitial nephritis.[3]
   d. Failure to isolate bacteria from the preponderance of cases of tubulo-interstitial nephritis indicates either that it is an uncommon cause or that lesions persist and progress after infection spontaneously resolves.

4. See Chapter 25, Pyelonephritis.

B. Drugs and chemicals.

1. Many drugs and chemicals that cause tubulo-interstitial disease in human beings have been identified (Table 18–1).
2. See Chapter 22, Acute Renal Failure: Ischemia and Chemical Nephrosis, for a description of some agents causing symptomatic acute tubulo-interstitial nephritis in dogs or cats.
3. A short time interval between exposure and development of signs may link drug or chemical exposure to development of tubulo-interstitial nephritis.
4. By contrast, slow, subtle development of lesions with chronic exposure may mask a cause-effect relationship between drug and chemical exposure and tubulo-interstitial nephritis.

C. Hereditary nephropathies.

1. Several hereditary nephropathies have histologic lesions consistent with primary tubulo-interstitial disease.
2. See Chapter 24, Congenital, Inherited, and Familial Renal Diseases.

D. Other causes.

1. Obstructive uropathy and hydronephrosis. (See Chapter 43, Physical Injuries to the Urinary Tract.)
2. Chronic hypercalcemia. (See Chapter 21, Canine and Feline Hypercalcemic Nephropathy.)
3. Transplantation rejection. (See Chapter 32, Clinical Renal Transplantation.)

E. Primary glomerulopathies versus primary tubulo-interstitial disease.

1. Diseases categorized as primary glomerulonephritis do not have lesions confined to glomeruli. Likewise, diseases categorized as primary tubulo-interstitial nephritis also may have glomerular lesions.
2. Although many theories exist (see Section III of

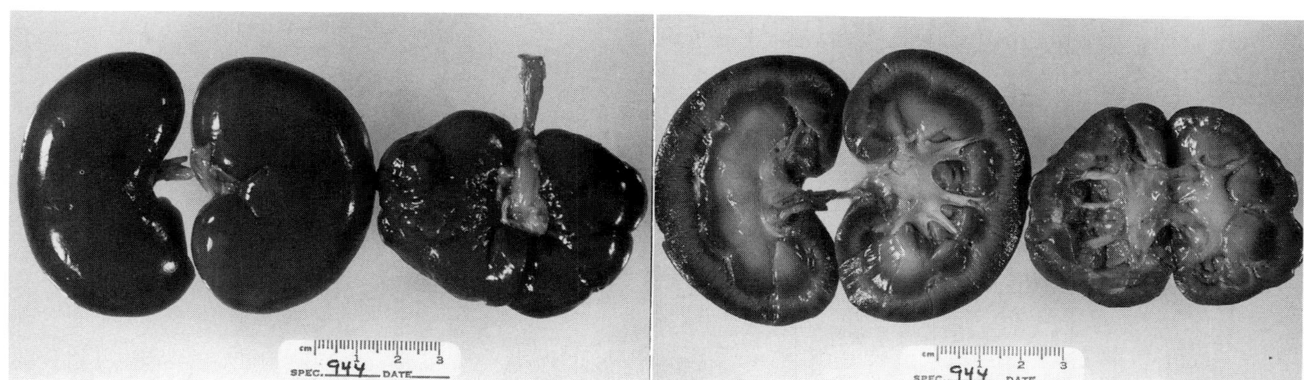

FIG. 18–2. Kidneys from a dog with bacterial nephritis induced unilaterally. The infected kidney is contracted **(A),** and the cortex is narrowed **(B).** Histologically, tubulo-interstitial nephritis was diagnosed.

TABLE 18–1.
DRUGS REPORTED TO CAUSE TUBULO-INTERSTITIAL NEPHRITIS IN HUMAN BEINGS*

Antibiotics	*Analgesics*
β-lactam antibiotics	Several NSAIDs
Penicillin	Aspirin
Methicillin	Phenacetin
Ampicillin	
Amoxicillin	*Other*
Several cephalosporins	Cimetidine
Sulfonamides	Allopurinol
Tetracycline	Phenobarbital
Erythromycin	Diazepam
Aminoglycosides	D-penicillamine
Kanamycin	Captopril
Gentamicin	
Diuretics	
Thiazides	
Furosemide	
Triamterene	
Diazepam	

*Documented cases of the same drugs, causing tubulo-interstitial nephritis in dogs and cats are absent, perhaps because of lack of surveillance.
NSAID = nonsteroidal anti-inflammatory drug.

this chapter), a factual picture of cause-effect relationships between glomerular and tubular lesions remains to be elucidated.

a. The predominant existing component is usually presumed to represent the primary problem, with the lesser component being a result of the major component.
b. No data refute the possibility, however, that the lesser component is self-limiting or regresses prior to discovery, yet nevertheless triggers the major component that leads to discovery of renal disease.

3. Studies on progression of renal failure in rats have incriminated glomerular capillary hypertension as a significant event in the development of glomerular lesions and of kidney damage. However, not all renal lesions of the tubulo-interstitium are explained by glomerular hemodynamic factors.

V. DIAGNOSIS OF PRIMARY TUBULO-INTERSTITIAL NEPHRITIS

A. Tubular deficits.

1. Because of disproportionately greater tubular damage than glomerular damage, clinical detection of primary tubulo-interstitial nephritis may be feasible by documenting disproportionately greater deficits in tubular functions.
2. Mild to moderate proteinuria in instances of severe primary renal failure suggest primary tubulo-interstitial nephritis.
3. Glucosuria, aminoaciduria, or inappropriately increased fractional excretion values for electrolytes suggest primary tubulo-interstitial nephritis and particularly proximal tubule lesions.
4. Hyposthenuria of renal origin suggests primary tubulo-interstitial nephritis and particularly distal tubule and collecting duct dysfunction.
5. Severe metabolic acidosis of renal origin with relative preservation of glomerular function suggests tubulo-interstitial disease.

B. Renal biopsy. Because morphologic findings are the basis of the diagnosis, renal biopsy should aid in diagnosis. (See Chapter 12, Canine and Feline Renal Biopsy.)

C. Limitations of diagnostic efforts.

1. Extrarenal causes of some of the preceding clinical signs must be eliminated from consideration.
2. As primary tubulo-interstitial nephritis progresses, the distinction between deficits in glomerular versus tubular functions narrows and finally disappears with end-stage renal disease.
3. Diagnosis of primary tubulo-interstitial nephritis should be considered a bridge to an etiologic diagnosis rather than a diagnosis in itself. Any specific therapeutic treatment that benefits the patient requires an etiologic diagnosis.

VI. TREATMENT OF PRIMARY TUBULO-INTERSTITIAL NEPHRITIS

A. Treatment is preferably based on an etiologic diagnosis.

B. Symptomatic and supportive treatment may be employed. (See Chapter 22, Acute Renal Failure: Ischemia and Chemical Nephrosis, and Chapter 28, Conservative Medical Management of Chronic Renal Failure.)

REFERENCES

1. Bohman S. The ultrastructure of the renal interstitium. In: Cotran RS, Brenner BM, Stein JH, eds. *Tubulointerstitial Nephropathies.* New York, New York: Churchill Livingstone; 1983.
2. Cameron JS. Tubular and interstitial factors on the progression of glomerulonephritis. *Pediatr Nephrol.* 1992;6:292-302.
3. Finco DR, Shotts EB, Crowell WA. Evaluation of methods for localizing urinary tract infection in the female dog. *Am J Vet Res.* 1979;40:707-712.
4. Howie AJ, et al. Distribution of immunoreactive Tamm-Horsefall protein in various species in the vertebrate classes. *Cell Tissue Res.* 1993;274:15-19.
5. Hoyer JR. Tubulointerstitial immune complex nephritis in rats immunized with Tamm-Horsefall protein. *Kidney Int.* 1980;17: 284-292.
6. Jones CL, Eddy AA. Tubulointerstitial nephritis. *Pediatr Nephrol.* 1992;6:572-586.
7. Krohn K, Mero M, Oksanen A, Sandholm M. Immunologic observations in canine interstitial nephritis. *Am J Pathol.* 1971; 65:157-168.
8. Kuncio GS, Neilson ER, Haverty T. Mechanisms of tubulointerstitial fibrosis. *Kidney Int.* 1991;39:550-556.
9. Low DG, Mather GW, Finco DR, Anderson NV. Longterm studies of renal function in canine leptospirosis. *Am J Vet Res.* 1967;28: 731-739.
10. McClusky RT. Immunologically mediated tubulo-interstitial nephritis. In: Cotran RS, Brenner BM, Stein JH, eds. *Tubulo-*

interstitial Nephropathies. New York, New York: Churchill Livingstone; 1983.

11. Nath KA. Tubulointerstitial changes as a major determinant in the progression of renal damage. *Am J Kidney Dis.* 1992;20:1-17.
12. Rentko VT, et al. Canine leptospirosis: A retrospective study of 17 cases. *J Vet Intern Med.* 1992;6:235-244.
13. Sato K, et al. Tubulointerstitial nephritis induced by Tamm-Horsefall protein sensitization in guinea pigs. *Virchows Arch [B].* 1990;58:357-363.
14. Truong LD, Farhood A, Tasby J, Gillum D. Experimental chronic renal ischemia: Morphologic and immunologic studies. *Kidney Int.* 1992;41:1676-1689.
15. Wehrmann M, Bohle A, Held H. Long-term prognosis of focal sclerosing glomerulonephritis. An analysis of 250 cases with particular regard to tubulointerstitial changes. *Clin Nephrol.* 1990;33:115-122.
16. Wright NG. Interstitial nephritis in the dog associated with infectious canine hepatitis virus. *Vet Rec.* 1970;86:92.
17. Yee J, Kuncio GS, Neilson EG. Tubulointerstitial injury following glomerulonephritis. *Semin Nephrol.* 1991;11:361-366.
18. Zager RA, Cotran RS, Hoyer JR. Pathologic localization of Tamm-Horsefall protein in interstitial deposits in renal disease. *Lab Invest.* 1988;38:52-57.

CHAPTER 19

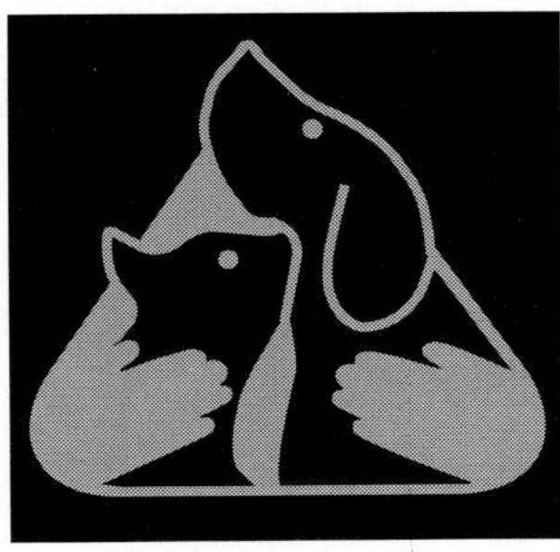

Pathophysiology and Management of Systemic Hypertension Associated with Renal Dysfunction

LINDA A. ROSS

I. NORMAL DETERMINANTS OF BLOOD PRESSURE

A. Physical determinants of blood pressure.

1. Blood pressure is equal to the product of cardiac output times the total peripheral resistance.
2. These two factors are each controlled by a complex interaction of neuroendocrine mechanisms.

B. Neuroendocrine control of blood pressure.

1. Neural control mechanisms
   a. The baroreceptor feedback system is most important in adjusting to short-term (minute-to-minute) changes in arterial pressure. Sensory receptors (baroreceptors) located in the wall of each internal carotid artery just above the bifurcation (carotid sinus) and in the aortic arch respond to changes in arterial pressure by altering neural input to the vasomotor center of the brain. The resulting changes in activity of the vasomotor center affect cardiac output and peripheral resistance to increase or decrease blood pressure appropriately.
   b. Chemoreceptors located in the carotid and aortic bodies sense oxygen content in blood. Their role in blood pressure control is significant only in hypoxic states, when their stimulation excites the vasomotor center of the brain.
   c. The central nervous ischemic response is activated only when blood pressure and flow to the brain are sufficiently low to cause ischemia of the neurons of the vasomotor center.[38]
2. Endocrine (humoral) control mechanisms
   a. Sympathetic activity stimulates the adrenal medulla to secrete epinephrine and norepinephrine. These catecholamines augment sympathetic activity by increasing heart rate and force of contraction and by causing vasoconstriction.
   b. Vasopressin is secreted by the pituitary gland in response to decreased blood pressure. Its actions include vasoconstriction and reduction of free water excretion by the kidney.
   c. The renin-angiotensin-aldosterone system has both short-term (via vasoconstriction) and long-term (via vascular volume) effects on the control of blood pressure. A decrease in blood pressure, or a decrease in sodium or chloride load or transport in the distal tubule, stimulates renin release. Renin cleaves angiotensinogen into angiotensin I, which in turn is converted to angiotensin II by a converting enzyme (ACE). Angiotensin II is a potent arteriolar vasoconstrictor and also stimulates secretion of aldosterone by the adrenal cortex. Aldosterone decreases sodium and water excretion by the kidney.[38]
   d. Atrial natriuretic factor (ANF) is a recently characterized polypeptide hormone formed

and stored in atrial myocytes and is released into the circulation in response to increased atrial filling. It acts by several mechanisms to cause a reduction in blood pressure.[7,8] The manner in which these actions are integrated and the role of ANF in blood pressure regulation remain under investigation.

(1). Administration of ANF causes marked natriuresis. The mechanisms for this natriuresis appear to be their effect on renal hemodynamics and their direct and indirect effects on tubular sodium reabsorption.[7]

(a). ANF causes a small increase in glomerular filtration rate (GFR) without an increase in renal blood flow. This effect is the result of glomerular efferent arteriolar vasoconstriction combined with afferent arteriolar dilation.[7,8,52,63]

(b). ANF inhibits sodium reabsorption in the medullary collecting duct. This has the effect of reducing medullary hypertonicity, which may interfere with the action of vasopressin.[8]

(2). ANF causes a decrease in renin secretion. Both direct and indirect mechanisms appear to play a role. The contribution of each under physiologic conditions continues to be investigated.[7,8]

(a). A direct cyclic guanosine monophosphate (GMP)-mediated effect occurs on the cells of the juxtaglomerular apparatus.[7,8]

(b). The increase in GFR induced by ANF increases sodium chloride delivery to the macula densa, thereby inhibiting renin secretion.[7,8]

(c). The afferent arteriolar dilation caused by ANF may increase hydraulic pressure at the juxtaglomerular apparatus.[7]

(d). ANF may inhibit sympathetic activity to the kidney, which reduces the stimulus for renin secretion.[8]

e. Recently the vascular endothelium has been recognized to play a role in the control of vascular tone, although our knowledge of the interaction of these factors is preliminary.

(1). Endothelium can release potent vasodilatory mediators, such as prostacyclin (PGI_2) and endothelium-derived relaxing factor (EDRF).[57,59]

(2). It can also release vasoconstrictive substances, including endothelin, platelet-derived growth factor, and platelet-activating factor.[49,59]

f. Several other hormones, including serotonin,[23] various neuropeptides,[71] kinins,[22] and kallikrein,[78] interact in the normal control of blood pressure.

II. PATHOPHYSIOLOGY OF HYPERTENSION

A. Primary (essential) hypertension.

1. This type of hypertension is the most common cause of increased blood pressure in humans,[47] but is uncommon in dogs and cats.[13,16-19,40,45,54,60]

2. Despite extensive research, the mechanisms responsible for initiating and sustaining the increase in blood pressure are not clear.

a. Theories include chronic volume expansion resulting from excess sodium intake in susceptible individuals, increased peripheral resistance resulting from centrally mediated neurogenic input, or decreased compliance of peripheral vessels.[65]

b. The kidney may bear the genetic message for the development of primary hypertension.

(1). Kidney cross-transplantation studies in different strains of genetically hypertensive rats have shown that hypertension "goes with the kidney," although the pathophysiologic mechanism for the hypertension varies between strains.[27]

(2). Some similar evidence exists in humans who have undergone kidney transplantation.[27]

c. Studies in one colony of dogs with spontaneous primary hypertension failed to show sodium sensitivity and suggested that the hypertension in these dogs was caused by some other mechanism.[19]

B. Secondary hypertension.

1. Secondary hypertension occurs when a disease alters one or more of the physical or neuroendocrine factors controlling blood pressure.

2. The hypertension found in dogs and cats with renal disease is most likely secondary in origin.

a. In dogs with chronic renal disease, the incidence of hypertension ranges from 50 to 93%.[24,26,42,69] This range may be attributed to different types of renal disease, varying methods of measurement of blood pressure, and different definitions of hypertension by the investigators. Two studies of dogs with familial renal disease did not find a significant difference in blood pressure between affected and normal dogs[35,66]; however, 70% of the affected dogs in 1 of these studies had eccentric cardiac hypertrophy at necropsy,[66] a finding that could be consistent with hypertension.

b. Two studies of cats with spontaneous renal disease have reported hypertension in 65%[51] and 61%[50] of affected animals. In two other reports of cats with hypertension, almost all had renal disease,[55,61] but the authors did not determine whether the hypertension was primary or secondary.

c. The incidence of hypertension in people with

renal parenchymal disease has been reported to range from 30 to 90%.[47,72]

III. ETIOPATHOGENESIS OF HYPERTENSION IN RENAL DISEASE

A. Acute renal failure.

1. Hypertension was reported in 39% of people with acute renal failure in a study.[15] The mechanism for such hypertension appears to be expanded extracellular fluid volume as the result of decreased urine production.[72]
2. Increases in blood pressure in dogs and cats with acute renal failure have not been reported.

B. Chronic renal disease.

The mechanism for the hypertension associated with chronic renal disease is not known.[47,48,72] Studies in experimental models of renal failure, as well as in people with renal disease, have noted abnormalities in several of the factors that control blood pressure (Table 19–1).[72] Perhaps a combination or interaction of these abnormalities is ultimately responsible for increased blood pressure; also, renal diseases of different etiopathogenesis might produce hypertension by different mechanisms.

1. Salt retention
   a. Decreased ability of the diseased kidneys to excrete sodium resulting in an increase in extracellular fluid volume has been reported.[72]
   b. The mechanism for decreased sodium excretion appears not to be caused by abnormal peritubular capillary physical forces, but more likely by neurohumoral factors affecting sodium excretion.[72]
   c. One report in dogs with chronic renal failure found a decrease in blood pressure when the dogs were fed a low-sodium diet,[24] thus suggesting that extracellular volume expansion may play a role.
2. Autonomic dysfunction
   a. Increased circulating levels of norepinephrine, as well as increased vascular responsiveness to circulating norepinephrine, have been reported in association with renal insufficiency.[72]
   b. The ability of renal denervation to prevent the onset of hypertension in experimental models of renal insufficiency is additional evidence for a neurogenic role in the pathogenesis of hypertension.[77]
3. Endocrine changes
   a. Renin-angiotensin-aldosterone system
      (1). Increased activity is not a consistent finding in people with renal parenchymal disease.[72]
      (2). Activation does appear to be the inciting cause of the increase in blood pressure associated with renal artery stenosis (renovascular hypertension).[72] This type of hypertension has not been documented in spontaneous disease in animals.
   b. Antihypertensive substances
      (1). The role of antihypertensive renomedullary lipid, a substance produced by renomedullary interstitial cells, has not been investigated in hypertensive renal disease.[72]
      (2). Decreased activity of the kallikrein-kinin system has been reported in hypertensive people with renal disease.[2]
      (3). Increased circulating ANF levels have been reported in people[72] and dogs[79] with renal disease. This increase has been suggested to be a physiologic response to increased blood pressure induced by other factors.
4. Cardiovascular function
   a. Data in people with renal disease[72] and dogs with experimental renal disease[37] suggest that increases in blood pressure in early renal disease result from expanded extracellular fluid volume and increased cardiac output.
   b. Later in the course of experimental renal disease in the dog, the increase in blood pressure is apparently sustained by an increase in total peripheral resistance.[37,38]
   c. The mechanism responsible for converting the increase in cardiac output to an increase in total peripheral resistance is not known, although recent research has led to speculation that endothelial factors, such as endothelin and EDRF, may play a role.[59]

TABLE 19–1.
FACTORS SUGGESTED TO PLAY A ROLE IN THE HYPERTENSION ASSOCIATED WITH RENAL DISEASE

Expanded extracellular fluid volume
Increased norepinephrine levels
Increased vascular responsiveness to norepinephrine
Activation of the renin-angiotensin-aldolsterone system
Decreased activity of kallikrein-kinin system
Increased cardiac output (early)
Increased total peripheral resistance (late)

IV. CLINICAL CARDIOVASCULAR CONSEQUENCES OF HYPERTENSION

A. Vascular disorders.

1. Sustained hypertension causes lesions in small arteries and arterioles, including hypertrophy and hyperplasia of the tunica media, loss of the internal elastic lamina, and fibrinoid necrosis (Fig. 19–1).[43,44]
2. These vascular lesions are responsible for much of the organ dysfunction associated with chronic hypertension.

B. Cardiac changes

1. Left ventricular hypertrophy occurs secondary to a chronic increase in arterial pressure.
2. The mechanism by which the hemodynamic

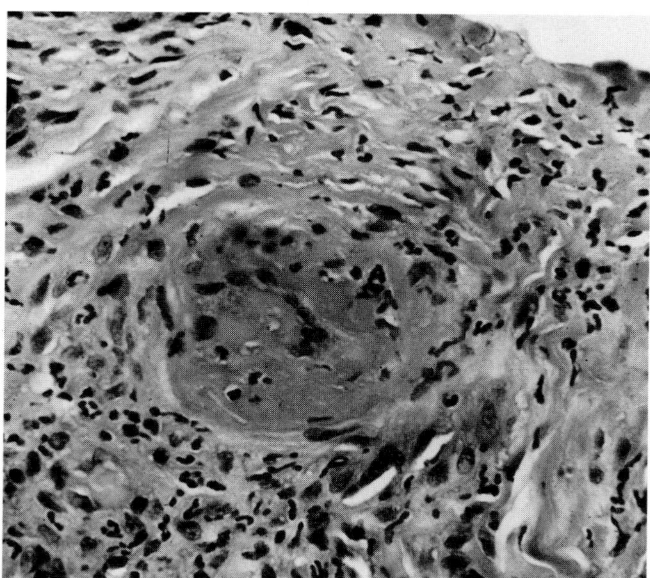

FIG. 19–1. Fibrinoid necrosis and obliteration of a small arteriole.

stimulus of pressure overload results in ventricular hypertrophy is not clear.[28]

3. Ventricular hypertrophy is rarely of sufficient degree to be associated with cardiac failure.

C. Ocular lesions.

1. Early retinal vascular changes include straightening and narrowing of the larger retinal vessels as the result of mild hypertension and dilated, tortuous vessels as the result of more severe increases in blood pressure.
   a. The straightening and narrowing are thought to represent vascular autoregulation (vasoconstriction) in response to the increase in blood pressure.
   b. The cause of the vasodilation is less clear, but may result from autoregulatory failure or hypertension-induced vascular damage.
2. "Cotton-wool" spots on the retina may be seen with mild to moderate hypertension.
   a. These spots are caused by ischemia of nerve fibers in the retina that results from arterial vasoconstriction or vascular disorder.
   b. The grayish-white appearance is caused by neuronal swelling and the accumulation of mitochondria and other axonal organelles at the borders of the lesion.
3. Retinal hemorrhages, exudates, and detachments may be seen with severe hypertension.
   a. Hemorrhages and exudates may result from vascular lesions that cause rupture of small arteries and arterioles or from exudation or plasma through the damaged vessel wall.
   b. Retinal detachments can occur as the result of exudation or edema.
4. Papilledema may be seen with severe hypertension.
   a. The pathogenesis is not clear.
   b. Axonal swelling may be the result of ischemia from vasoconstriction or vascular disease, or it may represent transmission of increased intracranial pressure.[32,33,36,76]

D. Renal effects.

1. Pathology
   a. The classic histologic lesion of hypertensive renal disease is fibrinoid necrosis of the afferent glomerular arterioles.[21,43,44]
   b. Focal and segmental glomerular proliferation and glomerulosclerosis may also occur.
   c. Differences in the renal lesions associated with hypertension may be species- or race-related. For example, Caucasian people with hypertensive renal disease have classic arteriolar lesions in their kidneys, whereas the glomeruli of African-American people more commonly show marked ischemic changes characterized by wrinkling of the glomerular membranes, shrinking of the glomerular tuft, and deposition of eosinophilic material in Bowman's space.[21]
2. Effect on progression of renal disease
   a. Several studies in rats indicate that the increased transcapillary glomerular capillary pressure (P_{GC}) (glomerular hyperfiltration) that occurs as the result of decreased quantities of nephrons plays a role in the development of glomerulosclerosis and the progression of renal disease.[3,5,6,72] (See Chapter 16, Pathophysiology of Renal Failure and Uremia.)
   b. Systemic hypertension with normal renal function does not necessarily result in glomerular hyperfiltration, because renal vascular autoregulation prevents transmission of the increased pressure to the glomerulus.[5,6]
      (1). In people, severe (malignant) hypertension is characterized by a rapid decline in renal function.
      (2). Some studies have shown a correlation between blood pressure and deterioration of renal function in people who initially had no clinical evidence of renal dysfunction.[68]
   c. With decreased quantities of nephrons, however, systemic hypertension may contribute to glomerular hyperfiltration.[5]
      (1). Indirect evidence for this hypothesis is the fact that reduction of blood pressure in hypertensive people with renal insufficiency is associated with slowing of the rate of decline of renal function.[12,20,67]
      (2). Similar data are not available for animals with spontaneous disease, although preliminary studies in dogs[54,69] and cats[51,55] do not support a correlation between

blood pressure and progression of renal disease.

V. MEASUREMENT OF BLOOD PRESSURE

A. Direct measurement.

1. Direct blood pressure measurement is considered the "gold standard" for accuracy.
2. The technique involves placing a needle or catheter into a peripheral artery, usually the femoral, and obtaining systolic and diastolic pressure readings via a transducer and recorder.

B. Indirect measurement.

1. Several studies have shown good correlation between direct and indirect blood pressure measurement as long as attention is paid to careful technique.[69]
2. The technique involves occluding a peripheral artery by a cuff surrounding the limb and determining blood flow through the artery by palpatory, auscultatory, or oscillometric methods following slow release of the occlusion.
3. With all methods, the average of at least three readings should be taken at several-minute intervals because of normal minute-to-minute variation in blood pressure caused by respiration, movement, and heart rate. A trend in serial readings dictates multiple readings until values stabilize.

C. Environment, attitude, technique.

1. Spurious blood pressure readings are commonplace if animals are excited, shivering, or moving.
2. Extreme attention to state of the patient and technique must be applied if meaningful readings are to be obtained.

VI. THERAPY

A. Goals.

1. To reduce blood pressure into the normal range without adversely affecting renal function.
2. To help to normalize glomerular hemodynamics to slow the progression of renal disease.

B. Sodium restriction.

1. Decreasing the sodium load reduces fluid retention and therefore extracellular volume.
2. Many commercial pet foods are relatively high in sodium,[53] and animals consuming these diets may be relatively volume expanded.
3. Changing the diet of dogs with renal disease from commercial food to food containing 0.23% sodium on a dry weight basis was shown to decrease mean blood pressure from 132 mm Hg to 108 mm Hg.[24,26]
4. Based on this information, all hypertensive dogs and cats with renal disease should be fed a diet restricted in sodium. Recommended dietary levels of sodium in this setting are 0.1 to 0.3% on a dry weight basis (10 to 40 mg/kg/d).[24,25,53]
5. Animals with renal failure have impaired ability to adjust excretion of sodium in response to sudden changes in dietary sodium intake.[80] Therefore, gradual (2 to 4 weeks) implementation of a sodium-restricted diet is recommended to avoid sodium and water depletion and the potential adverse effect on renal blood flow.

C. Pharmacologic options. Because the pathogenesis of the hypertension associated with renal failure in animals is not known, a recommendation of a specific drug to reduce blood pressure is not possible. One of two approaches to pharmacologic therapy may be used.

1. Stepwise therapy
   a. In this approach, antihypertensive therapy is administered in a logical order, beginning with those agents that have the mildest activity and fewest side effects.
   b. Each drug is administered for 1 to 2 weeks before its effectiveness in lowering blood pressure is determined.
   c. If a particular drug fails, a drug in the next class is selected rather than a different drug in the same class.
   d. The order of drug administration should follow that listed in the following sections, although it is somewhat empiric.
      (1). Diuretics
         (a). Diuretics act by causing sodium and water excretion and thereby reduce extracellular fluid volume. Direct vascular effects also are postulated to exist in humans.
         (b). Thiazide diuretics, such as chlorothiazide or hydrochlorothiazide, have been recommended as first-choice diuretics; however, animals with renal failure are generally refractive to their action.[26]
         (c). Potent loop diuretics, such as furosemide, are probably the first choice in animals with renal failure. However, they must be used cautiously because of the potential of producing excessive sodium and water loss, volume depletion, and subsequent decrease in renal function.
      (2). Beta-adrenergic antagonists
         (a). Propranolol is the most commonly used drug in this class.
         (b). The mechanism by which this class of drugs reduces blood pressure is not entirely known, but appears to involve reduction of cardiac output, inhibition of renin release, interference with central sympathetic activity, and/or presynaptic blockade of adrenergic neurons.[1,26,62]
         (c). Relative contraindications to their use include cardiac or pulmonary disease, because they can cause bradycardia, decreased cardiac output, and bronchospasm.[62]
      (3). Vasodilators
         (a). Vasodilators may be administered as

the sole pharmacologic agent or may be given in conjunction with diuretics and/or beta-adrenergic antagonists.

(b). Hydralazine acts directly on small arteries and arterioles to reduce vascular tone. As a result, it also stimulates reflex sympathetic increases in heart rate and cardiac output and enhances renin release; therefore, it usually must be administered in conjunction with a beta-adrenergic blocker and a diuretic.[14] For this reason, hydralazine is not recommended for animals with renal failure.

(c). Prazosin is an alpha-adrenergic receptor antagonist that causes dilation of both arterioles and veins without associated tachycardia or renin release. Although it is effective in lowering systemic blood pressure in dogs and cats,[14] prazosin does not appear to have an effect on P_{GC}.

(d). Calcium channel blocking (CCB) agents, such as verapamil, cause arteriolar vasodilation by inhibiting calcium transport through slow channels in smooth muscle cell membranes.[46]

(e). ACE inhibitors, such as captopril or enalapril, inhibit the conversion of angiotensin I to angiotensin II. The subsequent decrease in angiotensin II levels causes arteriolar dilation and venodilation, as well as suppresses aldosterone secretion, thereby resulting in increased sodium and water excretion.

2. Therapy to reduce systemic blood pressure and normalize intraglomerular hemodynamics
   a. Several studies have shown that antihypertensive therapy that is effective in lowering systemic blood pressure is not necessarily effective in normalizing intraglomerular hemodynamics (P_{GC}).[4,6,41] Renal disease may therefore continue to progress because of continuing glomerular hyperfiltration.
   b. Certain classes of antihypertensive drugs have been shown to be effective in reducing systemic blood pressure and P_{GC}.

(1). Angiotensin-converting enzyme inhibitors

(a). In rats with experimental renal injury and hypertension, treatment with ACE inhibitors is associated with normalization of P_{GC} as the result of vasodilation of the efferent glomerular arteriole, therefore preventing glomerular injury.[4,6,9,10,39,41,74,75]

(b). Although P_{GC} cannot be measured in humans, several clinical trials have suggested a decrease in the rate of decline in renal function and in proteinuria in patients receiving ACE inhibitors when they either were changed from nonACE inhibitor antihypertensive protocols or were compared to other patients on such protocols.[58,64,70,74]

(c). Although similar data in dogs and cats are not available, use of ACE inhibitors as antihypertensive therapy would seem logical based on these studies.

(1′). Captopril (1 to 2 mg/kg PO every 8 to 12 hours) or enalapril (0.5 mg/kg PO every 12 hours) may be used.

(2′). The dosage of either drug should be adjusted for the degree of renal impairment because both are excreted by the kidneys.

(3′). Clinically, enalapril may be preferred because it is associated with fewer side effects, such as anorexia and vomiting (personal observation).

(2). Calcium channel blocking agents

(a). CCB agents have been shown to be effective antihypertensive agents in humans with renal impairment and do not appear to affect renal function in the short term.[30]

(b). Conflicting experimental data exist regarding their long-term effect on renal function.[10,11]

(1′). In some studies, CCB agents caused preferential vasodilation of the afferent glomerular arteriole, thereby maintaining or increasing GFR and P_{GC}.[11,31,34,56,75]

(2′). In other studies, CCB agents caused a decrease in P_{GC}.[11,75]

(3′). In another report, administration of nifedipine reduced systemic blood pressure in rats with hypertension and decreased proteinuria and the percentage of injured glomeruli without decreasing P_{GC}, thus suggesting a nonhemodynamic mechanism of protection.[29]

(a′). Investigators also have suggested that CCB agents reduce glomerular injury and sclerosis by inhibiting compensatory renal hypertrophy.[30,31,34,73] (b′). Other mechanisms by which CCB agents might slow the progression of renal damage have been suggested to be the inhibition of formation of reactive oxygen products,[30,34] inhibition of the mitogenic effects of platelet-derived growth factor and platelet-activating factor, and modulation of mesangial entrapment of macromolecules.[34]

(c). Further studies are needed to resolve these differences so that clinical recommendations can be made.

REFERENCES

1. Allen TA. The treatment of hypertension. In: *Proceedings of the 4th Annual Veterinary Medical Forum*. American College of Veterinary Internal Medicine: 1986;3-105-3-107.
2. Almeida FA, et al. Malignant hypertension: A syndrome associated with low plasma kininogen and kinin potentiating factor. *Hypertension.* 1981;3:II-46-II49.
3. Anderson S, Meyer TW, Rennke HG, Brenner BM. Control of glomerular hypertension limits glomerular injury in rats with reduced renal mass. *J Clin Invest.* 1985;76:612-619.
4. Anderson S, Rennke HG, Brenner BM. Therapeutic advantage of converting enzyme inhibitors in arresting progressive renal disease associated with systemic hypertension in the rat. *J Clin Invest.* 1986;77:1993-2000.
5. Anderson S, Brenner BM. Role of intraglomerular hypertension in the initiation and progression of renal disease. In: Kaplan NM, Brenner BM, Laragh JH, eds. *The Kidney in Hypertension.* New York, New York: Raven Press; 1987:67-76.
6. Anderson S. Renal effects of converting enzyme inhibitors in hypertension and diabetes. *J Cardiovasc Pharmacol.* 1990; 15(suppl 3):S11-S15.
7. Atlas SA, Laragh JH. Atrial natriuretic factor and its involvement in hypertensive disorders. In: Laragh JH, Brenner BM, eds. *Hypertension: Pathophysiology, Diagnosis and Management.* New York, New York: Raven Press; 1990:861-884.
8. Ballermann BJ, Zeidel ML, Gunning ME, Brenner BM. Vasoactive peptides and the kidney. In: Brenner BM, Rector FC, eds. *The Kidney.* 4th ed. Philadelphia, Pennsylvania: WB Saunders Co; 1991:510-583.
9. Bauer JH, Gaddy P. Effects of enalapril alone, and in combination with hydrochlorothiazide, on renin-angiotensin-aldosterone, renal function, salt and water excretion, and body fluid composition. *Am J Kidney Dis.* 1985;6:222-232.
10. Bauer JH, Reams GP. Hypertension with co-existing renal disease. *J Human Hypertens.* 1990;4(suppl 5):27-34.
11. Benstein JA, Dworkin LD. Renal vascular effects of calcium channel blockers in hypertension. *Am J Hypertens.* 1990;3:305S-312S.
12. Bergstrom J, Alvestrand A, Bucht H, Gutierrez A. Progression of chronic renal failure in man is retarded with more frequent clinical follow-ups and better blood pressure control. *Clin Nephrol.* 1985;25:1-6.
13. Blanchard GL, et al. Primary essential hypertension in a Siberian husky dog. *Fed Proc.* 1979;38:1350. Abstract.
14. Bonagura JD, Muir W. Vasodilator therapy. In: Kirk RW, ed. *Current Veterinary Therapy IX.* Philadelphia, Pennsylvania: WB Saunders Co; 1986:329-333.
15. Bonomini V, Campieri C, Scolari MP, Vangelista A. Hypertension in acute renal failure. *Contrib Nephrol.* 1987;54:152-158.
16. Bovee KC, et al. Essential hereditary hypertension in dogs: A new animal model. In: *Proceedings of the 18th Annual Meeting of the American Society of Nephrology.* 1985;93A. Abstract.
17. Bovee KC, et al. Essential hereditary hypertension in dogs: A new animal model. *J Hypertens.* 1986;4(suppl 5):S172-S173.
18. Bovee KC, Littman MP, Crabtree BJ, Aguirre G. Essential hypertension in a dog. *J Am Vet Med Assoc.* 1989;195:81-86.
19. Bovee KC. Variance of blood pressure response to oral sodium intake in hypertensive dogs. In: *Proceedings of the 8th American College of Veterinary Internal Medicine Forum.* Washington, DC: May 1990;1128.
20. Brazy PC, Stead WW, Fitzwilham JF. Progression of renal insufficiency: Role of blood pressure. *Kidney Int.* 1989;35:670-674.
21. Campese VM, Karubian F. Renal consequences of salt and hypertension. *Semin Nephrol.* 1991;11(5):549-560.
22. Carretero DA, Scicli AG. Kinins as regulators of blood flow and blood pressure. In: Laragh JH, Brenner BM, eds. *Hypertension: Pathophysiology, Diagnosis and Management.* New York, New York: Raven Press; 1990:805-818.
23. Chalmers JP, Angus JA, Jennings GL, Minson JB. Serotonin and hypertension. In: Laragh JH, Brenner BM, eds. *Hypertension: Pathophysiology, Diagnosis and Management.* New York, New York: Raven Press; 1990:761-778.
24. Cowgill LD. Diseases of the kidney. In: Ettinger SJ, ed. *Textbook of Veterinary Internal Medicine.* 2nd ed. Philadelphia, Pennsylvania: WB Saunders Co; 1983:1793-1879.
25. Cowgill LD, Kallet AS. Recognition and management of hypertension in the dog. In: Kirk RW, ed. *Current Veterinary Therapy VIII.* Philadelphia, Pennsylvania: WB Saunders Co; 1983:1025-1028.
26. Cowgill LD, Kallet AJ. Systemic hypertension. In: Kirk RW, ed. *Current Veterinary Therapy IX.* Philadelphia, Pennsylvania: WB Saunders Co; 1986:360-364.
27. Cusi D, Bianchi G. The kidney in the pathogenesis of hypertension. *Semin Nephrol.* 1991;11(5):523-537.
28. Devereux RB. Hypertensive cardiac hypertrophy: Pathophysiologic and chemical characteristics. In: Laragh JH, Brenner BM, eds. *Hypertension: Pathophysiology, Diagnosis and Management.* New York, New York: Raven Press; 1990:359-377.
29. Dworkin LD, et al. Effects of nifedipine and enalapril on glomerular injury in rats with desoxycorticosterone-salt hypertension. *Am J Physiol.* 1990;259:F598-F604.
30. Dworkin LD. Impact of calcium entry blockers on glomerular injury in experimental hypertension. *Cardiovasc Drugs Ther.* 1990;4:1325-1330.
31. Dworkin LD. Effects of calcium channel blockers on experimental glomerular injury. *J Am Soc Nephrol.* 1990;1:S21-S27.
32. Editorial. Pathogenesis of retinopathy in malignant hypertension. *Br J Ophthalmol.* 1975;59:1.
33. Editorial. Pathogenesis of hypertensive retinopathy. *Br Med J.* 1975;1:700-701.
34. Epstein M. Calcium antagonists and renal hemodynamics: Implications for renal protection. *J Am Soc Nephrol.* 1991;2:S30-S36.
35. Finco DR. Familial renal disease in Norwegian Elkhound dogs: Physiologic and biochemical examinations. *Am J Vet Res.* 1976; 37:87-91.
36. Garner A, et al. Pathogenesis of hypertensive retinopathy: An experimental study in the monkey. *Br J Ophthalmol.* 1975; 59:3-44.
37. Guyton AC, et al. Salt balance and long-term blood pressure control. *Annu Rev Med.* 1980;31:15-27.

38. Guyton AC. *Textbook of Medical Physiology.* 7th ed. Philadelphia, Pennsylvania: WB Saunders Co; 1986:244-270.
39. Hall RL. Captopril slows the progression of chronic renal disease in partially nephrectomized rats. *Toxicol Appl Pharmacol.* 1985; 80:517-526.
40. Hamilton WF, et al. Blood pressure values in street dogs. *Am J Physiol.* 1939;128:233-237.
41. Jackson B, Debrevi L, Whitty M, Johnston CI. Progression of renal disease: Effects of different classes of antihypertensive therapy. *J Hypertens.* 1986;4(suppl 5):S269-S271.
42. Kallet A, Cowgill LD. Hypertensive states in the dog. [abstr]. In: *Proceedings of the American College of Veterinary Internal Medicine.* Salt Lake City, Utah: 1982;79.
43. Kashgarian M. Pathology of the kidney in hypertension. In: Kaplan NM, Brenner BM, Laragh JH, eds. *The Kidney in Hypertension.* New York, New York: Raven Press; 1987;3:77-89.
44. Kashgarian M. Hypertensive disease and kidney structure. In: Laragh JH, Brenner BM, eds. *Hypertension: Pathophysiology, Diagnosis and Management.* New York, New York: Raven Press; 1990: 389-398.
45. Katz JI, et al. Pathogenesis of spontaneous and pyelonephritic hypertension in the dog. *Circ Res.* 1957;5:137-143.
46. Keene BW, Hamlin RL. Calcium antagonists. In: Kirk RW, ed. *Current Veterinary Therapy IX.* Philadelphia, Pennsylvania: WB Saunders Co; 1986;340-342.
47. Kincaid-Smith P. Parenchymatous diseases of the kidney and hypertension. In: Genest J, ed. *Hypertension.* 2nd ed. New York, New York: McGraw Hill; 1983:989-1006.
48. Kincaid-Smith P, Whitworth JA. Pathogenesis of hypertension in chronic renal disease. *Semin Nephrol.* 1988;8:155-162.
49. King AJ, Marsden PA, Brenner BM. Endothelin: A potent vasoactive peptide of endothelial origin. In: Laragh JH, Brenner BM, eds. *Hypertension: Pathophysiology, Diagnosis and Management.* New York, New York: Raven Press; 1990:649-660.
50. Kobayashi DL, et al. Hypertension in cats with chronic renal failure or hyperthyroidism. *J Vet Intern Med.* 1990;4:58-62.
51. Labato MA, Ross LA. Diagnosis and management of hypertension. In: August JR, ed. *Consultations in Feline Internal Medicine.* Philadelphia, Pennsylvania: WB Saunders Co; 1991: 301-308.
52. Laragh SH. Atrial natriuretic hormone, the renin-aldosterone axis, and blood pressure—electrolyte hemostasis. *N Engl J Med.* 1985;313:1330-1340.
53. Lewis LD, Morris ML Jr, Hand MS. *Small Animal Clinical Nutrition.* 3rd ed. Topeka, Kansas: Mark Morris Associates; 1987.
54. Littman MP, Robertson JL, Bovee KC. Spontaneous systemic hypertension in dogs: Five cases (1981-1983). *J Am Vet Med Assoc.* 1988;193:486-494.
55. Littman MP. Spontaneous systemic hypertension in cats. In: *Proceedings of the 8th American College of Veterinary Internal Medicine Forum.* Washington, DC: May 1990;1128. Abstract.
56. Loutzenhiser R, Epstein M. Renal microvascular actions of calcium antagonists. *J Am Soc Nephrol.* 1990;1:S3-S12.
57. Luscher TF, Diederich D, Buhler FR, Vanhoutte PM. Interactions between platelets and the vessel wall: Role of endothelium-derived vasoactive substances. In: Laragh JH, Brenner BM, eds. *Hypertension: Pathophysiology, Diagnosis and Management.* New York, New York: Raven Press; 1990:637-648.
58. Mann J, Ritz E. Preservation of kidney function by use of converting enzyme inhibitors for control of hypertension. *Lancet.* 1987;2:622.
59. Marsden PA, Goligorsky MS, Brenner BM. Endothelial cell biology in relation to current concepts of vessel wall structure and function. *J Am Soc Nephrol.* 1991;1:931-948.
60. McCubbin JW, Corcoran AC. Arterial pressures in street dogs: Incidence and significance of hypertension. *Proc Soc Exp Biol Med.* 1953;84:130-131.
61. Morgan RV. Systemic hypertension in four cats: Ocular and medical findings. *J Am Anim Hosp Assoc.* 1986;22:615-621.
62. Muir W. Beta-blocking therapy in dogs and cats. In: Kirk RW, ed. *Current Veterinary Therapy IX.* Philadelphia, Pennsylvania: WB Saunders Co; 1986:343-346.
63. Needleman P, Greenwald JE. Atriopeptin: A cardiac hormone intimately involved in fluid, electrolyte, and blood-pressure homeostasis. *New Engl J Med.* 1986;314:828-834.
64. Opsahl JA, Abraham PA, Keane WF. Angiotensin-converting enzyme inhibitors in chronic renal failure. *Drugs.* 1990;39(suppl 2):23-32.
65. Page IH. *Hypertension Mechanisms.* New York, New York: Grune & Stratton; 1987.
66. Persson F, et al. Blood pressure in dogs with renal cortical hypoplasia. *Acta Vet Scand.* 1961;2:129-136.
67. Pettinger WA, Leeh C, Reisch J, Mitchell HC. Long term improvement in renal function after short term strict blood pressure control in hypertensive nephrosclerosis. *Hypertension.* 1989;13:766-772.
68. Rosansky SJ, Hoover DR, King L, Gibson J. The association of blood pressure levels and change in renal function in hypertensive and nonhypertensive subjects. *Arch Intern Med.* 1990;150: 2073-2076.
69. Ross LA. Hypertensive diseases. In: Ettinger SJ. *Textbook of Veterinary Internal Medicine.* 3rd ed. Philadelphia, Pennsylvania: WB Saunders Co; 1989;2047-2056.
70. Ruilope LM, et al. Converting enzyme inhibition in chronic renal failure. *Am J Kidney Dis.* 1989;13:120-126.
71. Said SI. Neuropeptides in blood pressure control. In: Laragh JH, Brenner BM, eds. *Hypertension: Pathophysiology, Diagnosis and Management.* New York, New York: Raven Press; 1990:791-804.
72. Smith MC, Dunn MJ. Hypertension due to renal parenchymal disease. In: Brenner BM, Rector FC, eds. *The Kidney.* 4th ed. Philadelphia, Pennsylvania: WB Saunders Co; 1991:1968-1996.
73. Sweeney C, Shultz P, Raij L. Interactions of the endothelium and mesangium in glomerular injury. *J Am Soc Nephrol.* 1990;1: S13-S20.
74. Tolins JP, Raij L. Angiotensin converting enzyme inhibitors and progression of chronic renal failure. *Kidney Int.* 1990;38(suppl 30):S-118-S-122.
75. Tolins JP, Raij L. Antihypertensive therapy and the progression of chronic renal disease. Are there renoprotective drugs? *Semin Nephrol.* 1991;11:538-548.
76. Tso MOM, Jampol LM. Hypertensive retinopathy, choroidopathy, and optic neuropathy of hypertensive ocular disease: A clinical and pathophysiologic approach to classification. In: Laragh JH, Brenner BM, eds. *Hypertension: Pathophysiology, Diagnosis and Management.* New York, New York: Raven Press; 1990: 433-465.
77. Vari RC, Freeman RH, Davis JO, Sweet WD. Role of renal nerves in rats with low-sodium one-kidney hypertension. *Am J Physiol.* 1986;250:H189-H194.
78. Vio CP. Renal kallikrein. In: Laragh JH, Brenner BM, eds. *Hypertension: Pathophysiology, Diagnosis and Management.* New York, New York: Raven Press; 1990:819-828.
79. Vollmar AM, Reusch C, Kraft W, Schulz R. Atrial natriuretic peptide concentration in dogs with congestive heart failure, chronic renal failure, and hyperadrenocorticism. *Am J Vet Res.* 1991;52:1831-1834.
80. Walser M. Nutrition in renal failure. *Annu Rev Nutr.* 1983;3: 125-154.

CHAPTER 20

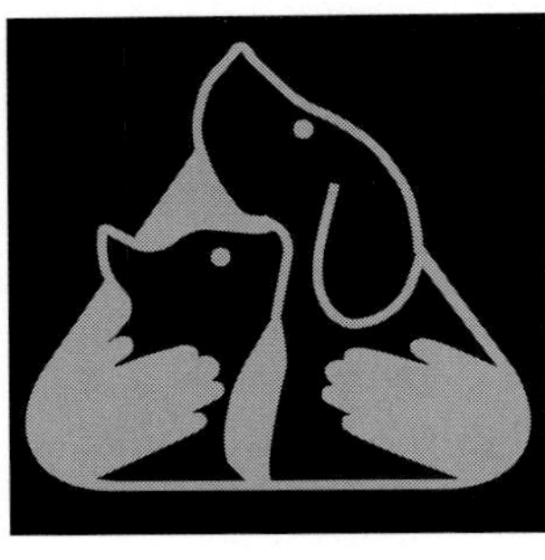

Renal Amyloidosis

STEPHEN P. DIBARTOLA

I. DEFINITION OF AMYLOIDOSIS

A. Amyloidosis refers to a diverse group of diseases characterized by the extracellular deposition of fibrils formed by polymerization of protein subunits with a specific biophysical conformation called the β-pleated sheet.[30,49]

B. This specific biophysical conformation is responsible for the unique optical and tinctorial properties of amyloid deposits, as well as their insolubility and resistance to proteolysis in vivo.

C. By routine light microscopy, amyloid deposits are extracellular and have a homogeneous, eosinophilic appearance when stained by hematoxylin and eosin.

D. Criteria for the diagnosis of amyloidosis.

1. Amyloid deposits demonstrate green birefringence after staining with Congo red when viewed under polarized light. The clinical diagnosis of amyloidosis is based on this pathologic finding. The biophysical conformation of the protein in question, and not its amino acid sequence, is responsible for this property.
2. Amyloid fibrils are variable in length, nonbranching, and 7 to 10 nm in width when viewed by transmission electron microscopy (Fig. 20–1).

E. Once stained with Congo red, amyloid deposits from patients with reactive (secondary) amyloidosis lose their affinity for Congo red after permanganate oxidation. This feature is useful in the preliminary differentiation of reactive from other types of amyloidosis. A notable exception is β_2-microglobulin, which also is permanganate sensitive. Amyloidosis associated with β_2-microglobulin occurs in human patients after long-term hemodialysis and has not been observed in domestic animals.[106]

II. CLASSIFICATION OF AMYLOID SYNDROMES

A. According to distribution of deposits.

1. Localized syndromes affect one organ and are uncommon in domestic animals
   a. Amyloidosis of the nasal meatus and ventral turbinates occurs in horses and is associated with epistaxis. This probably is an example of localized immunoglobulin-associated amyloidosis,[126] although one report is contradictory.[105]
   b. Amyloid deposits in pancreatic islet cells of domestic cats are characterized by the presence of a unique polypeptide hormone called islet amyloid polypeptide.[65,139]
2. Systemic syndromes affect more than one organ.
   a. Reactive.
   b. Immunoglobulin-associated.
   c. Heredofamilial.
      (1). Neuropathic (e.g., familial amyloid polyneuropathy).
      (2). Nonneuropathic (e.g., familial Mediterranean fever).

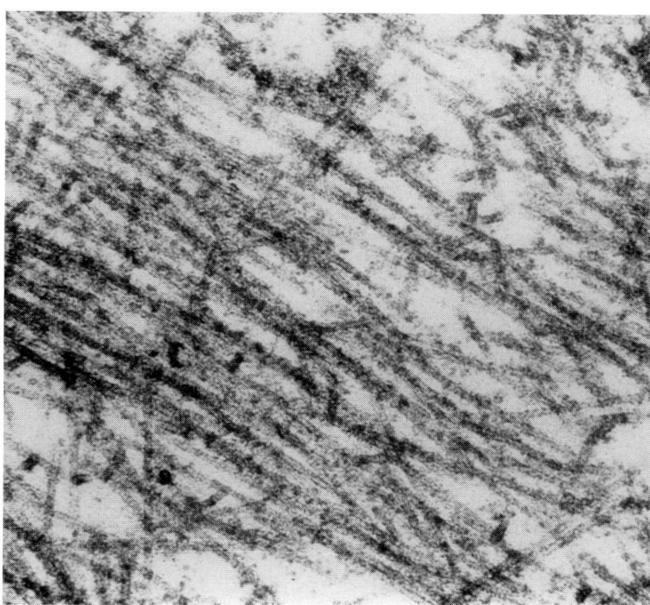

FIG. 20–1. Morphologic appearance of amyloid fibrils by transmission electron microscopy. (From Boyce JT, et al. Familial renal amyloidosis in Abyssinian cats. *Vet Pathol.* 1984;21:33-38.)

B. According to the responsible protein.

1. Reactive (secondary) amyloidosis is a systemic syndrome characterized by tissue deposition of amyloid A protein (AA amyloid). Naturally occurring systemic amyloidosis in domestic animals is an example of reactive amyloidosis. Familial amyloidosis in the Abyssinian cat and Shar pei dog is an example of reactive systemic amyloidosis.
2. Immunoglobulin-associated (primary) amyloidosis is characterized by tissue deposition of amino terminal fragments of immunoglobulin light chains (AL amyloid). It usually is systemic (e.g., amyloidosis complicating plasma cell dyscrasias), but also can be localized (e.g., solitary amyloid nodules in the skin, respiratory tract, and urogenital tract). This form of amyloidosis has been documented rarely in domestic animals.[21,48,104,126]
3. Prealbumin-associated amyloidosis may be systemic (e.g., familial neuropathic syndromes) or localized (e.g., senile cardiopathic syndromes). This type of amyloid has not been documented in veterinary medicine.
4. Other amyloid syndromes that have been documented only in human medicine include:
   a. β_2-microglobulin (hemodialysis-associated amyloidosis)
   b. Cystatin C or gamma trace protein (familial cerebrovascular hemorrhage)
   c. Procalcitonin (medullary carcinoma of the thyroid gland)
   d. Keratin (cutaneous amyloidosis)
   e. β protein (Alzheimer's disease, Down's syndrome)
   f. Atrial natriuretic factor (atrial amyloidosis)

III. PATHOPHYSIOLOGY OF REACTIVE SYSTEMIC AMYLOIDOSIS

A. Tissue deposits from animals with systemic amyloidosis contain AA amyloid, which is an amino terminal fragment of an acute-phase reactant called serum amyloid A protein (SAA).

1. AA amyloid has been characterized in several species of domestic animals.[16,17,36,64,66,73,114,115,132,133] In human beings and mice, AA amyloid contains 76 amino acids and has a molecular weight of 8.4 kd.
2. In all species studied to date, the amino acids at positions 33 to 45 are the same. An important functional role for this portion of the protein is suggested because this region has been strongly conserved during evolution.
3. The amino and carboxy terminal regions of AA amyloid show some variability among species.
   a. The protein in dogs, cats, and horses differs from that in mice and human beings in that an 8 amino acid insertion exists between positions 69 and 70 of the human protein[73,115] and a carboxy terminal extension of 10 amino acids exists in dog, cat, and horse proteins.
   b. In the cow, a 9 amino acid insertion in this region and a 6 amino acid carboxy terminal extension of the protein exist.[17]
4. In one study, three amino acid differences were found when the sequence of AA amyloid from a domestic cat with amyloidosis was compared to that reported for the Abyssinian cat.[66] The authors postulated that this sequence difference could explain the higher frequency of reactive systemic amyloidosis in the Abyssinian cat as compared with the lower frequency in other domestic cats.

B. SAA contains 104 amino acids and has a molecular weight of 12 kd.

1. SAA was first recognized by studying human serum, with antibodies directed against the amyloid fibril protein isolated from a patient with reactive systemic amyloidosis.[77]
2. Using plasma from a single human patient, 3 different SAA proteins have been characterized by amino acid sequence analysis and 3 corresponding DNA sequences have been detected.[43,72] Of these, 2 human SAA proteins (SAA2α and SAA2β) differ by only 1 amino acid residue, whereas the most abundant form in plasma (SAA1) differs by 7 and 8 positions (respectively) from the other 2 proteins. Thus, if the genes for SAA2α and SAA2β are alleles, at least 2 genetic loci for SAA exist in human beings. Alternatively, if each of the DNA sequences for SAA1, SAA2α, and SAA2β represents separate

genetic loci, 3 genes for SAA may exist in human beings.

3. SAA is one of several acute-phase reactants synthesized by the liver in response to tissue injury.[15,107,122,123]
   a. Cytokines (e.g., interleukin-1, tumor necrosis factor-α, interleukin-6) released from macrophages after tissue injury stimulate hepatocytes to synthesize and release SAA.[22,91,98,109,110,130]
   b. SAA is synthesized as a 14-kd precursor protein with an amino terminal signal peptide, which is cleaved at the time of release from the hepatocyte.[111]
   c. SAA released from hepatocytes binds to high-density lipoproteins (HDL_3), where it may displace apolipoproteins A-I, A-II, or C from lipoprotein particles.[29,60,93]
   d. SAA circulates complexed with HDL_3 and has an apparent molecular weight of approximately 180 kd. The SAA content of HDL may increase from 1 to greater than 25% after an inflammatory stimulus.[59]
   e. The increase in SAA after an inflammatory stimulus is the result of increased transcription of the SAA genes in hepatocytes and increased translation of the associated mRNA. The amount of mRNA for SAA present in hepatocytes increases 500- to 1000-fold after an inflammatory stimulus.[79]
   f. The normal serum concentration of SAA is approximately 1 mg/L, but its concentration increases 100- to 500-fold after tissue injury (e.g., inflammation, neoplasia, trauma, infarction).[10,84] SAA has an electrophoretic mobility in the α_1 to α_2 region.[95]
   g. The serum concentration of SAA begins to increase 2 to 4 hours after an inflammatory stimulus, peaks at 12 to 18 hours, and decreases to baseline by 36 to 48 hours if the inflammatory stimulus is removed.[12,110]
   h. When inflammation persists, SAA concentration remains increased.
4. SAA serves as the precursor of AA amyloid in tissues. This was demonstrated by experiments in which human SAA was injected intravenously into mice previously stimulated by casein administration to develop reactive amyloidosis. Human AA amyloid subsequently was identified immunohistochemically in the amyloid deposits of the affected mice.[63]
5. In mice, the three nonallelic genes for SAA (SAA1, SAA2, and SAA3) are expressed in various tissues.[80,136,138] A fourth DNA sequence for SAA apparently is transcription defective (i.e., a pseudogene).
   a. The genes for murine SAA1 and SAA2 are expressed predominantly in the liver. Some expression also is found in epithelial cells of the intestine and kidney.[86] The corresponding proteins are released in equal amounts from hepatocytes during an inflammatory response. In the mouse, SAA2 is selectively deposited as amyloid, whereas SAA1 is not.[62,87]
   b. mRNA for SAA3 is expressed in hepatocytes, but no corresponding protein has yet been detected in plasma. Therefore, a local function for this form of SAA is suspected.[129] The murine SAA3 gene is expressed in many extrahepatic tissues. The cells responsible for expression include adipocytes in many tissues, Leydig's cells in the testis, macrophages in the peritoneum, and parafollicular cells in the spleen.[11,86,97,101]
6. The distribution of SAA polymorphs in plasma does not seem to be influenced by the inflammatory stimulus or the presence or absence of amyloidosis.[85]
7. Leydig's cells and adrenocortical cells accumulate SAA, thus suggesting a role in local regulation of lipid or steroid metabolism.[88]
8. The mechanisms responsible for termination of SAA synthesis are not well understood.
   a. In the kidney, the small amount of SAA that is free in plasma is filtered by the glomeruli and reabsorbed by the proximal tubular cells, where it presumably is degraded to its constituent amino acids.[89]
   b. The liver also contributes to SAA degradation, and binding to HDL protects SAA from hepatic clearance.[9,46]
9. HDL containing SAA are cleared more rapidly from the circulation than are other lipoproteins. This observation and the fact that endotoxins bind to HDL have led to speculation that one function of SAA may be to confer a rapid clearance rate on HDL and thus to enhance the elimination of endotoxin or products of tissue injury from the body.[59,61]
10. Other studies have suggested an immunosuppressive function for SAA because it suppresses the antibody response to T cell-dependent antigens by interfering with T cell-macrophage interactions.[2,13,67]

C. Among the domestic animals, reactive amyloidosis is most common in the dog.[39] Reactive systemic amyloidosis appears to occur as a familial disease in the Shar pei dog.[42] It is uncommon in domestic cats, with the exception of the Abyssinian cat, in which reactive systemic amyloidosis is a familial disease.[19,26,36,37]

D. Kinetics of amyloid deposition.[70,71]

1. Predeposition phase
   a. SAA concentration is increased, but no amyloid deposits are observed during this phase.
   b. Colchicine administered during this phase may

prevent the formation of amyloid-enhancing factor (AEF).[20] This glycoprotein product of chronic inflammation appears in the spleen 48 hours before amyloid deposits are detected histologically and greatly shortens the time required for development of amyloidosis when administered to experimental animals.[4,70] AEF triggers the deposition phase, and macrophages containing large amounts of AEF are capable of processing SAA to AA amyloid in tissue culture.[108]

2. Deposition phase
   a. Rapid phase
      (1). The amount of amyloid in deposits increases rapidly during this phase.
      (2). Colchicine given during this phase delays, but does not prevent, tissue deposition of amyloid and decreases SAA concentration.
         (a). Colchicine impairs secretion of SAA from hepatocytes by binding to microtubules and preventing its release.[14]
         (b). Colchicine can prevent the development of reactive amyloidosis when given prophylactically to a patient population with a known high risk of reactive amyloidosis (i.e., human patients with familial Mediterranean fever).[140]
      (3). Dimethylsulfoxide (DMSO) given during this phase causes resolution of amyloid deposits and a persistent decrease in SAA concentration.[71]
   b. Plateau phase
      (1). Net deposition of amyloid changes little during this phase.
      (2). Neither colchicine nor DMSO is thought to be beneficial if given during this phase.[71]

E. Other components of amyloid with unknown roles.

1. Serum amyloid P (SAP) component
   a. SAP is a serum glycoprotein, related in structure to C-reactive protein, that is commonly found in amyloid deposits, regardless of their chemical type.[94]
   b. Its carbohydrate content may be responsible for the staining of amyloid deposits by periodic acid-Schiff and Lugol's iodine.[49]
   c. Some evidence exists of genetic differences in the DNA sequence for the SAP gene in patients with juvenile rheumatoid arthritis and amyloidosis as compared to patients with juvenile rheumatoid arthritis without amyloidosis and to normal human beings.[134] A recent study, however, found that this polymorphism did not serve as a genetic marker for reactive amyloidosis.[55]
   d. Alternatively, SAP may be nonspecifically bound to amyloid fibrils in a calcium-dependent manner.
2. Glycosaminoglycans (e.g., heparan sulfate, dermatan sulfate)
   a. Glycosaminoglycans are found in association with amyloid deposits, regardless of the chemical type of amyloid.[117]
   b. They may affect precursor processing, folding of amyloidogenic proteins to form a β-pleated sheet, or polymerization and deposition of amyloid fibrils.[78,116,118]
   c. Alternatively, they may be nonspecifically bound to the amyloid fibrils.
3. Fibronectin
   a. Fibronectin binds to macrophages and SAA.
   b. It may bind SAA to the surface of splenic macrophages during the early stages of amyloid deposition.[68]

F. Factors predisposing to development of reactive systemic amyloidosis.

1. Chronic inflammation and a prolonged increase in the concentration of SAA are necessary prerequisites for development of reactive amyloidosis, and the progression of amyloidosis in some human patients has been correlated with increased SAA concentrations.[45] Nevertheless, only a small percentage (< 10%) of individuals with chronic inflammatory disease develops amyloidosis. Thus, other factors must also be important in development of amyloidosis.
2. Amyloidogenic SAA polymorphs
   a. Murine SAA2 is selectively removed from the circulation and deposited as amyloid in mice with casein-induced amyloidosis.[62,87,136]
   b. Only one form of SAA appears to be deposited as AA amyloid in the mink.[82,121]
   c. On the other hand, amino acid sequences corresponding to more than one form of SAA have been detected in amyloid deposits from the thyroid gland of one human patient.[95]
3. Genetic factors
   a. The SJL amyloid-resistant mouse fails to develop amyloidosis because of defective expression of the SAA2 gene (i.e., this amyloidogenic SAA polymorph is not produced).[137]
   b. The resistance of the A/J mouse to amyloidosis is related to defective production of AEF.[47,58,102]
   c. Monocytes contain cell surface-associated serine proteases that initially degrade SAA to AA amyloid-like intermediates and then to soluble peptides.[75,76] In mice with casein-induced amyloidosis, Kupffer's cells degrade SAA to an AA amyloid-like intermediate, whereas Kupffer's cells from control mice degrade this intermediate further.[46] The second stage of the degradative process may be defective in some individuals and may be a predisposing constitutional factor to amyloidosis.

4. Acquired host variability in degradation
   a. Normal serum has AA amyloid degrading activity, which may be decreased in serum from patients with chronic inflammatory disease and in those with amyloidosis.[8,124,125] This activity is correlated with serum albumin concentration, and hypoalbuminemia in amyloidosis may contribute to decreased AA amyloid degrading activity.[83]
   b. Chronic inflammation may contribute to amyloidosis by increasing the concentration of other acute-phase proteins that are protease inhibitors (e.g., antitrypsin, antichymotrypsin).
   c. Chronic inflammation also provides for a persistent increase in SAA concentration, which may then act as a substrate for the formation of AA amyloid deposits.

G. No discernible associated inflammatory or neoplastic disease occurs in most dogs and cats with reactive systemic amyloidosis.[41,112] Diseases that have been observed in association with reactive systemic amyloidosis in the dog include:

1. Inflammatory diseases
   a. Systemic mycoses (e.g., blastomycosis, coccidioidomycosis)
   b. Chronic inflammatory or immune-mediated diseases (e.g., systemic lupus erythematosus, chronic pancreatitis)
   c. Chronic bacterial infections (e.g., osteomyelitis, bronchopneumonia, pyometra, pyelonephritis, chronic suppurative dermatitis, chronic suppurative arthritis, chronic peritonitis, chronic pleuritis caused by nocardiosis, chronic stomatitis)
   d. Chronic parasitic infections (e.g., dirofilariasis)
2. Neoplastic diseases
   a. Lymphosarcoma
   b. Other neoplasms
3. Other diseases
   a. Chronic insulin infusion in experimental dogs[1]
   b. Cyclic hematopoiesis in grey collie dogs[25,52]
   c. In an early study of Australian cats with amyloidosis, 6 of 7 had lesions of hypervitaminosis A associated possibly with a diet high in liver[27,28]

H. The cause of the specific tissue tropisms of different amyloid proteins is poorly understood.

1. Prealbumin: peripheral nervous system and heart.
2. AA amyloid: kidney, spleen, and liver.
3. AL amyloid: kidney, spleen, liver, tongue, heart, and musculoskeletal system.

I. The cause of species differences in the tissue tropisms of reactive amyloid deposits also is unknown.[131]

1. In the dog, AA amyloid deposits are most common in the kidney, and clinical signs are caused by renal failure and uremia. The spleen, liver, adrenal glands, and gastrointestinal tract also may be involved, but associated clinical signs are uncommon.
2. In the cat, widespread deposition of amyloid deposits occurs, but clinical signs are caused by renal failure and uremia.

IV. Signalment

A. Age

1. Most dogs and cats with renal amyloidosis are old at the time of diagnosis.
   a. The mean age of affected dogs was 9 years in 2 studies.[41,112] The range of ages was 1 to 15 years, with 91% older than 5 years in a study of 44 cases,[112] and was 2 to 14 years, with 85% older than 7 years in a study of 59 cases.[41]
   b. The mean age of affected cats is approximately 7 years.[28,33,57,81,92,103] The age range was 1 to 17 years, with 65% of reported cats older than 5 years.
2. The mean age of 127 Abyssinian cats with familial amyloidosis was 3.9 years (range, younger than 1 to 13 years), and 74% of these were 5 years of age or younger at the time of death or euthanasia.[33a]
3. The mean age of 14 Shar pei dogs with familial amyloidosis was 4 years (range, 1.5 to 6 years) at the time of death or euthanasia.[42]

B. Breed.

1. Beagles, collies, and walker hounds were at increased risk and German shepherd and mixed-breed dogs were at decreased risk for renal amyloidosis in one study.[41]
2. Glomerular amyloidosis has been reported in families of older beagle dogs,[18,56] and in one study, diabetes mellitus and hypothyroidism also were described.[56]
3. Systemic reactive amyloidosis occurs as a familial disease in the Abyssinian cat[19,26,36,37] and Chinese Shar pei dog.[42]
4. Amyloidosis also has been observed in a 1.5-year-old male Akita dog with polyarthritis.[33b] Amyloid deposits were observed in the kidney, liver, and gastrointestinal tract. The dog had proteinuria but was not in renal failure at the time of diagnosis.
5. Familial amyloidosis associated predominantly with thyroid and hepatic amyloid deposits has been observed in Siamese cats.[125a,141] Affected cats appeared at 1 to 4 years of age with cachexia and jaundice. Spontaneous hepatic rupture and hemorrhage also have been observed.[141] The deposits are sensitive to potassium permanganate oxidation, and this syndrome may represent another example of reactive amyloidosis.[125a]

C. Sex.

1. No sex predilection was apparent in one study of amyloidosis in dogs.[112]
2. Female dogs had a predilection for amyloidosis in another study of affected dogs.[41]
3. The female/male sex ratio for 119 affected Abyssinian cats was 1.6 (73 females, 46 males).[33a]

4. Of 14 affected Shar pei dogs, 10 were female and 4 were male.[42]

V. CLINICAL FINDINGS

A. The clinical findings in amyloidosis depend on the organs affected, the amount of amyloid present, and the reaction of the affected organs to the presence of the amyloid deposits.

B. In dogs and cats, amyloid deposits in the kidneys lead to progressive renal disease, and the observed clinical signs are those of chronic renal failure and uremia.

C. Amyloid deposits in other tissues usually do not cause clinical signs.

1. Thyroid and adrenal deposits in Abyssinian cats with familial amyloidosis do not cause endocrine dysfunction based on thyroid-stimulating hormone (TSH) and adrenocorticotropic hormone (ACTH) stimulation testing.[40]
2. Occasionally, hepatic involvement may be prominent and may lead to jaundice in affected Shar pei dogs; jaundice and hepatic hemorrhage have been observed in Siamese cats with familial amyloidosis.[141]
3. Rarely, pancreatic involvement can lead to maldigestion in affected Abyssinian cats.[33a]

D. History.

1. When no clear history of a predisposing disorder is apparent, the clinical findings are those of chronic renal failure and uremia. This presentation is most common in dogs and cats with renal amyloidosis. At the time of diagnosis, between 50 and 75% of dogs with amyloidosis have no history of a predisposing disease process, and most cats with amyloidosis have no detectable predisposing condition.
   a. Anorexia, lethargy, and weight loss are commonly observed in both dogs and cats.
   b. Polyuria and polydipsia are more commonly detected by owners of dogs than of cats, but occur in both species.
   c. Vomiting is more commonly observed in dogs than in cats.
   d. Diarrhea is relatively uncommon in both dogs and cats.
2. The animal may have signs of some underlying inflammatory or neoplastic disorder, but this is less common.
3. Clinical signs may result from thromboembolic phenomena, which may occur in as many as 40% of affected dogs.[113] This complication appears to be rare in affected cats.
   a. Dyspnea caused by pulmonary thromboembolism is most common.[113]
   b. Caudal paresis with thromboembolism of the iliac or femoral arteries also may occur (Fig. 20–2).[35]
   c. Other less common sites of thromboembolism[113] include:
      (1). Coronary arteries with sudden death caused by acute myocardial infarction.
      (2). Renal artery with flank pain and hematuria.
      (3). Mesenteric artery and portal vein thrombosis with acute abdominal crisis.
      (4). Splenic arteries without clinical signs.
      (5). Brachial artery with acute onset of lameness or without clinical signs.
4. If the patient develops ascites or subcutaneous edema as a result of the nephrotic syndrome, the animal may be examined for abdominal distention

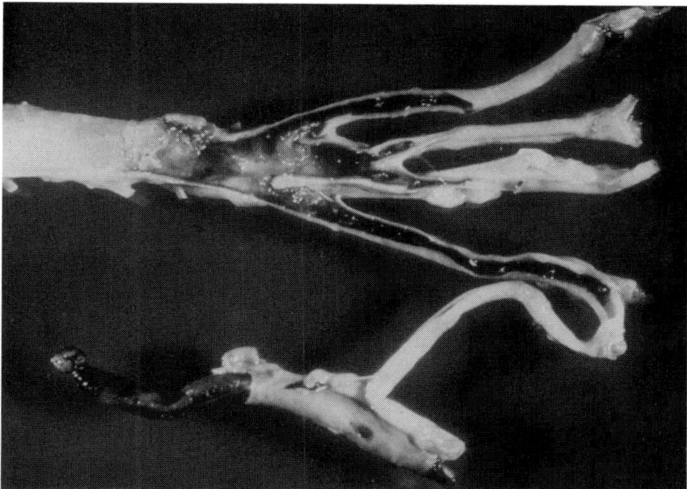

FIG. 20–2. Thrombi obstructing the terminal aorta, internal and external iliac arteries, and iliac vein in a dog with renal amyloidosis. The dog was examined by the veterinarian because of an acute onset of caudal paresis. (From DiBartola SP, Meuten DJ. Renal amyloidosis in two dogs presented for thromboembolic phenomena. *J Am Anim Hosp Assoc.* 1980;16:129-135.)

or swelling of the distal extremities, but these manifestations are relatively uncommon in dogs and cats with renal amyloidosis.

5. Occasionally, asymptomatic proteinuria may be detected on urinalysis during clinical evaluation of another medical problem.
6. Rarely, the animal may have signs compatible with uremia of apparently acute onset and may have oliguria. This manifestation mimics acute renal failure.

E. Physical examination findings are variable and usually are related to the presence of chronic renal failure.

1. Emaciation resulting from chronic weight loss.
2. Dehydration resulting from decreased water intake despite ongoing polyuria and vomiting, if present.
3. Dry, scaling haircoat caused by poor nutritional status.
4. Normal rectal temperature in most cases, but hypothermia if advanced renal failure is present.
5. Oral ulceration resulting from uremia.
6. The kidneys usually are small, firm, and irregular in affected cats, but the kidneys may be normal in size or slightly enlarged in affected dogs. Detection of slightly enlarged kidneys in some affected dogs has caused confusion with acute renal failure in some cases.
7. Other physical findings may be related to primary inflammatory (e.g., osteomyelitis, bronchopneumonia) or neoplastic disease processes.
8. Some affected Shar pei dogs have had a previous history of episodic joint swelling (usually the tibiotarsal joints) and high fever that resolve within a few days, regardless of treatment. This syndrome also has been observed in Shar pei dogs without documented amyloidosis and resembles familial Mediterranean fever in humans.[119]
9. Many affected Abyssinian cats have had severe gingivitis with loss of teeth, but this condition appears to be common in Abyssinian and Somali cats, regardless of the presence or absence of amyloidosis.[33a]
10. Ascites or subcutaneous edema occasionally may be found if classic nephrotic syndrome is present.
11. Signs of thromboembolism depend on the site of the thrombus (see previous section), but some dogs with thromboembolism do not have detectable clinical signs.[113]

VI. LABORATORY FINDINGS

A. Complete blood count findings in dogs[41] and cats[26,38] with renal amyloidosis are those of chronic renal failure.

1. Lymphopenia is common and is attributed to the stress of chronic disease.
2. Leukocytosis may indicate an underlying inflammatory disease or may be a manifestation of stress.
3. Nonregenerative anemia results primarily from lack of renal erythropoietin production, but shortened life span of the red cell and blood loss resulting from the hemorrhagic gastroenteritis of uremia also may contribute.
4. Plasma proteins
   a. Hypoproteinemia (< 6 g/dl) is observed in dogs with amyloidosis more commonly than is hyperproteinemia (> 8 g/dl). At the time of diagnosis, hypoproteinemia was observed in 24% of dogs with renal amyloidosis, whereas hyperproteinemia was observed in 8.5%.[41]
   b. Hypoproteinemia was observed in 5 of 14 Shar pei dogs with familial amyloidosis.[42]
   c. When present, hyperproteinemia may result from dehydration or chronic inflammatory disease.
   d. Hyperproteinemia caused by hyperglobulinemia is more common in cats with amyloidosis[33,103] and was observed in Abyssinian cats with familial amyloidosis.[26]

B. Chemistry.

1. Azotemia
   a. May be absent or mild at the time of diagnosis in approximately 50% of dogs with renal amyloidosis.[41,112]
   b. Commonly is observed at the time of diagnosis in cats with amyloidosis.[33,81,103]
   c. Commonly is present in Abyssinian cats and Shar pei dogs with familial amyloidosis.[26,42]
   d. Reflects prerenal (i.e., dehydration) and renal (i.e., chronic progressive renal disease with destruction of at least 75% of functional nephrons) factors when present.
2. Hyperphosphatemia parallels azotemia, is a result of decreased glomerular filtration rate (GFR), and indicates loss of at least 85% of functional nephrons.
3. Hypercholesterolemia
   a. Hypercholesterolemia is present in 75 to 95% of dogs with glomerular disease.[23,34]
   b. It is common in dogs with glomerular amyloidosis, and more than 85% of affected dogs had hypercholesterolemia in a study.[41]
   c. In cats, hypercholesterolemia is common in many types of renal disease and does not reliably predict glomerular disease. It occurred in more than 70% of cats with chronic renal disease in a study.[38]
   d. Hyperlipidemia occurs in a roughly inverse linear relationship to hypoalbuminemia in nephrotic syndrome, presumably as a result of increased hepatic synthesis of lipoproteins.[3]
4. Hypoalbuminemia
   a. Hypoalbuminemia occurs in most dogs and cats with renal amyloidosis.
   b. In dogs, severe loss of protein via the glomeruli probably is the most important factor.

(1). Other factors, however, must be involved because human patients treated by chronic ambulatory peritoneal dialysis lose more protein per day than do many patients with nephrotic syndrome, but the patients being dialyzed do not develop progressive hypoalbuminemia.[69]

(2). Hypoalbuminemia was found in 76% of dogs with glomerular disease,[34] in 70% of dogs with amyloidosis,[41] and in 32.5% of dogs with glomerulonephritis.[23] Thus, hypoalbuminemia may be somewhat more common in dogs with amyloidosis as compared to those with glomerulonephritis.

c. The mechanism of hypoalbuminemia may be somewhat different in affected cats than in dogs, because cats with medullary amyloidosis do not have large urinary losses of protein. The chronic inflammatory pattern observed on protein electrophoresis (i.e., polyclonal gammopathy) in affected cats indicates that the hypoalbuminemia may be reactive in nature. Albumin is a negative acute-phase reactant (i.e., its hepatic production decreases in response to inflammation).

5. Increased creatine kinase activity may be observed in some dogs with renal amyloidosis, possibly as a result of thromboembolism.
6. Increased liver enzyme activity (SAP, ALT) occurs in some dogs with renal amyloidosis for unknown reasons.
7. Hypocalcemia occurs in 50% of dogs with renal amyloidosis and is attributed to hypoproteinemia and a decreased protein-bound fraction of calcium.
8. Mild hyperglycemia occurs in some dogs with renal amyloidosis and is attributed to the insulin resistance of uremia.
9. Metabolic acidosis characterized by decreased serum bicarbonate concentration, high anion gap, and normal serum chloride concentration occurs in some dogs with amyloidosis and is attributed to uremia.
10. Hyperkalemia occasionally is observed, but the specific cause is not known.

C. Urinalysis.

1. Proteinuria in the absence of remarkable sediment findings is the hallmark of glomerular disease.
   a. Moderate to marked proteinuria is common in dogs with amyloidosis because of the predominant glomerular location of the deposits.[23,34,41]
   b. Proteinuria is mild or absent in animals with medullary amyloidosis that do not have concurrent glomerular involvement (e.g., most domestic cats with amyloidosis, at least 25% of Abyssinian cats with familial amyloidosis, and at least 33% of Shar pei dogs with familial amyloidosis). Thus, the absence of proteinuria does not rule out a diagnosis of amyloidosis, especially in Abyssinian and other domestic cats and in Shar pei dogs.
   c. Proteinuria usually is more severe in dogs with glomerular amyloidosis than in dogs with glomerulonephritis, but because individual variation is great, this finding cannot be relied on to make a diagnosis.
2. Impaired ability of the kidneys to concentrate urine is observed in most dogs and cats with amyloidosis.
   a. It reflects the osmotic diuresis typical of renal disease that has progressed to destruction of 67% or more of the renal parenchyma.
   b. Severe medullary amyloid deposition may contribute to defective concentrating ability by its physical presence and lead to early interference with urinary concentrating ability. Isosthenuria without proteinuria is common in cats with medullary amyloidosis.
3. Glucosuria may be observed in some affected animals in the presence of normal blood glucose concentration, but this finding is nonspecific and probably reflects altered proximal tubular function in the presence of chronic renal disease.[41]
4. Casts are observed in the urine of many dogs with renal amyloidosis.[41,112] Hyaline cylindruria classically is considered typical of glomerular disease, but in a recent study of dogs with glomerulonephritis, granular casts were more common than hyaline casts,[24] and in a retrospective study of amyloidosis in dogs, similar findings were observed.[41] In this study, hyaline, granular, and waxy casts all were observed.
5. Hematuria and pyuria may be observed but are uncommon unless a concurrent urinary tract infection exists.

D. Magnitude of urinary protein excretion.

1. Twenty-four-hour urinary protein excretion tends to be higher in dogs with glomerular amyloidosis than in dogs with glomerulonephritis, but because individual variation is great, this finding cannot be relied on for diagnosis.
   a. In 1 study, a mean value of 481.7 mg/kg/d (range, 350.8 to 533.7 mg/kg/d) was observed in 6 dogs with amyloidosis, whereas a mean value of 116.0 mg/kg/d (range, 7.5 to 526.1 mg/kg/d) was observed in 26 dogs with glomerulonephritis.[23]
   b. In an earlier study, a mean value of 506.9 mg/kg/d (range, 150.3 to 959.6 mg/kg/d) was observed in 6 dogs with amyloidosis, whereas a mean value of 164.7 mg/kg/d (range, 81.2 to 387.1 mg/kg/d) was observed in 11 dogs with glomerulonephritis.[34]
   c. In a recent study of dogs with amyloidosis, urinary protein losses were greater than 150 mg/kg/d in 9 dogs, 91 to 150 mg/kg/d in 4 dogs,

and less than 30 mg/kg/d (normal) in only 1 dog.[41]

2. Urine protein/creatinine ratios tend to be higher in dogs with glomerular amyloidosis as compared to those with glomerulonephritis, but because individual variation is great, this finding cannot be relied on for diagnosis.
   a. A mean urine protein/creatinine ratio of 22.5 (range, 11.17 to 46.65) was observed in 6 dogs with amyloidosis as compared to a ratio of 5.73 (range, 0.47 to 43.39) in 26 dogs with glomerulonephritis.[23]
   b. Urine protein/creatinine ratio was greater than 10 in 8 dogs, 2.0 to 9.9 in 7 dogs, and 0.41 to 1.9 in only 1 dog with amyloidosis in a recent retrospective study.[41]

E. Other laboratory tests.

1. Endogenous creatinine clearance was measured in 14 dogs with amyloidosis and was markedly low (< 0.5 ml/min/kg) in 4 dogs, moderately low (0.5 to 0.9 ml/min/kg) in 4 dogs, and mildly low (1.0 to 1.9 ml/min/kg) in 6 dogs.[41]
2. Microbiologic findings
   a. Urinary tract infection was documented in almost 40% of 18 dogs with amyloidosis.[41]
   b. Urinary tract infection should be ruled out, especially if pyuria is present.
   c. Urinary tract infection in dogs with amyloidosis may be incidental or may reflect chronic cystitis or pyelonephritis, either of which could contribute to development of reactive amyloidosis.

F. Radiographic findings.

1. Renal size typically is small in affected cats (< 2 times the length of the 2nd lumbar vertebra).
2. Renal size may be small (< 2.5 times the length of the 2nd lumbar vertebra), normal, or increased (> 3.5 times the length of the 2nd lumbar vertebra) in affected dogs.

VII. PATHOLOGIC FINDINGS

A. The pathologist must request a Congo red stain in addition to routine hematoxylin and eosin when submitting specimens, because small deposits of amyloid are easily missed in any organ. Substantial amounts of renal medullary amyloid can be missed on routine hematoxylin and eosin sections. Regardless of their chemical type, amyloid deposits appear green and birefringent when stained with Congo red and viewed under polarized light (Fig. 20–3).

B. Special studies, such as immunofluorescence, immunoperoxidase tests, and electron microscopy, help to characterize the lesions of glomerulonephritis, which may be subtle on light microscopy. Amyloid fibrils have a typical appearance on transmission electron microscopy (Fig. 20–1).

C. Evaluation of sections stained with Congo red before and after permanganate oxidation allows a presumptive diagnosis of AA amyloidosis versus other types, because AA amyloid loses its Congo red affinity after permanganate oxidation.[127,135] β_2-microglobulin-associated amyloid also is permanganate sensitive.[106] This form of amyloid has not yet been observed in veterinary medicine. (See Section III of this chapter.)

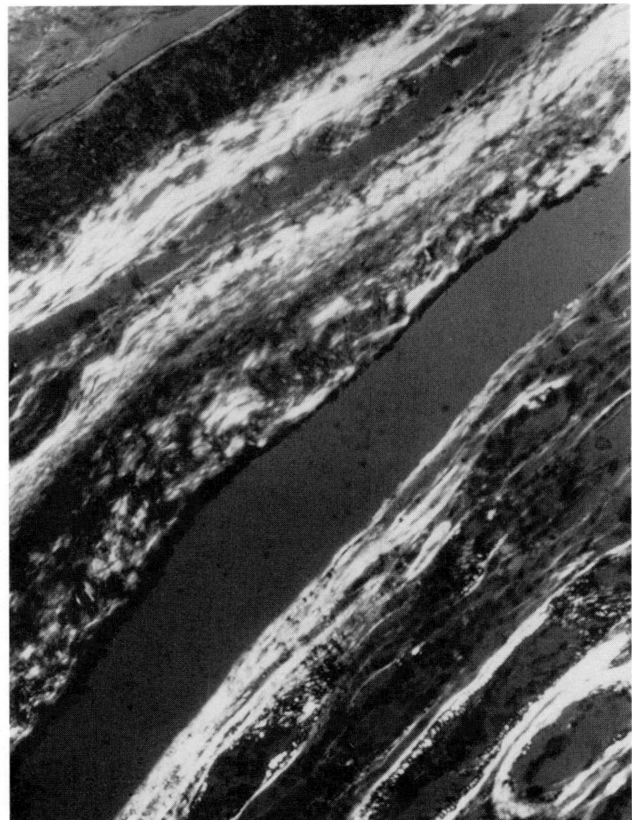

FIG. 20–3. Medullary amyloid deposits from a domestic cat with amyloidosis (Congo red stain). (Polarized light, 39×.)

D. Staining a gross specimen at necropsy with Lugol's iodine allows detection of large amounts of amyloid as bluish-black material. This stain is especially helpful for renal medullary deposits (Fig. 20–4).

E. A renal biopsy is necessary to differentiate glomerular amyloidosis from glomerulonephritis. This distinction is important because glomerulonephritis in dogs and cats may have a variable course characterized by clinical remission and stable renal function for several years, whereas amyloidosis generally is a progressive, fatal disease. Also, some aspects of therapy may differ between these two diseases. (See Section VIII of this chapter.)

1. In dogs other than Shar pei dogs, amyloidosis primarily is a glomerular disease and can be

diagnosed by renal cortical biopsy (Fig. 20–5). Early in the course of the disease, deposits are observed in the vascular pole of the glomerulus, in the glomerular capillary wall, and in the mesangium.

2. When medullary amyloidosis occurs without glomerular involvement in Abyssinian and other domestic cats (Fig. 20–3), results of renal cortical biopsies are negative for amyloidosis.
   a. Medullary amyloidosis without discernible glomerular involvement occurs in many domestic cats with amyloidosis, including at least 25% of Abyssinian cats with familial amyloidosis. Medullary amyloidosis without glomerular involvement also occurs in at least 33% of Shar pei dogs with familial amyloidosis.[42] In these cases, amyloidosis can be difficult to document clinically unless sufficient medullary tissue is obtained at the time of renal biopsy.
   b. In studies of human patients with medullary amyloidosis, the chemical structure of the AA amyloid was determined to be different from that in patients with glomerular amyloidosis.[132]
3. Other renal lesions
   a. Renal papillary necrosis may occur in cats and Shar pei dogs with medullary amyloidosis.
      (1). This lesion is thought to be caused by direct interference with blood flow to the inner medulla via the vasa recta by medullary amyloid deposits.
      (2). It can be observed grossly and in transverse histologic sections of affected kidney (Fig. 20–6).
   b. Chronic tubulo-interstitial lesions indicative of end-stage renal disease and of varying severity may be observed in dogs and cats with renal amyloidosis.
      (1). Interstitial fibrosis.
      (2). Lymphoplasmacytic inflammation.
      (3). Tubular atrophy.
      (4). Tubular dilatation.
      (5). Soft tissue mineralization.
      (6). Intratubular oxalates.
      (7). Protein casts.
      (8). Glomerular atrophy.
      (9). Glomerular sclerosis.
      (10). Periglomerular fibrosis.

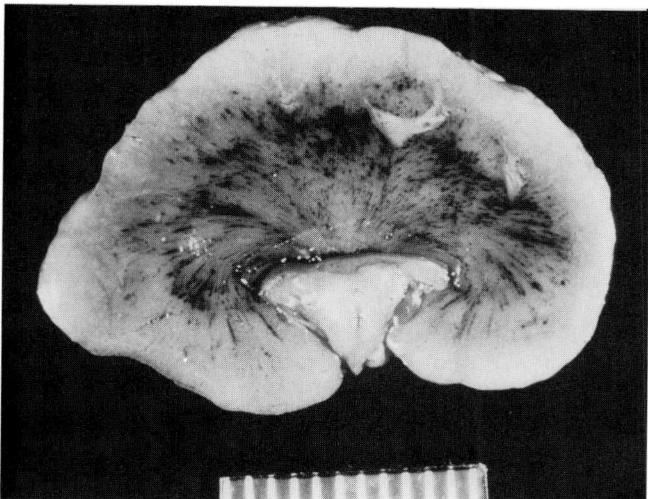

FIG. 20–4. Gross appearance of renal medullary amyloid deposits in an Abyssinian cat. (Lugol's iodine stain.) (From DiBartola SP, Rutgers HC. Diseases of the kidney. In: Sherding RG. *The Cat: Diseases and Clinical Management.* New York, New York: Churchill Livingstone; 1989:1378.)

F. Other organ involvement.

1. Most dogs with amyloidosis have predominantly renal involvement.[112] Small amounts of amyloid may be observed in spleen or liver and occasionally in the gastrointestinal tract, adrenal glands, and pancreas.
2. The extrarenal distribution of amyloid deposits in Abyssinian cats[37] and Shar pei dogs[42] with familial amyloidosis is wide and includes:
   a. Adrenal glands.
   b. Thyroid glands.
   c. Spleen.
   d. Liver.
   e. Myocardium.
   f. Gastrointestinal tract.
   g. Lymph nodes.
   h. Pancreas.
3. Tissue deposits in these extrarenal locations usually are clinically silent and cause no readily apparent problems for the host.

G. Thromboembolism.

1. This topic has been reviewed previously. (See Section V of this chapter.)
2. The most common site of thromboembolism in dogs with renal amyloidosis is the pulmonary artery.
3. This complication appears to be rare in cats with amyloidosis.

VIII. TREATMENT

A. Identify and effectively treat any underlying inflammatory or neoplastic predisposing disease process. Although such treatment rarely alters the course of the renal disease in animals with chronic renal failure and uremia secondary to renal amyloidosis, good medical practice dictates doing so.

B. Correct dehydration by appropriate fluid therapy.

C. Manage renal failure according to the principles of conservative medical treatment.

D. Experimental therapy for amyloidosis.

1. Dimethylsulfoxide (DMSO)
   a. Mechanisms by which DMSO may benefit patients with amyloidosis:
      (1). Solubilizing amyloid fibrils and allowing urinary excretion of subunit proteins. This

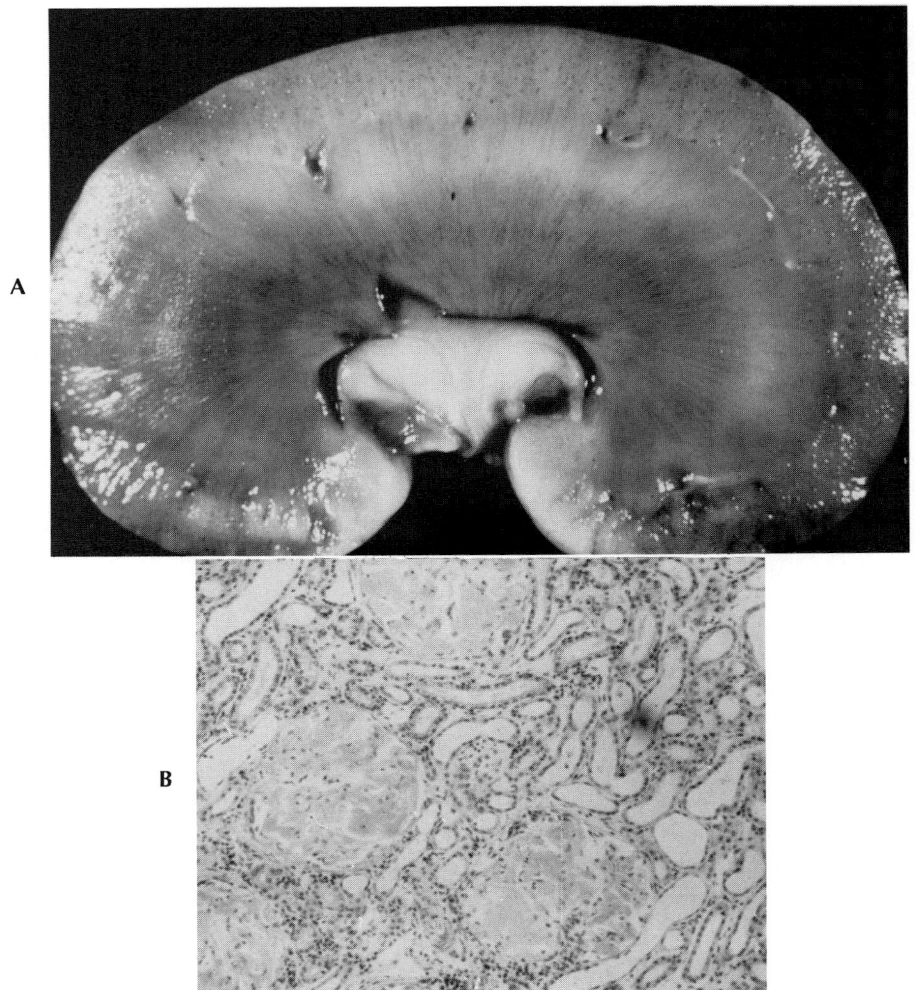

FIG. 20–5. Gross (Lugol's iodine, **A**) and microscopic (Congo red, **B**) appearance of glomerular amyloid deposits from a dog with renal amyloidosis.

mechanism is thought to be unlikely because the amount of amyloid in the kidneys of human patients who improved clinically after DMSO therapy was unchanged.[99,128]

(2). Reducing the concentration of the serum precursor protein SAA by the anti-inflammatory effect of DMSO.

(3). Reducing interstitial inflammation and fibrosis in the affected kidneys by the anti-inflammatory effect of DMSO. This effect may result in improvement of renal function and reduction in proteinuria.

b. Side effects of DMSO therapy

(1). Administration of DMSO results in nausea (in human patients) and an unpleasant garlic-like odor, which is thought to be caused by the metabolite dimethyl sulfite. These factors may lead to failure of owner compliance and to anorexia with decreased water consumption in the affected animal, thus worsening prerenal azotemia.

(2). Intravenous administration of DMSO can lead to transient hemoglobinuria, presumably a result of intravascular hemolysis.[33a] Hemolysis may result from diffusion of DMSO and water into erythrocytes.

(3). If undiluted, subcutaneous administration of DMSO may cause pain. I have diluted 90% DMSO 1:4 with sterile water before administering it subcutaneously.[33a]

(4). When given at a dose of 5 g/kg for 3 months, DMSO changed the refractive index and caused opacities of the lens in dogs.[53]

(5). Perivascular inflammation and local thrombosis may occur if undiluted DMSO is administered intravenously.[120]

c. Whether or not DMSO is beneficial in treatment of renal amyloidosis in dogs is controversial.
   (1). In 1 report,[120] 80 mg/kg DMSO was administered subcutaneously 3 times a week for 1 year and then topically for another year to a dog with glomerular amyloidosis. The magnitude of proteinuria decreased and serum albumin concentration increased to normal. After 2 years, GFR (estimated by endogenous creatinine clearance) was normal, but no pretreatment GFR estimate was available.
   (2). In another report,[32] 2 dogs with renal amyloidosis were treated with 125 mg/kg DMSO orally 2 times a day, using a 10% solution. Renal function and clinical condition improved for 9 months, but the magnitude of proteinuria did not change.
   (3). In another study of 4 dogs with renal amyloidosis, 300 mg/kg DMSO was given orally on a daily basis; 3 of the 4 dogs died of renal failure within 9 months of beginning therapy. The severity of amyloid deposition in the kidneys of these dogs was not affected by treatment.[53]
   (4). I have observed 14- and 20-month survival times in 2 dogs with renal amyloidosis treated with 90 mg/kg DMSO subcutaneously 3 times per week. Renal function and magnitude of proteinuria did not improve in these dogs, and both were in renal failure at the time of death. Of the 2 dogs, 1 died as a result of pulmonary thromboembolism.[33a]
d. The minimal toxicity of DMSO suggests that a therapeutic trial should be instituted in dogs and cats with stable renal amyloidosis, but the effectiveness of DMSO in this situation is uncertain.

2. Colchicine impairs the release of SAA from hepatocytes by binding to microtubules and preventing secretion[14] and may interfere with AEF production.[20]
   a. Colchicine prevents the development of amyloidosis in patients with familial Mediterranean fever and promotes stabilization of renal function in patients with nephrotic syndrome but without overt renal failure.[140] No evidence suggests, however, that it is beneficial once amyloidosis has resulted in renal failure.
   b. Colchicine is somewhat toxic in human pa-

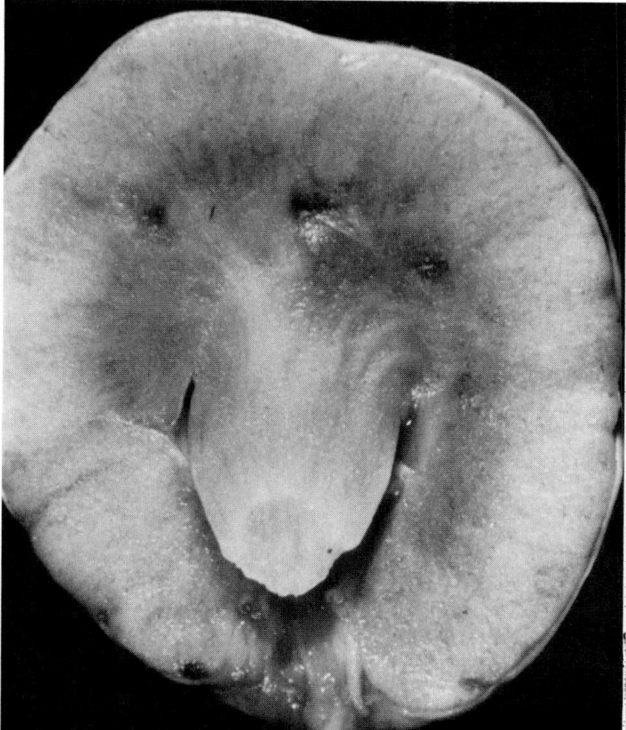

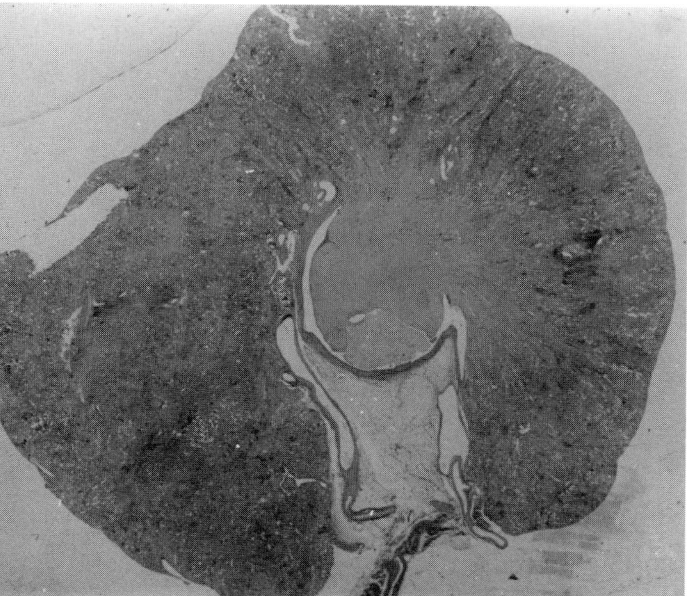

FIG. 20–6. Gross **(A)** and microscopic **(B)** appearance of papillary necrosis in an Abyssinian cat with renal medullary amyloidosis. (From DiBartola SP, Rutgers HC. Diseases of the kidney. In: Sherding RG. *The Cat: Diseases and Clinical Management.* New York, New York: Churchill Livingstone, 1989:1378.)

tients, and its side effects include vomiting, diarrhea, and nausea.

c. To my knowledge, there has been no experience with this drug in the treatment of dogs and cats with amyloidosis.

3. Mice with experimentally induced amyloidosis live longer when treated with vitamin C but have no change in the severity of their amyloid deposits.[5,6,100]

IX. COMPLICATIONS

A. Sodium retention and hypertension.

1. Hypertension has been observed to occur in 60% of dogs with renal disease and in 80% of dogs with glomerular disease.[31] Hypertension has been reported in 61% of cats with chronic renal failure.[74]
2. Affected dogs and cats may be examined for acute onset of blindness caused by retinal detachments and retinal hemorrhage.[7,54,90]
3. See Chapter 19, Pathophysiology and Management of Systemic Hypertension Associated with Renal Dysfunction, for information about the treatment of systemic hypertension in patients with renal failure.

B. Thromboembolism.

1. The pathophysiology of hypercoagulability in nephrotic syndrome appears to be multifactorial.
   a. Increased concentrations of coagulation factors I (fibrinogen), II, V, VII, VIII, and X may occur as a result of increased hepatic synthesis.
   b. Decreased concentrations of coagulation factors IX, XI, and XII may occur as a result of urinary loss.
   c. Decreased plasma concentration of antithrombin III occurs as a result of urinary loss and is one of the most important factors responsible for thromboembolism in nephrotic syndrome.[50] Antithrombin III is an inhibitor of coagulation factors, especially factor II.
   d. Platelet hyperaggregability occurs and may be aggravated by hypoalbuminemia.[51]
   e. Impaired fibrinolysis.
2. Treatment
   a. The main action of heparin is to potentiate the activity of antithrombin III. Heparin thus may be relatively ineffective in patients with nephrotic syndrome in which plasma concentrations of antithrombin III are abnormally low.[50] The dose of heparin is 150 to 250 IU/kg subcutaneously 2 to 3 times per day.
   b. Recently, a low dose of aspirin (0.5 mg/kg orally twice daily) has been reported to inhibit platelet aggregation in dogs more effectively than does a dose of 10 mg/kg orally once daily.[96] This treatment is unlikely to be harmful and may be beneficial in dogs with glomerular disease. Whether antiplatelet therapy is necessary in cats with glomerular disease is unclear, because the occurrence of thromboembolism in such cats is rare. If aspirin is used in affected cats, a standard dose of 25 mg/kg orally twice weekly should be safe.
   c. Warfarin blocks activation of vitamin K in the liver and prevents activation of clotting factors II, VII, IX, and X. Therapy with warfarin cannot be recommended at this time because of the risk of hemorrhage and lack of experience in veterinary medicine.

REFERENCES

1. Albisser AM, et al. Unanticipated amyloidosis in dogs infused with insulin. *Diabetes.* 1983;32:1092-1101.
2. Aldo-Benson M, Benson MD. SAA suppression of immune response *in vitro:* Evidence of an effect on T cell-macrophage interaction. *J Immunol.* 1982;128:2390-2393.
3. Appel GB, et al. The hyperlipidemia of the nephrotic syndrome: Relation to plasma albumin concentration, oncotic pressure, and viscosity. *N Engl J Med.* 1985;312:1544-1548.
4. Axelrad MA, et al. Further characterization of amyloid-enhancing factor. *Lab Invest.* 1982;47:139-146.
5. Baltz ML, et al. The failure of ascorbic acid to alter the induction or remission of murine amyloidosis. *Clin Exp Immunol.* 1984; 57:657-662.
6. Baltz ML, et al. Effect of vitamin C dietary supplementation on survival in amyloidosis. *Arthritis Rheum.* 1987;30:718-719.
7. Barclay SM, Riis RC. Retinal detachment and reattachment associated with ethylene glycol intoxication in a cat. *J Am Anim Hosp Assoc.* 1979;15:719-724.
8. Bausserman LL, Herbert PN. Degradation of serum amyloid A and apolipoproteins by serum proteases. *Biochemistry.* 1984;23: 2241-2245.
9. Bausserman LL, et al. Degradation of serum amyloid A by isolated perfused rat liver. *J Biol Chem.* 1987;262:1583-1589.
10. Benditt EP, Hoffman JS, Eriksen N. SAA, an apoprotein of HDL: Its structure and function. *Ann NY Acad Sci.* 1982;389:183-189.
11. Benditt EP, Meek RL. Expression of the third member of the serum amyloid A gene family in mouse adipocytes. *J Exp Med.* 1989;169:1841-1846.
12. Benson MD, et al. Kinetics of serum amyloid protein A in casein-induced murine amyloidosis. *J Clin Invest.* 1977;59: 412-417.
13. Benson MD, Aldo-Benson M. Effect of purified protein SAA on immune response *in vitro:* Mechanisms of suppression. *J Immunol.* 1979;122:2077-2082.
14. Benson MD, Kleiner E. Synthesis and secretion of serum amyloid protein A (SAA) by hepatocytes in mice treated with casein. *J Immunol.* 1980;124:495-499.
15. Benson MD: *In vitro* synthesis of the acute phase reactant SAA by hepatocytes. *Ann NY Acad Sci.* 1982;389:116-120.
16. Benson MD, Dwulet FE, DiBartola SP. Identification and characterization of amyloid protein AA in spontaneous canine amyloidosis. *Lab Invest.* 1985;52:448-452.
17. Benson MD, et al. A unique insertion in the primary structure of bovine amyloid AA protein. *J Lab Clin Med.* 1989;113:67-72.
18. Bowles M, Mosier DA. Renal amyloidosis in a family of beagles. *J Am Vet Med Assoc.* 1992;201:569-574.
19. Boyce JT, et al. Familial renal amyloidosis in Abyssinian cats. *Vet Pathol.* 1984;21:33-38.
20. Brandwein SR, et al. Effect of colchicine on experimental amyloidosis in two CBA/J mouse models. *Lab Invest.* 1985;52: 319-325.
21. Carothers MA, et al. Extramedullary plasmacytoma and immunoglobulin-associated amyloidosis in a cat. *J Am Vet Med Assoc.* 1989;195:1593-1597.

22. Castell JV, et al. Recombinant human interleukin-6 (IL-6/BSF-2/HSF) regulates the synthesis of acute phase proteins in human hepatocytes. *FEBS Lett.* 1988;232:347-350.
23. Center SA, et al. 24-Hour urine protein/creatinine ratio in dogs with protein-losing nephropathies. *J Am Vet Med Assoc.* 1985; 187:820-824.
24. Center SA, et al. Clinicopathologic, renal immunofluorescent, and light microscopic features of glomerulonephritis in the dog: 41 cases (1975-1985). *J Am Vet Med Assoc.* 1987;190:81-90.
25. Cheville NF. Amyloidosis associated with cyclic neutropenia in the dog. *Blood.* 1968;31:111-114.
26. Chew DJ, et al. Renal amyloidosis in related Abyssinian cats. *J Am Vet Med Assoc.* 1982;181:139-142.
27. Clark L, Seawright AA. Amyloidosis associated with chronic hypervitaminosis A in cats. *Aust Vet J.* 1968;44:584.
28. Clark L, Seawright AA. Generalised amyloidosis in seven cats. *Path Vet.* 1969;6:117-134.
29. Coetzee GA, et al. Serum amyloid A-containing human high density lipoprotein 3. *J Biol Chem.* 1986;261:9644-9651.
30. Cohen AS, Connors LH. The pathogenesis and biochemistry of amyloidosis. *J Pathol.* 1987;151:1-10.
31. Cowgill LD, Kallet AJ. Recognition and management of hypertension in the dog. In: Kirk RW, ed. *Current Veterinary Therapy VIII.* Philadelphia, Pennsylvania: WB Saunders Co; 1983:1026.
32. Cowgill LD. Diseases of the kidney. In: Ettinger SJ, ed. *Textbook of Veterinary Internal Medicine.* 2nd ed. Philadelphia, Pennsylvania: WB Saunders Co; 1983:1843.
33. Crowell WA, et al. Generalized amyloidosis in a cat. *J Am Vet Med Assoc.* 1972;161:1127-1133.
33a. DiBartola SP. Unpublished observations. Columbus, Ohio: 1982-1990.
33b. DeMorais H. Personal communication. Columbus, Ohio: 1990.
34. DiBartola SP, et al. Urinary protein excretion and immunopathologic findings in dogs with glomerular disease. *J Am Vet Med Assoc.* 1980;177:73-77.
35. DiBartola SP, Meuten DJ. Renal amyloidosis in two dogs presented for thromboembolic phenomena. *J Am Anim Hosp Assoc.* 1980;16:129-135.
36. DiBartola SP, et al. Isolation and characterization of amyloid protein AA in the Abyssinian cat. *Lab Invest.* 1985;52:485-489.
37. DiBartola SP, Tarr MJ, Benson MD. Tissue distribution of amyloid deposits in Abyssinian cats with familial amyloidosis. *J Comp Pathol.* 1986;96:387-398.
38. DiBartola SP, Rutgers HC, Zack PM, Tarr MJ. Clinicopathologic findings in 74 cats with chronic renal disease. *J Am Vet Med Assoc.* 1987;190:1196-1202.
39. DiBartola SP, Benson MD. Pathogenesis of reactive systemic amyloidosis. *J Vet Intern Med.* 1989;3:31-41.
40. DiBartola SP, Tarr MJ. Corticotropin and thyrotropin response tests in Abyssinian cats with familial amyloidosis. *J Am Anim Hosp Assoc.* 1989;25:217-220.
41. DiBartola SP, et al. Clinicopathologic findings in dogs with renal amyloidosis: 59 cases (1976-1986). *J Am Vet Med Assoc.* 1989; 195:358-364.
42. DiBartola SP, et al. Renal amyloidosis in related Chinese Shar pei dogs. *J Am Vet Med Assoc.* 1990;197:483-487.
43. Dwulet FE, Wallace DK, Benson MD. Amino acid structures of multiple forms of amyloid-related serum protein from a single individual. *Biochemistry.* 1988;27:1677-1682.
44. Reference omitted.
45. Falck HM, et al. Correlation of persistently high serum amyloid A protein and C-reactive protein concentrations with rapid progression of secondary amyloidosis. *Br Med J.* 1983;286: 1373-1456.
46. Fuks A, Zucker-Franklin D. Impaired Kupffer cell function precedes development of secondary amyloidosis. *J Exp Med.* 1985;161:1013-1028.
47. Gervais F, Hebert L, Skamene E. Amyloid-enhancing factor: Production and response in amyloidosis-susceptible and resistant mouse strains. *J Leukocyte Biol.* 1988;43:311-316.
48. Giesel O, Stiglmair-Herm M, Linke RP. Myeloma associated with immunoglobulin lamda-light chain derived amyloid in a dog. *Vet Pathol.* 1990;27:374-376.
49. Glenner GG. Amyloid deposits and amyloidosis: The beta fibrilloses. *N Engl J Med.* 1980;302:1283-1292, 1333-1343.
50. Green RA, Kabel AL. Hypercoagulable state in three dogs with nephrotic syndrome: Role of acquired antithrombin III deficiency. *J Am Vet Med Assoc.* 1982;181:914-917.
51. Green RA, et al. Hypoalbuminemia-related platelet hypersensitivity in two dogs with nephrotic syndrome. *J Am Vet Med Assoc.* 1985;186:485-488.
52. Gregory RS, Machado EA, Jones JB. Animal model: Amyloidosis associated with canine cyclic hematopoiesis in the gray Collie dog. *Am J Pathol.* 1977;87:721-724.
53. Gruys E, Sijens RJ, Biewenga WJ. Dubious effect of dimethylsulfoxide (DMSO) therapy on amyloid deposits and amyloidosis. *Vet Res Commun.* 1981;5:21-32.
54. Gwin RM, et al. Hypertensive retinopathy associated with hypothyroidism, hypercholesterolemia, and renal failure in a dog. *J Am Anim Hosp Assoc.* 1978;14:200-209.
55. Harats N, et al. Lack of association of a restriction fragment length polymorphism for serum amyloid P gene with reactive amyloidosis. *Arthritis Rheum.* 1989;32:1325-1327.
56. Hargis AM, et al. Relationship of hypothyroidism to diabetes mellitus, renal amyloidosis and thrombosis in purebred beagles. *Am J Vet Res.* 1981;42:1077-1081.
57. Hartigan PJ, Tuite M, McAllister H. Generalized amyloidosis in the domestic cat. *Ir Vet J.* 1980;34:1-4.
58. Hebert L, Gervais F. Apo-SAA1/apo-SAA2 isotype ratios during casein- and amyloid-enhancing-factor-induced secondary amyloidosis in A/J and C57BL/6J mice. *Scand J Immunol.* 1990;31: 167-173.
59. Hoffman JS, Benditt EP. Changes in high density lipoprotein content following endotoxin administration in the mouse. *J Biol Chem.* 1982;257:10510-10517.
60. Hoffman JS, Benditt EP. Secretion of serum amyloid protein and assembly of serum amyloid protein-rich high density lipoprotein in primary mouse hepatocyte culture. *J Biol Chem.* 1982;257:10518-10522.
61. Hoffman JS, Benditt EP. Plasma clearance kinetics of the amyloid-related high density lipoprotein apoprotein, serum amyloid protein (ApoSAA), in the mouse. *J Clin Invest.* 1983; 71:926-934.
62. Hoffman JS, et al. Murine tissue amyloid protein AA. NH_2-terminal sequence identity with only one of two serum amyloid protein (apoSAA) gene products. *J Exp Med.* 1984;159: 641-646.
63. Husebekk A, et al. Transformation of amyloid precursor SAA to protein AA and incorporation in amyloid fibrils *in vivo. Scand J Immunol.* 1985;21:283-287.
64. Husebekk A, et al. Characterization of bovine amyloid proteins SAA and AA. *Scand J Immunol.* 1988;27:739-743.
65. Johnson KH, et al. Islet amyloid, islet amyloid polypeptide and diabetes mellitus. *N Engl J Med.* 1989;321:513-518.
66. Johnson KH, et al. Amino acid sequence variations in protein AA of cats with high and low incidences of AA amyloidosis. *Comp Biochem Physiol [B].* 1989;94:765-768.
67. Kaminski NE, Holsapple MP. Inhibition of macrophage accessory cell function in casein-treated $B6C3F_1$ mice. *J Immunol.* 1987;139:1804-1810.

68. Kawahara E, et al. The role of fibronectin in the development of experimental amyloidosis. *Am J Pathol.* 1989;134:1305-1314.
69. Kaysen GA, et al. Mechanisms and consequences of proteinuria. *Lab Invest.* 1986;54:479.
70. Kisilevsky R, Boudreau L. Kinetics of amyloid deposition. I. The effects of AEF and splenectomy. *Lab Invest.* 1983;48:53-59.
71. Kisilevsky R, Boudreau L, Foster D. Kinetics of amyloid deposition. II. The effects of dimethylsulfoxide and colchicine therapy. *Lab Invest.* 1983;48:60-77.
72. Kluve-Beckerman B, Dwulet FE, Benson MD. Human serum amyloid A: Three hepatic mRNAs and the corresponding proteins in one person. *J Clin Invest.* 1988;82:1670-1675.
73. Kluve-Beckerman B, et al. Primary structures of dog and cat amyloid A proteins: Comparison to human AA. *Comp Biochem Physiol [B].* 1989;94:175-183.
74. Kobayashi DL, et al. Hypertension in cats with chronic renal failure or hyperthyroidism. *J Vet Intern Med.* 1990;4:58-62.
75. Lavie G, Zucker-Franklin D, Franklin EC. Degradation of serum amyloid A protein by surface-associated enzymes of human blood monocytes. *J Exp Med.* 1978;148:1020-1031.
76. Lavie G, Zucker-Franklin D, Franklin EC. Elastase-like proteases on the surface of human blood monocytes: Possible role in amyloid formation. *J Immunol.* 1980;125:175-180.
77. Levin M, Pras M, Franklin EC. Immunologic studies of the major nonimmunoglobulin protein of amyloid I. Identification and partial characterization of a related serum component. *J Exp Med.* 1973;138:373-380.
78. Linker A, Carney HC. Presence and role of glycosaminoglycans in amyloidosis. *Lab Invest.* 1987;57:297-305.
79. Lowell CA, Stearman RS, Morrow JF. Transcriptional regulation of serum amyloid A gene expression. *J Biol Chem.* 1986; 261:8453-8461.
80. Lowell CA, et al. Structure of the murine serum amyloid A gene family. *J Biol Chem.* 1986;261:8442-8452.
81. Lucke VM, Hunt VM. Interstitial nephropathy and papillary necrosis in the domestic cat. *J Pathol Bacteriol.* 1965;89:723-728.
82. Marhaug G, Husby G, Dowton SB. Mink serum amyloid A protein. *J Biol Chem.* 1990;265:10049-10054.
83. Maury CPJ, Teppo AM. Mechanism of reduced amyloid-A-degrading activity of serum of patients with secondary amyloidosis. *Lancet.* 1982;2(8292):234-237.
84. Maury CPJ. Reactive (secondary) amyloidosis and its pathogenesis. *Rheumatol Int.* 1984;5:1-7.
85. Maury CPJ, Ehnholm C, Lukka M. Serum amyloid A protein (SAA) subtypes in acute and chronic inflammation. *Ann Rheum Dis.* 1985;44:711-715.
86. Meek RL, Benditt EP. Amyloid A gene family expression in different mouse tissues. *J Exp Med.* 1986;164:2006-2017.
87. Meek RL, Hoffman JS, Benditt EP. Amyloidogenesis: One serum amyloid A isotype is selectively removed from the circulation. *J Exp Med.* 1986;163:499-510.
88. Meek RL, Eriksen N, Benditt EP. Serum amyloid A in the mouse: Sites of uptake and mRNA expression. *Am J Pathol.* 1989;135:411-419.
89. Miura K, Takahashi Y, Shirasawa H. Immunohistochemical detection of serum amyloid A protein in the liver and the kidney after casein injection. *Lab Invest.* 1985;53:453-463.
90. Morgan RV. Systemic hypertension in four cats: Ocular and medical findings. *J Am Anim Hosp Assoc.* 1986;22:615-621.
91. Moshage JH, et al. The effect of interleukin-1, interleukin-6 and its interrelationship on the synthesis of serum amyloid A and C-reactive protein in primary cultures of adult human hepatocytes. *Biochem Biophys Res Commun.* 1988;155:112-117.
92. Nakamatsu M, Goto M, Morita M. A case of generalized amyloidosis in the cat. *Jpn J Vet Sci.* 1966;28:259-265.
93. Parks JS, Rudel LL. Alteration of high density lipoprotein subfraction distribution with induction of serum amyloid A protein (SAA) in the nonhuman primate. *J Lipid Res.* 1985;26: 82-91.
94. Pepys MB, Baltz ML. Acute phase proteins with special reference to C-reactive protein and related proteins (pentaxins) and serum amyloid A protein. *Adv Immunol.* 1983;34:141.
95. Prelli F, Pras M, Frangione B. Degradation and deposition of amyloid AA fibrils are tissue specific. *Biochemistry.* 1987;26: 8251-8256.
96. Rackear DG, et al. The effect of three different dosages of acetylsalicylic acid on canine platelet aggregation. *J Am Anim Hosp Assoc.* 1988;24:23-26.
97. Ramadori G, Sipe JD, Colten HR. Expression and regulation of the murine serum amyloid A (SAA) gene in extrahepatic sites. *J Immunol.* 1985;135:3645-3647.
98. Ramadori G, et al. Interleukin-6, the third mediator of acute phase reaction, modulates hepatic protein synthesis in human and mouse. Comparison with interleukin 1β and tumor necrosis factor-α. *Eur J Immunol.* 1988;18:1259-1264.
99. Ravid M, et al. Prolonged dimethylsulfoxide treatment of 13 patients with systemic amyloidosis. *Ann Rheum Dis.* 1982;41: 587-592.
100. Ravid M, et al. Ascorbic acid induced regression of amyloidosis in experimental animals. *Br J Exp Pathol.* 1985;66:137-141.
101. Rokita H, et al. Differential expression of the amyloid SAA3 gene in liver and peritoneal macrophages of mice undergoing dissimilar inflammatory episodes. *J Immunol.* 1987;139:3849-3853.
102. Rokita H, et al. Serum amyloid A gene expression and AA amyloid formation in A/J and SJL/J mice. *Br J Exp Pathol.* 1989;70:327-335.
103. Saegusa S, et al. Concurrent feline immune-complex nephritis: Tubular-antigen positive and renal amyloidosis. *Arch Pathol Lab Med.* 1979;103:475-478.
104. Schwartzman RM. Cutaneous amyloidosis associated with a monoclonal gammopathy in a dog. *J Am Vet Med Assoc.* 1984; 185:102-104.
105. Shaw DP, Gunson DE, Evans LH. Nasal amyloidosis in four horses. *Vet Pathol.* 1987;24:183-185.
106. Shirahama T, et al. Histochemical and immunohistochemical characterization of amyloid associated with chronic hemodialysis as beta-2 microglobulin. *Lab Invest.* 1985;53:705-709.
107. Shirahama T, Cohen AS. Immunocytochemical study of hepatocyte synthesis of amyloid AA. *Am J Pathol.* 1985;118: 108-115.
108. Shirahama T, et al. Amyloid-enhancing factor-loaded macrophages in amyloid fibril formation. *Lab Invest.* 1990;62:61-68.
109. Sipe JD, et al. Detection of a mediator derived from endotoxin-stimulated macrophages that induces the acute phase serum amyloid A response in mice. *J Exp Med.* 1979;150:597-606.
110. Sipe JD, et al. The role of interleukin-1 in acute phase serum amyloid A (SAA) and serum amyloid P (SAP) biosynthesis. *Ann NY Acad Sci.* 1982;389:137-150.
111. Sipe JD, et al. Human serum amyloid A (SAA): Biosynthesis and postsynthetic processing of pre SAA and structural variants defined by complementary DNA. *Biochemistry.* 1985;24:2931-2936.
112. Slauson DO, Gribble DH, Russell SW. A clinicopathological study of renal amyloidosis in dogs. *J Comp Pathol.* 1970;80: 335-343.
113. Slauson DO, Gribble DH. Thrombosis complicating renal amyloidosis in dogs. *Vet Pathol.* 1971;8:352-363.
114. Sletten K, Husebekk A, Husby G. The amino acid sequence of

an amyloid fibril protein AA isolated from the horse. *Scand J Immunol.* 1987;26:79-84.

115. Sletten K, Husebekk A, Husby G. The primary structure of equine serum amyloid A (SAA) protein. *Scand J Immunol.* 1989;30:117-122.

116. Snow AD, Kisilevsky R. Temporal relationship between glycosaminoglycan accumulation and amyloid deposition during experimental amyloidosis: A histochemical study. *Lab Invest.* 1985;53:37-44.

117. Snow AD, Willmer J, Kisilevsky R. Sulfated glycosaminoglycans: A common constituent of all amyloids? *Lab Invest.* 1987;56:120-123.

118. Snow AD, et al. Characterization of tissue and plasma glycosaminoglycans during experimental AA amyloidosis and acute inflammation. *Lab Invest.* 1987;56:665-675.

119. Sohar E, et al. Familial Mediterranean fever: Survey of 470 cases and review of the literature. *Am J Med.* 1967;43:227-253.

120. Spyridakis L, et al. Amyloidosis in a dog: Treatment with dimethylsulfoxide. *J Am Vet Med Assoc.* 1986;189:690-691.

121. Syversen V, et al. The amino acid sequence of serum amyloid A (SAA) protein in mink. *Scand J Immunol.* 1987;26:763-767.

122. Takahasi M, et al. Ultrastructural evidence for the synthesis of serum amyloid A protein by murine hepatocytes. *Lab Invest.* 1985;52:220-223.

123. Tatsuta E, et al. Kinetics of SAP and SAA production by cultured mouse liver cells. *Ann NY Acad Sci.* 1982;389:467-470.

124. Teppo AM, Maury CPJ, Wegelius O. Characteristics of the amyloid A fibril-degrading activity of human serum. *Scand J Immunol.* 1982;16:309-314.

125. Teppo AM, Maury CPJ. Do serine proteases degrade amyloid fibrils? *Scand J Immunol.* 1983;18:363-366.

125a. Valentine, R. Personal communication. Boston, Massachusetts: 1990.

126. van Andel ACJ, Gruys E, Kroneman J. Amyloid in the horse: A report of nine cases. *Equine Vet J.* 1988;20:277-285.

127. van Rijswijk MH, van Heusden CWGJ. The potassium permanganate method: A reliable method for differentiating amyloid AA from other forms of amyloid in routine laboratory practice. *Am J Pathol.* 1979;97:43-54.

128. van Rijswijk MH, et al. Dimethylsulfoxide in the treatment of AA amyloidosis. *Ann NY Acad Sci.* 1983;389:67-83.

129. Webb CF, Tucker PW, Dowton SB. Expression and sequence analyses of serum amyloid A in the Syrian hamster. *Biochemistry.* 1989;28:4785-4790.

130. Weinstein JA, Taylor JA. Interleukin-1 and the acute phase response: Induction of mouse liver serum amyloid A mRNA by murine recombinant interleukin-1. *J Trauma.* 1987;27:1227-1232.

131. Westermark P, Sletten K, Eriksson M. Morphologic and chemical variation of the kidney lesions in amyloidosis secondary to rheumatoid arthritis. *Lab Invest.* 1979;41:427-431.

132. Westermark P, et al. AA-amyloidosis in dogs: Partial amino acid sequence of protein AA and immunohistochemical cross-reactivity with human and cow AA-amyloid. *Comp Biochem Physiol [B].* 1985;82:211-215.

133. Westermark P, et al. Bovine amyloid protein AA: Isolation and amino acid sequence analysis. *Comp Biochem Physiol [B].* 1986; 85:609-614.

134. Woo P, et al. A genetic marker for systemic amyloidosis in juvenile arthritis. *Lancet.* 1987;2(8562):767-769.

135. Wright JR, Calkins E, Humphrey RL. Potassium permanganate reaction in amyloidosis: A histologic method to assist in differentiating forms of this disease. *Lab Invest.* 1977;36: 274-281.

136. Yamamoto KI, Migita S. Complete primary structures of two major murine serum amyloid A proteins deduced from cDNA sequences. *Proc Natl Acad Sci USA.* 1985;82:2915-2919.

137. Yamamoto KI, Shiroo M, Migita S. Diverse gene expression for isotypes of murine serum amyloid A protein during acute phase reaction. *Science.* 1986;232:227-229.

138. Yamamoto KI, et al. Structural diversity of murine serum amyloid A genes: Evolutionary implications. *J Immunol.* 1987; 139:1683-1688.

139. Yano BL, Johnson KH, Hayden DW. Feline insular amyloid: Histochemical distinction from secondary systemic amyloid. *Vet Pathol.* 1981;18:181-187.

140. Zemer D, et al. Colchicine in the prevention and treatment of amyloidosis of familial Mediterranean fever. *N Engl J Med.* 1986;314:1001-1005.

141. Zuber M. Personal communication. Australia: 1990.

CHAPTER 21

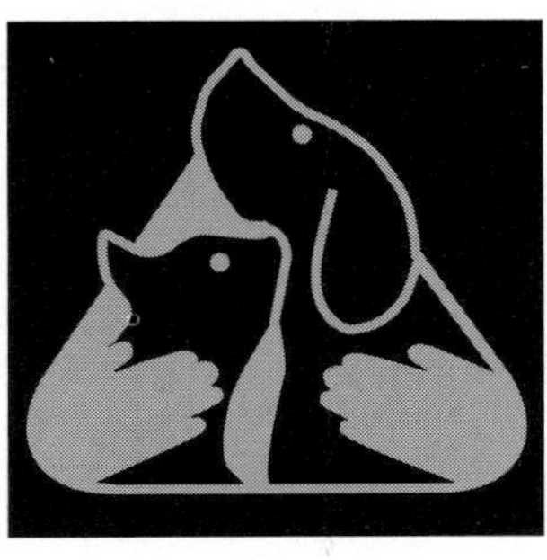

Canine and Feline Hypercalcemic Nephropathy

JOHN M. KRUGER
CARL A. OSBORNE

I. CLINICAL IMPORTANCE

A. Hypercalcemia is recognized as a frequent disorder of calcium metabolism in dogs and cats and comprises approximately 2 to 3% of total abnormal serum biochemical determinations.[30]

B. Calcium ion plays a central role in many fundamental physiologic processes; precise control of blood calcium concentration is essential to health. Hypercalcemia may profoundly disrupt cellular and organ function, resulting in severe renal, gastrointestinal, cardiovascular, and neurologic dysfunction. Of the many organ systems affected by hypercalcemia, the kidney appears to be particularly susceptible. Hypercalcemia-induced alterations in renal function and structure are linked to many, if not all, of the clinical manifestations observed in hypercalcemic patients. Because many renal effects induced by hypercalcemia are potentially reversible, early recognition and characterization of this problem with the goal of rapid therapeutic intervention are of great clinical significance.

C. There has been a concomitant increase in number, specificity, and efficacy of therapeutic agents or methods used for specific and symptomatic treatment of hypercalcemia. As new diagnostic and therapeutic methods become available, identification of specific applications and evaluation of their usefulness in the context of veterinary medicine are essential to minimize their misuse and to simplify and improve management of hypercalcemia and hypercalcemic nephropathy.

II. CAUSES OF HYPERCALCEMIA

A. Hypercalcemic of malignancy.

1. Nonparathyroid neoplasms, especially lymphomas, have been the most common cause of hypercalcemia in dogs and cats (Tables 21–1 and 21–2).[30,95] In a study, more than 40% of hypercalcemic dogs with classifiable disease were affected with some form of nonparathyroid neoplasia.[30]
2. Results of *in vivo* and *in vitro* studies in several species have identified two basic pathogenic mechanisms responsible for malignancy-associated hypercalcemia:
   a. Hypercalcemia caused by tumor-induced local osteolysis.
   b. Hypercalcemia caused by tumor-derived circulating factors stimulating generalized osteoclastic bone resorption (so-called "humoral hypercalcemia of malignancy").[15,21,95,106,121]
3. Hypercalcemia associated with malignancy may also involve both humoral and local pathogenic factors acting independently or in combination (Table 21–2).[15,121]

TABLE 21–1.
CHECKLIST OF CAUSES OF HYPERCALCEMIA IN DOGS*

Hypercalcemia of malignancy
  Lymphoid neoplasia
  Anal sac apocrine cell adenocarcinoma
Hypoadrenocorticism
Chronic renal failure
Hypervitaminosis D
  Iatrogenic
  Intoxication
Primary hyperparathyroidism
Infectious/inflammatory disorders
  Systemic fungal diseases
  Septic osteomyelitis

*Arranged in approximate order of decreasing likelihood of occurrence.

4. Humoral hypercalcemia of malignancy results from enhanced osteoclastic bone resorption mediated by systemically acting factors secreted by malignant cells (Table 21–2).[15,21,106,121] Although the role of increased bone resorption has been emphasized in the past, enhanced renal tubular calcium reabsorption appears to play a significant role in the pathogenesis of humoral hypercalcemia associated with some malignancies.[106,121]
   a. Recent studies in humans and dogs have identified several tumor-derived peptides that resemble parathyroid hormone (PTH) both in structure and physiologic properties.[15,21,99,101,121,124,150]
      (1). Like PTH, PTH-related peptides enhance osteoclastic bone resorption, promote distal renal tubular calcium reabsorption, inhibit proximal tubule phosphate reabsorption, and stimulate nephrogenous cyclic adenosine monophosphate (cyclic AMP) excretion.[15,21,95,106,121]
      (2). Unlike PTH, PTH-related peptides decrease osteoblastic bone formation, have limited ability to stimulate renal 1-α-hydroxylase activity, and do not cross-react with PTH antisera.[15,21,121]
      (3). Observations in hypercalcemic dogs with lymphoma and anal sac apocrine cell adenocarcinoma suggest that PTH-related peptides are the primary mediators of hypercalcemia associated with these neoplasms.[95,101,124,150,152]
   b. Tumor production of prostaglandin E_2, transforming growth factor, colony-stimulating factors, leukocyte cytokines, and 1,25-dihydroxyvitamin D may also play a role in the pathogenesis of some forms of humoral hypercalcemia of malignancy.[106,121]
      (1). Tumor-associated production of 1,25-dihydroxyvitamin D (calcitriol) appears to be responsible for hypercalcemia observed in a few human patients with lymphoma.[106,121]
      (2). Postaglandin E_2-mediated bone resorption has been hypothesized to play a role in hypercalcemia associated with several solid tissue tumors of humans and rodents.[106,121]
      (3). Increased serum concentrations of calcitriol or prostaglandin E_2 have not yet been observed in hypercalcemic dogs with lymphoma or anal sac apocrine cell adenocarcinoma.[70,100,101,152]
5. Hypercalcemia of malignancy may also result from tumor-induced local osteolysis.
   a. Primary or metastatic skeletal neoplasms may resorb bone directly, or may stimulate osteoclastic bone resorption via tumor secretion of prostaglandin E_2, interleukin-1, or tumor necrosis factor (Table 21–2).[15,95,106]
   b. Although tumor-induced local osteolysis is a common cause of hypercalcemia in humans, it appears to be an infrequently recognized cause of hypercalcemia in dogs and cats.[15,30,92,106]

B. Hypoadrenocorticism.

1. Hypoadrenocorticism has been the second most common disorder associated with hypercalcemia in dogs.[30] Hypercalcemia has been reported to occur in approximately 28 to 45% of dogs and 10% of cats with hypoadrenocorticism.[118,119,156]
2. Although exact mechanisms are unknown, hypercalcemia of hypoadrenocorticism may be attributable to increased calcium retention resulting from diminished glomerular filtration and enhanced renal calcium reabsorption secondary to volume contraction.[105,148] Other contributing factors include hemoconcentration, increased protein binding of calcium, and increased calcium complexing with plasma and ions, such as citrate and phosphate.[148]
3. Total plasma concentrations of calcium, protein, citrate, and phosphate were elevated in hypercalcemic adrenalectomized dogs; however, the ionized calcium concentration in plasma remained within normal range.[148]
4. The clinical significance of elevations in the nonionized calcium fraction in plasma requires further investigation.

C. Chronic renal failure.

1. Chronic renal failure has been uncommonly associated with hypercalcemia in dogs and cats.[30,31,38]
   a. Typically, total serum calcium concentrations have been normal to subnormal in patients with chronic renal failure; however, approximately 11 to 14% of dogs and cats developed hypercalcemia.[31,38]
   b. Paradoxically, dogs with hypercalcemia and chronic renal failure often had normal to de-

creased ionized calcium concentrations in serum despite elevations in total calcium.[31,108]

2. Hypercalcemia associated with chronic renal failure was first characterized in young dogs affected with severe familial renal disease.[20,52] Subsequently, hypercalcemia associated with chronic renal disease has been observed in dogs of all ages.[31]
3. The etiopathogenesis of hypercalcemia of chronic renal failure is most likely multifactorial, involving PTH-mediated increased bone resorption, decreased renal calcium excretion as a result of reduced nephron mass and glomerular filtration rate (GFR) increased intestinal calcium absorption as a result of enhanced target tissue sensitivity to calcitriol, and increased calcium complexing with anions.[31,52]
   a. Autonomous hypersecretion of PTH by the parathyroid gland is believed to play a central role in the pathogenesis of hypercalcemia of chronic renal failure.[31,52,90]
   b. The term tertiary hyperparathyroidism has been frequently used to define hypercalcemia associated with autonomous parathyroid function and hypercalcemia.[4,82,134] However, this term is most applicable to the development of an adenoma within hyperplastic parathyroid tissue.[4,90] Although parathyroid adenomas occasionally have been identified, hyperplasia has been the predominant parathyroid lesion observed in human patients with hypercalcemia of chronic renal failure.[4,82,90,137]
   c. Parathyroid gland hyperplasia is the characteristic finding in dogs with hypercalcemia

TABLE 21–2.
ETIOPATHOGENIC MECHANISMS OF HYPERCALCEMIA CAUSED BY NONPARATHYROID NEOPLASIA

Cause	Species		General Mechanisms
	Canine	Feline	
Hematologic malignancies			Proposed mechanisms incude:
Lymphoid			A. Humoral factors: increased generalized osteoclastic bone resorption[15,95,106,121]
Lymphoma[32,45,47,70,92,100,154,159]	+	+	1. PTH-related peptides
Multiple myeloma[92,94]	+	NR	2. Prostaglandin E_2
Myeloid			3. Calcitriol
Myeloproliferative disease[92,161]	+	+	4. Cytokines (osteoclast-activating factors)
Erythroleukemia[47]	NR	+	a. Interleukin-1
			b. Tumor necrosis factor
Nonhematologic malignancies			
Nonskeletal neoplasms			5. Transforming growth factors
Anal sac apocrine cell adenocarcinoma[99,101]	+	NR	6. Colony-stimulating factors
Squamous cell carcinoma[63,76]	+	+	B. Local factors[15,95,106]
Fibrosarcoma[92]	+	NR	1. Increased local osteoclastic bone resorption
Pulmonary epidermoid carcinoma[109]	+	NR	a. Prostaglandin E_2
Nasal adenocarcinoma[158]	+	NR	b. Cytokines
Cholangiocarcinoma[139]	+	NR	2. Pressure necrosis
Adenocarcinoma of exocrine pancreas[155]	+	NR	3. Direct resorption by cancer cells
Mammary adenocarcinoma[92]	+	NR	4. Direct resorption my macrophages
Interstitial cell tumor[92]	+	NR	
Seminoma[30]	+	NR	
Thyroid carcinoma[120,146]	+	+	
Thymoma[67]	+	NR	
Skeletal neoplasms			
Primary bone neoplasms[44]	+	NR	
Metastatic bone neoplasms			
Mammary gland adenocarcinoma[44,92]	+	NR	
Thyroid carcinoma[83]	+	NR	
Prostatic carcinoma[44]	+	NR	
Squamous cell carcinoma[76]	NR	+	
Liposarcoma[96]	+	NR	
Anal sac apocrine cell adenocarcinoma[99]	+	NR	

NR = not reported; PTH = parathyroid hormone.

caused by chronic renal failure.[52]

d. Hypercalcemia of chronic renal failure probably represents one extreme in the spectrum of secondary hyperparathyroidism in which disordered parathyroid growth is accompanied by loss of regulatory mechanisms controlling PTH secretion.[82,90]

(1). PTH secretion and synthesis are regulated by ionized calcium, calcitriol, and phosphorous concentrations in plasma.[16,49,90,91]

(a). Studies have demonstrated that PTH release is enhanced by decreases in ionized calcium and calcitriol concentrations in plasma.[16,49]

(b). Phosphate may directly stimulate PTH secretion by mechanisms independent of calcitriol or ionized calcium concentrations.[91]

(2). In patients with chronic renal failure, hyperphosphatemia, decreased renal production of calcitriol, and decreased ionized calcium concentration in plasma stimulate PTH secretion in an effort to maintain normal calcium homeostasis.[49,91] Low ionized calcium and calcitriol concentrations, hyperphosphatemia, and increased immunoreactive PTH (iPTH) levels have been observed in normocalcemic uremic dogs.[16,31,91] Similar findings have been observed in dogs with hypercalcemia caused by chronic renal failure.[31,108]

(3). Exact mechanisms by which hyperplastic parathyroid glands develop autonomous hypersecretion of PTH and subsequent hypercalcemia are not completely understood.

(a). Hypercalcemia has been hypothesized to develop as a result of an altered set point for plasma calcium concentration; the alteration is caused by changes in calcium transport by the parathyroid cell and in intracellular calcium concentration.[90,91]

(b). Changes in calcium metabolism by the parathyroid cell have been hypothesized to be mediated, at least in part, by reduced plasma calcitriol concentration, reduced quantities of calcitriol receptors in the parathyroid cell, and direct effects of hyperphosphatemia.[90,91]

D. Hypervitaminosis D.

1. Until recently, hypervitaminosis D was an uncommon cause of hypercalcemia in dogs and cats, and usually was associated with excess dietary or therapeutic vitamin D supplementation (Table 21–3).[10,28,39,40,46,51,54] However, availability of rodenticides containing vitamin D (0.075% cholecalciferol) has resulted in an increased detection of hypervitaminosis D.[28,39,40,53,64,104]
2. Cholecalciferol and other dietary vitamin D analogs undergo hepatic hydroxylation to form 25-hydroxyvitamin D (calciferol).[1] Formation of calciferol is primarily controlled by hepatic availability of its substrate, cholecalciferol.[1]
3. Renal 1-α-hydroxylase then converts calciferol to 1,25-dihydroxyvitamin D (calcitriol).[1]
   a. Calcitriol is the most potent vitamin D metabolite in terms of biologic activity and represents the primary metabolite involved in calcium homeostasis.[1,46]
   b. Renal 1-α-hydroxylase activity and formation of calcitriol are closely regulated by concentrations of PTH, calcitonin, calcitriol, and phosphorus.[1]
4. Because active metabolites of vitamin D stimulate intestinal calcium and phosphate transport, mobilize calcium from bone, and promote renal tubular reabsorption of calcium and phosphorus, excess vitamin D results in hypercalcemia, hyperphosphatemia, and dystrophic calcification of soft tissues.[1,39,40,46,64,133]
5. Although metabolites of cholecalciferol have minimal biologic activity at physiologic concentrations, high plasma concentrations of 25-dihydroxyvitamin D are capable of exerting direct effects on target tissues.[1,46,69]
   a. In a study, dogs receiving 10 mg/kg of body weight of cholecalciferol developed hypercalcemia and concurrent hyperphosphatemia within 12 to 36 hours after ingestion.[64]
   b. Toxicoses have also been reported in dogs receiving substantially lower doses (e.g., 1.5 to 3 mg/kg of body weight) of cholecalciferol.[39,59]

E. Primary hyperparathyroidism.

1. Primary hyperparathyroidism has been an uncommonly recognized cause of hypercalcemia in dogs and cats.[10,24,30,51]
2. Primary hyperparathyroidism is characterized by hypercalcemia resulting from excessive uncontrolled production of PTH by hyperplastic or neoplastic parathyroid glands (Table 21–3).[30,50,151]
   a. Solitary functional adenomas of the parathyroid gland have been the most common cause of primary hyperparathyroidism in dogs and cats.[24,30,51]
   b. Although parathyroid autonomy may result from abnormal proliferation of parathyroid cells, alterations in the set point at which ionized calcium is capable of suppressing PTH secretion may also have a role in the pathogenesis of primary hyperparathyroidism.[17,51,103]
3. Excess PTH enhances bone resorption and mobilization of calcium from bone by increasing osteocyte quantities and activity.[51,132,151]
4. In the kidney, excess PTH enhances distal tubular

calcium reabsorption, diminishes proximal tubular phosphate reabsorption, and stimulates 1-α-hydroxylase conversion of 25-Hydroxyvitamin D to calcitriol.[11,132,151] Calcitriol increases intestinal calcium and phosphate absorption and further enhances PTH-mediated osteoclastic bone resorption.[51,132,151]

5. In nonazotemic patients, the net effect of excess PTH is increased total and ionized calcium concentrations in serum with normal to decreased phosphorous concentrations in serum.[10,51,108,151]

F. Infectious and inflammatory disorders.

1. Hypercalcemia has been infrequently associated with chronic infectious or inflammatory disorders of humans, including sarcoidosis, pulmonary tuberculosis, beryIliosis, and systemic mycoses.[43,137] Similarly, hypercalcemia has been associated with blastomycosis, coccidiomycosis, and other chronic inflammatory disorders in dogs (Table 21–4).[43,44,144]
2. Recent studies in humans have revealed increased levels of calcitriol and abnormal vitamin D metabolism in patients with chronic granulomatous disease.[5,81,123]
   a. Based on findings that activated macrophages are capable of producing calcitriol when stimulated by gamma-interferon and interleukin-2, extrarenal production of calcitriol by activated macrophages has been hypothesized to be responsible for the hypercalcemia of granulomatous disorders.[5,9,81,86,123]
   b. Extrarenal production of calcitriol may be a factor in the pathogenesis of hypercalcemia associated with canine blastomycosis.[43] However, concentrations of vitamin D metabolites have not yet been determined in dogs with blastomycosis or other chronic inflammatory disorders.
3. Other mechanisms, such as localized bone reabsorption, may also account, at least in part, for hypercalcemia observed in these disorders.[43,44,144]

G. Miscellaneous causes of hypercalcemia.

1. Hypercalcemia occasionally has been associated with several additional pathologic and nonpathologic disorders of dogs and cats (Table 21–4).
2. These causes represent a diverse group of disorders for which the exact pathologic mechanisms responsible for hypercalcemia have yet to be defined.

III. CLINICAL MANIFESTATIONS

A. OVERVIEW.

1. Hypercalcemia may be associated with a wide variety of clinical signs that depend on interaction of one or more of the following:

TABLE 21–3.
ETIOPATHOGENIC MECHANISMS OF HYPERCALCEMIA CAUSED BY ENDOCRINOPATHIES

Cause	Species: Canine	Species: Feline	General Mechanism
Hyperparathyroidism			
Primary			Excess PTH secretion resulting in increased generalized bone resorption, increased renal tubular Ca reabsorption, and increased intestinal Ca absorption
Adenoma[10,24,51,151]	+	+	
Adenocarcinoma[10,51]	+	NR	
Familial[95]	+	NR	
Multiple endocrine neoplasia type IIa[120]	+	NR	
Secondary			
Chronic renal failure[20,31,38,52]	+	+	Exact mechanism unknown; increased bone resorption as a result of excess PTH; reduced renal Ca excretion; increased responsiveness to vitamin D; increased protein binding; increased anion complexing
Hypoadrenocorticism[118,119,156]	+	+	Exact mechanism unknown: reduced renal Ca excretion as a result of decreased GFR and enhanced renal tubular Ca reabsorption; increased plasma protein affinity for Ca; increased anion complexing
Hypervitaminosis D			Excess vitamin D promotes bone resorption, increases intestinal Ca absorption, and increases renal tubular Ca reabsorption
Rodenticides (cholecalciferol)[39,41,53,59,64,104]	+	+	
Pharmaceuticals (ergocalcitriol, dihydrotachysterol, calcitriol)[10,46,51]	+	+	
Plants *(Cestrum diurnum)*[44]	+	+	

CA = calcium; GFR = glomerular filtration rate; NR = not reported; PTH = parathyroid hormone.

TABLE 21–4.
ETIOPATHOGENIC MECHANISMS OF MISCELLANEOUS CAUSES OF HYPERCALCEMIA

Cause	Species		General Mechanism
	Canine	Feline	
Infectious or Inflammatory Disorders			Exact mechanism unknown: extrarenal production of calcitriol?; local osteolysis?
Blastomycosis[43]	+	NR	
Coccidiodomycosis[43]	+	NR	
Septic osteomyelitis[44]	+	NR	
Canine schistosomiasis[144]	+	NR	
Acute Renal Failure (diuretic phase)[18,44,89]	+	NR	Exact mechanism unknown: remobilization of Ca deposited after oliguric phase?; increased PTH?; increased calcitriol?
Hypothermia[125]	+	+	Exact mechanism unknown
Hyperproteinemia[29]	+	NR	Increased plasma protein binding
Laboratory Error[29]	+	+	Lipemia; detergents

Ca = calcium; NR = not reported; PTH = parathyroid hormone.

a. Local and systemic effects of the primary disorder.
b. Pathophysiologic effects of hypercalcemia.
c. Compensatory responses to alterations in normal homeostasis.

2. Clinical manifestations also reflect magnitude, duration, and progression of hypercalcemia.
3. Regardless of cause, clinical signs of hypercalcemia tend to be similar, and commonly involved in the urinary, gastrointestinal, cardiovascular, and neuromuscular systems (Table 21–5).

B. Urinary manifestations.

1. Alterations in renal function
   a. Impaired urine concentrating ability leading to polyuria and compensatory polydipsia are early manifestations of hypercalcemia in dogs.[48,51,93,99,115,154] Urine specific gravities of these patients are consistently less than 1.030, and usually less than 1.015.[51,99,154]
   b. In studies of induced acute hypercalcemia in dogs, the magnitude of polyuria was often disproportionately greater than would be predicted by the degree of azotemia and extent of renal morphologic changes.[48] These results suggest that, during early stages of hypercalcemia, factors other than those associated with renal failure secondary to nephrocalcinosis were involved in the pathogenesis of hypercalcemia-induced polyuria.[48]
   c. The pathogenesis of hypercalcemia-induced polyuria appears to involve derangements of normal urine concentrating mechanisms.
      (1). Although hypercalcemic patients typically consume excessive quantities of water, hypercalcemia-induced thirst (primary polydipsia) and suppressed antidiuretic hormone (ADH) secretion do not appear to play significant roles in the polyuria of hypercalcemia.[60] Studies in humans and rats have demonstrated that hypercalcemia-induced polyuria persists despite water restriction and administration of exogenous ADH.[34,60,128]
      (2). Hypercalcemia appears to antagonize adenylate cyclase in the renal medulla, resulting in reduced cyclic AMP concentrations

TABLE 21–5.
CLINICAL MANIFESTATIONS OF HYPERCALCEMIA

Urinary	Neuromuscular
Polyuria	Muscle weakness
Compensatory polydipsia	Muscle wasting
Azotemia	Twitching
Prerenal	Shivering
Primary renal	Stiff gait
Hypercalciuria	Depression
Hyperphosphaturia	Stupor
Sodium wasting	Coma
Magnesium wasting	Seizures
Glucosuria	
Nephrocalcinosis	**Cardiovascular**
Urolithiasis	Prolonged P-R intervall
Urinary tract infection	Shortened Q-T interval
	Ventricular arrhythmias
Gastrointestinal	Vasoconstriction
Anorexia	Hypertension
Vomiting	Endocardial calcification
Diarrhea	Arterial calcification
Constipation	
Weight loss	
Gastric calcification	
Intestinal calcification	

and subsequent blunting of collecting tubule responsiveness to ADH.[8,22,42]

(3). Calcium-induced renal resistance to ADH may also result from direct interference with ADH receptor binding.[22,42]

(4). Renal tubular resistance to ADH impedes transepithelial movement of water from collecting ducts into the medullary interstitium and reduces collecting duct permeability to urea.[126] The net effect is decreased renal water reabsorption and decreased urine osmolality.

(5). Diminished collecting duct responsiveness to ADH is further compounded by reduced medullary tonicity and disruption of medullary osmotic gradients.[60]

(a). Reduced medullary solute accumulation is probably related to decreased sodium and chloride reabsorption in the loop of Henle and to diminished collecting duct permeability to urea.[13,80,126,136,147]

(b). Concurrent increases in renal medullary blood flow and subsequent medullary washout appear to be important contributing factors in disruption of medullary osmotic gradients.[19,60]

(c). Studies of induced acute and chronic hypercalcemia in dogs have demonstrated a marked increase in renal medullary blood flow.[19]

(d). Exact mechanisms of hypercalcemia-induced increases in renal blood flow are unknown; however, calcium-induced synthesis of vasodilatory prostaglandins in the inner medulla may play a role.[162]

d. Elevations in serum calcium are frequently accompanied by variable reductions in GFR and variable increases in serum urea nitrogen (SUN) and serum creatinine (SC) concentrations.[51,64,115,133,153,154]

(1). Reductions in GFR and azotemia may result from prerenal factors, intrinsic renal factors, or combinations of both.[28,116,154]

(2). Hypercalcemia may directly alter renal hemodynamics and glomerular filtration.

(a). Studies in several species have demonstrated that moderate to severe hypercalcemia consistently produces reductions in GFR and renal blood flow as a result of renal vasoconstriction and a fall in the glomerular ultrafiltration coefficient.[23,33,48,58,74,87,110,160]

(b). Renal hemodynamic changes associated with hypercalcemia are potentially reversible; correction of hypercalcemia results in rapid restoration of GFR.[51,70,88,137]

(3). Other potentially reversible factors may account, at least in part, for increases in SUN and SC associated with hypercalcemia. In some patients, extracellular fluid (ECF) volume contraction resulting from diminished fluid intake and increased fluid losses (vomiting, diarrhea, and polyuria) may result in significant reductions in GFR and prerenal azotemia.[28,51,116] Correction of hypovolemia by fluid therapy usually results in restoration of GFR and rapid reduction in prerenal components of azotemia.[116]

(4). If hypercalcemia is persistent and severe, sustained renal vasoconstriction and nephrocalcinosis may lead to progressive intrinsic renal tubular injury and primary renal failure.[137] In this case, reversibility of reductions in GFR and primary renal azotemia ultimately depend on the degree of damage to the renal tubular cell and tubular basement membrane.[113,116]

e. Other renal tubular defects associated with hypercalcemic disorders in humans include metabolic acidosis secondary to proximal and distal defects in urine acidification mechanisms; metabolic alkalosis; renal sodium, potassium, magnesium, and phosphate wasting; hypercalciuria; aminoaciduria; and glucosuria.[137]

(1). In general, renal tubular defects have not been well characterized in hypercalcemic disorders of dogs and cats.

(2). Increased urine calcium concentrations and increased renal fractional calcium excretion values have been observed in association with several hypercalcemic disorders of dogs.[78,99,100,151,152] As serum calcium concentrations rise, filtered urine calcium increases proportionally and eventually overwhelms the calcium reabsorptive capacity of the distal renal tubules.[11] This hypercalciuric effect may occur despite distal tubular reabsorption of calcium enhanced by PTH or PTH-related peptide.[15,106,121,151,152]

(3). Increased urine phosphorous excretion has also been observed in hypercalcemic dogs with primary hyperparathyroidism, lymphosarcoma, and anal sac apocrine cell adenocarcinoma.[25,58,71,100,101,150,152,154] These patients were typically hypophosphatemic or normophosphatemic. Hyperphosphaturia observed in these disorders was most likely caused by decreased proximal tubule phosphate reabsorption resulting from the phosphaturic effects of PTH or PTH-related peptides or from direct tubular affects of hypercalcemia.[11,15,106,121,137]

(4). Transient glucosuria was observed in 2 of 18 dogs with vitamin D-induced hypercalcemia.[133] In humans, renal glucosuria has also been observed in patients with hypervitaminosis D and in patients with other vitamin D-related disorders, such as sarcoidosis.[44,143] The exact mechanism of hypercalcemia-associated renal glucosuria is unknown.

(5). In humans, hypercalcemic disorders have been associated with proximal and distal renal tubular acidosis and metabolic alkalosis.[137] Most of these disturbances result from alterations in handling of renal tubular bicarbonate and from defects in renal ammoniagenesis. Similar acid-base disturbances have not yet been reported in hypercalcemic dogs or cats.

2. Alterations in renal morphology
   a. Gross renal morphologic changes are most commonly associated with chronic or severe hypercalcemia.[6,115,133]
      (1). Kidneys may be normal to large, pale, and speckled or mottled, and may have a finely granular or pitted surface texture.[6,115,133,138,152]
      (2). As body fluids become supersaturated with calcium and phosphate, calcium phosphate ($CaHPO_4$) precipitates in kidneys as well as other soft tissues, including the heart, blood vessels, stomach, pancreas, lung, and thyroid and parathyroid glands.[64,99,115,133,154] Soft tissue mineralization is generally most pronounced when hypercalcemia is accompanied by concurrent hyperphosphatemia and the product of serum calcium concentration (mg/dl) multiplied by the serum phosphate concentration (mg/dl) exceeds 50.[28,99]
      (3). Gross evidence of mineralization may be observed as a distinctive white gritty band located adjacent to the corticomedullary junction.[6,99,115,133]
   b. In dogs, microscopic changes in renal structure vary with magnitude and duration of hypercalcemia.
      (1). Microscopic changes associated with acute or mild hypercalcemia are characterized by variable calcification, degeneration, and necrosis of tubular epithelium, and by formation of obstructing intertubular casts in the ascending loops of Henle, distal tubules, and collecting ducts.[23,48,133] Glomeruli and proximal tubules are usually normal in appearance.[23,133] Calcification of renal parenchyma is mild and randomly distributed, affecting primarily tubular epithelium and their basement membranes. Marked tubular dilatation of more proximal portions of the nephrons (intrarenal hydronephrosis) may be observed as a result of sloughing of tubular epithelium and cast formation.[23]
      (2). With severe or chronic hypercalcemia, the extent of tubular degeneration, necrosis, and obstruction and of renal parenchymal calcification is proportionately greater. Renal calcification is widespread, involving corticomedullary tubular epithelium and basement membrane, interstitial tissues, periglomerular capillary basement membranes, blood vessel walls, and Bowman's capsule.[6,23,64,115,133,154] Nephrocalcinosis may be concurrently associated with fibrosis and infiltration of interstitial tissues with mononuclear cells.[23,115,133,154] Glomerular lesions are usually mild, consisting of mild degeneration.[23,133]

3. Urolithiasis
   a. Hypercalciuria predisposes patients to formation of uroliths composed of calcium salts (calcium phosphate and calcium oxalate).[77-79,114]
   b. Hypercalcemic hypercalciuria caused by primary hyperparathyroidism is associated with formation of calcium-containing uroliths in approximately 50 to 80% of human patients.[157] In a series of 28 dogs, calcium-containing uroliths were reported in 28% of patients with primary hyperparathyroidism.[50] When present, uroliths were usually composed predominantly of calcium phosphate; uroliths composed of calcium oxalate occurred less frequently.[77-79,114]
   c. Other disorders causing hypercalcemic hypercalciuria (e.g., chronic granulomatous disease and hypercalcemia of malignancy) have infrequently been associated with urolithiasis in humans.[137] However, development of uroliths secondary to hypercalcemic disorders other than primary hyperparathyroidism has not yet been reported in dogs and cats.

4. Urinary tract infections (UTI)
   a. Primary hyperparathyroidism has been associated with bacterial UTI in humans.[129] Primary bacterial UTI and UTI secondary to urolithiasis have also been observed in approximately 30 to 40% of dogs with primary hyperparathyroidism.[10,50]
   b. Several hypercalcemia-induced abnormalities of the urinary tract, including renal insufficiency, formation of dilute urine, and concurrent urolithiasis, represent risk factors for bacterial UTI in dogs with primary hyperparathyroidism.[112] However, the question of whether or not hypercalcemia has direct ef-

fects on local or systemic urinary tract defense mechanisms in the host requires further investigation.

c. The prevalence of bacterial UTI in association with other hypercalcemic disorders of dogs is unknown.

C. Gastrointestinal manifestations.

1. Gastrointestinal signs are frequently observed in hypercalcemic dogs and cats (Table 21–5).[30,115,154]
2. The exact cause of these signs is obscure, but most likely represents combinations of functional and morphologic abnormalities of the gastrointestinal tract.
   a. Increased serum calcium concentration decreases excitability of gastrointestinal smooth muscle and promotes gastrointestinal mineralization.[8,28,65,115] Resultant gastric atony and ileus may account for, at least in part, inappetence, vomiting, diarrhea, and constipation observed in hypercalcemic dogs and cats.[8,28,51,115]
   b. Induced hypercalcemia has been associated with hypergastrinemia and gastric acid hypersecretion in cats, but not in dogs.[7] Hypergastrinemia and excess gastric acid are considered to be significant predisposing factors in the pathogenesis of gastric and duodenal ulceration observed in human patients with primary hyperparathyroidism.[7,137] As yet, gastrointestinal ulceration has not been observed in hypercalcemic dogs and cats.
   c. In humans, acute and chronic pancreatitis have been associated with primary hyperparathyroidism and other hypercalcemic disorders.[97,102,137,145] Although pancreatitis does not appear to be a clinically significant sequela of hypercalcemia in dogs and cats, induced acute hypercalcemia in cats results in increased pancreatic secretions, altered pancreatic duct permeability, and pancreatic acinar and ductal cell necrosis.[26,57] Similarly, increased pancreatic secretion and formation of intraductal precipitates have been observed in dogs.[140]

D. Neuromuscular manifestations.

1. Several neuromuscular abnormalities have been associated with hypercalcemia in dogs and cats (Table 21–5).[10,30,51,92,115,140,154]
2. The effects of hypercalcemia on skeletal muscle and nervous tissues are in large part attributable to alterations in membrane excitability.[130] Calcium ions inhibit voltage-dependent gaiting of cell membrane sodium-potassium channels, thereby resulting in decreased membrane permeability, impaired cellular excitability, and inhibition of nerve impulse propagation.[65,130]
3. Hypercalcemia may also induce seizure activity as a result of cerebral vasospasm, cerebral hemorrhage, or direct neurotoxicity.[75]

E. Cardiovascular manifestations.

1. Cardiovascular abnormalities associated with hypercalcemia are relatively uncommon in dogs and cats (Table 21–5).[10,51]
2. Marked elevations in plasma calcium concentrations prolong cardiac muscle transmembrane action potentials, thereby resulting in P-R interval prolongation, conduction disturbances, and ventricular arrhythmias.[51,56,107]
3. Hypercalcemia accelerates rate of ventricular repolarization and may result in a shortened Q-P interval.[56,107]
4. Hypercalcemia may induce myocardial ischemia and metastatic endometrial and myocardial calcification, which may account for cardiac abnormalities observed in some hypercalcemic patients.[64,99,127,133]
5. Systemic hypertension is a common clinical finding in human patients with hypercalcemia caused by primary hyperparathyroidism and vitamin D intoxication.[137] Studies of induced hypercalcemia in dogs have demonstrated increased vascular smooth muscle tension; vasoconstriction of coronary, renal, and peripheral limb arteriolar vascular beds; and increased arterial blood pressure.[58,66,127,133] However, the prevalence and clinical significance of hypercalcemia-induced increases in local and systemic vascular resistance in dogs and cats require further investigation.

IV. DIAGNOSTIC CONSIDERATIONS

A. Overview.

1. The finding of hypercalcemia in patients with azotemia, polyuria, and polydipsia, or with other hypercalcemia-related alterations in renal function or structure, is strongly suggestive of, but not conclusive for, hypercalcemic nephropathy.
2. Rarely, the combination of hypercalcemia and renal failure may be the result of autonomously hyperfunctioning hyperplastic parathyroid glands that develop secondarily to long-standing primary renal failure.[31,52]
3. Because most of the early functional abnormalities observed with hypercalcemia are reversible following correction of serum calcium concentration, rapid diagnosis and therapy are of great significance.
4. Identification of the cause(s) of hypercalcemia in dogs and cats and subsequent formulation of specific therapeutic plans depend on careful assessment of historical information, physical examination findings, and results of biochemical, radiographic, and histocytologic evaluations.

B. Laboratory findings.

1. In addition to biochemical determinations routinely employed in evaluating hypercalcemic patients (e.g., serum concentrations of calcium, inorganic phosphorus, urea nitrogen, creatinine, sodium, potassium, and chloride), other bio-

TABLE 21–6.
BIOCHEMICAL MEASUREMENTS USED IN DIFFERENTIATING CAUSES OF HYPERCALCEMIA IN DOGS

Laboratory Test	Sample Required	Comments	References
Total calcium	Serum	Measures total serum Ca (ionized, complexed, and protein bound); spurious values caused by lipemia, EDTA, and detergents	29,98
Ionized calcium	Serum*	Closely regulated by PTH; influenced by acid-base status; useful in interpretation of iPTH determinations	28,98,108
Inorganic phosphorus	Serum	Influenced by PTH and GFR; interpretation complicated by azotemia	29
Urea nitrogen	Serum	Evaluates renal functional status; influenced by prerenal, renal, and postrenal factors; necessary for interpretation of other laboratory data	29
Creatinine	Serum	Evaluates renal functional status; influenced by prerenal, renal, and postrenal factors; necessary for interpretation of other laboratory data	29
Sodium/potassium ratio	Serum	Values of less than 27 suggestive of, but not necessarily diagnostic for, hypoadrenocorticism	118,119,156
Chloride/inorganic phosphorous ratio	Serum	Values of less than 33 in humans with hyperparathyroidism; significant overlap reported between values for hyperparathyroidism, normal, and other causes of hypercalcemia; appears to be of limited diagnostic value in humans, invalid if azotemia present; not evaluated in dogs	2,51
Immunoreactive PTH	Serum*,† refrigerated at 4°C or frozen at −20°C	Quantitates concentrations of immunoreactive intact PTH or PTH peptide fragments; intact molecule, midmolecule, N-terminal, and C-terminal assays available; intact molecule assay measures biologically active form; intact molecule assay allows better differentiation of Ca disorders and is less affected by azotemia; intact molecule assay has been validated for dogs; sample requirements and normal ranges vary with laboratory and methodology employed.	12,108,141,142

Table 21–6 continued.

Ca = calcium; cyclic AMP = cyclic adenosine monophosphate; GFR = glomerular filtration rate; iPTH = immunoreactive parathyroid hormone; PTH = parathyroid hormone; PTHrP = parathyroid-related peptides; EDTA = ethylenediaminetetraacetic acid.

*Available through the Animal Health Diagnostic Laboratory, Endocrine Diagnostic Section, B629 West Fee Hall, Michigan State University, East Lansing, Michigan 44824-1316; phone (517) 353-0621.

†Available through the University of Minnesota Veterinary Diagnostic Laboratory, 1943 Carter Avenue, St. Paul, Minnesota 55108; phone (612) 625-9290.

TABLE 21–6. CONT'D
BIOCHEMICAL MEASUREMENTS USED IN DIFFERENTIATING CAUSES OF HYPERCALCEMIA IN DOGS

Laboratory Test	Sample Required	Comments	References
Nephrogenous cAMP	Urine (freeze at −20°C)	Calculated as difference between plasma cyclic AMP and total urinary cyclic AMP concentrations; value represents proximal renal tubular cycic AMP production; indirect measure of PTH or PTHrP; nephrogenous cyclic AMP significantly increased in hypercalcemic dogs with lymphoma and primary hyperparathyroidism; availability limited to major research centers	14,55,151,152
25-Hydroxyvitamin D	Serum*	Index of total body vitamin D stores; may be useful for diagnosis of vitamin D intoxication	46,69,73,108
1,25-Dihydroxyvitamin D	Serum	Major active form of vitamin D; elevations caused by PTH (but not PTHrP) excess and granulomatous disorders; decreased production with renal failure; availability limited to major research centers	9,69,101,151,152
Urine calcium excretion			
Total urinary excretion	24-hr urine	Measures net urinary excretion resulting from glomerular filtration and tubular reabsorption; determinations require atomic absorption spectrophotometry	37,62
Fractional clearance	Serum and urine	Evaluates renal tubular function in normal animals; interpretation complicated by hypercalcemia and renal failure	37
Urine phosphorous excretion			
Total urinary excretion	24-hr urine	Measures net urinary excretion resulting from glomerular filtration and tubular reabsorption	37
Fractional clearance	Serum and urine	Evaluates renal tubular function in normal animals; interpretation complicated by hyperphosphatemia and renal failure	37

chemical tests allow noninvasive evaluation of calcium homeostasis (Table 21–6).

2. Intact molecule iPTH, ionized calcium, and 25-hydroxyvitamin D determinations are commercially available to veterinarians by express mail, and may provide the most direct, useful, and cost-effective information concerning calcium homeostasis (Table 21–6).
3. Before samples are collected, laboratories should be asked for specific instructions regarding sample collection and handling and for information about normal values (Table 21–6).
4. Most causes of hypercalcemia in dogs and cats can readily be differentiated by combining findings from the history and physical examination with appropriate biochemical determinations. (See problem-specific data base and Tables 21–6 through 21–8.)

C. Radiographic and ultrasonic findings.

1. Hypercalcemic nephropathy has been rarely associated with radiographic evidence of renal mineralization.
   a. In studies of dogs with primary hyperparathyroidism and hypercalcemia of malignancy, renal mineralization was not radiographically apparent despite extensive microscopic evidence of renal parenchymal calcification.[6,10,116]
   b. Renal mineralization has been occasionally visualized radiographically in dogs with vitamin D intoxication.[39]

TABLE 21–7.
PROBLEM-SPECIFIC DATA BASE FOR HYPERCALCEMIC NEPHROPATHY

1. Hypercalcemia should be confirmed by determining serum calcium concentration in a venous blood sample. Blood samples should be allowed to clot at room temperature; they then are centrifuged for 10 minutes and immediately cooled to 4°C or frozen at −20°C within 2 hours of collection. When interpreting results, consider age, albumin concentration, presence of lipemia, and the possibility of laboratory error.
2. Obtain an appropriate history and perform a physical examination, including thorough examination of the rectum, perianal tissues, and lymph nodes for neoplasms.
3. Evaluate serum concentrations of inorganic phosphorus, total protein, albumin, urea nitrogen, creatinine, electrolytes (Na, K, Cl), and total bilirubin; determine alanine aminotransferase (ALT) and alkaline phosphatase (ALP) activities. Freeze an aliquot of serum at −20°C for possible future determinations of iPTH, ionized calcium, 25-hydroxyvitamin D, or other metabolites.
4. Perform a complete blood count
5. Perform a complete urinalysis. Freeze an aliquot of urine at −20°C for possible future determination of other metabolites.
6. Radiographically evaluate the thorax, abdomen, and their associated bony structures.
7. Ultrasonically evaluate the abdomen.
8. Formulate follow-up protocol to confirm or characterize tentative diagnoses.

2. Renal ultrasonography has proved to be a more sensitive means of detecting renal mineralization.[6,131]
   a. In humans, marked increases in the echogenicity of the renal cortex with concurrent accentuation of the corticomedullary junction are typical ultrasonic findings in hypercalcemic patients.[131]
   b. In three dogs with histologically confirmed hypercalcemic nephropathy, renal ultrasonography revealed mildly increased cortical echogenicity and a distinct narrow echogenic line at the corticomedullary junction.[6]
   c. Although significant renal tubular functional abnormalities may be present in hypercalcemic patients prior to microscopic and ultrasonic evidence of renal calcification, a normal renal ultrasonogram indicates potentially reversible disease and therefore may warrant a better prognosis.
3. Survey radiography and ultrasonography are also noninvasive means of identifying and differentiating various underlying causes of hypercalcemia in dogs and cats.
   a. Radiographic and ultrasonic evaluations of the thorax and abdomen are useful for identifying neoplastic or infectious/inflammatory processes not readily detected by physical examination.
   b. Skeletal radiographs may reveal local osteolysis resulting from neoplastic or infectious disorders of bone, or reveal variable degrees of generalized bone demineralization caused by primary hyperparathyroidism, chronic renal failure, or humoral hypercalcemia of malignancy.

TABLE 21–8.
LABORATORY ABNORMALITIES CHARACTERISTIC OF COMMON CAUSES OF HYPERCALCEMIA IN DOGS

Cause	SCa	iCa	SPO_4	Intact iPTH	25-OH Vit D	SUN or SCr	Na^+/K^+ Ratio	Reference
Hypercalcemia of malignancy	↑	↑	N, ↓*	N, ↓	N	N*	N	108,142
Hypoadrenocorticism	↑	N	N, ↑	Unk (N, ↓)†	Unk (N)	↑	↓	118,148,156
Chronic renal failure	↑	N, ↓	↑	↑	Unk (N)	↑	N	31,69,108
Vitamin D intoxication	↑	↑	N, ↑	↓	↑	N*	N	46,64,108,133
Primary hyperparathyroidism	↑	↑	N, ↓*	N, ↑	Unk (N)	N*	N	10,50,51,108,142

SCa = serum calcium; iCa = serum ionized calcium; SPO_4 = serum inorganic phosphorus; Intact iPTH = intact molecule immunoreactive parathyroid hormone; 25-OH Vit D = 25-hydroxyvitamin D; SUN = blood urea nitrogen; SCr = serum creatinine; Na^+ = serum sodium; K^+ = serum potassium; N = normal; ↑ = increased; ↓ = decreased; Unk = unknown.

*Values may be increased with reductions in glomerular filtration rate.

†Values in parentheses represent predictions based on logic and studies in other species.

(1). Severe generalized skeletal demineralization has not been a prominent feature in dogs with humoral hypercalcemia of malignancy, presumably because of its rapid clinical course.[116,154]

(2). Lack of skeletal abnormalities is typical of most dogs with primary hyperparathyroidism.[10,51] Severe generalized skeletal demineralization, pathologic fractures, and loss of the lamina dura have been reported only rarely in dogs with primary hyperparathyroidism.[85,116]

D. Renal biopsy.

1. Because hypercalcemic nephropathy may be associated with potentially reversible or irreversible renal injury, formulating effective therapeutic plans and establishing a meaningful prognosis may be facilitated by evaluation of renal biopsy specimens.
   a. If potentially reversible renal lesions are identified, the prognosis is more favorable, and vigorous specific and supportive therapy is justified.
   b. The extent to which renal lesions associated with hypercalcemic nephropathy are reversible depends on the severity and nature of the renal injury.[113,116]
      (1). Some renal lesions heal by tubular epithelial cell regeneration over a period of days to weeks; such lesions usually are confined to tubular epithelium and are characterized by viable tubular epithelial cells and intact basement membranes, and absence of concurrent irreversible renal disease.
      (2). Nephrons with severe lesions that disrupt tubular basement membranes are often irrevocably damaged.
      (3). We emphasize, however, that the degree of reversibility and functional compensation that occurs after renal injury may vary from patient to patient. Histologic examination alone is not a reliable index of these factors in every case. Both function and structure must be evaluated when attempting to assess the reversibility of renal injury caused by hypercalcemia.
2. Renal biopsy is generally contraindicated in patients with concomitant hemostatic abnormalities, hydronephrosis, renal cysts, or perirenal abscesses. In addition, findings of progressive polyuria and polydipsia, azotemia, isosthenuria, nonregenerative anemia, renal osteodystrophy, and abnormally small misshapen kidneys are indicative of chronic, generalized, irreversible, and progressive renal disease. Results of renal biopsy of such patients contribute little toward prognosis or formulation of specific therapy.

E. Problem-specific data base.

1. Using combined historical, physical, laboratory, radiographic, and ultrasonographic findings obtained from the initial data base (Table 21–7), most disease processes causing hypercalcemia in dogs and cats can be identified or at least localized to a specific anatomic region or organ system.[51,84]
2. Tentative diagnoses established from the initial data base should be confirmed or further characterized with additional laboratory evaluations or microscopic examination of biopsy materials obtained from lymph nodes, soft tissue mass lesions, bone, bone marrow, or other tissues.
3. Patients in which a cause for hypercalcemia is not obvious from the initial data base pose the greatest diagnostic challenge. Typically these patients may be classified into either of two basic scenarios:
   a. Patients that are hypercalcemic, hypo- or normophosphatemic, and nonazotemic (rule out occult neoplasia, primary hyperparathyroidism, or early vitamin D intoxication).
   b. Patients that are hypercalcemic, hyperphosphatemic, and azotemic (rule out occult neoplasia, primary hyperparathyroidism, advanced vitamin D intoxication, or primary renal disease).
4. Recent studies indicate that disorders represented by these two scenarios can be differentiated algorithmically by using results of assays for serum intact molecule iPTH, ionized calcium, and 25-hydroxyvitamin D (Fig. 21–1 and Table 21–8).[108,142]
5. All three of these assays have been validated in dogs and are available through several commercial laboratories.[108,141]
6. In nonazotemic dogs, primary hyperparathyroidism may be differentiated from hypercalcemia resulting from occult neoplasia or vitamin D intoxication by evaluating intact molecule iPTH concentrations (Fig. 21–1 and Table 21–8).[108,142]
   a. Dogs with primary hyperparathyroidism typically have high-normal to high concentrations of iPTH.
   b. The finding of low iPTH in a nonazotemic hypercalcemic dog without evidence of hypoadrenocorticism strongly suggests occult neoplasia or early hypervitaminosis D and warrants additional evaluation for these disorders.
7. In azotemic hypercalcemic dogs, differentiation of primary hyperthyroidism, occult neoplasia, vitamin D intoxication, and primary chronic renal failure may be accomplished by evaluating intact molecule iPTH, ionized calcium, and 25-hydroxyvitamin D (Fig. 21–1 and Table 21–8).[108,142]
   a. Azotemic dogs with primary hyperparathyroidism or primary chronic renal failure typically have high-normal to high intact molecule iPTH concentrations.
   b. Dogs with primary hyperparathyroidism have high ionized calcium concentrations, whereas

dogs with primary chronic renal failure typically have low to normal ionized calcium concentrations.

c. Hypercalcemic dogs with occult neoplasia or vitamin D intoxication typically have low intact molecule iPTH and high ionized calcium concentrations.

d. Dogs with vitamin D intoxication have high 25-hydroxyvitamin D concentrations, whereas dogs with occult neoplasia have normal 25-hydroxyvitamin D levels.

V. STRATEGIES FOR MANAGEMENT

A. Objectives.

1. The likelihood of regeneration and repair of the kidneys depends on the nature and magnitude of renal injury.[113] Once hypercalcemic nephropathy has progressed to a point where alterations in renal function and structure have resulted in uremia, no regime of therapy can eliminate renal lesions.[116]
2. The therapeutic goal, therefore, must be to support the patient until processes of regeneration, repair, and compensatory adaptation allow the kidney to regain sufficient function to re-establish and maintain an adequate degree of biochemical homeostasis.[115,116] This goal has been accomplished by:
   a. Controlling serum calcium concentrations.
   b. Minimizing deficits and excesses in fluid, electrolyte, and acid-base balance.

B. Treatment of underlying causes of hypercalcemia.

1. Initiation of specific therapy is the only consistently effective means of long-term management of hypercalcemia. Therefore, every effort should be made to identify the exact cause of underlying persistent hypercalcemia before therapy is begun.
2. Treatment of hypercalcemia-associated neoplasms utilizing surgical excision, chemotherapy, radiotherapy, immunotherapy, or other therapeutic methods eliminates the direct effects of neoplasia and the source of local or humoral factors (or both) responsible for excess bone resorption and hypercalcemia. Successful treatment of neoplasms associated with hypercalcemia is usually accompanied by reduction of serum calcium concentrations within several days.[28,70,88,154]
3. Correction of underlying metabolic, endocrine, inflammatory, iatrogenic, or toxicologic disorders also results in rapid correction of hypercalcemia.
   a. Proper treatment of adrenocortical insufficiency with replacement mineralocorticoids, glucocorticoids, and fluids is often the only action required to correct hypercalcemia.[118]
   b. Primary hyperparathyroidism should be corrected by surgical resection of the affected parathyroid glands.[50,51]
   c. Hypercalcemia that results from iatrogenic or toxicologic causes, especially vitamin D intoxication, is reversed by eliminating exogenous hypercalcemic agents.[46] However, certain vitamin D analogs (e.g., cholecalciferol) and their metabolites have long plasma half-lives. Therefore, their toxicologic effects persist for several weeks to months and necessitate long-term symptomatic therapy.[28,39,40,53]
   d. Treatment of systemic fungal diseases with fungicidal agents, such as amphotericin B, has been reported to lower serum calcium con-

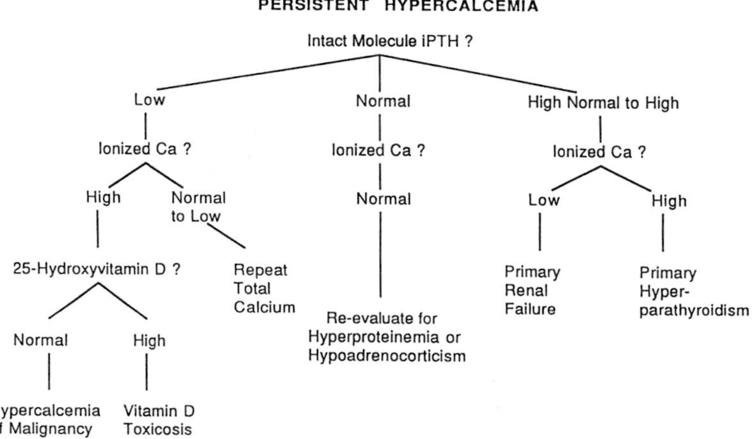

FIG. 21–1. Diagnostic algorithm for persistent hypercalcemia. The algorithm is based on observations and probabilities. Exceptions to these generalities may occur. Ca = calcium; iPTH =immunoreactive parathyroid hormone. (Adapted from Nachreiner RF, Refsal KR. The use of parathormone, ionized calcium and 25-hydroxyvitamin D assays to diagnose calcium disorders in dogs. In: *Proceedings of the 4th Annual Meeting of the Society for Comparative Endocrinology.* Washington, D.C.; 27-30:1990. Used with permission.)

centration in dogs with concurrent hypercalcemia.[43]

e. Treatment of septic osteomyelitis usually requires surgical debridement and antimicrobial therapy.[27]

C. Symptomatic treatment of hypercalcemia.

1. Overview
   a. Although specific therapy is the most effective means of successful long-term management of hypercalcemia, symptomatic therapy is often extremely important in the overall management of hypercalcemic patients.
   b. Symptomatic therapy temporarily reduces elevated serum calcium concentrations and often results in amelioration of cardiac, neurologic, and renal toxicity.
   c. Short-term control of hypercalcemia provides additional time for formulation and initiation of specific diagnostic and therapeutic plans.
   d. Premature, overzealous, or inappropriate symptomatic therapy may interfere with identification of specific causes and identification of concurrent but unrelated disorders. It may also expose patients to needless therapy and result in potentially life-threatening complications.
   e. Symptomatic therapy of hypercalcemia is primarily directed toward reducing serum calcium by one or more of the following methods[84]:
      (1). Increasing renal excretion of calcium.
      (2). Inhibiting bone resorption.
      (3). Altering the intravascular ionic distribution of calcium.
      (4). Promoting extrarenal loss of calcium.
   f. Many therapeutic agents are currently available for symptomatic treatment of hypercalcemia in dogs and cats, each with specific mechanisms of action, indications, limitations, and potential side effects (Tables 21–9 through 21–11).
   g. Unfortunately, no single pharmacologic agent is uniformly effective and safe, nor are any absolute guidelines available to indicate which therapeutic agents are most effective in a given hypercalcemic patient.
   h. The speed with which symptomatic therapy is initiated and the therapeutic agents employed depends on:
      (1). Etiopathogenesis.
      (2). Duration and magnitude of hypercalcemia.
      (3). Severity of associated clinical signs.
      (4). Concomitant metabolic, endocrine, hematologic, cardiovascular, or renal abnormalities.
   i. A combination of therapeutic manipulations is usually most effective, especially if the agents used are complementary or synergistic in their mechanisms of action.
2. Agents that enhance urinary calcium excretion
   a. Regardless of the severity of hypercalcemia, ECF volume expansion is an essential component of any therapeutic regime.
      (1). Volume contraction resulting from impaired renal sodium and water reabsorption, diminished fluid intake, and increased extrarenal fluid losses severely limits renal excretion of calcium.[3,28]
      (2). Expansion of ECF volume enhances renal calcium excretion by increasing glomerular filtration of calcium and by reducing proximal tubular reabsorption of calcium.[3,28,137]
      (3). Because sodium-dependent cotransport of calcium in the proximal tubule accounts for approximately 80% of renal calcium reabsorption, restoration of ECF volume decreases sodium reabsorption and effectively promotes renal calcium excretion.[11,137]
      (4). Dehydration should immediately be corrected by vigorous replacement therapy with 0.9% sodium chloride solution or other types of fluid electrolyte solutions suited to patient needs (Table 21–9).[28,84]
      (5). In patients with mild hypercalcemia (< 13.5 mg/dl), ECF volume expansion alone may result in normocalcemia.[28]
      (6). Overzealous fluid administration should be avoided in patients with hypertension, congestive heart failure, or other edematous disorders and in patients with preexisting hypokalemia or hypomagnesemia.[3]
   b. Patients with moderate to severe or with rapidly progressing hypercalcemia commonly require additional therapy to promote further renal calcium excretion (Tables 21–9 and 21–10).
      (1). Furosemide and other loop diuretics promote renal calcium excretion and enhance the calciuric effects of fluid therapy by inhibiting calcium reabsorption in the thick ascending limb of the loop of Henle.[3,28,111]
      (2). Because diuretic use in volume-contracted patients exacerbates hypercalcemia by accelerating fluid and electrolyte losses, correction of fluid and electrolyte deficits is an essential prerequisite to furosemide therapy.[3,111]
      (3). An optimal dosage of furosemide has not been determined for treatment of hypercalcemic dogs.[28]
      (4). In dogs with induced hypercalcemia, hourly administration of 5 mg/kg of furosemide in conjunction with aggressive fluid therapy resulted in substantial decreases in serum calcium concentrations.[28,111]

TABLE 21–9.
THERAPEUTIC AGENTS THAT ENHANCE URINARY CALCIUM EXCRETION

Therapeutic Agent	Approximate Dose and Route of Administration	Onset of Action*	Indications	Contraindications	Possible Adverse Effects	Comments	References
0.9% sodium chloride or other fluid that best suits patient needs	Hydration deficit plus 40 to 60 ml/kg IV infusion over 24 h	Rapid	Mild to severe hypercalcemia	Congestive heart failure; generalized edema; hypertension	Volume overload; hypokalemia; hypomagnesemia; hypernatremia	Restores and expands ECF volume; increases GFR; decreases renal tubular calcium resorption; enhances calcium and sodium excretion	3,28
Furosemide (Lasix, Hoechst-Roussel)	2 to 5 mg/kg IV q 1 to 12 h	Immediate	Moderate to severe hypercalcemia	Dehydration; hypovolemia	Volume depletion; hypokalemia; hypomagnesemia; hypochloremic alkalosis	Inhibits calcium resorption in ascending loop of Henle; rehydration prior to use essential	3,28,111

ECF = extracellular fluid; GFR = glomerular filtration rate; IV = intravenously.
*Approximate time to beneficial therapeutic effect; maximum effect may occur later; immediate = < 2 h; rapid = 3 to 12 h; delayed = > 2 days.

TABLE 21–10.
THERAPEUTIC AGENTS THAT INHIBIT BONE RESORPTION

Therapeutic Agent	Approximate Dose and Route of Administration	Onset of Action†	Indications	Contraindications	Possible Adverse Effects	Comments	References
Prednisolone	1 to 15 mg/kg PO q 12 h	Rapid to delayed	Moderate to severe hypercalcemia caused by steroid-responsive malignancy or vitamin D intoxication	Infectious disease; pancreatitis; hepatic insufficiency; renal failure; ulcerative colitis	Generalized catabolism, immunosuppression; pancreatitis; gastrointestinal ulceration; hepatopathy; myopathy; osteoporosis; others	Inhibits OAF, PGE_2, and vitamin D; decreases intestinal calcium absorption; promotes renal calcium excretion with chronic administration; direct neoplasm cytotoxicity	3,40,46,61, 70,92,95, 122,135
Calcitonin (Calcimar, USV Laboratories)	4 to 7 IU/kg SC q 6 to 8 h	Rapid	Mild to severe hypercalcemia when other therapy is ineffective or contraindicated	Hypersensitivity to calcitonin	Vomiting	Inhibits osteoclastic bone resorption; direct calciuric effect; transient response; limited experience in dogs	
Bisphosphonates							
Etidronate (Didronel, Norwich Eaton)	ND (20 mg/kg q 24 h PO, 7.5 mg/kg q 24 h IV)*	Delayed	Moderate to severe hypercalcemia when other therapy is ineffective or contraindicated; long-term management of chronic hypercalcemia	Hypersensitivity to biphosphonates	Osteomalacia (etidronate) pyrexia (pamidronate); diarrhea; hypocalcemia; hypophosphatemia; hypomagnesemia	Synthetic pyrophosphate analogs directly inhibit osteoclastic bone resorption; etidronate ineffective orally; pamidronate and Cl_2MBP very effective orally and intravenously; pamidronate potentially useful for chronic therapy; etidronate and pamidronate currently available; limited experience in dogs	3,95,138

Table 21–10 Continued.

Key: OAF = osteoclast activating factors; PGE_2 = prostaglandin E_2; EHDP = ethane-hydroxydiphosphonate; APD = amino-hydroxy-propylidine-diphosphonate; Cl_2MBP = dichloromethylene-biphosphonate; ND = not determined; D5W = 5% dextrose in water; PO = orally; SC = subcutaneously; IV = intravenously.

*Values in parentheses indicate approximate human doses.

†Approximate time to beneficial therapeutic effect; maximum effect may occur later; immediate = < 2 h; rapid = 3 to 12 h; delayed = > 2 days.

TABLE 21–10. CONT'D
THERAPEUTIC AGENTS THAT INHIBIT BONE RESORPTION

Therapeutic Agent	Approximate Dose and Route of Administration	Onset of Action†	Indications	Contraindications	Possible Adverse Effects	Comments	References
Bisphosphonates (continued)							
Pamidronate (investigational)	ND (18 mg/kg PO q 24 h for 6 days, then 3 mg/kg PO q 24 h maint, 0.9 to 1.3 mg/kg q 24 h IV)*	Delayed					See preceeding table
Mithramycin (Mithracin, Miles Laboratories)	ND (25 μg/kg IV in D5W slow infusion every 3 to 4 days for 3 to 4 weeks)*	Rapid	Moderate to severe hypercalcemia caused by glucocorticoid-resistant neoplasia that is unresponsive to other therapy	Renal failure; hepatic disease; hematologic disease	Nephrotoxicity; hepatotoxicity; thrombocytopenia; hypocalcemia; rebound hypercalcemia	Cytotoxic antibiotic; inhibits DNA-dependent RNA synthesis; unpredictable duration of effect; inconvenient administration; limited experience in dogs	3,92,95

Key: OAF = osteoclast activating factors; PGE_2 = prostaglandin E_2; EHDP = ethane-hydroxydiphosphonate; APD = amino-hydroxy-propylidine-diphosphonate; Cl_2MBP = dichloromethylene-biphosphonate; ND = not determined; D5W = 5% dextrose in water; PO = orally; SC = subcutaneously; IV = intravenously.

*Values in parentheses indicate approximate human doses.

†Approximate time to beneficial therapeutic effect; maximum effect may occur later; immediate = < 2 h; rapid = 3 to 12 h; delayed = > 2 days.

TABLE 21–11.
OTHER THERAPEUTIC AGENTS THAT AFFECT CALCIUM DISTRIBUTION

Therapeutic Agent	Approximate Dose and Route of Administration	Onset of Action*	Indications	Contraindications	Possible Adverse Effects	Comments	References
Sodium bicarbonate	Bicarbonate (mEq) = kg body wt × 0.3 × [desired plasma bicarbonate (mEq/L) – measured plasma bicarbonate (mEq/L)] or 1 mEq/kg IV every 10 to 15 min; maximum total dose of 4 mEq/kg	Immediate	Life-threatening hypercalcemic crisis	Alkalosis; congestive heart failure	Alkalosis; hypokalemia; paradoxical CSF acidosis; hypernatremia; ECF hyperosmolality; intracranial hemorrhage; coma; cardiac dysrhythmias	Decreases both ionized and total calcium in dogs; requires careful monitoring of acid-base status; temporary measure	28,68,98
Sodium EDTA	25 to 75 mg/kg/h	Immediate	Life-threatening hypercalcemic crisis	Renal failure	Acute renal failure; hypocalcemia	Complexes ionized calcium; calcium-EDTA excretion by the kidney; only indicated in emergency situations; temporary measure	28,117
Peritoneal dialysis	Low calcium or calcium-free dialysate IP	Rapid	Moderate to severe hypercalcemia with concurrent oliguric or anuric renal failure	Recent abdominal surgery; polycystic renal disease; abdominal neoplasia	Peritonitis	Technically demanding; short duration of response; efficacy has not been evaluated in the treatment of hypercalcemic dogs	28,71

CSF = cerebrospinal fluid; ECF = extracellular fluid; IV = intravenously; IP = intraperitoneally.
*Approximate time to beneficial therapeutic effect; maximum effect may occur later; Immediate = < 2 h; rapid = 3 to 12 h; delayed = > 2 days.

(5). Less rigorous protocols involving administration of furosemide at 8- to 12-hour intervals may be effective when combined with other therapeutic methods.[28]

(6). Unlike furosemide, thiazide-type diuretics and the potassium-sparing diuretic amiloride may decrease renal excretion of calcium and are therefore contraindicated.[35]

3. Agents that inhibit bone resorption. In patients with severe or rapidly progressing hypercalcemia associated with increased bone resorption, agents that inhibit bone resorption are indicated.
   a. Glucocorticoids are often highly effective in treatment of hypercalcemia associated with lymphoma or vitamin D intoxication (Table 21–10).[39,40,46,70,92,95]
      (1). Glucocorticoids may substantially alter lymphoid tissue structure; a definitive diagnosis should be established prior to glucocorticoid administration.[95]
      (2). In patients with hypercalcemia resulting from other causes, glucocorticoids have little or no therapeutic benefit; their usefulness should be weighed against their gluconeogenic effects in patients with severe renal failure.[116]
   b. The naturally occurring polypeptide hormone calcitonin inhibits bone resorption and enhances urinary calcium excretion (Table 21–10).[36,72]
      (1). Calcitonin is commonly used in human patients because of its rapid onset of action, high degree of efficacy, and few contraindications or adverse effects.[3]
      (2). Although calcitonin rapidly reduces serum calcium concentrations, its effects are transient, with most patients becoming refractory to this drug in 2 to 4 days.[3,36]
      (3). Calcitonin appears to be invaluable adjunctive therapy for the short-term management of patients with severe hypercalcemia.
      (4). Experiences with calcitonin in veterinary patients have been limited. In two reports of dogs with severe vitamin D intoxication, calcitonin successfully controlled hypercalcemia refractory to fluid, furosemide, and glucocorticoid therapy.[41,59]
   c. Bisphosphonates (synthetic analogs of bone pyrophosphates) are a new class of potentially useful therapeutic agents used for symptomatic treatment of hypercalcemia in humans and occasionally dogs.[3,95,138]
      (1). These agents are potent inhibitors of bone reabsorption because of their ability to inhibit growth and dissolution of calcium phosphate crystals and because of their direct effects of reducing osteoclast resorptive activity.[3]
      (2). Because of ease and flexibility of administration and few adverse effects, bisphosphonates have been used to manage a variety of hypercalcemic disorders in humans (Table 21–10).[3]
      (3). Etidronate and pamidronate are the only bisphosphonates currently approved for use in humans in the United States.[3,95] Because of limited gastrointestinal absorption, etidronate is most effective when administered intravenously (Table 21–10).[3] However, the safety and efficacy of etidronate have not been thoroughly evaluated in hypercalcemic dogs.[95,138]
      (4). Newer second-generation bisphosphonates, such as pamidronate, appear to be more effective, to be safer, and to allow greater flexibility in routes of their administration (Table 21–10).[3]
      (5). Second-generation bisphosphonates may be potentially useful for long-term management of hypercalcemia in veterinary patients.
   d. Mithramycin, a cytotoxic antibiotic, is a potent inhibitor of osteoclastic bone resorption (Table 21–10).[3]
      (1). Mithramycin has been successfully used on occasion to treat hypercalcemia in dogs with lymphoma or anal sac apocrine gland adenocarcinoma.[92,95]
      (2). Although highly effective, the potentially serious side effects of mithramycin (thrombocytopenia, hepatic and renal toxicity), its difficult administration, and its unpredictable duration of effect limit its use to hypercalcemic patients resistant to safer forms of therapy.[95]
   e. Other agents that inhibit bone resorption and that may be potentially useful for symptomatic treatment of hypercalcemic dogs include prostaglandin synthetase inhibitors, gallium nitrate, and gamma-interferon.[3,28,84,106]
      (1). Prostaglandin synthetase inhibitors (e.g., aspirin) inhibit prostaglandin E_2-mediated bone resorption.[3] Although initial reports on the efficacy of prostaglandin synthetase inhibitors were encouraging, subsequent studies have shown that these agents have limited utility in treating human patients with hypercalcemia of malignancy.[3,95]
      (2). Gallium nitrate, a new antihypercalcemic agent, is currently undergoing clinical studies in human patients.[3,149] However, its safety, efficacy, and clinical applicability in veterinary medicine must be evaluated before specific uses can be recommended.

(3). Gamma-interferon has been shown to be a powerful inhibitor of cytokine-induced bone resorption *in vitro*.[106] If similar effects can be demonstrated *in vivo*, gamma-interferon would be potentially useful for treatment of hypercalcemia caused by cytokine-producing neoplasms.

4. Agents that affect calcium distribution
   a. Therapeutic agents that alter the relative concentration of ionized calcium or promote extrarenal calcium excretion are usually reserved for emergency short-term management of hypercalcemic crises.[84]
   b. In the uncommon situation of the hypercalcemic crisis (severe hypercalcemia resulting in life-threatening cardiac dysfunction, neurologic dysfunction, or both), immediate attempts should be made to reduce plasma ionized calcium with intravenous sodium bicarbonate or sodium EDTA (Table 21–11).[28,68,98,117]
      (1). Both agents rapidly reduce plasma calcium concentration, but have short durations of effect (< 2 hours).[98,117]
      (2). Because sodium bicarbonate and sodium EDTA may be associated with significant adverse effects, their use requires continuous patient monitoring. They should be used only until less hazardous forms of antihypercalcemia therapy can be initiated.
   c. Peritoneal or pleural dialysis with calcium-free dialysate is potentially useful for symptomatic therapy of a hypercalcemic crisis, especially if concomitant renal failure has limited other therapeutic options.[28,71]

D. Treatment of renal failure.

1. When uremia caused by hypercalcemic nephropathy has developed, no regimen of therapy can eliminate the renal lesions. Renal damage, however, may heal spontaneously over a period of weeks if the hypercalcemic state is controlled or eliminated.[116]
2. The objective for patients with hypercalcemia-induced renal failure is to keep the patient alive until the body processes of regeneration, repair, and compensatory adaptation allow nephrons to regain sufficient function to re-establish and maintain an adequate degree of biochemical homeostasis. This goal may be accomplished by using therapeutic strategies designed to:
   a. Ameliorate clinical signs of uremia.
   b. Correct fluid, electrolyte, and acid-base imbalances.
   c. Provide adequate nutritional support.
   d. Avoid conditions that exacerbate or promote progressive renal dysfunction.

VI. PROGNOSIS

A. Because of the diversity of renal lesions associated with hypercalcemic nephropathy and the diversity of pathologic mechanisms associated with hypercalcemic disorders, short- and long-term prognoses for patients with hypercalcemic nephropathy are variable and often unpredictable. The probability of recovery of a given patient depends on:

1. The specific nature and reversibility of the primary disorder.
2. The magnitude of nephron injury.
3. The presence or absence of concurrent cardiac and neurologic dysfunction.
4. The availability of effective long-term therapy.

B. Patients with hypercalcemic nephropathy often need extensive supportive and symptomatic care. Consequently, every effort should be made to determine the reversibility of renal lesions, as well as the reversibility of the underlying cause of hypercalcemia.

C. The extent to which renal lesions associated with hypercalcemic nephropathy are reversible depends on the severity and character of damage to nephrons.[113,116]

1. Lesions confined to tubular epithelium heal by proliferation of viable epithelial cells, thus allowing tubular regeneration to take place over days to weeks.
2. Nephrons with more severe lesions involving disruption of tubular basement membranes are often irreversibly damaged. In this case, repair, regeneration, and compensatory adaptation of surviving nephrons may be insufficient to re-establish and maintain biochemical homeostasis.

REFERENCES

1. Allen TA, Weingand K. The vitamin D (calciferol) endocrine system. *Comp Cont Educ.* 1985;7:482-488.
2. Aro A, Pelkonen R, Sivula A. Hypercalcemia: Serum chloride and phosphate. *Ann Intern Med.* 1977;86:664.
3. Attie MF. Treatment of hypercalcemia. *Endocr Metab Clin North Am.* 1989;18:807-828.
4. Banergee SS, Faragher B, Hasleton PS. Nuclear diameter in parathyroid disease. *J Clin Pathol.* 1983;36:143-148.
5. Barbour GL, et al. Hypercalcemia in an anephric patient with sarcoidosis: Evidence for extrarenal generation of 1,25-dihydroxy vitamin D. *N Engl J Med.* 1981;305:440-443.
6. Barr FJ, et al. Hypercalcemic nephropathy in three dogs: Sonographic appearance. *Vet Radiol.* 1989;30:169-173.
7. Barreras RF. Calcium and gastric secretion. *Gastroenterology.* 1973;64:1168-1184.
8. Beck N, et al. Pathogenic role of cyclic AMP in the impairment of urinary concentrating ability in acute hypercalcemia. *J Clin Invest.* 1974;54:1049-1055.
9. Bell NH. Evidence that increased circulating 1,25-dihydroxy vitamin D is the probable cause for abnormal calcium metabolism in sarcoidosis. *J Clin Invest.* 1979;64:218-225.
10. Berger B, Feldman EC. Primary hyperparathyroidism in dogs: 21 cases (1976-1986). *J Am Vet Med Assoc.* 1987;191: 350-356.
11. Bijvoet OLM. Kidney function in calcium and phosphate metabolism. In: Avioli LV, Krane SM, eds. *Metabolic Bone Disease.* Vol 1. New York, New York: Academic Press Inc; 1977:49-140.
12. Blind E, et al. Two-site assay of intact parathyroid hormone in the investigation of primary hyperparathyroidism and other disorders of calcium metabolism compared with a midregion assay. *J Clin Endocrinol Metab.* 1988;67:353-360.

13. Booker BB, Galla JH, Luke RG. Effect of acute hypercalcemia on loop function. *Clin Res.* 1982;30:881A.
14. Broadus AE. Nephrogenous cyclic AMP as a parathyroid function test. *Nephron.* 1979;23:136-141.
15. Broadus AE, et al. Humoral hypercalcemia of cancer: Identification of a novel parathyroid hormone-like peptide. *N Engl J Med.* 1988;319:556-563.
16. Brown AJ, et al. 1,25$(OH)_2$D receptors are decreased in parathyroid glands from chronically uremic dogs. *Kidney Int.* 1989;35:19-23.
17. Brown EM, et al. Dispersed cells prepared from human parathyroid glands: Distinct calcium sensitivity of adenomas vs. primary hyperplasia. *J Clin Endocrinol Metab.* 1978;46:267-275.
18. Brown SA, Barsanti JA, Crowell WA. Gentamicin-associated acute renal failure in the dog. *J Am Vet Med Assoc.* 1985;7:686-690.
19. Brunette MG, Vary J, Carriere S. Hyposthenuria in hypercalcemia: The possible role of intrarenal blood flow redistribution. *Pflugers Arch.* 1974;350:9-23.
20. Burk RL, Barton CL. Renal failure and hyperparathyroidism in an Alaskan Malamute pup. *J Am Vet Med Assoc.* 1978;172:69-72.
21. Burtis WJ, et al. Humoral hypercalcemia of malignancy. *Ann Intern Med.* 1988;108:454-457.
22. Campbell BJ, Woodward G, Borgerg V. Calcium-mediated interactions between antidiuretic hormone and renal plasma membranes. *J Biol Chem.* 1972;247:6167-6175.
23. Carone FA, et al. The effects upon the kidney of transient hypercalcemia induced by parathyroid extract. *Am J Pathol.* 1960;30:77-103.
24. Carpenter JL, Andrews LK, Holzworth J. Tumors and tumor-like lesions. In: Holzworth J, ed. *Diseases of the Cat: Medicine and Surgery.* Philadelphia, Pennsylvania: WB Saunders; 1987:549.
25. Carrilo JM, Burk RL, Bode C. Primary hyperparathyroidism in a dog. *J Am Vet Med Assoc.* 1979;174:67-72.
26. Cates MC, et al. Acute hypercalcemia, pancreatic duct permeability, and pancreatitis in cats. *Surgery.* 1988;104:137-142.
27. Caywood DD. Osteomyelitis. *Vet Clin North Am [Small Anim Pract].* 1983;13:43-53.
28. Chew DJ, Carothers M. Hypercalcemia. *Vet Clin North Am [Small Anim Pract].* 1989;19:265-287.
29. Chew DJ, DiBartola SP. Diagnosis and pathophysiology of renal disease. In: Ettinger SJ, ed. *Textbook of Veterinary Internal Medicine.* Philadelphia, Pennsylvania: WB Saunders; 1989;1893-1961.
30. Chew DJ, Menten DJ. Disorders of calcium and phosphorus. *Vet Clin North Am [Small Anim Pract].* 1982;12:411-438.
31. Chew DJ, Nagode LA. Renal secondary hyperparathyroidism. In: *Proceedings of the 4th Annual Meeting of the Society for Comparative Endocrinology.* 1990; 17-26.
32. Chew DJ, et al. Pseudohyperparathyroidism in a cat. *J Am Anim Hosp Assoc.* 1975;11:46-52.
33. Chomdej P, Bell PD, Navar LG. Renal hemodynamic and autoregulatory responses to acute hypercalcemia. *Am J Physiol.* 1977;232:F490-F496.
34. Cohen SI, et al. Polyuria in hyperparathyroidism. *Q J Med.* 1957;26:423-431.
35. Costanzo LS. Localization of diuretic action in microperfused rat distal tubules: Ca and Na transport. *Am J Physiol.* 1985;248: F527-F535.
36. Deflos LJ, First BP. Calcitonin as a drug. *Ann Intern Med.* 1981;95:192-197.
37. DiBartola SP. Quantitative urinalysis including 24 hour protein excretion in the dog. *J Am Anim Hosp Assoc.* 1980;16:537-546.
38. DiBartola SP, et al. Clinicopathologic findings associated with chronic renal disease in cats: 74 cases (1973-1984). *J Am Vet Med Assoc.* 1987;190:1196-1202.
39. Dorman DC. Anticoagulant, cholecalciferol, and bromethalin-based rodenticides. *Vet Clin North Am [Small Anim Pract].* 1990; 20:339-351.
40. Dorman DC, Beasley VR. Diagnosis of and therapy for cholecalciferol toxicosis. In: Kirk RW, ed. *Current Veterinary Therapy X.* Philadelphia, Pennsylvania: WB Saunders; 1989:148-152.
41. Dougherty SA, Center SA, Dzanis DA. Salmon calcitonin as adjunct treatment for vitamin D toxicosis in a dog. *J Am Vet Med Assoc.* 1990;196:1269-1272.
42. Dousa TP, Valtin H. Cellular action of vasopressin in the mammalian kidney. *Kidney Int.* 1976;10:46-63.
43. Dow SW, et al. Hypercalcemia associated with blastomycosis in dogs. *J Am Vet Med Assoc.* 1986;188:706-709.
44. Drazner FH. Hypercalcemia in the dog and cat. *J Am Vet Med Assoc.* 1981;178:1252-1256.
45. Dust A, Norris AM, Valli VEO. Cutaneous lymphosarcoma with IgG monoclonal gammopathy, serum hyperviscosity and hypercalcemia in a cat. *Can Vet J.* 1982;23:235-239.
46. Dzanis DA, Kallfelz FA. Recent knowledge of vitamin D toxicity in dogs. In: *Proceedings of the 6th American College of Veterinary Internal Medicine Forum.* 1988;289-291.
47. Engleman RW, et al. Hypercalcemia in cats with feline leukemia virus-associated leukemia-lymphoma. *Cancer.* 1985;56: 777-781.
48. Epstein FH, et al. Changes in renal concentrating ability produced by parathyroid extract. *J Clin Invest.* 1959;38:1214-1221.
49. Feinfeld DA, Sherwood LM. Parathyroid hormone and 1,25$(OH)_2D_3$ in chronic renal failure. *Kidney Int.* 1988;33:1049-1058.
50. Feldman EC. Canine primary hyperparathyroidism. In: Kirk RW, ed. *Current Veterinary Therapy X.* Philadelphia, Pennsylvania: WB Saunders; 1989;985-987.
51. Feldman EC, Nelson RW. *Canine and Feline Endocrinology and Reproduction.* Philadelphia, Pennsylvania: WB Saunders; 1987; 328-356.
52. Finco DR, Rowland GN. Hypercalcemia secondary to chronic renal failure in the dog: A report of four cases. *J Am Vet Med Assoc.* 1978;173:990-994.
53. Fooshee SK, Forrester SD. Hypercalcemia secondary to cholecalciferol rodenticide toxicosis in two dogs. *J Am Vet Med Assoc.* 1990;196:1265-1268.
54. Forbes S, Nelson RW, Guptill L. Primary hyperparathyroidism in a cat. *J Am Vet Med Assoc.* 1990;196:1285-1287.
55. Fox J, Heath H III. Parathyroid hormone does not increase nephrogenous cyclic AMP excretion by the dog. *Endocrinology.* 1980;107:2124-2126.
56. Fox PR, Nichols CER. Cardiac involvement in systemic disease. In: Fox PR, ed. *Canine and Feline Cardiology.* New York, New York: Churchill Livingstone; 1988;565-587.
57. Frick TW, et al. Acute hypercalcemia induces acinar cell necrosis and intraductal protein precipitates in the pancreas of cats and guinea pigs. *Gastroenterology.* 1990;98:1675-1681.
58. Frohlich ED, Scott JB, Haddy FJ. Effect of cations on resistance and responsiveness of renal and forelimb vascular beds. *Am J Physiol.* 1962;203:583-587.
59. Garlock SM, Matz ME, Shell LG. Vitamin D_3 rodenticide toxicity in a dog. *J Am Anim Hosp Assoc.* 1991;27:356-360.
60. Goldfarb S, Agus ZS. Mechanism of the polyuria of hypercalcemia. *Am J Nephrol.* 1984;4:69-76.
61. Goodwin JS, et al. Mechanism of action of glucocorticosteroids: Inhibition of T cell proliferation and interleukin 2 production by hydrocortisone is reversed by leukotriene B4. *J Clin Invest.* 1986;77:1244-1250.
62. Gowans EMS, Fraser CG. Five methods for determining urinary calcium compared. *Clin Chem.* 1986;32:1560-1562.
63. Grain E, Walder EJ. Hypercalcemia associated with squamous

cell carcinoma in a dog. *J Am Vet Med Assoc.* 1982;181:165-166.

64. Gunther R, et al. Toxicity of a vitamin D_3 rodenticide to dogs. *J Am Vet Med Assoc.* 1988;193:211-214.
65. Guyton AC. *Textbook of Medical Physiology.* 8th ed. Philadelphia, Pennsylvania: WB Saunders Co; 1991:51-66.
66. Haddy FJ. Local effects of sodium, calcium, and magnesium upon small and large blood vessels of the dog forelimb. *Circ Res.* 1960;8:57-64.
67. Harris CL, et al. Hypercalcemia in a dog with thymoma. *J Am Anim Hosp Assoc.* 1991;27:281-284.
68. Hartsfield SM, Thurmon JC, Benson GJ. Sodium bicarbonate and bicarbonate precursors for treatment of metabolic acidosis. *J Am Vet Med Assoc.* 1981;179:914-916.
69. Haussler MR, McCain TA. Basic and clinical concepts related to vitamin D metabolism and action. *N Engl J Med.* 1977;297:974-983, 1041-1050.
70. Heath H, Weller RE, Mundy GR. Canine lymphosarcoma: A model for study of the hypercalcemia of cancer. *Calcif Tissue Int.* 1980;30:127-133.
71. Heyburn PJ, et al. Peritoneal dialysis in the management of severe hypercalcemia. *Br Med J.* 1980;280:525-526.
72. Hosking DJ, Gilson D. Comparison of the renal and skeletal actions of calcitonin in the treatment of severe hypercalcemia of malignancy. *Q J Med.* 1984;53:359-368.
73. Hughs MR, et al. Radioligand receptor assay for 25-hydroxyvitamin D_2/D_3 and 1 α, 25-dihydroxyvitamin D_2/D_3. Application to hypervitaminosis D. *J Clin Invest.* 1976;58:61-70.
74. Humes HD, et al. Influence of calcium on the determinants of glomerular ultrafiltration. *J Clin Invest.* 1978;61:32-40.
75. Ihle SL, Nelson RW, Cook JR. Seizures as a manifestation of primary hyperparathyroidism in a dog. *J Am Vet Med Assoc.* 1988;192:71-72.
76. Klausner JS, et al. Hypercalcemia in two cats with squamous cell carcinomas. *J Am Vet Med Assoc.* 1990;196:103-105.
77. Klausner JS, et al. Canine primary hyperparathyroidism and its association with urolithiasis. *Vet Clin North Am [Small Anim Pract].* 1986;16:227-239.
78. Klausner JS, O'Leary TP, Osborne CA. Calcium urolithiasis in two dogs with parathyroid adenomas. *J Am Vet Med Assoc.* 1987;191:1423-1426.
79. Klausner JS, Osborne CA. Canine calcium phosphate uroliths. *Vet Clin North Am [Small Anim Pract].* 1986;16:171-184.
80. Kokko JP, Rector FC Jr. Countercurrent multiplication system without active transport in inner medulla. *Kidney Int.* 1972;2: 214-223.
81. Kozeny GA, Barbato AL, Bausal VK. Hypercalcemia associated with silicone-induced granulomas. *N Engl J Med.* 1984;311: 1103-1105.
82. Krause MW, Hedinger CE. Pathologic study of parathyroid glands in tertiary hyperparathyroidism. *Human Pathol.* 1985; 16:772-784.
83. Krook L, Olsson SE, Rooney JR. Thyroid carcinoma in the dog: A case of bone-metastasizing thyroid carcinoma simulating hyperparathyroidism. *Cornell Vet.* 1960;50:247-260.
84. Kruger JM, Osborne CA, Polzin DJ. Treatment of hypercalcemia. In: Kirk RW, ed. *Current Veterinary Therapy IX.* Philadelphia, Pennsylvania: WB Saunders; 1986:75-90.
85. Legendre A, et al. Primary hyperparathyroidism in a dog. *J Am Vet Med Assoc.* 1976;168:694-696.
86. Lemann J, Gray RW. Calcitriol, calcium, and granulomatous disease. *N Engl J Med.* 1984;311:1115-1117.
87. Levi M, Ellis MA, Berl T. Control of renal hemodynamics and glomerular filtration rate in chronic hypercalcemia. *J Clin Invest.* 1983;71:1624-1632.
88. Lins LE. Reversible renal failure caused by hypercalcemia. *Acta Med Scand.* 1978;203:309-314.
89. Llach F, Felsenfeld AJ, Haussler MR. The pathophysiology of altered calcium metabolism in rhabdomyolysis-induced acute renal failure. *N Engl J Med.* 1981;305:117-123.
90. Lloyd HM, et al. The parathyroid glands in chronic renal failure: A study of their growth and other properties made on the basis of findings in patients with hypercalcemia. *J Lab Clin Med.* 1989;114:358-367.
91. Lopez-Hilker S, et al. Phosphorous restriction reverses hyperparathyroidism in uremia independent of changes in calcium and calcitriol. *Am J Physiol.* 1990;259:F432-F437.
92. MacEwen EG, Siegel SD. Hypercalcemia: A paraneoplastic disease. *Vet Clin North Am [Small Anim Pract].* 1977;7: 187-194.
93. Massry SG, Friedler RM, Coburn JW. Excretion of phosphate and calcium. *Arch Intern Med.* 1973;131:828-852.
94. Matus RE, et al. Prognostic factors for multiple myeloma in the dog. *J Am Vet Med Assoc.* 1986;188:1288-1292.
95. Matus RE, Weir EC. Hypercalcemia of malignancy. In: Kirk RW, ed. *Current Veterinary Therapy X.* Philadelphia, Pennsylvania: WB Saunders; 1989:988-993.
96. Meierhenry EF. Metastatic liposarcoma with extensive osteolysis in the dog. *J Am Anim Hosp Assoc.* 1974;10:478-481.
97. Meltzer LE, et al. Acute pancreatitis secondary to hypercalcemia of multiple myeloma. *Ann Intern Med.* 1962;57:1008-1012.
98. Meuten DJ. Hypercalcemia. *Vet Clin North Am [Small Anim Pract].* 1984;14:891-910.
99. Meuten DJ, et al. Hypercalcemia associated with an adenocarcinoma derived from the apocrine glands of the anal sac. *Vet Pathol.* 1981;18:454-471.
100. Meuten DJ, et al. Hypercalcemia in dogs with lymphosarcoma: Biochemical, ultrastructural and histomorphometric investigations. *Lab Invest.* 1983;40:553-562.
101. Meuten DJ, Segre GV, Kociba GJ. Hypercalcemia in dogs with adenocarcinomas derived from apocrine gland of anal sac: Biochemical and histomorphometric investigations. *Lab Invest.* 1983;48:428-435.
102. Mixter CA, Jr, Keynes M, Cope O. Further experience with pancreatitis as a diagnostic clue to hyperparathyroidism. *N Engl J Med.* 1966;266:265-272.
103. Monchik JM, et al. Nonautonomy of parathyroid hormone and urinary cyclic AMP in primary hyperparathyroidism. *Am J Surg.* 1977;133:498-505.
104. Moore FM, et al. Hypercalcemia associated with rodenticide poisoning in three cats. *J Am Vet Med Assoc.* 1988;193:1099-1100.
105. Muls E, et al. Etiology of hypercalcemia in a patient with Addison's disease. *Calcif Tissue Int.* 1982;34:523-526.
106. Mundy GR. The hypercalcemia of malignancy. *Kidney Int.* 1987;31:142-155.
107. Musselman EE. Electrocardiographic signs of adrenal cortical insufficiency with hypercalcemia in the dog. *Vet Med.* 1975;Dec: 1433-1437.
108. Nachreiner RF, Refsal KR. The use of parathormone, ionized calcium and 25-hydroxyvitamin D assays to diagnose calcium disorders in dogs. In: *Proceedings of the 4th Annual Meeting of the Society for Comparative Endocrinology.* 1990;27-30.
109. Nate LA, Patnaik AK, Lyman R. Hypercalcemia associated with epidermoid carcinoma in a dog. *J Am Vet Med Assoc.* 1980;176: 1253-1254.
110. Okahara T, et al. Effect of calcium on prostaglandin E_2 release in dogs. *Am J Physiol.* 1981;241:F77-F84.
111. Ong SC, et al. Effect of furosemide on experimental hypercalcemia in dogs. *Proc Soc Exp Biol Med.* 1974;145:227-233.
112. Osborne CA, Klausner JS, Lees GE. Urinary tract infections: Normal and abnormal host defense mechanisms. *Vet Clin North Am [Small Anim Pract].* 1979;9:587-609.

113. Osborne CA, Low DG, Finco DR. *Canine and Feline Urology*. Philadelphia, Pennsylvania: WB Saunders; 1972:127-134.
114. Osborne CA, Poffenbarger EM, Klausner JS. Etiopathogenesis, clinical manifestations, and management of canine calcium oxalate urolithiasis. *Vet Clin North Am [Small Anim Pract]*. 1986; 16:133-170.
115. Osborne CA, Stevens JB. Pseudohyperparathyroidism in the dog. *J Am Vet Med Assoc.* 1973;162:125-135.
116. Osborne CA, Stevens JB. Hypercalcemic nephropathy. In: Kirk RW, ed. *Current Veterinary Therapy VI*. Philadelphia, Pennsylvania: WB Saunders; 1977:1080-1087.
117. Partitt AM, Kleerekoper M. Clinical disorders of calcium, phosphorous and magnesium metabolism. In: Maxwell MH, Kleeman CR, eds. *Clinical Disorders of Fluid and Electrolyte Metabolism*. New York, New York: McGraw-Hill; 1980:947-1151.
118. Peterson ME, Feinman JM. Hypercalcemia associated with hypoadrenocorticism in sixteen dogs. *J Am Vet Med Assoc.* 1982;181:802-804.
119. Peterson ME, Greco DS, Orth DN. Primary hypoadrenocorticism in ten cats. *J Vet Intern Med.* 1989;3:55-58.
120. Peterson ME, et al. Multiple endocrine neoplasia in a dog. *J Am Vet Med Assoc.* 1982;180:1476-1478.
121. Ralston SH. The pathogenesis of humoral hypercalcemia of malignancy. *Lancet.* 1987;2:1443-1445.
122. Rapado A. Glucocorticoids and hypercalcemia. *Adv Exp Med Biol.* 1984;171:369-380.
123. Reichel H, et al. Regulation of 1,25-dihydroxyvitamin D_3 production by cultured alveolar macrophages from normal donors and from patients with pulmonary sarcoidosis. *J Clin Endocrinol Metab.* 1987;65:1201.
124. Rosol TJ, Capen CC. Pathogenesis of humoral hypercalcemia of malignancy. *Domestic Anim Endocrinol.* 1988;5:1-21.
125. Ross LA, Goldstein M. Biochemical abnormalities associated with accidental hypothermia in a dog and in a cat. In: *Proceedings of the Annual Meeting of the American College of Veterinary Internal Medicine*. St. Louis, Missouri; 66:1981.
126. Sands JM, Nonoguchi H, Knepper MA. Vasopressin effects on urea and H_2O transport in inner medullary collecting duct subsegments. *Am J Physiol.* 1987;253:F823-F832.
127. Scott JB, et al. Na^+, K^+, Ca^{++} and Mg^{++} action on coronary vascular resistance in the dog heart. *Am J Physiol.* 1961;203: 1095-1100.
128. Serros ER, Kirschenbaum MA. Prostaglandin-dependent polyuria in hypercalcemia. *Am J Physiol.* 1981;241:F224-F230.
129. Shane E, Bilezikian JP. Parathyroid carcinoma: A review of 62 patients. *Endocr Rev.* 1982;56:473-478.
130. Shelton GD, Cardinet GH. Pathophysiologic basis for canine muscle disorders. *J Vet Intern Med.* 1987;1:36-44.
131. Shuman WP, Mack LA, Rogers JV. Diffuse nephrocalcinosis: Hyperechoic sonographic appearance. *Am J Roentgenol.* 1981; 36:830-832.
132. Slatopolsky E, et al. Parathyroid hormone: Secretion, metabolism, and biological actions. *Semin Nephrol.* 1981;1:319-334.
133. Spangler WL, Gribble DH, Lee TC. Vitamin D intoxication and the pathogenesis of vitamin D nephropathy in the dog. *Am J Vet Res.* 1979;40:73-83.
134. St. Goar W. Case records of the Massachusetts General Hospital. Case 29. *N Engl J Med.* 1963;268:943-953.
135. Strumph M, Kowalski MA, Munday GR. Effects of glucocorticoids on osteoclast-activating factor. *J Lab Clin Med.* 1978;92: 772-778.
136. Suki WN, et al. The renal diluting and concentrating mechanism in hypercalcemia. *Nephron.* 1969;6:50-61.
137. Sutton RAL, Dirks JH. Calcium and magnesium: Renal handling and disorders of metabolism. In: Brenner BM, Rector FC, eds. *The Kidney*. Philadelphia, Pennsylvania: WB Saunders; 1986:568-569.
138. Thompson KG, et al. Primary hyperparathyroidism in German Shepherd dogs: A disorder of probable genetic origin. *Vet Pathol.* 1984;21:370-376.
139. Thompson MB, et al. Bile acid profile in a dog with cholangiocarcinoma. *Vet Pathol.* 1989;26:75-78.
140. Tiscornia O, et al. Analysis of the mechanism of action of calcium-induced exocrine pancreatic secretory changes in the dog. *Am J Gastroenterol.* 1975;63:293-298.
141. Torrance AG, Nachreiner R. Human-parathormone assay for use in dogs: Validation, sample handling studies, and parathyroid function testing. *Am J Vet Res.* 1989;50:1123-1127.
142. Torrance AG, Nachreiner R. Intact parathyroid hormone assay and total calcium concentration in the diagnosis of disorders of calcium metabolism in dogs. *J Vet Intern Med.* 1989;3:86-89.
143. Transbol I, Halver B. Relation of renal glycosuria and parathyroid function in hypercalcemic sarcoidosis. *J Clin Endocrinol Metab.* 1967;27:1193-1196.
144. Troy GC, et al. *Heterobilharzia americana* infection and hypercalcemia in a dog: A case report. *J Am Anim Hosp Assoc.* 1987;23:35-40.
145. Turner W. Acute pancreatitis after vitamin D. *Lancet.* 1966;1: 1423.
146. Turrel JM, et al. Thyroid carcinoma causing hyperthyroidism in cats: 14 cases (1981-1986). *J Am Vet Med Assoc.* 1988;193: 359-364.
147. Vanherweghem JL, et al. Effects of hypercalcemia on water and sodium excretion by the isolated dog kidney. *Pflugers Arch.* 1976;363:75-80.
148. Walser M, Robinson BHB, Duckett JW. The hypercalcemia of adrenal insufficiency. *J Clin Invest.* 1963;42:456-465.
149. Warrell RP Jr, et al. Gallium nitrate for acute treatment of cancer-related hypercalcemia: A randomized, double-blind comparison to calcitonin. *Ann Intern Med.* 1988;108:669-674.
150. Weir EC, Burtis WJ, Morris CA. Isolation of 16,000-dalton parathyroid hormone-like proteins from two animal tumors causing humoral hypercalcemia of malignancy. *Endocrinology.* 1988;123:2744-2751.
151. Weir EC, et al. Primary hyperparathyroidism in a dog: Biochemical, bone histomorphometric, and pathologic findings. *J Am Vet Med Assoc.* 1986;189:1471-1474.
152. Weir EC, et al. Humoral hypercalcemia of malignancy in canine lymphosarcoma. *Endocrinology.* 1988;122:602-608.
153. Weller RE, Hoffman W. Renal functions in dogs with hypercalcemia accompanying lymphosarcoma. In: *Proceedings of the Annual Meeting of the American College of Veterinary Internal Medicine.* 1981;68.
154. Weller RE, et al. Canine lymphosarcoma and hypercalcemia: Clinical laboratory and pathologic evaluation of twenty-four cases. *J Small Anim Pract.* 1982;23:649-658.
155. Weller RE, Pool RR, Hornof WJ. Paraneoplasia and hypercalcemia. *Calif Vet.* 1980;7:25-27.
156. Willard MD, et al. Canine hypoadrenocorticism: Report of 37 cases and review of 39 previously reported cases. *J Am Vet Med Assoc.* 1982;180:59-62.
157. Williams HE. Nephrolithiasis. *N Engl J Med.* 1974;290:33-38.
158. Wilson RB. Hypercalcemia associated with nasal adenocarcinoma in a dog. *J Am Vet Med Assoc.* 1983;182:1246-1247.
159. Yarrington JT, Hoffman WE, Macy D. Morphologic characteristics of the parathyroid and thyroid glands and serum immunoreactive parathyroid hormone in dogs with pseudohyperparathyroidism. *Am J Vet Res.* 1981;42:271-274.
160. Zawada ET, Terwee JA, McClung DE. Systemic and renal

vascular responses to dietary calcium and vitamin D. *Hypertension.* 1986;8:975-982.
161. Zenoble RD, Rowland GN. Hypercalcemia and proliferative, myelosclerotic bone reaction associated with feline leukovirus infection in a cat. *JAMA.* 1979;175:591-595.
162. Zenser TV, Herman CA, Davis BD. Effects of calcium and A23187 on renal inner medullary prostaglandin E_2 synthesis. *Am J Physiol.* 1980;238:E371-E376.

CHAPTER 22

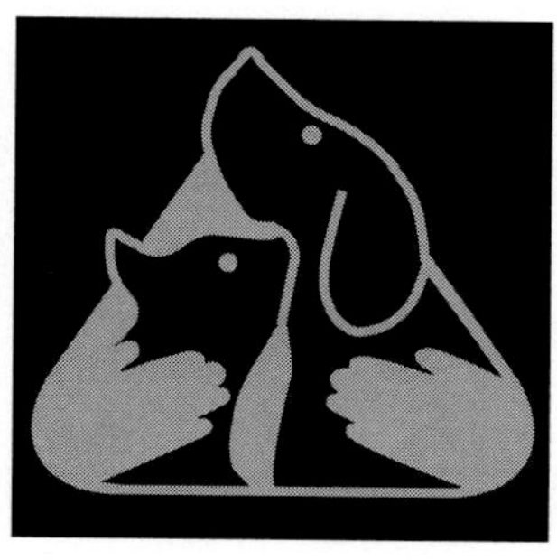

Acute Renal Failure: Ischemic and Chemical Nephrosis

GREGORY F. GRAUER
INDIA F. LANE

I. INTRODUCTION

A. Definition. Acute renal failure (ARF) results from an abrupt decline in glomerular filtration rate (GFR) and is usually caused by an ischemic or toxic insult. Ischemic or toxicant-induced injury frequently damages the metabolically active epithelial cells of the proximal tubules and thick ascending loops of Henle, causing impaired regulation of water and solute balance.

1. Damage to renal tubular cells occurs within hours or days.
2. Clinical signs associated with ARF include depression, lethargy, anorexia, vomiting, diarrhea, and dehydration.
3. Laboratory parameters often associated with ARF include azotemia, hyperphosphatemia, hyperkalemia, metabolic acidosis, and minimally concentrated or isosthenuric urine.

B. ARF is an important clinical syndrome because it is common and frequently results in death.[26] In some cases, after expensive and intense supportive care, ARF may be reversible and adequate renal function may be regained. Importantly, many cases of ARF are inadvertently caused iatrogenically. Prevention of ARF is possible in some cases by identifying patients at increased risk and either avoiding potential renal insults or utilizing prophylactic measures when those potential insults are necessary.

C. The kidneys are susceptible to ischemia and toxicants because of their unique anatomic and physiologic features.[22,135]

1. The large renal blood flow (approximately 20% of the cardiac output) results in increased delivery of blood-borne toxicants to the kidney as compared to other organs.
2. The renal cortex is especially susceptible to toxicant exposure because it receives 90% of the renal blood flow and contains the large endothelial surface area of the glomerular capillaries.
3. Within the renal cortex, epithelial cells of the proximal tubules and thick ascending loops of Henle are most frequently affected by ischemia and toxicant-induced injury because of their transport functions and high metabolic rates.[117] Hypoxia and decreased delivery of substrate associated with ischemia can decrease tubular cell adenosine triphosphate (ATP) stores, resulting in loss of membrane function, cell swelling, and death.
4. As water and electrolytes are reabsorbed from the glomerular filtrate, tubular epithelial cells may be exposed to increasingly high concentrations of toxicants.
5. Toxicants that are either secreted or reabsorbed by tubular epithelial cells (e.g., gentamicin) may accumulate in high concentrations within these

cells. Similarly, in the medulla, the countercurrent multiplier system may concentrate toxicants.

6. The kidneys also play a role in the biotransformation of many drugs and toxicants. Biotransformation usually results in the formation of metabolites that are less toxic than the parent compound; however, in some cases (e.g., oxidation of ethylene glycol to glycolate and oxalate), metabolites are more toxic.

II. ETIOLOGY

A. Ischemic injury occurs when renal blood flow is attenuated by decreased blood pressure or by renal vasoconstriction.[141] Decreased renal blood flow results in reduced amounts of oxygen and metabolic substrates presented to tubular cells, and this "cellular starvation" initiates a cycle of events.

1. The ATP energy pool is depleted rapidly and cellular transport mechanisms are affected, particularly the sodium/potassium and sodium/calcium ATPase pumps.
2. Increased intracellular concentrations of sodium result in extraction of plasma water and cell swelling, which occludes vascular and tubular lumens.[85]
3. Membrane damage results in excessive calcium influx into renal tubular epithelial cells.
   a. Calcium efflux from the cell by Ca-ATPase-dependent transport is depressed because of the depletion of energy sources; calcium processing by mitochondria and the endoplasmic reticulum is subsequently overwhelmed.[29,69,116,117,136]
   b. Increased intracellular calcium activates phospholipases, disrupts oxidative phosphorylation in mitochondria, and further constricts renal blood vessels.[69]
4. Persistent vasoconstriction and cell swelling create vascular stasis and platelet and red blood cell aggregation. Red blood cells are "trapped" in the vascular space, occluding as much as 30% of the blood supply to the renal cortex and creating further ischemic injury.[85]
5. Energy substrate delivery remains impaired and ATP restoration cannot occur. Decreased energy production also results in additional membrane damage and oxygen free radical formation.
6. Free radical scavengers are rapidly depleted, and damage caused by free radicals contributes to membrane and cellular defects.
7. Leukotrienes, thromboxane A_2, and other chemotactic factors result in infiltration of inflammatory cells and generation of additional inflammatory mediators and vasoactive chemicals.[30,85,109]

B. Potential ischemic events.

1. Shock
   a. Hypovolemic
   b. Hemorrhagic
   c. Hypotensive
   d. Septic
2. Decreased cardiac output
   a. Congestive failure
   b. Arrhythmias
   c. Cardiac arrest
   d. Cardiac tamponade
3. Deep anesthesia/extensive surgery
4. Trauma
5. Hyperthermia/hypothermia
6. Extensive cutaneous burns
7. Transfusion reaction
8. Renal vessel thrombosis/microthrombus formation/disseminated intravascular coagulation
9. Hyperviscosity/polycythemia syndromes
10. Nonsteroidal anti-inflammatory drug (NSAID) administration resulting in decreased renal prostaglandin formation

C. Nephrotoxicant-induced tubular injury is usually the result of direct effects on epithelial cells. Toxicants can attach at luminal or basolateral membrane sites or to intracellular organelles.[102] Cellular function is then disrupted by membrane and transport system damage, interference with energy production and cellular respiration, calcium influx, cell swelling, and cell death.[22,102] Toxicants that disrupt tubular function also indirectly affect glomerular function by tubuloglomerular feedback mechanisms, in which local generation of angiotensin II and other mediators leads to hemodynamic and mesangial cell alterations.[109] Nephrotoxic injury to the glomerulus includes the loss of capillary surface area (e.g., aminoglycosides), disruption of endothelial integrity and surface barriers by cationic substances (e.g., doxorubicin [Adriamycin], probenecid, protamine), and mesangial cell proliferation and hypertrophy (e.g., azathioprine, penicillamine).[22] Potential nephrotoxicants include:

1. Therapeutic agents
   a. Antimicrobials
      (1). Aminoglycosides
      (2). Cephalosporins
      (3). Polymyxins
      (4). Sulfonamides
      (5). Tetracyclines
      (6). Amphotericin B
   b. Anthelmintics-Thiacetarsamide
   c. Intravenous radiographic contrast agents[71]
   d. Anesthetics
      (1). Methoxyflurane
      (2). Enflurane
   e. Analgesics/NSAIDs
      (1). Aspirin
      (2). Acetaminophen
      (3). Ibuprofen
      (4). Phenylbutazone

f. Chemotherapeutic agents
(1). Cisplatin
(2). Methotrexate
(3). Daunorubicin
g. Gold salts
2. Heavy metals
a. Lead
b. Mercury
c. Cadmium
d. Chromium
e. Arsenic
f. Thallium
3. Organic compounds
a. Ethylene glycol
b. Carbon tetrachloride
c. Chloroform
d. Pesticides
e. Herbicides
f. Solvents
4. Pigments
a. Hemoglobin
b. Myoglobin
5. Snake venom/bee venom

D. Miscellaneous conditions that may result in ARF
1. Immune-mediated diseases
a. Glomerulonephritis/amyloidosis
b. Systemic lupus erythematosus
c. Vasculitis
2. Hypercalcemia
3. Infectious
a. Pyelonephritis
b. Leptospirosis
c. Borreliosis?
4. Urinary tract obstruction
5. Diabetes mellitus

III. PATHOPHYSIOLOGY

A. The induction phase is the time from the renal insult until the development of azotemia and defective urine concentrating capacity.
1. Therapeutic intervention at this time may prevent progression of renal damage and development of established ARF.
2. Clinical detection of the induction phase of ARF is difficult.
a. Cellular damage initially may be sublethal; however, without intervention, more and more cells sustain lethal injury.
b. Clinicopathologic signs may include a progressive decline in GFR and urine concentrating ability, and a progressive increase in proteinuria, enzymuria, and cylindruria.

B. The maintenance phase of ARF develops when renal tubular lesions are established. Reduced renal blood flow and GFR are common to all forms of ARF, although reductions in GFR are usually greater than the reduction in renal blood flow. At the individual nephron level, reduced GFR occurs in ARF as a result of a combination of tubular obstruction, tubular backleak, renal vasoconstriction, and decreased glomerular permeability.[115] The maintenance phase of ARF may last for 2 to 3 weeks.
1. Tubular obstruction[24]
a. Cellular debris or casts within the tubule may inspissate and obstruct flow of filtrate through the nephron.
b. Interstitial edema may compress and obstruct renal tubules.
2. Tubular backleak[122]
a. Backleak of filtrate occurs as a result of loss of tubular cell integrity, which allows filtrate to be abnormally "reabsorbed" from the tubular lumen into the renal interstitium.
b. Tubular backleak is facilitated by tubular obstruction and increased intratubular pressures proximal to the obstruction.
3. Afferent arteriolar vasoconstriction[66]
a. Vasoconstriction is often a physiologic response to decreased effective blood volume caused by hypovolemia or hypotension.
b. Decreased reabsorption by damaged proximal tubule segments results in increased solute delivery to the distal nephron and macula densa, thereby causing afferent glomerular arteriole constriction.
c. Efferent arteriolar vasodilatation may also contribute to decreased glomerular filtration pressure.
d. Intracellular calcium accumulation, which often occurs following ischemic or toxicant-induced cellular damage, disrupts renal vascular autoregulation and perpetuates constriction of afferent arterioles and mesangial cells.[117]
4. Decreased glomerular capillary permeability[66,114,143]
a. Swollen podocytes, alterations in endothelial cell fenestrae, and reduced glomerular capillary surface area can result in decreased GFR.
b. Aminoglycosides decrease both the number and the size of fenestrae in glomerular capillary endothelial cells, thereby decreasing the available surface area for ultrafiltration.[13]
c. Mesangial cell contraction stimulated by ischemia, toxicants, or thromboxane and/or angiotensin may also reduce filtration surface area.
5. The factors that predominate in patients with ischemia or toxicant-induced ARF are unknown and probably variable. A combination of these factors likely contributes to the decreased GFR of ARF.
6. Therapeutic intervention during the maintenance phase, although often life saving, usually does little to diminish existing renal lesions or improve renal function.

C. The recovery phase of ARF is associated with improved renal function. GFR increases as nephron repair and compensation occur, but

may not return to normal. Urine concentrating capacity may also remain impaired. Even if recovery is incomplete, adequate but subnormal function may be re-established.

1. Tubular lesions may be repaired if the tubular basement membrane is intact and sufficient viable epithelial cells are present.[87]
2. Although additional nephrons cannot be produced and irreversibly damaged nephrons cannot be repaired, functional and morphologic hypertrophy of surviving nephrons may adequately compensate for the decrease in nephron quantities.

D. Urine production in ARF is variable. Although oliguria was once considered the hallmark of ARF, in many instances urine production is normal or increased.

1. Nonoliguric ARF may occur with some nephrotoxicants (aminoglycosides, cisplatin) and milder ischemic events.[5]
2. Impaired tubular responses to antidiuretic hormone (ADH) can also contribute to nonoliguric ARF. Depressed responsiveness to ADH may result from reduced medullary hypertonicity, from the administration of diuretics, or from agents or conditions that interfere with ADH-receptor interaction (e.g., *Escherichia coli* endotoxemia, endogenous or exogenous glucocorticoids, and hypercalcemia).[6]

IV. SEVERAL RISK FACTORS HAVE BEEN IDENTIFIED THAT PREDISPOSE DOGS[21] AND HUMAN BEINGS[89] TO AMINOGLYCOSIDE-INDUCED ARF. THESE FACTORS MAY ALSO PREDISPOSE DOGS AND CATS TO OTHER TYPES OF TOXICANT-INDUCED ARF, AS WELL AS TO ARF INDUCED BY ISCHEMIA. ALTHOUGH PREVENTION OF ACCIDENTAL EXPOSURE TO NEPHROTOXIC AGENTS OUTSIDE THE HOSPITAL DEPENDS ON CLIENT EDUCATION AND ENVIRONMENTAL CONTROL, PREVENTION OF HOSPITAL-ACQUIRED ARF IS AIDED BY THE IDENTIFICATION OF PATIENTS AT RISK

A. Renal hypoperfusion significantly increases the risk of nephrotoxic and ischemic damage to the kidney.

1. Volume depletion is perhaps the most significant factor that predisposes patients to ARF and is often the only risk factor that can be corrected.[82,141] Volume depletion results in renal hypoperfusion, a decreased volume of distribution of nephrotoxic drugs, and decreased tubular flow. Decreased tubular flow potentiates tubular reabsorption, which can increase the intratubular and intracellular concentration of nephrotoxicants.[22]
2. Decreased cardiac output, decreased plasma oncotic pressure, increased blood viscosity, systemic vasodilatation, and decreased renal blood flow associated with decreased prostaglandin formation (e.g., administration of NSAIDs[99]) may also cause renal hypoperfusion.

B. Pre-existing renal disease and advanced age, which is often associated with some degree of decreased renal function, may alter the pharmacokinetics of administered drugs and increase the potential for nephrotoxicity.

1. Gentamicin clearance has been shown to be decreased in dogs with subclinical renal dysfunction that have undergone subtotal nephrectomy.[51] If possible, nephrotoxic drugs like gentamicin should be avoided in dogs with renal insufficiency. If they must be used, a decreased dosage and/or increased dosage interval should be employed.
2. Animals with renal insufficiency and/or advanced age may also have reduced urine concentrating ability and therefore a decreased ability to cope with prerenal influences.
3. Animals with renal insufficiency may be unable to produce adequate amounts of vasodilatory prostaglandins that help to modulate vasoconstriction.[35]
4. The hyperphosphatemia that can occur in patients with renal insufficiency may increase the risk of ARF.[147]

C. Electrolyte abnormalities

1. Sodium
   a. Low-sodium diets have been shown to enhance gentamicin nephrotoxicity, and oral sodium-loading strategies have been beneficial in reducing cortical gentamicin concentrations and mortality in rats.[16]
   b. The benefits of sodium loading may involve suppression of intrarenal and plasma renin activity and attenuation of early renin-angiotensin responses, although other manipulations to block renin or angiotensin effects are not uniformly protective after ARF is established.[82]
   c. Volume expansion secondary to high dietary sodium intake may protect the renal vasculature and may increase the volume of distribution of nephrotoxic drugs, thus reducing their effective serum and tissue concentrations.[16]
   d. Increased natriuresis, increased urine volume, and increased solute excretion prior to a potential renal insult may also be important.[132] Saline diuresis has been helpful prior to administration of some nephrotoxic agents (cisplantin,[92] amphotericin B[55]).
   e. Hyponatremia potentiates contrast-media-induced ARF in dogs.[83]
   f. Although sodium loading is not consistently protective against ARF, sodium depletion and hyponatremia should be avoided in patients receiving potential nephrotoxicants or undergoing elective anesthetic procedures.

2. Calcium and magnesium. Hypocalcemia and hypomagnesemia can enhance gentamicin-induced nephrotoxicity.
   a. Attachment, binding, and uptake of gentamicin in various tissues are inversely proportional to divalent cation concentration. Calcium and magnesium compete with gentamicin for anionic phospholipid membrane binding sites.[70,146] Dietary supplementation of calcium and magnesium has been shown to protect against gentamicin-induced nephrotoxicity in rats.[70,146]
   b. These cations also tend to decrease parathyroid hormone production and release, which decreases membrane phospholipid production and therefore gentamicin binding.[103]
3. Dietary potassium deficiency in dogs potentiates gentamicin nephrotoxicity,[20] possibly because potassium-depleted cells are more susceptible to necrosis. A side effect of high-dose gentamicin administration that has been observed in dogs is increased urinary excretion of potassium and resultant hypokalemia.[20] Increased urinary excretion of potassium possibly could result in potassium depletion (especially if combined with anorexia and/or vomiting) and increase the risk of gentamicin nephrotoxicity.
4. Diets that were deficient in calcium and potassium enhanced gentamicin nephrotoxicosis in horses.[118]

D. Concurrent use of potentially nephrotoxic drugs or drugs that may enhance nephrotoxicity.

1. Concurrent use of furosemide and gentamicin in dogs has been associated with increased risk for and severity of ARF.[1,104] Furosemide probably potentiates gentamicin-induced nephrotoxicity by causing dehydration and a reduction in volume of distribution and by increasing the renal cortical uptake of gentamicin. Fluid repletion minimizes the potentiation of furosemide on gentamicin nephrotoxicity in the dog.[1]
2. Anesthesia with methoxyflurane occasionally results in ARF in humans if the duration of exposure is prolonged. Nephrotoxicity of methoxyflurane is enhanced by the presence of dehydration or the concurrent use of nephrotoxic drugs.[88] Dogs appear to be more resistant to the effects of methoxyflurane exposure of short duration[101]; however, the administration of flunixin meglumine with methoxyflurane anesthesia has resulted in acute tubular necrosis.[86]
3. NSAIDs deserve consideration as risk factors for ARF and as potential nephrotoxicants.
   a. NSAIDs in single doses and with chronic use inhibit renal prostaglandin synthesis and decrease urinary prostaglandin excretion by inhibiting cyclo-oxygenase activity. Prostaglandins, particularly of the E and I series, serve important vasodilatory functions in the kidney and influence GFR and solute excretion.[35,99] Prostaglandins also modulate renin release, tubular ion transport, and water balance.[35]
   b. NSAID inhibition of prostaglandin synthesis in the normal kidney does not significantly impair renal function inasmuch as other regulatory mechanisms compensate for the loss of prostaglandin influence. In diseased kidneys, or with the addition of volume depletion or other stressors, the vasoconstrictor influences predominate, and a normal prostaglandin counterresponse is required.[99]
   c. Animals with subclinical renal insufficiency receiving NSAIDs become candidates for renal failure if volume depletion compromises renal hemodynamics. Dogs appear to be particularly sensitive to newer NSAIDs, such as ibuprofen or naproxen, which may result in gastrointestinal ulceration, vomiting, and renal failure.[75,121] Acute interstitial nephritis and papillary necrosis have also been reported secondary to NSAID administration.[99,111]
   d. Anesthesia, surgery, sodium or volume depletion, sepsis, congestive heart failure, nephrotic syndrome, and hepatic disease are situations in which renal function becomes more dependent on prostaglandin synthesis, and consequently, the susceptibility to NSAIDs in these situations is increased.[99]
4. Intravenous radiographic contrast agents may cause renal vasoconstriction and should be administered with care to patients under anesthesia or receiving NSAIDs or other potentially nephrotoxic drugs.

E. Critically ill patients, such as those suffering from shock, sepsis, and major organ system failure, are likely to require aggressive procedures and therapy, including anesthesia, surgery, and chemotherapeutics that are potentially damaging to the kidneys. Ironically, these critically ill patients are most at risk for developing ARF following such procedures and must be managed carefully to reduce this risk.

1. ARF is common in dogs with pyometra and *E. coli* endotoxin-induced urine concentrating defects. If fluid therapy is inadequate during anesthesia for ovariohysterectomy or during the recovery period, dehydration and decreased renal perfusion may result in ARF.
2. Trauma, extensive burns, pancreatitis, diabetes mellitus, and multiple myeloma are disorders associated with a high incidence of ARF in people.[141]
3. Metabolic acidosis enhances gentamicin nephrotoxicity in dog and rat experimental models.[20,68]
4. Additional clinical conditions that enhance the risk of ARF include vasculitis, fever, sepsis, liver

disease,[39,82] and prolonged surgery or anesthesia (surgical procedures in which the renal vasculature is occluded or disrupted result in a high incidence of ARF in humans[34,141]).

F. Risk factors are additive, and any complication occurring in high-risk patients increases the potential for ARF.

G. Knowledge of these predisposing risk factors should allow the clinician to assess the risk/benefit ratio in individual cases in which an elective anesthetic procedure is considered or use of potentially nephrotoxic drugs is suggested.[26]

V. DIAGNOSIS OF ARF. CLINICAL SIGNS ASSOCIATED WITH PRERENAL AND POSTRENAL AZOTEMIA ARE NONSPECIFIC AND MAY BE SIMILAR TO THOSE CAUSED BY RENAL FAILURE. ALTHOUGH INITIAL FLUID THERAPY MAY BE SIMILAR FOR NONRENAL AZOTEMIA AND RENAL FAILURE, SUBSEQUENT TREATMENT AND PROGNOSIS VARY GREATLY

A. Prerenal azotemia. Many extrarenal disorders can cause hypovolemia or hypotension that results in reduced renal perfusion, reduced glomerular filtration, and prerenal azotemia. Examples include dehydration, congestive heart failure, and hypoadrenocorticism.

1. In patients with prerenal azotemia, urine concentrating ability is usually maintained and hypersthenuric urine is produced (urine specific gravity ≥ 1.030 in dogs, ≥ 1.035 in cats).
2. The differentiation between prerenal and renal azotemia can be difficult if urine concentrating ability is impaired in patients with prerenal azotemia. Examples of conditions that may result in prerenal azotemia with concurrent urine concentrating defects include hypoadrenocorticism, pyometra, liver disease, hypotonic dehydration, and administration of diuretics.[45,130] Additional assessment of urine composition may be helpful in these circumstances.
   a. In patients with prerenal azotemia, urinary sodium concentration should be less than 10 to 20 mEq/L because sodium retaining capacity is intact. Urinary sodium concentrations greater than 25 mEq/L are suggestive of renal failure.[19,48,148]
   b. Urinary sodium concentrations can be variable in dogs; the fractional excretion of sodium

$$Fe_{Na} = \frac{Urine_{Na}}{Plasma_{Na}} \times \frac{Plasma_{Cr}}{Urine_{Cr}} \times 100\%$$

   is thought to be a more accurate reflection of sodium conservation. The FE_{Na} should be less than 1% in prerenal disorders with adequate tubular function. FE_{Na} values greater than 1% suggest renal failure.[19,48,148]
   c. Urine sodium concentrations and FE_{Na} values may not be accurate in sodium avid states, such as congestive heart failure, hepatic failure, or nephrotic syndrome. In these cases, retention of sodium may persist in the presence of tubular damage.[148]
   d. Other urinary indices supportive of prerenal azotemia include urine osmolality significantly greater than plasma osmolality (ratio > 5 to 6/1) and high urine-to-plasma creatinine ratios (> 20/1).[48]
   e. In human beings, urinary sodium excretion and urine-to-plasma creatinine values are combined to give a renal failure index (RFI). The RFI is determined by the following formula:

$$RFI = \frac{Urine_{Na}}{Urine_{Cr}/Plasma_{Cr}}$$ [48]

   RFI values greater than 1.0 are consistent with oliguric ARF, whereas RFI values less than 1.0 are indicative of prerenal azotemia.[19,48] However, in one group of human patients, RFIs were found to be unreliable indicators of ARF.[42]
3. Azotemia caused by prerenal conditions should resolve quickly with replacement of volume deficits and restoration of renal perfusion.

B. Postrenal azotemia.

1. Trigonal or urethral obstruction may lead to postrenal azotemia.
   a. Lower urinary tract obstruction should be considered if historical signs of stranguria, dysuria, or complete anuria are reported.[62]
   b. Obstruction of the urethra or bladder neck can usually be ruled out by the passage of a urinary catheter. This also provides an opportunity to obtain urine specimens for specific gravity determination and other analyses. Urine specific gravity is variable in patients with urinary tract obstruction. The urine sediment may contain crystals, red blood cells, and white blood cells.
   c. In some cases, positive contrast urethrography/cystography may be necessary to confirm a urethral obstruction.
2. Upper urinary tract obstruction should be considered when abdominal pain, abdominal masses, or a history of nephroliths are present. Unilateral obstruction of the renal pelvis or ureter, however, should not result in azotemia.
   a. Survey radiographs may be used to assess renal size, shape, and symmetry, and to rule out radiodense calculi and mass lesions.
   b. Renal ultrasonography may reveal hydronephrosis, hydroureter, nephroliths, or renal masses.
   c. Excretory urography or computed tomography may be necessary to completely rule out upper urinary tract disease.

3. Rupture of the urinary tract may result in postrenal azotemia and should be considered in cases of abdominal or pelvic trauma.
   a. Hematuria, swelling of the inguinal or perineal area, and/or ascites are signs suggestive of urine leakage.
   b. Peritoneal fluid with a creatinine concentration greater than serum creatinine measurements is supportive of urine leakage into the peritoneal cavity.
   c. Contrast radiography is the best way to confirm and localize the site of rupture.

C. **Acute versus chronic renal failure. A diagnosis of renal failure is generally made when azotemia is accompanied by isosthenuria (urine specific gravity 1.008 to 1.012) or by minimally concentrated urine (urine specific gravity 1.013 to 1.029 in dogs, 1.013 to 1.034 in cats). Inasmuch as the treatment and prognosis vary considerably between acute and chronic renal failure (CRF), differentiation of these two syndromes is important.**

1. Clinical findings commonly detected in ARF include:
   a. A young animal in good body condition without a history of previous illness is more likely to be suffering from ARF, unless the breed is known to have a high incidence of congenital/juvenile renal disease.
   b. A history of nephrotoxic drug use, toxicant exposure, trauma, or a potential ischemic insult may suggest ARF.
   c. The kidneys may be painful or enlarged in patients with ARF.
   d. The clinical signs associated with ARF are often more severe than those in the patient with CRF with the same level of dysfunction.
   e. Hyperkalemia and severe metabolic acidosis are more likely to occur in ARF; however, animals with nonoliguric ARF are less likely to be hyperkalemic.[5]
   f. Proteinuria, granular casts, renal epithelial cells, and debris are more likely to occur with acute renal damage.
2. Clinical findings commonly detected in CRF include:
   a. Historical or physical findings suggestive of CRF include previous weight loss, prior episodes of illness, polyuria, polydipsia, pale mucous membranes, and small, irregular kidneys.
   b. Nonregenerative anemia, normo- or hypokalemia, and mild metabolic acidosis may be more common in CRF.
   c. Dogs and cats with chronic renal insufficiency/failure may develop an apparently acute onset of clinical signs or an acute exacerbation of their disease ("acute on chronic" renal failure). The distinction between acute and chronic disease may require renal biopsy in these cases.

D. **Because therapeutic intervention is most successful when initiated in the induction phase of ARF, early recognition of renal dysfunction can be life saving. In humans, ARF has been defined by an increase in serum creatinine of 0.5 mg/dl/d for 2 consecutive days.[141] These relatively small changes are probably often missed or overlooked in veterinary patients. Frequent monitoring of serum creatinine in high-risk patients may allow earlier detection of prerenal or renal azotemia. However, monitoring additional criteria, as reviewed in the following, may allow detection of renal damage and dysfunction prior to the development of azotemia.**

1. Physical examination of the patient at risk for ARF should include assessment of cardiovascular function and hydration status.
   a. Pulse quality and hydration characteristics are outward indices of hemodynamic status.
   b. Frequent recording of body weight, packed cell volume, and plasma total solids may aid in the detection of subtle changes in hydration status.
   c. Direct or indirect blood pressure monitoring in critically ill patients helps to identify hypotensive patients, as well as to identify hypertensive patients, who may also be at increased risk for renal damage.
   d. Kidneys may become enlarged or painful if intracapsular swelling occurs following an acute insult.
2. Urine output should be monitored in all critically ill patients and objectively quantified in high-risk patients by utilizing a metabolic cage, intermittent catheterization, or a closed indwelling collection system.
   a. Normal urine output should be approximately 1 to 2 ml/h/kg body weight; significant increases or decreases from normal may signal the onset of ARF.
   b. Oliguria (< 0.27 ml/h/kg) or anuria (< 0.08 ml/h/kg)[43] requires prompt attention and treatment.
3. Urine appearance should be assessed at each collection for turbidity or gross hematuria, and the urine sediment should be examined daily for red blood cells, white blood cells, casts, renal epithelial cells, or cellular debris.
   a. The presence of low-molecular-weight proteins (which normally are freely filtered and then reabsorbed in the proximal tubules) in the urine (microproteinuria) may be an early marker of ARF. Beta$_2$-microglobulin and retinol binding protein assays have been used in human beings as early indicators of proximal tubular dysfunction.[108]
   b. In practice, the onset of proteinuria detected by semiquantitative (dipstick or turbidimetric) or quantitative (urine protein/creatinine ratio) methods may indicate early glomerular or tubular damage.

4. Urinary enzyme activity is a sensitive method of detecting early tubular damage.
   a. Such enzymes as gamma-glutamyl transpeptidase (GGT) and N-acetyl-beta-D-glucosaminidase (NAG) are too large to be normally filtered by the glomerulus. GGT and NAG enzymuria indicates cell leakage and is usually caused by tubular damage or necrosis.[60] Urinary GGT originates from the proximal tubular brush border, and NAG is present in the proximal tubule lysosomes.[60,123]
      (1). Urinary GGT activity was the earliest marker of renal damage/dysfunction in studies of gentamicin nephrotoxicity in dogs.[60]
      (2). Urinary NAG activity is also increased with tubular damage in early gentamicin nephrotoxicity and has also been investigated as an early marker for diabetic nephropathy in human beings.[123]
      (3). In a study of experimental organonitrile nephrotoxicity in rats, increases in urinary NAG correlated well with renal morphologic lesions that developed prior to the onset of azotemia.[58]
   b. Urinary amylase, lysozyme, beta-glucuronidase, lactic dehydrogenase, and aspartate aminotransferase activities have also been investigated in nephrotoxic models.[2,65,125]
   c. False-positive results can occur with severe glomerular damage, resulting in increased filtration of enzymes into the urine.
   d. False-negative results can occur after chronic damage and depletion of enzyme stores.[60]
   e. Interpretation of enzymuria is aided by baseline values obtained prior to a potential renal insult. Enzymuria is best quantitated by 24-hour urine collection; urine enzyme/creatinine ratios may be inaccurate in the presence of changing GFR.
5. The development of glucosuria or increases in the fractional excretion of sodium and chloride are additional early signals of tubular dysfunction.[54]

VI. GENERAL TREATMENT CONSIDERATIONS

A. Prerenal and postrenal factors contributing to renal dysfunction need to be quickly identified and treated.

B. If renal damage is suspected, all potentially nephrotoxic drugs should be discontinued.

1. If a toxic cause is suspected, nonspecific therapy to reduce further absorption of the agent should be instituted if appropriate.
   a. Induction of emesis or gastric lavage (best if performed within 2 hours of ingestion).
   b. Administration of activated charcoal and cathartics.
2. Specific antidotes should be administered if the toxicant is known, e.g., ethanol or 4-methylpyrazole for ethylene glycol.
3. Peritoneal dialysis can be used to decrease blood concentrations of dialyzable toxicants, e.g., ethylene glycol and gentamicin.

C. Underlying diseases should be identified and managed specifically if possible (e.g., hypoadrenocorticism, pyometra, hepatic disease).

D. Treatable intrinsic renal disorders (e.g., leptospirosis, pyelonephritis) should be identified and appropriate management initiated.

VII. GOALS OF TREATMENT

A. The goal of treatment of established ARF is correction of renal hemodynamic disorders and alleviation of water and solute imbalances to "buy time" for nephron regeneration and compensation.[19]

1. Tubular epithelial cells may be repaired and regenerate in nephrons that are not irreversibly damaged. An intact basement membrane and viable epithelial cells are thought to be necessary for tubular epithelial regeneration.[87]
2. Given time, viable nephrons will undergo hypertrophy and partially compensate for the decrease in nephrons.

B. Positive response to treatment.

1. Increase in glomerular filtration as evidenced by a decrease in serum creatinine concentrations.
2. Increase in urine production (if the patient appears in oliguric or anuric renal failure).
   a. An increase in urine production facilitates management of ARF by decreasing serum urea nitrogen and potassium concentrations (when tubular flow rates and volumes are increased, reabsorption of urea and potassium is decreased) and by lessening the tendency for overhydration to occur.
   b. In most cases, increased urine production occurs as a result of decreased tubular reabsorption of filtrate, not of an increase in glomerular filtration.

VIII. SPECIFIC TREATMENT RECOMMENDATIONS

A. Fluid therapy remains the mainstay of treatment for ARF. The goals of fluid therapy are to correct fluid and electrolyte imbalances, improve renal hemodynamics, and initiate a diuresis. The large volumes of fluid and rapid administration needed to treat ARF require that fluids be given by the intravenous route. Jugular catheters are preferred because they facilitate frequent blood sampling and infusion of hypertonic solutions, as well as supply access for central venous pressure (CVP) measurement.

1. Fluid deficits should be replaced intravenously during the first 4 to 6 hours of treatment. The fluid rate, however, should be reduced in animals with known or suspected cardiovascular dysfunction.

2. Solutions that can be utilized initially are 0.45% saline and 2.5% dextrose solutions or 0.9% saline solutions.
3. The amount of fluid required to restore extracellular fluid deficits can be calculated by multiplying the estimated percent dehydration by the patient's body weight in kilograms (e.g., 5% dehydration in a 10-kg dog: 0.05 × 10 kg = 0.5 kg = 0.5 L or 500 ml).[90]
4. During the rehydration phase, the animal should be carefully monitored for urine output and overhydration.
   a. Frequent assessment of body weight, CVP, packed cell volume, and plasma total solids helps to detect early overhydration.[74]
   b. Physical manifestations of overhydration include increased bronchovesicular sounds, tachycardia, restlessness, chemosis, and serous nasal discharge. Auscultation of overt crackles and wheezes is usually a late sign indicating established pulmonary edema.
   c. If overhydration occurs, the rate of fluid administration should be slowed and treatment with diuretics and/or vasodilators initiated.
5. If overhydration is not apparent after rehydration, further volume expansion may be helpful in improving urine flow.
   a. Volume expansion with an additional 3 to 5% body weight may facilitate rehydration and improve renal perfusion, because remaining deficits of this magnitude may be difficult to detect clinically.
   b. If volume expansion is attempted, close observation for signs of overhydration is necessary.
6. Significant decreases in serum creatinine concentration that may occur secondary to fluid therapy are usually associated with correction of prerenal dehydration.

B. Treatment of oliguria. Oliguria is defined as urine output less than 0.27 ml/kg/h[43]; however, after rehydration, urine output less than 1 to 2 ml/kg/h is inadequate. Additional pharmacologic manipulation with diuretics or vasodilators is necessary to initiate diuresis if oliguria persists after rehydration/volume expansion.

1. Furosemide (2 to 6 mg/kg, IV, 3 times a day) has been advocated as an initial treatment for oliguria in dogs and cats. Single, high-dose regimens (200 to 500 mg)[48] are utilized in human beings to initiate urine flow.
   a. Although furosemide is easy to administer, an infusion of mannitol or an infusion of dopamine in combination with furosemide is usually more effective than furosemide alone.[25,80]
   b. Furosemide has been shown to exacerbate gentamicin toxicity[1] and probably should be avoided in patients with ARF caused by aminoglycoside usage.
2. Osmotic diuretics
   a. Mannitol (10 or 20% solution) is administered at 0.5 to 1.0 g/kg as a slow bolus over 15 to 20 minutes.[74] Urine output should improve within 1 hour if the treatment is effective. A second bolus may be attempted, but the potential for volume overexpansion and complications, such as pulmonary and tissue edema, increases considerably.
      (1). As an osmotic agent, mannitol acts to increase tubular flow and to help to prevent tubular obstruction or collapse.[25,48]
      (2). Mannitol is also a weak renal vasodilator, an action that may be mediated by prostaglandins or atrial natriuretic peptide.[82]
      (3). Mannitol acts as a scavenger of oxygen-derived free radicals, which may form after ischemia and reperfusion.[48]
   b. Hypertonic (10 to 20%) glucose has been suggested as an alternative to mannitol.[47] Its effects in initiating tubular flow and urine output are similar to those of mannitol. These 10 to 20% dextrose solutions are easily formulated and also supply metabolizable energy. Hypertonic dextrose is administered at a dose of 25 to 50 ml/kg as an intermittent slow bolus over 1 to 2 hours, 2 to 3 times daily.[47]
      (1). A potential advantage of hypertonic glucose is that urine can be monitored early after initiating therapy, and thus the infusion can be stopped prior to the risk of overhydration if glucosuria is not present.
      (2). The presence of glucose in the urine, however, should not replace monitoring of urine output because glucosuria may occur without a significant increase in urine production.
   c. Mannitol is likely the superior choice because its other beneficial effects (vasodilation, free radical scavenging)[48] are not present with hypertonic glucose. Mannitol may also be a better osmotic agent, because it is not metabolized or reabsorbed by the renal tubules.
   d. Osmotic agents should not be used in overhydrated patients because they increase intravascular volume and may precipitate pulmonary edema.
3. Low-dose dopamine infusion (1 to 3 μg/kg/min) causes renal vasodilation and preserves renal and splanchnic blood flow.[98] Increases in glomerular filtration and sodium excretion may also occur.[48]
   a. When furosemide therapy is combined with dopamine infusion, the likelihood of inducing diuresis is enhanced.[80]
   b. Although the recommended dosage has minimal systemic effects, dopamine can be arrythmogenic, and electrocardiographic monitoring is advised. If an arrhythmia or tachycardia is observed, discontinuation of the dopamine in-

fusion should result in rapid resolution because the half-life of dopamine is extremely short.

C. Treatment of hyperkalemia. Serum potassium concentrations greater than 6.5 to 7.0 mEq/L can cause cardiac conduction disturbances (bradycardia, atrial standstill, idioventricular rhythms, ventricular tachycardia, fibrillation, and asystole) and electrocardiographic changes (peaked T waves, bradycardia, prolonged P-R intervals, widened QRS complexes, or the loss of P waves).[127,142]

1. Moderate hyperkalemia is primarily resolved with administration of potassium-free fluids (dilution) and improved urine flow (increased excretion).
2. Severe hyperkalemia (> 7 to 8 mEq/L) or hyperkalemia resulting in cardiotoxicity should be treated with agents that decrease serum potassium concentrations or counteract the effects of hyperkalemia on cardiac conduction.
   a. Sodium bicarbonate (0.5 to 2 mEq/kg IV over 20 to 30 minutes) helps to correct metabolic acidosis and lowers serum potassium concentration by exchanging intracellular hydrogen for potassium.[142]
   b. Glucose and insulin can also be used in emergency situations to increase intracellular shifting of potassium. Insulin is administered at a dose of 0.1 to 0.25 U/kg followed by a glucose bolus of 1 to 2 g/U of insulin given.[74] Blood glucose monitoring should be maintained for several hours following administration of insulin because hypoglycemia can occur.
   c. The cardiotoxic effects of excess potassium can be counteracted with 10% calcium gluconate (0.5 to 1.0 ml/kg IV over 10 to 15 minutes) without lowering the serum potassium.[142]
   d. The effects of these regimes are short-lived, and therapy to initiate and maintain diuresis is important to maintain potassium excretion and normokalemia.[90]

D. Treatment of metabolic acidosis. Mild to moderate metabolic acidosis commonly resolves with fluid therapy, and specific treatment is rarely necessary unless the blood pH is less than 7.10 to 7.15, or total CO_2 measures less than 10 to 12 mEq/L.

1. Bicarbonate requirements can be calculated utilizing the base deficit as determined from arterial blood, or an estimated base deficit (body weight [kg] × 0.5 × base deficit or [20 − total CO_2] = mEq bicarbonate required).[74]
2. Optimally, one-half the calculated bicarbonate dosage should be slowly administered intravenously over 15 to 30 minutes, and then acid-base parameters should be reassessed.[74]
3. Overzealous bicarbonate administration may result in ionized calcium deficits, paradoxic cerebrospinal fluid (CSF) acidosis, and cerebral edema.[74]

E. Maintenance fluid therapy. In nonoliguric ARF or once diuresis has been established, fluid therapy should be tailored to match urine volume and other losses, including insensible losses (e.g., water loss caused by respiration) and continuing losses (e.g., fluid loss caused by vomiting or diarrhea).

1. Insensible losses are estimated at 20 ml/kg/d. Insensible fluid losses may be increased in febrile patients.
2. Urine output is quantitated for 6- to 8-hour intervals, and that amount is replaced over an equivalent time period. Examples of total daily fluid maintenance needs for normal, oliguric, and polyuric patients follow.

	Normal	Oliguria	Polyuria
Insensible losses (ml/kg)	20	20	20
Urine output (ml/kg)	40	5	120
Total (ml/kg)	60	25	140

3. The volume of fluid loss caused by vomiting and/or diarrhea is estimated, and that amount is added to the 24-hour fluid needs of the patient.
4. If hyperkalemia is not present and diuresis has been established, polyionic maintenance fluids (e.g., lactated Ringer's solution, Normosol) should be utilized. In the recovery phase of ARF, urine volume and electrolyte losses can be great. Potassium supplementation may actually be necessary, especially if the patient is vomiting or anorexic.

Measured serum potassium concentration (mEq/L)	Amount of KCl (mEq) to be added to each liter of fluid
3.5-4.0	20
3.0-3.5	30
2.5-3.0	40
2.0-2.5	60
< 2.0	80

Do not exceed a potassium IV administration rate of 0.5 mEq/kg/h.

F. Supportive care.

1. Gastrointestinal complications are among the most frequent systemic signs in acute uremia. Nausea, anorexia, vomiting, hematemesis, diarrhea, and oral ulcerations are common.[33,94,124]
   a. Uremic stomatitis, characterized by oral ulcerations, discoloration or sloughing of the tip of the tongue, and fetid breath odor, is seen most frequently with chronic disease, but may also develop with severe acute uremia.

(1). The oral lesions may arise from the caustic effects of ammonia produced locally by the action of bacterial ureases, although the mucosal damage may be simply a manifestation of a more generalized disruption of gastrointestinal mucosa.[33,94]

(2). These effects are aggravated by periodontal disease in human beings, and good oral hygiene may reduce the severity of oral lesions.[94]

(3). Severe pain from oral ulceration may be relieved by the topical administration of lidocaine-containing compounds.

b. Hemorrhagic or ulcerative gastritis leading to anorexia and vomiting is commonly induced by uremia. Lesions may be caused by local irritation from high levels of ammonia or from an altered gastric mucosal barrier.[94,124] Renal failure also results in decreased clearance of gastrin, thus causing hypergastrinemia and increased gastric acid production, which exacerbates gastric lesions.[124] Pathologic findings include edema, mastocytosis, fibroplasia, and mineralization in the lamina propria, along with arteriolar lesions in the submucosa.[32]

(1). Vomiting caused by gastritis may be partially controlled by administration of histamine (H_2 receptor) blockers, such as cimetidine (5 to 10 mg/kg every 6 to 8 hours) or ranitidine (2 mg/kg every 8 to 12 hours), which reduce gastric hydrochloric acid production.

(2). Sucralfate (0.5 to 1.0 g every 6 to 8 hours), a gastrointestinal protectant, is administered to coat existing gastric and intestinal mucosal ulcerations. Sucralfate dissociates in the stomach to aluminum hydroxide and sucrose octasulfate, a viscous substance that complexes with gastrointestinal mucosa and preferentially adheres to ulcerated areas. Sucralfate also protects the mucosa from gastric acid penetration, inactivates pepsin, and adsorbs damaging bile acids.[96] Sucralfate can interfere with absorption of orally administered drugs and therefore should be given at least 1 hour after other medication.

c. The large and small bowel are also affected by increased serum urea concentrations. Diarrhea results from enterocolitis, partial malabsorption of proteins and carbohydrates, altered bile salt metabolism, and bacterial overgrowth.[18,33,94,124]

d. Vasculitis and coagulation abnormalities induced by uremia can create severe generalized gastrointestinal hemorrhage.[94,124] Hemorrhage into the gastrointestinal tract results in the digestion of plasma proteins and an increase in the concentration of blood urea nitrogen (BUN).

e. Vomiting also results from direct stimulation of the chemoreceptor trigger zone (CRTZ) by uremic toxins, such as guanidines.[94]

(1). Effects of these toxins can be reduced by administration of centrally acting antiemetics, such as metoclopramide (0.2 to 0.4 mg/kg every 6 to 8 hours, SQ), which acts at the CRTZ. Metoclopramide also works locally to facilitate gastric emptying and to decrease vomiting.

(2). Phenothiazine compounds, such as chlorpromazine, that act at both the emetic center and the CRTZ should probably be avoided unless adequate hydration and blood pressure have been restored, because alpha-adrenergic blockade can result in significant vasodilation and hypotension.

2. Critically ill uremic patients are highly susceptible to infection; infection is a major cause of death in human beings with renal failure.[19]

a. Depressed leukocyte function and depressed cellular immunity have been documented in human beings with renal failure.[4,53]

b. Production of chemotactic factors and polymorphonuclear chemotactic responses are depressed in uremia. Lymphocyte responses and quantities are also depressed.[4,53]

c. Defects in macrophage receptor functions and monocyte responsiveness have been documented in human beings with end-stage renal failure.[57,112]

d. Humoral immunity appears to be less significantly affected by uremia.[4,53]

e. Metabolic acidosis, altered mucosal barriers, and malnutrition also contribute to weakened host defenses.[18]

f. Prevention of infection is essential in uremic patients, and strict aseptic techniques should be utilized in the placement of vascular and urinary catheters, administration of parenteral medications, and care of any wounds.

(1). If urine output is in question, the use of metabolic cages or intermittent catheterization is preferred over indwelling urinary catheter placement, although indwelling closed systems may be required in some cases.

(2). If peritoneal dialysis is utilized, infection becomes an even greater concern, as peritonitis is a serious complication.[28,126] Careful attention to protocol and asepsis should be undertaken when peritoneal dialysis is utilized.

3. The bleeding tendency in uremic human beings is still not completely understood, but is characterized by an increased bleeding time and altered

platelet function. Uremic compounds produce defects in platelet aggregation, adhesiveness, and platelet factor 3 release in human beings; such defects are reversed by dialytic therapy.[4,53] Whole blood platelet aggregation, however, has been found to be normal in limited studies in uremic dogs.[50]

a. Hemorrhage is best managed by decreasing the severity of uremia, although some animals may require transfusions if significant blood loss occurs.
b. Administration of cryoprecipitate,[129] desmopressin (DDAVP),[133] and other vascular factors[41] has recently been shown to alleviate the bleeding tendency in some human beings with uremia.

4. Neurologic abnormalities associated with uremia include encephalopathic signs and peripheral neuropathy.[12,18,105]
   a. Uremic encephalopathy occurs in human beings when the GFR falls below 10% of the normal rate.[12] Clinical signs include sluggishness, confusion, disorientation, hallucinations, vertigo, ataxia, clonus, and centrally mediated anorexia, nausea, and vomiting.[12] In dogs, tremors, head bobbing, and seizures have been reported.[145]
      (1). Increases in calcium levels in the brain have been documented in human beings and dogs; it is speculated that increased cellular uptake of calcium is facilitated by parathormone (PTH).[12]
      (2). In rats, alterations in brain metabolism and energy use have also been observed, and uremic toxins other than PTH may play a role in the cause.[12]
   b. A peripheral neuropathy associated with uremia has also been observed in human beings, but is more likely to be clinically evident in chronic end-stage renal disease. This distal polyneuropathy is characterized by sensory changes in distal limbs and depressed distal reflexes. Motor nerve conduction velocities are variably reduced. Although similar electrophysiologic changes can be documented in human beings with ARF, clinical signs are usually not apparent.[12]
   c. Control of uremia is the best method of management of neurologic dysfunction. Seizures may be managed with low-dose diazepam as needed.
5. Nutritional support must be maintained in animals with ARF. Many animals cannot tolerate oral intake or cannot consume enough calories to compensate for severe illness. Ongoing catabolic processes then increase the burden of nitrogenous wastes presented to the kidneys.[46] Caloric requirements are met principally with carbohydrates. Required amino acids and proteins are provided, but in amounts that do not result in an excessive protein load on the damaged kidneys.[46]
   a. Ideally, protein should be supplied as amino acids; essential amino acid supplementation has been shown to improve survival in anephric dogs.[131]
   b. Suggested protein requirements for uremic dogs are 0.3 g/kg/d of a basic amino acid solution[46] or 2.2 g/kg/d total protein.
   c. Diets should be restricted in phosphorus, and intestinal phosphate binders may be needed to control hyperphosphatemia.
   d. Stomach tube, enteral, or parenteral feeding may be considered.[81,138]

G. Monitoring response to treatment.

1. A positive response to treatment includes:
   a. A significant decrease in azotemia associated with initial fluid therapy (correction of any prerenal component).
   b. Establishment of a diuresis and subsequent significant decreases in BUN, serum potassium, and metabolic acidosis.
   c. Control of nausea, vomiting, and gastrointestinal bleeding so that adequate caloric intake is maintained.
2. Increases in GFR (not associated with correction of pre- or postrenal complications) result from nephron repair and compensation and typically occur within 10 to 21 days in cases of reversible ARF.

H. Renal biopsy.

1. Histologic evaluation of renal tissue may be necessary in some cases of ARF to establish an accurate diagnosis and prognosis for return of renal function.
2. Indications for renal biopsy
   a. A definitive diagnosis is lacking.
   b. Significant and persistent proteinuria is present.
   c. Diffuse systemic disease is suspected.
   d. When conservative methods of treatment have failed.
      (1). Oliguria persists beyond 2 to 3 days of therapy.
      (2). Severe uremia or hyperkalemia persists for 5 to 7 days.
   e. Histologic assessment of reversibility is necessary to help to determine prognosis.
3. Histologic evidence of tubular regeneration and intact tubular basement membranes are considered good prognostic indicators of reversibility, whereas extensive tubular necrosis and interstitial mineralization with disrupted basement membranes are poor prognostic signs.[87]
4. In a series of human beings with ARF, renal biopsy results altered the diagnosis in 44% of cases in which a biopsy was obtained.[107] Specific therapy was altered in 37%, particularly when glomerular disease or interstitial nephritis was identified.[107]

5. Biopsies are most helpful when performed early in the course of treatment and should always be performed when intensive therapeutics, such as dialysis, are considered. A kidney biopsy can be easily obtained if a dialysis catheter is placed surgically.
6. A renal biopsy may be obtained at laparotomy, or alternatively, a keyhole technique and laparoscopic or ultrasound-guided percutaneous approaches may be used.[59,63,93,144] Various percutaneous and laparoscopic techniques appear to give similar adequate tissue samples,[144] and serious complications of biopsies are rare.
   a. Transient microscopic/gross hematuria is expected for 1 to 3 days postbiopsy.
   b. Severe hemorrhage is usually caused by poor biopsy technique. Subcapsular hemorrhage may result in renal hematoma formation and/or blood clot formation in the urinary bladder.
   c. Hydronephrosis and urine leakage are rare complications of renal biopsy.[72]
7. Coagulation parameters, including platelet count, activated clotting time, activated partial thromboplastin time (APTT), prothrombin time (PT), and bleeding time, should be performed prior to renal biopsy.

I. Peritoneal dialysis.

1. Dialytic therapy should be considered when initial fluid and diuretic therapy has not been successful in relieving oliguria or uremia.
2. Dialysis can also be utilized to manage overhydrated patients and to hasten elimination of certain toxicants.[97]
3. Peritoneal dialysis is expensive and labor intensive[28] and should not be undertaken without serious consideration of the financial and time commitment involved, as well as of the reversibility of renal damage/dysfunction (renal histologic findings).
4. The chances of catheter infection or peritonitis can be minimized by utilizing a few well-trained personnel in the dialysis procedure.
5. The specific procedures for peritoneal dialysis have been described elsewhere[97] and can be accomplished at 24-hour referral centers or teaching hospitals.

IX. POTENTIAL MECHANISMS OF PROTECTION AND EARLY INTERVENTION

A. Methods designed to protect the kidneys from acute insults attempt to prevent or interrupt the pathophysiologic events that result in ARF.[82] Goals of protective maneuvers are to:

1. Preserve or restore renal hemodynamics.
2. Increase solute excretion.
3. Minimize intratubular obstruction.
4. Enhance cellular recovery/repair.
5. Reduce toxicity of nephrotoxic agents.

B. Saline diuresis has been helpful prior to administration of some nephrotoxic agents (cisplatin,[92] amphotericin B[55]) because it causes volume expansion and increased natriuresis. Sodium depletion/hyponatremia clearly increases the risk of ARF.[16]

C. Diuretics and vasodilators.

1. Mannitol serves to increase intravascular volume, increase tubular flow, and prevent tubular obstruction or collapse. Mannitol also acts as a renal vasodilator, improving renal blood flow and GFR if given early in ARF.[25,48,77] The renal vasodilatory effects of mannitol may be mediated via prostaglandins[73] or by the release of atrial natriuretic hormone.[77] Hypertonic mannitol solutions help to reduce cellular swelling in ARF and thus prevent tubular obstruction and cell death. Cellular protection may also be afforded by free radical scavenging properties of mannitol and prevention of mitochondrial calcium accumulation.[25]
   a. Experimentally, mannitol has been protective in ischemic models of ARF[25,73,77] and in toxicant-induced models, including glycerol, methemoglobin, cisplatin and amphotericin B.[25]
   b. Clinically, mannitol is used in humans to protect against ARF during high-risk surgeries and intravenous radiocontrast procedures, and with the use of amphotericin B and cisplatin.[25]
2. Furosemide also acts to increase renal blood flow and tubular flow, but does not significantly influence GFR. Enhanced diuresis created by furosemide may resolve oliguria, but does not appear to affect recovery or survival in human beings.[25]
   a. Furosemide has been protective in ischemic renal failure models in rats,[40,76] but mixed results have been obtained with nephrotoxicants.
   b. Furosemide given after the induction of experimental ischemic ARF in dogs increases water and solute excretion but does not increase GFR.[95]
   c. Administration of furosemide in combination with gentamicin actually enhances nephrotoxicity, probably by creating volume depletion.[1]
3. Treatment with furosemide in combination with dopamine infusion appears to be more effective in inducing diuresis than does use of either agent alone.[80] The intravenous infusion of dopamine at low dosages (1 to 3 μg/kg/min) acts via renal dopaminergic receptors to increase renal blood flow, GFR, and sodium excretion in normal kidneys. Both furosemide and dopamine are most effective when administered early after the initiation of renal failure.
4. Other vasodilatory substances that have been used prophylactically or for early intervention in experimental models of ARF include beta-adrenergic antagonists,[31] synthetic vasodilatory

prostaglandins,[61] and thromboxane synthetase inhibitors.[15]

D. When aminoglycosides are used, monitoring of serum drug concentrations allows the clinician to tailor individual dosage regimens.

1. Nephrotoxicity increases with elevated trough serum levels (> 2 μg/mL for gentamicin, > 5 μg/mL for amikacin).[22]
2. Trough levels can be reduced by decreasing the dosage or increasing the dosage interval.[38]
3. Recent investigations suggest that increasing the dosage interval by a factor arithmetically related to serum creatinine or creatinine clearance values is the most effective means of reducing nephrotoxicity.[52,110]
4. Frequent dosing of gentamicin (every 8 hours) may be less efficacious and potentially more nephrotoxic than an equivalent total daily dosage given at 12-hour intervals.[52]
5. Vitamin B_6 supplementation has been shown to protect rabbits from gentamicin-induced nephrotoxicity.[44] Possible mechanisms of decreased nephrotoxicity include:
   a. Decreased binding of gentamicin to the tubular brush border.
   b. Increased synthesis of polyamines, which are essential for cell division and protein synthesis.

E. Recently, the time (8:00 a.m. versus 4:00 p.m.) of administration of cisplatin has been demonstrated to affect pharmacokinetics and nephrotoxicity in dogs.[64] Less toxicity was observed with the 4:00 p.m. dosing.

F. Dietary protein conditioning.

1. Feeding reduced dietary protein has been shown to improve renal function and survival rates in rats subjected to acute ischemic insults,[8,9] as well as to uranyl nitrate-,[10] puromycin-,[84] and gentamicin-induced[139] ARF. Low dietary protein intake may "downshift" renal work by reducing renal blood flow and GFR. Tubular metabolic work is also reduced, and therefore tubular uptake of gentamicin may be decreased.
   a. In an ischemic ARF model, 88% of rats receiving a 5% protein diet and all rats receiving a 0% protein diet survived, whereas only 31 and 7% of rats receiving normal or high-protein diets, respectively, survived.[8] Preconditioning with reduced protein diets required at least 1 week to be effective, and dietary manipulation immediately after the insult was not protective.[8,9]
   b. In rats given nephrotoxic dosages of gentamicin, preconditioning with a low-protein diet resulted in improved creatinine clearance, decreased enzymuria, and decreased renal cortical concentrations of gentamicin as compared to those in rats receiving normal or high-protein diets.[139]
   c. In another study, low dietary protein conditioning again improved survival in rats treated with gentamicin; however, significant protection was also provided by preconditioning the rats with a high-protein diet that was switched to low protein at the time of gentamicin administration.[7]
2. The effects of dietary protein conditioning may depend on the nephrotoxicant involved because high-protein intake is protective in models of mercuric chloride toxicity, even with short-term conditioning.[11]
3. If dietary protein conditioning could be shown to have renal protective effects in dogs, it may have important clinical implications. In some cases in which potentially nephrotoxic therapy is being considered (e.g., use of chemotherapy, analgesics, radiographic contrast agents, and certain antimicrobial agents) or in which potential renal hypoperfusion may exist (e.g., elective anesthetic procedures), delay of therapy may be possible while the patient is conditioned to a diet with a specific level of protein.

G. Atrial natriuretic peptide (ANP) counterbalances the vasoconstrictive activity of catecholamines and angiotensin II. ANP release results in vasorelaxation, diuresis, and natriuresis.[3] ANP appears to preserve renal blood flow and GFR during ischemia and volume depletion by causing afferent arteriolar vasodilation and possibly efferent arteriolar vasoconstriction.[49]

1. In a norepinephrine-induced ARF model in dogs, ANP infusion resulted in better protection of renal blood flow and creatinine clearance than did dopamine infusion, and elevations in systemic blood pressure and total vascular resistance were attenuated.[3]
2. In an ischemic ARF model in rats, ANP improved glomerular capillary pressure and afferent arteriolar blood flow as a result of a decrease in afferent arteriolar resistance.[37] In a similar but established ARF model in rats, ANP and dopamine increased and sustained GFR, as well as improved restoration of tubular function and structure.[36]
3. ANP preserved renal function in an experimental model of dogs with congestive heart failure receiving iodinated radiocontrast media intravenously.[83]
4. ANP infusion was not, however, found to be significantly more protective than mannitol in a clinical trial of high-risk human beings during angiography procedures.[77]

H. Calcium channel blockers (CCBs). Increased intracellular calcium concentrations secondary to ischemic or nephrotoxicant-induced injury cause membrane and cytoskeletal damage, deranged cellular metabolism, and sustained vasoconstriction in the injured kidney.[29,117]

1. CCBs exert a cytoprotective and vasodilatory effect if given prior to or early in the course of ischemia.[29,69,117]
2. In the normal animal, CCBs cause increases in renal blood flow, GFR, urine flow, and electrolyte excretion.[29] Hemodynamic alterations result from a decrease in afferent arteriolar resistance and are

accentuated if pre-existing vascular tone is high.[29]

3. In rats treated with amphotericin B, cotreatment with diltiazem ameliorated the rise in serum creatinine and the fall in GFR and renal blood flow observed in rats treated with amphotericin B alone.[128]
4. The protective mechanisms of CCBs in ARF may involve preservation of renal blood flow or cytoprotective effects, including the prevention of mitochondrial calcium overload and the prevention of reperfusion injury.[17,29,113,116]
5. In a model of ischemic injury in guinea pigs in which verapamil infusion was protective, the significant difference between treated and untreated animals was the preservation of magnesium concentrations in tissue.[140] Preservation of membrane integrity by interfering with the effects of calcium may prevent loss of magnesium in tissue.[140]
6. Experimentally, CCBs have been protective in ischemic ARF models in dogs.[23]
7. Protection in ischemic ARF models was best when CCBs were administered via arterial or intrarenal infusion both prior to and after the insult,[29,113] a characteristic that may limit their practicality and effectiveness in clinical ARF.
8. CCBs have also improved GFR in transplanted kidneys in dogs and are used clinically to help to prevent ARF in transplanted kidneys in humans.[113] CCBs apparently improve graft kidney function and may protect transplanted kidneys from cyclosporine toxicity[29]; however, improved graft survival has not been demonstrated.[113]
9. Although promising results have been observed in many experimental models, one must remember that CCBs may have profound systemic hypotensive and cardiodepressant effects that may decrease renal blood flow.

I. Free radical scavengers. Hypoxia, membrane damage, ATP degradation, and reperfusion can result in free radical formation that can create further membrane damage.[27,85,136] During ischemia, ATP in tissue is utilized rapidly, and adenosine degradation to hypoxanthine occurs. Xanthine dehydrogenase is converted to xanthine oxidase, which preferentially metabolizes hypoxanthine to free radicals. Xanthine oxidase formation is also enhanced by elevated intracellular calcium concentration. When oxygen reappears, a burst of free radical production occurs. Intermediates of oxygen, including superoxides, hydroxyl radicals, and singlet oxygen, are toxic to mitochondria and cell membranes.[27]

1. Free radical scavengers have been protective in ischemic models of ARF, as well as in ARF induced by aminoglycosides and glycerol.[91]
2. Increased lipid peroxidation and depressed glutathione peroxidase activity following renal ischemia were documented in rats fed a diet deficient in vitamin E and selenium, which are natural free radical scavengers.[134]
3. Superoxide dismutase, which metabolizes hydroxyl radicals to hydrogen peroxide, and allopurinol, which inhibits xanthine oxidase and reduces peroxide formation, have also been protective by reducing reactive oxygen metabolites in some models.[134] However, superoxide and hydroxyl radical scavengers did not attenuate renal dysfunction in a model of endotoxin-induced ARF in rats.[91]

J. Adenosine nucleotides. Elevations in adenosine concentrations in tissue occur following ATP degradation in renal ischemia, and infusion of adenosine into the interstitium of rat kidneys results in decreased GFR.[100] Adenosine may be responsible for tubuloglomerular feedback and renal vasoconstriction following ischemia.[119]

1. Adenosine receptor blockade with theophylline or aminophylline has reversed the effects of adenosine.[56,100]
2. Postischemic infusion of adenine nucleotides (ATP, ADP, AMP) combined with magnesium chloride in rats enhanced renal recovery, possibly by reducing adenine catabolism and adenosine production.[119] ATP with magnesium chloride may also protect the kidney from ischemia by promoting prostaglandin synthesis or by acting as an intracellular energy source; the influence of the magnesium source may also be important.[119]

K. Magnesium apparently plays a role in protection afforded by CCBs and may be influential in the effects of ATP-magnesium chloride infusion.[119,140]

1. High dietary magnesium intake is protective against gentamicin toxicity.[146]
2. Magnesium and calcium compete with gentamicin for binding sites at the renal tubular brush border.[70,146]

L. Glycine has been shown to exert protection against renal injury, although the mechanism of protection is obscure.

1. Glycine has improved renal function and reduced hypoxic renal injury in rats.[14,137]
2. Glycine infusion has reduced cisplatin nephrotoxicity in rats.[67]

X. PROGNOSIS. ONCE ARF IS ESTABLISHED, TREATMENT IS INTENSIVE AND COSTLY, PARTICULARLY IF DIALYTIC THERAPY IS CONSIDERED. WITH THE HIGH MORTALITY RATE ASSOCIATED WITH ARF, AN ACCURATE PROGNOSIS IS IMPORTANT PRIOR TO CONSIDERING AGGRESSIVE THERAPY

A. In general, nonoliguric ARF has a better prognosis than does oliguric ARF because typically uremia is less severe, hyperkalemia is less likely to be present, and the tendency for overhydration to occur is minimized.

B. Nephrotoxicant-induced ARF may have a better prognosis than ARF caused by ischemic episodes because tubular basement mem-

branes are more likely to remain intact following nephrotoxicant-induced damage.

C. Many prognostic factors have been investigated in human beings with ARF. Univariate and multivariate discrimination score systems exist to give a prognosis for survival in individual cases.[34,78,79,106]

1. Significant variables contributing to a poor prognosis include:
   a. Pre-existing cardiac disease, renal disease, or neoplasia.
   b. Acute trauma or pancreatitis.
   c. Complications, such as oliguria, respiratory failure, coma, and sepsis.[34,79,106]
2. The number of complications and number of organ systems failing also correlate with outcome.[34,78,106,120]
3. Mortality rates are highest in surgical patients (> 80%), primarily because of complications and multiple organ system failure.[34,78,141]
4. The severity of azotemia and the interval prior to instituting dialysis in the surgical patients were also important factors, thus emphasizing the need for early recognition and treatment.[34]
5. Age was a significant factor in several studies, with mortality increasing progressively in human patients older than 50 years of age.[34,141]
6. Overall, the conditions most frequently associated with mortality in several studies were hypotension, neurologic coma, and respiratory failure.[78,120]

D. The variables just listed can probably also be applied to veterinary medical patients as well. In general, the prognosis for dogs and cats with ARF is affected by:

1. The severity of renal dysfunction.
2. The response to treatment.
3. The extent of histologic damage.
4. Ability to manage problems of other organ systems.

E. In dogs and cats that survive to reach the recovery phase, adequate, but subnormal, renal function may be recovered.

REFERENCES

1. Adelman RD, et al. Furosemide enhancement of experimental gentamicin nephrotoxicity: Comparison of functional and morphological changes with activities of urinary enzymes. *J Infect Dis.* 1979;140:342-352.
2. Aderka D, Tene M, Graff E, Levo Y. Amylase-creatinine clearance ratio: A simple test to predict gentamicin nephrotoxicity. *Arch Intern Med.* 1988;148:1093-1096.
3. Aikawa N, Wakabayashi GO, Masakazu U, Shinozawa Y. Regulation of renal function in thermal injury. *J Trauma.* 1990;30:S174-178.
4. Anagnostou A, Kurtzman NA. Hematological consequences of renal failure. In: Brenner BM, Rector FC, eds. *The Kidney.* 3rd ed. Philadelphia, Pennsylvania: WB Saunders Co; 1986:1631-1656.
5. Anderson RJ, et al. Nonoliguric acute renal failure. *N Engl J Med.* 1977;296:1134-1138.
6. Anderson RJ, Schrier RW. Clinical spectrum of oliguric and nonoliguric acute renal failure. In: Brenner BM, Stein H, eds. *Acute Renal Failure.* New York, New York: Churchill Livingstone; 1980:3-4.
7. Andrews PM, Bates SB. Dietary protein as a risk factor in gentamicin nephrotoxicity. *Renal Failure.* 1987-88;10:153-159.
8. Andrews PM, Bates SB. Dietary protein prior to renal ischemia dramatically affects postischemic kidney function. *Kidney Int.* 1986;30:299-303.
9. Andrews PM, Bates SB. Dietary protein prior to renal ischemia and postischemic kidney function. *Kidney Int.* 1987;32(suppl 22):576-580.
10. Andrews PM, Bates SB. Effects of dietary protein on uranylnitrate-induced acute renal failure. *Nephron.* 1987;45:296-301.
11. Andrews PM, Chung EM. High dietary protein regimens provide significant protection from mercury nephrotoxicity in rats. *Toxicol Appl Pharmacol.* 1990;105:288-304.
12. Arieff AI. Neurologic manifestations of uremia. In: Brenner BM, Rector FC, eds. *The Kidney.* 3rd ed. Philadelphia, Pennsylvania: WB Saunders Co; 1986:1731-1758.
13. Avasthi PS, Evan AP. Glomerular permeability in aminonucleoside-induced nephrosis in rats. A proposed role of endothelial cells. *J Lab Clin Med.* 1979;93:266-276.
14. Baines AD, Shaikh N, Ho P. Mechanisms of perfused kidney cytoprotection by alanine and glycine. *Am J Physiol.* 1990;259: F80-F87.
15. Benabe JE, et al. Production of thromboxane A_2 by the kidney in glycerol induced acute renal failure in the rabbit. *Prostaglandins.* 1980;19:333-347.
16. Bennett WM, et al. Effect of sodium intake on gentamicin nephrotoxicity in the rat. *Proc Soc Exp Biol Med.* 1976;151:736-738.
17. Blau A, Shulman L, Eliahou HE. Calcium channel blockers and experimental acute renal failure. *Isr J Med Sci.* 1990;26:334-336.
18. Bovee KC. Metabolic disturbances of uremia. In: Bovee KC, ed. *Canine Nephrology.* Media, Pennsylvania: Harwal Publishing Co; 1984:555-612.
19. Brezis M, Rosen S, Epstein FH. Acute renal failure. In: Brenner BM, Rector FC, eds. *The Kidney.* 3rd ed. Philadelphia, Pennsylvania: WB Saunders Co; 1986:735-799.
20. Brinker KR, et al. Effect of potassium depletion on gentamicin nephrotoxicity. *J Lab Clin Med.* 1981;98:292-301.
21. Brown SA, Barsanti JA, Crowell WA. Gentamicin-associated acute renal failure in the dog. *J Am Vet Med Assoc.* 1985;186: 686-690.
22. Brown SA, Engelhardt JA. Drug-related nephropathies: Part I. Mechanisms, diagnosis and management. *Comp Cont Educ Pract Vet.* 1987;9:148-160.
23. Burke TJ, et al. Protective effect of intrarenal calcium membrane blockers before or after renal ischemia: Functional, morphological and mitochondrial studies. *J Clin Invest.* 1984; 74:1830-1841.
24. Burke TJ, et al. Ischemia and tubule obstruction during acute renal failure in dogs: Mannitol in protection. *Am J Physiol.* 1980;238:F305-314.
25. Burnier M, Schrier RW. Protection from acute renal failure. *Adv Exp Med Biol.* 1986;212:275-283.
26. Byrick RJ, Rose DK. Pathophysiology and prevention of acute renal failure: The role of the anaesthetist. *Can J Anaesth.* 1990;37:457-467.
27. Canavese C, Stratta P, Vercellone A. The case for oxygen free radicals in the pathogenesis of ischemic acute renal failure. *Nephron.* 1988;49:9-15.
28. Carter LJ, Wingfield WE, Allen TA. Clinical experience with peritoneal dialysis in small animals. *Comp Cont Educ Pract Vet.* 1989;11:1335-1343.

29. Chan L, Schrier RW. Effects of calcium channel blockers on renal function. *Annu Rev Med.* 1990;41:289-302.
30. Chatziantoniou C, Papanikloaou N. The role of prostaglandin and thromboxane synthesis by the glomeruli in the development of acute renal failure. *Eicosanoids.* 1989;2:157-161.
31. Chevalier RL, Finn WF. Effects of propranolol on postischemic acute renal failure. *Nephron.* 1980;25:77-81.
32. Cheville NF. Uremic gastropathy in the dog. *Vet Pathol.* 1979; 16:292-309.
33. Chew DJ, DiBartola SP. Diagnosis and pathophysiology of renal disease. In: Ettinger SJ, ed. *Textbook of Veterinary Internal Medicine.* 3rd ed. Philadelphia, Pennsylvania: WB Saunders Co; 1989:1893-1961.
34. Cioffi WG, Ashikaga T, Gamelli RL. Probability of surviving postoperative acute renal failure; development of a prognostic index. *Ann Surg.* 1984;200:205-211.
35. Clive DM, Stoff JS. Renal syndromes associated with nonsteroidal antiinflammatory drugs. *N Engl J Med.* 1984;310:563-571.
36. Conger JD, Falk SA, Hammond WS. Atrial natriuretic peptide and dopamine in established acute renal failure in the rat. *Kidney Int.* 1991;40:21-28.
37. Conger JD, Falk SA, Yuan BH, Schrier RW. Atrial natriuretic peptide and dopamine in a rat model of ischemic acute renal failure. *Kidney Int.* 1989;35:1126-1132.
38. Cooper K, Bennett WM. Nephrotoxicity of common drugs used in clinical practice. *Arch Intern Med.* 1987;147:1213-1218.
39. Cowgill LD. Acute renal failure. In: Bovee KC, ed. *Canine Nephrology.* Media, Pennsylvania: Harwal Publishing Co; 1984: 405-438.
40. DeTorrente A, et al. Effects of furosemide and acetylcholine in norepinephrine-induced acute renal failure. *Am J Physiol.* 1978;235:F131-F136.
41. DiPaolo N, et al. Bleeding tendency of chronic uremia improved by vascular factor. *Nephron.* 1989;52:268-272.
42. Durakovic Z, Durakovic A, Durokovic S. The lack of clinical value of laboratory parameters in predicting outcome in acute renal failure. *Renal Failure.* 1989-90;11:213-219.
43. English PB. Acute renal failure in the dog and cat. *Aust Vet J.* 1974;50:384-392.
44. Enriquez JI, et al. Effect of vitamin B_6 supplementation on gentamicin nephrotoxicity in rabbits. *Vet Hum Toxicol.* 1991;34: 32-35.
45. Feldman EC, Nelson RW. *Canine and Feline Endocrinology and Reproduction.* Philadelphia, Pennsylvania: WB Saunders Co; 1987:1-28.
46. Finco DR, Barsanti JA. Parenteral nutrition during a uremic crisis. In: Kirk RW, ed. *Current Veterinary Therapy VIII; Small Animal Practice.* Philadelphia, Pennsylvania: WB Saunders Co; 1983:994-996.
47. Finco DR, Low KG. Intensive diuresis in polyuric renal failure. In: Kirk RW, ed. *Current Veterinary Therapy VII; Small Animal Practice.* Philadelphia, Pennsylvania: WB Saunders Co; 1980: 1091-1093.
48. Finn WF. Diagnosis and management of acute tubular necrosis. *Med Clin North Am.* 1990;74:873-892.
49. Flier JS, Underhill LH. Atrial natriuretic hormone, the renin-aldosterone axis, and blood pressure electrolyte homeostasis. *N Engl J Med.* 1985;315:1330-1340.
50. Forsythe LT, Jackson ML, Meric SM. Whole blood platelet aggregation in uremic dogs. *Am J Vet Res.* 1989;50:1754-1757.
51. Frazier DL, Aucoin DP, Riviere JE. Gentamicin pharmacokinetics and nephrotoxicity in naturally acquired and experimentally induced disease in dogs. *J Am Vet Med Assoc.* 1988;192:57-63.
52. Frazier DL, Riviere JC. Gentamicin dosing strategies for dogs with subclinical renal dysfunction. *Antimicrob Agent Chemother.* 1987;31:1929-1934.
53. Fried W. Hematologic complications of chronic renal failure. *Med Clin North Am.* 1978;62:1363-1379.
54. Garry F, Chew DJ, Hoffsis GF. Urinary indices of renal function in sheep with induced aminoglycoside nephrotoxicosis. *Am J Vet Res.* 1990;51:420-427.
55. Gerkens JF, Branch RA. The influence of sodium status and furosemide on canine acute amphotericin B nephrotoxicity. *J Pharmacol Exp Ther.* 1980;214:306-311.
56. Gerkens JF, Heidemann HT, Jackson EK, Branch RA. Effect of aminophylline on amphotericin B nephrotoxicity in the dog. *J Pharmacol Exp Ther.* 1983;224:609-613.
57. Gibbons RA, Martinez OM, Garovoy MR. Altered monocyte function in uremia. *Clin Immunol Immunopathol.* 1990;56:66-80.
58. Gould DH, Fettman MJ, Daxenbichler ME, Bartuska BM. Functional and structural alterations of the rat kidney induced by the naturally occurring organonitrile 25-1-cyano-2-hydroxy-3,4 epithiobutane. *Toxicol Appl Pharmacol.* 1985;78: 190-201.
59. Grauer GF, Twedt DC, Mero KN. Evaluation of laparoscopy for obtaining renal biopsy specimens from dogs and cats. *J Am Vet Med Assoc.* 1983;183:677-679.
60. Greco DS, et al. Urinary gamma-glutamyl transpeptidase activity in dogs with gentamicin-induced nephrotoxicity. *Am J Vet Res.* 1985;46:2332-2335.
61. Grekas D, Kalekou H, Tourkantonis A. Effect of prostaglandin E_2 (PGE_2) in the prevention of acute renal failure in anesthetized dogs; in situ renal preservation. *Renal Failure.* 1989;11: 27-31.
62. Guly UM, Turney JH. Post-traumatic acute renal failure, 1956-1988. *Clin Nephrol.* 1990;34:79-83.
63. Hager DA, Nyland TG, Fisher P. Ultrasound-guided biopsy of the canine liver, kidney and prostate. *Vet Radiol.* 1985;26: 82-88.
64. Hardie EM, Page RL, Williams PL, Fischer WD. Effect of time of cisplatin administration on its toxicity and pharmacokinetics in dogs. *Am J Vet Res.* 1991;52:1821-1825.
65. Hardy ML, Hsu RC, Short CR. The nephrotoxic potential of gentamicin in the cat; enzymuria and alterations in urine concentrating ability. *J Vet Pharmacol Ther.* 1985;8:382-392.
66. Heller J, Horacek V. The cause of a depressed glomerular filtration rate after an ischemic insult: Whole kidney and superficial nephron study in the dog. *Pflugers Arch.* 1990;417: 360-364.
67. Heyman SN, et al. Protective action of glycine in cisplatin nephrotoxicity. *Kidney Int.* 1991;40:273-279.
68. Hsu CH, Kurtz TW, Easterling RE, Weller JM. Potentiation of gentamicin nephrotoxicity by metabolic acidosis. *Proc Soc Exp Biol Med.* 1974;46:894-897.
69. Humes HD. Role of calcium in pathogenesis of acute renal failure. *Am J Physiol.* 1986;250:F579-F589.
70. Humes HD, Sastrasinh M, Weinberg JM. Calcium is a competitive inhibitor of gentamicin-renal membrane binding interactions and dietary calcium supplementation protects against gentamicin nephrotoxicity. *J Clin Invest.* 1984;73:134-147.
71. Ihle SL, Kostolich M. Acute renal failure associated with contrast medium administration in a dog. *J Am Vet Med Assoc.* 1991;199:899-901.
72. Jeraj K, Osborne CA, Stevens JB. Evaluation of renal biopsy in 197 dogs and cats. *J Am Vet Med Assoc.* 1982;181:367-369.
73. Johnston PA, et al. Prostaglandins mediate the vasodilatory effect of mannitol in the hypoperfused rat kidney. *J Clin Invest.* 1981;68:127-133.
74. Kirby R. Acute renal failure as a complication in the critically ill

animal. *Vet Clin North Am (Small Anim Pract).* 1989;19:1189-1208.

75. Kore AM. Toxicology of nonsteroidal antiinflammatory drugs. In: Beasley VR, ed. *Toxicology of Selected Pesticides, Drugs, and Chemicals.* Philadelphia, Pennsylvania: WB Saunders Co; 1990: 419-430.
76. Kramer HJ, Schuurmann J, Wasserman C, Dusing R. Prostaglandin-independent protection by furosemide from oliguric ischemic renal failure in conscious rats. *Kidney Int.* 1980;17:455-464.
77. Kurnik BR, Weisberg LS, Cuttler IM, Kurnik PB. Effects of atrial natriuretic peptide versus mannitol on renal blood flow during radiocontrast infusion in chronic renal failure. *J Lab Clin Med.* 1990;116:27-35.
78. Liano F, et al. Easy and early prognosis in acute tubular necrosis: A forward analysis of 228 cases. *Nephron.* 1989;51:307-313.
79. Lien J, Chan V. Risk factors influencing survival in acute renal failure treated by hemodialysis. *Arch Intern Med.* 1985;145: 2067-2069.
80. Lindner A. Synergism of dopamine and furosemide in diuretic-resistant, oliguric acute renal failure. *Nephron.* 1983;33:121-126.
81. Lippert AC, Armstrong PJ. Parenteral nutritional support. In: Kirk RW, ed. *Current Veterinary Therapy X; Small Animal Practice.* Philadelphia, Pennsylvania: WB Saunders Co; 1989:25-30.
82. Mandal AK, Lightfoot BO, Treat RC. Mechanisms of protection in acute renal failure. *Circ Shock.* 1983;11:245-253.
83. Margulies KB, McKinley LJ, Cavero PG, Burnett JC. Induction and prevention of radiocontrast-induced nephropathy in dogs with heart failure *Kidney Int.* 1990; 38:1101-1108.
84. Marinides GN, Groggel GC, Cohen AH, Border WA. Enalapril and low protein diet reverse chronic puromycin aminonucleoside nephropathy. *Kidney Int.* 1990; 37:749-757.
85. Mason J. The pathophysiology of ischemic acute renal failure; a new hypothesis about the initiation phase. *Renal Physiol.* 1986;9:129-147.
86. Mathews K, Doherty T, Dyson D, Wilcock B. Renal failure in dogs associated with flunixin meglumine and methoxyflurane anesthesia. *Vet Surg.* 1987;16:323. Abstract.
87. Maxie MG. The urinary system. In: Jubb KV, Kennedy PC, Palmer N, eds. *Pathology of Domestic Animals.* 3rd ed. Orlando, Florida: Academic Press; 1985:343-411.
88. Mazze RI. Methoxyflurane nephropathy. *Environ Health Perspect.* 1976;15:111-119.
89. Meyer RD. Risk factors and comparisons of clinical nephrotoxicity of aminoglycosides. *Am J Med.* 1986;80:119-125.
90. Muir WM. DiBartola SP. Fluid therapy. In: Kirk RW, ed. *Current Veterinary Therapy VIII; Small Animal Practice.* Philadelphia, Pennsylvania: WB Saunders Co; 1983:28-40.
91. Nath KA, Paller MS. Dietary deficiency of antioxidants exacerbates ischemic injury in the rat kidney. *Kidney Int.* 1990;38: 1109-1117.
92. Ogilvie GK, et al. Evaluation of a short-term saline diuresis protocol for the administration of cisplatin. *Am J Vet Res.* 1988;49:1076-1078.
93. Osborne CA, et al. Percutaneous renal biopsy in the dog and cat. *J Am Vet Med Assoc.* 1967;151:1474-1480.
94. Osborne CA, Stevens JB, Polxin DJ. Gastrointestinal manifestations of urinary diseases. In: Anderson NV, ed. *Veterinary Gastroenterology.* Philadelphia, Pennsylvania: Lea & Febiger; 1980:681-704.
95. Papadimitriou M, Milionis A, Sakellariou G, Metaxas P. Effect of furosemide on acute ischemic renal failure in the dog. *Nephron.* 1978;20:157-162.
96. Papich MG. Medical therapy for gastrointestinal ulcers. In: Kirk RW, ed. *Current Veterinary Therapy X; Small Animal Practice.* Philadelphia, Pennsylvania: WB Saunders Co; 1989:911-918.
97. Parker HR. Peritoneal dialysis and hemofiltration. In: Bovee KC, ed. *Canine Nephrology.* Media, Pennsylvania: Harwal Publishing Co; 1984:723-754.
98. Parker S, et al. Dopamine administration in oliguria and oliguric renal failure. *Crit Care Med.* 1981;9:630-632.
99. Patrono C, Dunn MJ. The clinical significance of inhibition of renal prostaglandin synthesis. *Kidney Int.* 1987;32:1-12.
100. Pawlowska D, Granger JP, Knox FG. Effects of adenosine infusion into renal interstitium on renal hemodynamics. *Am J Physiol.* 1987;252:F678-682.
101. Pedersoli WM. Serum fluoride concentration, renal and hepatic function test results in dogs with methoxyflurane anesthesia. *Am J Vet Res.* 1977;38:949-953.
102. Porter GA, Bennett WM. Toxic nephropathies. In: Brenner BM, Rector FC, eds. *The Kidney.* Philadelphia, Pennsylvania: WB Saunders Co; 1981:2045.
103. Quarum ML, et al. Increasing dietary calcium moderates experimental gentamicin nephrotoxicity. *J Lab Clin Med.* 1984; 103:104-114.
104. Raisbeck MF. Fatal nephrotoxicosis associated with furosemide and gentamicin therapy in a dog. *J Am Vet Med Assoc.* 1983;183: 892-893.
105. Raskin NH, Fishman RA. Neurologic disorders in renal failure (part I). *N Engl J Med.* 1976;294:143-148.
106. Rasmussen HH, Pitt EA, Ibels LS, McNeil DR. Prediction of outcome in acute renal failure by discriminant analysis of clinical variables. *Arch Intern Med.* 1985;145:2015-2018.
107. Richet G. When should renal biopsy be done in acute uremia? *Kidney Int.* 1985;28(suppl 17):S152-S153.
108. Roberts DS, et al. Prediction of acute renal failure after birth asphyxia. *Arch Dis Child.* 1990;65:1021-1028.
109. Robinette JB, Conger JD. Angiotensin and thromboxane in the enhanced renal adrenergic nerve sensitivity of acute renal failure. *J Clin Invest.* 1990;86:1532-1539.
110. Rogers RA, Hanna AY, Riviere JE. Dose response studies of gentamicin nephrotoxicity in rats with experimental renal dysfunction. III. Effects of dosage adjustment method. *Res Commun Chem Pathol Pharmacol.* 1987;57:301-311.
111. Rubin SI. Nonsteroidal antiinflammatory drugs, prostaglandins, and the kidney. *J Am Vet Med Assoc.* 1986;188:1065-1068.
112. Ruiz P, Gomez F, Schrieber AD. Impaired function of macrophage Fc gamma receptors in end-stage renal disease. *N Engl J Med.* 1990;322:717-722.
113. Russell JD, Churchill DN. Calcium antagonists and acute renal failure. *Am J Med.* 1989;87:306-315.
114. Savin VJ, et al. Glomerular ultracoefficient after ischemic renal injury in dogs. *Circ Res.* 1983;53:439-447.
115. Schrier RW. Acute renal failure: Pathogenesis, diagnosis, and management. *Hosp Pract.* 1981;16:93-109.
116. Schrier RW. Role of calcium channel blockers in protection against experimental renal injury. *Am J Med.* 1991;90 (Suppl 5A):21S-25S.
117. Schrier RW, Arnold PE, Van Putten VJ, Burke TJ. Cellular calcium in ischemic acute renal failure: Role of calcium entry blockers. *Kidney Int.* 1987;32:313-321.
118. Schumacher J, et al. Effect of diet on gentamicin-induced nephrotoxicosis in horses. *Am J Vet Res.* 1991;52:1274-1278.
119. Siegel NJ, et al. Enhanced recovery from acute renal failure by the postischemic infusion of adenine nucleotides and magnesium chloride in rats. *Kidney Int.* 1980;17:338-349.
120. Smithies MN, Cameron JS. Can we predict outcome in acute renal failure? *Nephron.* 1989;51:297-300.
121. Spyridakis LK, Bacia JJ, Barsanti JA, Brown SA. Ibuprofen

toxicosis in the dog. *J Am Vet Med Assoc.* 1986;189:918-919.

122. Stein JH, Sorkin MI. Pathophysiology of a vasomotor and nephrotoxic model on acute renal failure in the dog. *Kidney Int.* 1976;10:S86-S93.
123. Stolarek I, Howey JE, Fraser CG. Biological variation of urinary N-acetyl-beta-D-glucosaminidase: Practical and clinical implications. *Clin Chem.* 1989;35:560-563.
124. Strombeck DR, Guilford WG. *Small Animal Gastroenterology.* 2nd ed. Davis, California: Stonegate Publishing Co; 1990.
125. Szczech GM, Carlton WW, Lund JE. Determination of enzyme concentrations in urine for diagnosis of renal damage. *J Am Anim Hosp Assoc.* 1974;10:1093-1096.
126. Thornhill JA. Therapeutic strategies involving antimicrobial treatment of small animals with peritonitis. *J Am Vet Med Assoc.* 1984;185:1181-1184.
127. Tilley LP. *Essentials of Canine and Feline Electrocardiography.* 2nd ed. Philadelphia, Pennsylvania: Lea & Febiger; 1985: 232-233.
128. Tolins JP, Raij L. Chronic amphotericin B nephrotoxicity in the rat: Protective effect of calcium channel blockade. *J Am Soc Nephrol.* 1991;2:98-102.
129. Triulzi DJ, Blumberg N. Variability in response to cryoprecipitate treatment for hemostatic defects in uremia. *Yale J Biol Med.* 1990;63:1-7.
130. Tyler RD, Qualls CW, Heald RD. Renal concentrating ability in dehydrated hyponatremia dogs. *J Am Vet Med Assoc.* 1987;191: 1095-1100.
131. Van Buren CT, et al. Effects of intravenous essential L-amino acids and hypertonic dextrose on anephric beagles. *Surg Forum.* 1972;23:83-84.
132. Vari RC, et al. Induction, prevention and mechanisms of contrast media induced acute renal failure. *Kidney Int.* 1988;33: 699-707.
133. Vigano GL, et al. Subcutaneous desmopressin (DDAVP) shortens bleeding time in uremia. *Am J Hematol.* 1989;31:32-35.
134. Walker PD, Shah SV. Reactive oxygen metabolites in endotoxin-induced acute renal failure in rats. *Kidney Int.* 1990;38:1125-1132.
135. Weening JJ. Mechanisms leading to toxin-induced impairment of renal function, with a focus on immunopathology. *Toxicol Lett.* 1989;46:205-211.
136. Weinberg J. The cell biology of ischemic renal injury. *Kidney Int.* 1991;39:476-500.
137. Weinberg JM, Davis JA, Abarzua M, Rajan T. Cytoprotective effects of glycine and glutathione against hypoxic injury to rat tubules. *J Clin Invest.* 1987;80:1446-1454.
138. Wheeler SL, McGuire BH. Enteral nutritional support. In: Kirk RW, ed. *Current Veterinary Therapy X; Small Animal Practice.* Philadelphia, Pennsylvania: WB Saunders Co; 1989:30-37.
139. Whiting PH, et al. The effect of dietary protein restriction on high dose gentamicin nephrotoxicity in rats. *Br J Exp Pathol.* 1988;69:35-41.
140. Widener LL, Mela-riker LM. Verapamil pretreatment preserves mitochondrial function and tissue magnesium in the ischemic kidney. *Circ Shock.* 1984;13:27-37.
141. Wilkes BM, Mailloux LU. Acute renal failure; pathogenesis and prevention. *Am J Med.* 1986;80:1129-1136.
142. Willard MD. Treatment of hyperkalemia. In: Kirk RW, ed. *Current Veterinary Therapy IX; Small Animal Practice.* Philadelphia, Pennsylvania: WB Saunders Co; 1987:94-101.
143. Williams RH, Thomas CE, Navar LG, Evan AP. Hemodynamic and single nephron function during the maintenance phase of ischemic acute renal failure in the dog. *Kidney Int.* 1981;19:503-515.
144. Wise LA, Allen TA, Cartwright M. Comparison of renal biopsy techniques in dogs. *J Am Vet Med Assoc.* 1989;195:935-939.
145. Wolf AM. Canine uremic encephalopathy. *J Am Anim Hosp Assoc.* 1980;16:735-738.
146. Wong NL, Magil AB, Dirks JH. Effect of magnesium diet in gentamicin-induced acute renal failure in rats. *Nephron.* 1989; 51:84-88.
147. Zager RA. Hyperphosphatemia: A factor that provokes severe acute renal failure. *J Lab Clin Med.* 1982;100:230-239.
148. Zarich SZ, Fang LST, Diamond JR. Fractional excretion of sodium; exceptions to its diagnostic value. *Arch Intern Med.* 1985;145:108-112.

CHAPTER 23

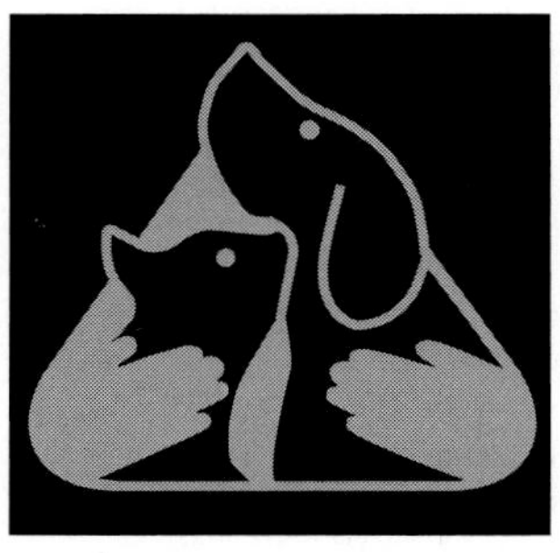

Cystic Diseases of the Kidney

JODY P. LULICH
CARL A. OSBORNE
DAVID J. POLZIN

I. RENAL CYSTS

Renal cysts may occur in association with inherited, developmental, or acquired diseases. Irrespective of the underlying condition, cysts are histologically similar (fluid-filled sacs lined by an epithelium[1]); however, their quantity, location, and clinical course may differ tremendously. For example, simple renal cysts may affect only one kidney and are usually clinically asymptomatic.[2] By comparison, polycystic kidney disease is characterized by multiple cysts that progressively crowd out normal parenchyma of both kidneys to the extent that renal function is impaired.[3,4] Some cysts communicate with glomeruli and collecting tubules, whereas others do not. Contrary to the view that many cysts are static structures, cysts are very dynamic. Studies in humans revealed that turnover of cyst fluid occurred as often as 20 times a day.[5]

Partly as a result of this diversity, no universally accepted method of classification for renal cysts exists. In this chapter, cysts have been classified based on the scheme proposed in 1987 by the Committee on Terminology, Nomenclature, and Classification, Section on Urology, American Academy of Pediatrics, in which the primary distinction is between genetic and acquired disorders.[6] Cystic disorders were further classified according to their clinical, radiologic, and pathologic features. Although inherited patterns of disease may be difficult to define for many veterinary patients, continuity of nomenclature between species aids communication and understanding of cyst formation, ultimately leading to improved understanding, diagnosis, and therapy.

A. Genetic cystic disorders of kidneys.

1. Overview. Many forms of genetically determined renal cystic disease occur in human beings (e.g., autosomal dominant polycystic kidney disease, autosomal recessive polycystic kidney disease, renal medullary cystic disease complex, and congenital nephrosis).[7] Polycystic kidney disease has been the only reported inherited cystic disease in companion animals.[8-11]
2. Polycystic Kidney Disease
   a. Polycystic kidney disease is a disorder in which significant portions of normally differentiated renal parenchyma are displaced by multiple cysts (Fig. 23–1).[6] Both kidneys are invariably involved, a phenomenon probably related to the inherited nature of this disorder.
   b. Lack of genealogic information often precludes

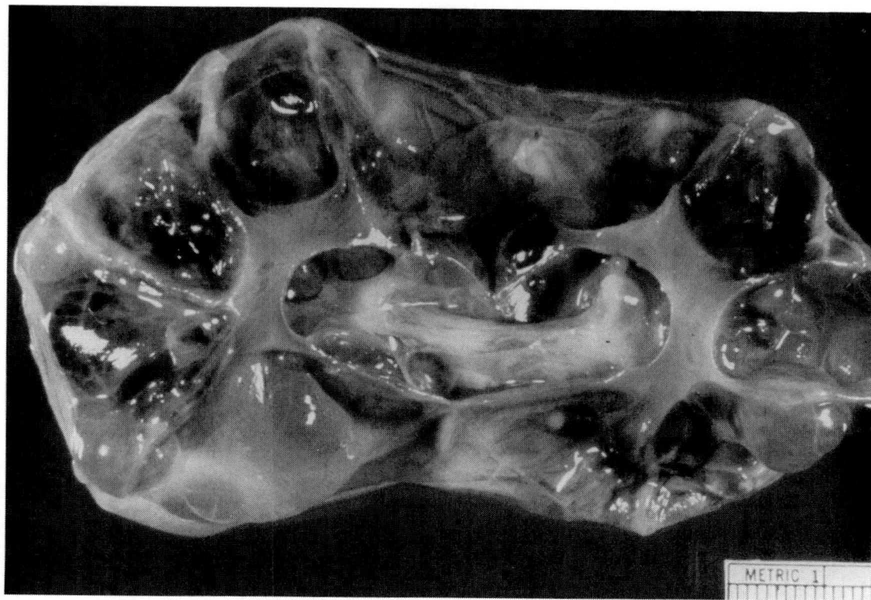

FIG. 23–1. Photograph of a sagittally sectioned polycystic kidney from a 10-year-old female domestic long-hair cat with renal failure.

a precise diagnosis of inherited polycystic kidney disease in most adult dogs and cats with multiple renal cysts.

c. As many as 75% of humans with polycystic kidney disease have hepatic cysts. Cysts have also been recognized in the pancreas, spleen, and thyroid gland in humans with polycystic kidney disease. Therefore, identification of cysts in other organs (liver, pancreas) may be helpful in the diagnosis of dogs and cats suspected of having polycystic kidney disease (Fig. 23–2). However, nonrenal organ involvement with cysts is not a requirement for diagnosis of polycystic kidney disease.

d. Persian and other long-haired varieties of cats have been the most common breeds identified with polycystic disease.[3,8] To our knowledge, cairn terriers and beagles have been the only canine breeds diagnosed with this disorder.[10,11] Beagle dogs with polycystic kidneys had only one kidney.[11] In addition to cats and dogs, polycystic kidney disease has been described in other species of animals, including mink, ferrets, rabbits, and rodents.[12]

e. Polycystic kidney disease has also been reported in many species without knowledge of a heritable pathogenesis.[3,13-16] To minimize confusion and possible misclassification, one should not use the term polycystic kidneys as a general term to describe kidneys with multiple cysts.

3. Glomerulocystic disease may have a familial tendency for affecting collie dogs; however, conclusive genetic transmission has not been proved.[17]

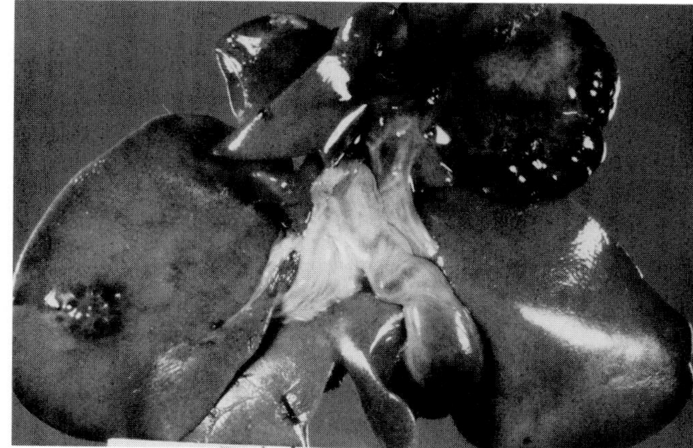

FIG. 23–2. Photograph of the liver of the cat with polycystic kidneys illustrated in Figure 23–1. Note cysts located in several hepatic lobes.

B. Acquired cystic disorders of kidneys.

1. Overview. Acquired cystic diseases of kidneys have been identified in dogs and cats with renal dysplasia, renal neoplasia, renal infection, and tubulo-interstitial nephritis.[18-21] In early stages, cystic disease is usually asymptomatic and detected inadvertently during ultrasonographic evaluation of the abdomen; in the later stages, cystic disease is often recognized during evaluation of the patient for causes of renal failure.

2. Cysts associated with chronic progressive renal disease.
   a. Renal cysts have been identified in the keeshond, cocker spaniel, and Yorkshire terrier with renal cortical hypoplasia, and in the Lhasa apso, Shih Tzu, Wheaton terrier, Doberman pinscher, and standard poodle with renal dysplasia.[18-20,22-24] Cystic lesions commonly reported with abnormalities in renal development include cortical cysts and cystic glomerular atrophy; however, cystic changes have also been recognized in other renal structures and locations of the kidney (Fig. 23–3).[21]
   b. Renal cysts have also been reported in association with primary renal neoplasia (embryonal nephroma and carcinoma).[25] A unique complex recognized primarily in the German shepherd dog is the combination of renal cystadenocarcinomas and nodular dermatofibrosis, a condition characterized by multiple collagenous nodules of the skin.[26,27]
   c. Common to the development of acquired renal cysts, irrespective of the underlying disorder, is the chronic progressive nature of underlying renal disease. However, whether or not chronic renal disease precedes cyst formation is not always clear. In fact, implementation of dialysis to prolong life in human patients with end-stage renal failure is followed by development of cysts.[12] Although cysts were once believed to result from dialysis, dialysis is now thought simply to extend the time during which cysts can develop. Nonetheless, because renal cysts have been described in association with nearly every type of chronic renal disease in humans, a popular hypothesis is that cysts develop as a consequence of chronic progressive renal insufficiency. According to this line of reasoning, epithelial hypertrophy of residual nephrons, in response to a progressive decline in renal function, gives way to epithelial hyperplasia. A combination of glomerular filtration and transepithelial secretion dilates the tubule with fluid. Focal proliferation of cells obstructs renal tubules and provides new tubular cells to allow expansion of cyst walls. Modulators hypothesized to stimulate cellular hyperplasia include parathyroid hormone, electrolyte abnormalities, vasopressin, cyclic adenosine monophosphate (cyclic AMP), and expression of protooncogenes.

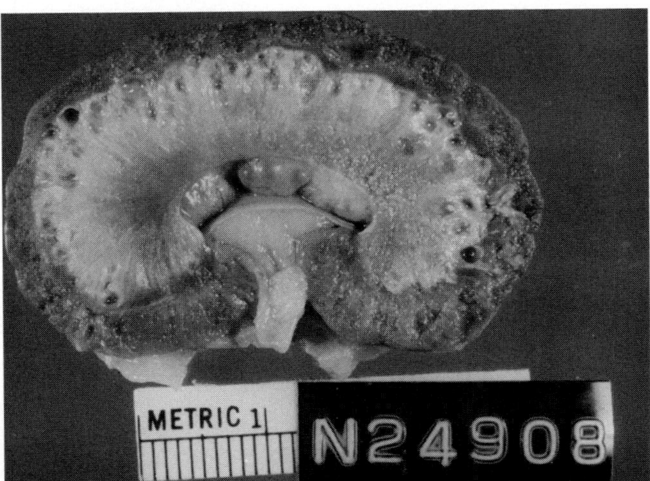

FIG. 23–3. Photograph of a sagittally sectioned kidney from a 5-year-old Shetland sheepdog with medullary cysts and chronic renal failure.

3. Cysts Induced By Chemicals
   a. Ingestion of diphenylthiazole, nordihydroguaiarectic acid, or diphenylamine by rats causes cysts to develop in otherwise normal kidneys.[12,28,29]
      (1). The severity of cyst formation caused by nordihydroguaiarectic acid accelerated when animals were exposed to normal enteric microbes or endotoxins.
      (2). Cysts caused by diphenylthiazole subside if the drug is discontinued.
      (3). Other examples of chemicals that induce cyst formation include trichlorophenoxyacetic acid, a defoliate agent used during the Vietnam War, and biphenyl, a chemical previously used to reduce fungus on citrus trees.[13]
      (4). Collectively, these findings indicate that chemically induced cyst formation can be modified by secondary factors, and that persistence of cysts requires continued exposure to cystogenic chemicals.
   b. The cystogenic potential of chemicals may also depend on the developmental stage of the kidney at the time of exposure. Although some chemicals promote cyst formation in fully developed kidneys, long-acting corticosteroids (9-fluoroprednisolone acetate and prednisolone tertiary butylacetate) only induced cysts in the kidneys of neonatal rabbits, hamsters, and rats.[30-32]
   c. Chemical cystogens appear to damage renal epithelium. The initial injury is then followed by focal tubular dilation and expansion. Chronic hypokalemia has been hypothesized to promote cyst formation in humans by a similar mechanism.[33]
4. Simple Renal Cysts. Solitary renal cysts unassociated with altered kidney function are called simple cysts.[6] Although once thought to be clinically inocuous, simple cysts have been associated with pain, hematuria, and infection. In humans, some simple cysts progressed in quantity and ultimately affected both kidneys.[2] The pathogenesis of simple

cysts is not completely known; however, in some cases, simple cysts may represent an early manifestation of multicystic diseases of kidneys.

C. Concepts of cyst origin and formation.

1. Postulated mechanisms that cause nephrons to undergo cystic change include the following:
   a. Morphologic Origins.
   Light microscopic and micropuncture studies in many animal species indicate that renal cysts are dilated segments of nephrons.[34]
   b. Renal Tubular Modifications.
      (1). The possibility of tubular obstruction as an initial event was hypothesized when researchers observed polyploid lesions in the funnel-shaped transition region between a cyst and a draining duct of normal renal tubular diameter.[35]
      (2). According to this hypothesis, once the renal tubule is obstructed, pressure-induced stretching or ballooning of tubular walls to cystic dimensions results from continued glomerular filtration and subsequent increases in hydrostatic pressure.
      (3). Although this scenario is plausible, it does not provide a complete explanation.
         (a). When hydrostatic pressure was measured in cysts, it was not elevated, and cells lining cysts were not reduced in height.
         (b). Ureteral obstruction usually results in hydronephrosis without renal cystic formation.
         (c). Thus, tubular stretching apparently could not have occurred as an isolated event. It must have been coupled with new growth of both cells and tubular basement membranes.
         (d). Perhaps cyst development occurs in obstructed tubules only when tubular cells are predisposed to divide at a lower threshold, possibly as a result of genetic predisposition, endogenous agents, or exogenous cystogenic chemicals. In fact, the concentration of epidermal growth factor measured in cyst fluid was high. Proto-oncogene expression was abnormally elevated in mice with autosomal recessive polycystic kidney disease.[7]
         (e). Tubular obstruction may not be necessary for cyst formation. Instead, obstruction could occur as a consequence of focally excessive cell growth of diffusely stimulated and hyperplastic tubular epithelium. This possibility is especially plausible for cysts that communicate with normal patent collecting ducts.
   c. Origin of Cyst Fluid. Although glomerular filtration is an obvious source of cyst fluid, active tubular secretion of fluid has also been postulated as a fundamental event in cyst formation.
      (1). Support for this concept stems from *in vitro* models that demonstrated formation of cyst-like spheres by transformed cells of the distal tubule cultured on collagen gel.[36]
      (2). In addition, fluid-filled cysts develop and grow in nonfunctioning end-stage polycystic kidneys and in severely dysplastic kidneys in the absence of connections to functioning glomeruli.
      (3). Localization of the sodium/potassium ATPase pump in epithelial cells lining cysts provided new information supporting the importance of altered tubular secretion.[37] In normal renal tubular cells, the sodium/potassium ATPase resides in the basolateral border. In transformed cells lining cysts, sodium/potassium ATPase is localized to the apical border.
   d. Summary
      (1). Renal cysts develop in pre-existing nephrons and collecting ducts, and can develop in the absence of distal tubular obstruction.
      (2). Although the exact pathogenesis is not known, three events are recognized as critically important:
         (a). Sustained tubular epithelial cell proliferation to accommodate tubular dilation.
         (b). Accumulation of cyst fluid derived from glomerular filtrate and/or transepithelial secretion of fluid and electrolytes.
         (c). Remodeling of the extracellular matrix adjacent to cysts to allow for expansion.
      (3). The stimulus for cellular hyperplasia and cyst filling, as well as the sequence of events, remains obscure; however, genetic, endogenous, and environmental factors appear to influence the process.
2. Clinical Correlates
   a. Because of the rapid turnover of cyst fluid, aspiration of fluid may only be a temporary means to control cystic disease.
   b. Genetic counseling should be beneficial in minimizing the occurrence of polycystic disease in affected families of cats and dogs.

D. Diagnostic considerations.

1. Overview
   a. Renal cysts often remain undetected until they have become of sufficient size and quantity to

contribute to renal failure or abdominal enlargement.[3]

b. In some instances, cysts are detected when investigating the underlying causes of hematuria, urinary infection, and renal disease.
c. Renal cysts are sometimes diagnosed during radiographic evaluation of the abdomen for nonrenal disorders.
d. Small solitary cysts are often first observed during postmortem evaluation of kidneys.
e. The insidious nature of renal cystic diseases may result from the slow growth rate of cysts and the ability of the kidneys to compensate until function is markedly reduced.
f. For these reasons, patients with renal cysts typically are clinically normal during initial stages of cyst formation and growth.

2. Physical Examination Findings
   a. Large cysts may be detected by abdominal palpation.
   b. Kidneys of cats with polycystic disease are often bosselated and markedly enlarged.
   c. Most renal cysts are not painful when palpated; however, acute secondary infection of cysts with bacteria may be associated with distention of the renal capsule and pain.
3. Radiography and ultrasonography
   a. Renal ultrasonography is the most widely accepted method for confirming a diagnosis of renal cysts in animals (Fig. 23–4).
      (1). Anechoic cavitating lesions characterized by sharply marginated smooth walls and distal enhancement are the criteria established for the diagnosis of renal cysts.[38]
      (2). Hypoechoic cystic cavities may be observed when cysts become infected with bacteria.
   b. Ultrasonography can also be used to detect cysts in other organs, a finding that is helpful in differentiating polycystic kidney disease from acquired multicystic disorders of kidneys.
   c. X-ray computed tomography is more sensitive for detecting smaller cysts than is ultrasonography.
   d. Survey radiography and intravenous urography are insensitive methods of confirming cystic disease until kidney size and contour become distorted by increases in cyst quantity and size.
4. Aspiration of Cyst Fluid
   a. Evaluation of fine-needle aspirates of the kidney may allow differentiation of cystic diseases from other diseases that result in kidney enlargement (e.g., neoplasia, mycosis, feline infectious peritonitis, pyelonephritis, and hydronephrosis).
   b. Cyst fluid may be clear, cloudy, or hemorrhagic, and may vary in character between different cysts from the same kidney.
   c. Analysis of the biochemical composition of cyst fluid may assist in differentiating the location of nephrons that have become cystic.[34,39]
      (1). Cysts derived from proximal nephron segments have solute concentrations similar to those of serum.
      (2). Cystic segments of functioning distal nephrons are expected to have lower concentrations of sodium, chloride, and total carbon dioxide and higher concentrations of potassium and creatinine, thus reflecting the secretory function of normal distal renal tubules.
   d. Bacterial infection of cysts may be verified by light microscopy of centrifuged cyst fluid and by culture of cyst fluid.
5. Concomitant Diseases.
   a. Detection of some diseases should arouse suspicion of concomitant cystic kidney disorders.
   b. Dermatofibrosis in German shepherd dogs is associated with renal cystadenocarcinomas.[26,27]
   c. Renal cysts were commonly found in the kidneys of a Dutch breed of setter (Drentse patrijshond) with red blood cell stomatocytosis and hypertrophic gastritis.[40]
   d. Polycystic kidney disease should be considered a possible cause for renal failure in Persian and other long-haired varieties of cats.
   e. Polycystic kidney disease was also recognized in Persian cats with neurovisceral mannosidosis associated with alpha-mannosidase deficiency.
   f. The kidneys of animals with hepatic cysts should be evaluated for concomitant renal cystic disease.
   g. Because some cystic diseases are inherited, detection of multiple cysts in a patient should

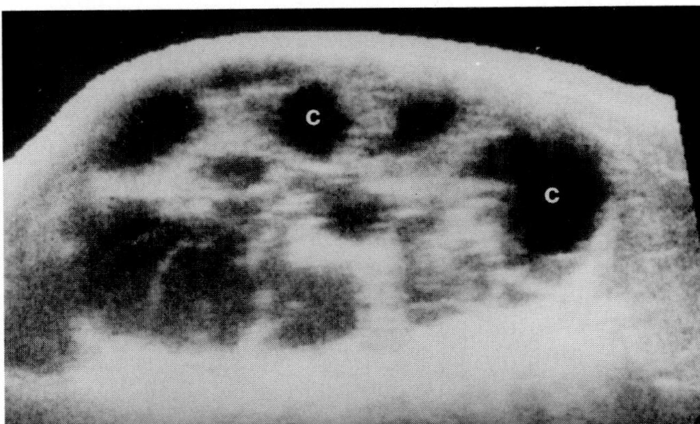

FIG. 23–4. Sagittal static-B ultrasonogram of a polycystic kidney from an 11-year-old male domestic long-hair cat. The multiple anechoic areas represent cysts (c).

prompt investigation for cysts in the kidneys of related animals.

E. Therapeutic considerations.

1. Overview. As with many chronic progressive diseases of the kidney, elimination of renal cysts and associated renal parenchymal lesions is usually not feasible. Inability to promote cyst regression is related to a current lack of knowledge concerning the specific cause and pathophysiology of cyst formation. Because inherited and congenital disorders may be impossible to reverse in mature kidneys, detection and intervention may be necessary at the time of renal organogenesis. Because such therapy is currently unavailable, therapy is often limited to minimizing the pathophysiologic consequences of renal cyst formation in kidneys (i.e., renal failure, renal infection, and hematuria).
2. Specific Therapy for Management of Cysts
   a. Spontaneous resolution of cysts has not been documented in dogs or cats; we suspect that it is uncommon.
   b. With time, most cysts increase in size and quantity, often compressing adjacent normal functioning parenchyma.[8]
   c. In some cases, reversal of the cystic condition has been observed following correction of putative cystogenic causes.
      (1). In humans, regression of uremia-associated renal cystic disease occurred after renal transplantation.[12]
      (2). Correction of hypokalemia and hyperaldosteronism in human patients resulted in a reduction in the quantity and size of medullary cysts in kidneys.[33]
      (3). Cystic changes induced by diphenylthiazole in kidneys of rats are completely reversed 4 to 8 weeks after withdrawal of diphenylthiazole from the diet.[29]
      (4). Reductions in cyst volume have also been achieved in humans by surgically removing part of the cyst wall and by percutaneous aspiration of cyst fluid.[41,42]
      (5). Percutaneous aspiration of fluid from large renal cysts can be performed to minimize compression of adjacent normal renal parenchyma. However, this procedure is impractical for kidneys with hundreds of cysts. Likewise, periodic aspiration of fluid (weekly to biweekly) is needed to maintain reduced cyst volume.
      (6). Percutaneous aspiration and instillation of bismuthphosphate has been effective in maintaining cyst reduction in humans with simple renal cysts.[43]
3. Managing Consequences of Cystic Disease
   a. Renal Failure. Renal failure is a common consequence of cystic diseases characterized by multiple cysts diffusely localized throughout both kidneys.[3] Progressive cyst enlargement compresses adjacent functioning renal parenchyma, ultimately leading to impaired renal function. Because of the reserve capacity of kidneys, solitary renal cysts are unlikely to alter function. When specific therapy promoting cyst regression is not feasible, therapy is directed at delaying the progression and consequences of renal failure. (See Chapters 27 through 32, which describe treatment of renal failure.) Reduction in the concentration of uremic toxins has been associated with reduction in progression of renal cyst enlargement in humans.[12] For large cysts thought to contribute to decreased renal perfusion or hypertension, percutaneous aspiration and decompression should be considered. Decompression via cyst aspiration may need to be repeated once cysts have resumed their original size.
   b. Renal Infection.
      (1). Bacterial infection of cysts has been observed in dogs and cats evaluated at our veterinary hospital. Infection was unilateral. Unless infection is accompanied by pyelonephritis, bacteria may not be observed in urine. Therefore, to minimize the possibility of overlooking a life-threatening but potentially reversible disease, one should consider parenchymal infection when renal cysts are associated with renal pain, fever, and leukocytosis, even in absence of bacteriuria. Increased cyst wall thickness and hypoechoic cyst cavities detected by ultrasonography are also indicative of bacterial infection. Confirmation of cyst infection requires aspiration and bacterial culture of cyst fluid. Little is known about the types of organisms that invade cysts in veterinary patients; however, we have observed *Escherichia coli* and staphylococcal urinary tract infections.
      (2). Treatment of infected cysts may require special consideration.
         (a). The acidic nature of cyst fluid and its containment by an epithelial barrier might inhibit the establishment of bactericidal concentrations of commonly used acidic antibiotics (e.g., cephalosporins and penicillins) within cysts.[44]
         (b). Alkaline lipid-soluble antibiotics (e.g., trimethroprim-sulfonamide combinations, enrofloxacin, chloramphenicol, tetracycline, and clindamycin), which penetrate epithelial barriers and become ionized and trapped in cyst lumens, have been recommended for humans with in-

fected cysts, and therefore should be considered for veterinary patients.[45]

(c). If possible, infected cysts should be drained by percutaneous aspiration. Antibiotics should then be injected into the cystic cavity.

(d). In more severe forms of disease, surgical drainage and/or nephrectomy may be required to resolve infection.

c. Hematuria. Visible hematuria may occur if cysts rupture into the renal pelvis. In humans, hematuria usually appears suddenly and persists for several days.[7] With persistent bleeding, other causes of hematuria should be investigated, including coagulation abnormalities, renal neoplasia, nephrolithiasis, and renal infection. Reduced physical activity may facilitate local hemostasis; however, specific therapy for hematuria is usually not needed. In the rare event that blood clots obstruct urine flow, surgery may be needed to restore renal function.

d. Pain. Pain is the most common symptom in humans with polycystic kidney disease.[7] The cause is often obscure. Occasionally, pain has been associated with rupture of cysts and release of their contents into perirenal tissues. Pain has not been commonly recognized in animals with renal cysts; however, this observation does not mean that pain does not occur. If renal pain is detected, renal infection should be considered when formulating therapy. In humans, some relief from cyst-induced renal pain has been achieved by percutaneous aspiration of fluid from large cysts. A similar approach would logically be helpful for veterinary patients.

e. Hepatic Cysts. Hepatic cysts have been reported in both dogs and cats with polycystic kidney disease.[3,8,10] Cysts developed from both bile ducts and within the hepatic parenchyma. In cats with polycystic kidney disease that we have evaluated, hepatic cysts were not associated with altered hepatic function. This finding may have resulted, at least in part, from the focal nature of hepatic cyst development as opposed to the diffuse cystic changes observed in kidneys. The observation of concomitant cysts in organs other than kidneys, however, supports the possibility of a generalized cyst-forming defect.

f. Others. Hypertension, erythrocythemia, and increased prevalence of renal neoplasia have been associated with renal cystic diseases in humans.[7,46-48] To our knowledge, these associations have not been reported in companion animals. If detected, cyst removal logically would provide appropriate relief. In the event that cystectomy is not feasible, however, antihypertensive agents can be used to control hypertension, and phlebotomy can be used to control erythrocythemia. Nephrectomy and, if needed, antineoplastic therapy can be used to manage renal neoplasia.

4. Goals for the Future

a. Because the severity of cyst formation was directly correlated to the presence of endotoxin in rats with acquired renal cysts, the benefits of antibiotics and other methods of endotoxin reduction need to be assessed.

b. Identification of pharmacologic agents that interfere with the accumulation of fluid (e.g., agents that selectively inhibit ATPase of cyst epithelial cells) or slow the rate of cellular proliferation is needed to minimize cyst expansion and progression of renal failure.

II. PERINEPHRIC PSEUDOCYST

A. Introduction.

1. Capsulogenic renal cyst,[49] capsular cyst,[50] pararenal pseudocyst,[51] capsular hydronephrosis,[52] perirenal cyst,[53] and perirenal pseudocyst[54] have been used to describe renomegaly caused by accumulation of fluid between renal parenchyma and the surrounding capsule. The renal capsule is loosely adhered to the kidney, except in the renal sinus where it is anchored to blood vessels and the renal pelvic recess.[55,56] By definition, a cyst is a filled sac lined by an epithelium. The renal capsule is a mesenchymally derived connective tissue cover and, therefore, devoid of an epithelial lining. Consequently, the collection of fluid between the kidney and its capsule is best described as a pseudocyst.

2. We found only seven reported cases of perirenal pseudocysts in the English literature since 1963.[49-51,53,54,57,58] All were in male cats. Of these, 2 cats were young adults and 5 cats were 8 years or older. Bilateral pseudocysts were reported in half of the cases; both young cats had unilateral disease. Between 1989 and 1993, perirenal pseudocysts were diagnosed in 3 cats and 1 dog at the Veterinary Teaching Hospital, University of Minnesota. In contrast to the previously reported cases, one cat was female, and all were older adults. The youngest cat was 11 years old, and the dog was 16 years old.

B. Etiology.

1. The cause of perirenal accumulation of fluid in cats is not known.

2. Evaluation of pseudocyst fluid may be helpful in understanding the pathophysiologic mechanisms responsible for fluid accumulation.

a. Accumulation of Transudate-Type Fluids.

(1). Increased capillary hydrostatic pressure and lymphatic obstruction are common mechanisms promoting formation of transudates.

(2). In four cats and one dog, evaluation of fluid aspirated via needle and syringe re-

TABLE 23–1.
COMPARISON OF SERUM, PSEUDOCYST, AND URINE CONCENTRATIONS OF UREA NITROGEN AND CREATININE FROM 10 CATS AND 1 DOG WITH PERIRENAL PSEUDOCYSTS

	Urea Nitrogen (mg/dl)/Creatinine (mg/dl)				
Species	**Serum**	**Right Pseudocyst**	**Left Pseudocyst**	**Urine**	**Reference**
Feline	NR	NOT CYSTIC	NR	NR	49
Feline	NR	NOT CYSTIC	NR	NR	50
Feline	6/NR	NR	NR	NR	53
Feline	39/NR	NR	NR	NR	51
Feline	37/2.3	2.2/40	2.2/40	NR	54
Feline	30/2.2	31.NR	NOT CYSTIC	NR	57
Feline	75/3.1	NR	NR	NR	58
Feline	39/2.4	41/2.5	NOT CYSTIC	NR	VTHUM
Feline	73/5.6	NR	NR	NR	VTHUM
Feline	54/4.5	58/4.5	56/4.3	> 150/122	VTHUM
Canine	16/1.2	NOT CYSTIC	NR/9	NR/85	VTHUM

NR = not reported; VTHUM = Veterinary Teaching Hospital, University of Minnesota.

vealed that it was consistent with a transudate (low protein concentration and low cellularity). In all five patients, the concentrations of creatinine and urea nitrogen in pseudocyst fluid were similar to the concentrations of these substances in serum (Table 23–1).

(3). The kidneys of these patients were smaller than normal. Those evaluated by light microscopy had evidence of renal fibrosis, and all four cats had renal failure.

(4). Logic suggests that underlying renal disease somehow contributed to pseudocyst formation. However, we have not determined whether progressive renal parenchymal contraction occluded lymphatics and blood vessels, thereby promoting transudation of fluid, or whether renal parenchymal compression from fluid within the pseudocyst promoted parenchymal fibrosis and impaired kidney function. In fact, the two events may not be related. Perirenal accumulation of transudate type of fluids can also result from ruptured renal cysts; however, renal cysts were not reported in any of the cases of perinephric pseudocysts.

b. Accumulation of Urine

(1). Uriniferous pseudocyst, sometimes referred to as a urinoma, represents extravasation of urine between the kidney and the renal capsule. Accumulation of perirenal urine indicates that the excretory pathway of the renal pelvis or proximal ureter has been disrupted.

(2). In one report of a cat with a perirenal pseudocyst, the concentration of urea nitrogen in pseudocyst fluid was eight times greater than the concentration in serum consistent with extravasation of urine.[53]

(3). In another report, a paraureteral urinoma in an 11-year-old dog was evaluated 3 weeks following ovariohysterectomy.[59] The ureter was assumed to have been crushed, transsected, or partially ligated during surgery.

c. Accumulation of Blood. Accumulation of blood in pseudocysts can result from external trauma, surgery, neoplastic erosion of blood vessels, rupture of aneurysms, or coagulopathies. Following hematoma formation, clot retraction, and lysis, a clear or light yellow fluid may remain between the kidney and capsule. None of the reported cases or those evaluated at our veterinary teaching hospital had pseudocyst characteristics consistent with perirenal bleeding.

3. Concomitant Renal Disease. Concomitant disease of affected kidneys was reported in many of the animals with pseudocysts. Six of seven cats evaluated were azotemic. The most common renal lesion was an irregular contour or interstitial fibrosis or both. One cat had small renal cysts and another had hydronephrosis.

4. Incidence in Cats Compared to that in Dogs. The fact that this disorder is rare in dogs is noteworthy. The difference in incidence between species may be related to the prominent network of subcapsular veins that is characteristic of feline kidneys.[55]

C. Diagnostic considerations.

1. In all reported cases, nonpainful enlargement of the abdomen was of primary concern to clients.

Laboratory findings at the time revealed either azotemia or no abnormalities.

2. Survey radiographs typically revealed a large abdominal mass of soft tissue density in the area normally occupied by the kidneys (Fig. 23–5). Excretory urograms revealed kidneys of normal or smaller-than-normal size surrounded by material of soft tissue density with a smooth external border. Obstruction of urine outflow, dilation of the excretory pathway, and extravasation of contrast medium were rare. Renal ultrasonography demonstrated normal or hyperechoic kidneys. The contents of the renal capsule were typically anechoic. The contents of the capsule may appear hypoechoic if blood or exudate separates the kidney from its capsule. Techniques not routinely performed that are likely to be of benefit include injection of contrast media into the space occupied by the capsule (Fig. 23–6), renal scintigraphy, and x-ray computed tomography.

D. Management.

1. Overview. Options for the management of perirenal pseudocysts include no treatment, periodic removal of fluid with the aid of a needle and syringe, or capsulectomy.
2. Surgical Therapy
   a. If surgical management of perirenal pseudocysts is being considered, other causes of renomegaly (polycystic kidney disease, hydronephrosis, neoplasia, and feline infectious peritonitis) should be eliminated by appropriate diagnostic procedures.
   b. Capsulectomy has been reported to be associated with a generally favorable outcome in three feline patients.[51,53,54] Removal of a unilateral perirenal pseudocyst by nephrectomy was associated with progressive renal dysfunction in one patient.[49]
   c. Peritoneal fenestration has been used to prevent development of lymphoceles following renal transplantation in humans.[60] This technique can be considered as an alternative to complete capsulectomy.
3. Paracentesis of Perinephric Pseudocysts. In one cat with bilateral perirenal pseudocysts and renal failure, we performed paracentesis every 7 to 14 days for 2 months. Removal of 100 to 150 mL of transudate from each pseudocyst was performed each period. Rate of fluid formation did not abate during this period. Following fluid removal, the cat became mildly depressed. We presumed that the cat became dehydrated as a result of

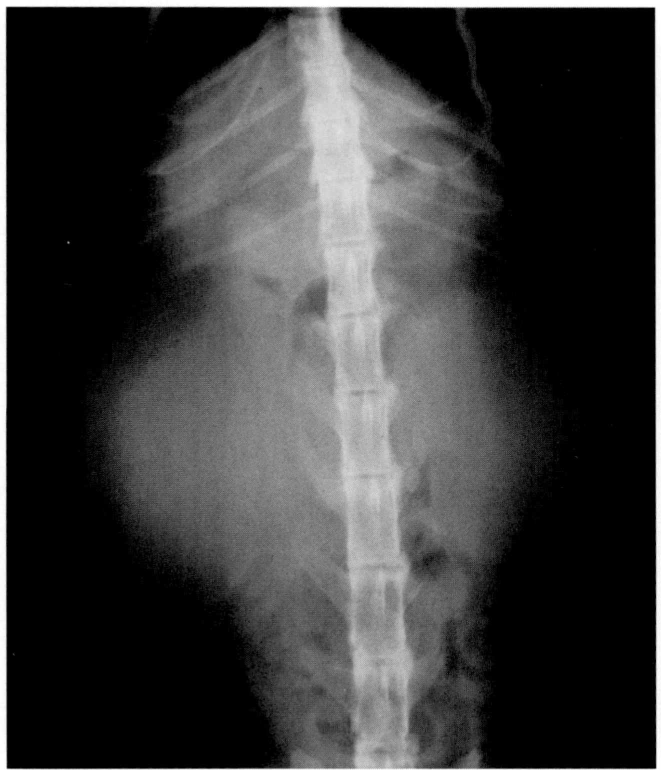

FIG. 23–5. Ventrodorsal survey abdominal radiograph of a 14-year-old female domestic long-hair cat illustrates bilateral renal enlargement caused by bilateral perirenal pseudocysts. This cat also had chronic renal failure.

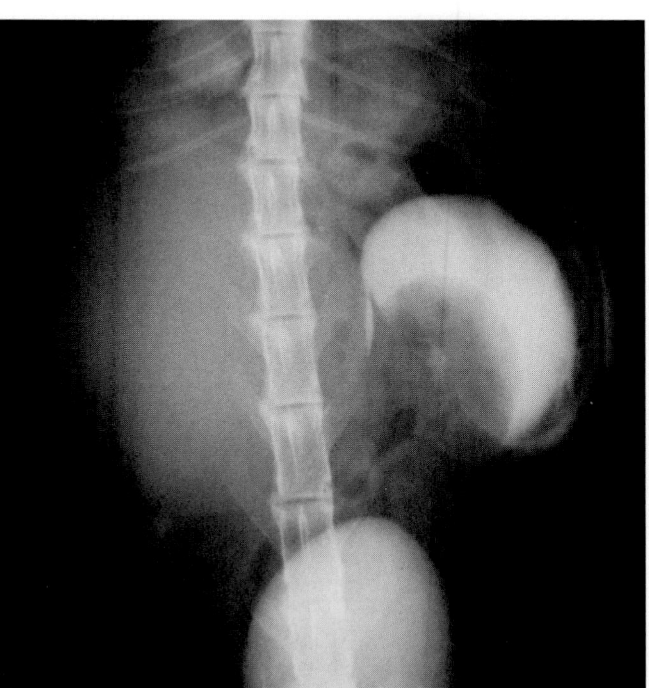

FIG. 23–6. Contrast perirenal cystogram of the left kidney illustrated in Figure 23–5. The radiograph was taken 1 hour after percutaneous injection of contrast media directly into the pseudocyst cavity. Note that the kidney lies within the cavity of the pseudocyst.

pseudocyst refilling. On occasion, paracentesis also resulted in hemorrhage into the pseudocyst. Based on these findings, we recognized the need to replace fluids removed by paracentesis with parenteral administration of physiologic solutions, especially in patients with renal failure. To minimize trauma to kidneys during paracentesis, one can use over-the-needle or through-the-needle catheters. The cutting needle can be removed once the pseudocyst has been penetrated.

4. Prognosis. The short-term prognosis appears to be favorable following capsulectomy in patients that have no evidence of renal dysfunction or only mild degrees of renal dysfunction. The long-term prognosis for patients with perirenal pseudocysts is not known because perirenal pseudocysts have not yet been determined to be in some way associated with underlying lesions in the renal parenchyma that may be progressive.

REFERENCES

1. *Stedman's Medical Dictionary.* 25th ed. Baltimore, Maryland: Williams & Wilkins; 1989:387.
2. Dalton D, Neiman H, Grayhack JT. The natural history of simple renal cysts: A preliminary study. *J Urol.* 1986;135: 905-908.
3. Lulich JP, Osborne CA, Walter PA, O'Brien TD. Feline idiopathic polycystic kidney disease. *Comp Cont Educ Pract Vet.* 1988;10: 1030-1040.
4. Franz KA, Reubi FC. Rate of functional deterioration in polycystic kidney disease. *Kid Int.* 1983;23:526-529.
5. Jacobsson L, Lindqvist B, Michaelson G, Bjerle P. Fluid turnover in renal cysts. *Acta Med Scand.* 1977;202:327-329.
6. Glassberg KI, et al. Renal dysgenesis and cystic disease of the kidney: A report of the Committee on Terminology, Nomenclature and Classification, Section on Urology, American Academy of Pediatrics. *J Urol.* 1987;138:1085-1092.
7. Welling LW, Grantham JJ. Cystic and developmental diseases of the kidney. In: Brenner BM, Rector FC, eds. *The Kidney.* Philadelphia, Pennsylvania: WB Saunders; 1992:1657-1694.
8. Biller DS, Chew DJ, DiBartola SP. Polycystic kidney disease in a family of Persian cats. *J Amer Vet Med Assoc.* 1990;196:1288-1290.
9. Cowgill LA, Hubbell JJ, Riley JC. Polycystic kidney disease in related cats. *J Am Vet Med Assoc.* 1979;175:286-288.
10. McKenna SC, Carpenter JL. Polycystic disease of the kidney and liver in the cairn terrier. *Vet Pathol.* 1980;17:436-442.
11. Fox MW. Inherited polycystic mononephrosis in the dog. *J Hered.* 1964;55:29-30.
12. Grantham JJ. Acquired cystic kidney disease. *Kid Int.* 1991;40: 143-152.
13. McQueen SD, Directo AC, Llorico BF. Bilateral congenital polycystic kidneys with vague symptomatology in a dog (a case report). *Vet Med/Small Anim Clin.* 1975;70:1167-1171.
14. Podell M, DiBartola SP, Rosol TJ. Polycystic kidney disease and renal lymphoma in a cat. *J Am Vet Med Assoc.* 1992;201:906-909.
15. Northington JW, Juliana MM. Polycystic kidney disease in a cat. *J Small Anim Pract.* 1977;18:663-666.
16. Battershell D, Garcia JP. Polycystic kidney in a cat. *J Am Vet Med Assoc.* 1969;154:555-565.
17. Chalifoux A. Glomerular polycystic kidney disease in a dog (blue merle collie). *Can Vet J.* 1982;23:365-368.
18. DiBartola SP, Davenport DJ, Chew DJ. Renal failure in young dogs. In: Kirk RW, ed. *Current Veterinary Therapy X, Small Animal Practice.* Philadelphia, Pennsylvania: WB Saunders Co; 1989: 1166-1173.
19. O'Brien TD, Osborne CA, Yano BL, Barnes DM. Clinicopathologic manifestations of progressive renal disease in Lhasa apso and Shih Tzu dogs. *J Am Vet Med Assoc.* 1982;180:658-664.
20. DiBartola SP, Chew DJ, Boyce JT. Juvenile renal disease in related standard poodles. *J Am Vet Med Assoc.* 1983;183: 693-696.
21. Picut CA, Lewis RM. Microscopic features of canine renal dysplasia. *Vet Pathol.* 1987;24:156-163.
22. Klopfer U, Neumann F, Trainin R. Renal cortical hypoplasia in a keeshond litter. *Vet Med/Small Anim Clin.* 1975;70:1081-1083.
23. Klopfer U, Nobel TA, Kaminiski R. A nephropathy similar to renal cortical hypoplasia in a Yorkshire terrier. *Vet Med/Small Anim Clin.* 1978;73:327-329.
24. Nash AS, Kelly DF, Gaskell CJ. Progressive renal disease in soft-coated Wheaten terriers: Possible familial nephropathy. *J Small Anim Pract.* 1984;25:479-487.
25. Nielsen SW, Moulton JE. Tumors of the urinary system. In: Moulton JE, ed. *Tumors in Domestic Animals.* 3rd ed. Berkeley, California: University of California Press; 1990:458-478.
26. Atlee BA, et al. Nodular dermatofibrosis in German shepherd dogs as a marker for renal cystadenocarcinoma. *J Am Anim Hosp Assoc.* 1991;27:481-487.
27. Lium B, Moe L. Hereditary multifocal renal cystadenocarcinomas and nodular dermatofibrosis in the German shepherd dog: Macroscopic and histologic changes. *Vet Pathol.* 1985; 22:447-455.
28. Gardner KD, et al. Endotoxin provocation of experimental renal cystic disease. *Kidney Int.* 1987;32:329-334.
29. Carone FA. Diphenylthiazole-induced renal cystis disease, rat. In: Jones TC, Mohr U, Hunt RD, eds. *Urinary System.* New York, New York: Springer-Verlag; 1986:262-267.
30. Perey DY, Herdman RC, Good RA. Polycystic renal disease: A new experimental model. *Science.* 1967;158:494-496.
31. Filmer RB, et al. Adrenal corticosteroid-induced renal cystic disease in the newborn hamster. *Am J Pathol.* 1973;72:461-472.
32. Crocker JF, et al. Steroid induced polycystic kidneys in the newborn rat. *Am J Pathol.* 1976;82:373-380.
33. Torres VE, et al. Association of hypokalemia, aldosteronism, and renal cysts. *N Engl J Med.* 1990;322:345-351.
34. Lang EK. Renal cyst puncture studies. *Urol Clin North Am.* 1987;14:91-102.
35. Evan AP, Gardner KD, Bernstein J. Polypoid and papillary epithelial hyperplasia: A potential cause of ductal obstruction in adult polycystic disease. *Kidney Int.* 1979;16:743-750.
36. McAteer JA, Evan AP, Gardner KD. Morphogenetic clonal growth of kidney epithelial cell line MDCK. *Anat Rec.* 1987;217: 229-239.
37. Wilson PD, et al. Reversed polarity of Na-K-ATPase: Mislocation to apical plasma membrane in polycystic kidney disease epithelia. *Am J Physiol.* 1991;260:F420-F430.
38. Walter PA, Johnston GR, Feeney DA, O'Brien TD. Applications of ultrasonography in the diagnosis of parenchymal kidney disease in cats: 24 cases (1981-1986). *J Am Vet Med Assoc.* 1988;192:92-98.
39. Ohkawa M, et al. Biochemical and pharmacodynamic studies of simple renal cyst fluids in relation to infection. *Nephron.* 1991; 59:80-83.
40. Slappendal RJ, et al. Familial stomatocytosis-hypertrophic gastritis, a newly recognized disease in the dog (Drentse patrijshond). *Vet Q.* 1991;13:30-40.
41. Rong Y, Yufeng C. Cyst decapitating decompression operation in polycystic kidney, preliminary report of 52 cases. *Chin Med J.* 1980;93:773-778.

42. Bennett WM, et al. Reduction of cyst volume for symptomatic management of autosomal dominant polycystic kidney disease. *J Urol.* 1987;137:620-622.
43. Holmberg G, Hietala SO. Treatment of simple cysts by percutaneous puncture and instillation of bismuth-phosphate. *Scand J Urol Nephrol.* 1989;23:207-212.
44. Muther RS, Bennett WM. Cyst fluid antibiotic concentrations in polycystic kidney disease: Differences between proximal and distal cysts. *Kidney Int.* 1981;20:519-522.
45. Schwab SJ, Bander SJ, Klahr S. Renal infection in autosomal dominant polycystic kidney disease. *Am J Med.* 1987;82:714-718.
46. Rosse WF, Waldmann TA, Cohen P. Renal cysts, erythropoietin, and polycythemia. *Am J Med.* 1963;34:76-81.
47. Navarro J, et al. Phlebotomy for polycythemia associated with acquired cystic renal disease in a patient in hemodialysis. *Nephron.* 1992;62:110-111.
48. Hughson MD, Buchwald D, Fox M. Renal neoplasia and acquired cystic kidney disease in patients receiving long-term dialysis. *Arch Pathol Lab Med.* 1986;110:592-601.
49. Ticer JW. Capsulogenic renal cyst in a cat. *J Am Vet Med Assoc.* 1963;143:613-614.
50. Kraft AM, Kraft CG. Renal capsular cyst in a domestic cat. *Vet Med Small Anim Clin.* 1970;65:692.
51. Mitten RA. Pararenal pseudocysts in a cat. *Iowa State Univ Vet.* 1978;40:65-67.
52. Osborne CA, Polzin DP, Feeney DA, Caywood DD. The urinary system: Pathophysiology, diagnosis, and treatment. In: Gourley IM, Vasseur PB, eds. *General Small Animal Surgery.* Philadelphia, Pennsylvania: JB Lippincott Co; 1985:522.
53. Chastain CB, Grier RL. Bilateral retroperitoneal perirenal cysts in a cat. *Feline Pract.* 1975;5:51-53.
54. Abdinoor DJ. Perinephric pseudocysts in a cat. *J Am Anim Hosp Assoc.* 1980;16:763-767.
55. Rosenzweig LJ. Anatomy of the cat. Dubuque, Iowa: Wm. C. Brown Publishers; 1990:190.
56. Evans HE, Christensen GC. *Miller's Anatomy of the Dog.* Philadelphia, Pennsylvania: WB Saunders Co; 1979:544-546.
57. Geel JK. Perinephric extravasation of urine with pseudocyst formation in a cat. *J South African Vet Assoc.* 1986;57:33-34.
58. Howe RS. What is your diagnosis? *J Am Vet Med Assoc.* 1991;198:471-472.
59. Tidwell AS, Ullman SL, Schelling SH. Urinoma (para-ureteral pseudocyst) in a dog. *Vet Radiol.* 1990;31:203-206.
60. Zaontz MR, Firlit CF. Pelvic lymphocele after pediatric renal transplantation: A successful technique for prevention. *J Urol.* 1988;139:557-559.

CHAPTER 24

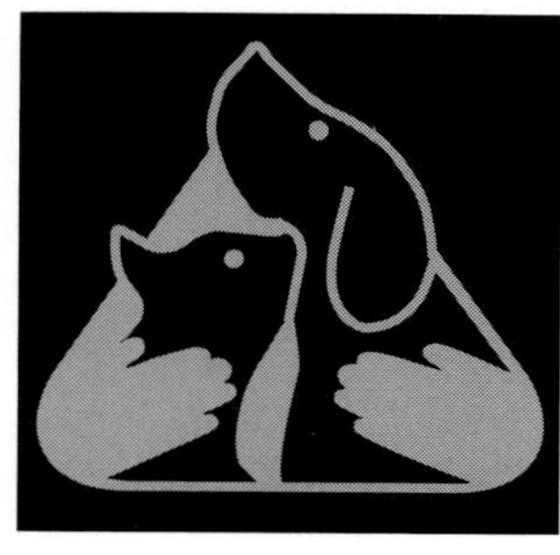

Congenital, Inherited, and Familial Renal Diseases

DELMAR R. FINCO

I. INTRODUCTION

A. Definitions.

1. Congenital.
   a. Congenital refers to the presence of a defect at birth.
   b. A congenital defect may have a genetic basis. In humans chromosomal disorders are known to cause a variety of defects, including several urinary tract anomalies.[15]
   c. Non-inherited causes of congenital defects also exist. Infectious agents, chemicals, and drugs can cause congenital lesions.
2. Inherited.[15]
   a. An inherited trait is derived from an ancestor as a consequence of transmission of genetic material (chromosomes) from progenitor to offspring.
   b. Chromosomes are composed in part of long strands of deoxyribonucleic acid (DNA). The linear arrangement of purine and pyrimidine bases in DNA determines the sequence of amino acids in the multitude of proteins synthesized by cells of the body.
   c. A gene is a segment of a chromosome that codes for a particular protein.
   d. Because chromosomes are paired, genes are also paired; the analogous genes at the same loci on the two chromosomes are called alleles.
   e. A homozygous individual has two identical alleles at a given locus, whereas a heterozygous individual has different alleles.
   f. A genetic defect that is expressed in both heterozygotes and homozygotes is a dominant trait, whereas a defect that is expressed only in homozygotes is a recessive trait.
   g. Incomplete penetrance is a phenomenon in which an apparently dominant trait is not expressed in every individual that carries the gene.
   h. Autosomal traits originate from genes other than the sex chromosomes, and are present in both sexes.
   i. Diseases due to defects of genes residing on the X (female sex) chromosome (sex-linked traits) are not expressed equally in both sexes. Like autosomal traits, however, they may be dominant or recessive.
      (1). A female who carries a dominant sex-linked trait has a 50% chance of transmitting that trait to any offspring, male or female. Affected males transmit such a trait to all female progeny, but to no male progeny.
      (2). If a sex-linked trait is recessive, all male offspring, but only the exceedingly rare homozygous female, are affected.
3. The term familial refers to a trait in a group of related individuals. Some familial diseases are

genetic, and others are acquired (e.g., via pathogens or toxin). A familial disease that may seem to be inherited could actually be acquired if all family members are exposed to a noxious agent.

B. Acquired versus inherited renal disease.

1. The causes of most renal disease in older dogs and cats are unknown.
   a. Because the disease is manifested long after birth, it often is assumed that it was acquired after birth and has no congenital or hereditary component.
   b. This assumption may or may not be correct. One form of polycystic renal disease of humans is known to be inherited, yet the clinical signs often do not emerge until 35 years of age or older.[29]
2. Chronic renal disease in young dogs and cats was rarely recognized until the 1950s.
   a. Because chronic renal failure had previously been considered to be an acquired disease of old pets, a shrunken kidney in a young animal was erroneously concluded to be the result of a congenital or an inherited anomaly.
   b. Part of the confusion about renal disease in young animals arose because of the presumption that a long period of time was required for a kidney to attain morphologic characteristics typical of "end-stage kidney." A decrease in kidney size and the development of lesions termed chronic by histologic evaluation are now known to develop in as little time as 60 days.[1,26]
3. Some reports of isolated cases of renal failure in young dogs ascribe congenital or inherited causes to the renal disease based solely on the finding of a shrunken kidney.[41,47,48,54,79] In retrospect, acquired disease was just as plausible in these patients.
4. Much remains to be learned about the role of genetics and developmental factors in renal diseases of dogs and cats. In this chapter, consideration is given to renal diseases of dogs and cats that have been reported as familial, inherited, or congenital diseases.

C. Types of congenital and hereditary disorders.

1. In humans, renal and lower urinary tract abnormalities are commonly associated with chromosomal disorders; however, no one renal anomaly is specific for one chromosomal disorder.[15]
2. In some hereditary diseases of humans that involve the kidneys, the damage is secondary to the accumulation in the kidneys of a toxic metabolite. In other instances, a circulating compound that is produced because of a metabolic dysfunction may injure renal tissue. In both instances, an enzyme deficit, with accumulation of an intermediate in a metabolic pathway, results in the disease.[15]
3. For many inherited renal diseases of humans, and for most of dogs, the biochemical basis of the lesion remains unknown.

D. Summary of embryonic and fetal development of the kidney.[45,66]

1. Three excretory organs develop serially during embryogenesis.
   a. Pronephros.
   b. Mesonephros.
   c. Metanephros.
2. The pronephros consists of pronephric tubules, which empty into the cloaca via paired pronephric ducts.
3. As mesonephric development begins, pronephric tubules degenerate, and mesonephric tubules gain entrance into the pronephric ducts. The pronephric ducts are now called the mesonephric ducts.
4. The mesonephric tubules serve briefly as excretory organs, but subsequently excretory function is assumed by structures formed from metanephric tissue.
5. A part of the mesonephric ducts eventually becomes the epididymis and ductus deferens in males. The same structures become the vestigial Gartner's ducts in females.
6. Mesonephric tissue also generates the Müllerian ducts, which form the oviducts and uterus in females but become vestigial structures in males.
7. In both sexes, outgrowth of the caudal portion of the mesonephric ducts acts as the ureteric bud. The development of these outgrowths is synchronous with the development of tubules from overlying metanephric tissue.
8. Tubular development from metanephric tissue proceeds in concert with branching of the ureteral buds. Tubules form, elongate, and join with the ureteral bud.
9. Glomeruli form from blood capillaries that invaginate into, or are surrounded by, the terminal end of the tubular structures.
10. Metanephric tissue is the source of the bulk of the renal tissue of mature animals. At maturity, the ureters, renal pelves, and collecting ducts are derived from the mesonephros, whereas the remainder of the tubular system and Bowman's space are derived from metanephric tissue.
11. Repeated divisions of the ureteric bud, and associated development of metanephric tubules, lead to the formation of several generations of nephrons during fetal development of the kidneys. Newer nephrons form more superficially in the cortex than do their predecessors. In newborn dogs and cats, nephrogenesis is incomplete, and immature structures can be seen in the subcapsular area.
12. Some malformations of the kidneys can be related to organogenesis.
    a. Failure of the pronephros to contribute the

mesonephric duct results in failure of the kidney to form because of the lack of ureteral buds. Abnormalities of the genital tract would also be anticipated, and even the adrenal gland and lung may be absent because the tissue of their origin lies close to the pronephros.

b. When abnormalities are restricted to the kidneys, the fault likely lies with budding of the mesonephric duct or with the metanephros. Faulty nephrogenesis may lead to renal agenesis, dysplasia, or hypoplasia.

c. Cranial migration and rotation of the kidneys occurs later in fetal development. Interference may lead to renal ectopia.

II. RENAL MALFORMATIONS

A. Anomalies of tissue mass.

1. Unilateral renal agenesis.

a. In cats, unilateral renal agenesis is reported rarely.

(1). A review of veterinary literature in 1975 uncovered reports of 20 cases of unilateral renal agenesis.[27]

(2). A review in 1987 tabulated 4 additional cases.[51]

(3). In cats, unilateral renal agenesis may occur more frequently in females and may affect the right side more frequently. Absence of the ureter, or absence of segments of the genital tract, also was reported.

b. Reports of unilateral renal agenesis in dogs are uncommon.[9,11,16,35,44,59,73,78,80,81]

(1). A relatively high prevalence was found in two colonies of research beagle dogs.[73,81]

(2). Another study concluded that the abnormality in beagle dogs was dysplasia rather than agenesis, because remnants of renal tissue were detected microscopically.[59]

c. Clinically, unilateral renal agenesis is asymptomatic unless associated extrarenal defects cause signs, or unless the opposite kidney is injured by acquired disease so that uremia develops. The condition is usually an incidental finding at autopsy or laparotomy. Detection of an anomalous genital tract during ovariohysterectomy warrants a search for unilateral renal agenesis.

d. Failure to visualize one kidney on survey radiographs or excretory urographs is not diagnostic of renal agenesis. Kidneys may be difficult to visualize, even with excretory urography, when a low glomerular filtration rate prevents sufficient filtration of contrast medium.

e. Based on studies of protein effects on dogs with uninephrectomy or greater reduction in renal mass,[23] no routine change in lifestyle is required for animals with unilateral renal agenesis. Any medical or surgical manipulation that put the remaining kidney at risk, however, should be avoided.

2. Bilateral renal agenesis.

a. Reports of bilateral renal agenesis are rare.[11]

b. This condition is fatal within the first few days of life, because no urine is formed.

3. Causes of renal agenesis.

a. In two colonies of beagle dogs, a high incidence of unilateral agenesis suggested that the abnormality was inherited.[73,81]

b. An instance of bilateral agenesis in two litters of a colony of Shetland sheepdogs suggested an inherited cause.[11]

c. Most reports of renal agenesis are of isolated cases, so information on inheritance cannot be assessed. Congenital, noninherited causes cannot be excluded.

4. Renal hypoplasia, renal cortical hypoplasia.

a. Renal hypoplasia describes formation of a smaller than usual mass of normal renal tissue.[46]

b. With this definition, the terms renal hypoplasia and renal cortical hypoplasia likely have been misused frequently when applied to shrunken end-stage kidneys in young animals.[12,19,41,47,69] This misnomer is significant, because it directs attention toward a congenital problem and away from changes in the kidney that may be acquired and thus subject to modification.

c. When the correct criteria for diagnosis are applied (remaining tissue morphologically normal), true cases of renal hypoplasia or renal cortical hypoplasia in dogs and cats are rare. Unfortunately, determining the true incidence of hypoplasia or cortical hypoplasia is complicated by the occurrence of acquired kidney lesions in dogs with reduced renal mass.

5. Excess tissue.

a. A supernumerary kidney is an extra mass of renal tissue that has no parenchymal connection with the definitive kidneys.[46]

b. This condition, extremely rare in humans, has not been reported in dogs or cats.

c. Renal and ureteral duplication have been reported in an English bulldog.[63]

(1). A common right renal artery supplied a single mass of renal tissue that was drained by two ureters, both of which emptied into the urinary bladder.

(2). Uroliths, urinary tract infection, and enlargement of one of the two right ureters were observed.

(3). The left kidney and ureter were normal.

B. Anomalies of position, form, and orientation.

1. Renal ectopia.

a. Renal ectopia refers to a congenital malposition of one or both kidneys. The kidneys normally

migrate craniad during fetal development and rotate so that the ureter exits the kidney medially rather than ventrally.
(1). Simple ectopia occurs when the ectopic kidney, ureter, and ureteral entrance into the urinary bladder are on the same side of the abdomen; crossed ectopia refers to transposition of the kidney or kidneys to the opposite side of the abdomen, so that the ureter crosses the midline before inserting into the bladder.
(2). Ectopic kidneys may be classified by location.
(a). Pelvic: within the pelvic canal.
(b). Iliac: in the iliac fossa.
(c). Abdominal: in the abdominal cavity.
b. Characteristics of 11 cases of renal ectopia in cats have been summarized.[51]
(1). No sex predilection existed (six males, four females).
(2). Both kidneys were ectopic in 7 of 11 cases.
(3). Pelvic, abdominal, and iliac sites of ectopia existed.
(4). Fusion (six cases), flattened shape (two cases), reduced size (two cases), and incomplete rotation (one case) were accompanying renal abnormalities.
(5). Other anomalies (renal vascular, cleft palate, and atresia, shortened ureters) existed in some cats.
c. Renal ectopia is rarely reported in dogs.[42]
2. Renal fusion.
a. Renal fusion refers to the joining of two kidneys by fully differentiated renal parenchyma.
b. This anomaly and renal ectopia often coexist.
c. The term horseshoe kidney is used to describe kidneys fused by a narrow band of tissue, so that the entire mass resembles a horseshoe.
d. Renal fusion has been described in both dogs[65] and cats[42] but is apparently rare.
3. Clinical significance of anomalies of position, form, orientation.
a. These anomalies usually do not affect survival, but they may be associated with extrarenal defects that do.
b. An anomaly such as horseshoe kidney may be detected by abdominal palpation and must be differentiated from extrarenal abdominal masses.
c. Nearly half of humans with horseshoe kidneys have symptoms related to partial urinary obstruction because of impaired ureteral outflow. Renal tumors may also be more prevalent in fused kidneys.[46]
d. Observations on dogs and cats are inadequate to allow clinical characterization.

C. Anomalies of differentiation.

1. Renal dysplasia.
a. Renal dysplasia refers to disorganized development resulting from arrested or anomalous cellular processes.
b. Causes.
(1). Causes consistent with this description have been described in association with infection of fetal cats with feline panleukopenia virus.[43]
(2). Puppies infected with canine herpesvirus had tubular and glomerular lesions consistent with dysplasia.[67]
(3). In humans, congenital ureteral obstruction leads to lesions of dysplasia.[46]
(4). In a necropsy study,[84] 0.3 to 4% of glomeruli were hypoplastic in 26.5% of 98 beagle dogs younger than 2 years. Of 140 dogs of other breeds (115 foxhounds), 25 also had hypoplastic glomeruli, but 16 of the 25 had canine distemper or pneumonia. The investigators concluded that the abnormality in "non-beagles" was influenced by disease.
(5). Familial renal disease in several breeds (e.g., Lhasa apso, Shih Tzu, standard poodles, soft-coated Wheaten terriers) has been described as dysplasia.[50,53,71] Although implications suggest that the dysplasia in these breeds is related to a primary error in renal maturation, this may not be the case. The morphologic findings described as dysplasia may represent a nonspecific response of the developing kidney to injury. The insult could be a circulating nephrotoxin, ischemia, or urinary obstruction, as already documented in humans.
2. Polycystic disease.
a. Renal cysts may have a congenital or hereditary basis, but many acquired causes exist as well.
b. See Chapter 23, Cystic Diseases of the Kidneys, for a review of polycystic disease.

III. FAMILIAL GENERALIZED RENAL DISEASES

A. Perspective.

1. Familial versus nonfamilial disease.
a. The term familial disease indicates simply that more than one member of a family has disease.
b. Signs of renal failure in two related animals does not mean that the cause of disease is the same for both.
c. Postnatal exposure of two related animals to a common nephrotoxin may result in renal failure in both, without a genetic basis for the disease.
2. For some of the generalized renal diseases subsequently described, sufficient data are available to conclude that the disease is inherited.
3. In other instances, whether the disease is congenital, inherited, or acquired is not possible to establish.

B. Norwegian elkhound dogs.

1. Evidence for familial disease.
   a. An initial study reported that 3 of 5 offspring from the breeding of an affected male to his dam developed renal failure before age 4 months.[24]
   b. Subsequent inbreeding of dogs with related pedigrees resulted in morphologic evidence of renal disease in 21 of 56 dogs[21,25]; however, no classic pattern of mendelian inheritance was discernible from these breeding trials.
   c. Pedigrees from Norwegian elkhound dogs throughout the United States that developed renal failure at a young age have been examined.[23] These findings suggest that more than a single line of dogs of this breed is afflicted with familial renal disease.
   d. The prevalence of renal disease in the Norwegian elkhound population is apparently quite low, but it has not been accurately determined.
2. Clinical characteristics.
   a. No unique clinical characteristics distinguish this disease from any other cause of chronic renal failure. History and physical examination are consistent with varying degrees of renal dysfunction.
   b. Dwarfing occurs when renal failure develops before physical maturity is attained (Fig. 24–1).
   c. Dogs that have hyposthenuria may drink a great quantity of water.
3. Laboratory characteristics.
   a. No unique hematologic, blood chemical, or radiologic findings have been reported with this disease that distinguish it from other causes of renal failure.
   b. Some dogs in the families studied had glucosuria, aminoaciduria, and hyposthenuria. The glucosuria and aminoaciduria occurred at a time when plasma glucose and amino acid concentrations were normal, suggesting multiple defects in proximal tubule reabsorption (Fanconi's syndrome).
   c. Urinalysis was negative or only mildly positive for protein.
4. Pathophysiology of the disease.[22]
   a. Study of dogs with this disease indicates that they were born with a normal number of histologically normal nephrons.[25]
   b. With time, progressive destruction of nephrons and shrinking of the kidney occurred, resulting in the development of end-stage kidneys.
   c. Studies clearly demonstrated that in Norwegian elkhound dogs this disease was not renal cortical hypoplasia.
   d. The severity of disease and the rate of progression were quite variable between dogs. In the colony studied, some dogs developed terminal renal failure when a few months of age, whereas others did not develop azotemia until 5 years of age. Because all dogs lived in the same environment, this variation appears to be an innate feature of the disease.
   e. No sex predilection for the disease was noted.
   f. Affected dogs did not have systemic hypertension.
   g. Total plasma calcium concentrations were normal in most dogs, ruling out hypercalcemia as a cause of the renal damage.
   h. Plasma, liver, and kidney amino acid profiles were similar in normal mongrel dogs and affected Norwegian elkhound dogs. Thus, this disease is not cystinosis, a disease described in humans in which the amino acid cystine accumulates in the kidneys.[15]
   i. Electron microscopic and immunofluorescence studies of kidney tissues from affected dogs did not suggest an immune system basis for the renal disease.
   j. Histologic and angiographic studies did not indicate the presence of primary vascular lesions in the dogs; however, a sharp line of demarcation between areas of involvement and apparently normal tissue was noted in some cases. This pattern was suggestive of a vascular basis for disease. The possibility of a vascular response to a potent vasoconstrictor, with subsequent ischemia, could not be eliminated.
   k. Limited attempts were made to demonstrate the presence of some transmissible agent. Injection of a homogenate of affected renal tissue into normal mongrel pups did not cause renal lesions.
5. Pathology.[25]
   a. Necropsy studies revealed extrarenal changes

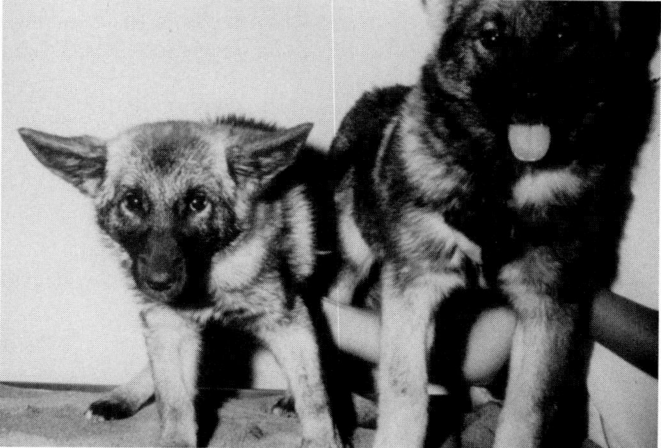

FIG. 24–1. Littermate Norwegian elkhound dogs about 3 months of age. The pup on the left had azotemia and renal failure, whereas renal function in the littermate on the right was normal.

typical of other causes of generalized renal failure.

b. Periglomerular fibrosis and, later, interstitial fibrosis were the earliest renal lesions seen histologically (Fig. 24–2).

c. Most affected glomeruli had hyperplasia and hypertrophy of parietal epithelial cells and some had thickening of the mesangium, but no changes occurred in the glomerular capillaries.

d. Small glomeruli were not observed in this disease, in contrast to the familial renal disease of some other breeds.

e. Interstitial fibrosis, in both cortex and medulla, was a prominent feature of the advanced stage of the disease.

f. Tubular changes were not observed by light microscopy early in the disease, but were apparent later in association with widespread interstitial fibrosis.

g. Microdissection of nephrons revealed sacculations in the distal tubules and collecting ducts of affected dogs (Fig. 24–3). Their significance is not known.

6. Diagnosis.
   a. On an individual case basis, there is no simple way to distinguish this familial renal disease from chronic renal failure of other causes.
   b. Presence of Fanconi's syndrome is suggestive of the familial disease, but it occurs in only a minority of cases, and acquired causes of Fanconi's syndrome are also known.[6]
7. Prognosis. The long-term prognosis is poor, but damage and progression vary considerably in affected dogs. Cases must be evaluated individually to assess the degree of renal dysfunction and the rate of progression of renal disease.

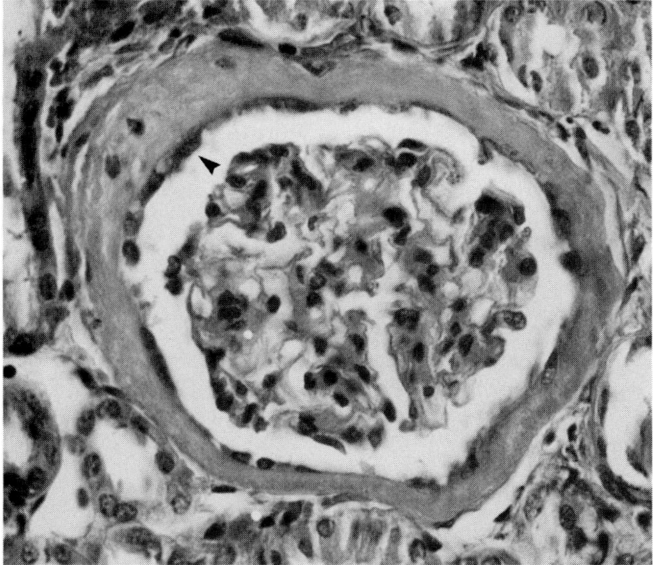

FIG. 24–2. Glomerulus from a Norwegian elkhound dog with familial renal disease. Note periglomerular fibrosis and the prominent parietal epithelial cells (arrow).

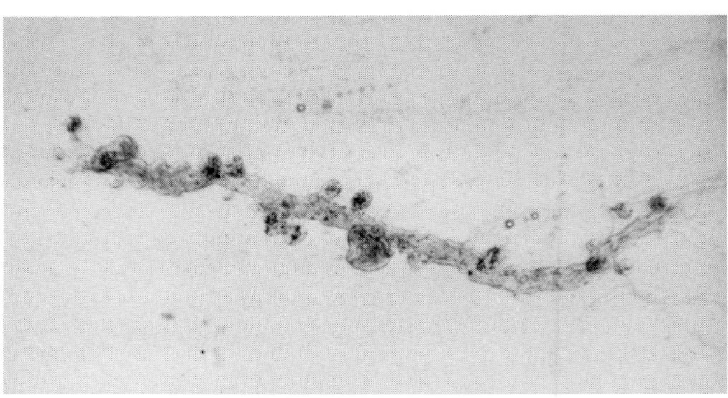

FIG. 24–3. Sacculations in nephrons dissected from Norwegian elkhound dogs with familial renal disease. The significance of this finding is unclear.

C. Cocker spaniel dogs.

1. Evidence for familial or hereditary disease.
   a. The results of necropsy studies on 40 cases of renal failure in cocker spaniel dogs 2 to 48 months of age were reported from Sweden.[49] The author concluded that the high incidence in cocker spaniels suggested a hereditary basis for the disease.
   b. Eight cases of familial nephropathy were reported in England[75]: in five of the cases at least one other member of the litter died from uremia. A charting of the genealogy of families revealed a distinct familial relationship over several generations, but a specific mode of inheritance could not be identified.
   c. Renal disease was reported in a litter of cocker spaniels.[40]
2. Clinical characteristics.
   a. Both sexes were affected with the disease.
   b. Disease was apparently unrelated to coat color, although one report[28] described it only in bicolored dogs.
   c. No clinical features of the disease distinguished it from chronic renal failure of other causes.
3. Laboratory characteristics.
   a. Some affected dogs had glucosuria but most did not.
   b. Proteinuria was persistent and marked.
   c. A high incidence of hyposthenuria occurred.
4. Pathophysiology.
   a. Investigators hypothesized that this disease was a result of formation of inadequate numbers of nephrons. The disease was called renal cortical hypoplasia, because end-stage kidneys had thin cortices.
   b. The disease has not been studied during its early phases. Considering that Norwegian elkhound dogs with familial renal disease ini-

tially have normal kidneys that later shrink with fibrosis, and that nonfamilial, presumably acquired renal diseases result in thin cortices, there is good reason to be skeptical of the cortical hypoplasia theory.

c. Blood pressure measurements made on affected dogs revealed normal values[68] or only modest elevations,[75] suggesting that hypertension did not play a primary role in the disease.

d. Investigators hypothesized that hypercalcemia caused renal injury, but subsequent studies indicated that normocalcemia existed.[69]

e. Fibrin deposition in glomeruli, in the absence of significant immunoglobulin G (IgG) or complement deposition, suggested a nonimmunologic mechanism of glomerular injury or occlusion.[75]

f. More recent studies suggest that cocker spaniels suffer from a familial disease in which the primary lesion is glomerulopathy,[48a] which may be similar to the defect in basement membrane formation subsequently described in Samoyed dogs.[49a] Whether a single familial disease exists in this breed or whether more exist is not clear.

5. Pathology.
   a. No unique extrarenal lesions have been described in this disease.
   b. In early studies, dogs were not examined before the onset of azotemia; thus, only lesions in advanced cases have been described.
      (1). One description of renal lesions with this disease emphasized renal calcification,[49] but this was probably a nonspecific change associated with advanced uremia.
      (2). Fibrin deposition and extravasation and fibrous thickening of Bowman's capsule have been described.[75]
   c. Splitting of basement membrane of glomerular capillary walls has been described.[49a]

D. Samoyed dogs.

1. Evidence for inherited disease
   a. Extensive breeding trials have been conducted to establish the genetic basis of this familial renal disease.[3,38]
   b. The pattern of inheritance is consistent with an X-linked dominant trait. The disease was overtly expressed in males, but genotype-positive females have renal lesions and may transmit the disease to male offspring even when mated to normal nonSamoyed males.
   c. One unexplained finding in the breeding trials was a preponderance of males in the litters of certain dams.
2. Clinical characteristics.[2,39]
   a. Affected males may develop signs of advanced uremia by 6 months of age.
   b. The body condition of carrier females is reported to be poorer than that of their normal littermates after 3 months of age, but they do not die of renal failure, as do affected males.
   c. No signs unique to this disease, compared to other causes of renal failure in immature dogs, have been reported.
3. Laboratory characteristics.[39]
   a. Urinalysis.
      (1). Proteinuria may be detected as early as 2 to 3 months of age, before the onset of clinical signs.
      (2). The 24-hour urinary protein excretion in 4 males varied from 32 to 185 mg/kg, whereas none was found by the same turbidometric method in normal dogs. Carrier females had proteinuria of about the same magnitude as that of affected males.
      (3). Urine electrophoresis revealed prealbumin, albumin, and globulins in smaller amounts, with some variation in relative amounts between dogs.
      (4). Urine specific gravity measurements in affected males were in the isosthenuria range at 4 months, although earlier values were 1.025.
      (5). Glucosuria occurred in some affected male dogs during periods of euglycemia. The occurrence of aminoaciduria and other defects in proximal tubule reabsorptive functions apparently was not examined.
      (6). Microscopic hematuria occurred in some affected dogs, but its presence was not as consistent as that of proteinuria.
   b. Blood chemical changes.
      (1). Hypoalbuminemia developed at 3 to 4 months of age and persisted thereafter in male dogs. Occasionally, carrier females developed mild, transient hypoalbuminemia.
      (2). Azotemia and other blood biochemical changes consistent with renal failure occurred only in affected male dogs.
      (3). Hypercholesterolemia was found in some affected male dogs, but not in others.
   c. No unique hematologic changes were associated with this disease.
4. Pathophysiology.
   a. Abnormalities in glomerular basement membrane (GBM) are believed to be the basis of this disease.[36,37]
      (1). Type IV collagen in GBM contains a domain identified as the NC1 domain. A part of this domain comprises Goodpasture's antigen, which is important in the development of Goodpasture's antiGBM disease in humans.
      (2). Humans with some forms of hereditary nephritis do not demonstrate the pres-

ence of Goodpasture's antigen, suggesting both structural and antigenic changes in the type IV collagen.

(3). Studies of the NC1 domain of type IV collagen from affected and carrier Samoyed dogs, and from normal mongrel dogs, suggest that structural changes present at birth in affected and carrier Samoyeds weaken the basement membrane and make it vulnerable to the high pressures of the glomerular capillaries.[76,77]

b. Extraglomerular renal capillaries do not develop lesions.

5. Pathology in affected males.
   a. Morphologic abnormalities typical of this disease have been studied at an early stage.
   b. Renal glomerular lesions have been noted by transmission electron microscopy as early as 1 month of age, when light microscopy was still normal. Lesions consisted of basement membrane duplication or splitting, with the accumulation of electron-dense particles between layers. Eventually, all glomerular capillaries are affected, and fusion of foot processes of glomerular epithelial cells occurs.
   c. The lesions become apparent by light microscopy when more advanced (4 to 5 months of age), and glomerulosclerosis becomes complete by age 8 to 10 months.
6. In carrier females, glomerular capillary lesions are similar to those in affected males, but the lesions apparently do not advance to the point of renal failure in females.

E. Doberman pinscher dogs.[13,56,70,82]

1. Evidence for familial or inherited disease.
   a. In the first report of the disease, pedigrees on nine affected dogs were traced to a common male.[82]
   b. No other information is available on the familial or inherited nature of renal disease in young Doberman pinscher dogs.
2. Clinical characteristics.
   a. No sex predilection is reported for this abnormality.
   b. Affected dogs develop the typical signs of renal failure between a few months of age and 5 years.
   c. No unique clinical signs distinguish this disease from other causes of chronic renal failure. A few dogs develop ascites or edema, apparently in association with hypoalbuminemia.
   d. In a study of 13 affected dogs, the right kidney was absent in 3 bitches, and the right uterine horn was absent from 1.[82] Such anomalies were not mentioned in the other series reported.
3. Laboratory characteristics.
   a. Urinalysis.
      (1). Dogs had mild to severe proteinuria; albumin was the sole urinary protein identified by electrophoresis in the few dogs studied.
      (2). Generalized renal failure led to impaired urine-concentrating ability.
      (3). Some dogs had glucosuria, but the study did not determine whether the cause was hyperglycemia or defective tubular glucose reabsorption.
      (4). Some dogs had hematuria and pyuria, but the study did not determine whether these were features of the disease or incidental to it.
   b. Blood chemical abnormalities.
      (1). Blood chemical findings that have been reported are consistent with chronic renal failure.
      (2). Hypercholesterolemia occurred consistently in affected dogs.
      (3). Some dogs had decreased total plasma protein concentration, presumably due to hypoalbuminemia.
   c. Hematologic studies.
      (1). Hematologic findings were typical of chronic generalized renal failure.
      (2). Results of blood coagulation studies were normal.
4. Pathology.
   a. Tissues available for study have been from dogs with uremia; thus, no information on the early lesions of the disease is currently available.
   b. Histologically, lesions are consistent with a membranoproliferative glomerulonephritis (see Fig. 17–2).
   c. Most cases studied have been negative for immunoreactants IgG, IgM, IgA, and complement. However, fluorescence was weakly positive in renal glomeruli from some dogs. This reaction was attributed to secondary immune complex formation *in situ* following leakage and entrapment of circulating antigens.[70]
   d. Electron micrographic studies of the GBM have demonstrated two distinct structural lesions in different dogs.
      (1). Multifocal, irregular thickening of the basement membrane with lamellation of the lamina densa.
      (2). Attenuation of the lamina densa of the thickened GBM with randomly dispersed collagen fibers at an intramembranous or subendothelial site.
      (3). Whether these distinctions represent subsets of the disease, limitations of sampling procedures for electron microscopy, or stages of disease is not apparent.
5. Pathophysiology.
   a. The lesions described in glomerular capillary basement membranes have prompted specu-

lation that the disease is the result of a developmental or metabolic defect in synthesis of GBM.[70]

b. No data to support this hypothesis are available at present.

F. **Basenji dogs.**[4-6,8,18,55,83]

1. Evidence for familial or inherited disease.
   a. Basenji dogs with generalized proximal tubule dysfunction (Fanconi's syndrome) have been reported.
   b. No evidence has been published indicating that the disease is inherited, but acquired causes of the disease have not been identified. Examination of pedigrees from several affected dogs revealed several common ancestors.[6]
2. Clinical characteristics.
   a. Dogs of either sex were affected.
   b. The disease does not seem to develop as early as some other familial renal diseases. The condition has not been reported in growing pups, and many reported cases involved dogs as old as 7 years.
   c. Dogs have been identified when routine urinalysis revealed glucosuria during periods of euglycemia.
   d. Some dogs were presented because of extreme polyuria. This sign may be present in the absence of azotemia, and it is probably related to a decrease in water reabsorption in the proximal tubules secondary to impaired solute reabsorption (osmotic diuresis).
   e. Anorexia, weight loss, and poor haircoat were reported; these signs may be related to electrolyte and acid-base abnormalities that occur in nonazotemic dogs secondary to proximal tubule dysfunction. They also may be related to uremia.
3. Laboratory findings.
   a. Laboratory findings reflect urinary losses associated with generalized dysfunction of renal proximal tubules, and with development of azotemia.
   b. Urinalysis often revealed glucosuria during euglycemia, and isosthenuria or hyposthenuria. Evaluation of urine for amino acids revealed generalized aminoaciduria.
   c. Blood chemical changes reflect the degree of proximal tubule dysfunction. In milder cases, blood chemicals were normal in concentration, but in severe cases, multiple electrolyte abnormalities occurred. Hypokalemia, hypobicarbonatemia, and hypophosphatemia may be sufficiently severe to cause clinical signs.
   d. Azotemia develops as the disease progresses.
4. Pathologic findings.
   a. Microscopic examination of kidneys of dogs with this disease revealed a spectrum of lesions. Karyomegaly of tubular cells was apparently the earliest lesion (Fig. 24–4). Tubular dilation, lymphocytic and plasma cell infiltration, glomerulosclerosis, and interstitial fibrosis also were noted.
   b. Acute papillary necrosis was observed in a few dogs, apparently the result of dehydration and acidosis that occurred because of inadequate replacement of urinary losses.

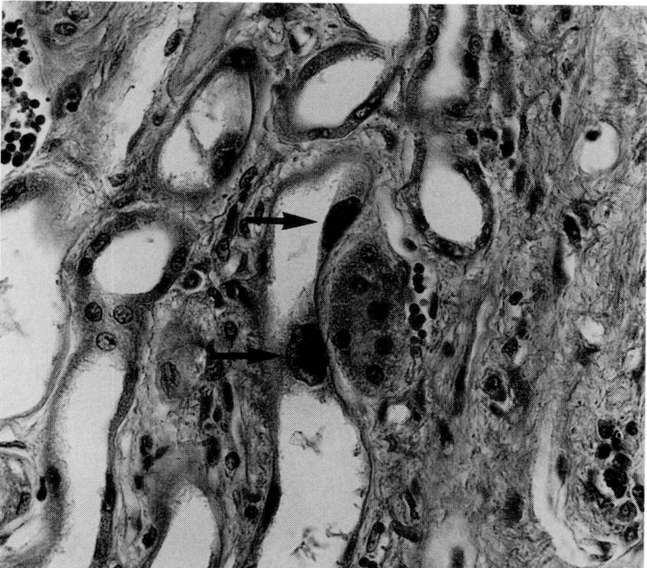

FIG. 24–4. Kidney from a basenji dog with Fanconi's syndrome. Note karyomegaly with hyperchromatism (arrows) of renal tubular epithelium.

5. Pathophysiology.
   a. The clinical and laboratory findings are related to the functional defects in the proximal tubules.
      (1). Study of brush border membrane vesicles indicates that sodium-dependent glucose transport is impaired in affected dogs.
      (2). Conversely, lysine transport is normal in the membrane vesicle system. This suggests defects at some other cellular site.
   b. The relation between the functional defects and the development of end-stage kidneys is unclear.
6. Treatment.
   a. No cure for this disease exists, but severe acid-base and electrolyte abnormalities may lead to early death if they are not rectified.
   b. Because of the renal leak, oral or parenteral administrations of electrolyte solutions are indicated to alleviate dehydration, acidosis, hypokalemia, or hypophosphatemia. Although treatment may not restore plasma values to normal, biochemical and clinical improvement may be achieved.

G. Lhasa apso and Shih Tzu dogs.[7,14,21,31,33a,34,62]

1. The familial renal diseases in Lhasa apso and Shih Tzu dogs currently are considered to have the same characteristics.
2. Evidence for familial or inherited disease.
   a. Limited breeding trials have established that some pups with renal disease are whelped from one or two affected parents. If inherited, the mode of inheritance seems complex. One study suggests an autosomal-dominant pattern with incomplete penetrance.[7] Another suggests simple recessive inheritance.[33a]
   b. Acquired factors in the disease have not been identified. Efforts to isolate canine herpesvirus from kidneys of pups with disease were not successful[23]; some histologic characteristics are common to this familial disease and herpes infection (juvenile glomeruli).[52,67]
3. Clinical characteristics.
   a. In cases reported, both sexes were affected.
   b. Many affected dogs had terminal uremia as early as a few months of age, but some affected dogs maintained relatively stable, mild renal dysfunction for years.
   c. Signs of disease were typical of chronic renal failure; no signs are unique to this disease.
   d. Impaired growth was observed in dogs affected with renal failure before physical maturity.
4. Laboratory characteristics.
   a. Laboratory findings were typical of renal failure.
   b. No findings unique to this disease have been reported.
5. Pathology.
   a. Grossly, some kidneys were diffusely affected. Others had areas of contraction resembling patterns of infarction.
   b. Histologically, lesions were sometimes generalized, but frequently a sharp line of demarcation separated an affected area from a relatively normal area. Radial streaks of fibrosis, and abnormal glomerular and tubular elements typified the affected areas.
   c. Small, juvenile glomeruli often were present in affected areas (Fig. 24–5). These glomeruli were distinctive to this familial disease, as compared with the familial diseases of Norwegian elkhound and cocker spaniel dogs.
   d. Morphologic studies have been made on dogs with advanced disease. Thus, identification of early lesions and determination of whether abnormalities existed at birth or were acquired have been difficult.
      (1). Three pups with a familial likelihood of the disease had unilateral nephrectomy performed at 3 to 4 weeks of age. Kidneys were histologically normal, including the expected, normal presence of juvenile glomeruli.[23]
      (2). Of the 3, 2 had azotemia at 4 months of age, and subsequent necropsy and histologic examination of the kidneys revealed advanced lesions.
      (3). These findings suggested that the renal lesions are not discernible at birth but become apparent or develop rapidly thereafter.[23]

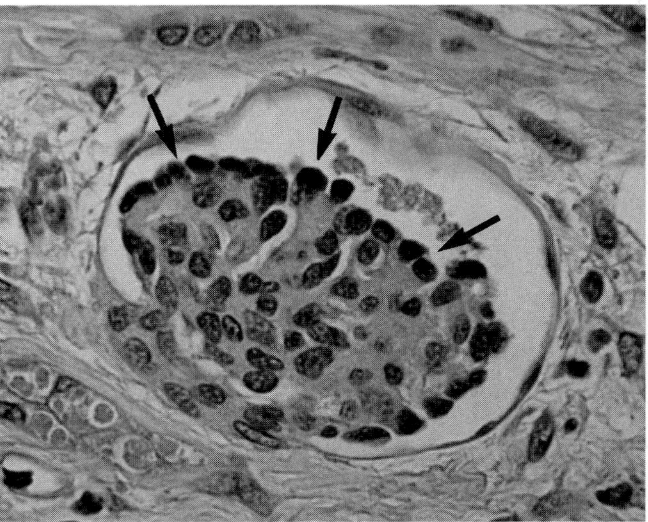

FIG. 24–5. Juvenile-appearing glomerulus from a chow chow dog. Note the closely packed nuclei located peripherally (arrows) and inconspicuous capillary lumens. Interstitial fibrosis also is present. Other breeds with familial renal disease, including Lhasa apso and Shih Tzu dogs, have the same findings.

   e. Examination of at least 100 glomeruli from wedge biopsies of Shih Tzu dogs after renal maturation but before development of advanced disease revealed that individual dogs varied in the quantities of juvenile glomeruli.[7]
      (1). Some dogs had no juvenile glomeruli.
      (2). In other dogs, greater than 15% of glomeruli were juvenile.
      (3). Repeat biopsy of dogs revealed no increase in percentage of juvenile glomeruli.
      (4). Examiners concluded that the percentage of juvenile glomeruli was a valid marker of disease and that wedge biopsy was a method of evaluating the renal status of dogs suspected of having renal disease.
   f. The histologic lesions in end-stage kidneys have been attributed to dysplasia.[72]
6. Pathophysiology.
   a. Hypertension–primary renal vascular disease.
      (1). Conflicting views exist on the role of hypertension in this disease.
      (2). One opinion is that the renal failure is caused by vascular lesions and systemic hypertension.

(3). Another view, based on direct measurement of systemic blood pressure in a limited number of cases, suggests that hypertension is not always present and that when present it is secondary to renal failure.[23]

b. The theory of a developmental abnormality (dysplasia) has been proposed.[72]

H. Standard poodle dogs.

1. Evidence for familial or inherited disease.
   a. Renal disease was reported in six offspring in two litters of standard poodle pups.
   b. The litters had the same sire but different dams; however, sire and dams were distantly related.[17]
2. Clinical characteristics.
   a. Both sexes were affected.
   b. Five affected dogs had uremia before 8 months of age; 1 developed uremia when 28 months of age.
   c. No clinical signs were unique to this disease.
3. Laboratory characteristics.
   a. Hypercholesterolemia was present in all affected dogs.
   b. In one of two dogs examined, urinary protein concentration was increased.
   c. Two dogs had moderate hypercalcemia.
4. Pathology.
   a. The end-stage kidneys available for examination had a variety of lesions.
   b. The histologic character of the lesions most resembled those of Lhasa apso and Shih Tzu dogs.

I. Soft-coated Wheaten terriers.[20,60]

1. Evidence for familial or inherited disease.
   a. Renal disease developed in two litters from the same parents.
   b. Renal disease was reported in seven young dogs, two of them littermates.
2. Clinical characteristics.
   a. Both sexes were affected.
   b. Affected dogs ranged in age from 1 to 30 months.
   c. No clinical signs seemed unique to this disease.
3. Laboratory characteristics.
   a. Laboratory findings were typical of the uremic syndrome.
   b. Proteinuria was mild or absent.
4. Pathology.
   a. The end-stage kidneys available for examination had a variety of lesions.
   b. One group concluded that lesions of dysplasia existed that seemed very similar to descriptions of kidneys from Lhasa apso and Shih Tzu dogs.[60]

J. Bull terriers.[32,33,61,74]

1. A chronic, familial nephropathy has been described in this breed.
2. Both sexes may be affected; the disease appears to be inherited as an autosomal-dominant trait.[32]
3. No unique clinical features of the disease have been described, but proteinuria appears to be a constant, early indicator of disease.[33]
4. Pathology.
   a. Early in the disease, lesions affect predominantly the glomeruli.
   b. Lesions described include segmental thickening of GBM, thickened Bowman's capsules, and adhesions between glomerular capillaries and Bowman's capsule. Thickening of tubular basement membrane also was described.[33]

K. Bernese mountain dogs.[72a]

1. A membranoproliferative glomerulonephritis was described in 16 females and 4 males of this breed.
2. Affected dogs were 2 to 5 years of age, and had signs of uremia. Some also had ascites or edema.
3. Proteinuria and hypoproteinemia were noted.
4. Investigators concluded that the disease may have a hereditary basis, but the presence of serum titers for *Borrelia burgdorferi* in 17 dogs suggested a possible role for this pathogen in development of the disease.

L. Other breeds of dogs.

1. Keeshonds: Uremia was reported, and end-stage kidneys were found at autopsy of all of a litter of five.[47]
2. Bedlington terriers: Three of nine pups from a litter developed uremia.[64]
3. Briards: Three pups from one litter developed uremia. Histologically, tubular dilatation was the prominent lesion.[30]
4. Chow chow dogs: Six young dogs that developed renal failure were studied. The clinical course was typical of progressive renal failure, and histologic lesions similar to lesions in Lhasa apso and Shih Tzu dogs were found (Fig. 24–4). Four of the six dogs were from two separate litters from the same parents, indicating the familial nature of the disease.[10]
5. Welsh corgi dogs and telangiectasia.
   a. A condition was described in eight red Pembroke Welsh corgi dogs that was characterized by marked hematuria.[57] Three of the dogs were euthanized or died because of the severe anemia.
   b. The condition appeared to be the result of anomalous development of blood vessels.
   c. No genealogic information was available, but none of the dogs were known to be related.
   d. Middle-aged to old dogs of both sexes were affected.
   e. Clinical characteristics.
      (1). Animals had a history of hematuria, but usually were clinically normal otherwise.
      (2). Occasionally, renal pain could be elicited, or a small, irregular kidney could be palpated.
   f. Laboratory characteristics.
      (1). Urinalysis revealed numerous red cells,

even when gross hematuria was not apparent.

(2). Excretory urography revealed renal reflux and distorted renal pelves in chronically affected dogs.

g. Pathology

(1). Bilateral renal involvement occurred consistently in six dogs necropsied. Red-black nodules existed both within the renal parenchyma and at subcapsular sites. Some kidneys exhibited hydronephrosis secondary to obstruction of the ureters with clots.

(2). Telangiectasia was present at extrarenal sites in most dogs as well. This finding suggests a generalized disease with renal signs (hematuria) prevailing because of the highly vascular nature of the kidneys, and because the kidneys provided a route for the exit of blood.

(3). Microscopically, the kidneys had some lesions that seemed secondary to the vascular anomalies. The vascular anomalies were characterized by multiple, cavernous, blood-filled spaces with simple endothelial lining and various amounts of blood and collagen in the lumens.

6. Cavalier King Charles spaniel: A single case of uremia in a 5-month-old female was reported, in which kidneys had juvenile glomeruli.[58]

M. Familial amyloidosis in Abyssinian cats.

1. See Chapter 20, Renal Amyloidosis, for a review of this disease of Abyssinian cats.

REFERENCES

1. Barber DL, Finco DR. Radiographic findings in induced bacterial pyelonephritis in dogs. *J Am Vet Med Assoc.* 1979;175:1183–1190.
2. Bernard MA, Valli VE. Familial renal disease in Samoyed dogs. *Can Vet J.* 1977;18:181–189.
3. Bloedow AG. Familial renal disease in Samoyed dogs. *Vet Rec.* 1981;108:167–168.
4. Bovee KC, et al. Spontaneous Fanconi syndrome in the dog. *Metabolism.* 1978;27:45–52.
5. Bovee KC, et al. The Fanconi syndrome in Basenji dogs: A new model for renal transport defects. *Science.* 1978;201:1129–1131.
6. Bovee KC, et al. Characterization of renal defects in dogs with a syndrome similar to the Fanconi syndrome in man. *J Am Vet Med Assoc.* 1979;174:1094–1099.
7. Bovee KC. Renal disease in Shi Tzu dogs. Personal communication, 1990.
8. Bovee KC, et al. Renal tubular defects of spontaneous Fanconi syndrome in dogs. In: *Animal Models of Inherited Metabolic Diseases.* New York, New York: Alan R Liss; 1982:435–447.
9. Brouwers J, Dewaele A. Contribution a l'étude de l'angenesie renale chez le chien et le chat. *Ann Med Vet.* 1960;V:229–231.
10. Brown C, et al. Suspected familial renal disease in Chow Chow dogs. *J Am Vet Med Assoc.* 1990;196:1279–1284.
11. Brownie CF, Tess MW, Prasad RD. Bilateral renal agenesis in two litters of Shetland sheepdogs. *Vet Hum Toxicol.* 1988;30:483–485.
12. Bruyere P, Posada GA, Gouffaux M. Hypoplasie du cortex renal chex le chien. *Ann Med Vet.* 1975;119:23–36.
13. Chew DJ, et al. Juvenile renal disease in Doberman pinscher dogs. *J Am Vet Med Assoc.* 1983;182:481–485.
14. Cottrell MB, Franklin JR. Congenital nephrosclerosis in a Lhasa apso. *Vet Med/Sm Anim Clin.* 1983;78:1221–1223.
15. Crawfurd MD. *The Genetics of Renal Tract Disorders.* New York, New York: Oxford University Press; 1988.
16. De Schepper J, et al. In-vivo diagnosis of right renal aplasia in a Pekingese bitch. *Vet Rec.* 1975;97:475.
17. DiBartola SP, Chew DJ, Boyce JT. Juvenile renal disease in related Standard Poodles. *J Am Vet Med Assoc.* 1983; 183:693–696.
18. Easley JR, Breitschwserdt EB. Glucosuria associated with renal tubular dysfunction in three basenji dogs. *J Am Vet Med Assoc.* 1976;168:938–943.
19. English PB, Winter H. Renal cortical hypoplasia in a dog. *Aust Vet J.* 1979;55:181–183.
20. Eriksen K, Grondalen J. Familial renal disease in soft-coated Wheaten terriers. *J Sm Anim Pract.* 1984;25:489–500.
21. Finco DR. Congenital and inherited renal disease. *JAAHA.* 1973;9:301–303.
22. Finco DR. Familial renal disease in Norwegian elkhound dogs: physiologic and biochemical examinations. *Am J Vet Res.* 1976; 37:87–91.
23. Finco DR. Unpublished data. The University of Georgia. 1992.
24. Finco DR, et al. Familial renal disease in Norwegian elkhound dogs. *J Am Vet Med Assoc.* 1970;156:747–760.
25. Finco DR, et al. Familial renal disease in Norwegian elkhound dogs: Morphologic examinations. *Am J Vet Res.* 1977;38: 941–947.
26. Finco DR, Shotts EB, Crowell WA. Evaluation of methods for localization of urinary tract infection in the female dog. *Am J Vet Res.* 1979;40:707–712.
27. Finco DR, Kneller SK, Crowell WA. Diseases of the Urinary System. In: Catcott, E.J., ed. *Feline Medicine and Surgery.* American Veterinary Publications; Santa Barbara, California: 1975: 251–302.
28. Freudiger U. Die kongenitale Nierenriderhypoplasie beim bunten Cocker Spaniel. *Schweiz Arch Tierheilk.* 1965;107: 547–566.
29. Grantham JJ, Gabow PA. Polycystic kidney disease. In: Schrier RW, Gottschalk CW, eds. *Diseases of the Kidney.* 4th ed. Boston, Massachusetts: Little, Brown; 1988:583–615.
30. Gysling C, Hagan A. Renale Dysplasie beim Briard (Berger de Brie) in vergleich zuanderen Nephropathien beim Hund. *Kleintier-praxis.* 1986;31:3–4, 6–8.
31. Hawe RS, Loeb WF. Caudal vaginal agenesis and progressive renal disease in a Shih Tzu. *J Am Anim Hosp Assoc.* 1984;20: 123–130.
32. Hood JC, et al. Hereditary nephritis in the bull terrier: Evidence for inheritance by an autosomal dominant gene. *Vet Rec.* 1990; 126:456–459.
33. Hood JC, et al. Proteinurias: an indicator of early renal disease in bull terriers with hereditary nephritis. *J Small Anim Pract.* 1991; 32:241–248.

33a. Hoppe A, et al. Progressive nephropathy due to renal dysplasia in Shih Tzu dogs in Sweden: a clinical pathological and genetic study. *J Small Anim Pract.* 1990;31:83–91.

34. Hoppe A, Swenson L. Progressive nephropathy in the Shih Tzu dog. *Sveriges Veterinharfhorbund.* 1986;38:190–197.
35. Jamkhedkar PP, Ajinkya SM. Unilateral agenesis of kidney and testicle in a dog. *Indian Vet J.* 1966;43:126–129.
36. Jansen B, et al. Animal model of human disease: Hereditary nephritis in Samoyed dogs. *Am J Pathol.* 1984;116:175–178.
37. Jansen BS, et al. Scanning electron microscopy of cellular and acellular glomeruli of male dogs affected with Samoyed hereditary glomerulopathy and a carrier female. *Can J Vet Res.* 1987; 51:475–480.
38. Jansen B, et al. Mode of inheritance of Samoyed hereditary

glomerulopathy: An animal model for hereditary nephritis in humans. *J Lab Clin Med.* 1986;107:551–555.
39. Jansen B, et al. Samoyed hereditary glomerulopathy: Serial, clinical and laboratory (urine, serum biochemistry and hematology) studies. *Can J Vet Res.* 1987;51:387–393.
40. Johnson ME, Denhart JD, Graber ER. Renal cortical hypoplasia in a litter of cocker spaniels. *JAAHA.* 1972;8:268–274.
41. Kaufman CF, Soirez RF, Tasker JP. Renal cortical hypoplasia with secondary hyperparathyroidism in the dog. *J Am Vet Med Assoc.* 1969;155:1679–1685.
42. Kaufmann ML, et al. Renal ectopia in a dog and a cat. *J Am Vet Med Assoc.* 1987;190:73–77.
43. Kilham L, Margolis G, Colby ED. Congenital infections of cats and ferrets by feline panleukopenia virus manifested by cerebellar hypoplasia. *Clin Invest.* 1967;17:465–480.
44. Kim Y, Yosida N, Yamada S. Congenital anomaly of the dog IV. A case of renal aplasia. *J Jpn Vet Med Assoc.* 1977;30:17–19.
45. Kissane JM. Development of the kidney. In: Heptinstall RH, ed. *Pathology of the kidney.* Vol I. Boston, Massachusetts: Little, Brown; 1974:51–68.
46. Kissane JM. Congenital malformations. In: Heptinstall RH, ed. *Pathology of the kidney.* Vol I. Boston, Massachusetts: Little, Brown; 1974:69–119.
47. Klopfer U, Neumann F, Trainin R. Renal cortical hypoplasia in a Keeshond litter. *Vet Med/Sm Anim Clin.* 1975;1081–1083.
48. Klopfer U, Nobel TA, Kaminski R. A nephropathy similar to renal cortical hypoplasia in a Yorkshire terrier. *Vet Med/Sm Anim Clin.* 1978;327–330.
48a. Koeman JP, et al. Zur familiaren Nephropathie der cocker spaniel. *Dtsch Tierarztl Wschr.* 1989;96:174–179.
49. Krook L. The pathology of renal cortical hypoplasia in the dog. *Nord Vet-Med.* 1957;9:161–176.
49a. Lees GE. Personal communication, 1993.
50. Lucke VM, et al. Chronic renal failure in young dogs—possible renal dysplasia. *J Small Anim Pract.* 1980;21:169–181.
51. Lulich JP, et al. Urologic disorders of immature cats. *Vet Clin North Am.* 1987;17:663–696.
52. Mandelli G, Cammarata M, Pecora E. Vestigial glomeruli in dog kidneys. *Atti Societa Italiana Della Scienze Veterinarie.* 1981;35: 616–617.
53. Mann PH, Bjotvedt G. Unilateral renal dysgenesis in a mongrel dog. *Comp Med Vet Sci.* 1966;30:301–303.
54. McIntee DP, Teale AJ. Renal cortical hypoplasia in a Swedish foxhound. *Vet Res.* 1973;93:260.
55. McNamera PD, et al. Cystinuria in dogs: Comparison of the cystinuric component of the Fanconi syndrome in basenji dogs to isolated cystinuria. *Metabolism.* 1989;38:8–15.
56. Miles CA, Feher RC, Cohen RD. Juvenile onset renal disease in Doberman pinschers. *Vet Med.* 1986;1106.
57. Moore FM, Thornton GW. Telangiectasia of Pembroke Welsh corgi dogs. *Vet Pathol.* 1983;20:203–208.
58. Murphy MG. Renal dysplasia in a Cavalier King Charles spaniel. *Irish Vet J.* 1989;42:96–97.
59. Murti GS. Agenesis and dysgenesis of the canine kidneys. *J Am Vet Med Assoc.* 1965;146:1120–1124.
60. Nash AS, Kelly DF, Gaskell CJ. Progressive renal disease in soft-coated Wheaten terriers: possible familial nephropathy. *J Sm Anim Pract.* 1984;25:479–487.
61. Nash AS, McCandlish IP. Chronic renal failure of young bull terriers. *Vet Rec.* 1986;118:735.
62. O'Brien TD, et al. Clinicopathologic manifestations of progressive renal disease in Lhasa apso and Shih Tzu dogs. *J Am Vet Med Assoc.* 1982;180:658–664.
63. O'Handley P, Carrig CB, Walshaw R. Renal and ureteral duplication in a dog. *J Am Vet Med Assoc.* 1979;174:484–487.
64. Oksanen A, Sittnikow K. Familjar nefropati med sekundar hyperparathyreoidism hos tre unghundar. *Nord Vet-Med.* 1972; 24:278–280.
65. Osborne CA. Congenital fusion of kidneys in a dog. *Vet Med.* 1972;67:39–42.
66. Patten BM. *Embryology of the pig.* New York, New York: Blakiston; 1948:197–211.
67. Percy DH, et al. Lesions in puppies surviving infection with canine herpesvirus. *Vet Pathol.* 1971;8:37–53.
68. Persson F, Persson S, Asheim A. Blood-pressure in dogs with renal cortical hypoplasia. *Acta Vet Scand.* 1961;2:129–136.
69. Persson F, Persson S, Asheim A. Renal cortical hypoplasia in dogs. A clinical study on uraemia and secondary hyperparathyroidism. *Acta Vet Scand.* 1961;2:68–84.
70. Picut CA, Lewis RM. Juvenile renal disease in the Doberman pinscher: Ultrastructural changes of the glomerular basement membrane. *J Comp Pathol.* 1987;97:587–596.
71. Picut CA, Lewis RM. Comparative pathology of canine hereditary nephropathies: An interpretive review. *Vet Res Commun.* 1987;11:561–581.
72. Picut CA, Lewis RM. Microscopic features of canine renal dysplasia. *Vet Pathol.* 1987;24:156–163.
72a. Reusch C, et al. A new familial membrano-proliferative glomerulonephritis in Bernese mountain dogs. Proceedings, 10th annual veterinary medical forum. American College of Veterinary Internal Medicine. 1992;10:803.
73. Robbins GR. Unilateral renal agenesis in the beagle. *Vet Rec.* 1965;77:1345.
74. Robinson WF, et al. Chronic renal disease in bull terriers. *Aust Vet J.* 1989;66:193–195.
75. Steward AP, Macdougall DF. Familial nephropathy in the cocker spaniel. *J Sm Anim Pract.* 1984;25:15–24.
76. Thorner P, et al. The NC1 domain of collagen Type IV in neonatal dog glomerular basement membranes: Significance in Samoyed hereditary glomerulopathy. *Am J Pathol.* 1989;134:1047–1054.
77. Thorner P, et al. Abnormalities in the NC1 domain of collagen Type IV in GBM in canine hereditary nephritis. *Kidney Int.* 1989;35:843–850.
78. Tuch VK, Matthiesen T. Einseitige Anomalie der niere beim Beagle. *Berl Munch Tierarztl Wschr.* 1978;91:365–367.
79. VanPelt RW, Sachtjen JF. Congenital unilateral renal hypoplasia complicated by chronic interstitial nephritis in a dog. *Vet Med.* 1973;68:745–748.
80. Verstraete A, et al. Unilaterale agenesie van de nier bij een hond en bij een kat. *Vlaams Diergeneeskundig Tijdschrift.* 1968;37:81–87.
81. Vymetal F. Case reports: Renal aplasia in beagles. *Vet Rec.* 1965;77:1344.
82. Wilcock BP, Patterson JM. Familial glomerulonephritis in Doberman pinscher dogs. *Can Vet J.* 1979;20:244–249.
83. Wright RP, Wright HJ. Paradoxic glucosuria (canine Fanconi syndrome) in two basenji dogs. *Vet Med.* 1984;79:199–202.
84. Yoon YH, Santamarina E. Hypoplastic renal corpuscles in the dog. *Toxicol Pathol.* 1979;7:1–5.

CHAPTER 25

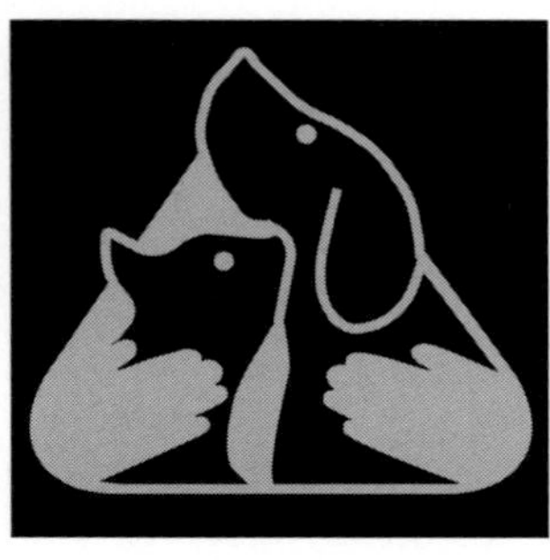

PYELONEPHRITIS

WAYNE A. CROWELL
LISA NEUWIRTH
MARY B. MAHAFFEY

I. DEFINITION

A. Tissues involved.

1. Pyelonephritis is inflammation of the renal pelvis and renal parenchyma. Inflammation of the pelvis alone is called pyelitis. Pyelitis is more common than pyelonephritis in dogs.[4,5]
2. The structures of the renal parenchyma that are involved in pyelonephritis may include papilla, medulla, and/or cortex, depending on the duration and severity of the inflammatory process.

B. Duration of pyelonephritis.

1. Acute pyelonephritis may involve only the pelvis and papilla. The initial renal infection and subsequent inflammatory process begin in the pelvis and papilla. This acute inflammatory reaction is characterized by neutrophil infiltration and necrosis (with areas of hemorrhage and fibrin exudate).
2. Chronic pyelonephritis is often the result of recurrent inflammatory episodes and generally involves the pelvis, papilla, medulla, and cortex. Histologically, pyelonephritis is a form of tubulointerstitial nephritis, because tubules and interstitium are the structures of the renal parenchyma involved. Fibrosis is invariably present and may be extensive, resulting in scarred, atrophic kidneys.

C. Agents (cause).

Bacteria are the most common cause of pyelonephritis, but fungi, viruses, and parasites are sometimes found in association with the bacterial infections.[9,11] Gram-negative bacteria are most frequently implicated in urinary tract infections,[21] and thus are the most common bacteria in pyelonephritis. Gram-negative bacteria (*Escherichia coli* in particular) are the predominant bacteria isolated from the urinary tracts of dogs with nosocomial infections.[31]

D. Route of infection.

1. Ascending infection. This is by far the most common route—and, by some definitions, the only route—of infection resulting in pyelonephritis (hematogenous routes would be termed embolic nephritis). The source of the infection may be any tissue in the lower urinary tract (ureter, bladder, prostate, urethra). The principal mechanism of the ascending infection is reflux of bacteria-contaminated urine from the lower tract up the ureter to the renal pelvis and papilla. This mechanism is reviewed in greater detail later.
2. Embolic infection. The renal parenchyma can be infected via bacterial emboli, resulting in a spectrum of renal inflammation (focal or diffuse, purulent or lymphoplasmacytic, mild or severe). This mechanism of infection initially results in

embolic nephritis, but occasionally the lesions progress and become indistinguishable from those of ascending pyelonephritis. This progression of inflammation must include the renal pelvis to be correctly termed pyelonephritis.

E. Renal involvement.

1. Unilateral. Because the infection may ascend via one or both ureters, one or both kidneys may be involved with pyelonephritis. The animal is often asymptomatic if only one kidney is affected. Unilateral pyelonephritis may be an incidental finding at necropsy.
2. Bilateral. Urinary tract infection that persists over time usually results in ascending infection in both kidneys. Bilateral pyelonephritis may progress to end-stage kidneys with azotemia and renal failure.

II. PREDISPOSING FACTORS

A. Anatomic abnormalities (causing obstruction and/or stasis).

1. Congenital lesions.
   a. Renal abnormalities. Structural abnormalities in the kidney itself have not been reported as a common predisposing factor in dogs or cats. Pigs and humans have complex (fused) papillae, whose conformation is predisposed to reflux of urine and, if the urine is contaminated, to subsequent pyelonephritis. These complex papillae have a "crater" conformation, which allows reflux of urine from the pelvis into the collecting ducts of the kidney through the central depression of the papillae. Complex papillae tend to be found on the poles of the kidney, and thus the poles are predisposed to inflammation and scarring.
   b. Ureteral abnormalities. Ectopic or misshapen ureters prevent normal expulsion of urine and are often associated with pyelonephritis. Ureters with abnormal sphincter apparati in the bladder are more likely to allow reflux of urine from the bladder into the ureter. These and other abnormalities reviewed in Chapter 35, Disorders of the Feline Lower Urinary Tract, predispose the associated kidney to pyelonephritis.
   c. Bladder abnormalities reviewed in Chapter 35, Disorders of the Feline Lower Urinary Tract, that predispose to bacterial cystitis or vesicoureteral reflux enhance the opportunity for ascending infection and pyelonephritis.
   d. Urethral abnormalities that cause abnormal excretion of urine or urine stasis or that predispose to bladder infection also increase the risk of urinary tract infection and the probability of ascending infection and subsequent pyelonephritis.
2. Acquired lesions.
   a. Fibrotic lesions. Scar tissue formed as a consequence of previous injury may predispose to abnormal urine excretion or reflux, and thus to ascending infection and pyelonephritis. Anastomosis of the ureter to the bladder in renal transplantation procedures occasionally causes formation of scar tissue and is associated with unilateral pyelonephritis.[6]
   b. Proliferative lesions. Neoplasms or granulomas may obstruct the urinary tract. This obstruction causes abnormal excretion or urine stasis. The resulting hydronephrosis and/or pyelonephritis may be unilateral or bilateral, depending on the site of the proliferative obstruction. Proliferative masses in the trigone of the bladder or the distal urinary tract may cause bilateral renal involvement,[15] whereas proliferative lesions in one ureter may affect only the associated kidney.
   c. Other lesions that cause obstruction or atony. Obstruction or impaired outflow of urine is associated with increased risk of renal infection.[13] Temporary ligation of one ureter (but not both) and subsequent intravenous injection of bacteria have been used experimentally to induce pyelonephritis in cats.[16] Unilateral renal infection occurs in the kidney with the ligated ureter. Bladder atony (associated with spinal cord injury) predisposes to pyelonephritis.

B. Functional and metabolic abnormalities (promoting bacterial contamination and/or growth).

1. Reflux.
   a. Vesicoureteral reflux. Retrograde flow of urine from the bladder into the ureter is termed vesicoureteral reflux. Such reflux may be primary (without detectable abnormalities) or secondary (resulting from infection, inflammation, obstruction, or anomalies). Iatrogenic vesicoureteral reflux may be induced by manual compression of the urinary bladder of dogs and cats.[7] Vesicoureteral reflux is reviewed further in Chapter 34, Ectopic Ureters and Ureteroceles. If the urine that refluxes is contaminated with bacteria, an ascending infection may result.
   b. Pyelotubular (intrarenal) reflux. Reflux of urine from the bladder to the ureter may be propelled upward in the ureter to the pelvis, where it may also enter the renal parenchyma. This retrograde passage of urine from the pelvis into the lumens of collecting ducts in the papilla is called pyelotubular reflux. If the urine is contaminated, renal infection may result. Pyelotubular reflux thus may be the end point of vesicoureteral reflux and the initiating factor in pyelonephritis.
2. Glucosuria. The presence of glucose in urine predisposes to urinary tract bacterial infection, and thus to pyelonephritis. Diabetes mellitus or other

conditions that predispose to glucosuria thus may be associated with pyelonephritis.

3. Papillary ischemia is often secondary to renal amyloidosis or nonsteroidal antiinflammatory drug therapy. Reduced blood flow or decreased perfusion of the papilla may result in necrosis. Loss of papillary tissue owing to necrosis reduces renal defenses against infection and thus predisposes to pyelonephritis. The abbreviated pathogenesis thus would be papillary ischemia followed by papillary necrosis, necrotic papillitis, and subsequent pyelonephritis. Unfortunately, papillary necrosis may also be a sequela of pyelonephritis. Thus, determining the chronology of papillary necrosis may be difficult (i.e., was it the cause or the effect?). Regardless, papillary necrosis is a serious renal lesion and should be anticipated when factors that may result in renal ischemia are present.
4. Immunosuppression. Dogs with hyperadrenocorticism may have increased susceptibility to urinary tract infections. Although the site of infection has not been established, pyelonephritis is feasible.[22]

C. Infection in the urinary tract.

1. Bladder infection and cystitis. Bacterial infection in the urinary bladder is frequently the source of infection that ascends to the kidney, resulting in pyelonephritis. The mechanism (as previously described) is vesicoureteral reflux and pyelotubular reflux of the contaminated urine from the bladder to the renal parenchyma.
2. Indwelling urinary catheters. Urinary tract infection and pyelonephritis are complications of indwelling urinary catheters,[2b] regardless of whether open or closed urine collection systems are used.
3. Prostate infection. Infection of the prostate can allow bacterial contamination of the urinary tract with subsequent infection of the bladder or kidney.

III. PATHOGENESIS

A. Infectious agents.

1. *E. coli* is the principal pathogen of pyelonephritis in dogs and cats. Experimental studies in humans have shown that type 1 fimbriate strains initiate more renal parenchymal scarring than do nonfimbriate strains.[30] Neutrophils are essential for this increased scarring, since the type 1 fimbriate strains increase neutrophilic protease activity and activation of the respiratory burst, with subsequent generation of toxic oxygen radicals.
2. Other gram-negative organisms. Cell wall components of gram-negative bacteria have several deleterious effects on renal function.[23] Two such effects are stimulation of vasoactive prostaglandin secretion and production of peptide mitogens by mesangial cells.

B. Renal invasion by the pathogen.

1. Pelvis. The specific means of entry of the infectious agent from the pelvis to the renal parenchyma is not completely understood in dogs or cats. Animals with calyces and multiple papillae may have compound papillae with flattening of the area cribrosa and may be predisposed to entrance of urine and bacteria into collecting ducts through these papillae.[26] Paired pelvic diverticulae, but not calyces, can be present in dogs or cats. (See Chapter 1, Applied Anatomy of the Urinary System with Clinicopathologic Correlation.) Spread of infection through the tip of the papilla and the ducts of Bellini has not been documented in dogs and cats.
2. Fornix. An early microscopic lesion seen following ascending infection of the kidney of the dog is inflammatory cells in the peripelvic tissue and the fornix. Whether the fornix is the initial site of penetration by ascending bacteria in dogs is not known.

C. Predisposing conditions in the papilla.

1. Hyperosmolality. Leukocyte function and complement activity are impaired in the papilla because of hyperosmolality.
2. Low oxygen tension. Decreased oxygen tension favors establishment and growth of certain bacteria in the medulla of the kidney. The inflammatory response is less, because of factors previously mentioned.

D. Leukocyte participation. Leukocytes are defenders against, and also promoters of, renal injury, depending on the initiating agent and associated factors, as described previously for fimbriated strains of *E. coli*. Injured or dying neutrophils may release lysosomal enzymes, which cause necrosis of adjacent tissue.

E. Progression of lesions.

1. Due to infectious agent.
   a. Experiments in monkeys demonstrated that invasion of the interstitium by *E. coli* increased thromboxane A_2 and plasma renin activity and decreased serum complement levels.[27] These findings indicate that renal infection is associated with renal vasoconstriction and ischemia.
2. Due to other factors.
   a. Tamm-Horsfall protein has been incriminated as a factor in the progression of pyelonephritis. Tamm-Horsfall protein normally lines the ascending loop of Henle and thus is isolated from lymphocytes and other mechanisms that normally recognize body protein as "self." When tubular injury occurs and Tamm-Horsfall protein enters the interstitium, it can act as an antigenic stimulus; authorities have speculated that it causes continued interstitial lymphoplasmacytic inflammation. Recently Tamm-Horsfall protein has been shown to activate the inflammatory response of neutrophils (including activation of neutrophil respiratory burst, neutrophil degranulation, generation of leukotriene, and activation of the alternative

pathway of complement).[14] This inflammatory response resulting from phagocytosis of Tamm-Horsfall protein by the neutrophils may cause severe renal damage and subsequent fibrosis.

b. Ischemia, regardless of cause, leads to tissue necrosis and fibrosis. Computed tomodensitometry recently has shown that human kidneys involved with acute pyelonephritis have areas of hypodensity, which were interpreted to be areas of ischemia. These areas subsequently developed cortical scars. The speculation was that these hypodense areas may result from intense vasoconstriction and ischemia induced by *E. coli* infection.[25a]

F. **Scarring.**

1. Pelvic scarring results from inflammation and necrosis in the papilla and renal pelvis. This scarring and subsequent deformation of the pelvis are the hallmarks of chronic pyelonephritis.
2. Scarring of the renal parenchyma is progressive and eventually results in small, atrophic kidneys or end-stage kidneys and renal failure. There are alterations in the type of collagen seen in the kidneys of cats with renal fibrosis resulting from pyelonephritis. Normal cat kidneys contain collagen of types I, IV, and V, but cat kidneys with scarring from pyelonephritis contain predominantly type I collagen.[24] This finding indicates that renal fibrosis in pyelonephritis "is not a passive compression of connective tissue with atrophy and collapse but rather an active process in which there are substantial alterations in the amounts of various collagen components."[24] Thus, scar formation is an active part of the pathogenesis of pyelonephritis.

G. **Atrophy.**

1. The shrinking of kidneys involved with pyelonephritis is the result of atrophy. Atrophy can be caused by necrosis or apoptosis. Atrophy associated with necrosis generally has more fibrosis than does atrophy associated with apoptosis. Apoptosis is the means by which tissues normally decrease in size, or involute. Apoptosis is the result of phagocytosis of cells in a tissue by adjacent cells of the same type. Thus, it is a miniature form of cannibalism. Because the cells are ingested without exposing cytoplasmic organelles to the extracellular environment (as would occur in necrosis), inflammation and scarring are minimal or absent.

H. **End-stage kidney. The preceding stages in the pathogenesis of pyelonephritis may progress to end-stage kidney.**

IV. DIAGNOSIS

A. **Clinical signs associated with pyelonephritis in dogs and cats are variable and nonspecific. Some animals may be asymptomatic, whereas others exhibit signs of septicemia. Acute pyelonephritis is often associated with fever, anorexia, lethargy, trembling, vomiting, and renal pain.[8,9] Animals with chronic pyelonephritis may be asymptomatic or exhibit polyuria and polydypsia. Uremia can occur after sufficient bilateral renal damage.**

B. **Laboratory studies.**

1. Urinalysis. Bacteriuria and pyuria indicate urinary tract infection but do not localize the infection to the kidneys. White blood cells, casts, and bacteriuria can support a diagnosis of bacterial pyelonephritis[1]; however, casts are rarely found in either naturally infected or experimentally infected dogs with pyelonephritis.[2a,3] Urine specific gravity may be low owing to loss of urine-concentrating ability. In bacterial pyelonephritis, the renal concentrating mechanism may be impaired by mechanisms unrelated to chronic renal failure. Studies in rats indicate that eicosanoids (prostaglandins) may play a role, because prostaglandin inhibitors reverse the concentration defect. Hyposthenuria and isosthenuria, which may exist in infected kidneys, are responsive to appropriate antibacterial therapy. Isosthenuria also may be detected because of chronic, generalized renal lesions that have resulted in diminution of functional renal mass. Isosthenuria of this cause is irreversible.[19,28]
2. Hemogram and serum chemistry. Leukocytosis may occur in dogs with acute pyelonephritis, but this finding is nonspecific because leukocytosis may be present in bacterial prostatitis as well. The presence of leukocytosis may help to rule out the bladder as the site of infection, because leukocytosis usually is not seen in cases of bacterial cystitis.[9] Serum chemistry may be normal. However, when pyelonephritis is bilateral and severe, azotemia and abnormalities in phosphorus, potassium, calcium, amylase, lipase, and acid-base balance are found.

C. **Urine bacterial culture. Quantitative bacterial culture of urine obtained by cystocentesis is the technique of choice to confirm the diagnosis of urinary tract infection; however, bacterial isolation does not localize the infection to the kidneys. Bladder washout, antibody coating of bacteria, and urinary enzymes have not been reliable for differentiation of upper tract and lower tract infection.[8] Conclusive diagnosis of pyelonephritis may be made from culture of urine obtained from the renal pelvis by percutaneous nephropyelostomy[20]; however, this procedure is invasive, not without risk, and requires fluoroscopy or ultrasonography.**

D. **Radiographic evaluation.**

1. Excretory urography is often used to detect pyelonephritis. Excretory urography is neither sensitive nor specific for pyelonephritis. In experimentally infected dogs, radiographic abnormalities associated with pyelonephritis included renal pelvic and proximal ureteral dilatation, decreased nephrographic opacity, and decreased pyelographic opac-

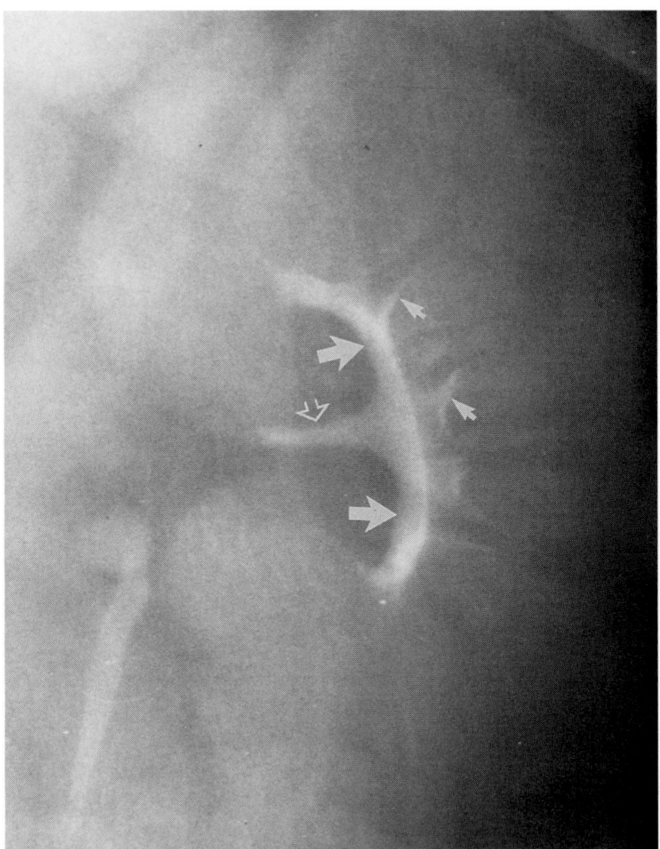

FIG. 25–1. Ventrodorsal radiographic view of a canine kidney made 40 minutes after intravenous injection of contrast medium for excretory urography. Dilatation of the renal pelvis (large arrows) with blunting of the renal pelvic recesses (small arrows) and mild dilatation of the proximal ureter (open arrow) indicate pyelonephritis.

ity.[2a,3,10,17] Renal pelvic diverticula were usually blunted, distorted, or not visualized (Fig. 25–1). Kidney size may be increased during acute pyelonephritis and may decrease progressively with progression of the disease.[2a,18] A negative excretory urogram does not rule out a diagnosis of pyelonephritis, because dogs with acute or chronic disease may have normal excretory urograms.

2. Ultrasonography, computed tomography (CT), and nuclear imaging. Ultrasonography can be used to detect renal pelvic, ureteral, and parenchymal abnormalities associated with pyelonephritis.[25b] Dilatation of the renal pelvis and proximal ureter, changes in parenchymal echogenicity, and increased prominence of the pelvic and ureteral mucosa suggest a diagnosis of pyelonephritis (Figs. 25–2 through 25–4). Ultrasonographic evaluation of the kidneys may be useful when excretory urography is contraindicated or otherwise unfeasible. CT and dimercaptosuccinic acid (DMSA) scans aid diagnosis of pyelonephritis in humans.[12,29] The usefulness of CT for detection of pyelonephritis in dogs and cats has not been established.

E. Renal biopsy. Histologic findings may not be diagnostic because of the small area of renal

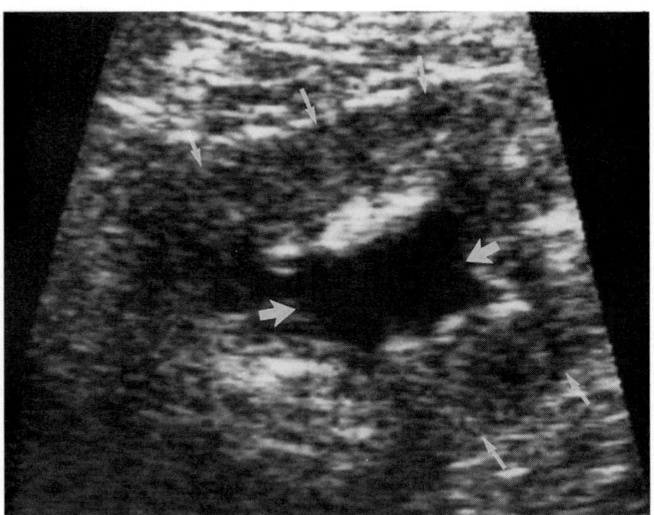

FIG. 25–2. Sagittal nephrosonogram of a dog with pyelonephritis. The renal pelvis (large arrows) is dilated and appears as a centrally located anechoic (black) space. The ventral aspect is to the top and the cranial is to the left. The ventral and dorsal margins of the kidney are outlined by the small arrows. The cranial margin is ill-defined, and the caudal pole is not included on the scan.

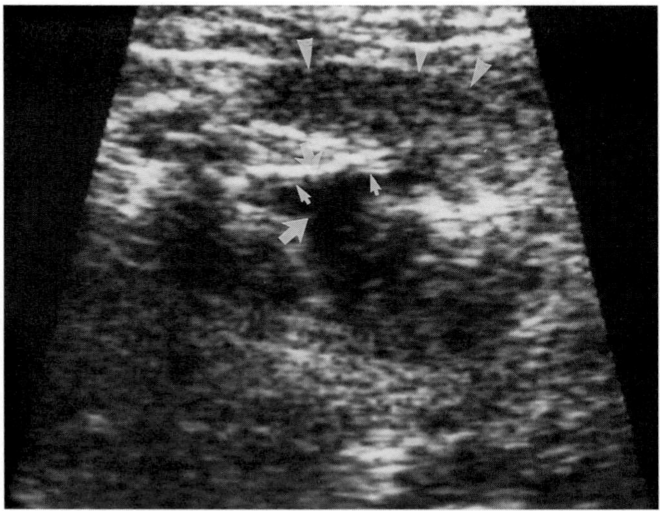

FIG. 25–3. Transverse nephrosonogram of the left kidney of a dog with pyelonephritis. The dilated renal pelvis and proximal ureter are seen as a central triangular, anechoic (black) area (large arrows). Increased echogenicity of the near field mucosal margin (small arrows) is seen as a white line. The ventral cortical margin is indicated by the arrowheads. Other renal margins either are not clearly delineated or are not present on the scan. The ventral aspect is to the top and the medial is to the left.

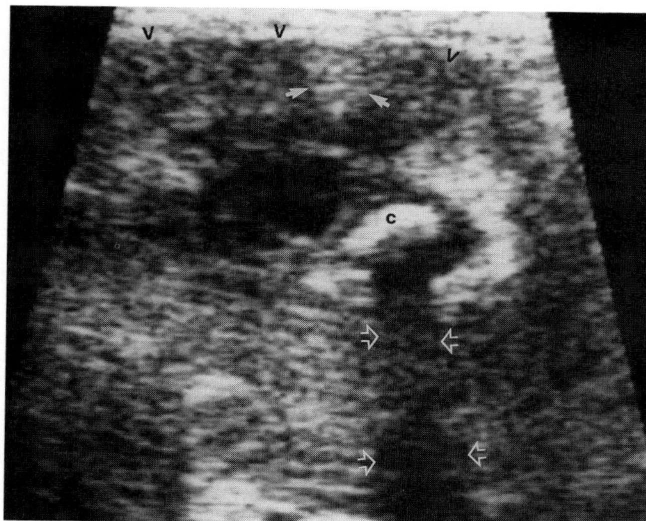

FIG. 25–4. Transverse nephrosonogram of the right kidney of a dog with pyelonephritis and a renal calculus. The calculus (c) is seen as a focal hyperechoic (white) structure with acoustic shadowing (open arrows). Focal renal pelvic dilatation is seen as an anechoic (black) space adjacent to and surrounding the calculus. A focal hyperechoic area (white arrows) within the renal cortex may be caused by fibrosis and scarring or inflammatory cell infiltration. The ventral cortical margin is indicated by the black arrowheads. Other renal margins either are not clearly delineated or are not present on this scan. The ventral aspect is to the top and the medial is to the right.

biopsy sampling. The deep medulla and pelvis are avoided during biopsy procedures, to prevent damage to large blood vessels in this area (with resultant severe hemorrhage) or to the pelvis (with subsequent urine leakage). Microscopic lesions of tubulo-interstitial nephritis that are compatible with pyelonephritis may be seen. In acute cases, a significant neutrophil component may be present. Interstitial fibrosis (including periglomerular fibrosis) may be present in chronic cases.

F. Necropsy.

1. Gross appearance. Kidneys involved with acute pyelonephritis are enlarged and may contain areas of hemorrhage and necrosis in the papilla, medulla, or cortex. Exudate may be present, but neutrophils are seldom present in sufficient quantities to be recognized as pus. Kidneys from animals with chronic pyelonephritis are often scarred, atrophic, and irregular. The pelvis usually lacks symmetry and may have scarred diverticula. Scars may also extend from the papilla upward to the cortex. The cortex may vary in thickness and even be absent in focal areas. One or both kidneys may be affected. If only one kidney is affected, the disease is usually an incidental finding.
2. Microscopic appearance. As reviewed under biopsy findings, the microscopic lesions are those of tubulo-interstitial nephritis. The cellular infiltrate is neutrophilic in acute or recurrent cases and lymphoplasmacytic in chronic cases. Necrosis may be extensive in acute cases and fibrosis extensive in chronic cases. Scar tissue may extend from the deep medulla to the outer cortex. The peripelvic tissue may contain variable numbers of inflammatory cells.

V. TREATMENT

A. Predisposing factors that contribute to continued or recurrent urinary tract infections should be eliminated. Anatomic defects, such as patent urachus and urachal diverticulum, can be surgically corrected. Calculi may be treated medically or surgically, as described in Chapter 41, Canine and Feline Urolithiases: Relationship of Etiopathogenesis to Treatment and Prevention. Sequestered infection in the urinary tract, which contributes to renal infection (i.e., prostate infection, bladder infection), must be eradicated through proper medical therapy. Urine culture and sensitivity should be used to determine the proper antibiotic regimen. The chosen antibiotic should be capable of medullary diffusion and be transferred from the blood or urine to the renal interstitium. Survey and contrast radiography, as well as ultrasonography of the urinary tract, can be useful in detecting predisposing factors for pyelonephritis.

B. Elimination of infection. Pyelonephritis and other associated chronic urinary tract infections can be difficult to eliminate. Antibiotics should be selected on the basis of results of urine culture and sensitivity. The therapeutic regimen should include factors reviewed in Chapter 40, Bacterial Infections of the Canine and Feline Urinary Tract. Duration of therapy is often long, usually 4 weeks or more. Urine culture and sensitivity tests are recommended after therapy starts, to ensure effectiveness of the chosen antibiotic. After therapy is discontinued, urine culture and sensitivity should be repeated monthly for several months to detect recurrence of infection. Animals with end-stage kidneys as a result of chronic pyelonephritis should be given supportive therapy, as described in Chapter 28, Conservative Medical Management of Chronic Renal Failure. Nephrectomy can be performed if only one kidney is involved and the remaining kidney has sufficient function. Prophylactic therapy may be needed for animals that suffer frequent reinfections. In some animals, urinary tract infection cannot be cured and therapy should be directed at controlling clinical signs.

REFERENCES

1. Allen TA, Jaenke RS. Pyelonephritis in the dog. *Compend Contin Educ Pract Vet.* 1985; 7:421–428.

2a. Barber DL, Finco DR. Radiographic findings in induced bacterial pyelonephritis in dogs. *J Am Vet Med Assoc.* 1979; 175:1183–1190.

2b. Barsanti JA, Shotts EB, Crowell WA, Finco DR, Brown J. Effect of therapy on susceptibility to urinary tract infection in male cats with indwelling urethral catheters. *J Vet Intern Med.* 1992; 6:64–70.

3. Biery DN: Upper urinary tract. In: O'Brien TR, ed. *Radiographic diagnosis of disorders in the dog and cat.* Philadelphia, Pennsylvania: WB Saunders; 1978; 481–542.

4. Christie BA. Occurrence of vesicoureteral reflux and pyelonephritis in apparently normal dogs. *Invest Urol.* 1973; 10:359–366.

5. Crowell WA, Finco DR. Frequency of pyelitis, pyelonephritis, renal perivasculitis and renal infarction in dogs. *Am J Vet Res.* 1975; 36:111–114.

6. Crowell WA, Finco DR, Rawlings CA, Barsanti JA, Rao RN. Lesions in dogs following renal transplantation and immunosuppression. *Vet Pathol.* 1987; 24:124–128.

7. Feeney DA, Osborne CA, Johnston GR. Vecisocureteral reflux induced by manual compression of the urinary bladder of dogs and cats. *J Am Vet Med Assoc.* 1983; 182:795–797.

8. Finco DR. Evaluation of methods of localization of urinary tract infection in the female dog. *Am J Vet Res.* 1979; 40:707.

9. Finco DR, Barsanti JA. Bacterial pyelonephritis. *Vet Clin North Am/Small Anim Pract.* 1979; 9:645–660.

10. Fuller WJ. Case report: subacute pyelonephritis with a nonvisualized nephrogram. *J Am Anim Hosp Assoc.* 1976; 12: 509–513.

11. Ginder DH. Urinary tract infection and pyelonephritis due to *Escherichia coli* in dogs infected with canine adenovirus. *J Infect Dis.* 1974; 129:715–719.

12. Goldraich NP, Ramos OL, Goldraich IH. Urography versus DMSA scan in children with vesicoureteral reflux. *Pediatr Nephrol.* 1989; 3:1–5.

13. Heptinstall RH. Urinary tract infection, reflux, and pyelonephritis. In: Heptinstall RH, ed. *Pathology of the Kidney.* 3rd ed. Boston, Massachusetts: Little, Brown; 1983:1257–1322.

14. Horton JK, Davies M, Topley N, Thomas D, Williams JD. Activation of the inflammatory response of neutrophils by Tamm-Horsfall glycoprotein. *Kidney Int.* 1989; 37:717–726.

15. Jergens AE, Miles KG, Turk Margaret. Bilateral pyelonephritis and hydroureter associated with metastatic adenocarcinoma in a dog. *J Am Vet Med Assoc.* 1988; 193:961–963.

16. Kelly DF, Lucke VM, McCullagh KG: Experimental pyelonephritis in the cat. 1. Gross and histological changes. *J Comp Pathol.* 1979; 89:125–139.

17. Kneller SK. Role of the excretory urogram in the diagnosis of renal and ureteral disease. *Vet Clin North Am/Small Anim Pract.* 1971; 4:843–861.

18. Lees GA, Rogers KS. Diagnosis and localization of urinary tract infection. In: Kirk RW, ed. *Current veterinary therapy IX.* Philadelphia, Pennsylvania: WB Saunders; 1986:1118.

19. Levinson SP, Levinson ME. Effect of indomethacin and sodium meclofenamate on the renal concentrating defect in experimental enterococcal pyelonephritis in rats. *J Lab Clin Med.* 1976; 88:958.

20. Ling GV. Percutaneous nephropyelocentesis and nephropyelostomy in the dog: a description of the technique. *Am J Vet Res.* 1979; 40:1605.

21. Ling GV, Biberstein EL, Hirsch DC. Bacterial pathogens associated with urinary tract infections. *Vet Clin North Am.* 1979; 9:617–630.

22. Ling GV, Stabenfeldt GH, Comer KM, Gribble DH, Schechter RD. Canine hyperadrenocorticism: pretreatment clinical and laboratory evaluation of 117 cases. *J Am Vet Med Assoc.* 1979; 174:1211–1215.

23. Lovett DH, Bursten SL, Gemsa D, Bessler W, Resch K, Ryan JL. Activation of glomerular mesangial cells by gram-negative bacterial cell wall components. *Am J Pathol.* 1988; 133:472–484.

24. McCullagh KG, Bishop KA, Lucke VM, Kelly DF. Experimental pyelonephritis in the cat: 3. Collagen alterations in renal fibrosis. *J Comp Pathol.* 1983; 93:9–25.

25a. Meyrier A. Long-term risks of acute pyelonephritis. *Nephron.* 1990; 54:197–201.

25b. Neuwirth L, Mahaffey M, Crowell W, Selcer B, Barsanti J, Cooper R, Brown J. Comparison of excretory urography and ultrasonography for detection of experimentally induced pyelonephritis in dogs. *Am J Vet Res.* 1993; 54:660–669.

26. Ransley PG, Risdon RA. Renal papillary morphology and intrarenal reflux in the young pig. *Urol Res.* 1975; 3:105–115.

27. Roberts JA. Pathogenesis of pyelonephritis. *J Urol.* 1983; 129: 1102–1106.

28. Ronald AR, Cutler RE, Turck M. Effect of bacteriuria on the renal concentrating mechanism. *Ann Intern Med.* 1969; 70:723.

29. Smellie JM, Shaw PJ, Prescod NP, Bantock HM. Tc-99m Dimercaptosuccinic acid (DMSA) scan in patients with established radiological renal scarring. *Arch Dis Child.* 1988; 63:1315–1319.

30. Topley N, Steadman R, Mackenzie R, Knowlden JM, Williams JD. Type 1 fibriate strains of *Escherichia coli* initiate renal parenchymal scarring. *Kidney Int.* 1989; 36:609–616.

31. Wise LA, Jones RL, Reif JS. Nosocomial canine urinary tract infections in a veterinary teaching hospital (1983 to 1988). *J Am Anim Hosp Assoc.* 1990; 26:148–152.

CHAPTER 26

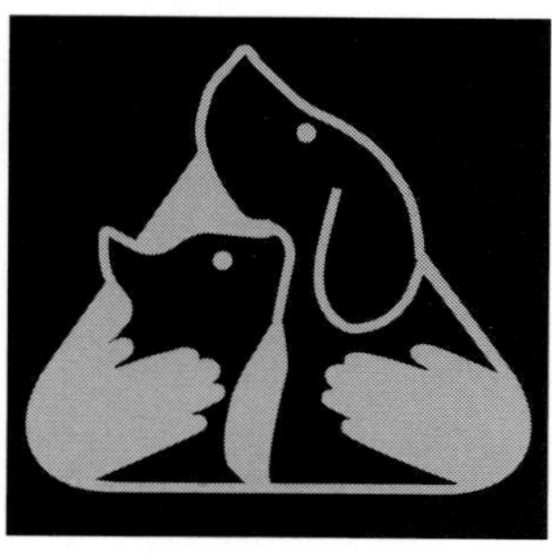

Renal Manifestations of Polysystemic Diseases

S. DRU FORRESTER
GEORGE E. LEES

I. SPECTRUM OF RENAL INVOLVEMENT IN POLYSYSTEMIC DISEASES

A. Renal disorders that can be caused by polysystemic diseases.

1. Each of the major clinical syndromes of renal disease can be secondary to systemic or polysystemic extrarenal diseases or a primary renal disease.
2. The major clinical syndromes of renal disease are:
   a. Acute renal failure.
   b. Chronic renal failure.
   c. Nephrotic syndrome.
   d. Renal tubular defects.
   e. Subclinical urine abnormalities.
3. See Chapter 3, Fundamentals of the Practice of Veterinary Nephrology and Urology, for a general description of each of these major clinical syndromes of renal disease.

B. Mechanisms of renal injury in polysystemic diseases.

1. A limited number of mechanisms are responsible for the renal effects of polysystemic diseases. Although many different primary diseases can have secondary renal involvement, the pathogenic mechanisms for associated renal injury are few.
2. Causes of renal lesions in polysystemic diseases include:
   a. Direct injury by infectious agents.
   b. Immune-mediated injury.
   c. Hemodynamically mediated injury.
   d. Direct injury by substances.

C. Sites of renal injury in polysystemic diseases.

1. The spectrum of sites where renal lesions may be produced is even more limited than the spectrum of mechanisms that may cause secondary renal lesions.
2. The limited number of possible sites of action for mechanisms of renal injury causes their effects to be revealed as vascular and/or glomerular renal disease or as tubulo-interstitial renal disease.

II. DISEASES ASSOCIATED WITH DIRECT RENAL INJURY BY INFECTIOUS AGENTS (TABLE 26–1)

A. Systemic infectious diseases often cause renal injury, but such injury usually is produced by immune-mediated events (see the following).

B. Few of the organisms that cause infectious diseases of dogs and cats are known to cause direct renal injury, and not all these injuries are clinically important.

1. During the initial phase of canine adenovirus 1 (CAV-1) infection, (e.g., infectious canine hepatitis) virus replicates in and injures glomerular endothelial cells.[45]
2. This injury may help to cause the mild, transient proteinuria seen during early stages of CAV-1 infection; however, it plays a minor, probably inconsequential, role in producing the

TABLE 26–1
DISEASES ASSOCIATED WITH DIRECT RENAL INJURY BY INFECTIOUS AGENTS

Vascular injury
- Glomerular endothelial cells: Infectious canine hepatitis (CAV-1)
- Renal involvement in generalized vasculitis: Canine herpesvirus (neonatal infection), leptospirosis, canine ehrlichiosis, Rocky Mountain spotted fever, brucellosis

Tubulointerstitial injury
- Tubular epithelial cells: Leptospirosis, infectious canine hepatitis (CAV-1), encephalitozoonosis
- Interstitial nephritis: Leptospirosis, infectious canine hepatitis (CAV-1), encephalitozoonosis, Lyme borreliosis, brucellosis
- Granulomatous interstitial nephritis: Feline infectious peritonitis, histoplasmosis, blastomycosis, cryptococcosis, coccidioidomycosis, disseminated aspergillosis, candidiasis, protothecosis, tuberculosis

general clinical illness caused by infectious hepatitis.

C. **Most examples of clinically important renal vascular injuries in systemic infections reflect involvement of the kidneys in a more generalized vasculitis, sometimes with intravascular coagulation.**
1. Systemic infectious diseases that may cause generalized vasculitis leading to significant renal injury include neonatal canine herpesvirus infection,[17] leptospirosis,[43,74] Rocky Mountain spotted fever,[44] canine ehrlichiosis,[35,88] and brucellosis.[18]
2. Renal failure is more likely to be a prominent clinical feature of illness in animals with leptospirosis or Rocky Mountain spotted fever than in animals with the other disorders listed.

D. **Infectious agents sometimes cause tubulointerstitial renal disease.**
1. Infectious agents that localize in renal tubular epithelial cells include leptospires, CAV-1, and the microsporidian *Encephalitozoon cuniculi.*[86]
   a. These organisms are shed in the urine of infected animals because of their ability to persist and replicate in renal tubular epithelium.
   b. Direct or indirect contact with organism-laden urine from infected animals is an important method of transmission for each of these pathogens.
2. Acute or chronic interstitial nephritis, which may or may not cause renal failure, may be associated with leptospirosis, Lyme borreliosis,[41] infectious canine hepatitis, and encephalitozoonosis.
3. Modified live-virus vaccines containing CAV-1 may cause subclinical interstitial nephritis and persistent shedding of virus in urine.
4. Dogs with brucellosis also may have mild interstitial nephritis, and organisms may be recovered from their urine; however, these organisms are thought to come from the prostate gland and epididymis.
5. Leptospirosis is the single most important infectious cause of renal disease in dogs. (See Chapter 18, Primary Tubulo-Interstitial Diseases of the Kidney, for a detailed description of this disorder.)

E. **Granulomatous interstitial nephritis may occur in association with feline infectious peritonitis (FIP),[2] blastomycosis,[62] histoplasmosis,[4] cryptococcosis,[85] coccidioidomycosis,[3] disseminated aspergillosis,[25,55] candidiasis,[46] protothecosis,[89] or tuberculosis.[47]**
1. Renal involvement is common in cats with FIP, although most affected cats do not develop signs of renal failure.
2. Other organs are more often involved in patients with disseminated blastomycosis, histoplasmosis, cryptococcosis, or coccidioidomycosis; however, the kidneys are occasionally affected.
3. Disseminated aspergillosis often involves the kidneys as well as other organs; organisms often are isolated from urine of affected dogs.[25]
4. Systemic candidiasis is an uncommon disease, but renal lesions are often found in affected patients.

III. DISEASES ASSOCIATED WITH IMMUNE-MEDIATED RENAL INJURY

A. **General perspectives.**
1. Immune-mediated events probably are the most frequent and clinically important causes of renal injury associated with polysystemic disease.
   a. Immune mechanisms can produce tubulointerstitial or vascular renal lesions, but immune-mediated glomerular lesions are most numerous and best-characterized.
   b. Renal manifestations of systemic diseases usually occur as a result of glomerular disease, most (but not all) of which are immune-mediated.
2. Pathogenesis of immune-mediated renal diseases involves mainly humoral mechanisms leading to renal injury, but a possible role for cellular immune mechanisms has been increasingly recognized in recent years.[21,94]
   a. In immune complex disease, antibodies interact in dynamic equilibrium with soluble intravascular antigens to form immune complexes. Biologically active immune complexes usually form in the presence of mild excess of antigen compared to antibodies. When immune complexes escape clearance by the mononuclear phagocytic system, they circulate and may accumulate in various glomerular structures (e.g., mesangium, capillary wall, basement membrane) as well as in renal vessels, tubular basement membranes, or interstitial sites. Immune complexes also can form locally (i.e., *in situ*) when soluble antigen and antibody inde-

pendently arrive at these sites. Regardless of whether immune complexes form in the circulation or *in situ*, the antigen's solubility permits diffusion of the antigen away from the immune deposit and affects dynamics of antigen-antibody interaction at the site of immune injury.

b. In antiglomerular basement membrane disease, lesions arise because of accumulation of antibody with specificity for insoluble basement membrane antigens. The antigen may be a naturally occurring component of the structure, or it may have become fixed or planted in the basement membrane after originating elsewhere. In either case, the antigen's insolubility makes kinetics of antigen-antibody interaction at the site of immune injury much different from those of immune complex disease.

c. Once antibodies combine with soluble or insoluble antigens in renal tissues, a variety of mechanisms of tissue injury may be set in motion. Some of these mechanisms are induced by antibody deposition alone, whereas others involve formation of complement membrane attack complexes, inflammatory cells from the circulation, or effects mediated by resident mesangial cells.

d. See Chapter 17, Primary Diseases of Glomeruli, for a more thorough description of mechanisms of glomerular diseases.

3. Morphologic expression of glomerular disease is diverse.

   a. Based on their appearance, glomerular lesions generally are classified as proliferative (mesangial) glomerulonephritis, membranous glomerulonephritis, membranoproliferative (mesangioproliferative) glomerulonephritis, minimal change disease, glomerulosclerosis, or amyloidosis. (See Chapter 17, Primary Diseases of Glomeruli, for a detailed description of morphologic characteristics of these glomerular lesions.)

   b. Amyloidosis is an example of direct renal injury by a substance (see the following).

   c. Some forms of glomerulosclerosis are thought to be caused by hemodynamically mediated renal injury (see the following).

   d. For all the other listed forms of glomerular disease, immune-mediated mechanisms are known or suspected to be responsible for producing renal lesions.

4. Clinical classification of glomerular disease depends on whether or not an underlying extrarenal disorder also is recognized.

   a. Whenever any of the listed glomerular lesions (including their subsets and variants) are found in patients who have only renal disease (with or without systemic manifestations of renal disease), the associated illness generally is categorized and described as a primary glomerular disease.

   b. However, a similar spectrum of glomerular lesions occurs in some patients who have systemic (nonrenal) primary diseases (Table 26–2). The renal manifestations of illnesses in these patients are categorized as secondary glomerular diseases.

B. Systemic lupus erythematosus (SLE) is the most prominent and clinically important ex-

TABLE 26–2
DISORDERS ASSOCIATED WITH SECONDARY GLOMERULAR DISEASES IN DOGS AND CATS

Dogs	Cats
Inflammatory	
SLE	SLE
Polyarthritis	Pancreatitis
Pancreatitis	Cholangiohepatitis
Chronic dermatitis	
Infectious	
Infectious canine hepatitis	Feline leukemia virus
Brucellosis	Feline infectious peritonitis
Pyometra	Polyarthritis *(Mycoplasma)*
Bacteremia	
Chronic bacterial infections	
Borreliosis	
Rocky Mountain spotted fever	
Ehrlichiosis	
Dirofilariasis	
Hepatozoonosis	
Leishmaniasis	
Trypanosomiasis	
Neoplastic	
Lymphoma	Lymphoma
Leukemia (myeloid, lymphocytic)	Mastocytosis
Mastocytosis	
Primary erythrocytosis	
Carcinoma	
Heredofamilial	
Bull terrier	
Bernese mountain dog	
Chinese Shar pei (amyloidosis)	
Doberman pinscher	
Samoyed	
Drug-Induced	
Trimethoprim-sulfadizine	
Hydralazine	
Corticosteroids	
Corynebacterium parvum immunotherapy	
Miscellaneous	
Hepatic disease (cirrhosis)	Erythrocytosis (left-to-right shunts)
Hyperadrenocorticism	
Diabetes mellitus	

ample of a noninfectious polysystemic disorder that may cause secondary glomerular disease.

1. SLE is a polysystemic disease of unknown cause, characterized by a diverse assortment of clinical manifestations and a variety of "autoantibodies."
   a. Fundamental cause(s) of SLE are incompletely understood. Development of the disease involves complex interactions of the immune system with genetic, environmental, infectious, and hormonal factors.[77] Humans and animals with SLE have major aberrations of humoral and cellular immune function that lead to inappropriate synthesis of antibodies with specificity for antigens that are normal components of the individual's cells and tissues (so-called, autoantibodies). With ongoing exposure of the immune system to "self" antigens (or antigens that cross-react with "self" antigens) and with formation of antibodies against these antigens, an abundance of immune complexes may be produced.
   b. The clinical manifestations of SLE are expressions of immune complex disease. Deposition of circulating antigen-antibody complexes or formation *in situ* of such complexes stimulates a variety of immune effector and amplifier mechanisms that cause inflammation and injury to adjacent tissue. Clinical manifestations thus vary according to location, extent, intensity, and duration of both immune complex deposition and inflammation. Factors that control these determinants of clinical expression of SLE are ill-understood.
2. SLE has been reported in dogs and cats.[30,48,57,77] The total number of cases of SLE in dogs and cats that appear in published reports depends on the criteria chosen to confirm a diagnosis of SLE (see the following). Nonetheless, reported cases of canine SLE that are reasonably well documented are fewer than 300, and reported cases of feline SLE are fewer than 20. Thus, SLE is much less thoroughly characterized in dogs and cats than in humans.
3. General features of SLE in dogs.
   a. Most dogs are 2 to 9 years old when SLE is diagnosed (average age, 6 years); however, SLE has been reported in dogs of all ages.[48,77]
   b. Although early investigators suggested that SLE was more common in females (partly because such is the case in humans), results of formal studies of occurrence of SLE in dogs indicate either no gender predilection or evidence of significantly greater risk for SLE reproductively intact males.[48,57,77]
   c. Available data about breed predilections for development of SLE are inconsistent. Early reports suggested that German shepherds and poodles were at increased risk for SLE. Formal studies of the prevalence of canine SLE have suggested increased risk for Shetland sheepdogs, collies, and beagles (but not German shepherds or poodles)[77] or for German shepherds (but not other breeds).[57]
   d. Clinical manifestations of SLE are diverse (Table 26–3). The frequency of specific signs may be influenced by interests and expertise of clinicians contributing cases to reports (e.g., dermatologists may be more likely to see dogs with cutaneous manifestations of SLE); however, several generalities are supported by the findings of multiple investigators. Nonerosive polyarthritis is the most common clinical expression of SLE in dogs.[30,48,57,77] Cutaneous lesions also occur frequently; however, dermatologic changes associated with SLE are pleo-

TABLE 26–3
PRINCIPAL MANIFESTATIONS OF CANINE SYSTEMIC LUPUS ERYTHEMATOSUS

Finding	Prevalence (%)
Autoantibody tests	
ANA	54–97
LE cell preparation	15–93
Coombs' reaction	22–37
Musculoskeletal	
Polyarthritis	39–77
Polymyositis	4–8
Integumentary	33–54
Dermatitis	10–26
Alopecia	19–45
Mucocutaneous ulcers	16–27
Oral ulcers	4–39
Footpad lesions	23
Hematologic	53
Anemia	35–60
Nonregenerative	12–31
Hemolytic	8–23
Thrombocytopenia	8–24
Leukopenia	10–28
Leukocytosis	29–33
Nephropathic	50
Proteinuria	46–55
Azotemia	14
Thoracic*	10–31
Neurologic†	4–25
Miscellaneous others	
Fever	31–67
Lymphadenopathy	28–29
Anorexia	40
Diarrhea	28
Vomiting	19

*Thoracic findings include pleuritis, pleural effusion, myocarditis, pericarditis, cardiac murmur, and respiratory disease.

†Neurologic findings include seizures, abnormal behavior, and suspected cases of polyneuropathy.

Data from references 48,56,57,76.

morphic. Dogs with SLE often have hematologic abnormalities. Anemia is common, although hemolytic anemia occurs less frequently than nonregenerative anemia, even when Coombs' test is positive. Thrombocytopenia may occur, but it is not found in most cases. Similarly, leukopenia may occur, but leukocytosis is seen more often. Proteinuria is observed in about half of all dogs with SLE, but azotemia is less common. In addition to joints, skin, blood, and kidneys, immune complex disease affecting other tissues may contribute to clinical expression of SLE in dogs. These sites include skeletal muscle, cardiac muscle, pericardium, pleura, lung, meninges, and peripheral nerves. Although these tissues are affected less frequently, associated clinical manifestations often are quite important in affected individuals.

4. Nephropathy associated with SLE (lupus nephropathy).
   a. Clinical and pathologic features of nephropathy in dogs and cats with SLE have been characterized in too few animals to formulate meaningful generalizations. For comparative purposes, information regarding nephropathy that occurs in humans with SLE is provided here; however, caution must be exercised in applying this information to dogs and cats. The extent to which lupus nephropathy in dogs and cats is clinically or pathologically similar to lupus nephropathy in humans is unknown.
   b. Prevalence of nephropathy in humans with SLE depends on methods and criteria used to define the existence of the condition. Overt clinical evidence of nephropathy is found at the time of diagnosis in about two thirds of human beings with SLE.[37] If light microscopic examination of renal biopsy or postmortem specimens is included, renal lesions are found in about 90% of cases. However, evidence of renal involvement emerges in virtually all cases if special immunofluorescence and electron microscopic studies are done.
   c. The basic immune system abnormality that characterizes lupus nephropathy is accumulation or deposition of immunoglobulin and complement components in the mesangium. This basic lesion often is a background upon which more severe changes are superimposed. Immune deposits may form or accumulate in glomerular capillary walls as well as in the mesangium. Local glomerular reaction and contributions by cells from circulating blood combine to produce varying patterns of glomerular injury seen by light microscopy.
   d. Glomerular lesions of lupus nephropathy are pleomorphic and have been classified.[37] Each class of lesion has its own distinctive combination of light microscopic, immunopathologic, and ultrastructural changes, and several classes include variant subtypes. Additionally, assorted vascular, tubular, and interstitial changes may contribute to the appearance of lupus nephropathy. Detailed characteristics of various morphologic forms of human lupus nephropathy have been described.[37]
   e. More than one morphologic form of glomerular injury may be found at any one time or sequentially during the course of disease in a single patient, or the pattern of morphologic change may remain the same. In humans with SLE, correlation between the morphologic pattern of renal injury observed in biopsies and the clinical features of associated illness is only approximate.
   f. Therapeutic decisions and prognostic judgments, however, may be aided by light microscopic evaluation of renal biopsy specimens (Table 26–4). In humans with lupus nephropathy, lesions indicating that the underlying disease is active may also indicate potential for reversibility with aggressive treatment, whereas lesions indicating chronicity are associated with a poorer prognosis.[37]

TABLE 26–4
LIGHT MICROSCOPIC INDICATORS OF DISEASE ACTIVITY AND CHRONICITY IN HUMAN LUPUS NEPHROPATHY[37]

Lesions Indicating Activity	Lesions Indicating Chronicity
Glomerular changes: hypercellularity, fibrinoid necrosis, karyorrhexis, cellular crescents, wire loops, hyaline thrombi, leukocyte infiltration	Glomerulosclerosis Fibrous crescents Interstitial fibrosis Tubular atrophy
Tubulo-interstitial changes: Mononuclear infiltration	

5. Diagnosis of SLE requires fulfillment of multiple criteria.
   a. In general, diagnosis of SLE rests on the existence of three basic conditions: 1) an active disease process that is known (or can be presumed) to be an expression of immune complex disease, 2) autoantibodies, and 3) absence of other identifiable conditions (e.g., chronic infection) that might produce immune complex formation.
   b. According to some definitions of SLE, manifestations of immune complex disease must be found in multiple organ systems. Using this definition, however, means that SLE cannot be

conclusively diagnosed at the outset of illness in some patients because the disease in these individuals appears in just one system at first; evidence of multisystem involvement that justifies diagnosis of *systemic* lupus erythematosus in these individuals develops only as the passage of time permits full expression of their disease. Other definitions of SLE permit diagnosis of the condition with single organ system involvement (e.g., polyarthritis) and clear evidence of excess autoantibody production (e.g., antinuclear antibody).

c. Because of diverse clinicopathologic manifestations of SLE and the multitude of different ways they can be combined in a single patient, diagnosis of SLE often is difficult to make with confidence. In actual practice, SLE is diagnosed by "weighing the evidence." The greater the total number of findings attributable to SLE (and for which there is no better explanation), the more likely is the diagnosis of SLE to be correct. Published guidelines for diagnosis of SLE generally provide a list of possible findings and state the minimum number (or combination) of findings sufficient to support a diagnosis (Table 26–5).

d. The autoantibody most characteristic of SLE is antinuclear antibody (ANA), which is a broad class of immunoglobulins that reacts with components of cell nuclei.
   (1). The ANA titer is considered the screening test of choice when SLE is suspected.
      (a). Results are positive in as many as 90% of dogs with SLE.
      (b). Findings are relatively constant from day to day.
      (c). It is more likely to remain positive after initiation of corticosteroid therapy than is the lupus erythematosus (LE) cell test.
   (2). A variety of methods are used to detect ANA; laboratory-specific reference values are needed to interpret test results with confidence.
   (3). Positive ANA titers may be generated by disorders other than SLE (e.g., infectious, inflammatory, or neoplastic diseases); however, the value generally is not as markedly elevated.[56]
   (4). Sometimes when a diagnosis of SLE is otherwise well supported, the ANA test result is negative; this may occur in 10 to 25% of dogs with SLE. Dogs with polyarthritis, anemia, or thrombocytopenia and dermatologic lesions have a high probability, however, of having SLE, even in the absence of ANA.[57]
   (5). Several patterns of nuclear fluorescence may be observed in patients with SLE, including peripheral (rim), homogeneous (diffuse), speckled, and nucleolar. Although homegeneous fluorescence has been reported to be most common in dogs,[30,77] the speckled pattern occurred most often in one study.[56] In human patients, some correlation exists between the pattern of fluorescence and the type of immune-mediated disease; however, the significance of the pattern of fluorescence in veterinary patients is unknown.

e. The LE cell test may provide supportive evidence when SLE is suspected.
   (1). It is performed by incubating clotted blood from a patient and looking for formation of LE cells *in vitro*. LE cells are phagocytic cells that contain degraded nuclear material opsonized by ANA. Rarely, synovial fluid from patients with SLE contains LE cells.
   (2). The LE cell test is considered less reliable than an ANA titer for diagnosis of SLE in dogs.
      (a). LE cells must be differentiated from tart cells, which are neutrophils that have phagocytosed intact nuclei.
      (b). The LE cell test is more likely to be negative as a result of corticosteroid therapy than is the ANA titer.
      (c). Results of the LE cell test may vary from day to day; therefore, the test should be repeated several times before the result is considered negative.
      (d). Like the ANA titer, the LE cell test may be positive in conditions other than SLE.

6. Treatment of SLE primarily involves administration of immunosuppressive drugs.
   a. In the authors' experience, many dogs respond favorably to treatment with corticosteroids (e.g., prednisone) alone.

TABLE 26–5
CRITERIA FOR DIAGNOSIS OF SLE*

Major Signs	Minor Signs
Nonerosive polyarthritis	Fever
Glomerulonephritis	Myositis
Dermatitis	Myocarditis
Hemolytic anemia	Pericarditis
Thrombocytopenia	Pleuritis
	Lymphadenopathy
	Hepatosplenomegaly

*A diagnosis of SLE is made when there is a positive ANA titer and two major signs or one major sign and 2 minor signs.
Data from references 48 and 57.

(1). Administer an induction dose of 1 to 2 mg/kg orally every 12 hours until there is significant clinical improvement.

(2). Gradually decrease the dose to 0.5 to 1 mg/kg given on alternate days.

b. If adequate control is not gained using corticosteroids alone, or if the patient experiences undesirable side effects, additional immunosuppressive therapy may be administered together with prednisone.

(1). Administer azathioprine (Imuran) to dogs, 2.2 mg/kg orally every 48 hours; continue prednisone on alternate days. Monitor the hemogram every 2 weeks for 8 weeks and then monthly to detect signs of azathioprine toxicosis (leukopenia, thrombocytopenia).

(2). Alternatively, administer cyclophosphamide (Cytoxan) at 50 mg/m^2 orally every other day or once daily for 4 consecutive days per week. Monitor the hemogram weekly for evidence of myelosuppression and urinalysis for signs of sterile, hemorrhagic cystitis. The likelihood of developing cystitis may be reduced by administering prednisone and cyclophosphamide on the same day in the morning.

c. Consider gradually discontinuing immunosuppressive therapy if the patient's condition is stable for 6 months.

7. The ideal therapeutic management of dogs and cats with SLE-associated glomerular disease has not been determined. (See Chapter 17, Primary Diseases of Glomeruli, for a more detailed review of treatment of glomerulonephritis.)

a. The use of corticosteroids in dogs with glomerulonephritis is controversial; however, controlled studies that prove or disprove their efficacy are lacking. A retrospective study of 41 dogs with glomerulonephritis showed that corticosteroids (0.5 to 1.1 mg/kg) were not beneficial in 5 dogs and, in some instances, were detrimental.[20]

b. In humans with SLE, long-term effects of corticosteroids on survival and renal disease are unknown.[37] Use of the lowest possible dosage of corticosteroids is generally recommended; administration of cytotoxic drugs (cyclophosphamide, azathioprine) may allow smaller dosages of corticosteroids to be given.

c. Until results of further studies are available, specific treatment of glomerular disease associated with SLE in dogs and cats should probably be reserved for patients with histologic evidence of glomerulonephritis.[90]

(1). Administering azathioprine and/or cyclophosphamide may be preferable to using corticosteroids, especially in azotemic patients.

(2). Monitoring of treatment should include periodic evaluation of serum chemistries and quantitation of urine protein loss, either by determining urine protein/creatinine ratio or 24-hour urine protein excretion. (See Chapter 9, Urinary Protein Loss, and Chapter 10, Evaluation of Renal Functions.) Alter treatment in patients with progressive azotemia and/or increased proteinuria. Remember that, as renal failure progresses and glomerular filtration rate declines, urinary protein excretion decreases. Therefore, monitoring creatinine clearance may be a better indicator of therapeutic efficacy than is urinary protein excretion in these patients.

8. The prognosis for patients with SLE is guarded because the outcome is unpredictable.

a. Remissions and relapses are common. Some patients may have complete resolution of their disease, whereas others may require periodic immunosuppressive treatment for the remainder of their lives.

b. Patients with hemolytic anemia and thrombocytopenia may not respond to corticosteroids alone; they may require additional immunosuppressive therapy.[30]

c. Patients with SLE should be monitored closely for secondary infections and treated aggressively.

d. If glomerular disease progresses to renal failure in SLE patients, the prognosis declines.

C. Many infectious diseases (bacterial, viral, fungal, rickettsial, protozoal) may be associated with secondary glomerular diseases in dogs and cats (see Table 26–2).[54,64,70] In most instances, the pathogenesis of glomerular disease involves deposition of immune complexes in glomeruli.

1. Dirofilariasis may be associated with *in situ* immune complex formation as well as deposition of preformed immune complexes.

a. At present, formation of immune complexes *in situ* has been shown in experimental studies only and not in cases of naturally occurring disease.

b. Dogs experimentally infected with *Dirofilaria immitis* infective larvae develop membranoproliferative glomerulonephritis characterized by glomerular basement membrane thickening, mesangial proliferation, and intramembranous electron-dense deposits (antigen-antibody complexes).[19,40,42] Other findings include granular and linear fluorescence of glomerular capillary walls, characteristic of deposition of preformed immune complexes, and formation *in situ* of immune complexes, respectively.[42]

c. In addition to immune-mediated glomerular

disease, other factors may potentially contribute to renal disease in dogs with dirofilariasis[69]:
  (1). Decreased renal perfusion secondary to congestive heart failure.
  (2). Decreased glomerular filtration rate caused by decreased oncotic pressure from hypoalbuminemia.
  (3). Renal tubular damage associated with vena caval syndrome.
    (a). Ischemia secondary to disseminated intravascular coagulation.
    (b). Hemoglobinuria associated with intravascular hemolysis.
  (4). Although the incidence is unknown, some dogs with dirofilariasis develop glomerular amyloidosis, which contributes to renal dysfunction.[69]

d. Dirofilariasis is diagnosed by identifying microfilaria of *D. immitis* (Knott's test) or finding a positive serum antigen test.

e. Treatment of glomerular disease associated with dirofilariasis in dogs includes supportive and specific measures.
  (1). Supportive care, including rehydration and correction of other prerenal factors (e.g., congestive heart failure), should be instituted initially.
  (2). Administration of adulticide (thiacetarsemide) and microfilaricide drugs may cause marked improvement in renal function (i.e., decreased severity of urinary protein loss and hypoalbuminemia). Correction of all prerenal factors is important in preventing arsenic-induced renal failure.
  (3). Administration of immunosuppressive drugs is not recommended, pending controlled studies that document their efficacy in patients with dirofilariasis. Potential complications include:
    (a). Protein catabolism and worsening azotemia.
    (b). Worsening glomerulonephritis.
    (c). Increased glomerular deposition of amyloid.

2. Bacterial endocarditis can predispose to immune complex glomerulonephritis.
  a. In humans with bacterial endocarditis, glomerulonephritis usually develops when diagnosis and treatment are delayed.[37] The most common abnormality detected by light microscopy is a focal and segmental proliferative glomerular lesion. At one time, glomerulonephritis was thought to be secondary to embolic disease; however, this is no longer presumed to be the case.
  b. In three studies, approximately 17% of dogs with endocarditis were reported to have glomerulonephritis.[14,80,87] The significance of glomerular disease in the pathogenesis of renal disease in these patients is unknown. Embolic disease is probably an important factor that contributes to development of renal failure in dogs with endocarditis (see the following review of renal hypoperfusion).

3. Infectious diseases associated with glomerulonephritis in cats include feline leukemia virus infection, polyarthritis caused by *Mycoplasma gatae* infection, and FIP.[49,67] In a study of cats with histologically confirmed FIP, glomerulonephritis was diagnosed in 70% of 85 cases.[49]

D. Neoplasms may be associated with glomerulonephritis.[20,26,38,52,53,68,72,93]

1. In a study of dogs with naturally occurring glomerulonephritis, 17 of 42 cases (40%) had associated neoplasia; lymphoma was the most common (9 cases), followed by carcinoma (4 cases), leukemia (2 cases), and mastocytosis (2 cases).[68]
2. Glomerular disease usually is only a part of the overall clinical illness, although some patients may have clinical signs referable to significant proteinuria.
3. Prevalence of glomerular disease in dogs with neoplasia is unknown; however, in a study of 29 dogs with mastocytosis, 69% had glomerulitis at necropsy.[52] Pathologic findings included pericorpuscular infiltration of plasma cells, focal accumulations of an amorphous eosinophilic material in glomerular capillary basement membranes, and thickening of Bowman's capsule.
4. Some patients may develop glomerular disease secondary to treatment of neoplasia (see the following).[63]
5. Paraneoplastic disorders (e.g., hyperviscosity syndrome, erythrocytosis) could potentially cause glomerulopathy.[72]

E. Heredofamilial glomerular disease has been observed in dogs (see Table 26–2).[5,22,27,29,75,92] (For a more detailed review of these disorders, please see Chapter 24, Congenital, Inherited, and Familial Renal Diseases.)

F. Administration of certain drugs may be associated with glomerular disease.

1. Glucocorticoid excess, from either administration of corticosteroids or spontaneous hyperadrenocorticism, may predispose to development of glomerulonephritis.[20] Glucocorticoids may affect the solubility of immune complexes and delay clearance of complexes by the reticuloendothelial system.
2. A presumed glomerulopathy characterized by hypoalbuminemia and proteinuria occurred after administration of trimethoprim-sulfadiazine to one dog.[39] Other adverse effects associated with trimethoprim-sulfadiazine include polymyositis, focal retinitis, fever, anemia, leukopenia, and

thrombocytopenia. Doberman pinschers appear to be at risk for these adverse events, although other breeds may be affected.[39,61,91]

3. Administration of *Corynebacterium parvum* as adjuvant immunotherapy for a dog with cutaneous melanoma was associated with proliferative glomerulonephritis and chronic active hepatitis.[63]
4. Experimental administration of hydralazine to dogs was associated with signs of systemic involvement, including anemia, hyperglobulinemia, leukopenia, positive LE cell tests, and glomerulonephritis.[24]
5. Several drugs have been associated with glomerular disease in humans and should be considered potential causes of glomerulopathy in dogs and cats. These include gold salts, D-penicillamine, allopurinol, captopril, and nonsteroidal anti-inflammatory drugs.[37]
6. Vaccination has not been linked to glomerular diseases in dogs and cats, but this should be considered if historical and clinical findings suggest a cause-and-effect relationship.

IV. DISEASES ASSOCIATED WITH HEMODYNAMICALLY MEDIATED RENAL INJURY

A. Hemodynamically mediated injury generally has been considered an infrequent cause of clinically apparent renal disease in veterinary patients, although its importance is being recognized, especially in relation to its role in progression of chronic renal disease.[6,31,50,73]

1. Altered renal hemodynamics may occur with hyperperfusion (i.e., hyperfiltration) or hypoperfusion (i.e., hypofiltration).
2. Within the kidney, injury may affect glomeruli or tubules.
   a. Glomerulosclerosis is the end result of glomerular hyperfiltration.
   b. Acute tubular necrosis may occur secondary to inadequate renal perfusion.

B. Renal blood flow (RBF) and glomerular filtration rate (GFR) are regulated by complex and incompletely understood mechanisms.

1. The kidneys are capable of maintaining RBF and GFR at relatively constant values, despite changes in renal perfusion pressure. This phenomenon is called autoregulation.
2. Although changes in efferent (postglomerular) arteriolar resistance may contribute to autoregulation, maintenance of RBF and GFR primarily occurs via changes in afferent (preglomerular) arteriolar resistance.
3. Vasoconstriction of the afferent arteriole causes decreased RBF and GFR, whereas arteriolar vasodilation increases RBF and GFR.
4. For a complete review of renal autoregulatory mechanisms, see Chapter 2, Applied Physiology of the Kidney.

C. Disorders associated with hyperperfusion have been recognized infrequently in veterinary patients, although recent experimental studies have focused on the role of glomerular hyperfiltration in dogs with renal disease.[9,10,73]

1. Hyperfiltration has been documented in numerous experimental studies using renal ablation (i.e., remnant kidney model).[6,9,50,73]
   a. Early studies performed in rats revealed that after significant loss of renal function, surviving nephrons underwent structural and functional changes, including increased single-nephron GFR (i.e., hyperfiltration), increased glomerular capillary pressure (i.e., glomerular hypertension), and glomerular hypertrophy.[50,78] These changes lead to progressive glomerulosclerosis and nephron loss, which is characteristic of progressive renal disease in rats.
   b. Experimental studies have confirmed that glomerular hyperfiltration and hypertension occur in dogs and are associated with glomerular lesions.[9,10,11,73] However, the role of hyperfiltration in progression of canine renal failure has not been clearly established.[12,13]
2. Systemic hypertension may contribute to progression of renal disease by causing hyperfiltration and secondary glomerulosclerosis.
   a. In patients with normal renal function, afferent arteriolar activity generally prevents glomerular hypertension; however, systemic hypertension may contribute to glomerular hyperfiltration in patients with decreased amounts of nephrons.
   b. Hypertension often leads to chronic renal failure in humans, and antihypertensive therapy slows progression to end-stage renal failure.[16] Thus, although not proved in dogs and cats, systemic hypertension more than likely would contribute to the severity or the progressive nature of renal disease.
   c. For additional information on hypertension, see Chapter 19, Pathophysiology and Management of Systemic Hypertension Associated with Renal Dysfunction.
3. Diabetes mellitus frequently is associated with renal disease in humans. Diabetic nephropathy frequently is not recognized in veterinary patients, perhaps because of their shorter life span as compared with that of humans. The following brief review of diabetic nephropathy in humans is presented for comparative purposes.
   a. Insulin-dependent diabetes mellitus is characterized initially by increased GFR (hyperfiltration), which eventually progresses to glomerulosclerosis and renal failure in approximately 20 to 50% of diabetic humans.[51]
   b. Newly diagnosed diabetic patients have increased GFR, which may be 20 to 50% greater than normal. Their kidneys are also enlarged.

c. The cause of hyperfiltration and subsequent glomerulosclerosis is unknown, but it is thought to be associated with several factors.[31,37,51] Control of hyperglycemia by administration of insulin is associated with return of GFR to normal values in young diabetic patients.[51]

d. Onset of clinical diabetic nephropathy is defined as detection of protein in urine by routine dipstick analysis. In general, these patients have lived with diabetes mellitus for 10 to 30 years before diabetic nephropathy has been diagnosed.

e. The hallmark of the diabetic glomerulosclerotic lesion is generalized increase in mesangial matrix, usually accompanied by diffuse thickening of glomerular capillary walls.[51]

4. Miscellaneous conditions and drugs that cause glomerular hyperperfusion include high-protein diet, administration of amino acid solutions (hyperaminoacidemia) or glucose solutions (hyperglycemia), and drug therapy (α_2 antagonists, calcium channel blockers, dopamine).[8,11] A glomerulopathy characterized by glomerular hypertrophy and mesangial proliferation was diagnosed in a young kitten with a right-to-left cardiac shunt.[79] Suggested causes of glomerular disease in this case included hypoxia, polycythemia, hyperviscosity, and increased capillary blood flow.

D. Renal hypoperfusion can occur in a variety of situations, including systemic disorders, such as hypovolemia, decreased cardiac output, vasodilation, renal vasoconstriction, and thromboembolic disease (Table 26–6).[7,8,76,84] Renal hypoperfusion appears to be a less common cause of renal injury in veterinary patients than in humans; however, with increased use of certain pharmacologic agents (nonsteroidal anti-inflammatory drugs, angiotensin-converting enzyme inhibitors), prevalence of this type of renal injury may increase.

1. General perspectives.
   a. In patients with normal renal function, renal hypoperfusion usually is manifested as prerenal azotemia, which resolves rapidly following correction of the underlying cause.
   b. In contrast, patients with abnormal renal autoregulatory mechanisms (i.e., pre-existing renal disease) are more likely to sustain renal injury as a result of renal hypoperfusion.
2. Disorders associated with hypovolemia or low cardiac output may cause renal hypoperfusion. Patients with normal renal function rarely experience significant renal injury in these situations; however, intravascular volume and cardiac output should be corrected rapidly to avoid permanent renal injury, especially in patients with pre-existing renal disease.
3. Increased renal vascular resistance (i.e., renal vasoconstriction) may result from several disorders, of which the most clinically important is administration of drugs.[8]
   a. Angiotensin-converting enzyme inhibitors, such as captopril and enalapril, block production of angiotensin II, which causes efferent arteriolar dilation and decreased GFR.
   b. Administration of nonsteroidal anti-inflammatory drugs, such as aspirin, ibuprofen, and flunixin meglumine, reduces local production of renal vasodilatory prostaglandins, resulting in afferent arteriolar constriction and decreased GFR.[7] These drugs may cause acute renal failure, especially in patients with pre-existing renal disease or hypovolemia.[84]
   c. Amphotericin-B presumably causes afferent arteriolar constriction via tubuloglomerular feedback.

TABLE 26–6
DISORDERS ASSOCIATED WTH RENAL HYPOPERFUSION

Hypovolemia
- Dehydration: Vomiting, diarrhea, third space disorders (ascites, edema)
- Hypoalbuminemia
- Hemorrhage
- Hypoadrenocorticism

Decreased cardiac output
- Congestive heart failure: Mitral insufficiency, Cardiomyopathy
- Pericardial disease
- Cardiac arrhythmias

Renal vasoconstriction
- Sympathetic stimulation
- Hepatorenal syndrome
- Myoglobinuria
- Hemoglobinuria (intravascular hemolysis)
- Hypercalcemia
- Drugs: Angiotensin-converting enzyme inhibitors (captopril, enalapril), nonsteroid anti-inflammatory drugs (aspirin, ibuprofen), amphotericin B

Systemic vasodilation
- Anaphylaxis
- Inhalation anesthesia
- Septicemia
- Heat stroke
- Drugs (arteriolar dilators)

Thromboembolic disease
- Bacterial endocarditis
- Disseminated intravascular coagulation
- Nephrotic syndrome: Amyloidosis, glomerulonephritis

Hyperviscosity syndrome
- Polycythemia vera
- Hyperglobulinemia: Multiple myeloma, chronic lymphocytic leukemia, macroglobulinemia

4. Disorders associated with systemic vasodilation (e.g., heat stroke) may cause renal injury and acute renal failure in veterinary patients.[60]
5. Systemic thromboembolism may affect the renal vasculature, leading to hypoperfusion and renal injury.
   a. Septic emboli from left-sided bacterial endocarditis may cause renal infarction and acute renal failure.[14,32,80,87] The kidney is one of the most common organs that may be infarcted in dogs with bacterial endocarditis. In 1 study, approximately 75 to 80% of dogs had evidence of renal infarcts at necropsy.[14,80] Although the incidence of renal infarction is high, only 10% of dogs with bacterial endocarditis developed acute renal failure.[14]
   b. Renal vessel thrombosis also may occur in patients with systemic coagulopathies and disorders associated with a hypercoagulable state, such as nephrotic syndrome.[28,81] Acute renal failure may occur in dogs with disseminated intravascular coagulation, presumably secondary to thrombosis and renal ischemia (personal observation).
6. Conditions that cause hyperviscosity (i.e., increased red cell mass or hyperglobulinemia) can potentially lead to renal hypoperfusion and injury, although this possibility has not been documented in veterinary patients.

V. DISEASES ASSOCIATED WITH RENAL INJURY BY SUBSTANCES

A. General concepts.

1. Polysystemic diseases can cause renal injury mediated by pigments (myoglobin, hemoglobin), crystals (oxalate, calcium), and insoluble proteins (amyloid, Bence Jones proteins).
2. The site and type of renal injury vary with the substance involved.
   a. Acute tubular necrosis may occur in association with pigment nephropathies and injury secondary to crystal formation. (See Chapter 21, Canine and Feline Hypercalcemic Nephropathy, for a complete review of this disorder.)
   b. Renal injury secondary to amyloidosis varies with species and breed.
      (1). Amyloid deposits in dogs usually cause protein-losing glomerulopathy, although significant medullary amyloidosis occurs in the Chinese Shar pei.[27]
      (2). Medullary amyloid deposition in cats progresses to chronic renal failure, and sometimes papillary necrosis.
      (3). Please see Chapter 20, Renal Amyloidosis, for a complete review of this disorder.
   c. In humans, immunoglobulin light chains (i.e., Bence Jones proteins) may act as a direct tubular toxin, or they may precipitate within tubular lumens, causing intrarenal obstruction.[82]

TABLE 26–7
DISORDERS ASSOCIATED WITH MYOGLOBINURIA AND HEMOGLOBINURIA IN DOGS AND CATS

Myoglobinuria
Crush injuries (severe muscle trauma)
Hypokalemia (experimental)
Severe hypophosphatemia (experimental)
Status epilepticus
Exertional rhabdomyolysis
Malignant hyperthermia
Myositis
Hemoglobinuria
Immune-mediated hemolytic anemia
Babesiosis
Heinz body hemolytic anemia: Acetaminophen toxicosis (cats), onions, benzocaine, vitamin K_3, methylene blue, phenazopyridine
Incompatible blood transfusion
Severe hypophosphatemia (< 1 mg/dl)
Phosphosfructokinase deficiency (English springer spaniel, cocker spaniel)
Zinc toxicosis
Copper toxicosis (hepatic copper storage disease)
Heat stroke
Heartworm caval syndrome
Disseminated intravascular coagulation
Hemangiosarcoma
Splenic torsion

B. Rarely are pigments associated with clinically significant renal injury in dogs and cats.

1. Myoglobinuria generally is secondary to rhabdomyolysis, a rare condition in dogs and cats.[1,36,58,59,83]
   a. Severe muscle injury and necrosis cause leakage of myoglobin, which is poorly protein bound and therefore rapidly filtered through glomeruli into the urine.
   b. A single case report describes acute renal failure in a dog secondary to seizure-induced rhabdomyolysis.[83] Renal histologic lesions consisted primarily of acute tubular necrosis.
   c. Electrolyte disturbances may potentiate rhabdomyolysis and myoglobinuria, especially in patients with pre-existing muscle disease.
      (1). Muscle necrosis has been produced experimentally in dogs as a result of concurrent potassium depletion and electrically stimulated muscle exercise.[58]
      (2). Experimentally induced hypophosphatemia (< 1.0 mg/dl) has been shown to cause rhabdomyolysis in dogs.[59]
2. Hemoglobinuria is more common than myoglobinuria and usually is associated with disorders that cause intravascular hemolysis (Table 26–7).
3. The mechanism by which pigments cause acute

renal failure is unknown, but it appears to depend on extracellular fluid volume and urine pH.[34]

a. Both myoglobin and hemoglobin are dissociated to ferrihemate (hematin) and a globin moiety at or below a urine pH of 5.6.[1]
b. Hematin is suspected to be the toxic component of pigment-induced nephropathy. Intravenous administration of hematin to dogs causes severe tubular necrosis.[1]
c. Nephrotoxicosis is apparently most likely to develop when either myoglobinuria or hemoglobinuria occurs with disorders that decrease urine pH and renal perfusion (e.g., dehydration, hypovolemia, acidosis).[34]

4. Pigment-induced renal injury should be suspected when acute renal failure occurs in patients with disorders that are associated with myoglobinuria and hemoglobinuria (see Table 26–7).
   a. Urinalysis findings include reddish-brown urine and positive occult blood reaction (dipstick analysis) in the absence of hematuria. Other findings may include cylindruria and isosthenuria or minimally concentrated urine (specific gravity < 1.025).
   b. Evaluation of serum color may help to distinguish which pigment is present; with hemoglobinuria serum, usually is pink, whereas with myoglobinuria it is clear.
   c. Serum activities of creatine kinase, lactic dehydrogenase, alanine aminotransferase, and aspartate transaminase usually are increased in patients with myoglobinuria.
   d. Evidence of intravascular hemolysis (e.g., regenerative anemia, autoagglutination) should be sought if hemoglobinuria is suspected.
5. Treatment of pigment-induced renal disease is aimed at correcting the underlying cause. In addition, supportive care should be given to patients with acute renal failure. (See Chapter 22, Acute Renal Failure: Ischemic and Chemical Nephrosis, and Chapter 28, Conservative Medical Management of Chronic Renal Failure, for a more detailed review of treatment.)

C. Multiple myeloma often is associated with renal disease in humans[23,33,82] and it may be in veterinary patients also.[15,66,71]

1. Renal histologic findings in dogs with multiple myeloma include proteinaceous tubular casts as well as interstitial accumulation of plasma cells.[15,66,71] "Myeloma kidney" of humans, characterized by dense eosinophilic tubular casts that contain paraproteins, albumin, and immunoglobulin,[33] has not been described in veterinary patients.
2. Renal failure in human myeloma patients often occurs in association with Bence Jones proteins, although not all patients with renal failure have Bence Jones proteinuria.
3. Other factors that may contribute to renal injury in human and veterinary patients with multiple myeloma include dehydration, hypercalcemia, and systemic infection.[33]
4. Diagnosis of multiple myeloma is based on the finding of at least two of four criteria:[65]
   a. Monoclonal hyperglobulinemia.
   b. Plasma cell infiltration of bone marrow.
   c. Immunoglobulin light chains (Bence Jones proteins) detected by immunoelectrophoresis of urine.
   d. Multiple osteolytic skeletal lesions.
5. Treatment includes chemotherapy for multiple myeloma[65] and medical management if renal failure is present. To lessen the likelihood of renal injury, associated abnormalities, such as dehydration, infection, and hypercalcemia, should be promptly corrected.

REFERENCES

1. Anderson WAD, Morrison DB, Williams EF. Pathologic changes following injections of ferrhemate (hematin) in dogs. *Arch Pathol.* 1942; 33:589–602.
2. Barlough JE, Stoddart CA. Feline coronaviral infections. In: Greene CE, ed. *Clinical Microbiology and Infectious Diseases of the Dog and Cat.* Philadelphia, Pennsylvania: WB Saunders; 1990.
3. Barsanti JA. Coccidioidomycosis. In: Greene CE, ed. *Infectious Diseases of the Dog and Cat.* Philadelphia, Pennsylvania: WB Saunders; 1990.
4. Barsanti JA. Histoplasmosis. In: Greene CE, ed. *Clinical Microbiology and Infectious Diseases of the Dog and Cat.* Philadelphia, Pennsylvania: WB Saunders; 1983.
5. Bernard MA, Vali VE. Familial renal disease in Samoyed dogs. *Can Vet J.* 1977; 18:181–189.
6. Brenner BM, Meyer TW, Hostetter TH. Dietary protein intake and the progressive nature of renal disease: The role of hemodynamically mediated glomerular injury in the pathogenesis of progressive glomerular sclerosis in aging, renal ablation, and instrinsic renal disease. *N Engl J Med.* 1982; 302:652–659.
7. Brown SA. Renal effects of nonsteroidal anti-inflammatory drugs. In: Kirk RW, ed. *Current Veterinary Therapy.* Vol 10. Philadelphia, Pennsylvania: WB Saunders; 1989.
8. Brown SA, Barsanti JA, Finco DR. Effects of vasoactive agents on kidney function. In: Kirk RW, Bonagura JD, eds. *Kirk's Current Veterinary Therapy.* Vol 11. Philadelphia, Pennsylvania: WB Saunders; 1992.
9. Brown SA, Finco DR, Crowell WA, et al. Single-nephron adaptations to partial renal ablation in the dog. *Am J Physiol.* 1990; 258:F495–F503.
10. Brown SA, Finco DR, Crowell WA, et al. Dietary protein intake and the glomerular adaptations to partial nephrectomy in dogs. *J Nutr.* 1991; 121:S125–S127.
11. Brown SA, Navar LG. Single-nephron responses to systemic administration of amino acids in dogs. *Am J Physiol.* 1990; 259:F739–F746.
12. Brown SA. Dietary protein restriction: Some unanswered questions. *Semin Vet Med Surg.* 1992; 7:237–243.
13. Brown SA, Crowell WA, Barsanti JA, et al. Beneficial effects of dietary mineral restriction in dogs with marked reduction of functional renal mass. *J Am Soc Nephrol.* 1991; 1:1169–1179.
14. Calvert CA. Valvular bacterial endocarditis in the dog. *J Am Vet Med Assoc.* 1982; 180:1080–1084.

15. Campbell KL, Latimer KS. Polysystemic manifestations of plasma cell myeloma in the dog: A case report and review. *J Am Anim Hosp Assoc.* 1985; 21:59–66.
16. Campese VM, Karubian F. Renal consequences of salt and hypertension. *Semin Nephrol.* 1991; 11:549–560.
17. Carmichael LE, Greene CE. Canine herpesvirus infection. In: Greene CE, ed. *Infectious Diseases of the Dog and Cat.* Philadelphia, Pennsylvania: WB Saunders; 1990.
18. Carmichael LE, Greene CE. Canine brucellosis. In: Greene CE, ed. *Infectious Diseases of the Dog and Cat.* Philadelphia, Pennsylvania: WB Saunders; 1990.
19. Casey HW, Splitter GA. Membranous glomerulonephritis in dogs infected with *Dirofilaria immitis. Vet Pathol.* 1975; 12:111–117.
20. Center SA, Smith CA, Wilkinson E, et al. Clinicopathologic renal immunofluorescent and light microscopic features of glomerulonephritis in the dog: 41 cases (1975–1985). *J Am Vet Med Assoc.* 1987; 190:81–90.
21. Chew DJ, DiBartola SP. Diagnosis and pathophysiology of renal disease. In: Ettinger SJ, ed. *Textbook of Veterinary Internal Medicine.* Philadelphia, Pennsylvania: WB Saunders; 1989.
22. Chew DJ, et al. Juvenile renal disease in Doberman pinscher dogs. *J Am Vet Med Assoc.* 1983; 182:481–485.
23. Cohen DJ, Sherman WH, Osserman EF, et al. Acute renal failure in patients with multiple myeloma. *Am J Med.* 1984; 76:247–256.
24. Commens P. Experimental hydralazine disease and its similarity to disseminated lupus erythematosus. *J Lab Clin Med.* 1956; 47:444–454.
25. Day MJ, Penhale WJ, Eger CE, et al. Disseminated aspergillosis in dogs. *Aust Vet J.* 1986; 63:55–59.
26. DiBartola SP, Rutgers HC, Zack PM, et al. Clinicopathologic findings associated with chronic renal disease in cats: 74 cases (1973–1984). *J Am Vet Med Assoc.* 1987; 190:1196–1202.
27. DiBartola SP, Tarr MJ, Webb DM, et al. Familial renal amyloidosis in Chinese Shar pei dogs. *J Am Vet Med Assoc.* 1990; 197:483–487.
28. DiBartola SP, Tarr ML, Parker AT, et al. Clinicopathologic findings in dogs with renal amyloidosis: 59 cases (1976–1986). *J Am Vet Med Assoc.* 1989; 195:358–364.
29. DiBartola SP, Davenport DJ, Chew DJ. Renal failure in young dogs. In: Kirk RW, ed. *Current Veterinary Therapy.* Vol. 10. Philadelphia, Pennsylvania: WB Saunders; 1989.
30. Drazner FH. Systemic lupus erythematosus in the dog. *Compend Contin Educ Pract Vet.* 1980; 11:243–254.
31. Dunn BR, Anderson S, Brenner BM. The hemodynamic basis of progressive renal disease. *Semin Nephrol.* 1986; 6:122–138.
32. Ellison GW, King RW, Calderwood-Mays M. Medical and surgical management of multiple organ infarctions secondary to bacterial endocarditis in a dog. *J Am Vet Med Assoc.* 1988; 193:1289–1291.
33. Fer MF, McKinney TD, Richardson RL, et al. Cancer and the kidney: Renal complications of neoplasms. *Am J Med.* 1981; 71:704–718.
34. Flamenbaum W, Gehr M, Gross M, et al. Acute renal failure associated with myoglobinuria and hemoglobinuria. In: Brenner BM, Lazarus JM, eds. *Acute Renal Failure.* Philadelphia, Pennsylvania: WB Saunders; 1983.
35. Forrester SD, Lees GE. Acute renal failure associated with systemic infectious disease. In: Kirk RW, Bonagura JD, eds. *Kirk's Current Veterinary Therapy.* Philadelphia, Pennsylvania: WB Saunders; 1992.
36. Gannon JR. Exertional rhabdomyolysis (myoglobinuria) in the racing greyhound. In: Kirk RW, ed. *Current Veterinary Therapy.* Vol 7. Philadelphia, Pennsylvania: WB Saunders; 1980.
37. Glasscock RJ, Cohen AH, Adler SG, et al. Secondary glomerular diseases. In: Brenner BM, Rector FC, eds. *The Kidney.* 4th ed. Philadelphia, Pennsylvania: WB Saunders; 1991.
38. Glick AD, Horn RG, Holscher M. Characterization of feline glomerulonephritis associated with viral-induced hematopoietic neoplasms. *Am J Pathol.* 1978; 92:321–327.
39. Giger U, Werner LL, Millichamp NJ, et al. Sulfadiazine-induced allergy in six Doberman pinschers. *J Am Vet Med Assoc.* 1985; 186:479–484.
40. Grauer GF. Glomerulonephritis. *Semin Vet Med Surg.* 1992; 7: 187–197.
41. Grauer GF, Burgess EC, Cooley AJ, et al. Renal lesions associated with *Borrelia burgdorferi* infection in a dog. *J Am Vet Med Assoc.* 1988; 193:237–239.
42. Grauer GF, Culham CA, Cooley AJ, et al. Clinicopathologic and histologic evaluation of *Dirofilaria immitis*–induced nephropathy in dog. *Am J Trop Med Hygiene.* 1987; 37:588–596.
43. Greene CE, Shotts EB. Leptospirosis. In: Greene CE, ed. *Infectious Diseases of the Dog and Cat.* Philadelphia, Pennsylvania: WB Saunders; 1990.
44. Greene CE, Breitschwerdt EB. Rocky Mountain spotted fever and Q fever. In: Greene CE, ed. *Infectious Diseases of the Dog and Cat.* Philadelphia, Pennsylvania: WB Saunders; 1990.
45. Greene CE. Infectious canine hepatitis and canine acidophil cell hepatitis. In: Greene CE, ed. *Infectious Diseases of the Dog and Cat.* Philadelphia, Pennsylvania: WB Saunders; 1990.
46. Greene CE, Chandler FW. Candidiasis. In: Greene CE, ed. *Infectious Diseases of the Dog and Cat.* Philadelphia, Pennsylvania: WB Saunders; 1990.
47. Greene CE. Mycobacterial infections. In: Greene CE, ed. *Infectious Diseases of the Dog and Cat.* Philadelphia, Pennsylvania: WB Saunders; 1990.
48. Grindem CB, Johnson KH. Systemic lupus erythematosus: Literature review and report of 42 new canine cases. *J Am Anim Hosp Assoc.* 1983; 19:489–503.
49. Hayashi T, Ishida T, Fujiwara K. Glomerulonephritis associated with feline infectious peritonitis. *Jpn J Vet Sci.* 1982; 44:909–916.
50. Hostetter TH, Olson, Rennke HG, et al. Hyperfiltration in remnant nephrons: A potentially adverse response to renal ablation. *Am J Physiol.* 1981; 241:F85–F93.
51. Hostetter TH. Diabetic nephropathy. In: Brenner BM, Rector FC, eds. *The Kidney.* 4th ed. Vol II. Philadelphia, Pennsylvania: WB Saunders; 1991.
52. Hottendorf GH, Nielsen SW. Pathologic report of 29 necropsies on dogs with mastocytoma. *Vet Pathol.* 1968; 5:102–121.
53. Jeraj KP, Hardy R, O'Leary TP, et al. Immune complex glomerulonephritis in a cat with renal lymphosarcoma. *Vet Pathol.* 1985; 22:287–290.
54. Johnson ME, DiBartola SP, Gelberg HB. Nephrotic syndrome and pericholangiohepatitis in a cat. *J Am Anim Hosp Assoc.* 1983; 19:191–196.
55. Kabay MJ, Robinson WF, Huxtable CRR, et al. The pathology of disseminated *Aspergillus terreus* infection in dogs. *Vet Pathol.* 1985; 22:540–547.
56. Kass PH, Strombeck DR, Farver TB, et al. Application of the log-linear model in the prediction of the antinuclear antibody test in the dog. *Am J Vet Res.* 1985; 46:2336–2339.
57. Kass PH, Farver TB, Strombeck DR, et al. Application of the log-linear and logistic regression models in the prediction of systemic lupus erythematosus in the dog. *Am J Vet Res.* 1985; 46:2340–2345.
58. Knochel JP, Schlein EM. On the mechanism of rhabdomyolysis in potassium depletion. *J Clin Invest.* 1972; 51:1750–1758.
59. Knochel JP, Barcenas C, Cotton JR, et al. Hypophosphatemia and rhabdomyolysis. *J Clin Invest.* 1978; 62:1240–1246.

60. Krum SH, Osborne CA. Heatstroke in the dog: A polysystemic disorder. *J Am Vet Med Assoc.* 1977; 170:531–535.
61. Lees GE, Rogers KS, Troy GC. Polyarthritis associated with sulfadiazine administration in a Labrador retriever dog. *Southwest Vet.* 1986; 37:13–17.
62. Legendre AM. Blastomycosis. In: Greene CE, ed. *Infectious Diseases of the Dog and Cat.* Philadelphia, Pennsylvania: WB Saunders; 1990.
63. Leifer CE, Page RL, Matus RE, et al. Proliferative glomerulonephritis and chronic active hepatitis with cirrhosis associated with *Corynebacterium parvum* immunotherapy in a dog. *J Am Vet Med Assoc.* 1987; 190:78–80.
64. Lucke VM. Glomerulonephritis in the cat. *Vet Annu.* 1982; 22:270–278.
65. MacEwen EG, Hurvitz AI. Diagnosis and management of monoclonal gammopathies. *Vet Clin North Am.* 1977; 7:119–132.
66. Miller C, Fish MB, Danelski TF. IgA multiple myeloma with multi-system manifestations in the dog: A case report. *J Am Anim Hosp Assoc.* 1982; 18:53–56.
67. Moise NS, Crissman JW, Fairbrother JF. Mycoplasma gateae arthritis and tenosynovitis in cats: Case report and experimental production of the disease. *Am J Vet Res.* 1983;44:16–21.
68. Murray M, Wright NG. A morphologic study of canine glomerulonephritis. *Lab Invest.* 1974; 30:213–221.
69. Osborne CA, Hammer RF, O'Leary TP, et al. Renal manifestations of canine dirofilariasis. In: *Proc American Heartworm Symposium.* Veterinary Medical Publishing Co; Edwardsville, Kansas: 1981: 67–92.
70. Osborne CA, Vernier RL. Glomerulonephritis in the dog and cat: A comparative review. *J Am Anim Hosp Assoc.* 1973; 9:101–127.
71. Osborne CA, Perman V, Sautter JH, et al. Multiple myeloma in the dog. *J Am Vet Med Assoc.* 1968; 153:1300–1319.
72. Page RL, Stiff ME, McEntee MC, et al. Transient glomerulonephropathy associated with primary erythrocytosis in a dog. *J Am Vet Med Assoc.* 1990; 196:620–622.
73. Polzin DJ, Leininger JR, Osborne CA, et al. Development of renal lesions in dogs after 11/12 reduction of renal mass. *Lab Invest.* 1988; 58:172–183.
74. Rentko VT, Clark N, Ross LA, et al. Canine leptospirosis: A retrospective study of 17 cases. *J Vet Intern Med.* 1985; 6:235–244.
75. Reusch C, Liehs M, Bren G, et al. A new familial membranoproliferative glomerulonephritis in Bernese mountain dogs. *J Vet Intern Med.* 6:120, 1992 (abstr).
76. Schelling JR, Linas SL: Hepatorenal syndrome. *Semin Nephrol.* 1990; 10:565–570.
77. Scott DW, Walton DK, Manning TO, et al. Canine lupus erythematosus. I. Systemic lupus erythematosus. *J Am Anim Hosp Assoc.* 1983; 19:461–479.
78. Shimamura T, Morrison AB. A progressive glomerulosclerosis occurring in partial five-sixths nephrectomized rats. *Am J Pathol.* 1975; 79:95–106.
79. Shirota K, Saitoh Y, Une Y, et al. Glomerulopathy in a cat with cyanotic congenital heart disease. *Vet Pathol.* 1987; 24:280–282.
80. Sisson D, Thomas WP. Endocarditis of the aortic valve in the dog. *J Am Vet Med Assoc.* 1984; 184:570–577.
81. Slauson DO, Gribble DH. Thrombosis complicating renal amyloidosis in dogs. *Vet Pathol.* 1971; 8:352–363.
82. Solomon A. Clinical implications of monoclonal light chains. *Semin Oncol.* 1986; 13:341–349.
83. Spangler WL, Muggli FM. Seizure-induced rhabdomyolysis accompanied by acute renal failure in a dog. *J Am Vet Med Assoc.* 1978; 172:1190–1194.
84. Spyridakis LK, Bacia JJ, Barsanti JA, et al. Ibuprofen toxicosis in a dog. *J Am Vet Med Assoc.* 1986; 188:918–919.
85. Stampley AR, Barsanti JA. Disseminated cryptococcosis in a dog. *J Am Anim Hosp Assoc.* 1988; 24:17–21.
86. Szabo JR, Pang V, Shadduck JA. Encephalitozoonosis. In: Greene CE, ed. *Infectious Diseases of the Dog and Cat.* Philadelphia, Pennsylvania: WB Saunders; 1990.
87. Toboada J, Palmer GH. Renal failure associated with bacterial endocarditis in the dog. *J Am Anim Hosp Assoc.* 1989; 25:243–251.
88. Troy GC, Forrester SD. Canine ehrlichiosis. In: Greene CE, ed. *Infectious Diseases of the Dog and Cat.* Philadelphia, Pennsylvania: WB Saunders; 1990.
89. Tyler DE. Protothecosis. In: Greene CE, ed. *Infectious Diseases of the Dog and Cat.* Philadelphia, Pennsylvania: WB Saunders; 1990.
90. Vaden SL, Grauer GF. Medical management of canine glomerulonephritis. In: Kirk RW, Bonagura JD, eds. *Kirk's Current Veterinary Therapy.* Philadelphia, Pennsylvania: WB Saunders; 1992.
91. Werner LL, Bright JM. Drug-induced immune hypersensitivity disorders in two dogs treated with trimethoprim sulfadiazine: Case reports and drug challenge studies. *J Am Anim Hosp Assoc.* 1983; 19:783–790.
92. Wilcock BP, Patterson JM. Familial glomerulonephritis in Doberman pinscher dogs. *Can Vet J.* 1979; 20:244–249.
93. Willard MD, Krehbiel JD, Schmidt GM, et al. Serum and urine protein abnormalities associated with lymphocytic leukemia and glomerulonephritis in a dog. *J Am Anim Hosp Assoc.* 1981; 17:381–386.
94. Wilson CB. The renal response to immunologic injury. In: Brenner BM, Rector FC, eds. *The Kidney.* 4th ed. Philadelphia, Pennsylvania: WB Saunders; 1991.

CHAPTER 27

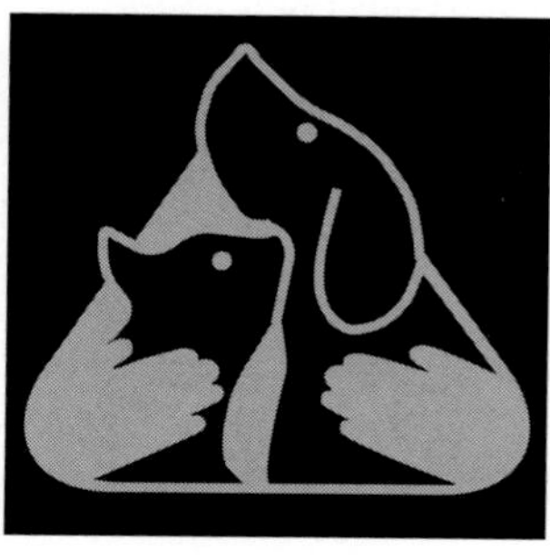

Prognosis of Renal Disease, Renal Failure, and Uremia

DAVID J. POLZIN
CARL A. OSBORNE

I. DEFINITIONS

A. Prognosis.

1. Prognosis is a forecast as to the prospect of recovery from a disease as indicated by the nature and clinical signs of the disease.
2. With regard to renal failure, short-term and long-term prognoses are helpful.
   a. Short-term prognosis refers to the probability of amelioration of signs and survival during the first several days or weeks of illness.
   b. Long-term prognosis refers to the probability of progressive derangements in renal structure and function resulting in uremia and death over the subsequent months to years.
   c. Prognoses should be offered in the context of outcomes with and without treatment.
3. Ideally, prognoses should be provided in quantitative terms. However, quantitative data on prognoses are often not available. Because use of qualitative terms for prognoses has been correctly criticized as being ambiguous,[1] guidelines defining commonly used quantitative terms are provided in Table 27-1.[2]

B. See Chapter 16, Pathophysiology of Renal Failure and Uremia.

II. MULTIPLE FACTORS INFLUENCE THE PROGNOSIS OF PATIENTS WITH RENAL FAILURE. AMONG THE MOST IMPORTANT FACTORS ARE ETIOPATHOGENESIS OF RENAL FAILURE, SEVERITY OF RENAL FAILURE, REVERSIBILITY OF RENAL LESIONS, AND THE PROGRESSIVE NATURE OF THE RENAL DISEASE. NO SINGLE FACTOR CONSISTENTLY PROVIDES AN ADEQUATE BASIS FOR PROGNOSIS; ACCURATE PROGNOSIS REQUIRES CONSIDERATION OF ALL THESE FACTORS.

A. Etiopathogenesis of renal failure.

1. Prerenal and postrenal renal failure and uremia
   a. Early correction of prerenal and postrenal renal failure occurring in the absence of primary renal failure should be expected to result in complete resolution of uremia without significant renal injury. Prognosis depends largely on the reversibility and biologic behavior of the primary disease process responsible for inducing prerenal or postrenal renal failure. Development of renal injury secondary to prerenal or postrenal causes may adversely affect the prognosis.
   b. Diagnosis of prerenal renal failure is usually established on the basis of the medical history, physical examination, and urinalysis. Except with certain glomerulopathies, primary renal failure can usually be excluded by demonstrating that urine specific gravity values exceed 1.030 in azotemic dogs and 1.035 in azotemic cats.
   c. Diagnosis of postrenal renal failure can usually

TABLE 27–1
DEFINITION OF PROGNOSTIC TERMS

Term	Prediction of Recovery (%)
Excellent	75–100
Good	50–75
Guarded	50
Poor	25–50
Grave	0–25

(From Osborne C, Lulich J. Prognosis: Guidelines for sentencing patients. In: Kirk R, Bonagura J, eds. *Current Veterinary Therapy XI: Small Animal Practice.* Philadelphia, Pennsylvania: WB Saunders Co; 1992:2-5.)

be established on the basis of the physical examination or by radiography.

d. The contribution of prerenal causes to azotemia can often be established by monitoring the response to therapy designed to correct the prerenal cause (e.g., fluid therapy to correct dehydration or hypovolemia [Fig. 27-1]).

2. Primary renal failure

a. Knowledge that azotemia results from primary renal failure does not provide an adequate basis for prognosis because the prognosis of primary renal failure is variable, depending on the cause of renal injury.[3] Knowledge of the etiopathogenesis of primary renal failure contributes greatly to establishing prognosis. For example, acute tubular necrosis induced by gentamicin nephrotoxicity typically does not progress to chronic renal failure. Patients that survive the acute episode of renal failure often recover fully. In contrast, renal amyloidosis is almost invariably a progressive disease that ultimately leads to death of the patient. Specific therapy for active renal disease may profoundly affect both short-term and long-term prognoses. Unfortunately, the cause of primary renal failure commonly remains obscure. In such instances, other factors must be considered in establishing a prognosis.

b. Diagnosis of primary renal failure is accomplished by eliminating prerenal and postrenal causes for azotemia. Inadequate urine concentration in an unobstructed, azotemic patient suggests primary renal failure. Further support for the diagnosis may be provided by radiography, ultrasonography, and renal biopsy.

B. Severity of renal failure.

1. Magnitude of azotemia

a. Prognoses should not be established on the basis of a single determination of blood urea nitrogen (BUN) or serum creatinine (SC). Although the assumption that prognosis should be inversely related to the magnitude of azotemia appears logical, this assumption can be misleading. Concentrations of BUN and SC may be influenced by prerenal, postrenal, and nonrenal factors that may be correctable. The severity of underlying renal dysfunction can only be established after eliminating the effects of these other factors.

b. Serial determination of BUN and SC may provide useful information in establishing response to therapy and progressivity and reversibility of renal lesions. These factors are of substantially greater prognostic significance than is the magnitude of azotemia per se.

c. No specific values exist for BUN or SC above which the prognosis can reliably be stated to be hopeless.

(1). No specific values exist for BUN or SC that indicate irreversible renal injury in patients with acute renal failure. Reversibility of acute renal failure is best established by determining response to therapy (Fig. 27-1). In selected cases, renal biopsy may be used as a guide to reversibility of primary renal injury.

(2). No specific values exist for BUN or SC that indicate that renal failure will be progres-

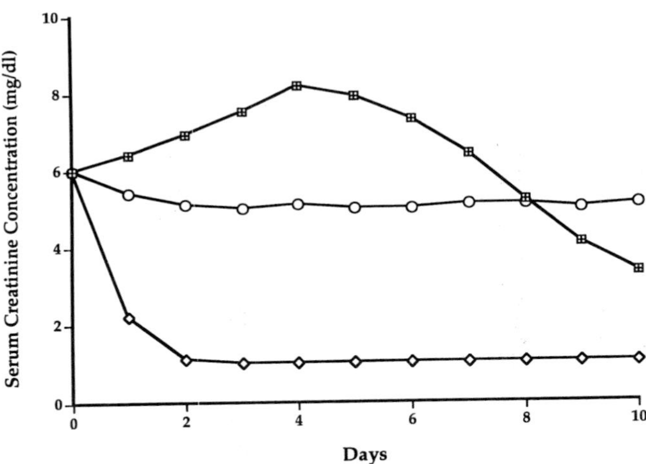

FIG. 27–1. The effect of intravenous fluid therapy on serum creatinine concentrations in three dehydrated azotemic dogs (sufficient fluid is administered on day 0 to correct dehydration and circulating fluid volume depletion). Correcting volume depletion caused by dehydration rapidly and completely corrects azotemia in dogs with prerenal azotemia (diamonds). Azotemia may progress despite correction of prerenal factors in dogs with acute renal failure caused by acute tubular necrosis (squares), but azotemia may later decline because of reversibility of the primary renal injury. Azotemia in dogs with chronic renal failure may improve somewhat after correction of the prerenal component of azotemia induced by dehydration (circles), but azotemia persists as a result of irreversible primary renal failure.

sive or that symptomatic, supportive, and palliative therapy cannot ameliorate clinical signs. The progressive nature of renal failure and response to therapy must be determined individually for each patient.

2. Urine output
   a. In patients with acute renal failure, pathologic oliguria usually indicates severe renal injury and is a negative prognostic indicator.
      (1). Given sufficient supportive care and time, some patients with oliguric acute renal failure recover adequate renal function.
      (2). Pathologic oliguria must be differentiated from physiologic oliguria that results from prerenal causes, usually volume contraction. Physiologic oliguria that resolves when the cause for poor renal perfusion is corrected is not associated with a negative prognosis.
   b. Nonoliguria generally indicates less severe renal injury than does oliguria in patients with acute renal failure and should generally be interpreted as a favorable prognostic finding in this setting.
   c. Pathologic oliguria detected during the end stage of chronic renal failure is typically a grave prognostic sign.
3. Clinical signs of uremia
   a. Severity of uremic signs is often a relatively good predictor of short-term prognosis. Patients without clinical signs of uremia usually have a good to excellent short-term prognosis. Patients with severe clinical signs of uremia typically have a poor short-term prognosis.
   b. When signs of uremia are present, one should determine whether clinical signs can be ameliorated and renal function can be therapeutically improved before establishing the short-term prognosis. A uremic crisis often occurs in patients with chronic renal failure as a consequence of superimposed acute renal failure or prerenal or postrenal conditions. If treatment improves renal function and ameliorates clinical signs of uremia, the short-term prognosis may be upgraded from guarded to good.

C. Reversibility of renal lesions.

1. Depending on the extent and severity of renal lesions, acute renal failure may be a reversible condition. Reversibility of the loss of renal function may result from healing of primary renal injuries and from compensatory adaptations in structure and function that may develop in the days to weeks following acute renal injury. Compensatory adaptations are largely complete within 2 to 3 months after acute renal injury. Reversibility is best established by serial monitoring of renal function, but findings obtained by renal biopsy may also provide useful prognostic information in this setting.
2. Chronic renal failure is an irreversible condition; patients do not "recover" from chronic renal failure. However, renal function may improve and clinical signs may be ameliorated by correcting prerenal or postrenal factors, treating active renal disease, and eliminating complicating conditions, such as urinary tract infection. Unlike acute renal failure, the capacity for compensatory adaptations has already been largely exhausted in chronic renal failure. Thus, prognosis for patients with chronic renal failure does not refer to recovery of normal renal function.

D. Progressive nature of renal failure.

1. A progressive decline in renal function appears to occur in at least some patients with chronic renal failure. The long-term prognosis for patients with chronic renal failure is therefore largely determined by the progressive nature of the patient's disease. Progression may be influenced by the underlying renal disorder, complications of renal failure (e.g., systemic hypertension, urinary tract infection), compensatory renal adaptations, and treatment.
2. Establishing the long-term outcome of chronic renal failure in dogs and cats is complicated by lack of knowledge concerning the natural course of specific primary renal diseases in these species and by the frequency with which an etiopathologic diagnosis is not established. Therefore, the course of renal failure should be established for each individual patient by serially monitoring renal function (over months to years). Renal function may remain stable or only slowly decline in some dogs and cats with chronic renal failure. However, decrements in renal function may occur in a progressive predictable pattern or in an unpredictable step-wise pattern. Thus, stable renal function over several months may not exclude the possibility of further decline in renal function later.
3. A pattern of progressively declining renal function does not typically occur subsequent to clinical recovery from acute tubular necrosis unless renal damage is largely irreversible and chronic renal failure ensues.

REFERENCES

1. Crow S. Usefulness of prognoses: Qualitative versus quantitative designations. *J Am Vet Med Assoc.* 1985;187:700-703.
2. Osborne C, Lulich J. Prognosis: Guidelines for sentencing patients. In: Kirk R, Bonagura J, eds. *Current Veterinary Therapy XI: Small Animal Practice.* Philadelphia, Pennsylvania: WB Saunders; 1992:2-5.
3. Finco D. Prognosis of renal failure. In: Kirk R, ed. *Current Veterinary Therapy VI.* Philadelphia, Pennsylvania: WB Saunders; 1977: 1130-1133.

CHAPTER 28

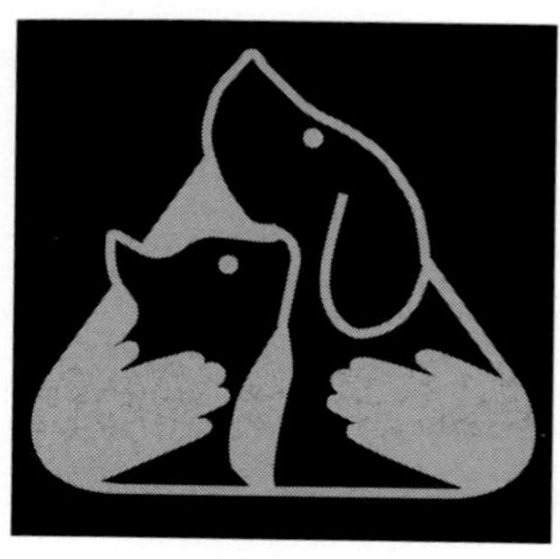

Conservative Medical Management of Chronic Renal Failure

DAVID J. POLZIN
CARL A. OSBORNE

I. CONSERVATIVE MEDICAL MANAGEMENT OF CHRONIC RENAL FAILURE (CRF) CONSISTS OF SUPPORTIVE, SYMPTOMATIC, AND PALLIATIVE THERAPY DESIGNED TO MINIMIZE THE CLINICAL AND PATHOPHYSIOLOGIC CONSEQUENCES OF REDUCED RENAL FUNCTION

A. The goals of conservative medical management of patients with chronic primary renal failure are to: 1) ameliorate clinical signs of uremia; 2) minimize disturbances associated with excesses or losses of water, electrolytes, vitamins, and minerals; 3) support adequate nutrition; and 4) slow progression of renal failure.

1. These goals are best achieved when therapeutic recommendations are individualized to patient needs based on clinical and laboratory findings.
2. Because CRF is dynamic and often progressive, serial clinical and laboratory assessment of the patient, and subsequent modification of the therapy in response to changes in the patient's condition, is an integral part of conservative medical management.
3. Conservative medical management is intended for patients with compensated CRF. It is not intended for patients unable to eat or accept oral medications because of severe uremia.
4. The components of conservative medical management are summarized in Table 28-1.

B. Conservative medical management is most beneficial when combined with specific therapy directed at correcting the primary cause of renal disease.

1. Specific therapy of renal disease consists of therapy designed to slow or stop development of renal lesions by influencing the etiopathogenic processes responsible for the lesions.
2. Although determining the initiating disease process in dogs and cats with CRF is frequently difficult or impossible, the value of formulating specific therapy based on an etiologic/pathologic diagnosis should not be overlooked.
   a. Progression of renal lesions, and thus renal failure, may be slowed or stopped by therapy designed to eliminate active renal diseases.
      (1). Because renal lesions responsible for CRF are largely irreversible, they cannot be completely reversed or eliminated by specific therapy.
      (2). Diagnostic efforts directed especially at detecting treatable renal diseases should be performed prior to formulating plans for conservative medical management.
      (3). Nonrenal conditions (i.e., prerenal and postrenal causes) that may aggravate or precipitate uremic crises should be sought and corrected.

TABLE 28–1
COMPONENTS OF CONSERVATIVE MEDICAL MANAGEMENT OF CHRONIC RENAL FAILURE

Restrict dietary protein intake
Minimize uremic anorexia
Correct metabolic acidosis
Correct hypokalemia
Correct hyperphosphatemia
Correct hypocalcemia
Correct calcitriol deficit
Minimize arterial hypertension
Correct and prevent dehydration
Correct anemia of chronic renal failure
Modify drug dosages when appropriate
Limit progression of renal failure
Monitor patient response to treatment and modify therapy as needed

II. MODIFYING DIETARY PROTEIN INTAKE

A. The rationale for restricting protein intake of patients with CRF is based on the premise that controlled reduction of nonessential proteins results in decreased production of nitrogenous wastes with consequent amelioration of clinical signs.

1. Loss of renal function is associated with accumulation of a wide variety of nitrogen-containing compounds in the body.
   a. Many nitrogenous waste products of protein catabolism are excreted primarily by glomerular filtration.
   b. Retention of these metabolic wastes may be further aggravated by impaired tubular secretion and by extrarenal factors that promote renal hypoperfusion and increased catabolism of body tissues.
2. Because these nitrogen-containing compounds are derived almost entirely from protein degradation, their production decreases when dietary protein intake is limited.
3. Although a direct cause-and-effect relationship has not been proved in many instances, investigators generally believe that retained protein catabolites contribute significantly to production of uremic signs and many of the laboratory abnormalities found in patients with renal failure.[1-6]
   a. Clinical signs of uremia appear to be related to blood urea nitrogen concentrations, a clinical marker of retained proteinaceous catabolites.
   b. Uremic symptoms can be induced in well-dialyzed humans with CRF by adding urea to the dialysate bath so that blood urea nitrogen concentrations remain greater than 140 mg/dl for 1 week.[7]
   c. In human patients with CRF treated by hemodialysis, maintaining blood urea nitrogen concentrations close to 50 mg/dL has been shown to be associated with fewer complications than does maintaining blood urea nitrogen concentrations at approximately 90 mg/dL.
4. Reducing dietary protein intake may also ameliorate signs of uremia by mechanisms other than limiting uremic toxins.
   a. Reducing protein intake usually limits phosphorus intake and therefore may ameliorate hyperphosphatemia, renal secondary hyperparathyroidism, renal osteodystrophy, and their associated clinical manifestations.
   b. Severity of polyuria and polydipsia is often moderated by reducing protein intake because solute diuresis caused by proteinaceous waste products, particularly urea, is limited.[8]
   c. Protein restriction may limit the severity of anemia of CRF and its associated clinical signs because proteinaceous waste products can inhibit hematopoiesis, promote hemolysis, and promote blood loss by causing gastrointestinal ulcerations and impairing platelet function; however, excessive protein restriction may limit hematopoiesis.
   d. Because hydrogen ions are a by-product of catabolism of some proteins, protein restriction may minimize metabolic acidosis.
5. By formulating diets that contain a reduced quantity of high-quality protein and adequate nonprotein calories, many signs associated with uremia may be reduced in severity or eliminated, even though renal function remains essentially unchanged.

B. The decision as to when to intervene with dietary therapy in patients with CRF is based, in part, on the severity of renal dysfunction and clinical consequences of CRF present in the patient.

1. Little controversy exists as to the value of reducing protein intake when overt clinical signs of CRF are present.
   a. Onset of the earliest clinical signs of CRF varies in dogs and cats, but often occurs when serum creatinine concentrations exceed 1.5 to 2.5 times the upper limit of normal.
   b. Protein restriction is likely to be more readily accepted by the patient when initiated prior to onset of more advanced gastrointestinal and neurologic signs of CRF.
2. The therapeutic value of dietary protein restriction is less clear in the absence of clinical signs of CRF.
   a. The principal justification for protein restriction in early or incipient renal failure has been to limit progression of CRF.[9,10]
      (1). Early therapeutic intervention with protein restriction may forestall onset of signs of uremia.
      (2). Although contradictory data exist, dietary protein restriction may modulate devel-

opment of renal lesions in dogs and cats.[11-14]

b. Moderate protein restriction early in the course of CRF does not appear to be harmful; however, excessive protein restriction may have adverse nutritional consequences and should generally be avoided.[15,16]

C. Appropriate dietary protein intake should be individualized to the metabolic needs of the patient.

1. Initially, dogs with mild to moderate CRF should be fed a diet providing at least 13% of gross energy as protein.
2. Initially, cats with CRF should be fed a diet containing at least 21% of gross energy as protein.
   a. Cats have significantly higher dietary protein requirements compared to those of dogs.[17]
   b. The higher protein requirement for cats reflects reduced efficiency of anabolic utilization of dietary protein in cats compared to that in other species.
      (1). Cats do not appear to have a higher requirement for one or more essential amino acids.
      (2). A significant portion of the protein cats eat is used as a source of calories.
   c. Reduced-protein diets formulated for dogs are not appropriate for cats.
3. Optimum dietary protein requirements for dogs and cats with CRF have not been established.
   a. The minimum dietary requirement for an ideal protein (a protein that is 100% digestible and has a biologic value of 100%) has been reported to be approximately 4% of gross energy for normal adult dogs (12% in puppies) and 9% for normal adult cats (22% in kittens).[18]
   b. Because uremia is a catabolic state characterized by a variety of abnormalities in protein metabolism, protein requirements in uremic patients may be increased compared to those in normal individuals.[1,10,19]
      (1). Metabolic acidosis has been shown to impair protein metabolism in CRF in some species, an effect that may occur even with mild acidosis.[1]
      (2). Metabolic acidosis inhibits adaptive responses to dietary protein restriction and increases protein requirements in patients with CRF by increasing amino acid oxidation and protein breakdown.[1]
      (3). Monitoring for and correction of metabolic acidosis may be especially important when protein intake is limited in patients with CRF.
   c. Albuminuria, hematuria, and gastrointestinal hemorrhage may also increase dietary protein requirements.
4. The goal of modifying protein intake is to minimize clinical signs of uremia while maintaining adequate nutrition.
   a. This goal can only be achieved by monitoring the patient's response to diet therapy via serial assessment of renal function, clinical response, and nutritional status.
   b. If evidence of protein malnutrition occurs (hypoalbuminemia, anemia, weight loss, or loss of body tissue mass), dietary protein should gradually be increased until these abnormalities are corrected.
      (1). After initiating protein restriction, serum albumin concentrations may decline and then stabilize at a lower serum concentration.
      (2). This decline in serum albumin usually represents loss of some portion of the labile protein pool; patients remain in negative nitrogen balance until albumin concentrations stabilize.
      (3). Although inconclusive, evidence available from other species suggests that loss of these labile protein stores is probably not harmful for most patients.[20]
   c. If limiting protein intake fails to adequately ameliorate clinical and biochemical manifestations of uremia, dietary protein intake may be cautiously reduced further.
      (1). The decision to reduce dietary protein further must be based primarily on clinical assessment of the patient.
      (2). Dietary protein should not be reduced for the sole purpose of attaining a prescribed reduction in serum urea nitrogen concentration.
      (3). Dietary protein intake should generally not be reduced below 18 to 20% of calories as protein in cats.[17]
   d. The clinician should strive to achieve the best attainable compromise between the impact of diet on the biochemical and clinical manifestations of uremia, renal function, and prevention of malnutrition.
5. Consumption of adequate nonprotein calories is important to minimize catabolism of protein for energy.
   a. Calorie intake should be adjusted to maintain stable, normal body weight.
   b. Excessive fat and calorie intake appears to promote renal injury in some rodents and should therefore probably be avoided.[21-27]

III. TREATMENT OF UREMIC ANOREXIA

A. Uremic anorexia can often be overcome once the underlying causes for the anorexia are recognized.

1. Reduction in the palatability of renal failure diets is commonly incriminated as a major factor leading to inappetance.
   a. Although modification of diets so that they contain reduced quantities of protein, phosphorus, sodium, and acid metabolites is a cornerstone of therapeutic regimens for renal

failure, many patients with renal failure may refuse to eat some or all of such diets offered to them.

b. Although reduced palatability is often attributed to reduction in dietary protein, sodium, and phosphorus, the observation that patients with renal failure often selectively eat diets containing unrestricted quantities of these ingredients suggests that poor palatability of diets is not the only factor involved.

2. Anorexia often results from toxic and metabolic consequences of CRF.[28,29]
   a. Anorexia may be the primary abnormality prompting owners of dogs and cats with renal failure to seek the assistance of veterinarians. In a retrospective study of clinical manifestations of renal failure in 132 cats performed at the University of Minnesota, anorexia was observed by owners in 80% of the patients.[30]
   b. A complete diagnostic evaluation of the patient should be performed in anorexic patients to identify metabolic derangements that may promote anorexia and require therapy.
   c. Toxic and metabolic consequences of CRF that may contribute to uremic anorexia include uremic gastritis, hypokalemia, metabolic acidosis, dehydration, anemia, and possibly hyperparathyroidism.[28,31]
3. Because nutritional support is the cornerstone of long-term management of patients with renal failure, management must encompass a plan to minimize inappetance.
   a. If catabolic patients with renal failure do not consume their daily requirements of dietary nutrients, further catabolism characterized by metabolism of endogenous proteins for energy will follow.
   b. Catabolism of endogenous proteins, in turn, augments production of protein catabolic wastes, which further contribute to anorexia.

B. Ameliorating uremic nausea and vomiting.

1. Uremic vomiting is mediated locally and centrally.
   a. Local factors include gastritis, forced foods and fluids, and intolerance to some medications.
   b. Central factors consist of stimulation of the medullary emetic chemoreceptor trigger zone by circulating uremic toxins (e.g., methylguanidine) and intolerance to some medications.
2. Hypergastrinemia-induced anorexia, nausea, and vomiting may be ameliorated by administration of H_2-receptor antagonists, such as cimetidine or ranitidine.
   a. Anorexia, nausea, and vomiting are in part related to gastric hyperacidity induced by hypergastrinemia.
   b. For dogs, cimetidine is commonly administered intravenously or orally at a dose of 5 mg/kg every 8 to 12 hours. After 2 to 4 weeks of oral therapy at this dosage, 5 mg/kg are given once daily for 2 to 3 weeks prior to withdrawal.
   c. In cats, an initial dose of 2.5 to 5.0 mg/kg given every 8 to 12 hours is commonly used.
   d. Cimetidine given intravenously may be diluted with saline and slowly given over a 2-minute period to minimize bradycardia.
   e. Because cimetidine may interfere with the hepatic metabolism of such drugs as diazepam and propranolol by p450 enzymes, ranitidine is sometimes chosen as an alternative.
      (1). Ranitidine is more potent than cimetidine, and has less effect on hepatic p450 enzymes.
      (2). Ranitidine is commonly given orally or intravenously at a dose of 2 to 4 mg/kg every 12 hours.
   f. Because cimetidine and ranitidine depend on renal excretion for elimination, the lower end of the dosage ranges should be considered.
3. In addition to or as an alternative to H_2-receptor antagonists, sucralfate may be given to create a protective layer over the gastric mucosal surface.
   a. In an acid environment, sucralfate becomes charged and binds to gastric proteins of the opposite charge, thereby minimizing back diffusion of hydrochloric acid and pepsin into the stomach wall.
   b. The empirically established dose of sucralfate for dogs is 0.25 to 1.0 g every 8 to 12 hours.
   c. Because sucralfate may interfere with the action of other orally administered drugs, these drugs should be given approximately 30 minutes prior to the administration of sucralfate.
   d. Caution should also be used if consideration is being given to using sucralfate for extended periods, because significant elevations in serum aluminum concentration may occur.
4. As an alternative or supplement to H_2-receptor antagonists and sucralfate, metoclopramide may be given to minimize the action of uremic toxins on the medullary emetic chemoreceptor trigger zone.
   a. An empirically established oral dose of metoclopramide is 0.2 to 0.4 mg every 6 to 8 hours.
   b. Injectable metoclopramide may be given at a dose of 1.0 to 2.0 mg/kg every 24 hours.
   c. The lower dosages are preferred because metoclopramide is eliminated by the kidneys.
   d. Signs of metoclopramide overdosage include drowsiness, disorientation, tremors, muscle hypertonia, and reduction in seizure thresholds.

C. Preventing drug-induced anorexia, nausea, and vomiting.

1. Patients in renal failure may be intolerant to side effects of many drugs (e.g., captopril, enalapril, trimethoprim-sulfa, digoxin, and tetracyclines).
2. Some drugs may contribute to anorexia by impairing taste or smell (e.g., ampicillin, sulfas,

tetracyclines, aminoglycosides, allopurinol, d-penicillamine, and captopril).

3. The manufacturer's recommendations and description of side effects should be reviewed before giving any drug to a patient in renal failure.
4. Because many patients with renal failure are intolerant to drugs, they should not be routinely given with the philosophy that they might help but will do no harm.

D. Correcting and preventing vitamin B deficiency.

1. Patients with renal failure are at risk for vitamin B deficiency as a result of decreased appetites, vomiting, diarrhea, and perhaps losses associated with polyuria.
   a. Uremic human beings tend to develop deficiencies of water-soluble vitamins, especially folate and pyridoxine.[32]
   b. Deficiencies of thiamin and niacin may result in anorexia.
2. Administration of supplemental vitamin B as therapy for anorexia in CRF is logical, but its efficacy has not been established in dogs and cats.
   a. No data support the notion that consumption of vitamin B in excess of daily requirements stimulates appetite.
   b. The daily vitamin B requirement of normal cats is estimated to be 6 to 8 times greater than that of dogs.
   c. If multiple-vitamin supplements are used, caution must be used not to give excessive quantities of fat-soluble vitamins.

E. Improving dietary palatability and acceptance.

1. Because preference for new flavors and textures of food may be a learned response for some dogs and cats, dietary changes should be made gradually over a period of 1 to 2 weeks.
   a. In patients that are especially selective in their eating habits, changes may require a longer period for adaptation.
   b. If the patient refuses to completely accept the recommended diet, partial compliance with modified diets (i.e., a mixture of the modified formulation with the patient's preferred diet) is probably better than no dietary modification.
   c. If the patient is hospitalized, continuation of the patient's favorite foods may be preferable to making a sudden change in diet.
2. Patient acceptance of the modified diet will likely be enhanced by careful selection of the diet formulation and optimum presentation of the food.
   a. When obtaining the medical history, special emphasis should be placed on the dietary history, especially in relation to patient food preferences.
   b. New diets should have the same texture and flavor as preferred diets.
   c. Warming food to just below body temperature may improve its palatability.
   d. If dry foods are selected, addition of warm water may be of benefit.
   e. Offering fresh aromatic food is sometimes helpful.
   f. Be sure that the nasal passages are open.
3. The possibility that food aversion may develop should be considered.
   a. If a patient with renal failure is given a diet designed for long-term management of renal failure at a time when nausea or vomiting is present, aversion to that food may develop.
   b. Food aversion is most likely to occur if nauseated patients are force fed or if painful sample collection or drug administration is associated with feeding.
   c. In general, unpalatable drugs should not be mixed with regular food or water.
   d. To minimize the possibility of aversion to renal failure diets designed for long-term use, one should not offer them to patients with renal failure until the underlying causes contributing to anorexia, nausea, and vomiting are minimized or eliminated.
   e. Consider using a temporary diet formulation during recovery from uremic crises to avoid inducing dietary aversions to the long-term renal failure diet to be used.
4. Flavoring agents may be used to enhance the palatability of diets.
   a. Suggested options for flavoring agents include animal fat, butter, dehydrated cottage cheese, garlic, bouillon, clam juice, brewer's yeast, and carnitine.
   b. Enteral nutrition liquids designed for renal failure may also be used as flavoring agents.
5. Patients with renal failure that are anorexic or nauseated should be given small quantities of food several times each day.
   a. Minimizing distention of the stomach may minimize gastric secretions and the feeling of nausea.
   b. Consumption of smaller quantities of food minimizes postprandial elevation of absorbed nutrients, including protein catabolites.
6. Placing small quantities of palatable food in the mouth or on the patient's paws may stimulate a licking response, which, in turn, may stimulate neural and humoral mechanisms that normally stimulate appetite.
7. The feeding environment should also be considered when managing renal patients with anorexia.
   a. Timid animals should not be hospitalized in noisy wards with heavy traffic.
   b. Loud and persistent barking may be especially stressful to cats.
   c. Food should be placed in wide bowls or flat saucers so that tactile whiskers are not adversely stimulated.

d. A comfortable environmental temperature should be maintained.

8. Rewarding patients at the time of feeding may be helpful.
   a. Owners may play an important role by providing a reassuring voice and gentle hand.
   b. Partially anorexic cats may begin to eat if gently stroked at the time a meal is offered.

F. Administration of pharmacologic appetite stimulants.

1. Although manufacturers of veterinary anabolic agents state that these drugs improve appetite, no data support this claim in dogs or cats with renal failure. In a 6-week study in moderately azotemic dogs with induced renal failure, anabolic agents had no beneficial effect on food intake, body weight, nitrogen balance, or lean body mass.[33]
2. No data support a long-term beneficial effect of glucocorticoids in uremic dogs or cats.
   a. Glucocorticoids enhance catabolism, impair the repair of gastric mucosa, and enhance glomerular hyperfiltration.
   b. Although they may enhance appetite, this effect does not translate into weight gain.
3. Benzodiazepine derivatives, such as diazepam and oxazepam, are known to stimulate appetite in a variety of species.
   a. They appear to be most effective in patients with partial anorexia.
   b. The objective is to stimulate the appetite of the patient in a "jump-start" fashion, so that licking and chewing will stimulate normal humoral and neural appetite mechanisms.
   c. Diazepam may be given orally, intramuscularly, or intravenously, but is most effective when given at an intravenous dose of 0.2 mg/kg with a maximum dose of 5 mg/patient. Diazepam may be given twice per day.
   d. Oxazepam is available only for oral administration. It is commonly given at a dose of 2.5 mg/cat.
   e. Care must be taken not to use excessive dosages of these drugs in depressed patients.

IV. TREATMENT OF METABOLIC ACIDOSIS

A. Potential benefits of alkalization therapy in patients with CRF include:

1. Ameliorating signs of anorexia, lethargy, nausea, vomiting, muscle weakness, and weight loss that may be caused by uremic acidosis.[34]
2. Preventing the catabolic effects of metabolic acidosis on protein metabolism in patients with CRF, thereby promoting adaptation to dietary protein restriction.[1,19,35,36]
3. Minimizing the potential adverse effects of increased renal ammoniagenesis on self-perpetuation of progressive renal failure.[37]
4. Enhancing the patient's capacity to adapt to additional acid stress resulting from such factors as diarrhea, dehydration, or respiratory acidosis.[28]
5. Limiting skeletal damage (demineralization and inhibited skeletal growth) resulting from bone buffering.[38]
6. Rectifying or preventing the adverse effects of severe acidosis on the cardiovascular system (impaired myocardial contractility and enhanced venoconstriction).[34]

B. Because even mildly reduced plasma bicarbonate concentrations may promote some of the adverse effects of chronic metabolic acidosis, oral alkalization therapy is probably indicated when serum bicarbonate (or total carbon dioxide) concentration declines below the established normal range for the laboratory.[35]

1. Appropriate reference ranges are equipment- and method-specific, and therefore, published ranges for therapeutic goals must be extrapolated with caution.
   a. Because of inherent differences in sample collection and analytic methods, a substantial systematic difference may exist between blood bicarbonate concentrations determined by blood gas analysis performed on anaerobically collected whole blood samples and serum total CO_2 concentrations determined using autoanalyzers on serum samples.
   b. When blood collection tubes are not fully filled or are left exposed to air while awaiting analysis, the vacuum or air above the tube can draw CO_2 out of the serum, thereby falsely lowering CO_2 concentrations.
2. Problems associated with clinical determination of acid-base status may have resulted in artifactually expanded reference ranges and clinician mistrust of the accuracy of total CO_2 determinations, thereby causing an underappreciation of the true prevalence of metabolic acidosis in CRF.

C. Oral sodium bicarbonate is the most commonly used alkalinizing agent for patients with metabolic acidosis of CRF.

1. Because the effects of gastric acid on oral sodium bicarbonate are unpredictable, the dosage should be individualized for each patient.
2. The suggested initial dose of sodium bicarbonate is 8 to 12 mg/kg given every 8 to 12 hours.
   a. Sodium bicarbonate may be administered as tablets, as powder (mixed with food), or as a solution.
   b. A solution containing approximately 84 mg of sodium bicarbonate per milliliter (1 mEq/mL) of solution can be prepared by adding 2.5 oz of sodium bicarbonate to 1 qt of water (84 mg added to 1 L of water).
      (1). This solution may be stored capped and refrigerated for several months.
      (2). This solution may be administered at a starting dose of 1 to 1.5 mL/10 kg.
      (3). The solution may be administered orally by syringe or mixed with the food.

(4). Some patients find the taste of sodium bicarbonate solutions unappealing.

D. Potassium citrate is a useful alkalinizing agent that limits sodium intake and provides supplemental potassium.[30]

1. Potassium citrate may be administered orally at a dose of 40 to 60 mg/kg every 12 hours.
2. Because citrate may promote intestinal absorption of aluminum, it should be used with caution in patients receiving concurrent therapy with aluminum-containing phosphate binding agents or sucralfate.
3. Alkalinizing agents should be given in several smaller doses rather than in a single large dose to minimize fluctuations in blood pH.
4. The patient's response to alkalization therapy should be determined by measuring blood bicarbonate or serum (plasma) total CO_2 concentrations 10 to 14 days after initiating therapy.
   a. Ideally, blood should be collected just prior to administration of the drug.
   b. Dosage of alkalinizing agents should be adjusted so that blood bicarbonate (or serum total CO_2) concentrations are maintained between 18 and 24 mEq/L.
   c. Urine pH is often insensitive as a means of assessing the need for or the response to treatment and is not recommended for these purposes.

E. Alkalization therapy should be used with caution in some patients.

1. Increasing blood pH in the presence of hypocalcemia may precipitate tetany.
2. Administration of sodium-containing drugs should be minimized or avoided in patients with congestive heart failure, nephrotic syndrome, hypertension, oliguria, or volume overload.
   a. Sodium bicarbonate may not promote fluid retention to the same extent as does sodium chloride.[39-41]
   b. Nonetheless, development of edema or progressive rise in arterial pressure that occur after initiating therapy with sodium bicarbonate may indicate sodium intolerance.
   c. Sodium-free alkalinizing agents, such as calcium acetate, carbonate, lactate, or citrate or potassium citrate, may be considered for use in patients that appear to be sodium intolerant.
   d. Citrate-containing alkalinizing agents may promote intestinal absorption of aluminum when aluminum-based intestinal phosphate binding agents are used concurrently. (See Section VI B of this chapter.)
   e. Care should be taken to avoid iatrogenic metabolic acidosis.

F. Extrarenal factors may exacerbate uremic acidosis and should be identified and corrected.

1. Unexpectedly severe metabolic acidosis should prompt consideration of possible extrarenal acidosis superimposed on uremic acidosis.
2. Factors that may promote metabolic acidosis in patients with renal failure include:
   a. Administration of certain drugs, including urinary acidifiers, salicylates, and hyperalimentation solutions.
   b. Feeding diets designed to produce acid urine.
   c. Dehydration.
   d. Severe diarrhea.
   e. Hyporeninemic hypoaldosteronism.
3. The need for alkalization therapy in patients receiving such therapy should be evaluated after withdrawing the potentially responsible drug or diet.

G. Acid-base status of the patient should be monitored at appropriate intervals to assess adequacy of or need for therapy.

1. Blood bicarbonate or serum (plasma) total CO_2 concentrations should be evaluated at least every 3 to 4 months for patients receiving alkalization therapy.
2. Changes in renal function, as well as extrarenal factors, may influence the patient's need for alkalization therapy.
   a. Reducing dietary protein intake may limit the quantity of dietary acid consumed while simultaneously limiting substrate available for renal ammoniagenesis and hydrogen ion excretion.[42]
   b. Because phosphate is the predominant buffer involved in excretion of hydrogen ions as urinary titratable acid, excessive dietary phosphate restriction and use of phosphate binding agents may promote metabolic acidosis by limiting urine phosphate excretion.[43]
   c. Dietary restriction of phosphate may enhance tubular reabsorption of HCO_3^- in dogs, whereas dietary restriction of sodium may inhibit tubular reabsorption of HCO_3^- in dogs.[44]
   d. Although the clinical importance of these effects for dogs and cats with spontaneous CRF is unclear, they emphasize the need to monitor patient response to treatment.

V. TREATMENT OF HYPOKALEMIA

A. Hypokalemia is a relatively frequent complication of renal failure, with a reported incidence of 19% in a clinical study of feline renal failure.[30]

1. Although an association between renal failure and development of hypokalemia has been confirmed in cats, the mechanism of hypokalemia has not been established.[45,46]
   a. Studies performed in our laboratory have confirmed that renal failure is a risk factor for development of hypokalemia in cats.[46]
   b. Studies have suggested that hypokalemia may result from excessive urinary potassium excretion and that increasing urinary potassium losses may represent "a basic renal physiologic response" to decreased renal function in cats.[45]
   (1). However, 24-hour urinary potassium ex-

cretion did not appear to be increased in cats with experimentally induced CRF, even among cats that developed hypokalemia.[46]

(2). Fractional excretion of potassium is increased in most cats with CRF, but this increase is usually adaptive rather than pathologic.[46]

(3). Diagnosis of excessive or inappropriate kaliuresis should be based on measurement of 24-hour urine potassium excretion determinations.

c. Uncontrolled preliminary findings suggest that chronic ingestion of a potassium-deficient diet may induce primary renal failure in cats.[47]

2. Inadequate dietary potassium intake may be an important factor promoting hypokalemia in CRF.[45]
   a. Increasing dietary protein intake has been shown to increase potassium requirements in cats.[48]
   b. Acidifying diets and chronic metabolic acidosis may promote hypokalemia.[49,50]

B. Hypokalemia has been associated with myopathy and renal functional impairment.

1. The cardinal sign of hypokalemia, regardless of cause, is generalized muscle weakness.[51] Cats with hypokalemia often have profound cervical ventroflexion and difficulty ambulating.
2. Chronic potassium depletion also appears to impair renal function in cats.[49]
   a. Persistent potassium depletion may promote metabolic acidosis, which may enhance urinary potassium losses, thereby promoting hypokalemia and additional decline in renal function.
   b. Renal function usually improves with potassium supplementation and restoration of normokalemia.
3. Hypokalemia may also promote mild cardiac rhythm disturbances.

C. Potassium replacement therapy is indicated for cats with hypokalemia, even in absence of clinical signs of hypokalemia.

1. Oral administration is the safest and preferred route of administration for potassium replacement therapy.
   a. Parenteral administration is more likely to induce iatrogenic hyperkalemia.
   b. Parenteral therapy is generally reserved for patients requiring emergency reversal of hypokalemia or for patients that cannot or will not accept oral therapy.
2. Potassium gluconate is generally regarded as the potassium salt of choice for replacement therapy.[50]
   a. Potassium may be administered orally as potassium gluconate in a palatable powder form (Tumil-K, Daniels Pharmaceuticals, Inc., St. Petersburg, Florida), potassium gluconate elixir (Kaon Elixir, Adria Laboratories, Columbus, Ohio), or potassium citrate solution (Polycitra-K, Willen Drug, Baltimore, Maryland).
   b. Potassium chloride is generally avoided as a source of potassium in cats because its use may be associated with anorexia and vomiting; it also fails to provide additional alkalinization.
   c. Depending on the size of the cat and severity of hypokalemia, potassium gluconate is given initially at a dose of 2 to 6 mEq/cat/d.[50]
   d. Muscle weakness usually resolves within 1 to 5 days after initiating parenteral or oral potassium supplementation.
   e. Potassium dosage should thereafter be adjusted based on the clinical response of the patient and on serum potassium determinations performed during the initial phase of therapy.
      (1). Serum potassium concentrations should be monitored every 24 to 48 hours during the initial phase of therapy.
      (2). Serum potassium concentrations should be monitored every 7 to 14 days during the maintenance phase of therapy.

D. Routine supplementation of all cats with CRF has been advocated, regardless of serum potassium concentrations.[50]

1. The goal of such therapy is to prevent or correct hypokalemia-induced renal dysfunction.
2. The safety and efficacy of this approach have not been evaluated.

E. Diets that are acidifying and restricted in magnesium content may promote hypokalemia, and should therefore generally be avoided in cats with CRF.

F. Intensive fluid therapy during uremic crises, particularly with potassium deficient fluids, may promote hypokalemia even in cats that have not previously experienced hypokalemia.

1. Serum potassium concentrations should be monitored during fluid therapy, and maintenance fluids should be supplemented with potassium chloride to prevent inducing hypokalemia (concentrations of 13 to 20 mEq/L are appropriate for maintenance fluids).
2. Fluids generally should be administered in such a manner that allows the intravenous delivery of potassium at a rate no greater than 0.5 mEq/kg/h.

G. Potassium depletion and metabolic acidosis may promote potentially fatal reductions in plasma taurine concentrations in cats.[50]

VI. TREATMENT OF HYPERPHOSPHATEMIA

A. Minimizing phosphorus retention and hyperphosphatemia is important because it may:

1. Limit renal secondary hyperparathyroidism and renal osteodystrophy.[34,52]
   a. Minimizing phosphorus retention enhances renal calcitriol production and decreases parathyroid hormone (PTH) values.
      (1). Minimizing phosphorus retention and hyperphosphatemia decreases renal intracellular phosphate concentrations.

(2). Reduced renal intracellular phosphorus concentration increases renal 1α-hydroxylase activity, which in turn increases conversion of 25-hydroxycholecalciferol (25-$(OH)D_3$) to 1,25-dihydroxycholecalciferol (calcitriol), the most metabolically active form of vitamin D.

(3). Increased calcitriol activity minimizes renal secondary hyperparathyroidism by directly inhibiting PTH release and by increasing plasma calcium concentration.[53]

(4). Reducing serum phosphorus may also reduce PTH by a mechanism independent of the levels of calcitriol or ionized calcium.[54]

b. Preventing phosphorus retention by reducing phosphate intake in proportion to the decrease in glomerular filtration rate (GFR) has been shown largely to prevent renal secondary hyperparathyroidism in dogs.[52,55,56]

c. Clinical studies in human beings indicate that dietary phosphorus restriction in patients with mild CRF can reduce PTH levels and improve the skeletal calcemic response to PTH.[57]

d. In addition to skeletal disease, hyperparathyroidism may promote soft tissue mineralization, soft tissue necrosis, encephalopathy and peripheral neuropathy, leukocyte malfunction, hyperlipidemia, anemia, deranged carbohydrate metabolism, anorexia, and abnormal myocardial function.[53,58]

2. Slow progression of renal failure.

a. Dietary phosphorus restriction appears to limit progression of renal failure and enhance survival in dogs with markedly reduced renal function, regardless of dietary protein intake.[59,60]

b. Phosphorus restriction has been shown to limit renal mineralization in cats with induced CRF, but renal function remained unchanged in this study.[61]

c. The protective effect of phosphorus restriction on progressive renal dysfunction has been hypothesized to result from precipitation of phosphorus salts within the renal parenchyma.[62]

3. Minimize soft tissue mineralization.[58]

a. Tissues that may be affected by mineralization include the kidneys, blood vessels, and brain.

b. Acute uremia of 3 days' duration results in marked increase in mineral content in brains of dogs.[63]

B. Phosphorus retention and hyperphosphatemia are managed by restricting dietary phosphate intake, oral administration of intestinal phosphate binding agents, or a combination of these methods.

1. Phosphorus is absorbed from the gastrointestinal tract, primarily the duodenum and jejunum, and excreted primarily by the kidneys.

a. Renal excretion of phosphorus reflects the net effect of glomerular filtration and tubular reabsorption.

b. Reduced GFR in CRF results in phosphorus retention and subsequent hyperphosphatemia.

c. Authors have suggested that optimum control of hyperphosphatemia would be achieved by reducing dietary phosphorus intake "in proportion" to the decrease in GFR.[55]

2. The ultimate goal of therapy is to prevent or minimize renal secondary hyperparathyroidism and its various adverse consequences.

a. Normalization of serum phosphorus concentrations is an economically acceptable and clinically useful therapeutic end point.

(1). Normalization of serum phosphorus concentration should not be interpreted to indicate that plasma PTH activity is within normal limits.

(2). Although the clinical efficacy of normalizing serum phosphorus concentrations in limiting the adverse consequences of phosphorus retention in dogs and cats with CRF is unproved, this approach remains the most practical end point for phosphate restriction therapy in most patients.

b. Monitoring plasma PTH activity directly measures effectiveness of therapy.

(1). PTH measurements are expensive to attain and have not been proved superior to monitoring of serum phosphate concentrations in dogs and cats with renal failure; therefore, they are rarely utilized as the end point of therapy.

(2). Determination of serum PTH activity may be considered after serum phosphorus has been normalized to determine the need for additional therapy to control hyperparathyroidism.

c. Use of fractional excretion of phosphorus has been advocated as a therapeutic end point because it may serve as a clinical estimate of plasma PTH activity.[64]

(1). Fractional excretion of phosphorus may be calculated from serum and urine concentrations of phosphorus and creatinine determined from simultaneously collected serum and urine samples.

(2). Fractional excretion of phosphorus is calculated as follows:

$$FE_P = [P_{Urine}][Cr_{Serum}]/[P_{Serum}][Cr_{Urine}]^*$$

(3). Fractional excretion of phosphorus is typically less than 0.1 in normal dogs.

*P_{Urine} = urine phosphorus concentration; Cr_{Serum} = serum creatinine concentration; P_{Serum} = serum phosphorus concentration; Cr_{Urine} = urine creatinine concentration.

(4). Fractional excretion values of less than 0.3 have been advocated as evidence of adequate control of phosphorus retention in dogs with renal failure.[42,64,65]

(5). Whether fractional excretion of phosphorus provides a therapeutic advantage over serum phosphate concentration as an end point for establishing effectiveness of therapy designed to limit phosphorus retention has not been determined.

(6). Fractional excretion of phosphorus may not always reflect plasma PTH activity.[66]

(7). One researcher has reported that fractional excretion of phosphorus is a relatively insensitive indicator of the extent of hyperparathyroidism in dogs with CRF.[67]

3. Reducing dietary phosphorus intake is the first step toward limiting phosphorus retention in CRF.
   a. The need for dietary phosphorus restriction should be established after correcting dehydration or other prerenal causes for hyperphosphatemia.
   b. Dietary phosphorus restriction is an important and effective first step toward normalizing phosphate balance because:
      (1). It may normalize serum phosphorus concentrations in mild to moderate CRF.
      (2). It reduces the quantity of phosphorus that must be bound by intestinal phosphorus binding agents.
   c. Because proteinaceous foods are the major dietary phosphorus sources, protein-restricted diets are usually low in phosphorus content.[68]
      (1). Typical commercial dog foods contain approximately 1 to 2% phosphorus on a dry matter basis and provide about 2.7 mg/kcal or more of phosphorus.
      (2). Modified protein diets designed for dogs with renal failure may contain as little as 0.13 to 0.28% phosphorus on a dry matter basis and provide about 0.3 to 0.5 mg/kcal of phosphorus.
      (3). Typical commercial cat foods contain from 1 to 4% phosphorus on a dry matter basis and provide about 2.9 mg/kcal or more of phosphorus.
      (4). Modified protein diets designed for cats with renal failure may contain as little as 0.5% phosphorus on a dry matter basis and provide about 0.9 mg/kcal of phosphorus.
      (5). Although reduced-protein diets are generally reduced in phosphorus content, a reduction in protein intake is not always necessary to reduce phosphorus intake.
   d. Unfortunately, as renal failure becomes more advanced, dietary protein/phosphorus restriction alone often fails to prevent hyperphosphatemia.
   e. Serum phosphorus concentrations should be determined after the patient has been consuming the phosphorus-restricted diet for about 2 to 4 weeks.
      (1). Samples obtained for determinations of serum phosphorus concentration should be collected after a 12-hour fast to avoid postprandial effects.[69]
         (a). Feeding may increase serum phosphorus concentrations by as much as 1 to 2 mg/dL over fasting values.
         (b). Postprandial lipemia may increase serum phosphorus concentrations by several milligrams per deciliter.
      (2). Sample hemolysis should be avoided because red blood cells contain substantial quantities of phosphorus.
      (3). When hyperphosphatemia persists despite dietary phosphorus restriction, administration of intestinal phosphorus binding agents should be considered.

4. Phosphorus binding agents should be used in conjunction with dietary phosphorus restriction when dietary therapy alone fails to reduce serum phosphorus concentrations to within the normal range.
   a. Intestinal phosphorus binding agents render ingested phosphorus and the phosphorus contained in saliva, bile, and intestinal juices nonabsorbable.[70]
      (1). Because the primary goal is limiting absorption of phosphorus contained in the diet, administration of phosphorus binding agents should be timed to coincide with feeding.
      (2). These agents are best administered with or mixed into the food, or just prior to each meal.
   b. Dietary phosphorus intake should be reduced before initiating therapy with intestinal phosphorus binding agents to reduce the quantity of phosphorus that must be bound.
      (1). High dietary phosphorus content may greatly limit the effectiveness of phosphorus binding agents, or substantially increase the dosage required to achieve the desired therapeutic effect.
      (2). Administration of 1500 to 2500 mg of aluminum carbonate to dogs with moderate CRF failed to consistently correct hyperphosphatemia when dogs were fed diets containing greater than 1.0% phosphorus on a dry matter basis.[71]
      (3). Phosphorus binding agents appear to be ineffective in controlling hyperphosphatemia when dietary phosphorus intake exceeds 2.0 g/d in humans.[70]
   c. Currently available phosphorus binding agents include aluminum-based and calcium-based compounds.

(1). Aluminum-containing intestinal phosphorus binding agents include aluminum hydroxide, aluminum carbonate, and aluminum oxide.
(a). These drugs are available over the counter from most pharmacies as antacid preparations (Table 28-2).
(b). They are available as liquids, tablets, or capsules.
(c). Capsules are less effective than liquids, but patient compliance may be better with tablets and capsules.[58]
(d). Although quite effective for binding phosphorus, an important disadvantage of long-term use of aluminum-containing antacids in humans with CRF has been development of aluminum toxicity.
(1′). Aluminum contained in phosphorus binding antacids may be absorbed from the intestinal tract and accumulate in various tissues of the body, such as bone and brain.[70]
(2′). Encephalopathies, microcytic anemia, and bone disease (particularly osteomalacia) related to aluminum toxicity have been extensively reported in human patients treated with these drugs.
(3′). The potential for toxicity of aluminum salts in dogs and cats has been confirmed, but clinical evidence of toxic accumulation of aluminum has not been reported in these species.[71-73]
(e). Aluminum salts may be more effective than calcium salts in binding intestinal phosphorus.

TABLE 28–2
INTESTINAL PHOSPHORUS BINDING AGENTS

Drug	Approximate Dosage*
Aluminum-containing phosphorus binding agents	
Aluminum hydroxide	30 to 90 mg/kg/d
Aluminum carbonate	30 to 90 mg/kg/d
Aluminum oxide	30 to 90 mg/kg/d
Calcium-containing phosphorus binding agents	
Calcium acetate	60 to 90 mg/kg/d
Calcium carbonate	90 to 150 mg/kg/d

*This dosage represents the starting dosage. Dosage should be adjusted on the basis of serial evaluation of response to therapy (see text).

(2). Calcium salts, such as calcium acetate, calcium carbonate, or calcium citrate, may be highly effective as phosphorus binding agents.[58]
(a). Calcium-based phosphate binding agents do not entail the risk of aluminum toxicity that accompanies use of aluminum-based phosphorus binding agents.
(b). Unfortunately, calcium-based products may promote clinically significant hypercalcemia; therefore, serum calcium concentrations must be carefully monitored intermittently when using these drugs.
(c). Calcium carbonate and calcium acetate may be used concurrently with aluminum-based binding agents to limit dosages required of both drugs, thereby reducing risks of hypercalcemia and aluminum toxicity.
(1′). For patients with marked hyperphosphatemia, therapy may begin with aluminum-based phosphorus binding agents.
(2′). A calcium-based phosphorus binder may be added as serum phosphorus concentrations are reduced toward normal.
(d). Calcium citrate may promote absorption of aluminum and should therefore not be used in concert with aluminum-based binding agents.
(e). Calcium acetate is the most effective calcium-based phosphorus binding agent, as well as the agent least likely to induce hypercalcemia because it releases the least amount of calcium compared to the amount of phosphorus it binds.
(f). Calcium-based phosphorus binding agents must be administered with meals both to enhance the effectiveness of phosphorus binding and to minimize absorption of calcium and the risk of hypercalcemia.
(g). Administration of calcium-based phosphorus binding agents between meals promotes absorption of calcium and increases the risk of inducing hypercalcemia.
(h). Some calcium carbonate preparations may not be effective because they fail to dissolve well in the gastrointestinal tract; this possibility may be investigated by examining the stool or radiographing the abdomen for evidence of undissolved tablets.

(i). Aluminum-containing phosphorus binding agents may be preferred over calcium-containing agents in patients that appear with hypercalcemia (confirmed by measuring ionized calcium concentrations) or develop hypercalcemia during therapy with calcium-containing agents.[69]

(3). A combination of aluminum and calcium salts may be given to bind dietary phosphorus while minimizing the potential adverse consequences of both forms of intestinal phosphorus binding agents.

(a). Initially, aluminum salts may be given with the goal of more rapidly reducing the magnitude of hypercalcemia.

(b). Once serum phosphorus concentration has been stabilized, calcium salts may be used to maintain reduced serum phosphorus concentrations.

(4). Sucralfate, a complex polyaluminum hydroxide salt of sulfate used primarily for treatment of gastrointestinal ulcerations, may be effective in binding phosphorus within the intestine.[64]

d. Dosage of phosphorus binding agents should be individualized so that serum phosphorus concentrations are normalized.

(1). An initial dose of 30 to 90 mg/kg/d has been recommended for aluminum-based phosphorus binding agents.

(2). An initial dose of 60 to 90 mg/kg/d has been recommended for calcium acetate, and 90 to 150 mg/kg/d have been recommended for calcium carbonate.

(3). A dose of approximately 100 mg/kg/d divided into 2 or 3 doses has been suggested as an appropriate starting dose for aluminum- or calcium-based phosphorus binding agents when serum phosphorus concentration exceeds 6.0 mg/dl.[69]

(4). The effect of therapy should be monitored by serial evaluation of serum phosphorus concentrations at about 10- to 14-day intervals.

(a). Initially, serum phosphorus concentrations may decrease slowly because of the large pool of accumulated phosphorus requiring excretion.[69]

(b). Serum phosphorus concentrations are usually returned to normal within a few weeks.[69]

(5). Dosage should be increased until serum phosphorus concentrations are reduced to or near normal.

(6). Dosage of calcium-based phosphorus binding agents should be decreased if serum calcium concentrations exceed normal limits; additional aluminum-based agents should be used in these patients if hyperphosphatemia persists.

(7). Thereafter, serum calcium and phosphorus concentrations should be monitored every 4 to 6 weeks or as needed.

e. Overzealous use of phosphorus binding agents may induce hypophosphatemia.

(1). The likelihood of hypophosphatemia is particularly enhanced when both dietary phosphorus restriction and intestinal phosphorus binding agents are used before investigating the impact of diet alone.

(2). Severe hypophosphatemia and phosphorus depletion may cause debility, weakness, and anorexia, which may be confused with signs of uremia.

(3). In addition, phosphorus depletion may aggravate bone disease and even cause osteomalacia.

(4). Constipation and vomiting may also occur with higher dosages of most intestinal phosphorus binding agents.

f. Administration of cimetidine and other H_2 histamine receptor antagonist drugs has been advocated as a means of suppressing PTH secretion in CRF.[64]

(1). However, cimetidine does not reduce intact PTH levels as measured by aminoterminal PTH determinations and therefore appears to be of no value in therapy or prophylaxis of renal secondary hyperparathyroidism.[74,75]

(2). Cimetidine apparently lowers the concentration of inactive forms of PTH, such as those measured by carboxy-terminal or midmolecule PTH assays, by limiting hepatic production or hastening renal clearance of these degradation products of intact PTH molecules.

VII. TREATMENT OF HYPOCALCEMIA

A. Hypocalcemia was detected in about 10% of dogs with CRF in a study; however, when evaluated by determining ionized calcium concentrations in blood, 40% of the dogs were hypocalcemic.[53]

B. Oral calcium supplements may be used to augment the amount of calcium available for absorption, thereby ameliorating hypocalcemia and suppressing hyperparathyroidism.[58]

1. Intestinal malabsorption of calcium is common in CRF, but can be overcome by increasing dietary calcium intake.[76]
2. Because increasing calcium intake may elevate serum calcium concentration and thereby reduce serum PTH activity, calcium supplementation may play an important role in preventing or ameliorating renal osteodystrophy and systemic toxicities resulting from hyperparathyroidism.

3. The optimum time for initiating calcium supplementation during the course of CRF is uncertain.
   a. Early initiation of calcium supplementation may prevent renal osteodystrophy and other manifestations of renal secondary hyperparathyroidism.
   b. Calcium supplementation is not without hazards.
      (1). Oral calcium supplementation may induce hypercalcemia.
      (2). Gastrointestinal disturbances are a common side effect of oral calcium supplements, particularly when administered in large doses.
   c. Because of increased risk of inducing extraskeletal mineralization, calcium supplementation should generally be withheld until serum phosphate concentrations are normalized.
   d. Oral calcium supplementation should be considered in patients with:
      (1). Hypocalcemia.
      (2). Clinical, radiographic, or histologic evidence of renal osteodystrophy.
      (3). Inadequate dietary calcium intake.
4. Oral administration of a variety of calcium salts may be used to improve calcium balance.
   a. Calcium carbonate may be the preferred calcium salt in many patients with CRF because it contains a high fraction of calcium and is inexpensive, tasteless, and usually well tolerated.[58]
      (1). Calcium carbonate is also useful because of its alkalinizing properties.
      (2). Initially, calcium carbonate should be administered at a dose of 100 mg/kg/d.
   b. Calcium may also be supplied as calcium lactate, calcium gluconate, or calcium glubionate.
      (1). Elemental calcium constitutes 40% of calcium carbonate, 12% of calcium lactate, 8% of calcium gluconate, and 6% of calcium glubionate.
      (2). Dosages of calcium preparations should be calculated based on supplying equimolar amounts of elemental calcium.
      (3). Systemic acid-base balance should be considered when selecting the calcium salt to be used; calcium carbonate and calcium lactate may be useful in patients with metabolic acidosis, but are undesirable in alkalemic patients.
      (4). Calcium chloride should generally not be used for calcium supplementation in patients with CRF because of its acidifying properties.[76]
   c. To maximize calcium absorption, one should administer calcium salts in small quantities throughout the day.
      (1). Administration of one or two large doses is likely to be substantially less effective and more likely to induce complications, such as gastrointestinal side effects.
      (2). Administration of calcium carbonate with meals that contain large quantities of phosphate should be avoided because the phosphorus binding effect will limit calcium absorption.
   d. Dosage of calcium carbonate should be individualized according to response.
      (1). A goal of therapy is to maintain serum calcium concentrations (ideally, serum ionized calcium activities) within the normal range.
      (2). Serum calcium and phosphorus concentrations should be monitored at least every 7 to 14 days until patient response has been established.
      (3). Long-term calcium and phosphorus concentrations and renal function should be monitored at least monthly for patients receiving oral calcium supplements.
      (4). If hypercalcemia develops, therapy should be stopped until calcium levels return to normal; calcium therapy may then be resumed at one-half the previous dosage.
         (a). Although often clinically silent, hypercalcemia may be revealed as polyuria (less apparent in patients with renal failure), nausea, anorexia, vomiting, or lethargy.
         (b). Hypercalcemia has been reported to worsen hypertension in humans with renal failure.[58,76]

VIII. CALCITRIOL THERAPY

A. Calcitriol (1,25 dihydroxycholecalciferol) production is impaired in patients with CRF.

1. Calcitriol deficiency plays a pivotal role in development of renal secondary hyperparathyroidism and renal osteodystrophy in patients with CRF. (Consult Chapter 16, Pathophysiology of Renal Failure and Uremia.)
2. Calcitriol is produced by the kidneys through 1α-hydroxylation of 25-hydroxycholecalciferol.
3. Phosphorus restriction initially enhances calcitriol production, but as renal failure progresses, phosphorus restriction alone ultimately fails to prevent renal secondary hyperparathyroidism, thus necessitating vitamin D supplementation for complete PTH suppression.
   a. In mild renal failure, calcitriol deficiency results predominantly from the inhibitory effects of phosphorus retention on renal 1α-hydroxylase activity. Dietary phosphorus restriction may be effective in minimizing renal secondary hyperparathyroidism during this phase.
   b. In more advanced renal failure, loss of viable renal tubular cells limits calcitriol synthetic

capacity. Calcitriol supplementation is typically required to correct renal secondary hyperparathyroidism in these patients.

B. **Administration of calcitriol rapidly and effectively suppresses renal secondary hyperparathyroidism in dogs and humans because it does the following[53,58,77]:**
   1. Binds to specific receptors with parathyroid secretory cells and directly blocks PTH synthesis and secretion.
   2. Lowers the set point for calcium to inhibit PTH secretion and prevents or reverses parathyroid gland hyperplasia.
   3. Increases gastrointestinal calcium absorption and ionized calcium concentrations in blood, which act synergistically with increased calcitriol levels in blood to inhibit PTH secretion and synthesis.

C. **Although potentially beneficial in patients with CRF, calcitriol therapy must be undertaken with great caution because hypercalcemia is a frequent and potentially serious complication of calcitriol therapy.[58]**
   1. Calcitriol therapy does not directly impair renal function, but sustained calcitriol-induced hypercalcemia can result in reversible or irreversible reduction in GFR.
   2. Hypercalcemia reportedly occurs in 30 to 57% of humans treated with calcitriol.
   3. Chew and colleagues reported that hypercalcemia was an uncommon side effect in dogs with CRF when calcitriol was administered at low dosages.[77]
      a. Hypercalcemia was reported to occur when calcitriol therapy was combined with calcium-containing phosphorus binding agents.
      b. Hypercalcemia resolved when oral calcium carbonate therapy was terminated.
   4. Because hyperphosphatemia enhances the tendency for calcitriol therapy to promote renal mineralization and injury, serum phosphate concentration must be normalized before initiating calcitriol therapy.
   5. In general, patients should not receive calcitriol therapy unless serum calcium and phosphate concentrations will be carefully monitored throughout treatment.

D. **Calcitriol (Rocaltrol Capsules, 0.25 μg and 0.50 μg; Roche Laboratories, Nutley, New Jersey) is the recommended form of vitamin D replacement therapy for patients with CRF.**
   1. An important advantage of calcitriol therapy in CRF is that it does not require renal activation for maximum efficacy.
   2. Dogs and cats appear to require dosages of calcitriol lower than those recommended for humans (on a per weight basis).[53]
      a. Nagode and colleagues have recommended a dose of 1.5 to 3.5 ng/kg/d given orally to dogs with CRF.[53]
      b. Preliminary findings suggest similar dosages may be effective in cats with CRF as well.
      c. Brown and colleagues have recommended a dose of 6.6 ng/kg given orally once daily.[78]
      d. Calcitriol may enhance intestinal absorption of calcium and phosphorus and therefore should not be given with meals.
   3. Serum calcium concentrations must be monitored during therapy with calcitriol to prevent hypercalcemia.
      a. Hypercalcemia may develop at any point during therapy with calcitriol.
      b. The rapid onset of action of calcitriol (about 1 day) and short duration of action (half-life < 1 day) permits rapid control of unwanted hypercalcemia, but early detection of hypercalcemia is indicated to limit the extent of renal injury.
   4. The recommended end point of calcitriol therapy is normalization of PTH activity.
   5. In addition to its beneficial effect on divalent ion metabolism, improvement in clinical signs has been reported in dogs with CRF given calcitriol.[53]
   6. Capsules containing appropriate dosages of calcitriol for use in dogs and cats may be custom-made by some pharmacies.[77]

E. **Although not recommended, vitamin D can alternatively be administered as 1α-hydroxyvitamin D or 25-hydroxyvitamin D (calcidiol).**
   1. The vitamin D analog 1α-hydroxyvitamin D (DHT [dihydrotachysterol tablets], 0.125, 0.2, and 0.4 mg, [Roxane, Columbus, Ohio; and Hytakerol] capsules, 0.125 mg, and oral solution, 0.25 mg/mL, Winthrop, New York, New York) was recommended for treatment of patients with renal failure before calcitriol became commercially available.
      a. Dihydrotachysterol requires hepatic 25-hydroxylation for maximum biologic activity, but it does not undergo and presumably does not require renal 1α-hydroxylation for maximal biologic activity.
      b. It is highly active in patients with renal failure, and in humans, therapeutic results with calcitriol and 1α-hydroxyvitamin D are similar.[58]
      c. When used in combination with oral calcium supplementation in dogs with renal failure, dosage is reported to be 0.03 mg/kg/d for 2 days, then 0.02 mg/kg/d for 2 days, then 0.01 mg/kg/d as a maintenance dose.[79]
      d. In contrast to calcitriol, therapeutic response to dihydrotachysterol may require 1 week of therapy, and reversal of hypercalcemia may require several days.
   2. Despite an apparent block in 1-hydroxylation, calcidiol may also be effective in suppressing hyperparathyroidism and preventing or reversing renal osteodystrophy.[52,58]
      a. In a study in uremic children, calcidiol in-

creased bone formation more effectively than did 1α-hydroxyvitamin D.[80]

b. Administration of pharmacologic dosages of calcidiol to uremic dogs or anephric humans has been shown to return calcitriol levels to normal, thus suggesting the presence of an extrarenal source of 1α-hydroxylase, which is effective in the presence of elevated levels of calcidiol.[81]

c. Hypercalcemia may be a greater concern with calcidiol because of its greater effective half-life compared to that of calcitriol.

F. Regardless of the vitamin D preparation selected, optimum dosage must be determined for each patient on the basis of serial evaluation of PTH activities and serum calcium and phosphorus concentrations.

1. If initially elevated, serum alkaline phosphatase activities may also provide some guidance as to the impact of therapy on skeletal lesions.
2. Initially, serum calcium and phosphorus concentrations should be evaluated at 24- to 48-hour intervals until an appropriate dosage is determined.
3. Because the onset of hypercalcemia after initiation of vitamin D therapy is unpredictable, and may occur after days to months of treatment, continued monitoring of serum calcium, phosphorus, and creatinine concentrations is necessary to detect hypercalcemia, hyperphosphatemia, or deteriorating renal function before irreversible renal damage ensues.
4. If hypercalcemia develops, treatment should be stopped completely rather than reducing the dosage.
5. Therapy may be reinstituted with a reduced dosage after serum calcium concentration returns to normal.
6. Administration of vitamin D is not recommended if serum calcium and phosphate concentrations cannot be monitored.

IX. TREATMENT OF SYSTEMIC HYPERTENSION IN PATIENTS WITH CRF

A. Systemic hypertension appears to be a common complication of CRF.

1. CRF appears to be the most common cause of systemic hypertension in dogs and cats.
2. Hypertension has been reported to occur in about 60 to 65% of cats with CRF.[82,83]
3. Hypertension has been reported to occur in 50 to 93% of dogs with CRF.[84,85]
4. Hypertension may occur even more frequently with primary glomerulopathies.
5. Hypertension complicates the clinical course of most humans with CRF.[86]

B. Sustained hypertension may be associated with serious cardiovascular, ocular, neurologic, and renal complications.

1. Hypertension reportedly results in hypertrophy and muscular hyperplasia of arteriolar walls, fibrinoid necrosis, loss or fragmentation of the internal elastic lamina, hyalinization, myoarteritis, and capillary occlusion.[83,85,87]
   a. These lesions primarily occur in small arteries and arterioles.
   b. Hypertension-induced end-organ injury results, at least in part, from ischemia, decreased tissue perfusion, and hemorrhage subsequent to these vascular lesions.
   c. Epistaxis may be a clinical manifestation of hypertensive vascular disease.
2. Left ventricular hypertrophy and cardiomegaly are commonly recognized in hypertensive dogs and cats.[87,88]
   a. In one report, mitral insufficiency secondary to hypertensive cardiac changes resulted in systolic heart murmurs in 57% of dogs and 42% of cats with hypertension.[87]
   b. Sustained hypertension may promote heart failure, particularly in patients with preexisting cardiac disease.[88]
3. Ocular complications are among the more easily detected clinical effects of hypertension.
   a. Clinical signs may include acute blindness, retinal detachment, hyphema, retinal hemorrhage, reduced pupillary light reflexes, anterior uveitis, or glaucoma.[83,85]
   b. Retinal examination should be routinely performed on all dogs and cats with CRF.
      (1). Retinal lesions may include hemorrhage, detachment, edema, arterial tortuosity, and papilledema.
      (2). Subclinical hypertensive retinopathy may be relatively common among cats with renal hypertension.[89]
   c. Retinal lesions may be reversible with therapy.[87]
4. Hypertensive encephalopathy appears clinically as seizures, depression, behavioral changes, and dementia.
   a. Neurologic signs are typically sudden in onset.
   b. Clinical signs may result from cerebral arteriosclerosis and intracerebral hemorrhages.[90-92]
5. Current evidence in humans suggests that poorly controlled hypertension may cause renal disease and failure or hasten the decline in renal function in patients with pre-existing renal disease.[86,93-95]
   a. Hypertensive renal lesions similar to those observed in hypertensive humans have been observed in dogs.[83]
      (1). Hypertensive glomerular lesions may include glomerulosclerosis, atrophy, proliferative glomerulitis, hyalinization, capillary occlusion, and fibrinoid necrosis.[85,87]
      (2). Hypertensive renal vascular lesions may also cause renal tubular degeneration and interstitial fibrosis.[85]
   b. Hypertension may promote renal injury by

promoting nephrosclerosis with consequent ischemic renal injury or by direct glomerular capillary injury subsequent to intraglomerular hypertension.[93]

C. Diagnosis of systemic hypertension should be based on determination of arterial blood pressure.

1. Blood pressure should be routinely determined in dogs and cats with renal disease by using either direct or indirect methods.[85,96]
2. Normal values for blood pressure may vary with the method used (Table 28-3).
3. Diagnosis of hypertension should generally be based on results of at least three independent determinations of blood pressure that are free of excitement- or anxiety-induced artifacts.
   a. Values consistently greater than approximately 160/95 mm Hg may indicate hypertension in dogs and cats.[83,91,97]
   b. Based on statistical evaluation of a population of 102 normal dogs, Remillard and colleagues determined that pressures in the range of 183 to 202/102 to 113 mm Hg should be interpreted as "borderline hypertension," whereas values greater than 202/113 mm Hg represent definitive hypertension.[98]
   c. Evidence of hypertensive organ damage supports a diagnosis of systemic hypertension.
4. Studies using 24-hour monitoring of arterial blood pressures have indicated that intermittent, short-term determinations of blood pressure may not provide a reliable method for establishing a diagnosis of systemic hypertension.[97]

D. Therapy designed to reduce blood pressure should be considered for dogs and cats with blood pressures consistently greater than 180/100 mm Hg.

1. Justification for treatment of hypertension in dogs and cats remains controversial because of limited data concerning normal blood pressure values, sequelae of long-term hypertension, and beneficial and adverse effects of antihypertensive therapy.
2. When therapy is deemed appropriate, the goal of antihypertensive therapy should be to lower arterial pressure to about 160/100 mm Hg or less or mean arterial pressure to 120 mm Hg or less (i.e., defined as "effective therapy").
   a. The goal of antihypertensive therapy in humans with renal parenchymal disease is to reduce systolic pressures to less than 150 mm Hg and to reduce diastolic pressures to about 85 to 90 mm Hg.[93]
   b. Normalizing blood pressure often reverses many of the acute ocular manifestations of hypertension, but the effect of such therapy on the renal, neurologic, or cardiovascular manifestations of hypertension in dogs and cats with CRF has not been determined.
   c. Antihypertensive therapy is not without risk.
      (1). Overzealous therapy may promote hypotension, volume depletion, and additional renal injury.
      (2). Pharmacologic management of hypertension also entails risks of drug reactions.

TABLE 28–3
NORMAL VALUES FOR BLOOD PRESSURE IN DOGS AND CATS

Dogs

Systolic	Mean	Diastolic	Method	Number of Dogs	Reference
144±27	110±21	91±20	Oscillometric	73	145
147±28	104±17	83±15	Oscillometric	102	98
155±26	N/A	74±14	Doppler	45	84
155±27	N/A	73±14	Direct	45	84
138	103	90	Oscillometric	24	146
148±16	102±9	87±8	Direct	N/A	85

Cats

Systolic	Mean	Diastolic	Method	Number of Cats	Reference
118±11	N/A	84±12	Doppler	33	82
123	97	81	Oscillometric	6	146
171±22	149±24	123±17	Direct	10	147

N/A = not available.

3. Specific guidelines for treatment of systemic hypertension have not been established for dogs and cats.
   a. Until clinical data concerning effectiveness of various forms of therapy become available, therapy should be formulated based on the pathophysiologic mechanisms thought to be responsible for development of hypertension in patients with renal failure.
   b. Therapy should be directed primarily at limiting extracellular fluid volume expansion and counteracting the vasoconstrictor effects of angiotensin II and norepinephrine.[93,95]
      (1). Hypertension of renal parenchymal failure results primarily from increased production of vasoconstrictors (predominantly angiotensin II and norepinephrine) and volume expansion resulting from salt retention.
      (2). Decreased production of renal vasodilators (prostanoids) may also contribute.
   c. Therapy should be initiated in a step-wise fashion beginning with nonpharmacologic therapy (sodium restriction and obesity control) followed by pharmacologic therapy if necessary.
4. Because salt retention appears to be central to the pathogenesis of hypertension in renal parenchymal failure, sodium restriction is indicated for patients with CRF.
   a. Sodium intake should be reduced to about 0.3% of the diet or less (canine maintenance requirement for sodium is about 0.06% of diet).
   b. Patients with CRF adapt to a wide range of dietary sodium intakes; however, adaptation may occur gradually.
      (1). Changes in sodium intake should generally be made gradually over a period of 1 to 2 weeks or more.
      (2). Abrupt changes in dietary sodium may be associated with transient imbalances between intake and urine loss.
      (3). Too rapid a reduction in sodium intake may reduce extracellular fluid volume, thereby leading to poor renal perfusion and further reduction in renal function; recent studies, however, have failed to support this concern.[99]
      (4). Response to adjustments in dietary sodium may be determined by monitoring body weight, hydration, and renal function during, and for several weeks after, the reduction in dietary sodium.
         (a). Progressive loss of body weight, progressive azotemia, and/or dehydration suggest that the patient may be unable to adapt to reduced sodium intake.
         (b). In this event, a more gradual and lesser reduction of sodium intake may be considered.
   c. Whether sodium restriction alone is effective in normalizing systemic hypertension in dogs and cats with CRF is unclear.
      (1). Salt restriction alone has been reported to produce mild reductions in blood pressure.[85]
      (2). Others have reported that sodium restriction alone either failed to reduce blood pressures or inconsistently reduced blood pressures in dogs.[67,87]
   d. Without sodium restriction, administration of some antihypertensive drugs, such as beta-adrenergic antagonists and vasodilators, may lead to sodium retention, extracellular fluid volume expansion, and attenuation of the antihypertensive effects of the drugs.[93,100]
   e. Studies in humans and rats suggest that the anion with which sodium is associated greatly influences the propensity to promote hypertension.[39-41]
      (1). Sodium bicarbonate is less likely to promote hypertension compared to sodium chloride.
      (2). The effect of sodium-containing drugs on blood pressure should be determined by monitoring blood pressure before and after implementing such therapy.
5. Pharmacologic management of hypertension should be considered when sodium restriction alone has proved ineffective in maintaining blood pressures of 160/100 mm Hg or less.
   a. In patients with mild to moderate renal failure, antihypertensive therapy should ideally be effective as monotherapy (i.e., using a single drug), cause minimal side effects, promote regression of left ventricular hypertrophy (or prevent its development), and limit progression of renal failure.[93]
   b. Therapy should also minimize expense and demands on the client.[85]
   c. Angiotensin-converting enzyme (ACE) inhibitors, calcium channel blockers (CCBs), and beta-adrenergic antagonists appear to fit the needs of patients with renal failure most favorably and should be regarded as first-choice drugs.[93]
   d. Drug therapy should only be used when the effect of therapy can be monitored by serial determinations of blood pressure.
      (1). Antihypertensive therapy should be administered at the lowest effective dosage with the dosage titrated according to blood pressure response (Table 28-4).[93]
      (2). Hypotension is usually the first sign that drug dosage needs to be reduced.[95]

TABLE 28–4
ANTIHYPERTENSIVE DRUGS USED IN DOGS AND CATS

Generic Name	Proprietary Name	Dosage	Reference
ACE Inhibitors:			
Captopril	Capoten	0.5–2.0 mg/kg PO q 8–12 h	92
Enalapril	Vasotec	0.25–3.0 mg/kg PO q 12–24 h	91
Lisinopril	Prinivil	0.4–2.0 mg/kg PO q 24 h (dogs)	91
Calcium Channel Blocker:			
Diltiazem	Cardizem	0.5–1.5 mg/kg PO q 8–12 h (dogs) 1.0–2.25 mg/kg PO q 8–12 h (cats)	92
Beta-adrenergic antagonists:			
Propranolol	Inderal	5–80 mg PO q 8–12 h to maximum of 200 mg/d (dogs)	91
		2.5–5.0 mg PO q 8–12 h (cats)	91
Atenolol	Tenormin	2 mg/kg PO q 24 h	91
Diuretics:			
Chlorothiazide	Diuril	20–40 mg/kg PO q 12–24 h	85
Furosemide	Lasix	0.5–2.0 mg/kg PO q 8–24 h	91
Hydrochlorothiazide	HydroDIURIL	1–5 mg/kg PO q 12 h	91
Alpha-adrenergic antagonist:			
Prazosin	Minipress	0.25–2.0 mg PO q 8–12 h (dogs) 0.25–1.0 mg PO q 8–12 h (cats)	92
Vasodilators:			
Hydralazine	Apresoline	1–2 mg/kg PO q 12 h	85
Nitroprusside	Nipride	3–10 mg/kg/min IV	85

(From Polzin DJ, et al. Treatment of chronic renal failure. In: Ettinger S, Feldman E, eds. *Textbook of Veterinary Internal Medicine*. Philadelphia, Pennsylvania: WB Saunders Co; 1995:1734-1760.)

e. Therapy should begin with a single antihypertensive drug.
   (1). Response to therapy should be determined after 7 to 14 days by measuring blood pressure.
   (2). If therapy has not reduced blood pressure to the target range within 2 to 4 weeks, therapy may be changed in 1 of 3 ways:[85]
      (a). Dosage of the current drug may be increased to a higher but nontoxic level.
      (b). The drug may be discontinued and therapy begun with another class of drug.
      (c). A second drug may be added to the treatment regimen.

6. ACE inhibitors have been advocated as first-choice monotherapy to control hypertension in humans with renal failure.
   a. ACE inhibitors are the antihypertensive agents most likely to protect against hypertension-induced renal injury.[86]
      (1). ACE inhibitors may limit hypertensive renal injury by lowering both systemic blood pressure and intraglomerular pressure.[86,101]
         (a). Intraglomerular pressure is determined by the balance between efferent and afferent resistance.
         (b). Angiotensin II promotes intraglomerular hypertension by preferentially enhancing efferent vascular resistance.
         (c). ACE inhibitors reduce efferent resistance, thereby lowering intraglomerular pressure by blocking conversion of angiotensin I to angiotensin II.
      (2). The uniqueness of ACE inhibitors in limiting intraglomerular hypertension has been questioned.[102]
      (3). ACE inhibitors may require concurrent sodium restriction for maximal effectiveness.[100]
   b. ACE inhibitors have been reported to be effective in management of hypertension in dogs.[87,103]
   c. ACE inhibitors may have an increased rate of side effects in patients with CRF, but careful monitoring and dosage adjustments may limit these effects.[95]
      (1). Hypotension and renal injury have occurred with captopril therapy, particularly in patients with concurrent congestive heart failure.[87]

(2). Toxicity of enalapril in dogs is essentially limited to nephrotoxicity; however, toxicity purportedly occurs at levels higher than those achievable with clinically employed dosages, even in renal failure.[104]
(3). ACE inhibitors may promote hyperkalemia.
(4). Captopril and enalapril are excreted by the kidneys; dosage should be modified according to their effects on blood pressure.
(5). Use of ACE inhibitors may be associated with anorexia.

7. Calcium channel blocking agents (CCBs) are commonly used for management of hypertension in human patients with CRF, but their use in treatment of hypertension in dogs and cats with CRF is limited.
   a. CCBs promote vasodilation by inhibiting calcium transport into vascular smooth muscle cells.
   b. CCBs have proved to be effective antihypertensive agents for humans with CRF, but the value of these agents in limiting progressive renal injury is not well established.[86]
      (1). Long-term effects of CCBs on the course of CRF are not known in humans, dogs, or cats.[86]
         (a). Because renal vasodilatory effects of CCBs preferentially reduce afferent vascular resistance, CCBs do not generally reduce intraglomerular pressure.
         (b). Even if systemic pressures are reduced by CCBs, intraglomerular pressures may remain elevated.
         (c). Although some studies suggest CCBs may slow progression of CRF in humans, evidence that CCBs provide a renoprotective effect in hypertensive patients with CRF remains limited.
      (2). Whether CCBs reduce proteinuria in patients with CRF is unclear.
   c. Potential adverse effects of CCBs include hypotension, edema, conduction disturbances, heart failure, and bradycardia.
   d. Because CCBs have negative ionotropic and chronotropic effects, they should not be combined with beta-adrenergic antagonists, which also limit cardiac output.
8. Beta-adrenergic antagonists are effective in management of some patients with hypertension, but their mechanism of action remains controversial.
   a. Antihypertensive effects of beta-blockers may result from decreased cardiac output or renin release, or from effects on the central nervous system or peripheral beta-receptors.
   b. Serious side effects with beta-adrenergic antagonists are unusual.
      (1). Beta-adrenergic antagonists may promote sodium and water retention; thus, combination therapy with diuretics may be appropriate.
      (2). Beta-adrenergic antagonism may limit renin production, thereby promoting hyperkalemia.
      (3). Because of their negative ionotropic effects, beta-antagonists should not be used in combination with CCBs.
      (4). Propranolol may promote bronchospasm in patients with pulmonary disease.
   c. Atenolol, a cardioselective beta-blocker, may be preferred to propranolol, a nonselective beta-blocker, because it may be administered once daily and appears to be relatively free of side effects.[87]
9. Diuretics ameliorate hypertension by reducing extracellular fluid volume and through their vasodilatory actions.[95]
   a. Thiazide diuretics are commonly used as first-choice monotherapy for mild hypertension in humans.
      (1). They may be used in combination with other antihypertensive drugs for severe or refractory hypertension.
      (2). Thiazides are often ineffective in patients with moderate to advanced renal failure.
   b. Furosemide is likely to be more effective than are thiazides in limiting hypertension in patients with moderate to advanced renal failure.[83]
   c. Diuretic therapy should generally be combined with dietary sodium restriction.
   d. Potential adverse side effects of diuretic therapy include extracellular fluid volume depletion, hyponatremia, hypokalemia, and hypercalciuria (with furosemide).
10. Alpha-adrenergic antagonists ameliorate hypertension by promoting vasodilation and decreasing peripheral resistance.
   a. Prazosin appears to be moderately effective in limiting hypertension in dogs with CRF.[83]
   b. Administration of prazosin may be associated with a short-lived hypotension following the first dose ("first dose effect").
   c. Efficacy of alpha-agonists may be limited by salt retention in some patients with renal failure, thereby necessitating addition of a diuretic to the therapeutic regimen.[93]
11. Vasodilators act directly on smooth muscles of the vasculature via incompletely understood mechanisms to decrease peripheral resistance.
   a. Hydralazine has been used effectively to limit hypertension in dogs and cats.

b. Because they may cause sodium retention and reflex tachycardia, such vasodilators as hydralazine often require additional therapy with a diuretic and/or sympatholytic drug.[93]

X. SUPPLEMENTAL FLUID THERAPY

A. Fluid balance in patients with polyuric renal failure is maintained by compensatory polydipsia.

1. When water consumption fails to balance water loss caused by polyuria, dehydration and renal hypoperfusion may ensue, thereby precipitating a uremic crisis.
2. Continued dehydration and renal hypoperfusion may induce ischemic renal injury.
3. Fresh, clean, unadulterated water should be available in adequate quantities at all times to minimize the likelihood of insufficient fluid intake.

B. Fluid supplementation may be indicated when patients with CRF fail to consume sufficient water to prevent volume depletion.

1. Flavored liquids, such as clam juice or tuna broth, may be used to promote additional fluid consumption.
   a. Such fluids should generally be used as a supplement to fluid consumption, not as a substitute for water consumption.
   b. The impact of the mineral and electrolyte content of such supplemental fluids should be considered.
2. When voluntary fluid intake is inadequate to prevent dehydration, supplemental fluids may be administered subcutaneously at home by the owner.
3. Chronic administration of lactated Ringer's solution or normal saline as the principal maintenance fluid source may cause hypernatremia because these fluids fail to provide sufficient electrolyte-free water.
4. Patients with polyuric renal failure frequently fail to consume adequate quantities of water when hospitalized.
   a. When negative body water balance characterized by rapid loss in body weight, loss of skin pliability, and/or hemoconcentration occurs, supplemental fluids should be given orally or parenterally.
   b. In selected patients, prophylactic fluid therapy during periods of hospitalization may be prudent.

XI. TREATMENT OF ANEMIA OF CHRONIC RENAL FAILURE. CONSULT CHAPTER 29, MEDICAL MANAGEMENT OF THE ANEMIA OF CHRONIC RENAL FAILURE

XII. MODIFYING DRUG DOSAGES IN PATIENTS WITH RENAL FAILURE

A. Nephrotoxic drugs and drugs requiring renal excretion should generally be avoided in patients with renal failure.

1. Drugs normally excreted by the kidneys tend to accumulate in patients with renal failure.
   a. Renal drug clearance is reduced in renal failure, thus prolonging drug half-life.
   b. Distribution, protein binding, and hepatic biotransformation of drugs may be altered in renal failure.[105]
2. Excessive drug accumulation promotes an increased rate of adverse drug reactions and nephrotoxicity.
3. The potential risks and benefits associated with use of nephrotoxic drugs and drugs requiring renal excretion should always be considered before initiating therapy with such drugs in patients with CRF.
4. Careful clinical and laboratory monitoring for toxicosis and desired pharmacologic effect is essential.
5. If drugs requiring renal excretion must be administered to patients with renal failure, dosage regimens should be adjusted to compensate for decreased organ function.

B. Because drug accumulation in patients with CRF is primarily a result of reduced renal drug clearance, dosage adjustments should be made according to changes in drug clearance.[28,105,106]

1. Changes in renal drug clearance are usually assumed to parallel changes in GFR.
2. Drug clearance may be estimated by measuring serum creatinine concentrations or, more accurately, by measuring creatinine clearance (C_{cr}).
3. Although C_{cr} is the preferred measure of renal dysfunction for modifying drug therapy in CRF, serum creatinine concentration is the more universally available measure of renal dysfunction.
   a. Although the relationship between serum creatinine concentration and C_{cr} is not linear, the reciprocal of serum creatinine concentration may be used to approximate C_{cr} when serum creatinine concentration is less than 4 mg/dl.[105]
   b. This rule of thumb overestimates C_{cr} when serum creatinine concentration exceeds 4 mg/dl.
   c. Serum urea nitrogen concentration is influenced by many extrarenal factors and does not provide an accurate basis for modifying drug dosage regimens.
   d. Despite the increased expense and effort involved, we recommend using C_{cr} as the basis for modifying drug dosage schedules whenever possible. (This recommendation is particularly relevant when a potentially nephrotoxic drug must be administered.)

C. Dosage of antimicrobial drugs may be modified according to three general patterns, depending on the fraction of the drug eliminated by the kidneys (Table 28-5): 1) doubling the dosing interval or halving the drug dosage in patients with severe reduction in renal function, 2)

TABLE 28–5
DRUG DOSAGE MODIFICATIONS FOR PATIENTS WTH RENAL FAILURE

Drug	Route(s) of Excretion*	Nephrotoxicity	Dosage Adjustment in Renal Failure†
Amikacin	R	yes	Pr
Amoxicillin	R	no	D/I
Amphotericin B	O	yes	Pr
Ampicillin	R,(H)	no	D/I
Cephalexin	R	no	C_{cr}
Cephalothin	R,(H)	no(?)	C_{cr} or D/I
Clindamycin	H,(R)	no	N
Chloramphenicol	H,(R)	no	N,A
Cyclosphosphamide	H,(R)	no	N
Corticosteroids	H	no	N
Dicloxacillin	R,(H)	no	N
Digoxin	R,(O)	no	Pr
Doxycycline	GI,(R)	?	N
Furosemide	R	no(?)	N
Gentamicin	R	yes	Pr
Heparin	O	no	N
Kanamycin	R	yes	Pr
Neomycin	R	yes	C/I
Nitrofurantoin	R	no	C/I
Penicillin	R,(H)	no	D/I
Propranolol	H	no	N
Streptomycin	R	yes	C_{cr}
Sulfisoxazole	R	yes	C_{cr}
Tetracycline	R,(H)	yes	C/I
Tobramycin	R	yes	Pr
Trimethoprim/sulfamethoxazole	R	yes	C_{cr},A

*Routes of excretion: R = renal; H = hepatic; GI = gastrointestinal; O = other (minor route in parentheses).
†Dosage modification: N = normal; D/I = half dose or double dosage interval (in severe renal dysfunction); C_{cr} = adjust according to C_{cr} (see text); Pr = precise dosage modification (see text—adjust according to K_f); C/I = contraindicated; A = avoid in advanced renal failure.
(From Polzin DJ, et al. Diseases of the kidneys and ureters. In: Ettinger SJ, ed. *Textbook of Veterinary Internal Medicine.* Philadelphia, Pennsylvania: WB Saunders Co; 1989:1963-2046.)

increasing the dosage interval according to ranges of C_{cr} values, and 3) precise dosage modification.[105]

1. Modifying drug administration by doubling the dosing interval or halving the drug dosage is reserved for drugs that are relatively nontoxic.
2. When modifying drug according to ranges of C_{cr}, dosing interval is increased two-fold when C_{cr} is between 1.0 and 0.5 mL/min/kg, three-fold when C_{cr} is between 0.5 and 0.3 mL/min/kg, and four-fold when C_{cr} is less than 0.3 mL/min/kg.
3. Some relatively toxic antimicrobial drugs that are excreted solely by glomerular filtration (particularly aminoglycoside antibiotics) require precise dosage modification according to the dosage fraction.[105]
   a. The dosage fraction (K_f) is calculated as the patient's percentage reduction in C_{cr} (i.e., the ratio of patient C_{cr} to normal C_{cr}):

$$K_f = (\text{patient } C_{cr}/\text{normal } C_{cr})$$

   b. Dosage regimens can be adjusted by decreasing the normal dosage or increasing the normal dosage interval in direct proportion to K_f:
      (1). For drugs excreted entirely by glomerular filtration, increases in dosage intervals may be calculated by dividing the normal dosing interval by K_f:

$$\text{Modified modified dose interval} = (\text{normal dose interval}/K_f)$$

      (2). For drugs excreted entirely by glomerular filtration, dosage reductions may be determined by multiplying the normal dose by K_f:

$$\text{modified dose reduction} = (\text{normal dosage} \times K_f)$$

   c. For drugs requiring such precise dosage modification, increased-interval fixed-dosage regimens appear to result in less nephrotoxicity than do fixed-interval reduced-dosage methods.

d. A combination of dosage reduction and interval extension has been recommended for animals with severe renal dysfunction ($C_{cr} < 0.7$ mL/min/kg).

e. A normogram is available for calculating dosages and dosage intervals for these patients.[105]

D. Another means of adjusting drug dosage in patients with CRF is to monitor plasma drug concentrations.

1. Based on knowledge of specific therapeutic ranges and toxic levels of the drug, dosage may be adjusted according to measured plasma drug concentrations.[107]
2. Use of therapeutic drug concentrations for monitoring therapy is particularly advisable if toxic drugs, such as aminoglycosides, must be administered to patients with CRF.

XIII. LIMITING PROGRESSION OF RENAL FAILURE

A. Reducing dietary protein intake.

1. Although results of numerous studies of rats with induced renal injury and of humans with spontaneous CRF suggest that progression of CRF may be slowed by reducing dietary protein intake, limiting protein intake has not been proved to limit progression of CRF in dogs and cats.[12,13,108,109]

a. Reducing protein intake limits glomerular capillary hypertension, glomerular hypertrophy, proteinuria, glomerular sclerosis, and progression of renal failure in rats.[110,111]

b. The effects of reducing protein intake on renal function, renal structure, and progression of renal failure are less well established in dogs and cats.

(1). GFR of dogs and cats with induced renal failure is substantially reduced by limiting dietary protein intake.[108,109]

(2). Whether dietary protein restriction lowers GFR by limiting the extent of glomerular hypertension and hypertrophy or by some other mechanism is unclear.[112]

(3). Reducing protein intake does limit renal enlargement in dogs and cats and glomerular hypertrophy in cats.[109,113]

(4). Feeding a moderately restricted protein diet (16% dry matter) to dogs with 15/16 reduction in renal mass did not prevent development of glomerular capillary hypertension and glomerular hypertrophy; however, the effects of higher or lower protein intakes on glomerular capillary pressures and glomerular enlargement were not determined.[112]

(5). Reducing protein intake is generally associated with reduced proteinuria in both dogs and cats with induced CRF; however, this reduction may represent a hemodynamic event, glomerular injury, or a combination of these effects.[108,114]

(a). Glomerular lesions develop in dogs with reduced renal mass, but unlike in rats, reducing protein intake has not been shown to limit development of these lesions in dogs.[12,113]

(b). Reducing protein intake largely prevented development of glomerular lesions in cats with induced CRF, but interpretation of these findings was complicated by reduced food consumption by cats fed the lower-protein diet.[109]

(6). Studies on the impact of dietary protein intake on progression of renal failure have been somewhat contradictory.

(a). Limiting dietary protein intake did not appear to influence progression of renal failure in dogs following 15/16 nephrectomy.[12]

(b). In a prospective study on the management of spontaneous canine renal failure, dogs fed a diet providing moderately restricted intakes of protein and phosphorus appeared to survive longer than did dogs fed a standard maintenance dog food.[16]

(1′). The apparent beneficial effects of protein restriction in this study may have resulted from the beneficial metabolic effects of protein restriction in patients with CRF.

(2′). On the other hand, arterial hypertension is reportedly a common complication of spontaneous renal failure in dogs, whereas only minor increases in blood pressure develop in the partial nephrectomy model of renal failure in dogs.

(3′). Because consumption of high-protein diets may promote glomerular injury and progression, in part by impairing renal autoregulation and exposing the glomerular capillaries to increased systemic pressures, the relationship between dietary protein intake and progressive renal injury may be obscured in the absence of arterial hypertension.

(c). A diet with reduced quantities of protein, phosphorus, calcium, and lipid was shown to limit glomerular basement membrane splitting in Samoyed dogs with spontaneous canine X-linked hereditary nephritis, a primary glomerulopathy.[13]

(1′). Dogs fed this modified protein diet (containing 13.5% protein dry matter basis) survived 53% longer than did dogs fed a 23% protein maintenance diet.

(2′). Because the renal-sparing effects of this dietary modification appeared to be primarily related to the effect on glomerular injury, phosphorus intake probably was not responsible for the beneficial effects of the diet.

(3′). Patients with glomerular injury may benefit from dietary protein restriction to a greater degree than do patients with primarily tubulo-interstitial disease.

(d). Despite the apparent adverse effect of high-protein feeding on renal disorders in cats with induced renal failure, high-protein feeding was not associated with a progressive loss of renal function.[109,115]

2. The therapeutic role for protein restriction in limiting decline in GFR and prolonging survival of dogs and cats with spontaneous CRF remains unclear.
   a. The primary indication for protein restriction is to limit the metabolic consequences of renal failure; an added benefit in terms of limiting progression may or may not exist.
   b. If or when protein restriction is indicated is unclear in dogs and cats that do not require protein restriction to limit clinical consequences of uremia.
   c. Nonuremic patients with primary glomerulopathies may benefit from dietary protein restriction.
      (1). Studies have shown that high dietary protein intake may have an adverse effect on the magnitude of proteinuria and protein nutrition in human patients with nephrotic syndrome.[116]
      (2). Because the role of protein restriction in limiting progression and improving nutrition in dogs and cats with spontaneous glomerulopathies is yet to be determined, protein restriction should be undertaken with caution and careful monitoring of the patient's response to therapy.

B. Limiting dietary phosphorus intake.

1. Restricting dietary phosphorus intake (to 0.4 to 0.5% dry matter basis) has been shown to retard the decline in GFR and enhanced survival in dogs with moderate induced CRF (mean plasma creatinine concentrations approximately 3 to 4 mg/dL).[12,59,60]
   a. These beneficial effects of phosphorus restriction did not require protein restriction, nor were they enhanced by dietary protein restriction.[12]
   b. The adverse effect of dietary phosphorus, hyperphosphatemia, and hyperparathyroidism on progressive renal dysfunction has been hypothesized to result from precipitation of phosphorus salts within the renal parenchyma.[62]
      (1). Renal mineralization leads to inflammation, scarring, and subsequent loss of nephrons.
      (2). In the canine studies referred to previously, a substantial increase in renal phosphorus content and a massive increase in renal calcium content were detected after 2 years of renal failure.[12]
         (a). However, dietary phosphorus intake (0.4 versus 1.5% dry matter basis) did not influence the concentrations of calcium or phosphorus in renal tissue.
         (b). Nonetheless, dogs dying of uremia in these studies had greater renal mineralization and fibrosis than did dogs surviving the study.
         (c). The mechanisms by which phosphorus restriction improved survival in these dogs are unclear, but the authors hypothesized a role for extrarenal mechanisms.
      (3). Phosphorus restriction may also retard progression of CRF by: 1) minimizing renal intracellular calcium concentrations, thus preventing calcium-mediated cellular injury, 2) inhibiting renal cell injury by reducing cellular energy metabolism, 3) influencing abnormalities of lipid metabolism associated with uremia, 4) suppressing immune responsiveness, or 5) influencing glomerular hypertension.[117]
2. Phosphorus restriction has also been shown to limit renal mineralization in cats with induced CRF, but renal function remained unchanged in this study.[61]
3. Although these preliminary findings support the practice of limiting phosphorus intake for patients with renal failure, clinical studies confirming the efficacy of such therapy in improving survival of dogs and cats with spontaneous renal failure are needed.

C. Dietary calorie intake.

1. Food restriction, and particularly energy restriction, has been shown to improve the outcome of several forms of experimental renal disease in rodents.[24,26]
   a. Restricting carbohydrate, fat, and mineral (except for calcium and phosphorus) intake retarded growth and prevented development of end-stage renal disease in rats with reduced renal mass, regardless of whether or not protein intake was restricted.[27]
   b. Renal injury may have been ameliorated in rats fed calorie-restricted diets as a result of limited renal growth and hypertrophy.

c. Because dietary protein restriction is often associated with reduced food consumption, the question has been raised as to whether the apparent benefit of dietary protein restriction in limiting renal injury in rats may in fact have resulted from calorie and mineral restriction.

(1). Restricting protein without restricting any other dietary component failed to retard growth or to prevent development of glomerular sclerosis.[27]

(2). In a similar study, protein restriction was found to have an independent role in limiting renal injury, but the beneficial effects of calorie restriction were substantially greater than the benefits of protein restriction.[24]

2. Studies on the role of food or calorie intake on progression of renal failure in dogs and cats have not been reported.
3. Whereas limiting food/calorie intake is probably not a practical means of preserving renal structure and function for dogs and cats, the prudent course may be to: 1) avoid overfeeding and obesity in dogs and cats with CRF, and 2) attempt to modify calorie intake to attain optimum body weight.

D. Dietary lipids.

1. Evidence from studies in rodents suggests a role for dietary lipids in modulating progression of renal disease.[118-121]

a. The mechanisms responsible for these modulating effects may be related to renal eicosanoid production and plasma lipid concentrations.

b. The composition of dietary lipids may influence systemic blood pressure, blood lipid composition, platelet aggregation, blood viscosity, the immune system, and fibrinolytic activity.[121]

c. Although conflicting data exist, accumulation of lipid macromolecules in the mesangium, especially cholesterol and cholesterol esters, has been hypothesized to contribute to mesangial cell injury and to stimulate production of mesangial matrix, thus promoting glomerular sclerosis.[122,123]

(1). A close correlation seems to exist between the lipid status of the glomerulus and the presence or absence of macrophages.[23,124]

(2). Glomeruli experiencing mesangial deposits of antibody or macromolecules release a lipid chemoattractant specific for monocytes.

(3). Macrophages, which comprise a major portion of atherosclerotic plaque in humans, may contribute to or modulate many of the processes thought to contribute to progressive renal injury: release of platelet-derived growth factor (a mesangial cell mitogen), interleukin-1 (a mesangial cell activator), and cytokines that induce the leukocyte adhesion proteins on endothelial cells and membrane-bound procoagulant activity on endothelial cells.[124]

2. Diets rich in linoleic acid, an omega-6 fatty acid, have been found to ameliorate progression of renal disease in rats with reduced renal mass.[119]

a. Linoleic acid, which occurs in high proportions in fats derived from plant sources, is the immediate precursor of arachadonic acid, the substrate for eicosanoid production.

b. Diets rich in linoleic acid could theoretically enhance renal eicosanoid production, thereby providing a renoprotective effect.

(1). However, enhanced renal production of PGE_2 could exacerbate intraglomerular hypertension, which could be injurious to the glomerulus.[22]

(2). Nonetheless, feeding a diet high in linoleic acid to rats with subtotal renal ablation increased GFR and renal plasma flow, and reduced blood pressure, proteinuria, and glomerular lesions.[119]

(3). The beneficial effects of high linoleate intake appear to be additive with the beneficial effect of reduced protein diets in this model.[125]

c. Dietary linoleic acid did not appear to affect the clinical course of mice with immune-mediated renal disease.[126]

3. Fish oil-enriched diets have been shown to be beneficial in reducing proteinuria in certain immune-mediated renal diseases in mice and humans.[120]

a. Omega-3 fatty acids, including eicosapentaenoic acid and docosahexaenoic acid, appear to be the active components responsible for many of the beneficial effects of fish oil.

(1). Because omega-3 fatty acids are poor substrates for cyclo-oxygenase, increased dietary omega-3 fatty acids inhibit production of arachadonic acid-derived cyclo-oxygenase metabolites, and thus may exert an antiplatelet effect, reduce production of biologically active thromboxane, and, perhaps, lower blood pressure.[120]

(2). However, impaired prostaglandin production may be detrimental because adequate production of renal prostaglandins, specifically PGE_2 and PGI_2, is important for maintaining glomerular filtration.

b. Fish oil diets appear to accelerate deterioration of renal function and structure in rats with nonimmune-mediated renal disease induced by surgical ablation of renal tissue.[120]

4. Plasma lipid (cholesterol and triglycerides) concentrations appear to influence development and progression of renal disease.

a. Renal disease in humans is associated with abnormalities in lipid metabolism revealed as elevated serum concentrations of low-density lipoproteins, total cholesterol, and triglycerides.[127]

b. High-cholesterol diets have been shown to induce hyperlipidemia and renal failure in rats.[128]

c. Although a role for lipids in modifying development and progression of renal disease has not been established for dogs and cats, dogs maintained on a moderately reduced protein/low phosphorus/moderately reduced fat diet after marked reduction of renal mass developed glomerular lesions and loss of renal function, which were directly related to elevations of plasma triglyceride and total cholesterol.[59]

5. The effects of altering dietary lipids on progression of spontaneous or experimental renal disease in dogs and cats are currently under investigation.
   a. As is evident from the studies just described, dietary lipids may influence progression of different forms of renal disease in different ways, depending on the mechanism of renal injury.
   b. Generalizations concerning formulation of dietary lipids for patients with renal failure are not yet possible.

E. Calcitriol therapy.

1. Chronically elevated levels of PTH may promote progression of renal failure.[129-131]
   a. PTH is hypothesized to promote intracellular deposition of calcium in the renal parenchyma.
   b. Calcitriol administration may slow progression of CRF by minimizing hyperparathyroidism, thereby limiting development of nephrocalcinosis.
2. Although renal mineralization is a well-recognized phenomenon in canine and feline CRF, renal secondary hyperparathyroidism and nephrocalcinosis have not been proved to cause progression of CRF in dogs or cats.
   a. Preliminary evidence suggests that calcitriol therapy may slow progression of renal failure in dogs.[129]
   b. Controlled studies are needed to confirm the safety and long-term value of calcitriol in limiting progression of renal failure in dogs and cats.

F. Minimizing metabolic acidosis and hypokalemia.

1. Metabolic acidosis is theorized to play a role in progression of renal failure because it may increase renal ammoniagenesis.
   a. Although total renal ammonium excretion may decline with CRF (decreased total renal mass), the capacity of each individual nephron to increase ammonium production is very high, and this renal response to chronic metabolic acidosis is retained until CRF is advanced.
      (1). Renal ammoniagenesis may be augmented in chronic metabolic acidosis, hypokalemia, subtotal renal ablation, diets high in protein, diabetic nephropathy, and antioxidant (vitamin E or selenium) deficiency.
      (2). All these states are associated with the induction or progression of renal failure in an experimental model or clinical disease state.[132]
   b. Elevated intrarenal ammonia concentrations have been proposed to be one of the common pathways whereby diverse renal insults result in similar pathologic manifestations of renal injury.[132]
      (1). High levels of ammonium may promote renal injury by activating the third component of complement by the alternate pathway.
         (a). Complement-mediated renal inflammation results in tubulo-interstitial damage suspected of promoting progression of renal disease.
         (b). Prevention of metabolic acidosis by dietary supplementation with sodium bicarbonate has been shown to prevent the development of tubulo-interstitial lesions in rats with induced CRF.[37]
      (2). Increased ammoniagenesis may also contribute to progression by promoting renal hypertrophy.
         (a). High ammonia levels promote growth of renal cells in culture.
         (b). Increased urine osmolarity (reflecting increased workload of interstitium to generate gradients for excretion) induces renal hypertrophy and progression of CRF. Either acidosis or a high-protein diet would augment ammonium production, thereby contributing added solutes and requiring increased urine concentration.[133]
2. Chronic potassium depletion has been shown to cause renal disease, termed hypokalemic nephropathy, in rats and humans, and has been implicated as a cause for renal disease in cats.[45,47]
   a. In rats and humans, the kidneys are enlarged, proximal tubular cells become vacuolated tubulo-interstitial inflammatory lesions develop, and urine concentrating ability is lost; hypokalemic nephropathy can progress to end-stage renal disease if the potassium depletion is not corrected.
      (1). Renal vasoconstriction associated with increased thromboxane and prostaglandin levels is thought to be important in the pathogenesis of hypokalemic nephropathy.
      (2). Increased renal ammonia production, enhanced by hypokalemia, may also pro-

mote ammonium-mediated renal damage as previously described.[134]

b. A syndrome of hypokalemic nephropathy exists in cats, but appears to be somewhat different from hypokalemic nephropathy as described in humans and rats.[45,47]
   (1). Feeding of high-protein diets with relatively low dietary potassium content seems to promote potassium depletion in cats.
   (2). Metabolic acidosis exacerbates the condition, possibly by increasing renal and fecal potassium excretion.
   (3). Whether pre-existing renal impairment is a prerequisite for the development of hypokalemic nephropathy in cats is unclear.

G. Antihypertensive therapy.

1. Arterial hypertension is thought to promote glomerular injury and progression of CRF at least in part from free transmission of elevated systemic pressures to the glomerulus with resultant glomerular capillary hypertension.[86]
   a. In normal kidneys, systemic hypertension does not necessarily result in glomerular hypertension.
   b. Although the normal glomerular hemodynamic response to elevations in renal perfusion pressure is vasoconstriction with an increase in preglomerular resistance (autoregulation), arterial hypertension can cause glomerular hypertension when renal autoregulation is impaired, as may be the case in patients with CRF.
2. Hypertensive glomerular injury may also result from nonhemodynamic mechanisms, including glomerular hypertrophy, intrarenal activation of the alternative complement pathway, increased metabolic activity in surviving nephrons, increased mesangial macromolecular traffic, and activation of the coagulation system.[86]
3. Nephrologists generally accept that treatment of arterial hypertension in humans with renal disease can slow or even arrest development of progressive renal insufficiency.[86]
   a. Results of a recent clinical study on treatment of hypertension in humans with CRF were interpreted to suggest that aggressive control of blood pressure with a target blood pressure level significantly less than the routinely accepted level may be necessary to limit progressive renal damage.[135]
   b. Certain antihypertensive drugs appear to preserve renal function better than do other antihypertensive agents that may be equally effective at normalizing systemic blood pressures.[86]
      (1). Studies in rodents and humans have suggested that converting enzyme inhibitors (CEIs) possess a unique renoprotective effect on progressive glomerular injury.[86,135-137]
         (a). The renoprotective effect is associated with the normalization of both systemic and glomerular capillary pressures that results from renal vasodilation, predominantly of the efferent arteriole.
         (b). Although other antihypertensive agents may prove effective in reducing systemic blood pressure, glomerular capillary pressures may remain elevated, thus exposing the glomerulus to continuing hypertensive injury.
         (c). Therapy with CEIs has also been shown to have an antiproteinuric effect, an effect that may provide a direct therapeutic advantage over other antihypertensive agents.
         (d). No data exist on the impact of CEIs in limiting progressive renal injury in dogs and cats.
            (1′). Because of the potential advantages delineated here, we have generally selected enalapril as our initial drug for management of arterial hypertension in dogs and cats.
            (2′). Enalapril appears to be generally safe and well tolerated in dogs and cats with CRF when used judiciously and with appropriate monitoring.
      (2). A recent study comparing the renoprotective effects of the CEI captopril and the CCB nifedipine found both drugs had similar benefits in slowing the rate of progression of renal insufficiency in human patients.[135]
         (a). CCBs are effective antihypertensive agents in human patients with CRF and do not appear to have adverse short-term effects on renal function.[86]
         (b). CCBs do not reduce glomerular capillary pressures or proteinuria, nor do they appear to limit glomerulosclerosis.
            (1′). The CCB may actually increase proteinuria and promote glomerulosclerosis.
            (2′). Reductions in systemic pressures induced by CCBs are balanced by reduced afferent arteriolar resistance, thus maintaining elevated intraglomerular capillary pressures.
            (3′). CCBs may lower systemic blood pressure without conferring a renoprotective effect of hemodynamic origin.

(4′). Preliminary findings suggest that the seemingly adverse hemodynamic effects of CCBs may not be harmful or that other beneficial effects of these agents modulate the adverse hemodynamic effects.[138]

(c). The renoprotective effects are probably not hemodynamically mediated.

(1′). Studies in rats with subtotal renal ablation have indicated that the renoprotective effects of CCBs may be associated with their ability to limit renal calcium content.[139]

(2′). Mechanisms known or postulated to mediate the renoprotective actions of CCBs include reducing systemic blood pressure, reducing renal hypertrophy, modulating mesangial traffic of macromolecules, inhibiting mitogenic effects of platelet-derived growth factor and of thrombin, scavenging toxic oxygen-free radicals, reducing metabolic activity of remnant kidneys, and ameliorating uremic nephrocalcinosis.[138]

(d). Experience with CCBs in treatment of dogs and cats with CRF is limited, and the role of these agents in modulating progression of renal failure is unclear.

(1′). These agents may have a role as supplemental or alternative therapy when arterial hypertension fails to respond to CEI therapy alone.

(2′). Studies on the safety and efficacy of CCBs in dogs and cats with CRF are needed to formulate recommendations concerning their use as renoprotective agents.

4. Convincing data linking systemic or glomerular hypertension to progressive renal injury in dogs and cats have not been generated.
   a. Whether treatment of arterial hypertension for the purpose of preserving renal structure and function can be justified in dogs and cats at this time is therefore controversial.
   b. We have observed a few dogs with markedly elevated systemic blood pressures, rapidly progressive renal failure, and renal lesions compatible with hypertension-induced renal injury. These findings suggest that, at least in some dogs, hypertension may have adverse renal consequences.
   c. Additional studies are needed to establish the clinical significance of arterial hypertension and its role in progressive renal injury in dogs and cats.

XIV. MONITORING PATIENTS WITH CRF

A. Response to treatment should be monitored at appropriate intervals so that treatment can be individualized to the specific, and often changing, needs of the patient.

B. The database obtained before initiation of conservative medical management should be used as a baseline for comparison of the patient's progress.

1. This evaluation should be repeated at appropriate intervals, which vary according to specific needs of the patient.
   a. Immediately following initiation of therapy, patients should be monitored every 2 to 4 weeks to assess the response to therapy.
   b. The frequency of evaluation may vary depending on severity of renal dysfunction, complications present in the patient, and response to treatment.
   c. Certain forms of therapy, such as administration of recombinant human erythropoietin (rHuEPO), may also necessitate more frequent patient monitoring.
2. Recommendations for monitoring are summarized in Table 28-6.

C. Serial assessment of renal function may be used to determine a more accurate prognosis and to assess the impact of therapy on progression of renal failure.

1. On the basis of this information, therapy may be modified to better achieve the important therapeutic goal of slowing or stopping progressive deterioration of renal function.
2. Several methods for determining progression of renal dysfunction are available, but all have certain intrinsic disadvantages.
   a. Serial measurement of endogenous or exogenous C_{cr} provides a reliable measure of changes in GFR.[140,141]

      (1). Such studies are inconvenient, highly variable, and may be associated with the risk of catheter-induced urinary tract infection.

      (2). In addition, incomplete urine collections may constitute an important error in clearance calculations.
   b. Single-injection techniques using a plasma disappearance curve may also be used to determine GFR serially.[142]
   c. Monitoring serial changes in the reciprocal or logarithm of the serum creatinine concentration is commonly performed to provide an estimate of changes in renal function during long-term therapy of CRF in humans.[143]

      (1). In humans with CRF, one of these two relationships is typically found to be linear.

      (2). This technique is reportedly only useful

TABLE 28–6
GUIDELINES FOR MONITORING PATIENTS WITH CHRONIC RENAL FAILURE

Test	Purpose
History	To assess response to therapy; to ascertain compliance with recommendations and owner-perceived problems with therapy; to detect communication problems with the client; to detect new problems or complications; to encourage client compliance
Physical examination	To detect new problems or complications; to assess hydration; to assess nutritional status and well-being of the animal
Body weight	To assess nutritional and hydration status
Serum creatinine concentration	To assess severity and progression of renal dysfunction; to detect concomitant prerenal and postrenal azotemia
Blood urea nitrogen concentration	To assess compliance with dietary recommendations; to detect concomitant prerenal and postrenal azotemia
Urinalysis	To detect urinary tract infection; to detect changes in urine sediment or urine chemistries suggestive of active or changing renal lesions that may warrant specific therapy or changes in therapy; to monitor proteinuria
Serum phosphorus concentration	To determine success of dietary phosphorus restriction; to adjust dosages of intestinal phosphorus binders
Serum calcium concentration	To assess need for and to adjust dosage of calcium supplements and vitamin D
Serum albumin concentration	To assess nutritional status; important for monitoring impact of urinary protein loss in patients with glomerulopathies; necessary for interpretation of serum calcium values and assessment of influence on protein-bound drugs
Total CO_2 concentration	To assess need for alkalinization therapy; necessary for adjusting dosage of alkalinization therapy
Packed cell volume or complete blood count	To assess response to therapy for anemia; may also be useful to assess nutritional status
Urine culture	Indicated: (1) if urinalysis supports possible urinary tract infection, (2) to confirm that previously detected and treated urinary tract infections have been successfully eradicated, (3) as routine part of follow-up studies in patients with recurrent urinary tract infections and CRF

(From Polzin DJ, et al. Diseases of the kidney and ureters. In: Ettinger SJ, ed. *Textbook of Veterinary Internal Medicine.* Philadelphia, Pennsylvania: WB Saunders Co; 1989:1963-2046.)

when serum creatinine concentrations exceed about 3 mg/dL in humans.

(3). Preliminary studies in dogs suggest that reciprocal of serum creatinine concentration versus time may be linear in this species as well.[144]

(4). Use of these techniques is controversial in human patients and requires validation in dogs and cats.

REFERENCES

1. Mitch WE. Dietary protein restriction in patients with chronic renal failure. *Kidney Int.* 1991;40:326-341.
2. Kelly R, Mitch W. Creatinine, uric acid, and other nitrogenous waste products: Clinical implication of the imbalance between their production and elimination in uremia. *Semin Nephrol.* 1983;3:286-294.
3. Johnson W. Does elevated blood urea participate in the pathogenesis of the uremic syndrome? *Semin Nephrol.* 1983;3:265-272.
4. Campbell R. Polyamines, uremia, and anemia. *Semin Nephrol.* 1983;3:273-285.
5. Massry S, Kopple J. Uremic toxins: What are they? How are they identified? *Semin Nephrol.* 1983;3:263-264.
6. Keshaviah P, Kjellstrand C. Middle molecules: Do they exist? Are they toxic? *Semin Nephrol.* 1983;3:295-305.
7. Johnson W, et al. Effects of urea loading in patients with far-advanced renal failure. *Mayo Clin Proc.* 1972;47:21-29.
8. Polzin D, et al. Effects of modified protein diets in dogs with chronic renal failure. *J Am Vet Med Assoc.* 1983;183:980-986.
9. Brenner BM, et al. Dietary protein intake and the progressive nature of kidney disease: The role of hemodynamically mediated glomerular injury in the pathogenesis of progressive glomerular sclerosis in aging, renal ablation, and intrinsic renal disease. *N Engl J Med.* 1982;307:652-659.
10. Polzin D, et al. Dietary management of canine and feline chronic renal failure. *Vet Clin North Am: [Small Anim Pract].* 1989;19:539-560.
11. Polzin DJ, et al. Effect of modified protein diets in dogs and cats with chronic renal failure: Current status. *J Nutr.* 1991;121:S140-144.
12. Finco D, et al. Effects of dietary phosphorus and protein in dogs with chronic renal failure. *Am J Vet Res.* 1992;53:2264-2271.
13. Valli VEO, et al. Dietary modification reduces splitting of

glomerular basement membranes and delays death due to renal failure in canine X-linked hereditary nephritis. *Lab Invest.* 1991;65:67-73.

14. Adams L, et al. Influence of dietary protein on renal function and morphology in cats with 5/6 nephrectomy. *Lab Invest.* 1994;70:347-357.
15. Polzin D, et al. Influence of modified protein diets on nutritional status of dogs with experimental chronic renal failure. *Am J Vet Res.* 1983;44:1694-1702.
16. Barsanti J, Finco D. Dietary management of chronic renal failure in dogs. *J Am Anim Hosp Assoc.* 1985;21:371-376.
17. Burger I, et al. The protein requirement of adult cats for maintenance. *Feline Pract.* 1984;14:8-14.
18. Lewis L, et al. *Small Animal Clinical Nutrition III.* Topeka, Kansas: Mark Morris Associates; 1987:1-16.
19. May R, et al. Mechanisms for defects in muscle protein metabolism in rats with chronic uremia: The influence of metabolic acidosis. *J Clin Invest.* 1987;79:1099-1103.
20. Mitch W, Walser M. Nutritional therapy of the uremic patient. In: Brenner B, Rector F, eds. *The Kidney.* Philadelphia, Pennsylvania: WB Saunders Co; 1991:2186-2222.
21. Kasiske B, et al. Lipids and the kidney. *Hypertension.* 1990;15: 443-450.
22. Brown S. Dietary lipids and progressive renal disease in the dog. In: *Proceedings of the 16th Waltham/OSU Symposium.* Columbus, Ohio: Kal Kan Foods; 1992.
23. Kasiske BL, et al. Renal injury of diet-induced hypercholesterolemia in rats. *Kidney Int.* 1990;37:880-891.
24. Masoro E, et al. Dietary modulation of the progression of nephropathy in aging rats: An evaluation of the importance of protein. *Am J Clin Nutr.* 1989;49:1217-1227.
25. Masoro E, Yu B. Diet and nephropathy. *Lab Invest.* 1989;60: 165-167.
26. Tapp DC, et al. Food restriction retards body growth and prevents end-stage renal pathology in remnant kidneys of rats regardless of protein intake. *Lab Invest.* 1989;60:184-195.
27. Tapp D, et al. Protein restriction or calorie restriction? A critical assessment of the influence of selective calorie restriction on the progression of experimental renal disease. *Semin Nephrol.* 1989;9:343-353.
28. Polzin DJ, et al. Diseases of the kidneys and ureters. In: Ettinger SJ, ed. *Textbook of Veterinary Internal Medicine.* Philadelphia, Pennsylvania: WB Saunders Co; 1989:1963-2046.
29. Osborne C, et al. Management of anorexia associated with renal failure. In: *Proceedings Tenth Annual Veterinary Medical Forum.* San Diego, California: American College of Veterinary Internal Medicine; 1992.
30. Lulich J, et al. Feline renal failure: Questions, answers, questions. *Compendium Cont Educ Pract Vet.* 1992;14:127-152.
31. Polzin D. Spectrum of clinical and laboratory abnormalities in uremia. In: Kirk R, ed. *Current Veterinary Therapy X.* Philadelphia, Pennsylvania: WB Saunders Co; 1989:1133-1138.
32. Kopple J. Chronic renal failure: Nutritional and nondialytic management. In: Glassock R, ed. *Current Therapy in Nephrology and Hypertension, 1984-85.* St. Louis, Missouri: CV Mosby Co; 1984:252-260.
33. Finco D et al. Effects of an anabolic steroid on acute uremia in the dog. *Am J Vet Res.* 1984;45:2285-2288.
34. Rose BD. *Clinical Physiology of Acid-Base and Electrolyte Disorders.* 3rd ed. New York, New York: McGraw-Hill; 1989:501-555.
35. Mitch WE. Dietary protein restriction in chronic renal failure: Nutritional efficacy, compliance, and progression of renal insufficiency. *J Am Soc Nephrol.* 1991;2:823-831.
36. Hara Y, et al. Acidosis, not azotemia, stimulates branched-chain amino acid catabolism in uremic rats. *Kidney Int.* 1987;32: 808-814.
37. Nath KA, et al. Pathophysiology of chronic tubulo-interstitial disease in rats: Interactions of dietary acid load, ammonia, and complement component C3. *J Clin Invest.* 1985;76:667-675.
38. Litzow JR, et al. The effect of treatment of acidosis on calcium balance in patients with chronic azotemic renal disease. *J Clin Invest.* 1967;46:509-513.
39. Husted FC, et al. Sodium bicarbonate and sodium chloride tolerance in chronic renal failure. *J Clin Invest.* 1975;56: 414-419.
40. Kurtz TW, et al. "Salt-sensitive" essential hypertension in men. Is the sodium ion alone important? *N Engl J Med.* 1987;317: 1043-1048.
41. Weinberger MH. Sodium chloride and blood pressure. *N Engl J Med.* 1987;317:1084-1086.
42. Polzin DJ, Osborne CA. The importance of egg protein in reduced protein diets designed for dogs with renal failure. *J Vet Intern Med.* 1988;2:15-21.
43. Schwartz WB. On the mechanism of acidosis in chronic renal disease. *J Clin Invest.* 1959;38:39.
44. Schmidt RW, Gavellas G. Bicarbonate reabsorption in experimental renal disease: Effects of proportional reduction of sodium or phosphate intake. *Kidney Int.* 1977;12:393-402.
45. Dow SW, et al. Potassium depletion in cats: Renal and dietary influences. *J Am Vet Med Assoc.* 1987;191:1569-1575.
46. Adams LG, et al. Comparison of fractional excretion and twenty-four hour urinary excretion of sodium and potassium in clinically normal cats and cats with induced chronic renal failure. *Am J Vet Res.* 1991;52:718-722.
47. DiBartola S, et al. Development of chronic renal disease in cats fed a commercial diet. *J Am Vet Med Assoc.* 1993;202: 744-751.
48. Hills D, et al. Potassium requirement of kittens as affected by dietary protein. *J Nutr.* 1982;112:216-222.
49. Dow SW, et al. Effects of dietary acidification and potassium depletion on acid-base balance, mineral metabolism and renal function in adult cats. *J Nutr.* 1990;120:569-578.
50. Dow S, Fettman M. Renal disease in cats: The potassium connection. In: Kirk R, Bonagura J, eds. *Current Veterinary Therapy XI.* Philadelphia, Pennsylvania: WB Saunders Co; 1992:820-822.
51. Dow SW, et al. Potassium depletion in cats: Hypokalemic polymyopathy. *J Am Vet Med Assoc.* 1987;191:1563-1568.
52. Rutherford WE, et al. Phosphate control and 25-hydroxycholecalciferol administration in preventing experimental renal osteodystrophy in the dog. *J Clin Invest.* 1977;60: 332-341.
53. Nagode L, Chew D. The use of calcitriol in treatment of renal disease of the dog and cat. In: *Proceedings Purina International Nutrition Symposium.* Orlando, Florida: Ralston Purina Co; 1991.
54. Delmez JA, Slatopolsky E. Hyperphosphatemia—Its consequences and treatment in patients with chronic renal disease. *Am J Kidney Dis.* 1992;19:303-317.
55. Slatopolsky E, et al. On the prevention of secondary hyperparathyroidism in experimental chronic renal disease using "proportional reduction" of dietary phosphorus intake. *Kidney Int.* 1972;2:147-.
56. Slatopolsky E, Bricker N. The role of phosphorus restriction in the prevention of secondary hyperparathyroidism in chronic renal disease. *Kidney Int.* 1973;4:141-.
57. Llach F, Massry S. On the mechanism of prevention of secondary hyperparathyroidism in moderate renal insufficiency. *J Clin Endocrinol Metab.* 1985;61:601-606.
58. Coburn J, Slatopolsky E. Vitamin D, parathyroid hormone, and the renal osteodystrophies. In: Brenner B, Rector F, eds. *The Kidney.* Philadelphia, Pennsylvania: WB Saunders Co; 1991: 2036-2120.

59. Brown SA, et al. Beneficial effects of dietary mineral restriction in dogs with marked reduction of functional renal mass. *J Am Soc Nephrol.* 1991;1:1169-1179.
60. Finco D, et al. Effects of phosphorus/calcium-restricted and phosphorus/calcium-replete 32% protein diets in dogs with chronic renal failure. *Am J Vet Res.* 1992;53:157-163.
61. Ross LA, et al. Effect of dietary phosphorus restriction on the kidneys of cats with reduced renal mass. *Am J Vet Res.* 1982;43: 1023-1026.
62. Lau K. Phosphate excess and progressive renal failure: The precipitation-calcification hypothesis. *Kidney Int.* 1989;36: 918-937.
63. Areiff A, Massry S. Calcium metabolism of brain in acute renal failure. *J Clin Invest.* 1974;53:387.
64. Mikiciuk MG, Thornhill JA. Control of parathyroid hormone in chronic renal failure. *Compendium Cont Educ [Small Anim].* 1989;11:831-836.
65. Finco DR. The role of phosphorus restriction in the management of chronic renal failure of the dog and cat. In: *Proceedings 7th Kal Kan Symposium for the Treatment of Small Animal Diseases.* Columbus, Ohio; 1983.
66. Parfitt AM, et al. Reduced phosphate reabsorption unrelated to parathyroid hormone after renal transplantation: Implications for the pathogenesis of hyperparathyroidism in chronic renal failure. *Mineral Electrolyte Metab.* 1986;12:356-362.
67. Hansen B, et al. Clinical and metabolic findings in dogs with chronic renal failure fed two diets. *Am J Vet Res.* 1992;53: 1992.
68. Lewis L, et al. *Small Animal Clinical Nutrition.* Topeka, Kansas: Mark Morris Associates; 1987:8-12.
69. Chew D, et al. Phosphorus restriction in the treatment of chronic renal failure. In: Kirk R, Bonagura J, eds. *Current Veterinary Therapy XI.* Philadelphia, Pennsylvania: WB Saunders Co; 1992:853-857.
70. Massry S. Prevention and treatment in divalent ion metabolism in renal failure. *Semin Nephrol.* 1986;6:114-121.
71. Finco DR, et al. Effects of three diets on dogs with induced chronic renal failure. *Am J Vet Res.* 1985;46:646-653.
72. Henry D, et al. Parenteral aluminum administration in the dog: II. Induction of osteomalacia and effect on vitamin D metabolism. *Kidney Int.* 1984;25:36-75.
73. Goodman W, et al. Parenteral aluminum administration in the dog: I. Plasma kinetics, tissue levels, calcium metabolism, and parathyroid hormone. *Kidney Int.* 1984;25:362-369.
74. Fiore C, et al. Long-term effects of histamine-H2 receptor antagonists on serum parathyroid hormone in chronic renal failure. *Clin Endocrinol.* 1985;23:277-282.
75. Cunningham J, et al. Effect of histamins H_2-receptor blockade on parathyroid status in normal and uremic man. *Nephron.* 1984;38:17-21.
76. Sherwood L. Vitamin D, parathyroid hormone, and renal failure. *N Engl J Med.* 1987;316:1601-1603.
77. Chew D, Nagode L. Calcitriol in treatment of chronic renal failure. In: Kirk R, Bonagura J, eds. *Current Veterinary Therapy XI.* Philadelphia, Pennsylvania: WB Saunders Co; 1992: 857-860.
78. Brown S, et al. Medical management of canine chronic renal failure. In: Kirk R, Bonagura J, eds. *Current Veterinary Therapy XI.* Philadelphia, Pennsylvania: WB Saunders Co; 1992: 842-847.
79. Plumb D: *Veterinary Drug Handbook.* White Bear Lake, Minnesota: PharmaVet Publishing; 1991.
80. Witmer G, et al. Effects of 25-hydroxycholecalciferol on bone lesions of children with terminal renal failure. *Kidney Int.* 1976;10:395.
81. Halloran B, et al. Plasma vitamin D metabolite concentration in chronic renal failure: Effect of oral administration of 25-hydroxy D_3. *J Clin Endocrinol Metab.* 1984;59:1063-1069.
82. Kobayashi D, et al. Hypertension in cats with chronic renal failure or hyperthyroidism. *J Vet Intern Med.* 1990;4:58-62.
83. Ross L: Hypertensive disease. In: Ettinger S, ed. *Textbook of Internal Medicine.* Philadelphia, Pennsylvania: WB Saunders Co; 1989:2047-2056.
84. Weiser M, et al. Blood pressure measurement in the dog. *J Am Vet Med Assoc.* 1977;171:364-368.
85. Cowgill L, Kallet A. Systemic hypertension. In: Kirk R, ed. *Current Veterinary Therapy IX.* Philadelphia, Pennsylvania: WB Saunders Co; 1986:360-364.
86. Tolins J, Raij L. Antihypertensive therapy and the progression of chronic renal disease: Are there renoprotective drugs? *Semin Nephrol.* 1991;11:538-548.
87. Littman M, et al. Spontaneous systemic hypertension in dogs: Five cases (1981-1983). *J Am Vet Med Assoc.* 1988; 193:486-494.
88. Atkins C. The role of noncardiac disease in the development and precipitation of heart failure. *Vet Clin North Am.* 1991;21: 1035-1080.
89. Stiles J, et al. The prevalence of retinopathy in hypertensive cats with systemic hypertension and chronic renal failure or hyperthyroidism. In: *J Am Anim Hosp Assoc.* 1994;30:564-570.
90. Littman M. Spontaneous systemic hypertension in cats. *J Vet Intern Med.* 1990;4:126A.
91. Littman M. Update: Treatment of hypertension in dogs and cats. In: Kirk R, Bonagura J, eds. *Current Veterinary Therapy XI.* Philadelphia, Pennsylvania: WB Saunders Co; 1992: 838-841.
92. Ross L. Endocrine hypertension. In: Kirk R, Bonagura J, eds. *Current Veterinary Therapy XI.* Philadelphia, Pennsylvania: WB Saunders Co; 1992:309-313.
93. Smith M, Dunn M. Hypertension due to renal parenchymal disease. In: Brenner B, Rector F, eds. *The Kidney.* Philadelphia, Pennsylvania: WB Saunders Co; 1991:1968-1996.
94. Campese V, Bigazzi R. The role of hypertension in the progression of renal diseases. *Am J Kidney Dis.* 1991;17:43-47.
95. Kincaid-Smith P, Whitworth J. Pathogenesis of hypertension in chronic renal disease. *Semin Nephrol.* 1988;8:155-162.
96. Dimski D, Hawkins E. Canine systemic hypertension. *Compendium Cont Educ Vet.* 1988;10:1152-1159.
97. Bovee K. Current status of hypertension in the dog. In: *Proceedings of the 16th Annual Waltham/OSU Symposium for the Treatment of Small Animal Disease.* Columbus, Ohio: Kal Kan Foods; 1992.
98. Remillard R, et al. Variance of indirect blood pressure measurements and prevalence of hypertension in clinically normal dogs. *Am J Vet Res.* 1991;52:561-565.
99. Greco D, et al. Effect of dietary sodium intake on glomerular filtration rate in partially nephrectomized dogs. *Am J Vet Res.* 1994;55:152-159.
100. Terzi F, et al. Renal effect of antihypertensive drugs depends on sodium diet in the excision remnant kidney model. *Kidney Int.* 1992;42:354-363.
101. Anderson S, et al. Antihypertensive therapy must control glomerular hypertension to limit glomerular injury. *J Hypertens.* 1986;4:S242-S244.
102. Dworkin L, et al. Renal vascular effects of antihypertensive therapy in uninephrectomized SHR. *Kidney Int.* 1989;35: 790-798.
103. Bovee K, et al. Essential hypertension. *J Am Vet Med Assoc.* 1989;195:81-86.
104. MacDonald J, et al. Renal effects of enalapril in dogs. *Kidney Int.* 1987;31:S-148-S-153.
105. Riviere J. Calculation of dosage regimes of antimicrobial drugs

in animals with renal and hepatic dysfunction. *J Am Vet Med Assoc.* 1984;185:1094-1097.
106. Lazarus J, Hakim R. Medical aspects of hemodialysis. In: Brenner B, Rector F, eds. *The Kidney.* Philadelphia, Pennsylvania: WB Saunders Co; 1991:2223-2298.
107. Neff-Davis C. Clinical monitoring of drug concentrations. In: Davis L, ed. *Manual of Therapeutics in Small Animal Practice.* New York, New York: Churchill-Livingstone; 1985:633-655.
108. Churchill J, et al. The influence of dietary protein intake on progression of chronic renal failure. *Semin Vet Med Surg [Small Anim].* 1992;7:244-250.
109. Adams L, et al. Influence of dietary protein/calorie intake on renal morphology and function in cats with 5/6 nephrectomy. *Lab Invest.* 1994;70:347-357.
110. Klahr S. Effects of protein intake on the progression of renal disease. *Annu Rev Nutr.* 1989;9:87-108.
111. Hostetter T. The hyperfiltering glomerulus. *Med Clin North Am.* 1984;62:387-398.
112. Brown SA, et al. Dietary protein intake and the glomerular adaptations to partial nephrectomy in dogs. *J Nutr.* 1991;121: S125-S127.
113. Polzin DJ, et al. Development of renal lesions in dogs after 11/12 reduction of renal mass: Influences of dietary protein intake. *Lab Invest.* 1988;58:172-183.
114. Neugarten J, et al. Dietary protein restriction and glomerular permselectivity in nephrotoxic serum nephritis. *Kidney Int.* 1991;40:57-61.
115. Adams L, et al. Effects of dietary protein restriction in clinically normal cats and cats with induced chronic renal failure. *Am J Vet Res.* (in press): 1993.
116. Kaysen G, et al. Effect of dietary protein intake on albumin homeostasis in nephrotic patients. *Kidney Int.* 1986;29:1986.
117. Lumlertgul D, et al. Phosphate depletion arrests progression of chronic renal failure independent of protein intake. *Kidney Int.* 1986;29:658-666.
118. Glomset J. Fish, fatty acids, and human health. *N Engl J Med.* 1985;312:1253-1254.
119. Heifets M, Morrissey J. Effect of dietary lipids on renal function in rats with subtotal nephrectomy. *Kidney Int.* 1987;32: 335-341.
120. Scharschmidt L, et al. Effects of dietary fish oil on renal insufficiency in rats with subtotal nephrectomy. *Kidney Int.* 1987;32:700-709.
121. Barcelli U, Pollak V. Is there a role for polyunsaturated fatty acids in the prevention of renal disease and renal failure? *Nephron.* 1985;41:209-212.
122. Moorehead J, et al. Lipid nephrotoxicity in chronic progressive glomerular and tubulo-interstitial disease. *Lancet.* 1982;ii: 1309-1311.
123. Rayner H, et al. The role of lipids in the pathogenesis of glomerulosclerosis in the rat following subtotal nephrectomy. *Eur J Clin Invest.* 1990;20:97-104.
124. Schreiner G: Pathways leading from glomerular injury to glomerulosclerosis. In: Gurland H, Morgan J, Wetzels E, eds. *Immunologic Perspectives in Chronic Renal Failure. Contributions in Nephrology.* Basel: Karger; 1990:1-18.
125. Ito Y, et al. A low protein-high linoleate diet increases glomerular PGE_2 and protects renal function in rats with reduced renal mass. *Prostaglandins Leukotrienes Med.* 1987;28:277-284.
126. Hurd E, et al. Prevention of glomerulonephritis and prolonged survival in New Zealand black/New Zealand white$_{F1}$ hybrid mice fed an essential fatty acid-deficient diet. *J Clin Invest.* 1981;67:476-485.
127. Moorehead J, et al. The role of abnormalities of lipid metabolism in the progression of renal disease. In: Mitch W, ed. *The Progressive Nature of Renal Disease.* New York, New York: Churchill Livingstone; 1986:133-148.
128. Grone H, et al. Induction of glomerulosclerosis by dietary lipids. *Lab Invest.* 1989;60:433-446.
129. Nagode L, Chew D. Nephrocalcinosis caused by hyperparathyroidism in progression of renal failure: Treatment with calcitriol. *Semin Vet Med Surg [Small Anim].* 1992;7:202-220.
130. Hirschel-Scholz S, et al. Protection from progressive renal failure and hyperparathyroid bone remodeling by WR-2721. *Kidney Int.* 1988;33:934-941.
131. Klahr S, Slatopolksi E. Toxicity of parathyroid hormone in uremia. *Annu Rev Med.* 1986;37:71-78.
132. Nath K, et al. Increased ammoniagenesis as a determinant of progressive renal injury. *Am J Kidney Dis.* 1991;17:654-657.
133. Bankir L, et al. Possible role of vasopressin and urine concentrating process in the progression of chronic renal failure. *Kidney Int.* 1989;36 (suppl 27):S32-S37.
134. Tolins JP, et al. Hypokalemic nephropathy in the rat: Role of ammonia in chronic tubular injury. *J Clin Invest.* 1987;79:1447-1458.
135. Zucchelli P, et al. Long-term comparison between captopril and nifedipine in the progression of renal insufficiency. *Kidney Int.* 1992;42:452-458.
136. Keane W, et al. Angiotensin converting enzyme inhibitors and progressive renal insufficiency. Current experience and future directions. *Ann Intern Med.* 1989;111:503-516.
137. Kamper A, et al. Effect of enalapril on the progression of chronic renal failure. A randomized controlled trial. *Am J Hypertens.* 1992;5:423-430.
138. Epstein M. Calcium antagonists and the kidney: Implications for renal protection. *Kidney Int.* 1992;36(suppl):S66-S72.
139. Harris D, et al. Verapamil protects against progression of experimental chronic renal failure. *Kidney Int.* 1987;31:41-46.
140. Finco DR, et al. Exogenous creatinine clearance as a measure of glomerular filtration rate in dogs with reduced renal mass. *Am J Vet Res.* 1991;52:1029-1032.
141. Finco D, et al. Simple, accurate method for clinical estimation of glomerular filtration rate in the dog. *Am J Vet Res.* 1981;42: 1874-1877.
142. Fettman M, et al. Single-injection method for evaluation of renal function with 14C-inulin and 3H-tetraethylammonium bromide in dogs and cats. *Am J Vet Res.* 1985;46:482-486.
143. Mitch W. The influence of the diet on the progression of renal insufficiency. *Annu Rev Med.* 1984;35:249-264.
144. Allen T, et al. A technique for estimating progression of chronic renal failure in the dog. *J Am Vet Med Assoc.* 1987;190: 866-868.
145. Coulter D, Keith J. Blood pressures obtained by indirect measurement in conscious dogs. *J Am Vet Med Assoc.* 1984;184: 1375-1378.
146. Edwards N. Non-invasive blood pressure measurements in the clinical setting. In: *Proceedings 8th Annual ACVIM Forum.* Washington, DC; American College of Veterinary Internal Medicine; 1990.
147. Gordon D, Goldblatt H. Direct percutaneous determination of systemic blood pressure and production of renal hypertension in the cat. *Proc Soc Exp Biol Med.* 1967;125:177.

CHAPTER 29

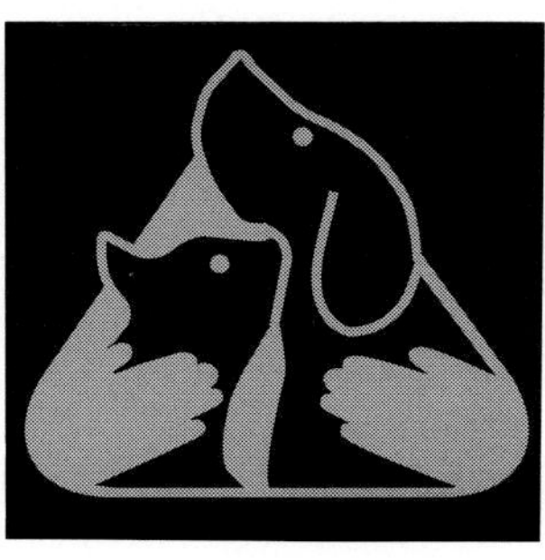

Medical Management of the Anemia of Chronic Renal Failure

LARRY D. COWGILL

I. ROLE OF ANEMIA IN THE MANIFESTATIONS OF THE UREMIC SYNDROME

A. Development of anemia.

An association between progression of renal insufficiency and the development of anemia is well established in human patients.[3,30,43,64] Anemia is also a feature of chronic renal failure in dogs and cats.[22,28,49,55,78,95] Figure 29–1 illustrates the inverse correlation between hematocrit and serum creatinine in these species.

1. The scattering of the observations about the regression curves is the result of differences in the stages and causes of renal failure in individual animals and of clinical variations among patients. In an individual patient, however, the progression of anemia is a predictable and inevitable consequence of the uremic syndrome.
2. When recently surveyed, dogs and cats with renal insufficiency demonstrated a decline in hematocrit by an average of 0.15 percentage points and 0.17 percentage points per day, respectively.[22]

B. Clinical significance of anemia.

1. The significance of anemia for the clinical manifestations of uremia in companion animals has been ill-understood. Reluctance to transfuse uremic animals to maintain a normal red blood cell mass and the inability to control the biochemical consequences of renal failure by dialysis have prevented disassociation of these influences on the clinical expression of renal failure. Consequently, the contributions of anemia *per se* to the manifestations of chronic renal failure have been consolidated with other polysystemic consequences of uremia. Only recently has anemia been recognized as an important contributor to the clinical disability characteristic of end-stage renal disease (ESRD). Table 29–1 lists many characteristics that may be ascribed, specifically or in large part, to anemia in uremic humans and companion animals.
2. In animal patients in which anemia was corrected independently of changes in azotemia, the signs of inappetence, weakness, fatigue, lethargy, cold intolerance, and apathy, which characterize the uremic syndrome in dogs and cats, significantly improved.[19,20] Importantly, resolution of anemia in these animals promoted dramatic improvement in their overall clinical well-being. Anemia should no longer be regarded as an inevitable feature of ESRD that is conveniently tolerated and therapeutically ignored. Its resolution promotes clinical and behavioral benefits that facilitate the medical management and significantly allay the morbidity of renal failure in companion animals.

II. PATHOPHYSIOLOGY OF ANEMIA IN CHRONIC RENAL FAILURE

A. Causal factors.

1. The causes of anemia during the progression of renal failure are multifactorial.

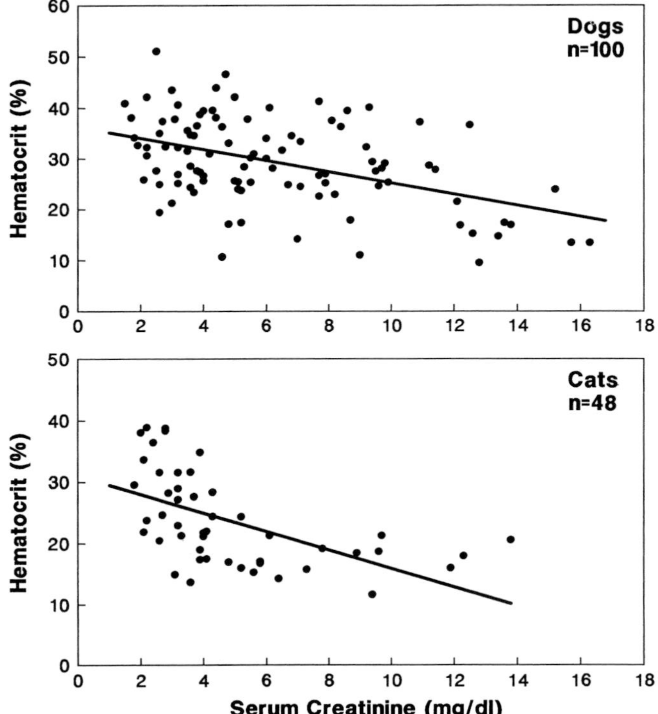

FIG. 29–1. Relationship of hematocrit and the severity of renal failure (serum creatinine) in dogs (upper panel) and cats (lower panel) with naturally occurring renal disease. (Cowgill LD. Erythropoietin: Its use in the treatment of chronic renal failure in dogs and cats. *Proceedings of the 15th Waltham OSU Symposium.* Kal Kan Foods; Vernon, California: 1991:66–67.)

TABLE 29–1
CLINICAL FEATURES ATTRIBUTABLE TO ANEMIA IN ESRD

Uremic humans	
Fatigue	Anorexia
Angina	Insomnia
Shortness of breath	Poor sexual performance
Muscular weakness	Cardiomegaly
Poor hair growth	Depression
Poor hair texture	Poor skin color
Uremic dogs and cats	
Inappetence	Cold intolerance
Weakness	Behavioral apathy
Fatigue	Decreased affection
Lethargy	Increased sleep

2. It is now generally agreed that bone marrow failure from the lack or insufficient production of erythropoietin by the residual renal mass is the most significant contributor.
3. Shortened red blood cell lifespan, uremic inhibitors of erythropoiesis, external blood loss, nutritional deficiencies, and marrow fibrosis variably contribute to and foster the anemia.[34,39]

B. Erythropoietin.

Erythropoietin is the principal regulatory hormone for red blood cell production by the bone marrow.[39,56] It stimulates committed erythroid progenitor cells to differentiate and to mature into red blood cells.[31] Erythropoietin also promotes hemoglobin synthesis and release of reticulocytes into the circulation.[56]

1. The kidney is the principal site of erythropoietin production, but small contributions may come from the liver in most species.[10,56]
2. In contrast to other species, in dogs, the kidneys may be the sole site of erythropoietin production.[69–71]
3. Progressive destruction of functional renal parenchyma results in a relative or absolute deficiency of erythropoietin and, subsequently, in erythroid hypoplasia of the bone marrow. When sensitive methods are applied to assay erythropoietin in human uremic patients, serum concentrations are generally low or normal, though occasionally higher-than-normal levels are detected.[12,33,64,80,87] Regardless of the absolute concentration, serum erythropoietin concentrations in human uremic patients are always lower than measurements from patients with comparable anemia and normal renal function. Therefore, uremia is associated with either a relative or an absolute deficiency of erythropoietin.[12,33,36,64,80,87]
4. Results of evaluation of serum erythropoietin concentrations in dogs with both experimentally induced and spontaneous renal failure support a similar pathogenesis for the anemia accompanying renal failure in canines.[31,48,49]
   a. Dogs with surgically induced remnant kidneys developed anemia coincident with reduced basal erythropoietin concentrations and decreased erythroid stimulation to acute blood loss.[76] Similarly, in dogs with naturally occurring chronic renal failure, serum erythropoietin concentrations are in the low-to-normal range and inappropriately below measurements in nonuremic dogs with a comparable degree of anemia.[48,49,55]
   b. Corrected reticulocyte counts are predictably low, and bone marrow cytology in uremic animals reveals normal or increased myeloid/erythroid (M/E) ratios characteristic of erythropoietin deficiency and erythroid hypoplasia.

C. Decreased red blood cell life span.

1. Shortened survival and hemolysis of red blood cells in the uremic milieu have been regarded as a potential contributor to the anemia of chronic renal failure.[16,37,39,42] The responsible factors are unknown but appear to be inherent in the uremic environment and not to intrinsic defects of the cells *per se*.[16,47] A correlation between red cell

survival and protein intake and blood urea nitrogen (BUN) has been reported,[85] but red blood cell survival is not corrected consistently by hemodialysis, thus discrediting a role for low-molecular-weight uremia toxins in the process.

2. Hyperparathyroidism is a consistent feature of progressive renal insufficiency, and parathyroid hormone has been implicated in the shortened red blood cell survival in both human uremic patients[7,61,62] and dogs with experimental renal failure.[4] However, in a small population of dogs with spontaneous renal failure, parathyroid hormone concentration did not correlate with the severity of the anemia or with increased erythrocyte osmotic fragility.[55] From these results *in vivo* the contributions of parathyroid hormone to development of anemia in dogs remain unresolved.

D. Uremic inhibitors of erythropoiesis.

1. There has been continued controversy and speculation that serum of uremic individuals contains inhibitors of erythropoiesis that contribute directly to the anemia.[12,34,64,82]
2. The bulk of speculation is based on findings that uremic serum inhibits *in vitro* proliferation of erythroid progenitor cells and heme synthesis and on the correlation of these effects with the degree of renal failure and anemia *in vivo*.[13,25,64,74,75,94]
   a. Many substances accumulated in renal failure, including parathyroid hormone, "middle molecules," and spermine, have been implicated in this inhibitory effect; however, it remains unclear how specific the effects of these substances may be for erythropoiesis.[25,39,64]
   b. Improvements in the anemia and reduced inhibition of erythroid progenitors *in vitro* result from the initiation of dialysis in some patients and is cited as evidence for these effects.[42,74]
   c. The identity and significance of uremic inhibitors remain undefined. The recent availability and therapeutic application of recombinant human erythropoietin have demonstrated clearly that the effects of putative inhibitors can be surmounted in the face of adequate erythropoietin stimulation.[33,39,41]
   d. At best, uremic inhibitors contribute only minimally to the pathogenesis of anemia and remain subordinate to the deficiency of kidney-derived erythropoietin.

E. External blood loss.

1. A bleeding tendency is a common feature of uremia, and blood loss from overt hemorrhage, dialyzer losses, or occult gastrointestinal bleeding can contribute significantly to the anemia.
2. Bleeding tendencies in animals are characterized clinically by ecchymoses, prolonged buccal mucosal bleeding times, hematemesis, fecal occult blood, and melena.[17]
3. Evidence of iron deficiency or sudden and inappropriate increases in the BUN/creatinine ratio suggest gastrointestinal bleeding.

F. Miscellaneous.

1. Iron deficiency, myelofibrosis, and aluminum toxicity from excessive use of intestinal phosphate binding preparations may incidentally contribute to the anemia.
2. Primary blood disorders, including immune-mediated hemolytic anemia, haemobartonellosis, angiopathic anemia, hypersplenism or excessive blood sampling, also may augment the anemia.

G. Summary.

1. Anemia is a complex and important component of chronic renal failure in dogs and cats.
2. The relative significance and contributions of its varied causes differ in each patient; the degree of anemia depends on their collective impact.
3. Appropriate replacement of erythropoietin can effectively mask all other contributors to the anemia.
4. In the absence of adequate erythropoietin, amelioration of the other contributors at best, can improve the anemia only slightly.

III. MANAGEMENT OF ANEMIA IN CHRONIC RENAL FAILURE

A. General considerations.

1. Nutritional deficiencies.
   a. Prolonged deficiencies of protein, selected vitamins, and minerals can significantly impair erythropoiesis, and such conditions should be resolved to maximize the erythropoietic potential of the patient.[54,78] Failure to correct any of these nutritional inadequacies interferes with therapeutic attempts to resolve the anemia.
   b. Establishing adequate calorie and nitrogen intake is a lofty but essential therapeutic goal. Intensive diuresis and institution of a nitrogen-restricted diet to reduce azotemia may promote better nutrition and improve the anemia.[77,78] Excessive restriction of dietary protein can promote protein malnutrition and further exacerbate the anemia.[77]
   c. Vitamin B_{12}, folic acid, niacin, and vitamin B_6 are required for normal erythropoiesis, synthesis of hemoglobin, and iron metabolism.[54] Although deficiencies of these vitamins have not been described in dogs and cats with ESRD, their generally poor nutritional status could predispose them to such deficiencies.[68] Water-soluble vitamin supplements, including B-complex, folate, and niacin, should be provided routinely.
2. Iron depletion.
   a. Many dogs and cats with anemia of chronic renal failure have a serum iron concentration below reference values and transferrin saturation below 15% (Cowgill, unpublished observations).
   b. These abnormalities are rarely recognized, be-

cause iron measurements are seldom included in diagnostic evaluations, and microcytosis and hypochromasia, which characterize iron deficiency anemia, are an uncommon feature of chronic renal failure.

c. Iron deficiency may occur from inadequate iron intake or blood loss from gastrointestinal bleeding.

d. Serum iron and total iron-binding capacity (TIBC) should be measured in all azotemic patients with anemia.[86]

(1). When deficiencies are demonstrated, treatment should be initiated with oral ferrous sulfate at 100 to 300 mg/day in dogs and 50 to 100 mg/day in cats.[60]

(2). Adjustments to the initial dosage should be made to maintain serum iron, TIBC, and erythrocyte indices within normal ranges. Iron supplements should be maintained for a minimum of 3 months, and thereafter until iron adequacy is established.

3. Gastrointestinal hemorrhage.

a. Gastrointestinal hemorrhage is an important source of blood loss in uremic animals. The potential for bleeding increases with the degree of azotemia, which promotes both gastrointestinal ulceration and bleeding tendencies. A BUN/creatinine ratio excessive for the patient's protein intake[17] or a ratio greater than 40 may indicate active gastrointestinal bleeding.

b. Treatment is directed at lessening the azotemia with a protein-restricted diet appropriate for the degree of renal insufficiency.[33] (See Chapter 28, Conservative Medical Management of Chronic Renal Failure.)

c. Histamine H_2–receptor antagonists have been advocated for uremic gastritis and gastric ulceration associated with hypergastrinemia and gastric hyperacidity.[89]

(1). For dogs, cimetidine is administered orally at 5 mg/kg every 8 to 12 hours for 2 to 4 weeks. The dosage is then adjusted to 5 mg/kg once daily for 2 to 3 weeks before complete withdrawal. For cats, the initial dosage is 2.5 to 5.0 mg/kg every 8 to 12 hours.

(2). Alternatively, oral ranitidine may be substituted in both dogs and cats, at 2.2 to 4.4 mg/kg every 12 hours.

(3). Evidence of the efficacy of this therapy in the presence of occult gastrointestinal bleeding is indicated by reductions in the BUN/creatinine ratio.

d. Sucralfate is an antiulcer drug that forms an adherent complex on gastric ulcers to create a protective barrier against excessive gastric acidity. Its efficacy in animals with uremic gastritis is untested, but it may help to prevent gastric hemorrhage and mucosal damage. For dogs, the dose is 0.5 to 1.0 g every 8 to 12 hours, orally. For cats, sucralfate is administered at 0.25 g every 8 to 12 hours orally.

B. Blood transfusion.

1. Transfusion of whole blood or packed red blood cells has been the most direct and effective therapy for anemia in animals with renal insufficiency. Although blood transfusion is effective and clearly indicated, it has many disadvantages that limit its usefulness.

a. Practical disadvantages.

(1). Limited availability of adequate blood resources.

(2). Reduced life span of transfusion products in uremic patients.

(3). High cost of long-term blood replacement therapy.

(4). Development of donor incompatibilities and complications with repeated transfusions.

(5). Inability to optimally restore red cell mass to normal with routine blood product administration.

b. These constraints have effectively prohibited transfusion therapy as long-term management of chronic renal failure in dogs and cats.

2. Many patients with moderate uremia can maintain a hematocrit in the mid 20% range, and their condition is stable enough to preclude transfusion therapy. As the hematocrit approaches 20%, they inevitably show signs of anorexia, fatigue, weakness, fainting, or seizures, which may warrant treatment by blood transfusion. Blood transfusion should be performed only with compatible blood products.

a. Canine blood donors should test negative for groups DEA–1.1, –1.2, and –7.

b. Blood groups of cats are less completely characterized, but serious blood type incompatibilities are described.[5,50] Naturally occurring alloantibodies in cats that promote severe incompatibility reactions justify routine typing of recipient and donor blood before transfusion.[50] These recommendations are particularly justified in many purebred and outbred cats, for which the prevalence of type B blood is greater.[50]

c. Only cross-matched compatible blood products should be administered, owing to the requirement for repeated transfusions and the potential for sensitization of the recipient to mistyped donors. If possible, fresh blood should be used to provide optimal cell survival and oxygen transfer capacity. Properly stored blood can be administered, if necessary, with little compromise of efficacy.

d. The changes in hematocrit anticipated following transfusion of a 250-mL unit of blood to

TABLE 29–2
ANTICIPATED CHANGE IN HEMATOCRIT (%) PER UNIT OF TRANSFUSED BLOOD IN DOGS AND CATS*

Donor HCT (%)	Recipient's Weight (kg)					
Dogs	5	10	15	20	25	30
35	19	10	6	5	4	3
40	22	11	7	5.5	4	4
45	25	13.5	8	6	5	4
Cats	2	3	4	5	6	7
30	13	8.5	6	5	4.5	4
35	15	10	7.5	6	5	4
40	17	11	8.5	7	6	5

*Calculations based on formulae by Weiss[95] and 250-mL and 60-mL units for dogs and cats, respectively.

dogs or a 60-mL unit of blood to cats from donors with varying hematocrits can be estimated from Table 29–2. It is not essential—indeed, hazardous—to correct the hematocrit to normal ranges with blood transfusion. Target hematocrit values approaching 25 to 30% are usually adequate and achievable.

e. The rate of blood administration depends on the clinical condition of the animal. Generally, infusion of 10 mL/kg body weight per hour is well tolerated. Excessively rapid blood infusion may promote volume overload, vomiting, respiratory distress, or congestive heart failure.
f. For most uremic animals with no recent history of hemorrhage, administration of packed red blood cells is preferable to whole blood because a greater red cell mass can be provided with less risk of volume overload.

3. The complications of blood transfusion must be considered in concert with the necessity for blood supplementation.
   a. Acute or immediate incompatibility reactions may exhibit urticaria, hypotension, restlessness, respiratory distress, vomiting, hemolysis, tachycardia, shivering, vocalization, disseminated intravascular coagulation, or acute renal failure.[5,50,90]
      (1). Acute transfusion reactions should be managed by immediate cessation of blood infusion and symptomatic support of ventilation, cardiovascular instability, and shock.[5,51]
      (2). Less severe immediate reactions, including shivering, fever, vomiting, and urticaria, can be treated with antihistamines or corticosteroids (dexamethasone sodium phosphate at 4 to 6 mg/kg or prednisolone sodium succinate at 30 to 35 mg/kg).
   b. Circulatory overload may occur in patients given an excessive volume of blood or repeated transfusions. Clinical signs include vomiting, urticaria, systemic hypertension, pulmonary edema, or congestive heart failure. When chronic transfusion therapy is contemplated, substitution of packed red blood cells for whole blood can minimize these untoward effects.
   c. Iron overload is a common complication in human patients receiving hemodialysis who require regular transfusion therapy.[36,39,57] Uremic animals are rarely given sufficient blood replacement for iron overload to be clinically significant. Iron overload requires mobilization and removal of parenchymal iron stores with chelating agents like desferrioxamine or repeated phlebotomy in combination with recombinant erythropoietin administration.[36,57]
4. For selected patients who require immediate, short-term correction of red blood cell mass to alleviate acute hemorrhage or to facilitate the management of chronic renal failure, blood transfusion remains the most efficient and effective therapy. For long-term resolution of anemia, chronic blood transfusion has been supplanted by erythropoietin replacement therapy, which provides more efficacious and protracted resolution for the anemia (see Section D, Recombinant Human Erythropoietin, on the following pages).

C. Androgenic hormones.

1. Androgenic hormones have an established influence on erythropoiesis in humans and animals. Adult males typically have higher hematocrit, hemoglobin concentration, and red blood cell count than do adult females or castrated or prepubescent males.[23,83] As a consequence, androgens have been employed empirically to ameliorate a variety of anemias, including the anemia of ESRD.[11,15,23,67,72,83]
2. The efficacy of androgenic hormones for the anemia of renal insufficiency remains controversial. Erythropoietic responses often require prolonged periods of drug administration. Demonstrated responses are often minimal and must be carefully balanced with the adverse effects of these hormones.[15,23,52,72,83] Clinical effects in humans are variable and depend on the nature of the study population, the severity of the anemia, the androgen preparation used, concurrent diseases, and the design of the clinical trial.
3. Three major classes of androgens have been employed in uremic humans.
   a. Testosterone esters (testosterone propionate, testosterone enanthate, testosterone cypionate, and mixed testosterone esters) produce inconsistent increases in red blood cell mass, hematocrit, hemoglobin, and red blood cell count and decrease transfusion dependency in treated humans.[66,84,93] In general, the response to injectable testosterone esters is favorable.

The majority of human patients demonstrate at least a 5% increase in hematocrit, and in occasional patients, responses exceed 15%.[84]

b. Nortestosterone esters (nandrolone phenylpropionate, nandrolone decanoate) are synthetic androgens with relatively high anabolic-to-androgenic activity. In general, their hematologic properties are similar to injectable testosterone esters, but they are used preferentially in humans to minimize the virilizing effects of androgen therapy. In controlled clinical trials, patient groups given nandrolone demonstrate consistent increases in hematocrit, hemoglobin, and red blood cell mass.[11,15,29,72,96] However, individual patients show variable responses and may prove refractory to nandrolone therapy.[11,15,29,72,96] In general, these preparations require months of continuous administration to promote clinical responses.

c. The 17α-alkylated androgens are another group of synthetic drugs with high anabolic to androgenic activity. Their oral administration provides an attraction over other preparations with high anabolic activity. The effect of 17α-alkylated androgens on the anemia of humans with renal failure is inconstant and highly individualized; they seem to be less efficacious than injectable preparations.[35,72]

4. The mechanisms by which androgens stimulate erythropoiesis are only partially understood.
   a. Evidence clearly shows that androgens increase both renal and extrarenal erythropoietin secretion, and that their erythropoietic response depends in part on this secretory effect.[11,15,67] Their efficacy is generally greater in the presence of remnant kidneys; however, the site specificity for erythropoietin production may vary with the type of androgen and the species of animal.[83]
   b. Androgens or their metabolites may stimulate erythroid progenitors directly to increase both the pool of erythroid-committed cells and their sensitivity to erythropoietin.
   c. Androgens may have concomitant stimulatory effect on heme synthesis, independent of influences on erythropoietin production.
5. Androgenic steroids also influence erythrocyte metabolism, in addition to their direct and indirect effects on erythropoiesis. The concentration of 2,3-diphosphoglycerate (2,3-DPG) in erythrocytes is consistently increased when androgens are administered to patients with ESRD.[11,52,83]
   a. The increase in erythrocyte 2,3-DPG potentiates tissue-oxygen delivery by decreasing hemoglobin-oxygen affinity and shifting the oxygen equilibrium curve to the right.
   b. Results of a recent study of dialysis patients treated with nandrolone for 6 months indicated that its effect on red blood cell 2,3-DPG concentrations may be transient and not accompanied by significant changes in hemoglobin-oxygen affinity.[52] Moreover, any improvements in red blood cell mass and oxygen-carrying capacity may be offset entirely by concurrent increases in basal metabolic rate and oxygen requirements. Such tradeoff effects could offset any benefits of androgenic steroids for improving physical performance in uremic patients.[52]
6. Androgen therapy must be provided with knowledge of the likelihood of benefits, known or potential side effects, and cost of therapy. Major side effects relate to the virilizing and anabolic properties of these drugs and their hepatotoxicity.
   a. Virilism is a negligible consequence of androgen therapy for veterinary therapeutics, but it represents the most consistent adverse effect in humans.
      (1). Masculinization effects are most pronounced in women and children. Acne, flushing of the skin, deepening of the voice, changes in external genitalia, hirsutism, and baldness occur in both sexes. Amenorrhea and clitoral enlargement occur in women, and priapism, prostatomegaly, and impotence occur in adult males.[83]
      (2). The risks of masculinizing side effects can be reduced by the use of nortestosterone derivatives or 17α-alkylated androgens with greater anabolic-androgenic activity.
   b. Increases in serum creatinine, weight gain, and fluid retention develop variably, owing to the anabolic properties of androgens to promote nitrogen retention and muscle development. The BUN/creatinine ratio is likely to decrease in patients treated with androgens, but abrupt withdrawal of therapy could exacerbate the azotemia.
   c. Androgen therapy, especially with the 17α-alkylated derivatives, has been associated with hepatic toxicity and alteration of hepatic function.[83] Toxic signs include increases in serum transaminases, bilirubin, and triglycerides, and sulfobromophthalein retention. Hepatic failure and development of hepatic neoplasia have also been reported.
   d. The expense of therapy (including office visits) and pain associated with parenteral administration must be considered in the therapeutic plan. Greater efficacy and reduced potential for hepatotoxicity favor the use of injectable androgens.[72,83] In most circumstances clients can be instructed to administer injectable preparations at home, to obviate excessive office visits.
7. No systematic evaluation of androgen therapy for anemia in dogs or cats with ESRD has been

conducted. The authors' experience with anabolic steroids has been disappointing, regardless of the preparation used. The lack of apparent benefit may relate to the duration of therapy and aspects of uremia unique to animals.

a. The long treatment intervals required for documented efficacy in humans often exceed the life expectancy of many animals with renal failure.
b. Uncorrected nutritional deficiencies, progressive uremia, occult blood loss, and underlying disease may prevent responses comparable to those seen in human patients whose uremia is controlled by maintenance dialysis.
c. The plausible lack of significant extrarenal production of erythropoietin in dogs may further impair their responsiveness to these hormones.[69,71]

8. The lack of substantive support for a therapeutic role for androgenic steroids in the anemia of chronic renal failure in companion animals prohibits explicit endorsement of their use. Androgen administration must be predicated theoretically on experiences in human medicine or on their possible anabolic effect. In view of the clinical consequences of progressive anemia, a therapeutic trial of androgenic steroids may be warranted for animal patients for which other and more effective forms of therapy are unsuitable (see Section D, Recombinant Human Erythropoietin, which follows).
   a. Androgen therapy should be considered when the hematocrit falls below 30% in dogs and 25% in cats or when signs of progressive anemia become apparent. Patients with less severe anemia may respond better to androgen administration than those with severe anemia.
   b. Injectable androgens appear to be superior to oral preparations in stimulating erythropoietic responses.[23,72] In dogs and cats, virilizing side effects should not preclude selection of less expensive preparations with lower anabolic to androgenic activities. Nandrolone decanoate, nandrolone phenylpropionate, testosterone enanthate, and testosterone propionate have demonstrated efficacy in human patients with ESRD and may be the most appropriate for animals when their use seems justified.
   c. Table 29–3 lists recommended initial dosages for companion animals.[27,78] Efficacy should be assessed at monthly intervals. Failure to attain a 3 to 5 percentage point increase above the baseline hematocrit after 3 months of treatment necessitates evaluation for other causes of anemia (external blood loss, iron deficiency, nutritional deficiencies, progressive azotemia). At this stage, doubling the initial dosage should be considered.[23,78] If a significant increase in hematocrit is not achieved after 6 months of therapy, a further dosage increase, the selection of another androgen preparation, or the use of an alternative form of therapy (intermittent transfusion or recombinant human erythropoietin, see the following) must be considered.
   d. Patients treated with androgens should be evaluated at regular intervals, to assess efficacy and to monitor clinical and laboratory signs of virilism and hepatotoxicity.

TABLE 29–3
INITIAL RECOMMENDED DOSES FOR ANDROGENIC STEROIDS IN DOGS AND CATS

Drug Name	Recommended Dosage[27,78] (mg/kg/wk, intramuscular)
Testosterone propionate	2.2
Testosterone enanthate	4–7
Nandrolone deconoate	1–5
Nandrolone phenylpropionate	1

D. Recombinant human erythropoietin.

1. Development and manufacture.
   a. Recombinant human erythropoietin (r-HuEPO) is a product of modern biotechnology. The human genome is probed to identify, and then isolate, the specific segments of DNA that code for the erythropoietin molecule. The gene is then expressed in a cell system *in vitro*, to produce erythropoietin.[31,53,59]
   b. The essential steps involved in this process are depicted in Fig. 29–2.
      (1). Isolation, purification, and molecular sequencing of native human erythropoietin.
      (2). Production of DNA probes capable of reacting with nucleotide sequences complementary to the erythropoietin peptide.
      (3). Isolation of gene segments that react with the DNA probes, and insertion (transfection) of the intact erythropoietin gene into an immortalized mammalian cell system capable of transcribing the gene sequence for erythropoietin.
      (4). Harvesting, purification, and characterization of the transcription products produced by the cultured cells.
   c. The recombinant protein contains 165 amino acids and has a molecular weight of approximately 34,000 daltons. It has the same primary structure as human urinary erythropoietin and is a faithful molecular and biologic replica of the native hormone.[31,32]
2. Efficacy in uremic humans.
   a. A relative or absolute deficiency of erythropoietin is the principal cause of anemia associated with chronic progressive renal failure. Predict-

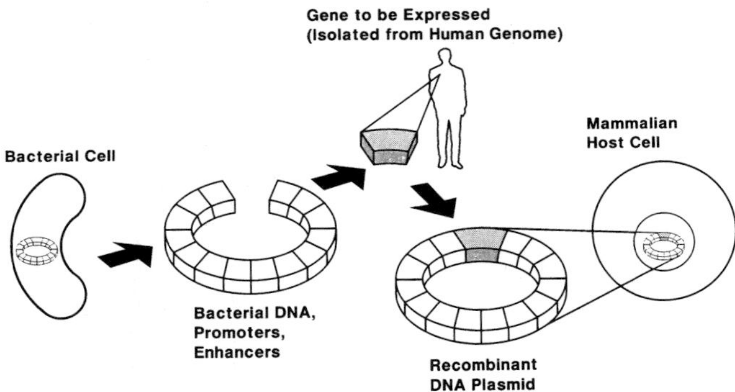

FIG. 29–2. General steps involved in the cloning of the human erythropoietin gene. (Courtesy of Amgen, Inc., Thousand Oaks, California.)

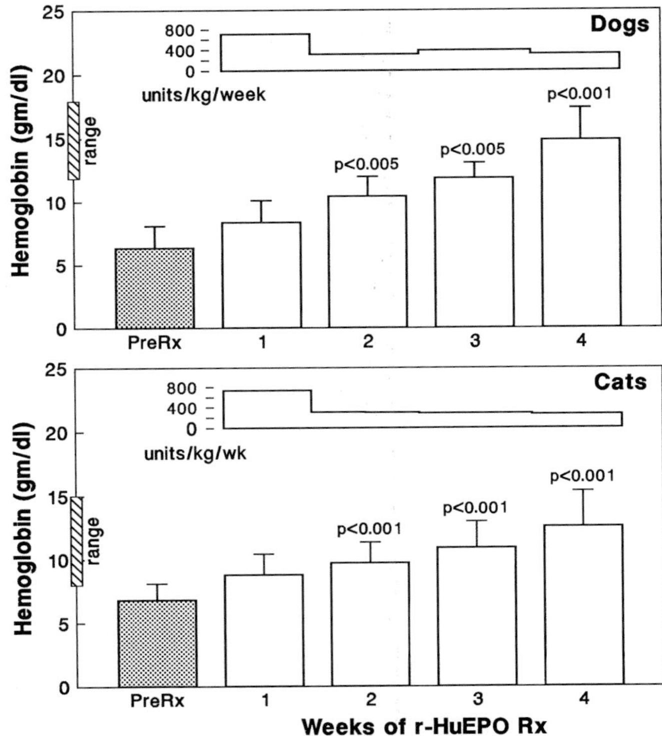

FIG. 29–3. Change in hemoglobin before and during treatment of 6 uremic dogs (upper panel) and 11 uremic cats (lower panel) with r-HuEPO for 4 weeks. Each bar represents the mean ± SE hemoglobin. The insert above the bars represents the average weekly dosage of r-HuEPO administered subcutaneously. The shaded areas on the vertical axes depict the respective reference ranges.

ably, adequate replacement of erythropoietin could resolve the anemia and effectively compensate for other contributions promoted by the uremia. The recent development and availability of r-HuEPO has revolutionized the ability to treat this consistent and inevitable consequence of progressive renal failure.

(1). Clinical trials involving thousands of human patients have overwhelmingly documented that r-HuEPO effectively reverses anemia and transfusion dependency in virtually all patients, regardless of the cause of their renal failure or their need for maintenance dialysis.[2,6,9,34,39–41,44,46,88]

(2). Recombinant HuEPO normalizes the hematocrit, hemoglobin concentration, and red blood cell counts in a dose-dependent manner, with either intravenous or subcutaneous administration.[1,6,8,9,33,41,65]

(3). Along with the hematologic benefits, human patients report improvement in their sense of well-being, appetite, strength, exercise and work capacity, sleep habits, hair growth, cognitive functions, psychologic health, and sexual performance.[24,26,40,45,63,73,97]

3. Efficacy of r-HuEPO for red blood cell production in dogs and cats.
   a. The erythropoietin molecule has been remarkably conserved among species, and r-HuEPO has been shown to stimulate red cell precursors *in vitro* and erythropoiesis *in vivo,* in nonhuman species, including cats and dogs. These observations suggest that r-HuEPO could be an important adjunct to the conservative management of renal failure in companion animals, as it has become in human uremic patients.
   b. Critical evaluation of the application of r-HuEPO in dogs and cats has been limited. Its efficacy, safety, and utility in dogs and cats with naturally occurring chronic renal failure has been assessed in a preliminary clinical investigation.[19–22] Subsequently, a multicenter national investigation of r-HuEPO replacement therapy in dogs and cats with renal failure has been implemented,* and a scattering of case reports have appeared on the subject.[49,79]
   c. Available information reveals that, in both dogs and cats, r-HuEPO promotes initial reticulocytosis and rapid, progressive, and significant increases in hematocrit, red blood cell count, and hemoglobin concentration to reference ranges within 2 to 3 weeks of therapy (Fig. 29–3).[19,22]
   d. Positive rates of red blood cell production can be recognized within the first week of treatment. In a preliminary clinical trial, the reticulocyte count increased significantly, from 0.35

*A Multicenter Clinical Trial of r-HuEPO therapy for the anemia of dogs and cats with naturally occurring renal failure was sanctioned in 1990 under the auspices and sponsorship of Amgen Inc., Thousand Oaks, California.

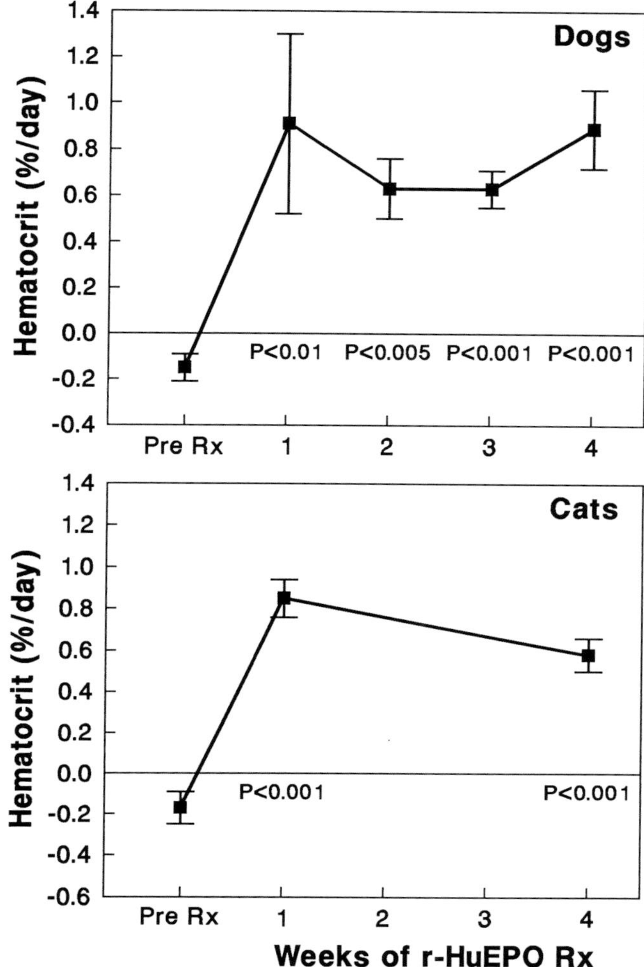

FIG. 29–4. Rate of change of hematocrit before and during treatment with r-HuEPO for 4 weeks in uremic dogs (upper panel) and uremic cats (lower panel). Note the conversion from a negative rate of change, which is consistent with progressive anemia in the pretreatment period, to the strongly positive production of red blood cells with r-HuEPO therapy.

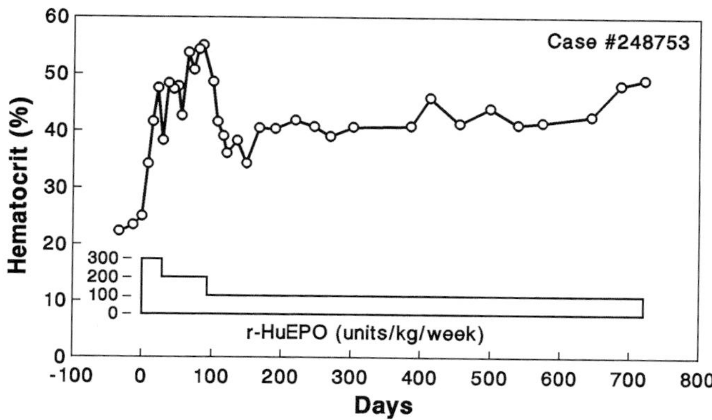

FIG. 29–5. Changes in hematocrit following r-HuEPO administration to a uremic cat illustrate both initial and long-term efficacy. The insert depicts the initial and maintenance subcutaneous doses during therapy.[21] Note that polycythemia resulted from the initial thrice-weekly dosing and the stability of the hematocrit with once-weekly administration in the long-term maintenance period. (Modified from Cowgill LD. Erythropoietin: Its use in the treatment of chronic renal failure in dogs and cats. *Proceedings of the 15th Waltham OSU Symposium.* Kal Kan Foods; Vernon, California: 1991:68.)

to 4.62% in dogs and from 0.12 to 2.96% in cats, during the first week of therapy.[22] Reticulocyte production is transient and generally unrecognized beyond 2 to 3 weeks of treatment. Also, the magnitude of reticulocytosis is modest compared to that seen in hemolytic or acute blood loss anemia.

e. As illustrated in Figure 29–4, r-HuEPO dramatically reverses the progression of the anemia (negative rate of change in hematocrit) and stimulates an increase in hematocrit approaching 1 percentage point per day.
f. Administration of r-HuEPO has no consistent effect either on leukocyte or platelet count or on leukocyte distribution in dogs, although transient increases in platelet count may be recognized in individual patients. Transient thrombocytosis may be seen also in cats during the initial phases of treatment.[20–22]
g. The M/E ratio of bone marrow aspirates decreases, reflecting the conversion from erythroid hypoplasia to an active proliferative state early during the course of therapy. The initial improvement in red blood cell mass achieved with r-HuEPO therapy can be sustained indefinitely in the majority of patients (Fig. 29–5).
h. Clinical experiences with r-HuEPO in dogs and cats with naturally occurring renal failure substantiate that its erythropoietic and clinical effects are comparable to those recognized in human uremic patients.

4. Influence of r-HuEPO on clinical well-being.
   a. Striking improvements in the clinical appearance of uremic animals are observed after r-HuEPO therapy, and concurrent erythropoietic responses. The changes are analogous to the rehabilitation and improved clinical well-being reported in human patients.[24,26,40,45,73] The most compelling of these attributes is a consistent boost in appetite and a willingness to eat therapeutic diets.[20,21,79] In many patients, appetite improves in advance of the erythropoietic responses, suggesting a direct mechanism.
   b. Increased activity level, playfulness, weight gain (typically 10 to 12%), increased physical strength, and decreased sleep requirements are regularly documented as the anemia resolves.[20,21,79]

(1). Changes in behavior, increased affection, and reappearance of old habits and grooming patterns are regularly described in feline patients and are exhibited frequently in treated dogs.
(2). Fewer patients display better tolerance to cold and increased alertness.

c. Collectively, these responses confirm that anemia contributes importantly to the signs of inappetence, weakness, fatigue, lethargy, cold intolerance, and "behavioral apathy" that characterize uremia in dogs and cats.
d. The short- and long-term efficacy of erythropoietin replacement to resolve the anemia and improve well-being are unparalleled by any other method of therapy, and this therapeutic response reinforces the necessity to address the anemia in the therapeutic approach to renal failure in companion animals.

5. Complications of r-HuEPO therapy.
   a. The efficacy of r-HuEPO for resolving the erythroid hypoplasia and secondary complications of anemia in uremic animals must be tempered by predictable and theoretic adverse effects associated with its administration.
      (1). Some adverse effects are expected consequences (pathophysiologic adaptations) of the increased red blood cell mass in patients that have become acclimated to a chronic anemic or hypoxic state.
      (2). The immunologic heterology of r-HuEPO for dogs and cats and its formulation in human serum albumin (HSA) confer the risk of local and systemic allergic reactions.
   b. In human patients, the most consistent and notable adverse effects of r-HuEPO therapy are 1) systemic hypertension, 2) iron deficiency, 3) hyperkalemia, 4) seizures, and 5) clotting in the hemodialyzer and in the vascular access.[14,38,39,46,58,91,92] These complications are secondary to the effects of the increased red blood cell mass. Adverse effects inherent to the drug *per se* are limited to diffuse myalgia and headache occurring transiently in a small percentage of patients or normal volunteers.[6,40,88] No immune-mediated consequences or anti–r-HuEPO antibodies have been recognized in human patients, a finding that is consistent with the identity of the recombinant protein being identical to that of the native erythropoietin.
   c. Preliminary clinical experiences have revealed a variety of adverse events coincident with r-HuEPO treatment in dogs and cats, including 1) development of anti–r-HuEPO antibodies, 2) refractory anemia or erythroid hypoplasia, 3) polycythemia, 4) seizures, 5) injection discomfort, 6) systemic hypertension, 7) iron depletion, and 8) skin reactions.[20,21,49]

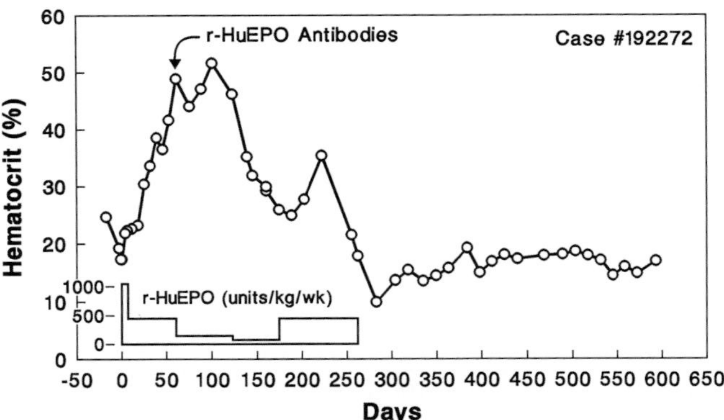

FIG. 29–6. Changes in hematocrit following r-HuEPO administration and anti–r-HuEPO antibody production in a uremic cat. Note the rapid, r-HuEPO–unresponsive decline in hematocrit with the appearance of the antibodies. With disappearance of the antibodies, hematocrit returned to the pretreatment value.

      (1). Development of anti–r-HuEPO antibodies is the most frequent and important adverse effect of r-HuEPO therapy. The clinical repercussions are rapidly progressive and profound declines in hematocrit, red cell count, and hemoglobin concentration and extreme hypoplasia of the bone marrow that is unresponsive to r-HuEPO administration. The onset, duration, and intensity of the anemia and bone marrow failure correspond to the appearance of these binding antibodies.[30] Figure 29–6 illustrates the course of such a misadventure in a cat.
         (a). The incidence of antibody formation has not been determined precisely, but it may approach 20 to 50% of treated animals.[20,21]
         (b). It occurs with similar frequency in dogs and cats. The onset is variable from the start of treatment and independent of intravenous or subcutaneous routes of r-HuEPO administration (L.D. Cowgill, unpublished observations).
         (c). Presumably, as the antibody titer increases, its binding to r-HuEPO (and to native erythropoietin) nullifies their mitogenic effects on the erythroid progenitor cells, promoting the erythroid hypoplastic state. In lieu of specific measurement of anti–r-HuEPO antibodies, their appearance can be predicted by an increase in the M/E ratio of bone marrow aspirates from affected animals. In general, an M/E ratio greater than 8/1 to 10/1 in a patient receiving r-HuEPO is con-

sistent with antibody conversion and warrants cessation of therapy.

(d). The development of anti–r-HuEPO antibodies in dogs and cats has tempered initial expectations for its application to dogs and cats. Antibody production appears to be reversible with discontinuation of r-HuEPO; however, the rapidity and extent of recovery from the resulting anemia depend on antibody titer, its metabolic clearance, and the ability of the animal to secrete erythropoietin. Generally, affected patients recover to their pretreatment hematologic status or to a level of erythropoiesis commensurate with native erythropoietin production (Fig. 29–6).

(2). Polycythemia may be associated with rigid dosing schedules or failure to adequately monitor the therapeutic response (see Fig. 29–5). Flexible dosing and proper monitoring should obviate this complication, although no clinical sequelae have been attributed specifically to the induced polycythemia.

(3). Seizures were identified in 3 of 17 (18%) animals with no history of convulsive tendencies.[20] The seizures were associated with severe azotemia and/or systemic hypertension in each case, but the precise cause of the seizures remains unknown.

(4). Systemic hypertension is being investigated currently as part of a large multicenter clinical trial. In an earlier trial involving fewer patients, administration of r-HuEPO was associated with the onset and exacerbation of systemic hypertension or increased requirement for antihypertensive medication in two of six dogs and three of five cats with progressive renal failure (L. D. Cowgill, personal observations).

(a). Development or exacerbation of systemic hypertension is one of the most frequent consequences of r-HuEPO therapy in human patients.[14,38,58,91]

(b). Chronic adaptations to anemia appear to impair appropriate vasodilator responses, as blood volume is increased and cardiac output is reduced.[39,58] Increased blood viscosity could exacerbate peripheral vascular resistance but is unlikely to be requisite for the changes in blood pressure.[39,81]

(c). Hypertension does not relate to the dosage of r-HuEPO or to the rate of change in hematocrit value.[39]

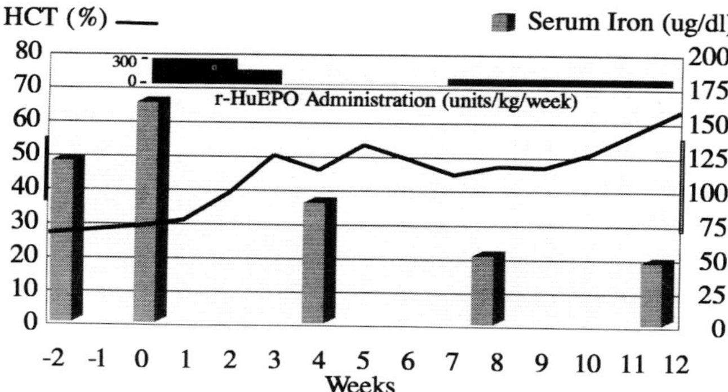

FIG. 29–7. Changes in hematocrit and serum iron following r-HuEPO administration to a uremic dog without iron supplementation. The insert depicts the initial and maintenance dose of r-HuEPO, and the shaded areas on the vertical axes represent the reference ranges. Note the progressive fall in serum iron with the onset of the erythropoietic response.

(5). Acute allergic reactions, revealed as cellulitis, cutaneous or mucocutaneous reactions, fever, and arthralgia, are uncommon sequelae of r-HuEPO therapy. An allergic basis for these reactions could not be demonstrated by intradermal skin testing with the formulated products, HSA, or pure r-HuEPO; however, all clinical manifestations resolved within days of discontinuing r-HuEPO therapy in affected patients.[20]

(6). Iron depletion is a potential concern in all animals treated with r-HuEPO. Many uremic animals have a low serum iron concentration and percent transferrin saturation before starting erythropoietin replacement therapy. The erythropoietic response fostered by r-HuEPO requires massive mobilization of iron from tissue stores to support hemoglobin synthesis. In patients inadequately supplemented with iron, the demands may exceed available tissue stores and promote iron depletion (Fig. 29–7). Depletion of transferable iron blunts or halts the erythropoietic response and may exacerbate of the anemia.

(7). Acute anaphylactic reactions have been observed in toxicity studies in experimental dogs receiving large doses of r-HuEPO. To date, no such reactions have been reported from clinical trials in uremic animals.

6. Application and interim recommendations for r-HuEPO use in uremic dogs and cats.

a. Indications.

(1). Formulations of r-HuEPO (epoetin alfa [Epogen, Amgen Inc., Thousand Oaks,

California; PROCRIT, Orth Biotech, Raritan, New Jersey] and epoetin beta [MAROGEN, Chugai-Upjohn, Inc., Rosemont, Illinois]) are currently available to veterinarians and are prescribed with increasing frequency for a variety of hematologic disorders in animals. However, r-HuEPO is not licensed for use in animals, and to date, guidelines for its use in animals with anemia of chronic renal failure have been extrapolated from recommendations for human patients and from preliminary clinical trials in dogs and cats. Its therapeutic benefits are consistent and profound, but the potential for adverse effects must be confronted realistically in risk-versus-benefit decisions about its use. The optimal dosage and route of administration for human patients are subject to ongoing debate and modification.[1] The following recommendations for dogs and cats should be regarded only as tested references until its indications, efficacy, and safety have been more explicitly documented.

(2). Erythropoietin replacement is indicated for any uremic patient that demonstrates hypoproliferative anemia and the attendant consequences of weakness, fatigue, inappetence, apathy, cold intolerance, or altered behavior. These signs become more apparent as the hematocrit approaches 30% for dogs and 25% for cats, but they vary considerably in individual patients. The clinical benefits of correcting even a mild degree of anemia with r-HuEPO can be dramatic, but the risks of therapy must be carefully balanced against the disability of the patient and the projected clinical gains.

(a). For patients with mild to moderate anemia and no obvious disability, a cautious approach is indicated, and the risks and benefits must be carefully evaluated.

(b). If the anemia is moderate to profound (hematocrit <30% in dogs and <25% in cats) and associated with overt clinical signs, the risks of treatment are generally warranted and the results beneficial. Pet owners should be counseled about the rationale, benefits, and potential adverse effects of r-HuEPO therapy and should provide informed consent for its administration.

(c). Both blood pressure and serum iron should be measured before starting r-HuEPO therapy. More than 60% of patients with renal disease have systemic hypertension,[18] and perhaps 15 to 25% of uremic patients have a low serum iron concentration. Until systemic hypertension or iron deficiency are corrected, r-HuEPO should be withheld.

b. Dosage and route of administration.

(1). In both dogs and cats, r-HuEPO therapy is initiated at 100 U/kg body weight by subcutaneous injection 3 times per week. This dosage promotes an effective erythropoietic response in most animals.[21,22]

(a). The initial dosage is maintained until the target hematocrit (between 37 and 45% for dogs and 30 to 40% for cats) is achieved.

(b). Once the lower target is reached, the dosage interval is reduced to twice weekly, to prevent overshooting the target range.

(c). If the hematocrit approaches the upper target value, the dosage interval is further reduced to once weekly, to prevent polycythemia.

(d). The dosage schedule is further modified as required, between one and three times weekly to maintain the hematocrit within the target range.

(e). If adequate control cannot be achieved with these treatment intervals, dosage may be increased by 25 to 50 U/kg. In general, the dosing intervals should not exceed thrice weekly or be less than once weekly.

(2). The maintenance dosage that sustains the hematocrit value within the target range must be established individually for each patient by judicious adjustment of the dosage and/or interval of administration and adequate surveillance of the patient's responses. Usually, a dose between 75 and 100 U/kg once or twice weekly is sufficient (Fig. 29–5).

(3). If the target hematocrit is not attained by 8 to 12 weeks of thrice-weekly therapy, the dosage may be increased by 25 to 50 U/kg every 3 to 4 weeks until the target is achieved. Failing an adequate initial response, or if the patient becomes unresponsive to r-HuEPO, a thorough evaluation for iron deficiency, external blood loss, hemolytic processes, concurrent infectious, inflammatory, or neoplastic diseases, or the development of anti–r-HuEPO antibodies that could diminish or prevent erythropoiesis should be performed.

(a). Owing to the finite lag between dosage modifications and responses in hematocrit, neither dosage nor interval of administration should be adjusted more frequently than every 3 weeks. More frequent dosage adjustments may result in large fluctuations of hematocrit, the tendency to "chase" the volatile excursions with dosage adjustments, and failure to achieve a smooth transition to a maintenance dosage.

(b). Rapid decreases in hematocrit following usual dosage reductions may indicate anti–r-HuEPO antibody formation and should prompt further evaluation of the patient.

(4). Treatment should be withheld temporarily if the hematocrit exceeds reference ranges. Once it is re-established at the upper limit of the target range, treatment should be reinstituted with smaller dosages.

c. Iron supplementation.

(1). The effective erythropoiesis promoted by r-HuEPO significantly affects iron homeostasis. The rapid demand for iron can deplete iron stores and promote iron depletion (Fig. 29–7). Consequently, all patients treated with r-HuEPO should be supplemented with iron, to prevent this complication and to foster the therapeutic response.

(2). Serum iron concentrations, total iron binding capacity (TIBC), and percent transferrin saturation should be normalized before initiating r-HuEPO therapy by administration of ferrous sulfate, orally, at 100 to 300 mg per day for dogs and 50 to 100 mg per day for cats.[60,86]

(3). Maintenance iron therapy should be provided daily with oral ferrous sulfate or multivitamin preparations that contain ferrous sulfate in similar dosages.

d. Monitoring the therapeutic response.

(1). The potency of r-HuEPO and the requirement for lifelong therapy necessitate regular evaluation of the patient to ensure maximal therapeutic efficacy and to identify untoward effects of treatment.

(2). Hematocrit should be monitored weekly until it is established within the target range for at least 4 weeks. Thereafter, a complete blood count should be performed at monthly or bimonthly intervals to ensure adequacy of the erythropoietic response and to monitor for adverse hematologic reactions.

(a). A sudden decrease in hematocrit or development of anemia in the presence of adequate dosages of r-HuEPO and normal iron metabolism may signal development of anti–r-HuEPO antibodies. A bone marrow aspirate that demonstrates severe erythroid hypoplasia is consistent with this development and contraindicates further r-HuEPO administration.

(b). Antibody formation is unpredictable but commonly is evident after 4 to 16 weeks of therapy.

(3). Serum iron, TIBC, and erythrocyte indices (mean corpuscular volume, mean corpuscular hemoglobin, mean corpuscular hemoglobin concentration) should be monitored 3 to 4 weeks after starting r-HuEPO therapy and then monthly or bimonthly for the duration of treatment. This precaution is taken to assess disorders of iron metabolism and the adequacy of iron supplementation.

(4). Systemic blood pressure should be determined by direct or indirect methods at least monthly during the initiation phase of therapy and monthly or bimonthly thereafter, to monitor for development or exacerbation of hypertension.[18]

(5). Pain, inflammation, or discoloration at injection sites should be evaluated regularly, to ascertain if the patient is allergic or sensitive to the drug.

e. Cessation of therapy.

(1). The r-HuEPO therapy should be discontinued if any of the following adverse events are recognized:

(a). Polycythemia.

(b). Fever, anorexia, joint pain, cellulitis, or cutaneous or mucosal ulceration, which may indicate systemic or local sensitivity to r-HuEPO or bacterial contamination of the product when multiple-dose use is prescribed. As currently formulated, the commercial preparations are intended for single-dose use and contain no antimicrobial preservatives. Because multiple-dose use usually is prescribed for animals, careful instruction of the client in handling precautions and aseptic technique is required.

(c). Development of anti–r-HuEPO antibodies, as predicted by serum tiers, sudden (r-HuEPO nonresponsive) drop in hematocrit, or profound erythroid hypoplasia (high M/E ratio in bone marrow aspirate).

(d). Onset or exacerbation of systemic hypertension that is refractory to antihypertensive therapy.

IV. SUMMARY

A. Hypoproliferative anemia is a predictable and serious complication of progressive renal failure and contributes significantly to the overall morbidity and debilitation of the uremic state in animals.

B. The pathogenesis of the anemia of chronic renal failure is multifactorial, but, clearly, bone marrow failure from the deficient production of erythropoietin by the diseased kidneys is pivotal and the most influential cause.

C. Until recently, there was no satisfactory therapy to resolve the anemia, and consequently the significance of its contributions to the uremic syndrome was overlooked.

D. Today, the anemia of chronic renal failure can be explicitly corrected with r-HuEPO, and the clinical debility generally attributable to excretory insufficiency can be lessened or ameliorated.

E. Anemia must no longer be regarded as an intractable consequence of the uremic syndrome and should be managed as conscientiously as the other polysystemic features of uremia.

REFERENCES

1. Abraham PA, St Peter WL, Redic-Kill KA. Controversies in determination of epoetin (recombinant human erythropoietin) dosages. *Clin Pharmacokinet.* 1992;22: 409–415.
2. Adamson JW, Eschbach JW. Treatment of the anemia of chronic renal failure with recombinant human erythropoietin. *Annu Rev Med.* 1990;41:349–360.
3. Adamson JW, Eschbach J, Finch CA. The kidney and erythropoiesis. *Am J Med.* 1968;44:725–733.
4. Akmal M, Telfer N, Ansari AN, et al. Erythrocyte survival in chronic renal failure. Role of secondary hyperparathyroidism. *J Clin Invest.* 1985;76:1695–1698.
5. Auer LA, Bell K. Feline blood transfusion reactions. In: Kirk RW, ed. *Current Veterinary Therapy. Small Animal Practice.* 9th ed. Philadelphia, Pennsylvania: WB Saunders, Co, 1986.
6. Bennett WM. A multicenter clinical trial of epoetin-beta for anemia of end-stage renal disease. *Am Soc Nephrol.* 1991;1: 990–998.
7. Bogin E, Massry SG, Levi J, et al. Effect of parathyroid hormone on osmotic fragility of human erythrocytes. *J Clin Invest.* 1982; 69:1017–1025.
8. Bommer J, Barth H-P, Zeier M, et al. Efficacy comparison of intravenous and subcutaneous recombinant human erythropoietin administration in hemodialysis patients. *Contemp Nephrol.* 1991;88:136–143.
9. Bommer J, Kugel M, Schoeppe W, et al. Dose-related effects of recombinant human erythropoietin on erythropoiesis. Results of a multicenter tiral in patients with end-stage renal disease. *Contemp Nephrol.* 1988;66:85–93.
10. Bondurant MC, Koury MJ. Anemia induces accumulation of erythropoietin mRNA in the kidney and liver. *Molec Cell Biol.* 1986;6:2731–2733.
11. Buchwald D, Argyres S, Easterling RE, et al. Effect of nandrolone decanoate on the anemia of chronic hemodialysis patients. *Nephron.* 1977;18:232–238.
12. Caro J, Brown S, Miller O, et al. Erythropoietin levels in uremic nephric and anephric patients. *Lab Clin Med.* 1979;93:449–458.
13. Caro J, Erslev AJ. Uremic inhibitors of erythropoiesis. *Semin Nephrol.* 1985;5:128–132.
14. Casti S, Passerini P, Campise MR, et al. Benefits and risks of protracted treatment with human recombinant erythropoietin in patients having haemodialysis. *Br Med J.* 1987;295:1017–1020.
15. Cattran DC, Fenton SSA, Wilson DR, et al. A controlled trial of nandrolone decanoate in the treatment of uremic anemia. *Kidney Int.* 1977;12:430–437.
16. Chaplin H, Mollison PL. Red cell life-span in nephritis and hepatic cirrhosis. *Clin Sci.* 1953;12:351–360.
17. Cowgill LD. Diseases of the kidney. In: Ettinger SJ, ed. *Textbook of Veterinary Internal Medicine.* 2nd ed. Vol 2. Philadelphia, Pennsylvania: WB Saunders; 1983.
18. Cowgill LD, Kallet AJ. Systemic hypertension. In: Kirk RW, ed. *Current Veterinary Therapy. Small Animal Practice.* 9th ed. Philadelphia, Pennsylvania: WB Saunders; 1986:360–364.
19. Cowgill LD, Feldman B, Levy J, et al. Efficacy of recombinant human erythropoietin (r-HuEPO) for anemia in dogs and cats with renal failure. *J Vet Intern Med.* 1990;4:126.
20. Cowgill LD. Clinical experience and use of recombinant human erythropoietin in uremic dogs and cats. *Proceedings of the 9th American College of Veterinary Internal Medicine Forum.* New Orleans, Louisiana: 1991;147–149.
21. Cowgill LD,. Erythropoietin: Its use in the treatment of chronic renal failure in dogs and cats. *Proceedings of the 15th Annual Waltham/OSU Symposium.* Kal Kan Foods, Inc; Vernon, California: 1992:65–71.
22. Cowgill LD. Application of recombinant human erythropoietin in dogs and cats. In: Kirk RW, Bonagura JD, eds. *Current Veterinary Therapy. Small Animal Practice.* 11th ed. Philadelphia, Pennsylvania: WB Saunders; 1992.
23. Dainiak N. The role of androgens in the treatment of chronic renal failure. *Semin Nephrol.* 1985;5:147–154.
24. Delano BG. Improvements in quality of life following treatment with r-HuEPO in anemic hemodialysis patients. *Am J Kidney Dis.* 1989;14 (Suppl 1):14–18.
25. Delwiche F, Segal GM, Eschbach JW, et al. Hematopoietic inhibitors in chronic renal failure: Lack of in vitro specificity. *Kidney Int.* 1986;29:641–648.
26. Deniston OL, Luscombe FA, Buesching DP, et al. Effects of long-term epoetin beta therapy on the quality of life of hemodialysis patients. *ASAIO Trans.* 1990;36:M157–M160.
27. Dennis JS. Anabolic steroids: Their potential in small animals. *Comp Contin Ed.* 1990;12:1403–1410.
28. DiBartola SP, Rutgers HC, Zack PM, et al. Clinicopathologic findings associated with chronic renal disease in cats: 74 cases (1973–1984). *J Am Vet Med Assoc.* 1987;190:1196–1202.
29. Doane BD, Fried W, Schwartz F. Response of uremic patients to nandrolone decanoate. *Arch Intern Med.* 1975;135:972–975.
30. Dr. Joan Egrie, Amgen, Thousand Oaks, CA, personal communication, 1991.
31. Egrie JC, Browne JK, Lai P, et al. Characterization of recombinant monkey and human erythropoietin. In: Stammatoyannopoulos G, Neinhuis AW, eds. Experimental Approaches for the Study of Hemoglobin Switching. New York, New York: Alan R Liss, 1985.
32. Egrie JC, Strickland TW, Lane J, et al. Characterization and biological effects of recombinant human erythropoietin. *Immunobiology.* 1986;172:213–224.
33. Erslev AJ. Erythropoietin. *N Engl J Med.* 1991;324:1339–1344.
34. Eschbach JW. The anemia of chronic renal failure: Pathophysiology and the effects of recombinant erythropoietin. *Kidney Int.* 1989;35:134–148.
35. Eschbach JW, Adamson JW. Improvement in the anemia of

chronic renal failure with fluoxymesterone. *Ann Intern Med.* 1973;78:527–532.

36. Eschbach JW, Adamson JW. Anemia in renal disease. In: Schrier RW, Gottschalk CW, eds. *Diseases of the Kidney.* 4th ed. Vol III. Boston, Massachusetts: Little, Brown; 1988.
37. Eschbach JW, Adamson JW. Recombinant human erythropoietin: Implications for nephrology. *Am J Kidney Dis.* 1988;11: 203–209.
38. Eschbach JW, Adamson JW. Guidelines for recombinant human erythropoietin therapy. *Am J Kidney Dis.* 1989;14 (Suppl 2):2–8.
39. Eschbach JW, Adamson JW. The pathophysiology and treatment of the anemia of chronic renal failure. In: Gonick HC, ed. *Current Nephrology.* Vol 14. St. Louis, Missouri: Mosby–Year Book; 1991.
40. Eschbach JW, Abdulhadi MH, Browne JK, et al. Recombinant human erythropoietin in anemic patients with end-stage renal disease. Results of a phase III multicenter clinical trial. *Ann Intern Med.* 1989;111:992–1000.
41. Eschbach JW, Egrie JC, Downing MR, Browne JK, Adamson JW. Correction of the anemia of end-stage renal disease with recombinant human erythropoietin. Results of a combined phase I and II clinical trial. *N Engl J Med.* 1987;316:73–78.
42. Eschbach JW, Funk D, Adamson J, Kuhn J, Scribner BH, Finch CA. Erythropoiesis in patients with renal failure undergoing chronic dialysis. *N Engl J Med.* 1967;276:653–658.
43. Eschbach JW, Haley NR, Adamson JW. The anemia of chronic renal failure: Pathophysiology and effects of recombinant erythropoietin. *Contrib Nephrol.* 1990;78:24–37.
44. Eschbach JW, Kelly MR, Haley NR, et al. Treatment of the anemia of progressive renal failure with recombinant human erythropoietin. *N Engl J Med.* 1989;321:158–163.
45. Evans RW, Rader B, Manninen DL, et al. The quality of life of hemodialysis recipients treated with recombinant human erythropoietin. *JAMA.* 1990;263:825–830.
46. Fisher JW, et al. Statement on the clinical use of recombinant erythropoietin in anemia of end-stage renal disease. *Am J Kidney Dis.* 1989;14:163–169.
47. Freedman MH, Cattran DC, Saunders EF. Anemia of chronic renal failure: Inhibition of erythropoiesis by uremic serum. *Nephron.* 1983;35:15–19.
48. Giger U. Serum erythropoietin concentrations in polycythemic and anemic dogs. *Proceedings of the 9th American College of Veterinary Internal Medicine Forum.* New Orleans, Louisiania: 1991.
49. Giger U. Erythropoietin and its clinical use. *Compend Contin Ed Pract Vet.* 1992;14:25–34.
50. Giger U. The feline AB blood group system and incompatibility reactions. In: Kirk RW, Bonagura JD, eds. *Current Veterinary Therapy. Small Animal Practice.* 11th ed. Philadelphia, Pennsylvania: WB Saunders; 1992.
51. Haskins SC. Shock. The pathophysiology and management of circulatory collapse states. In: Kirk RW, ed. *Current Veterinary Therapy. Small Animal Practice.* 8th ed. Philadelphia, Pennsylvania: WB Saunders; 1983.
52. Hendler ED, Solomon LR. Prospective controlled study of androgen effects on red cell oxygen transport and work capacity in chronic hemodialysis patients. *Acta Haematol.* 1990;83:1–8.
53. Jacobs D, Shoemaker C, Rudersdorf R, et al. Isolation and characterization of genomic and cDNA clones of human erythropoietin. *Nature.* 1985;313:806–810.
54. Jain NC. Depression or hypoproliferative anemias. In: Jain NC, ed. *Schalm's Veterinary Hematology.* 4th ed. Philadelphia, Pennsylvania: Lea & Febiger; 1986.
55. King LG, Giger U, Diserens D, et al. Anemia of chronic renal failure in dogs. *J Vet Intern Med.* 1992;6:264–270.
56. Krantz SB. Erythropoietin. *Blood.* 1991;77:419–434.
57. Lazarus JM, Hakim RM, Newell J. Recombinant human erythropoietin and phlebotomy in the treatment of iron overload in chronic hemodialysis patients. *Am J Kidney Dis.* 1990;16: 101–108.
58. Levin N. Management of blood pressure changes during recombinant human erythropoietin therapy. *Semin Nephrol.* 1989;9 (Suppl 2):16–20.
59. Lin FK, Suggs S, Lin C-H, et al. Cloning and expression of the human erythropoietin gene. *Proc Natl Acad Sci USA.* 1985;82: 7580–7584.
60. Mahaffey EA. Disorders of iron metabolism. In: Kirk RW, ed. *Current Veterinary Therapy. Small Animal Practice.* 9th ed. Philadelphia, Pennsylvania: WB Saunders; 1986.
61. Malachi T, Bogin E, Gafter U, et al. Parathyroid hormone effect on the fragility of human young and old red blood cells in uremia. *Nephron.* 1986;42:52–57.
62. Massry SG. Pathogenesis of the anemia of uremia: Role of secondary hyperparathyroidism. *Kidney Int.* 1983;24 (Suppl 16):S-204–S-207.
63. Mayer G, Thum J, Cad EM, et al. Working capacity is increased following recombinant human erythropoietin treatment. *Kidney Int.* 1988;34:525–528.
64. McGonigle RJS, Wallin JD, Shadduck RK, et al. Erythropoietin deficiency and inhibition of erythropoiesis in renal insufficiency. *Kidney Int.* 1984;25:437–444.
65. McMahon FG, Vargas R, Ryan M, et al. Pharmacokinetics and effects of recombinant human erythropoietin after intravenous and subcutaneous injections in healthy volunteers. *Blood.* 1990; 76:1718–1722.
66. Mirahmadi MK, Vaziri ND, Gorman JT. Controlled evaluation of hemodialysis patients on nandrolone decanoate (ND) vs testosterone enanthate (TE) (androgens and dialysis patients). *Trans Am Soc Artif Intern Organs.* 1979;25:449–453.
67. Mirand EA, Gordon AS, Wenig J. Mechanism of testosterone action in erythropoiesis. *Nature.* 1965;206:270–272.
68. Mitch WE, Walser M. Nutritional therapy of the uremic patient. In: Brenner BM, Rector FC, eds. *The Kidney.* 3rd ed. Vol 2. Philadelphia, Pennsylvania: WB Saunders; 1989.
69. Murphy GP, Mirand EA, Kenny GM, et al. Extrarenal and renal erythropoietin levels in human beings and experimental animals in the intact, anephric or renal allotransplanted state. *J Urol.* 1970;103:686–691.
70. Neats JP, Heuse AF. Effects of anaemic anoxia on erythropoiesis of nephrectomized dogs. *Nature.* 1962;195:190.
71. Neats JP, Heuse A. Effects of anemic hypoxia on erythropoiesis of normal and uremic dogs with or without kidneys. *J Nucl Med.* 1964;5:471–479.
72. Neff MS, Goldberg J, Slifkin RF, et al. A comparison of androgens for anemia in patients on hemodialysis. *N Engl J Med.* 1981;304: 871–875.
73. Nissenson AR. Recombinant human erythropoietin: Impact on brain and cognitive function, exercise tolerance, sexual potency, and quality of life. *Semin Nephrol.* 1989;9 (Suppl 2):25–31.
74. Ohno Y, Rege AB, Fisher JW, et al. Inhibitors of erythroid colony-forming cells (CFU-E and BFU-E) in sera of azotemic patients with anemia of renal disease. *J Lab Clin Med.* 1978;92: 916–923.
75. Petrites-Murphy MB, Pierce KR, Fisher JW. Effect of incorporation of serum from dogs with renal impairment on canine erythroid bone marrow cultures. *Am J Vet Res.* 1989;50:1537–1543.
76. Petrites-Murphy MB, Pierce KR, Lowry SR, et al. Role of parathyroid hormone in the anemia of chronic terminal renal dysfunction in dogs. *J Vet Res.* 1989;50:1898–1905.
77. Polzin DJ, Osborne CA, Stevens JB, et al. Influence of modified

protein diets on the nutritional status of dogs with induced chronic renal failure. *Am J Vet Res.* 1983;44:1694–1702.

78. Polzin D, Osborne C, O'Brien T. Diseases of the kidneys and ureters. In: Ettinger SJ, ed. *Textbook of Veterinary Internal Medicine.* 3rd ed. Philadelphia, Pennsylvania: WB Saunders; 1989.
79. Polzin DJ, Osborne CA. The use of erythropoietin in chronic renal failure. *Adv Small Anim Med Surg.* 1990;3(1):1–3.
80. Radtke HW, Claussner A, Erbes PM, et al. Serum erythropoietin concentration in chronic renal failure: Relationship to degree of anemia and excretory renal function. *Blood.* 1979;54:877–884.
81. Raine AEG. Hypertension, blood viscosity, and cardiovascular morbidity in renal failure: Implications of erythropoietin therapy. *Lancet.* 1988;1:97–100.
82. Segal GM, Eschbach JW, Egrie JC, et al. The anemia of end-stage renal disease: Hematopoietic progenitor cell response. *Kidney Int.* 1988;33:983–988.
83. Shahidi NT. Androgens and erythropoiesis. *N Engl J Med.* 1973; 289:72–80.
84. Shaldon S, Koch KM, Oppermann F, et al. Testosterone therapy for anaemia in maintenance dialysis. *Br Med J.* 1971;3:212–214.
85. Shaw AB. Haemolysis in chronic renal failure. *Br Med J.* 1967; 2:213–216.
86. Smith JE. Iron metabolism in dogs and cats. *Compend Contin Ed Pract Vet.* 1992;14:39–43.
87. Sun CH, Ward HJ, Paul WL, et al. Serum erythropoietin levels after renal transplantation. *N Engl J Med.* 1989;321:151–157.
88. Sundal E, Kaeser U. Correction of anaemia of chronic renal failure with recombinant human erythropoietin: Safety and efficacy of one year treatment in a European multicenter study in 150 haemodialysis-dependent patients. *Nephrol Dial Transplant.* 1989;4:979–987.
89. Thornhill JA. Control of vomiting in the uremic patient. In: Kirk RW, ed. *Current Veterinary Therapy. Small Animal Practice.* 8th ed. Philadelphia, Pennsylvania: WB Saunders; 1983.
90. Turnwald GH, Pichler ME. Blood transfusion in dogs and cats part II. Administration, adverse effects, and component therapy. *Comp Contin Ed.* 1985;7:115–124.
91. van de Borne P, Tielemans C, Vanherweghem JL, et al. Effect of recombinant human erythropoietin therapy on ambulatory blood pressure and heart rate in chronic haemodialysis patients. *Nephrol Dial Transplant.* 1992;7:45–49.
92. Van Wyck DB. Iron management during recombinant human erythropoietin therapy. *Am J Kidney Dis.* 1989;14 (Suppl 2):9–13.
93. von Hartitzsch B, Kerr DNS, Morley G, et al. Androgens in the anaemia of chronic renal failure. *Nephron.* 1977;18:13–20.
94. Wallner SF, Vautrin RM. Evidence that inhibition of erythropoiesis is important in the anemia of chronic renal failure. *J Lab Clin Med.* 1981;97:170–178.
95. Weiss DJ. Therapy for disorders of erythropoiesis. In: Kirk RW, ed. *Current Veterinary Therapy. Small Animal Practice.* 9th ed. Philadelphia, Pennsylvania: WB Saunders; 1986.
96. Williams JS, Stein JG, Ferris TF. Nandrolone decanoate therapy for patients receiving hemodialysis. *Arch Intern Med.* 1974;134: 289–292.
97. Wolcott DL, Marsh JT, LaRue A, et al. Recombinant human erythropoietin treatment may improve quality of life and cognitive function in chronic hemodialysis patients. *Am J Kidney Dis.* 1989;14:478–485.

C H A P T E R 30

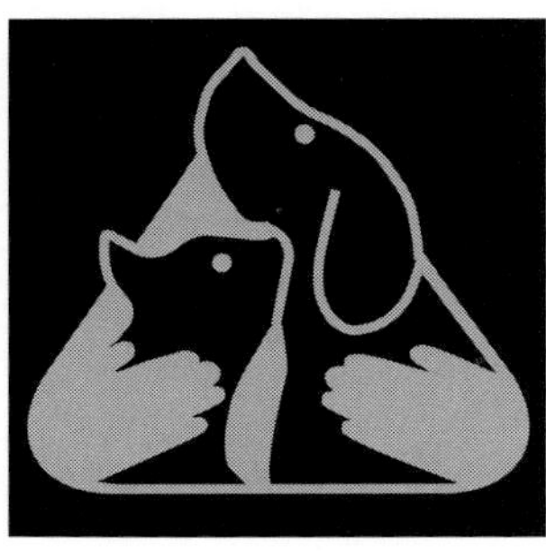

Drug Therapy during Renal Disease and Renal Failure

J. E. RIVIERE
SHELLY L. VADEN

I. INTRODUCTION

A. Renal and hepatic elimination determine the concentration-time profile of most drugs used in veterinary medicine. If routine dosage regimens are used in animals with renal failure, drugs eliminated primarily by renal mechanisms will accumulate.

B. If a drug is toxic, the dosage regimen must be adjusted to avoid intoxication. People with a blood urea nitrogen (BUN) greater than 40 mg/dL have 2.5 times the rate of adverse drug reactions when compared to that of the normal population.[94]

C. The purposes of this chapter are to outline principles of drug disposition in renal disease, drug dosage modification techniques, and effects of dialysis on drug disposition and to provide specific recommendations for dosage regimens for dogs with impaired renal function. Guidelines are largely extrapolated from human uremic patients because the literature available on drug therapy in dogs is sparse.

II. PRINCIPLES OF DRUG DISPOSITION

A. Overview.

1. For any drug to be therapeutically effective, it must reach its site of action at a rate and in an amount sufficient to elicit the desired response. The therapeutic effect of most drugs, especially antimicrobial agents, correlates more closely with plasma concentration than with total dose administered.
2. The final plasma concentration of a drug depends on the rate and extent of absorption, the nature of its distribution throughout the body, its binding to plasma proteins and tissue, the extent of its biotransformation, and the rate and routes of elimination.
3. An approach used to study the disposition of a drug is to model the body as a system of theoretic compartments, thereby allowing the formulation of mathematical models that describe the behavior of the drug over time.[9,62,86,87] Each compartment contains some fraction of the administered dose. The size or volume of these compartments is reflected by the kinetics of the entry of the drug into and the exit of the drug from each area.
4. A drug is absorbed from an extravascular site (subcutaneous, intramuscular, gastrointestinal) into the blood, or central compartment, and subsequently is distributed to other compartments. The drug is eventually eliminated from the central compartment by renal and nonrenal mechanisms (Fig. 30–1).
5. Rate constants can be used to characterize the fraction of drug that is absorbed (K_a), transferred between compartments (K_{21}, K_{12}, K_{31}, K_{13}) or cleared by an elimination organ (K_{el}) per unit of time.

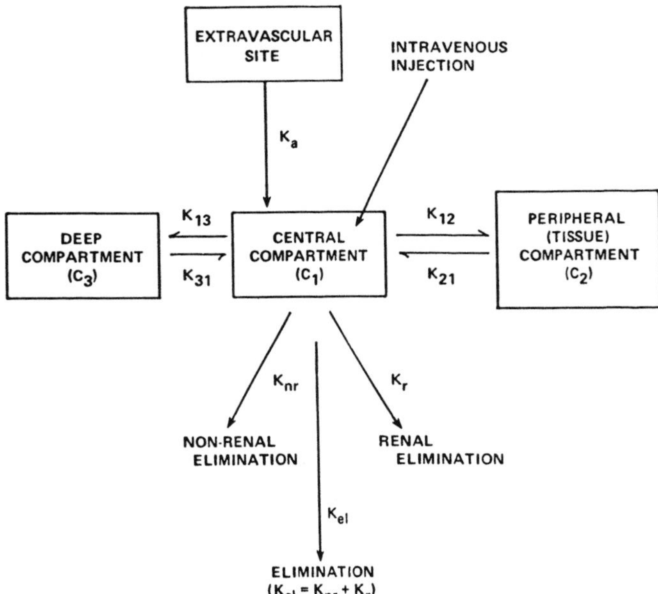

FIG. 30–1. Open three-compartment pharmacokinetic model depicting drug disposition. The rate constants describing these processes are K_a for absorption; K_{12}, K_{21}, K_{13}, and K_{31} for distribution; and K_{el} for elimination. Distribution between C_1 and C_3 occurs more slowly than between C_1 and C_2.

a. The primary determinants of these rate constants are the biochemical and physical properties of the drug, the regional blood flow, and the physical nature of the compartments. If the drug is given intravenously directly into the central compartment, K_a would be 0.
b. If the magnitude of K_{13} and K_{31} is less than that of K_{12} and K_{21}, the rate of transfer into and out of compartment 3 would be slower than the rate into and out of compartment 2. Compartment 3 would be termed a "deep" compartment, associated with prolonged elimination and possible accumulation.
c. K_{el} is the algebraic sum of its two components: renal (K_r) and nonrenal (K_{nr}). K_{nr} is usually a result of hepatic biotransformation.

6. The volume of distribution (Vd) is defined as the volume of fluid that would be required to contain the total amount of drug in the body uniformly distributed at a concentration equal to that in the plasma. Thus,

$$Vd = D/C(0) \qquad \text{(equation 1)}$$

where D is the administered dose and C(0) is the concentration of drug in plasma just after giving an intravenous bolus dose.

a. Thus, Vd enables the clinician to relate dose to expected plasma concentration.
b. The magnitude of this volume depends on the degree of drug binding to plasma proteins and tissue and on the number of compartments into which the drug distributes. Vd is the sum of the volumes of the individual compartments.
c. Because total blood concentration of drug is measured, yet only free drug is available for distribution to the tissues, an inherent error exists in the estimation of Vd when total concentrations are employed.

7. Total body clearance (Cl_B) is the volume of serum cleared of drug by all possible mechanisms per unit time.
a. Cl_B can be partitioned into renal and nonrenal parts, such that

$$Cl_B(\text{mL/min}) = Cl_r + Cl_{nr} \qquad \text{(equation 2)}$$

where Cl_r is the renal, and Cl_{nr} is the nonrenal, drug clearance.
b. Changes in body clearances can be induced by altering the function of the excretory organs.
c. All clearances are normally expressed in terms of body weight or surface area.

8. The half-life of a drug (t½) is used to describe the amount of time required for the body to eliminate 50% of drug present. It is a function of both clearance and volume of distribution such that

$$t½ = 0.693Vd/Cl_B = 0.693/K_{el} \qquad \text{(equation 3)}$$

where

$$K_{el} = Cl_B/Vd \qquad \text{(equation 4)}$$

and 0.693 equals the $\ln_2$.

B. Pharmacokinetic alterations of renal disease.

1. Clearance
a. Many drugs are eliminated primarily by the renal excretion of unmetabolized, pharmacologically active drug and may accumulate during renal failure. Table 30–1 summarizes how renal disease can influence drug disposition, activity, and toxicity.[25,31,39,65,70,74,83,91]
b. Drugs are cleared by the kidney through the processes of glomerular filtration, active tubular secretion and reabsorption, and nonionic passive tubular reabsorption. The total renal clearance and renal elimination rate constant, K_r, is determined by the sum of these processes.[21,69,96,102]
c. Glomerular filtration is a unidirectional process that removes nonprotein-bound drugs from the blood. The magnitude of this process de-

TABLE 30–1
EFFECTS OF RENAL INSUFFICIENCY ON DRUG DISPOSITION, ACTIVITY, AND TOXICITY

Altered gastrointestinal drug absorption
Decreased renal clearance with accumulation of parent drug or active metabolites
Altered rate of biotransformation
- Reduced hepatic metabolism
- Reduced first-pass effect with increased oral bioavailability

Decreased protein binding
Altered volume of distribution
Altered electrolyte balance associated with drug therapy and impaired electrolyte homeostasis
- Sodium overload (ampicillin, carbenicillin, cephalothin, and penicillin G)
- Potassium overload (penicillin G)
- Magnesium overload (antacids and laxatives)

Altered drug disposition and activity secondary to
- Acid-base disturbances (weak acids and bases)
- Fluid imbalance

Subtherapeutic antimicrobial urine concentrations
- Decreased renal excretion
- Dilutional effect of isosthenuria

Enhanced drug activity or toxicity secondary to synergy with uremic complications
- Hemorrhagic disorders
- Gastrointestinal irritation
- Neurologic disturbances

TABLE 30–2
EXAMPLES OF DRUGS UNDERGOING RENAL TUBULAR SECRETION AND REABSORPTION

Acids	Bases
Acetazolamide (A,P)	Amphetamine (P)
p-Aminohippurate (A)	Chloroquin (P)
Cephalexin (A)	Diphenhydramine (P)
Chlorothiazide (A,P)	Dopamine (A)
Chlorpropamide (A)	Ephedrine (P)
Ciprofloxacin (A)	Fenfluramine (P)
Clavulinic acid (A)	Hexamethonium (A)
Dapsone (A)	Histamine (A)
Ethacrynic acid (A)	Isoproterenol (A,P)
Furosemide (A)	Morphine (A)
Glucoronides (A)	Neostigmine (A)
Hippurates (A)	Opiates (P)
Indomethacin (A)	Phenothiazine (P)
Methotrexate(A)	Procainamide (A,P)
Nitrofurantoin (P)	Procaine (A)
Penicillin (A,P)	Quinidine (A,P)
Phenolsulfonphthalein (A,P)	Tetraethylammonium (A)
Phenylbutazone (A,P)	Thiamine (A)
Probenecid (A,P)	Trimethoprim (A,P)
Salicylic acid (A,P)	
Spironolactone (A)	
Sulfonamides (A,P)	

A = active tubular secretion or reabsorption; P = passive tubular reabsorption (nonionic back diffusion).

pends on the extent of drug protein binding and the glomerular filtration rate (GFR).

d. Active tubular secretion and reabsorption is a bidirectional process, although the primary orientation is from blood to tubular filtrate.
   (1). This saturable, carrier-mediated process is energy dependent and described by the laws of Michaelis-Menton enzyme kinetics.
   (2). The limited capacity of this process means that tubular secretion remains constant above certain blood concentrations, despite further increases in blood concentration. At subsaturation, clearance of actively secreted substances depends on renal plasma flow.
   (3). The magnitude of this process is not affected by protein binding.
   (4). The two distinct secretory pathways are in the pars recta of the proximal renal tubule—one for acids and one for bases. Table 30–2 lists acidic and basic drugs that are actively and passively excreted by the tubules.[83]
   (5). Drugs competing for tubular transport sites function as reversible, competitive inhibitors. For example, probenecid or phenylbutazone inhibits penicillin secretion.[105]
   (6). Agents secreted by the acid transport system may produce biphasic effects, inhibiting secretion at low concentrations and reabsorption at high concentrations. Salicylate inhibition of uric acid secretion follows this pattern.[106]
   (7). Damage to renal tubules impairs the ability of the kidneys to clear drugs and their conjugates by active tubular processes.

e. Nonionic passive tubular reabsorption or back diffusion is the third mechanism of renal clearance. Lipid-soluble nonionized drugs are reabsorbed into the blood.
   (1). This process depends on urine flow rate and pH and on the lipid solubility of the nonionized drug.
   (2). Ionization is a function of the pKa of the drug and the pH of the tubular fluid. Weak acids are reabsorbed at low urinary pH, whereas weak bases are reabsorbed at high urinary pH. Such conditions as renal tubular acidosis modify renal clearance by enhancing reabsorption of acidic drugs and decreasing reabsorption of basic drugs.[67]

(3). When the urine flow rate is low, the time for back diffusion is greater. Concentrated tubular fluid also facilitates diffusion.

(4). These principles are utilized while treating salicylate intoxication in dogs. Alkaline diuresis decreases salicylate reabsorption by ion trapping and increased urinary flow rate.

(5). Small changes in urinary pH or urine flow rate do not significantly contribute to altered drug clearance in healthy dogs. However, with decreased tubular loading of drug secondary to reduced GFR, altered urinary pH could further reduce overall drug clearance.

2. Protein binding
   a. The pharmacologic effect of most drugs depends on the concentration of free drug in plasma.[58]
   b. A marked reduction in protein binding of some drugs can occur in uremia. This reduction can have profound effects on drug disposition and activity if the fraction of total bound drug is greater than 90% and the free drug has a relatively small volume of distribution.[3,4,28,32,53,64,72-75]
   c. Uremic toxins, such as free fatty acids, amino acids, and unidentified small dialyzable organic acids, may induce conformational changes in albumin, thereby altering the binding sites. These toxins could also compete for binding sites or alter the affinity of the binding site for the drug.[29]
   d. When significant proteinuria is present, hypoalbuminemia can contribute to the binding defect.
   e. In general, protein binding of acidic drugs is decreased in uremia, whereas that of basic drugs is normal or only slightly decreased. Examples of drugs that have decreased protein binding in human uremic patients are benzylpenicillin, diazepam, dicloxacillin, pentobarbital, phenobarbital, phenylbutazone, phenytoin, salicylate, sulfonamides, thiopental, thyroxine, and warfarin.[65]
   f. Drugs cleared by glomerular filtration show an increased clearance, although tubular reabsorption may counterbalance this effect.
3. Volume of distribution
   a. During uremia, reduced protein binding of drugs that are normally highly protein bound results in increased free-drug concentration and increased Vd.[64,65]
   b. Distribution changes have also been documented with drugs that are not significantly protein bound. Vd of digoxin and diazepam decreases, whereas Vd of some aminoglycosides has been shown to increase. The decreased Vd of digoxin is in part the result of decreased binding to the kidney, liver, and myocardium. Dialysis can increase the Vd of some drugs.[42,46,79,82]
   c. Some estimates of Vd have a mathematical dependence on the magnitude of K_{el}. Estimates of Vd (i.e., Vd_{SS}) that are independent of K_{el} should be used so that true volume changes in renal disease states can be detected.[76]
   d. The clinical significance of altered Vd with renal failure is not known, and dosage adjustment regimens generally do not account for the alteration. True estimates of the magnitude of Vd can only be obtained through an analysis of drug time-concentration profiles in the blood.
4. Biotransformation
   a. Changes in the biotransformation of drugs during renal failure have been documented, although sharp contrasts exist among species.[39,64,65,71,73]
   b. Hepatic enzyme activity (including p450) is reduced from 71 to 26% in rats with chronic renal failure.[39]
   c. Glycine conjugation, acetylation, and hydrolysis reactions are slowed in uremia. Uremia does not appear to alter microsomal oxidation, reduction, glucuronide synthesis, sulfate conjugation, or methylation pathways.[71,73]
   d. Decreased biotransformation can result in decreased K_{nr} and drug accumulation. The nonrenal clearance of captopril, cimetidine, cortisol, cefonicid, cefotaxime, cilastatin, imipenem, metaclopromide, moxalactam, and procainamide is reduced in human uremic patients.[65]
   e. A study of pentobarbital disposition in nephrectomized dogs did not detect a different drug t½ than that measured in controls.[26]
   f. In humans, renal insufficiency can lead to the accumulation of active metabolites of drugs eliminated by biotransformation, thereby resulting in intoxication and enhanced drug activity. Examples of such drugs are doxorubicin, allopurinol, cephalothin, cephapirin, chlorpropamide, digitoxin, lidocaine, mephobarbital, primidone, procainamide, and some sulfonamides.[31]
   g. Reduced hepatic metabolism associated with renal insufficiency leads to increased oral bioavailability of propranolol and dihydrocodeine. An enhanced pharmacodynamic response is associated with dihydrocodeine but not with propranolol.
5. Other
   a. The administration of antibiotics containing sodium or potassium could result in electrolyte overload. Magnesium intoxication could result from administration of antacids and laxatives.[78]
   b. Penicillin and carbenicillin, functioning as nonreabsorbable anions in the distal tubules,

could cause excessive loss of hydrogen and potassium ions.

c. Acidemia favors dissociation of salicylate and phenobarbital, thereby leading to increased concentrations of the drugs in the brain. Acidemia also decreases sensitivity of adrenergic receptors.[83]

d. Altered blood-brain barrier function in uremia can lead to increased cerebrospinal fluid concentrations of some drugs, including opiates, barbiturates, and tranquilizers. Decreased protein binding of these drugs accentuates the effect.[83]

e. Renal failure results in decreased renal excretion of antimicrobial drugs, thereby making the treatment of urinary tract infections difficult. Prolonged polyuric states can further decrease antibiotic concentrations in the urine. Concentrations of antibiotics in renal parenchyma are lower in severely diseased kidneys than in normal kidneys.[13,60,105,113]

f. Uremic complications may synergistically potentiate drug toxicity. Examples include administration of anticoagulants to patients with uremia-induced bleeding disorders and urinary acidifiers to patients with metabolic acidosis.

g. The antianabolic activity of tetracycline and the catabolic action of corticosteroid hormones may worsen the degree of azotemia.

h. The rate and extent of gastrointestinal drug absorption can be affected by vomiting, diarrhea, mucosal edema, altered gastrointestinal motility, and the coadministration of oral antacids and gastrointestinal protectants. Decreased blood perfusion and dehydration may impair drug absorption from alimentary, muscular, and subcutaneous sites.[65]

III. DRUG DOSAGE MODIFICATIONS IN RENAL DISEASE

A. Pharmacokinetics.

1. Predictions of drug disposition during renal failure are based on the assumptions that renal drug clearance directly correlates with clinical measures of GFR, that the intact nephron hypothesis holds true, and that a relative glomerulotubular balance is present.[18]

2. Renal clearance is thus a linear function of GFR whether the drug is cleared by glomerular or tubular mechanisms, and

$$Cl_r = M \times GFR \qquad \text{(equation 5)},$$

where M is a proportionality constant.

3. It follows that

$$Cl_B = M \times GFR + Cl_{nr} \qquad \text{(equation 6)}.$$

4. If equation 6 is divided by Vd, the following relationship results:

$$K_{el}(\text{ml/min}) = K_r + K_{nr} = M' \times GFR + K_{nr} \qquad \text{(equation 7)}.$$

a. This equation describes a straight line with slope M' and y-axis intercept K_{nr}. Thus, K_{el} represents the fraction of the distribution volume of a drug cleared per unit time. For a one-compartment model, K_{el} is equivalent to K, the slope of the plasma concentrations–time profile plotted on semilogarithmic graph paper (x-axis = time, y-axis = natural logarithm of plasma concentration).

b. The relationship defined in equation 7 has been shown to hold for most drugs studied when GFR has been estimated by creatinine clearance.

c. This relationship is graphically depicted in Figure 30–2. The three drugs shown all have the same K_{nr}.

(1). The first is primarily cleared by nonrenal mechanisms. As creatinine clearance decreases, K_{el} remains relatively stable (solid line).

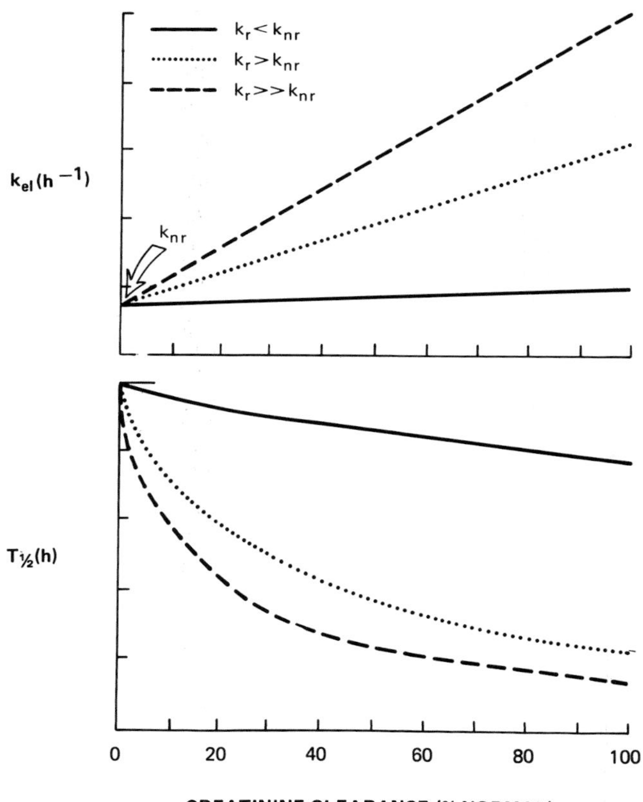

FIG. 30–2. Relationship between creatinine clearance and elimination rate constant (K_{el}) or half-life ($t^{1/2}$). The three drugs depicted depend on renal elimination (K_r) to varying degrees.

(2). The second drug is eliminated from the body by renal and nonrenal mechanisms. Decreases in creatinine clearance result in a steady decline in K_{el} until K_{el} equals K_{nr} at a creatinine clearance of 0 (dotted line).

(3). In the third drug, primarily eliminated by renal mechanisms, decreases in creatinine clearance result in great decreases in K_{el}, with K_{el} still approaching K_{nr} (broken line). If the drug were eliminated solely by renal mechanisms, K_{el} would equal 0 in the functionally anephric patient.

5. GFR can also be related to the elimination t½ of a drug by the following equation:

$$t\tfrac{1}{2}\ (\text{min}) = \frac{0.693 \times Vd}{Cl_B} = \frac{0.693}{K_{el}} = \frac{0.693}{K_r + K_{nr}}$$

(equation 8).

A plot of GFR versus t½ for the same three drugs is depicted in the lower half of Figure 30–2. This plot is clinically applicable because most dosage regimens are expressed in terms of t½.

a. For the drug that is eliminated primarily by nonrenal mechanisms, t½ remains relatively constant over varying degrees of renal function.

b. However, if drug is excreted by renal mechanisms, t½ is stable until creatinine clearance is 30 to 40% of normal, at which point t½ drastically increases. In general, dosage adjustment in renal failure is only necessary when greater than two thirds of renal function is lost.

c. If a drug is excreted almost entirely by the kidneys, t½ approaches infinity as creatinine clearance approaches 0.

6. An alternative method used to relate GFR to t½ of drugs primarily eliminated by renal mechanisms is through the use of a dose fraction (K_f), defined as

$$K_f = \frac{\text{Abnormal creatinine clearance}}{\text{Normal creatinine clearance}} = \frac{Cl_B(\text{abnormal})}{Cl_B(\text{normal})}$$

(equation 9)

B. Dosage regimens.

1. The goal of dosage modification regimens is to maintain comparable plasma drug concentrations in animals with and without normal renal function. The approach in this section is to modify dosage regimens that are appropriate in normal animals in proportion to decreases in renal function estimated by the dose fraction.[10,11,30,80,83,91,104]

2. This method assumes the following:

a. A standard loading dose is administered.

b. Drug absorption, volume of distribution, protein binding, extrarenal elimination, and tissue sensitivity (dose-response relation) are unchanged.

c. Creatinine clearance is directly correlated to drug clearance.

d. Renal function remains relatively constant over time.

3. Normal dosage regimens are adjusted according to the dose fraction by two basic procedures.

a. The first method, termed "constant-interval, dose-reduction," reduces the dose (D) by a factor of the dose fraction. The dose interval (T) is the same as that used in the healthy animal.

$$D_{\text{renal failure}} = D_{\text{normal}} \times K_f$$
$$T_{\text{renal failure}} = T_{\text{normal}}$$

(equation 10)

(1). This method results in peak concentrations that are lower than and trough concentrations that are greater than those seen in healthy patients dosed by the usual method. Periods of subtherapeutic concentrations do not exist (Fig. 30–3).

(2). This method is preferred for drugs with a low therapeutic index for which the toxic and therapeutic plasma concentrations are close.

b. The second method, referred to as the "constant-dose, interval-extension method," extends the dosage interval by the inverse of

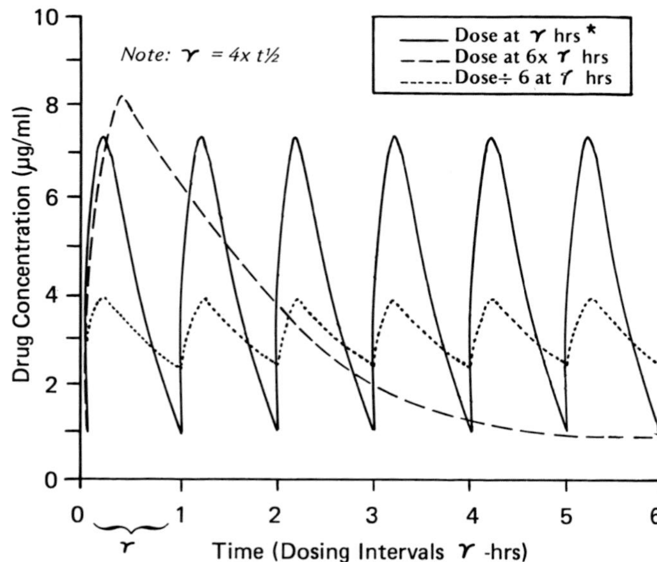

FIG. 30–3. Comparison of constant dose (broken line) and constant interval (dotted line) regimens in renal failure (Cl_{cr} = one-sixth usual) with a normal dosage regimen (solid line) in a healthy patient (asterisk).

the dose fraction, a value referred to as the "dose-interval multiplier."

$$T_{\text{renal failure}} = T_{\text{normal}} \times (1/K_f)$$
$$D_{\text{renal failure}} = D_{\text{normal}}$$

(equation 11)

(1). This regimen produces peak and trough concentrations similar to those seen in the healthy patient; however, prolonged periods of potentially subtherapeutic serum concentrations exist (Fig. 30–3).

(2). This method is more convenient because the drug can be administered less frequently. It is also easier for drugs that are available in fixed-dosage forms.

c. One study in human uremic patients demonstrated accumulation of ampicillin and cephalexin when dosages were adjusted on the basis of creatinine clearance alone; such findings suggest that these methods may be inappropriate for drugs for which clearance depends on active tubular secretion. A complex method using both creatinine clearance and phenolsulfonphthalein excretion was utilized to formulate a nomogram for dosing cephalexin.[48] Similar data are not available for the dog.

d. The clinician should determine if drug toxicity is correlated to peak, trough, or average plasma concentrations and then should select a regimen that balances efficacy against potential toxicity.

4. The most effective means of maintaining a constant plasma concentration of a drug is by continuous infusion at a constant rate.

5. In chronic renal failure, the nephron has undergone compensatory hypertrophy, and each individual surviving nephron is exposed to a greater tubular load of drug per unit of whole kidney GFR than is a nephron in a healthy animal. Even if a drug dosage is appropriately reduced according to decreased GFR, the nephrotoxic potential of a drug could be greater in the patient with renal failure.[77]

6. The ultimate goal of dosage adjustment as stated at the beginning of this section can be further defined as maintaining a constant product of ($t\frac{1}{2} \times D/T$) in healthy dogs and those with renal failure. When this product is held constant, the average steady-state plasma concentration of drug remains unchanged.

a. A constant steady-state plasma concentration is achieved by the use of the dose fraction to compensate for the decreased $t\frac{1}{2}$ in the following manner:

$$(t\tfrac{1}{2} \times D/T)_{\text{normal}} = K_f \times (t\tfrac{1}{2} \times D/T)_{\text{renal failure.}}$$

(equation 12)

b. This method represents a compromise between the constant-dose, interval-extension method and the constant-interval, dose-reduction method of dosage adjustment.

7. With repeated drug administration, accumulation occurs until steady-state plasma concentrations are achieved in approximately 4 to 5 $t\frac{1}{2}$. The prolonged $t\frac{1}{2}$ in dogs with renal failure would cause excessive delay in attaining steady-state concentration. Therefore, an appropriate loading dose should always be administered so that the therapeutic concentration of a drug is immediately attained.[83,87,100]

a. With the constant-interval, dose-reduction method, loading is accomplished by giving the usual dose initially, followed by the calculated reduced dose.

b. If the constant-dose method is used, the initial two doses should be given according to the usual interval and the following doses given at the prolonged interval.

8. The previous equations hold for drugs that are only eliminated by the kidney, because the dose fraction adjusts dosages as if K_{nr} equaled 0. For drugs undergoing biotransformation, a measure of the nonrenal percent of clearance is necessary.

a. This portion can be estimated by knowledge of the fraction of the absorbed dose of drug that is excreted unchanged in the urine (f).

b. The constant-interval method then becomes

$$D_{\text{renal failure}} = D_{\text{normal}} \times (f \times (K_f - 1) + 1);$$
$$T_{\text{renal failure}} = T_{\text{normal.}}$$

(equation 13)

c. For the constant-dose, increased-interval method,

$$T_{\text{renal failure}} = T_{\text{normal}} \times \frac{1}{(f \times (K_f - 1) + 1)};$$
$$D_{\text{renal failure}} = D_{\text{normal.}}$$

(equation 14)

d. The fraction excreted unchanged in urine is not currently available for animals for most drugs. If it is relatively small, then K_r is less than K_{nr} and $t\frac{1}{2}$ will remain relatively stable, thus avoiding the need to adjust dosages.

9. When creatinine clearance is not available, the inverse of serum creatinine (mg/dL) has been used to predict the fraction of renal failure that has been lost. This relationship between $t\frac{1}{2}$ and serum creatinine may not hold for serum creatinine levels greater than 4 mg/dL.[80,102]

10. The most accurate method of adjusting dosage regimens in renal failure is to calculate a dose, administer it, and monitor the resultant peak and trough serum concentrations by direct assay.

Individualized pharmacokinetic profiling could then be employed.[35] The main advantage is that dosage can be constantly adjusted so that changes in parameters assumed constant in the previous formulas will be detected.

11. The following points by Anderson and coworkers should serve as guidelines for drug treatment during impaired renal function.[2]
    a. Do not use drugs unless definite indications are present.
    b. If the dosage regimen of a drug in renal failure has been determined in a well-controlled study, this regimen should be followed in preference to the previously described general formulas.
    c. When a drug has not been studied but some information on its characteristics, such as the percentage of its excretion in an unchanged form by the kidney, is available, the previous formulas can be used to make an estimate of the proper dosage in renal failure.
    d. If an assay procedure for the drug is available, the periodic measurement of blood concentrations of the drug is advisable for any schedule.
    e. Careful clinical monitoring for toxicity and pharmacologic effect is mandatory in all cases.
12. When possible, the clinician should select a drug that is biotransformed by the liver or excreted in the bile rather than eliminated unchanged by the kidneys. For example, digitoxin could be selected instead of digoxin, chloramphenicol instead of gentamicin, or a barbiturate or inhalant anesthetic instead of ketamine.

IV. DIALYSIS

A. Peritoneal dialysis and hemodialysis increase the clearance of some drugs.[40,41,45,47,59,98,101] Total body clearance can be modified to include all possible clearance mechanisms, such that

$$Cl_B(mL/min) = Cl_r + Cl_{nr} + Cl_d \quad \text{(equation 15)}$$

B. If t½ before and during dialysis is known, the overall elimination constant can be calculated from similar blood concentration-time plots, and equation 4 may be used to calculate total body clearance in dialysis from the elimination constant and Vd. Total body clearance could then be used to calculate the amount of drug removed during dialysis by the following:

$$\text{Drug recovery (mg)} = Cl_B(mL/min) \times C_{ss}(mg/ml) \times \text{duration dialysis (min)}, \quad \text{(equation 16)}$$

where C_{SS} = steady-state plasma concentration.

C. When this estimate of total body clearance during dialysis is obtained, dose fraction is determined by the following:

$$K_f = \frac{Cl_B}{\text{Normal creatinine clearance}} \quad \text{(equation 17)}$$

D. Total body clearance is the average daily clearance and reflects time on and off dialysis. Dose fraction, analogous to dose fraction in renal failure without dialysis, can then be used directly in equations 10 and 11.

E. The preferred method is to calculate the amount of drug lost during a dialysis period according to equation 16 and to give this dose post dialysis. The normal dose fraction is then used for interdialysis dosing.

1. If Vd is unknown, but t½ before and after dialysis is available, the fraction of drug removed during dialysis (F) can be calculated.

$$F' = \frac{t½\,(\text{before}) - t½\,(\text{dialysis})}{t½\,(\text{before})}$$

$$F = F' \times [1 - e^{[-0.693/t½\,(\text{dialysis}) \times \text{dialysis (min)}]}] \quad \text{(equation 18)}$$

2. Dialyzer clearance can also be calculated solely for the dialysis process independent of body clearance mechanisms.
   a. With peritoneal dialysis,

$$Cl_d\,(ml/min) = \frac{C_D \times V}{C_P \times \text{dialysis duration (min)}} \quad \text{(equation 19)}$$

   where C_D is the concentration of drug in the dialysate fluid after exchange, V is the total dialysate drainage volume, and C_P is the plasma concentration of drug at the midpoint of dialysis.

   b. When long dwell periods of dialysate are used during peritoneal dialysis, appreciable amounts of drug may move from the dialysate fluid to the blood, thereby reducing total body clearance.[51]
   c. Hemodialysis and hemofiltration clearance can be calculated according to the relationship

$$Cl_d\,(ml/min) = \frac{Q \times (C_{in} - C_{out})}{C_{in}} \quad \text{(equation 20)}$$

   where Q is the flow of blood through the dialyzer, C_{in} is the concentration of drug in the plasma entering the dialyzer, and C_{out} is the concentration of drug in the plasma exiting the dialyzer.

3. Some discrepancies in dialyzer clearance values obtained occur when the plasma concentration of a drug is not representative of total blood concentration. This discrepancy results because the concentration of drug is measured for plasma, whereas the flow is measured for blood. Adjustments based on hematocrit can be made, or blood concentrations can be separated into erythrocyte and plasma water concentrations.
4. When a significant amount of drug is removed by dialysis, a normal loading dose should be administered after dialysis.

V. SPECIFIC RECOMMENDATIONS FOR ANTIMICROBIAL AGENTS

A. Introduction.

1. Many antimicrobial agents are primarily excreted by the kidneys. In addition, many are nephrotoxic.
2. The selected dosage regimen should minimize toxicity and maximize efficacy.
3. Controversy exists over the efficacy of constant-dose versus constant-interval regimens.
   a. For bactericidal antibiotics, peak concentrations are important, and periods of subinhibitory levels may be beneficial by allowing for postantibiotic effects. Subtherapeutic intervals may also be responsible for breakthrough bacteremia. Area under the plasma concentration-time curve may be the most important factor for all antimicrobial drugs.[11,12,83]
   b. Bacteriostatic drugs should be given according to a constant-interval regimen so that subinhibitory levels are not encountered.
   c. High peak concentrations obtained in fixed-dose regimens facilitate drug entry into the tissue, yet high-trough concentrations obtained in fixed-interval regimens tend to maintain effective tissue levels.[83]
   d. If the drug is effective over a large concentrations range, the end result of the two methods may not differ.

B. Aminoglycosides.

1. The aminoglycosides are eliminated primarily by glomerular filtration; 90% of the intravenous dose can be recovered in the urine after 24 hours.[36,83]
2. The remainder accumulates within the renal cortex, resulting in the formation of a deep tissue compartment.[88,89,105]
   a. This process has been documented to occur to varying degrees with most aminoglycosides.
   b. The $t\frac{1}{2}$ of accumulation ranges from 30 to 150 hours in all species studied.
   c. High cortical drug concentrations have been linked to nephrotoxicity in humans and animals.
   d. Renal cortical gentamicin and amikacin concentrations were decreased despite elevated serum concentrations in people with prerenal azotemia.
3. Increased Vd of aminoglycosides has been documented in some cases of renal insufficiency in humans and dogs.[36]
4. Aminoglycosides are generally poorly absorbed from the gastrointestinal tract, yet ototoxicity and increased serum concentrations have been seen after oral administration of neomycin to patients with renal insufficiency.
5. Nebulization of gentamicin to dogs with normal renal function did not produce detectable serum concentrations.[84] Irrigation of potentially absorptive surfaces with any of the aminoglycosides should be done with caution in the face of renal insufficiency.
6. Aminoglycosides produce three primary toxic syndromes: nephrotoxicity, ototoxicity, and neuromuscular blockade.
   a. Major risk factors for nephrotoxicity are prior renal insufficiency, concurrent exposure to other nephrotoxins (i.e., furosemide), hypovolemia, metabolic acidosis, and dosage regimens producing peak gentamicin concentrations greater than 12 µg/ml or trough concentrations greater than 2µg/ml.[24,37,83,90] An increment increase of 1 µg/mL in amikacin peak and trough concentrations over 48 hours may predict the appearance of renal toxicity.
   b. Nephrotoxicity is reversible if the tubular basement membrane is not severely damaged.
   c. Of the commonly employed drugs, neomycin is the most toxic, followed by amikacin, kanamycin, gentamicin, and tobramycin. Streptomycin is not nephrotoxic at therapeutic dosages.
   d. Ototoxicity in humans is irreversible and predisposed by excessive daily dosages, prior renal insufficiency, and peak concentrations greater than 10 µg/mL or trough concentrations greater than 3 µg/mL.
7. The pharmacokinetic behavior of amikacin, gentamicin, kanamycin, sisomicin, and tobramycin is similar in normal and impaired renal function. When renal function is stable, the total body clearance can be predicted reasonably well from creatinine clearance.[35,83]
8. Dosage regimens can be constructed using equations 9 and 11. The constant-dose, increased-interval method is less likely to produce nephrotoxicosis than is the fixed-interval method of dosage adjustment or continuous infusion.[81]
9. A nomogram employing the constant-dose, increased-interval method for aminoglycoside dosage in dogs with impaired renal function can be constructed as shown in Figure 30–4.[22,66]
   a. To avoid excessively high peak concentrations, the nomogram incorporates a correction fac-

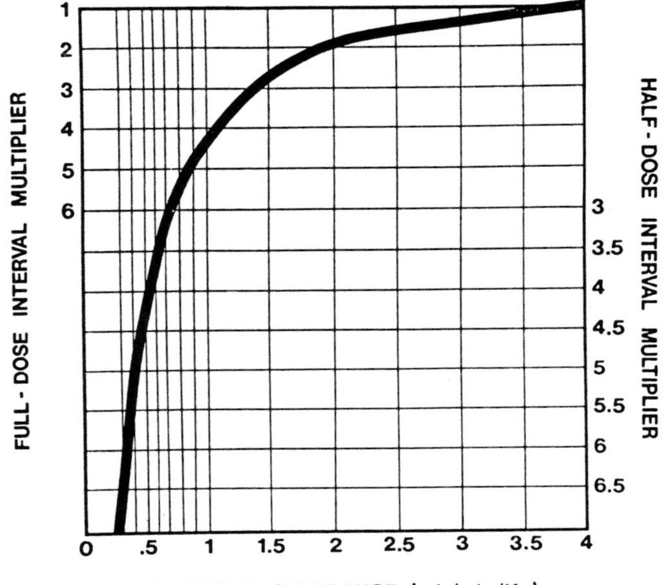

FIG. 30–4. Nomogram for aminoglycoside dosage in dogs with renal insufficiency. The constant-dose, increased-interval method of dosage adjustment is employed. The normal-dose interval is multiplied by the dose interval multiplier according to creatinine clearance. The left scale assumes a normal dose is administered; the right scale assumes half the normal dose. Examples are: $Cl_{cr} = 2$, administer normal dose every 2 intervals; $Cl_{cr} = 0.5$, administer ½ normal dose every 4 intervals.

tor to decrease the dosage by half when the predicted interval is greater than six times normal.

b. This nomogram was verified using data obtained from dogs with spontaneous renal failure and from surgically nephrectomized dogs.
c. This nomogram should be applicable for amikacin, gentamicin, kanamycin, sisomicin, and tobramycin administrations.[83]

10. Single daily dose regimens have been recommended for use in humans and dogs. These regimens result in prolonged subtherapeutic concentrations that can lead to breakthrough bacteremia.
11. Whenever aminoglycosides are administered, baseline renal function tests should be conducted.
12. Dialysis is generally efficient in removing aminoglycosides and can be a viable therapeutic intervention. Gentamicin clearance in hemodialysis correlates well with creatinine clearance.
    a. Hemodialysis for 8 to 12 hours decreases the total body burden of drug by as much as 50%, whereas peritoneal dialysis is considerably less efficient.[23,43,95]
    b. If specific clearance data are available, equations 16 and 20 should be employed.

C. Cephalosporins.

1. Cephalosporins are eliminated primarily by the kidney, and dosage modifications are required when creatinine clearance falls to less than 15 to 20% of normal.
2. Hepatic metabolism of some cephalosporins is significant, thus making dosage adjustments unnecessary. The oral cephalosporin cefaclor is primarily metabolized in the dog, and dosage adjustments are not necessary.[14,97]
3. Such cephalosporins as cefazolin demonstrate decreased protein binding and increased Vd in uremia in humans; however, cefazolin is highly protein bound in humans (80%) compared to dogs (20 to 30%). The decrease in protein binding is probably not an important consideration for the dog.
4. Cephalothin hydrolysis is depressed in renal failure, whereas the metabolites of cephalothin and cephapirin (desacetyl compounds) accumulate in renal insufficiency. Desacetylcephalothin is significantly less active biologically than is the parent compound.
5. Most cephalosporins are relatively nontoxic, the exception being cephaloridine.[8]
    a. Cephaloridine is less toxic in dogs than in other animals.
    b. Nephrotoxicity is potentiated by excessive dosage, prior renal insufficiency, furosemide, and possibly aminoglycosides.
    c. Some studies have indicated that nephrotoxicity is enhanced by a single dose of cephaloridine, rather than divided daily doses.
6. Dosage adjustments can be made relatively simply as shown in Table 30–3. For cephalosporins excreted by the kidney, equations 10 and 11 can be employed.
7. For most cephalosporins, 6 to 8 hours of hemodialysis removes 40% of the body stores, whereas 24 to 36 hours of peritoneal dialysis (cefamandole excluded) removes 20% of a dose.[1]

D. Penicillins.

1. Excretion of penicillins is primarily by active tubular secretion when renal function is normal. Hepatic biotransformation and fecal excretion become important during renal failure.[83]
2. The isoxazolyl penicillins, cloxacillin, dicloxacillin, oxacillin, and nafcillin, are eliminated primarily by hepatic metabolism and do not require dosage adjustments in renal insufficiency.
3. Penicillin G, penicillin V, methicillin, amoxicillin, and carbenicillin have increased t½ during renal insufficiency, and dosage intervals should be extended as indicated in Table 30–3.[50]
4. A full dose of ampicillin, amoxicillin, or carbenicillin should be given after hemodialysis, but supplementation is not required with peritoneal dialysis.[44]

TABLE 30–3
SPECIFIC RECOMMENDATIONS FOR DOSAGE ADJUSTMENTS IN PATIENTS WITH RENAL FAILURE

Drug	Elimination Route	Dosage Adjustment in Renal Failure	Amount of Drug Removed During Dialysis
Antimicrobial Agents			
Aminoglycosides			
Amikacin*	Renal†	Nomogram‡ or equations 9 and 11	
Gentamicin	Renal	Nomogram or equations 9 and 11	
Kanamycin	Renal	Nomogram or equations 9 and 11	H 50%
Neomycin	—	Contraindicated	
Sisomicin	Renal	Nomogram or equations 9 and 11	P 20%
Streptomycin	Renal	Mild: DIM = 2 Severe: DIM = 3-4	
Tobramycin	Renal	Nomogram or equations 9 and 11	
Cephalosporins			
Cephalexin	Renal	IE or	
Cefazolin	Renal	Cl_{cr} > 1; DIM = 1	
		Cl_{cr} 0.5-1.0; DIM = 2	H: 40%
		Cl_{cr} 0.3-0.5; DIM = 3	P: 20%
		Cl_{cr} < 0.3; DIM = 4	
Cephalothin	Renal, hepatic§	Cl_{cr} < 0.5; DIM = 2	
Cefamandole	Renal, hepatic	Cl_{cr} < 0.5; 0.5 dose	H: mild P: negligible
Cefaclor	Hepatic, renal	No adjustment necessary	H: 30% P: mild
Cefoxitin	Renal	DIM	H: significant P: mild
Penicillins			
Dicloxacillin	Hepatic	No change	H, P: negligible
Oxacillin	Hepatic	No change	H, P: negligible
Methicillin	Renal, hepatic	Cl_{cr} < 0.5; 0.5 dose or DIM = 2	H, P: negligible
Penicillin G	Renal, hepatic	Cl_{cr} < 0.5; 0.5 dose or DIM = 2	H: 10-20% P: none
Penicillin V	Renal, hepatic	Cl_{cr} < 0.5; 0.5 dose or DIM = 2	H: 10-20% P: none
Ampicillin	Renal, hepatic	Cl_{cr} < 0.5; 0.5 dose or DIM = 2	H: 80% P: mild
Amoxicillin	Renal, hepatic	Cl_{cr} < 0.5; 0.5 dose or DIM = 2	H: 80% P: mild
Carbenicillin	Renal, hepatic	Cl_{cr} < 0.5; 0.5 dose or DIM = 2	H: 80% P: mild
Ticarcillin	Renal, hepatic	Cl_{cr} < 0.5; 0.5 dose or DIM = 2	H: significant P: significant
Imipenem/cilastatin	Renal, hepatic	DIM or DR	H: significant P: 24-32%
Clavulinic acid	Renal	DIM	H, P: significant
Sulfonamides			
Sulfisoxazole	Renal, hepatic	Cl_{cr} < 1; DIM = 2-3	H: 80-90% P: significant
Trimethoprim-sulfamethoxazole	Renal, hepatic	Do not use if Cl_{cr} < 1	H: significant
Tetracyclines			
Doxycycline	Hepatic, renal	No change	H, P: negligible
All others	Contraindicated		
Quinolones			
Ciprofloxacin	Renal, hepatic	Other, DR	H: some P: minimal
Norfloxacin	Renal, hepatic	Other, DR	H: none P: unknown
Enrofloxacin	Renal, hepatic	Other, DR	H, P: unknown

Table 30-3 continued.

H = hemodialysis (6-10 hours); P = peritoneal dialysis (24-36 hours); DIM = dosage interval multiplier; IE = interval extension (equation 11); Cl_{cr} creatinine clearance (ml/min/kg); DR = dose reduction (equation 10).

*Human data.

†Renal = filtration, secretion.

‡Nomogram = Figure 30–4.

§Hepatic = biliary secretion and biotransformation.

TABLE 30–3 CONT'D
SPECIFIC RECOMMENDATIONS FOR DOSAGE ADJUSTMENTS IN PATIENTS WITH RENAL FAILURE

Drug	Elimination Route	Dosage Adjustment in Renal Failure	Amount of Drug Removed During Dialysis
Miscellaneous			
Chloramphenicol	Hepatic	No change; avoid in severe renal failure	H: 20% P: negligible
Clindamycin	Hepatic	No change	H, P: negligible
Erythromycin	Hepatic, renal	No change	H, P: negligible
Lincomycin	Hepatic, renal	Cl_{cr} < 0.5; DIM = 3	H, P: negligible
Methenamine mandelate	Contraindicated		
Metronidazole	Hepatic, renal	No change	H: significant
Nitrofurantoin	Contraindicated		
Vancomycin	Renal	IE	H, P: negligible
Antifungal Agents			
Amphotericin	Hepatic	0.5 dose in renal failure	H, P: negligible
5-Fluorocytosine	Renal	IE	H: 80-90%
Ketoconazole	Hepatic	No change	P: negligible
Immunosuppressive and Antineoplastic Agents			
Bleomycin	Renal	Decrease dose	H: insignificant
Cyclophosphamide	Hepatic, renal	DIM = 2 in severe renal failure	H: 40% P: unknown
Methotrexate	Renal	0.5 dose in severe renal failure	H: significant P: minimal
Cisplatin	Renal, hepatic	Increase interval	H: significant
Azathioprine	Nonrenal	DIM = 2 in severe renal failure	H: significant
Cytosine arabinoside	Nonrenal	No change	
Doxorubicin	Hepatic, renal	No change	
5-Fluorouracil	Hepatic, renal	No change	H: significant
Vincristine	Hepatic	No change	
Cyclophosphamide	Hepatic	None	H, P: unknown
Cardioactive Agents			
Digoxin	Renal, hepatic	Decrease dose 50% for 50 mg/dL Increase in serum urea nitrogen	H, P: none
Digitoxin	Hepatic, renal	No change	H, P: Insignificant
Procainamide	Renal, hepatic	Cl_{cr} < 0.5; DIM = 2	
Dolbutamine	Hepatic	No change	H, P unknown
Lidocaine	Hepatic	No change	H, P: none
Propranolol	Hepatic, extrahepatic	No change	H, P: none
Atenolol	Renal	DR or IE	H: moderate
Quinidine	Hepatic	No change	H, P: moderate
Enalapril	Renal, hepatic	DR and IE	H, P: significant
Captopril	Renal, hepatic	DR and IE	H: significant
Verapamil	Hepatic	None	H: none
Diltiazem	Heaptic	None	H, P: unknown
Miscellaneous Agents			
Aspirin	Renal, hepatic	No change	H, P: significant
Cimetidine	Renal	DR or IE	H: significant
Diazepam	Hepatic, renal	No change	H, P: minimal
Furosemide	Renal, hepatic	No change	H: insignificant
Heparin	Hepatic	No change	H, P: minimal
Morphine	Hepatic	No change	
Omeprazole	Hepatic	No change	H: insignificant
Pentazocine	Hepatic	No change	
Phenobarbital	Hepatic, renal	Severe: DIM = 2	H, P: significant
Phenylbutazone	Hepatic, renal	No change	H, P: probably minimal
Phenytoin	Hepatic	No change	H: none
Primidone	Hepatic, renal	Severe: DIM = 2-3	H: significant removal
Theophylline	Renal, hepatic	No change	
Valproic acid	Hepatic	No change	
Warfarin	Hepatic	No change	

5. Dose-related toxicity associated with penicillins is rare.
   a. Oxacillin, methicillin, and ampicillin have been associated more often with interstitial nephritis in humans and dogs than have other penicillins.
   b. Caution must be exercised to avoid sodium and potassium overload when administering sodium carbenicillin, sodium penicillin, and potassium penicillin.

E. Sulfonamides.

1. Sulfonamides have been associated with interstitial nephritis and interrenal crystal deposition. The risk of crystal formation is lessened with the use of more soluble, shorter-acting drugs, such as sulfamethoxazole and sulfisoxazole.[20]
2. Sulfonamides are often used to treat urinary tract infections; however, decreased renal function can severely decrease urinary levels of drugs.[61] Trimethoprim-sulfamethoxazole achieves adequate urinary concentrations in renal failure.
3. Sulfonamides are cleared by active tubular secretion, and the $t\frac{1}{2}$ increases with renal insufficiency.[103]
4. Renal failure drastically affects the protein binding of the sulfonamides, with a resultant increase in Vd.
5. Biotransformation of some of these drugs is also affected in uremia.
6. The normal dose should be halved and the interval doubled in severe renal failure.
7. The short-acting sulfonamides are readily dialyzed, and treatment should be repeated after hemodialysis.
8. Because of the ready availability of alternative drugs that are less toxic, sulfonamides should only be used when absolutely necessary.

F. Tetracyclines.

1. The use of tetracyclines with renal insufficiency should be avoided because their catabolic effects may exacerbate azotemia and because they are potentially nephrotoxic. Only doxycycline can safely be used with renal failure because antianabolic effects have not been associated with its use.[5,49]
2. Tetracycline can cause a fatty metamorphosis of the liver that may lead to hepatic failure.
3. A toxic degradation product of outdated tetracyclines has caused Fanconi's syndrome.
4. Hemodialysis and peritoneal dialysis are ineffective in removing significant quantities of tetracyclines.

G. Quinolones.

1. Ciprofloxacin and norfloxacin are eliminated by proximal tubular secretion, with 30 to 70% of the administered dose being recovered in the urine. The renal clearance of these drugs is reduced during renal failure.[7,16]
2. Only a few side effects are associated with the quinolones, but these may be more common in renal failure. The most common side effects are related to the gastrointestinal and central nervous systems, although ciprofloxacin has been associated with interstitial nephritis.
3. The dosage should be reduced in severe renal failure.
4. Hemodialysis removes only moderate amounts of ciprofloxacin, whereas peritoneal dialysis removes a small amount. Norfloxacin is not appreciably removed by hemodialysis.[92,93]
5. Nalidixic acid is not efficacious in the presence of renal failure.

H. Miscellaneous antimicrobial agents.

1. The urinary tract antiseptics, nitrofurantoin and methenamine mandelate, are not efficacious in the presence of renal failure.[20]
   a. Nitrofurantoin is associated with polyneuropathy and pulmonary infiltrates, and methenamine mandelate can result in systemic acidosis.
   b. Their use in renal failure is not justified when other agents are available.
2. The polymyxin antibiotics, polymyxin B and colistimethate (colistin, polymyxin E), are associated with nephrotoxicosis, peripheral neuropathy, and respiratory arrest in humans.[27]
   a. Polymyxin B is contraindicated with renal failure.
   b. Colistimethate is less nephrotoxic than polymyxin B, but at therapeutically effective dosages, azotemia, cylindruria, and proteinuria can occur. Dosages should be adjusted using a constant-interval technique as in equation 10.
3. Vancomycin is associated with ototoxicity and possibly nephrotoxicity in humans. Results of studies in laboratory animals and dogs are contradictory. Renal insufficiency appears to increase the incidence of toxicosis.
   a. If therapy with vancomycin is essential, as in the case of resistant group D streptococcal infections, dosage interval should be increased as determined by equation 11 or a predetermined dosing chart.[19]
   b. Dialysis is inefficient in removing the drug.
4. Administration of erythromycin and clindamycin to patients with renal failure does not require dosage adjustment because these drugs are eliminated primarily by nonrenal mechanisms.[55]
   a. They are not removed by dialysis.
   b. Renal failure is a risk factor for ototoxicity of erythromycin in human uremic patients.
5. Lincomycin undergoes significant renal elimination; however, dosage adjustments are only necessary in severe renal insufficiency because of its low toxicity. Lincomycin is not removed by dialysis.
6. Information is not available on the toxicity of tylosin in renal failure or on its ability to be

removed by dialysis. It is eliminated by hepatic and renal mechanisms.

7. Chloramphenicol is primarily eliminated by hepatic biotransformation, and dosage adjustment would not seem to be necessary.
   a. Metabolites accumulate and intoxication can occur in the presence of severe renal insufficiency in humans.
   b. Chloramphenicol should be avoided in dogs until definitive studies are conducted.
   c. Chloramphenicol is not removed by peritoneal dialysis but is moderately eliminated by hemodialysis.

VI. SPECIFIC RECOMMENDATIONS FOR ANTIFUNGAL AGENTS

A. Flurocytosine.

1. Flurocytosine is primarily eliminated by glomerular filtration. Dosage should be adjusted in renal failure according to equation 10.
2. The drug is effectively removed with hemodialysis, and a full dose should be given post dialysis.[15]
3. Hepatic and myeloid toxic side effects have been reported.

B. Amphotericin.

1. Amphotericin possesses unusual pharmacokinetic properties, that make accurate recommendations of dosage in renal insufficiency difficult.
2. The major side effect of the drug is nephrotoxicosis.
   a. Toxicity may be minimized by insuring adequate hydration and possibly by concurrent mannitol administration.[85]
   b. The nephrotoxicity has been reported to be synergistic with gentamicin.
3. Amphotericin is a colloid and is not removed by dialysis.[15]
4. Amphotericin should not be used in dogs with renal failure.

C. Ketoconazole.

1. The maximum serum concentration of ketoconazole is reduced in human uremic patients when compared to controls.[52]
2. Protein binding is reduced in the uremic state.
3. Ketoconazole is not appreciably removed by peritoneal dialysis.[52]

VII. SPECIFIC RECOMMENDATIONS FOR IMMUNOSUPPRESSIVE AND ANTINEOPLASTIC AGENTS

A. Corticosteroids.

1. Long-term, high-dose corticosteroid therapy should be avoided in renal failure because of the catabolic action of the drug.
2. An exception is the use of corticosteroids and other immunosuppressive drugs to treat specific glomerulonephropathies.

B. Bleomycin.

1. Bleomycin is excreted primarily by glomerular filtration and accumulates in renal insufficiency.
2. Dosage should be substantially reduced in severe renal failure.

C. Cyclophosphamide.

1. Cyclophosphamide is metabolized in the liver. Active alkylating metabolites are excreted by the kidney, accumulate in renal failure, and can produce toxicosis.
2. Dosages should be decreased in severe renal failure by increasing dosage interval to prevent metabolite accumulation and intoxication.
3. Cyclophosphamide is readily removed by hemodialysis.[101]

D. Methotrexate.

1. Methotrexate is actively excreted by the renal tubules and accumulates in renal insufficiency.[68]
2. Its pharmacokinetic disposition is described by a three-compartment model with a terminal tissue accumulation phase. As much as 90% of a dose is excreted within 48 hours.
3. A 7-hydroxylated nephrotoxic metabolite can be detected in plasma following high-dose therapy.
4. Dosage should be halved in severe renal failure.

E. Cisplatin.

1. Cisplatin is a potent tubular nephrotoxin in dogs and is excreted by both hepatic and renal mechanisms.
2. A two-compartment pharmacokinetic model characterizes its disposition.
3. Renal failure can affect the distribution of the drug because protein binding is greater than 90%.
4. Renal function must be carefully monitored throughout therapy.
5. Nephrotoxicity is revealed by azotemia, hypochlorremia, and proteinuria and appears more likely in normal human patients when the dose is administered at relatively close intervals. Long-term accumulation studies at subtoxic dosage levels have not been performed for verification.
6. In normal renal function, intravenous hydration therapy with mannitol or concurrent furosemide administration has been recommended to minimize toxicity.
7. The concurrent administration of other nephrotoxins with cisplatin should be done with extreme caution. Carboplatin should be used instead of cisplatin in the presence of pre-existing renal insufficiency.

F. Doxorubicin produces a dose-dependent toxic nephropathy that can exacerbate pre-existing renal disease. However, dosage adjustment does not appear to be necessary.

G. Mitomycin and streptozocin are also potent nephrotoxins.

1. Recommendations for usage in renal insufficiency are not available.
2. If possible, these agents should be avoided in severe renal failure.

VIII. SPECIFIC RECOMMENDATIONS FOR CARDIOACTIVE AGENTS

A. Digitalis glycosides.

1. The disposition of digoxin in the dog is described by a 3-compartment model with a terminal-phase t½ of 28 to 39 hours.[6]
2. The elimination t½ of digoxin increases and the volume of distribution decreases in dogs with renal failure, thereby resulting in plasma digoxin concentrations that are higher than expected.
   a. A longer period of time is required to attain steady-state concentrations owing to the increased t½.
   b. Creatinine clearance does not consistently predict digoxin t½ in the dog.
   c. The use of urea clearance of serum urea nitrogen appears useful in predicting dosage modification in dogs.[54]
3. Hemodialysis, hemofiltration, and peritoneal dialysis are not effective in removing digoxin because the large fraction of drug is not present in the central compartment.[41]
4. The incidence of adverse reactions secondary to digoxin administration is increased in human patients with renal disease.
5. Digitoxin is primarily excreted by hepatic biotransformation to cardioinactive or only slightly active metabolites, with a fraction metabolized to digoxin.
6. The t½ of digitoxin does not change in renal failure and steady state is attained more rapidly.
7. Digitoxin is the cardiac glycoside of choice for renal disease.
8. Digitoxin is not removed well by dialysis.

B. Angiotensin-converting enzyme inhibitors.

1. The clearance of captopril is reduced in parallel to reductions in GFR in the early stages of renal failure. With severe renal impairment, the nonrenal clearance is also reduced.[33,34]
2. The peak serum concentrations of captopril and its conjugates are increased in uremic patients.
3. A sustained fall in both diastolic and systolic blood pressures occurs following captopril administration to uremic patients, with the maximal response at 6 hours (compared to 30 minutes in normal patients).
4. High dosages of captopril can cause renal failure in dogs.
5. In severe renal failure, both the dosage and frequency of administration should be reduced.
6. Hemodialysis effectively removes lisinopril, enalapril, and captopril.[56]

C. Procainamide.

1. Procainamide is actively secreted and passively reabsorbed by the kidney.[38]
2. Its total body clearance appears independent of urinary pH and flow.
3. Dosage interval should be doubled in severe renal failure.

IX. MISCELLANEOUS AGENTS

A. Aspirin.

1. Aspirin is hydrolyzed to salicylic acid, which undergoes passive tubular reabsorption.
2. Alkaline urine increases excretion, whereas acidic urine decreases excretion.
3. Short courses of standard dosages can be administered without adverse consequences.

B. Phenylbutazone.

1. Phenylbutazone is highly protein bound, the extent of which may be affected during renal failure.
2. The high degree of protein binding of this drug precludes it from being dialyzed to any significant extent.

C. The dosage interval of primidone should be doubled or tripled because the metabolite phenobarbital accumulates.

D. Phenytoin and valproic acid show decreased protein binding in severe renal failure.[17,57]

E. Furosemide.

1. The pharmacokinetics of furosemide are altered in anephric patients with increased Vd and K_{nr} and decreased protein binding. Accumulation is not expected.[99]
2. Furosemide is eliminated in the kidney by active tubular secretion and has an intratubular site of action.
3. Dosage adjustment is not needed to enhance efficacy or avoid accumulation.
4. Furosemide can potentiate the toxicity of other therapeutic agents, such as aminoglycosides. Furosemide is ototoxic.
5. Excessive use can result in extracellular fluid depletion and exacerbation of the renal failure.
6. Creatinine and urea nitrogen excretion is not influenced by furosemide. Patients should not be given furosemide to enhance the elimination of creatinine and urea.

REFERENCES

1. Ahern MJ, Cohen SL. Pharmacokinetics of cefamandole in patients undergoing hemodialysis and peritoneal dialysis. *Antimicrob Agents Chemother.* 1976;10:457.
2. Anderson RJ, Gambertoglio JG, Schrier RW. Fate of drugs in renal failure. In: Brenner BM, Rector FC, eds. *The Kidney.* Philadelphia, Pennsylvania: WB Saunders Co; 1976:1911.
3. Andreasen F. Protein binding of drugs in plasma from patients with acute renal failure. *Acta Pharmacol Toxicol.* 1973;32:417.
4. Andreasen F. The effect of dialysis on the protein binding of drugs in the plasma of patients with acute renal failure. *Acta Pharmacol Toxicol.* 1974;34:284.
5. Aronson AL. Pharmacotherapeutics of the newer tetracyclines. *J Am Vet Med Assoc.* 1980;176:1061.
6. Aronson JK. Clinical pharmacokinetics of digoxin 1980. *Clin Pharmacokinet.* 1980;5:137.
7. Arrigo G, et al. Pharmacokinetics of norfloxacin in chronic renal failure. *Int J Clin Pharmacol Ther Toxicol.* 1985;23(9):491-496.

8. Atkinson RM, Currie JP, Davis B. Subacute toxicity of cephaloridine to various animal species. *J Toxicol Appl Pharmacol.* 1966;8:407.
9. Baggot JD. Some aspects of clinical pharmacokinetics in veterinary medicine I and II. *J Vet Pharmacol Ther.* 1978; 1:5, 111.
10. Benet LZ, Sheiner LB. Design and optimization of dosage regimens; pharmacokinetic data. In: Gilman AG, et al., eds. *Goodman and Gilman's The Pharmacological Basis of Therapeutics.* 6th ed. New York, New York: Macmillan; 1980:1675.
11. Bennett WM, et al. Drug prescribing in renal failure: Dosing guidelines for adults. *Am J Kidney Dis.* 1983;3:155-193.
12. Bennett WM, et al. Guidelines for drug therapy in renal failure. *Ann Intern Med.* 1977;86:754.
13. Bergan T, Brodwall EK, Dyri A. Renal excretion of gentamicin in chronic pyelonephritis. *Acta Med Scand.* 1971;189:1.
14. Berman SJ, et al. Pharmacokinetics of cefaclor in patients with end stage renal disease and during hemodialysis. *Antimicrob Agents Chemother.* 1978;14:281.
15. Block ER, et al. Fluorocytosine and amphotericin B. Hemodialysis effects of the plasma concentration and clearance. *Ann Intern Med.* 1974;80:613.
16. Boelaert J, et al. The pharmacokinetics of ciprofloxacin in patients with impaired renal function. *J Antimicrob Chemother.* 1985;16:87-93.
17. Brewster D, Muir NC. Valproate plasma protein binding in the uremic condition. *Clin Pharmacol Ther.* 1980;27:76.
18. Bricker NS, Morrin PF, Kine SW Jr. The pathologic physiology of chronic Bright's disease. An exposition of the "intact nephron hypothesis." *Am J Med.* 1960;28:77.
19. Brown DL, Mauro LS. Vancomycin dosing chart for use in patients with renal impairment. *Am J Kidney Dis.* 1988;11: 15-19.
20. Brumfit W, Hamilton-Miller JMT. Sulfonamides, trimethoprim sulfamethoxazole, nalidixic acid, oxalinic acid, methenamine and nitrofurans. In: Kagan BM, ed. *Antimicrobial Therapy.* Philadelphia, Pennsylvania: WB Saunders Co; 1980:137.
21. Cafruny EJ. Renal tubular handling of drugs. *Am J Med.* 1977;62:490.
22. Chan RA, Benner EF, Hoeprich PD. Gentamicin therapy in renal failure: A nomogram for dosage. *Ann Intern Med.* 1972; 76:773.
23. Christopher TG, et al. Gentamicin pharmacokinetics during hemodialysis. *Kidney Int.* 1974;6:38.
24. Colburn WA, et al. A model for the prospective identification of the prenephrotoxic state during gentamicin therapy. *J Pharmacokinet Biopharm.* 1978;6:179.
25. Davis LE. Drug therapy in renal disorders. In: Kirk RW, ed. *Current Veterinary Therapy.* vol 7. Philadelphia, Pennsylvania: WB Saunders Co; 1980:1114.
26. Davis LE, et al. Elimination kinetics of pentobarbital in nephrectomized dogs. *Am J Vet Res.* 1973;34:231.
27. Davis SD. Polymyxins, colistin, vancomycin and bacitracin. In: Kagan BM, ed. *Antimicrobial Therapy.* Philadelphia, Pennsylvania: WB Saunders Co; 1980:77.
28. Dayton PG, Israili ZH, Perel JM. Influence of binding on drug metabolism and distribution. *Ann NY Acad Sci.* 1973; 226:172.
29. Depner TA, Gulyassy TA. Plasma protein binding in uremia: Extraction and characterization of an inhibitor. *Kidney Int.* 1980;18:86.
30. Dettli L. Individualization of drug dosage in patients with renal disease. *Med Clin North Am.* 1974;58:977.
31. Drayer DE. Active drug metabolites and renal failure. *Am J Med.* 1977;62:486.
32. Dromgoole SH. The binding capacity of albumin and renal disease. *J Pharmacol Exp Ther.* 1974;191:318.
33. Drummer OH, et al. The pharmacokinetics of captopril and captopril disulfide conjugates in uraemic patients on maintenance dialysis: Comparison with patients with normal renal function. *Eur J Clin Pharmacol.* 1987;32:267-271.
34. Duchin KL, et al. Elimination kinetics of captopril in patients with renal failure. *Kidney Int.* 1984;25:942-947.
35. Frazier DL, Riviere JE. Gentamicin dosing strategies for dogs with subclinical renal dysfunction. *Antimicrob Agent Chemother.* 1987;31:1929-1934.
36. Frazier DL, Aucoin DP, Riviere JE. Gentamicin pharmacokinetics and nephrotoxicity in naturally acquired and experimentally induced disease in dogs. *J Am Vet Med Assoc.* 1988;192: 57-63.
37. Frazier DL, et al. Increased gentamicin nephrotoxicity in normal and diseased dogs administered identical serum drug concentration profiles: Increased sensitivity in subclinical renal dysfunction. *J Pharmacol Exp Ther.* 1986;239:946-951.
38. Galeazzi RL, et al. The renal elimination of procainamide. *Clin Pharmacol Ther.* 1976;19:55.
39. Gibson TP. Renal disease and drug metabolism: An overview. *Am J Kidney Dis.* 1986;8:7-17.
40. Gibson TP, Atkinson AJ Jr. Effect of changes in intercompartment rate constants on drug removal during hemoperfusion. *J Pharm Sci.* 1978;67:1178.
41. Gibson TP, et al. Hemoperfusion removal of digoxin from dogs. *J Lab Clin Med.* 1978;91:673.
42. Gierke KD, et al. Digoxin disposition kinetics in dogs before and during azotemia. *J Pharmacol Exp Ther.* 1978;205:459.
43. Goetz DR, et al. Prediction of serum gentamicin concentrations in patients undergoing hemodialysis. *Am J Hosp Pharm.* 1980; 37:1077.
44. Greenberg PA, Sanford JP. Removal and absorption of antibiotics in patients with renal failure undergoing peritoneal dialysis. *Ann Intern Med.* 1967;66:465.
45. Gwilt RP, Perrier D. Plasma protein binding and distribution characteristics of drugs as indices of hemodialyzability. *Clin Pharmacol Ther.* 1978;24:154.
46. Gyselynck A, Forrey A, Cutler R. Pharmacokinetics of gentamicin: Distribution and plasma and renal clearance. *J Infect Dis.* 1971;124:S70.
47. Handelman WA, Schrier RW. Influence of renal impairment and dialysis. In: Kagan BM, ed. *Antimicrobial Therapy.* Philadelphia, Pennsylvania: WB Saunders Co; 1980:481.
48. Hori R, et al. A new dosing regimen in renal insufficiency: Application to cephalexin. *Clin Pharmacol Ther.* 1985;38:290-295.
49. Houin G, et al. The effects of chronic renal insufficiency on the pharmacokinetics of doxycycline in man. *Br J Clin Pharmacol.* 1983;16:245-252.
50. Humbert G, et al. Pharmacokinetics of amoxicillin. Dosage nomogram for patients with impaired renal function. *Antimicrob Agents Chemother.* 1979;15:28.
51. Janick DM, et al. Pharmacokinetic modeling of bidirectional transfer during peritoneal dialysis. *Clin Pharmacol Ther.* 1986; 40:209-218.
52. Johnson RJ, et al. Ketoconazole kinetics in chronic peritoneal dialysis. *Clin Pharmacol Ther.* 1985;37:325-329.
53. Jusko WJ. Pharmacokinetics in disease states changing protein binding. In: Benet LZ, ed. *Effects of Disease States on Drug Pharmacokinetics.* Washington, DC: Academy of Pharmaceutical Sciences; 1976:99.
54. Jusko WJ, Szefler SJ, Goldfarb AL. Pharmacokinetic design of digoxin dosage regimens in relation to renal function. *J Clin Pharmacol.* 1974;16:525.

55. Kanfer A, et al. Changes in erythromycin pharmacokinetics induced by renal failure. *Clin Nephrol.* 1987;27(3): 147-150.
56. Kelly JG, et al. Pharmacokinetics of lisinopril, enalapril and enalaprilat in renal failure: Effects of haemodialysis. *Br J Clin Pharmacol.* 1988;26:781-786.
57. Kinniburgh DW, Boyd ND. Phenytoin binding to partially purified albumin in renal disease. *Clin Pharmacol Ther.* 1981; 29:203.
58. Kunin CM, et al. Influence of binding on the pharmacologic activity of antibiotics. *Ann NY Acad Sci.* 1973;226:214.
59. Lee CS, Marbury TC, Benet LZ. Clearance calculations in hemodialysis: Application to blood, plasma, and dialysate measurements for ethambutol. *J Pharmacokinet Biopharm.* 1980;8:69.
60. Ling GV. Treatment of urinary tract infections. *Vet Clin North Am.* 1979;9:795.
61. Ling GV, Ruby AL. Trimethoprim in combination with a sulfanamide for oral treatment of canine urinary infections. *J Am Vet Med Assoc.* 1979;174:1003.
62. Loughnan PM, et al. The two-compartment open-system kinetic model: A review of its clinical implications and applications. *J Pediatr.* 1976;88:869.
63. Madias NE, Harrington JT. Platinum nephrotoxicity. *Am J Med.* 1978;65:307.
64. Maher JF. Pharmacokinetics in patients with renal failure. *Clin Nephrol.* 1984;21:39-46.
65. Matzke GR, Keane WF. Drug dosing in patients with impaired renal function. In: DiPiro JT, et al., eds. *Pharmacotherapy: A Pathophysiologic Approach.* New York, New York: Elseviere; 1989.
66. McHenry MC, et al. Gentamicin dosages for renal insufficiency. Adjustments based on endogenous creatinine clearance and serum creatinine concentration. *Ann Intern Med.* 1974;74:192.
67. Milne MD. Influence of acid-base balance on efficacy and toxicity of drugs. *Proc R Soc Med.* 1965;58:961.
68. Patel DD, et al. Methotrexate excretion patterns and renal toxicity after intravenous injection or arterial infusion. *Arch Surg.* 1969;98:305.
69. Prescott LF. Mechanisms of renal excretion of drugs. *Br J Anaesth.* 1972;44:246.
70. Reeves DS. The effect of renal failure on the pharmacokinetics of antibiotics. *J Antimicrob Chemother.* 1988;21:9-16.
71. Reidenberg MM. Kidney disease and drug metabolism. *Med Clin North Am.* 1974;58:1059.
72. Reidenberg MM. The binding of drugs to plasma proteins and the interpretation of measurements of plasma concentrations of drugs in patients with poor renal function. *Am J Med.* 1977;62:466.
73. Reidenberg MM. The biotransformation of drugs in renal failure. *Am J Med.* 1977;62:482.
74. Reidenberg MM, Affrime M. Influence of disease on binding of drugs to plasma proteins. *Ann NY Acad Sci.* 1973;226:115.
75. Reidenberg MM, Drayer DE. Drug therapy in renal failure. *Annu Rev Pharmacol Toxicol.* 1980;20:45.
76. Riegelman S, Loo J, Rowland M. Concept of a volume of distribution and possible errors in evaluation of this parameter. *J Pharm Sci.* 1968;57:128.
77. Riviere JE. A possible mechanism for increased susceptibility to aminoglycoside nephrotoxicity in chronic renal disease. *N Engl J Med.* 1982;307:252.
78. Riviere JE. Checklist of hazardous drugs in patients with renal failure. In: Kirk RW, ed. *Current Veterinary Therapy VIII.* Philadelphia, Pennsylvania: WB Saunders Co; 1983.
79. Riviere JE. Paradoxical increase in aminoglycoside body clearance in renal disease when volume of distribution increases. *J Pharm Sci.* 1982;71:720.
80. Riviere JE, Coppoc GL. Dosage of antimicrobial drugs in patients with renal insufficiency. *J Am Vet Med Assoc.* 1981; 178:70.
81. Riviere JE, et al. Pharmacokinetics and comparative nephrotoxicity of fixed-dose versus fixed-interval reduction of gentamicin dosage in subtotal nephrectomized dogs. *Toxicol Appl Pharmacol.* 1984;75:496-509.
82. Riviere JE, et al. Gentamicin pharmacokinetic changes in acute canine nephrotoxic glomerulonephritis. *Antimicrob Agents Chemother.* 1981;20:387.
83. Riviere JE, Davis LE. Renal handling of drugs in renal failure. In: Bovee KC, ed. *Canine Nephrology.* Media, Pennsylvania: Harwal Publishers; 1984:643-685.
84. Riviere JE, et al. Gentamicin aerosol therapy in 18 dogs: Failure to induce detectable serum concentrations of the drug. *J Am Vet Med Assoc.* 1981;179:166.
85. Rosch M, Pazin GJ, Fireman P. Reduction of amphotericin B nephrotoxicity with mannitol. *JAMA.* 1976;235:1995.
86. Rowland M, Benet LZ, Graham GG. Clearance concepts in pharmacokinetics. *J Pharmacokinet Biopharm.* 1973;1:123.
87. Rowland M, Tozer TN. Clinical pharmacokinetics: Concepts and applications. Philadelphia, Pennsylvania: Lea & Febiger; 1980.
88. Schentag JJ, et al. Gentamicin tissue accumulation and nephrotoxic reactions. *JAMA.* 1978;240:2067.
89. Schentag JJ, Jusko WJ. Renal clearance and tissue accumulation of gentamicin. *Clin Pharmacol Ther.* 1977;22:364.
90. Schentag JJ, et al. Aminoglycoside nephrotoxicity in critically ill surgical patients. *J Surg Res.* 1979;26:270.
91. Senior DF. Drug therapy in renal failure. *Vet Clin North Am.* 1979;9:805.
92. Shalit I, et al. Pharmacokinetics of single-dose oral ciprofloxacin in patients undergoing chronic ambulatory peritoneal dialysis. *Antimicrob Agents Chemother.* 1986;30(1): 152-156.
93. Singlas E, et al. Pharmacokinetics of ciprofloxacin tablets in renal failure; influence of haemodialysis. *Eur J Clin Pharmacol.* 1987;31:589-593.
94. Smith JW, Seidl LG, Cluff LE. Studies on the epidemiology of adverse drug reactions. V. Clinical factors influencing susceptibility. *Ann Intern Med.* 1966;65:629.
95. Somani P, et al. Unidirectional absorption of gentamicin from the peritoneum during continuous ambulatory peritoneal dialysis. *Clin Pharmacol Ther.* 1982;32:113.
96. Steele TH, Rieselbach RE. The renal handling of urate and other organic anions. In: Brenner BM, Rector FC, eds. *The Kidney.* Philadelphia, Pennsylvania: WB Saunders Co; 1976:442.
97. Sullivan HP, et al. Metabolism of ^{14}C cefaclor, a cephalosporin antibiotic, in three species of laboratory animals. *Antimicrob Agents Chemother.* 1976;10:630.
98. Thornhill JA. Peritoneal dialysis in the dog and cat. An update. *Comp Cont Educ Pract Vet.* 1981;3:20.
99. Traeger A, et al. Pharmacokinetic and pharmacodynamic effects of furosemide in patients with impaired renal function. *Int J Clin Pharmacol Ther Toxicol.* 1984;22(9):481–486.
100. van Rossum JM. Pharmacokinetics of accumulation. *J Pharm Sci.* 1968;57:2162.
101. Wang LH, et al. Clearance and recovery calculations in hemodialysis: Application to plasma, red blood cell, and dialysate measurement for cyclophosphamide. *Clin Pharmacol Ther.* 1981;29:365.
102. Welling PG, Craig WA. Pharmacokinetics in disease states

modifying renal function. In: Benet LZ, ed. *Effects of Disease States on Drug Pharmacokinetics.* Washington, DC: Academy of Pharmaceutical Sciences; 1976:155.

103. Welling PG, et al. The pharmacokinetics of trimethoprim and sulfamethoxazole in normal subjects and in patients with renal failure. *J Infect Dis.* 1973;128:S556.

104. Welling PG, Craig WA, Kunin CM. Prediction of drug dosage in patients with renal failure using data derived from normal subjects. *Clin Pharmacol Ther.* 1975;18:45.

105. Whelton A, Walker WG. Intrarenal antibiotic distribution in health and disease. *Kidney Int.* 1974;6:131.

106. Yu TF, Gutman AB. Study of the paradoxical effects of salicylate in low, intermediate and high dosage on the renal mechanism for excretion of urate in man. *J Clin Invest.* 1959;38:1298.

CHAPTER 31

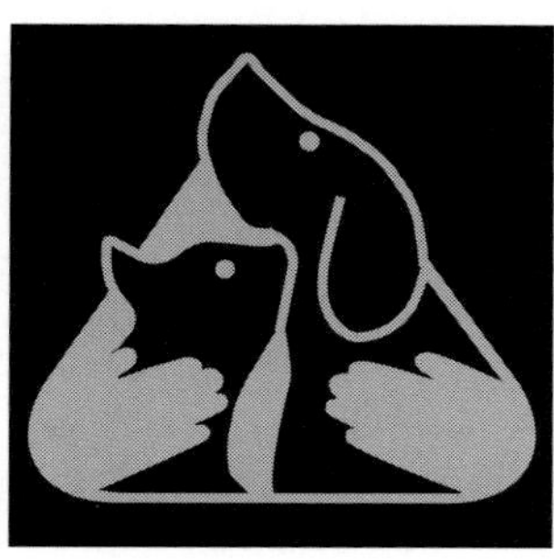

Application of Peritoneal Dialysis and Hemodialysis in the Management of Renal Failure

LARRY D. COWGILL

I. INDICATIONS FOR DIALYSIS THERAPY

A. Definition and rationale.

1. Dialysis is a therapeutic process designed to remove toxic solutes from body fluids and to normalize endogenous solutes whose aberrant concentrations disrupt physiologic processes and threaten the patient's life. Its principal application is in the management of uremia to remove accumulated "uremia toxins" and to correct alterations of electrolyte and hydrogen ion balance and disorders of fluid metabolism that occur with renal failure. Dialysis replaces many of the excretory functions of failing kidneys and helps to restore homeostasis to patients with severe kidney failure. Peritoneal dialysis and hemodialysis are the most common dialysis techniques. Even though they are technically diverse techniques, patient selection and the principles and objectives of therapy are fundamentally the same.
2. Dialysis therapy is indicated when the manifestations of renal failure cause severe morbidity or the risk of death (Table 31–1).
   a. In animals, acute renal failure is the prevailing indication for dialysis.[6,23,10] Dialysis should be instituted when conventional therapy is inadequate to alleviate azotemia and fluid and electrolyte disturbances, or to promote appropriate diuresis. When started timely, dialysis can stabilize the patient until the damaged kidneys regain effective excretory capability. If dialysis is not initiated, patients with acute uremia frequently die before renal repair can occur.
   b. Chronic, end-stage renal disease is the principal application of dialysis therapy in human medicine. Approximately 150,000 patients with end-stage renal disease are maintained by dialysis in the United States.[16] Though end-stage renal disease is clearly an indication for dialysis therapy in dogs and cats, technical and economic constraints have restricted its use in veterinary medicine.
      (1). Improvements in dialysis techniques and delivery systems, increasing sophistication of veterinary practice, and advances in the management of chronic renal failure now make intermittent dialysis a realistic adjunct to the conservative management of end-stage renal disease in companion animals.[10]
      (2). Short-term dialysis is useful for preoperative support and conditioning of renal transplant candidates, extending the available pool of suitable patients and reducing the risks of surgery.[10] Dialysis support can be provided during periods of acute transplant rejection, to sustain the animal until the rejection episode is over.
   c. Dialysis is uniquely indicated for management of acute poisoning when the toxin is "dialyz-

TABLE 31–1
INDICATIONS FOR DIALYAIS THERAPY IN ANIMALS

Acute renal failure
Failure of fluid administration, diuretics, or vasodilator therapy to initiate adequate diuresis
Failure of conventional therapy to control the biochemical and clinical manifestations of acute uremia
Life-threatening fluid overload
Life-threatening electrolyte or acid-base disturbance
BUN ≥100 mg/dL; serum creatinine ≥10 mg/dL
Clinical course refractory to conservative therapy for more than 24 hours
Chronic renal failure
Azotemia and uremic signs unresponsive to dietary and medical therapy
BUN ≥90 mg/dL; serum creatinine ≥8 mg/dL
Miscellaneous
Severe pulmonary edema
Acute poisoning or drug overdose

able." Rapid and effective clearance of the toxin from the body can prevent or minimize its harmful effects.

d. The ultrafiltration capabilities of dialysis permit removal of excessive fluid in overload conditions associated with life-threatening pulmonary edema or congestive heart failure.

B. Therapeutic objectives.

1. In acute uremia, dialysis sustains the patient's life, providing time for the native kidneys to repair themselves and resume adequate function. The outcome goals are to minimize azotemia and correct life-threatening fluid, electrolyte, and acid-base imbalances.
   a. Azotemia and retained "uremia toxins" promote anorexia, nausea, vomiting, diarrhea, lethargy, hypothermia, and gastrointestinal hemorrhage, signs that characterize acute uremia. Removal of these solutes by dialysis alleviates these signs and reduces morbidity associated with acute renal failure.
   b. Dialysis therapy facilitates implementation of parenteral alimentation and intensive diuresis. Without an exogenous mechanism to maintain fluid balance and dissipate the fluid loads associated with these therapies, overhydration results and they quickly become contraindicated.
2. For chronic renal failure, the objective of dialysis is to boost the limited excretory capacity of the animal by removing solute and water. Lessening azotemia decreases gastrointestinal disturbances, permits feeding a less restricted diet, promotes better nutritional status (increased appetite, decreased weight loss, improved hair coat and skin condition), and makes the patient a more acceptable pet.

   The efficacy of dialysis therapy can be assessed by kinetic evaluation of urea balance.[12,37] Although urea is considered to be relatively nontoxic, its appearance and accumulation in the body reflect the retention of other uremia toxins of greater clinical significance. Dialysis can be prescribed to achieve a time-averaged urea concentration that predictably ameliorates the clinical symptoms.[13,17]
3. In animals exposed accidentally or iatrogenically to toxicants, the goal of dialysis therapy is to promote rapid and complete elimination of the toxin from the body to forestall its toxic effects (Fig. 31–1). Secondarily, it supports renal function when the toxicant is nephrotoxic.

C. Physical principles.

1. In its clinical application, dialysis is a process by which the composition of blood is altered by interaction of plasma water with an artificial solution, the *dialysate,* across an interposed limiting membrane. Endogenous solutes and uremia toxins undergo diffusive and convective movement from blood through the membrane into the dialysate along outwardly directed gradients established by the dialysis procedure. The amount of solute transferred is determined by (1) the concentration gradient for each solute across the membrane, (2) the diffusivity of the solute, (3) permeability characteristics of the membrane, (4) the time allocated for dialysis, and (5) the amount of ultrafiltration. Although the membrane, the dialysate, and the mechanics of peritoneal dialysis and hemodialysis are fundamentally different, the same physical principles govern these therapies.
2. Diffusion of solutes across dialysis membranes results from their molecular motion and random collision with dialysis membranes. The more frequently these collisions occur, the greater is the probability that solutes will encounter a diffusion pore and pass through the membrane. The frequency of membrane interaction is related directly to the concentration of solutes on each side of the membrane. If a concentration of a solute, such as urea, is 100 times greater in blood than in dialysate, the relative movement of urea into dialysate is proportionately greater than its movement in the opposite direction. Thus, net movement of urea from blood to dialysate results. As the difference in concentration of a solute across the membrane is diminished, the respective bidirectional movements approximate each other and net diffusion dissipates. When the concentration of solute is identical on each side of the membrane, filtration equilibrium is achieved (the bidirectional fluxes become equal) and net diffusion is nil.
   a. Filtration equilibrium is desirable to prevent loss of important plasma solutes, such as so-

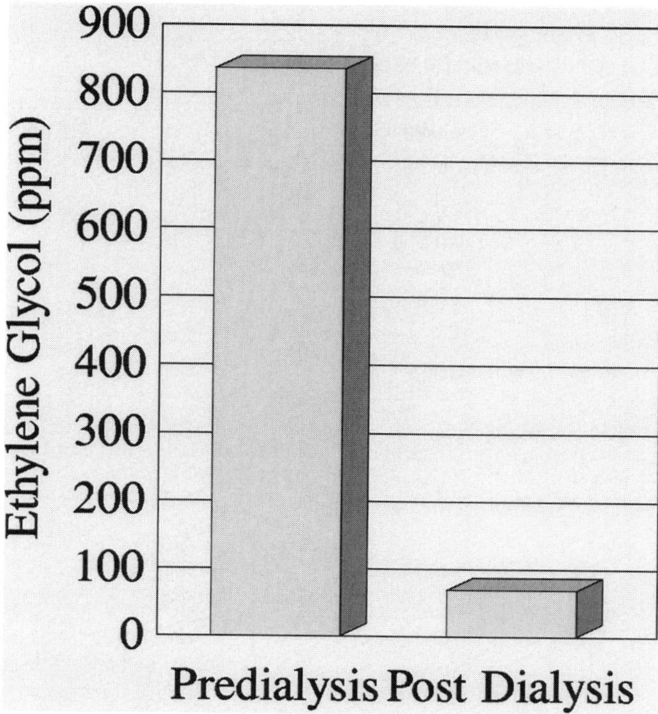

FIG. 31–1. Change in serum ethylene glycol concentration in a Shar Pei treated with 3 hours of hemodialysis following exposure to antifreeze 30 hours before treatment. The single dialysis treatment substantially reduced the serum concentration of ethylene glycol and reduced its toxic effects. ppm = parts per million.

dium, calcium, and chloride, during dialysis. The dialysate is formulated so that the concentration of these solutes is equivalent to their plasma concentration, thus eliminating the diffusion gradient and net transmembrane transfer (Table 31–2).

b. Net addition of solutes (like bicarbonate) from the dialysate into the blood is also possible by formulating the dialysate with a higher concentration of these solutes. Dialysis is thus able to replenish solutes depleted by uremia (see Table 31–2).

The diffusivity of a solute is influenced directly by it molecular weight and size. Molecular motion is inversely related to molecular weight and size. Solutes with low molecular weight, like urea (60 daltons), diffuse faster than larger solutes like creatinine (113 daltons) or vitamin B_{12} (1352 daltons). Correspondingly, the plasma concentrations of larger solutes change more slowly during dialysis than do those of smaller solutes (see Table 31–2).

c. The area available for diffusion and the resistance of the membrane to solute transfer directly influence solute diffusion.

(1). The larger the effective surface area for dialysis is, the more solute can be transferred during a given dialysis session. The maximal available surface area for peritoneal dialysis is fixed by the size of the animal, but it can be reduced by incomplete distribution of dialysate in the peritoneal cavity. With hemodialysis, the surface area of dialyzers varies, and it can be adjusted to meet the dialysis requirements of the animal.

(2). The dialysis membrane itself imposes intrinsic resistances to solute transport. The resistance is caused by the relative thickness of the membrane and the size and distribution of its diffusion channels. Thick membranes with small, narrow pores and low pore density offer much resistance to diffusion. The size of the diffusion pores also determines which solutes (i.e., of what molecular weight) can pass through the membrane.

(a). Hemodialyzers have finite pore sizes and a molecular weight cutoff for diffusion. Cellulosic membranes are the most restrictive, permitting only limited passage of molecules greater than 1000 daltons. Synthetic membrane, high-flux dialyzers are designed with large pores and are especially thin, to provide little resistance

TABLE 31–2
CHANGES IN SERUM SOLUTES DURING HEMODIALYSIS IN A DOG

	Predialysis	Postdialysis	Change (%)
Urea nitrogen (mg/dL)	101	11	–89
Creatinine (mg/dL)	15.6	3.1	–80
Inorganic phosphate (mg/dL)	16.8	4.3	–74
Calcium (mg/dL)	17.8	11.9	–33
Total carbon dioxide (mmol/L)	13.0	29.0	+123
Sodium (mmol/L)	150	144	–4
Potassium (mmol/L)	7.3	4.1	–40
Chloride (mmol/L)	106	107	+0.9

Values were obtained from a 25-kg Labrador retriever with chronic renal amyloidosis undergoing twice weekly hemodialysis treatments. The dialysis prescription included a 0.6 m^2 dialyzer, blood flow rate of 500 mL/min, dialysate flow at 500 mL/min, and session length of 5 hours. The composition of the dialysate was sodium, 155 mmol/L (1 hour), 150 mmol/L (2 hours), 145 mmol/L (last 3 hours); potassium, 3.0 mmol/L; bicarbonate, 35 mmol/L; calcium, 3.0 mmol/L; magnesium, 0.78 mmol/L; chloride, 117 to 107 mmol/L; acetic acid, 4.0 mmol/L; and dextrose, 200 mg/dL.

and greater permeability to molecules in the 500- to 5,000-dalton range.

(b). The resistance of the peritoneal membrane to large-molecular-weight solutes, and even to some proteins, is markedly less as compared with that of hemodialyzers. This characteristic permits more efficient removal of many large uremia toxins but also promotes loss of plasma proteins. The resistance of the peritoneal membrane is also influenced by disease. Peritonitis decreases its resistance and increases the magnitude of albumin loss.

3. The second mechanism for solute removal is *convective transport* associated with ultrafiltration. Ultrafiltration is a process for fluid transfer across semipermeable membranes, and in conventional hemodialysis and peritoneal dialysis, it is used to eliminate fluid accumulation associated with renal failure. Ultrafiltration is accomplished as water is forced through the membrane by either hydrostatic (hemodialysis) or osmotic (peritoneal dialysis) pressure gradients. As water is forced through the membrane, solutes capable of passing through the ultrafiltration channels are transported simultaneously by the process of solvent drag in quantities close to their plasma concentrations. Ultrafiltration is used in high-efficiency hemodialysis and specialized dialysis procedures like hemofiltration, to enhance removal of large-molecular-weight solutes independently of their gradient-dependent diffusion.
   a. In hemodialysis, ultrafiltration is achieved by imposing a hydrostatic pressure gradient across the dialyzer membrane. This is effected by positively directed pressure on the blood side of the membrane and generation of negative pressure on the dialysate side. The transmembrane pressure that produces ultrafiltration is the algebraic sum of the two pressures.
   b. The ability of a membrane to transport water is determined by its hydraulic permeability and is quantitated by its ultrafiltration coefficient (K_{UF}). K_{UF} is expressed in milliliters per hour per millimeter of mercury and varies among types of dialyzers. The product of K_{UF} and the average transmembrane pressure in the dialyzer determines the rate of ultrafiltration, expressed in milliliters per hour. Conventional dialyzers used for animals have K_{UF} values between 2.0 and 4.5 mL/hr/mm Hg, and are capable of fluid removal rates approaching 2 L/hr.
   c. For peritoneal dialysis, ultrafiltration is accomplished by inducing a transmembrane osmotic pressure gradient created by the presence of hypertonic dextrose in the dialysate. Until the dextrose achieves diffusion equilibrium with plasma, the imposed gradient promotes fluid and solute flux into the dialysate.

D. Patient selection.

1. The technical and manpower demands of dialysis, its expense, and the limited availability of facilities that support dialysis therapy make it problematic. However, if the decision to start dialysis is delayed unnecessarily, the potential benefit to the patient is diminished. General guidelines for patient selection and indications for dialysis therapy are outlined in Table 31–1.
2. For acute uremia, selection criteria include likelihood of reversible renal injury in animals with clinical signs that cannot be controlled adequately during the repair process by conservative measures alone.

a. When effective diuresis cannot be initiated or maintained with appropriate fluid replacement, osmotic or chemical diuretics, and renal vasodilators, patients with severe oliguria or anuria should start dialysis immediately. If these initial treatments fail, additional drugs or excessive fluid loads are unlikely to be beneficial. Protracted attempts with conservative therapies are contraindicated because they delay the start of dialysis and predispose the animal to life-threatening iatrogenic fluid imbalances that are not easily resolved.
b. Dialysis should be provided to animals with uremic signs (vomiting, diarrhea, seizures) and acid-base or electrolyte abnormalities that cannot be effectively controlled with medical therapy.
c. To alleviate the morbidity and mortality of acute uremia, dialysis is indicated for animals in which the blood urea nitrogen (BUN) value exceeds 100 mg/dL, or in which the serum creatinine level exceeds 10 mg/dL. In all cases, dialysis should be considered as a therapeutic option if the clinical course is refractory to supportive therapy for longer than 24 hours. Longer delays cause clinical deterioration that may be impossible to reverse.
d. If the facilities or technical expertise to begin dialysis therapy are not available, the patient should be transferred *immediately* to a referral center where it can be performed.

3. In end-stage renal failure, the efficacy of conventional dietary and medical therapy to alleviate the clinical consequences of uremia is limited. For these patients, intermittent dialysis therapy reduces azotemia and clinical signs of uremia and makes the patients more acceptable pets.[10]

   Dialysis is most beneficial for animals in which BUN exceeds 90 mg/dL or in which serum creatinine exceeds 8 mg/dL. At this stage of uremia, medical therapy alone has limited efficacy and the clinical consequences of uremia become profound.
4. Dialysis is also indicated for animals (uremic or nonuremic) with fluid overload that produces life-threatening pulmonary edema or congestive heart failure. With ultrafiltration, the fluid burden can be alleviated independent of renal excretory capacity.
5. Dialysis is very effective for acute poisoning or drug overdose, if the offending toxin is readily dialyzable (Fig. 31–2). Removal of the toxin by dialysis reduces exposure to the poison or its toxic metabolites, decreasing its clinical effects. Dialysis is sometimes an option for initial management of poisoned animals. Selection criteria include history or known exposure to a dialyzable toxin, persistence of a significant blood toxin concentration, and lack of an effective medical antidote.

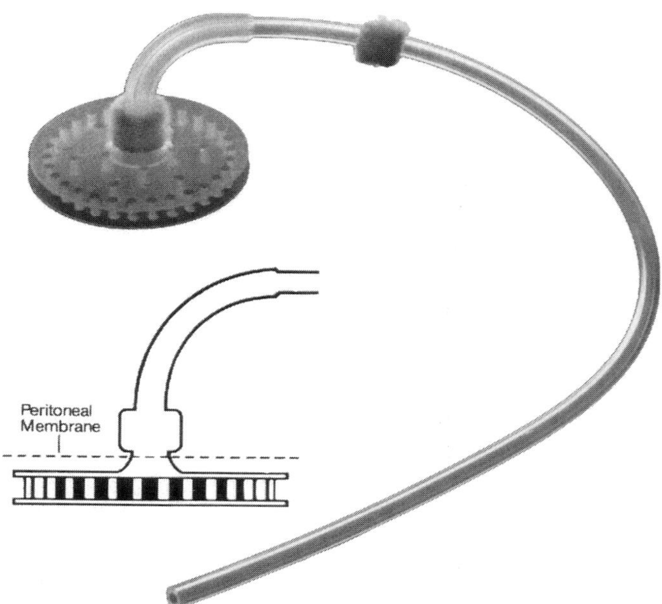

FIG. 31–2. Column-disk catheter for peritoneal dialysis of dogs and cats. (Lifecath, Quinton Instrument Company, Seattle, Washington.)

II. PERITONEAL DIALYSIS

A. Theoretic basis.

1. Peritoneal dialysis is a seemingly straightforward procedure in which dialysate is instilled into the abdominal cavity. Then, by diffusive and convective transport, toxic wastes and excess fluid are transferred from plasma to equilibrate with the dialysate across the limiting barrier of the peritoneal lining. The peritoneal limiting membrane is more complex than the artificial barriers of hemodialyzers. It is composed of the capillary endothelium and basement membrane, loose connective tissue, and the mesothelial surface of the peritoneum.
2. Because peritoneal blood flow, surface area, and permeability are relatively fixed, concentration gradients between plasma and the dialysate are the principal driving forces for solute transfer. As fresh dialysate is placed in the peritoneal cavity, gradient-directed diffusion proceeds from blood to the dialysate, until the two fluids achieve concentration equilibrium, at which point net transport ceases.
   a. Smaller-molecular-weight solutes like urea diffuse more quickly across the peritoneal barrier and, thus, reach equilibrium more rapidly than do larger solutes like creatinine or vitamin B_{12}.[33]
   b. Unlike hemodialyzer artificial membranes, the peritoneal membrane of mammals is less restrictive to the passage of large molecular solutes and macromolecules. This is advanta-

geous for removal of middle– and large-molecular-weight uremia toxins, which are difficult to clear with conventional hemodialyzers; however, the same property permits the undesirable loss of plasma proteins into the dialysate.

3. Ultrafiltration is driven by osmotic gradients imposed across the peritoneal membrane by high concentrations of glucose in the dialysate. The osmotic pressure exerted by glucose draws water from blood into the dialysate; however, these effects are transient. As dextrose is absorbed from the dialysate, its osmotic effect dissipates and the volume of ultrafiltrate diminishes exponentially with time. Ultrafiltration also promotes convective removal of solute and contributes to the mass transfer rate for solutes during peritoneal dialysis.

B. Delivery.

1. Peritoneal dialysis catheters.
   a. The catheter is both the heart and the Achilles heel of peritoneal dialysis. The conduit between the external environment and the peritoneal cavity, the catheter permits delivery of fresh dialysate into the peritoneal cavity and drainage of the "equilibrated fluid" at the end of the dwell time. To work satisfactorily, the catheter system must 1) possess efficient fluid inflow and outflow characteristics, 2) be biocompatible, 3) resist infection of the peritoneal cavity and the subcutaneous tunnel, and 4) retard leakage at the peritoneal interface.
      (1). Some conventional catheters consist of fenestrated silicone tubes of straight, curved, or coiled configuration. Others use a column-disk architecture (see Fig. 31–1). Dacron velour cuffs are bonded to the catheter at the peritoneal and cutaneous exit sites, to prevent fluid leakage and descending bacterial contamination and to provide fibrous anchors to retard catheter displacement. Straight and coiled Tenckhoff catheters are the most popular for human patients,[21] whereas the column-disk catheter has become the most popular for dogs.[11,23]
      (2). Development of the Tenckhoff catheter and other hybrid fenestrated silicone tube catheters made long-term peritoneal dialysis feasible in humans with end-stage renal disease. Their performance in, and suitability for, dogs and cats has been disappointing.[33,40,41] Although initial flow characteristics are satisfactory, within days of placement, flow rates diminish, fluid recovery rates dwindle, and the catheters become nonfunctional. In both dogs and cats, drainage failure is usually caused by obstruction of the catheter with omentum or fibrin.[41] To continue dialytic therapy, the obstructed catheter must be replaced by another, which may likewise become blocked.
      (3). The column-disk design appeared to resist these complications and has been advocated for use in dogs and cats. The catheter is surgically positioned in the caudal abdominal cavity to prevent interaction with the omentum and bowel. Two Dacron velour cuffs seal the peritoneal exit site and immobilize the cutaneous perforation.[4,36,40,41,44]
         (a). The large fluid channels associated with column-disk geometry facilitate rapid input and output fluid flow rates without generating excessive flow velocity and suction associated with fenestrated catheters.[3] These characteristics prevent attraction of omentum and bowel loops to the catheter and obstruction of the drainage ports.
         (b). The column-disk catheter has improved delivery of peritoneal dialysis to animals, but it is still susceptible to outflow obstruction by the omentum.[11,36] For maximal performance and longevity of the catheter, partial omentectomy is recommended at the time of catheter placement.[4,6] Omentectomy is performed by pulling the omentum through the peritoneal placement incision and then cross-ligating and excising the retracted pedicle.[4,6]
         (c). When the catheter is used immediately after placement, it should be tested to ensure that a tight peritoneal seal has been achieved and that there are no leaks. Initially, large volumes of dialysate should be avoided, to minimize intraperitoneal pressure. Heparin, 100 to 500 U/L, is often added to the dialysate for 3 to 7 days following placement, to minimize occlusion of the catheter by fibrin clots.
         (d). The dialysis catheter is a major source of the complications, frustration, and morbidity associated with peritoneal dialysis. Leakage of dialysate, drainage failure, and infection are the most frequent and important complications.
            (1′). Pericatheter leakage of dialysate from the exit site or into the subcutaneous tissues of dependent portions of the body occurs frequently. The incidence and

degree of leakage are greater with temporary, trochar-type catheters, which are not intended for peritoneal dialysis but often are used in emergencies. Dacron velour cuffs make a better peritoneal and abdominal seal, but do not function effectively when catheters are used immediately following placement. Leakage may be minimized by securing the exit point of the catheter in a superior position or by decreasing the volume of dialysate per exchange. In some cases, the catheter site must be explored surgically, to tighten the tissue seal or reinsert the catheter in a different location. The subcutaneous accumulation of dialysate can be sufficient to require cessation of dialysis.

(2′). Drainage failure results most often from attachment or infiltration of the catheter by omentum or from blockage of the fenestrations by fibrin plugs. Drainage failure prevents adequate recovery of dialysate and promotes progressive weight gain and hypervolemia, which may require suspension of dialysis. If omentum or bowel loop attachment causes outflow failure, attempts can be made to reposition Tenckhoff-type catheters deeper into the pelvic canal, away from the omentum, by manipulating the catheter tip with a metal stylet. With longstanding obstruction, the omentum must be surgically stripped from the catheter or the catheter must be replaced. Thus, a partial omentectomy is preferable at the time of initial catheter placement, to minimize these complications. Outflow obstruction of column-disk catheters requires partial omentectomy and replacement of the catheter.

(3′). Infection of the exit site or the subcutaneous tunnel is a frequent problem in animals, owing to the difficulty of maintaining a sanitary environment. Such infections may progress to peritonitis or systemic infection. Superficial infections associated with redness, swelling, and exudate should be treated with daily catheter care. Hair should be clipped to provide a wide margin around the catheter. Crusts, debris, dirt, and scabs should be removed by gentle cleansing with antiseptic soap, and the site should be dried, treated with topical povidone-iodine ointment, and covered with sterile gauze. Systemic antibiotics, selected on the basis of bacterial culture and antimicrobic susceptibility tests, are indicated for persistent exit site or tunnel infections. Antibiotics should be continued 2 weeks if a beneficial effect is observed. Resistant infections may require surgical removal of the subcutaneous cuff(s) or the entire catheter.

2. Peritoneal dialysate. Renewed utilization of peritoneal dialysis in human patients with end-stage renal failure has increased availability of ready-to-use dialysis solutions. Peritoneal dialysate has more exacting manufacturing requirements than does hemodialysate. It must be sterile, pyrogen free, and biologically inert, and must be formulated to remove uremic solutes and excessive fluid from the patient, to correct acidosis, and to supply solutes depleted by uremia.

Peritoneal dialysate is a polyionic solution with the approximate electrolyte composition of plasma. Ready-to-use dialysate formulated for humans is generally suitable for animals and more convenient and safer to use than dialysate formulated from solutions intended for intravenous administration.

a. Typical formulations for ready-to-use solutions are listed in Table 31–3. Sodium and potassium concentrations vary; they may be selected to meet the precise requirements of individual patients.

(1). The sodium concentration of dialysate is frequently lower than the serum sodium concentration. This accelerates sodium transport and obviates the tendency for hypernatremia associated with ultrafiltration.

(2). Standard solutions for peritoneal dialysis contain no potassium. Although suitable for patients with acute renal failure, these solutions might induce hypokalemia and negative potassium balance in animals without elevated potassium concentrations. Therefore, potassium chloride

TABLE 31–3
COMPOSITION OF STANDARD SOLUTIONS FOR PERITONEAL DIALYSIS

Product Name	Dextrose (%)	Na^+ (mEq/L)	K^+ (mEq/L)	Ca^{++} (mEq/L)	Mg^{++} (mEq/L)	Cl^- (mEq/L)	Lactate (mEq/L)	Osm (mOsm/L)
Dianeal* PD-1 with 1.5% dextrose	1.5	132		3.5	1.5	102	35	347
Dianeal* PD-1 with 2.5% dextrose	2.5	132		3.5	1.5	102	35	398
Dianeal* PD-1 with 3.5% dextrose	3.5	132		3.5	1.5	102	35	448
Dianeal* PD-1 with 4.25% dextrose	4.25	132		3.5	1.5	102	35	486
Impersol† LM with 1.5% dextrose	1.5	132		3.5	0.5	96	40	346
Impersol† LM with 2.5% dextrose	2.5	132		3.5	0.5	96	40	396
Impersol† LM with 3.5% dextrose	3.5	132		3.5	0.5	96	40	447
Impersol† LM with 4.25% dextrose	4.25	132		3.5	0.5	96	40	485
Dialyte‡ Pattern LM with 1.5% dextrose	1.5	131		3.5	0.5	94	40	345
Dialyte‡ Pattern LM with 2.5% dextrose	2.5	131.5		3.5	0.5	94	40	395
Dialyte‡ Pattern LM with 4.25% dextrose	4.25	131.5		3.5	0.5	94	40	485

*Dianeal, Baxter Healthcare Corp., Renal Division, McGaw Park, Illinois 60015.
†Impersol, Fresenius USA, Inc., Walnut Creek, California 94598.
‡Dialyte, McGaw, Inc., Irvine, California 92713.

should be added to achieve a dialysate concentration of 2 to 4 mmol/L.

(3). Lactate is used as the standard bicarbonate-generating base, in lieu of bicarbonate, which is unstable in ready-to-use solutions. Usual lactate concentrations are 35 to 45 mmol/L, to promote sufficient bicarbonate generation to correct existing base deficits. Because animals with concurrent hepatic insufficiency may be unable to metabolize lactate adequately, they may require a solution containing bicarbonate. Acetate, which is the usual base-generating anion in nonbicarbonate hemodialysis concentrates, may cause peritoneal damage, causing loss of ultrafiltration efficiency with prolonged use. Thus, it is not generally used.

b. Peritoneal dialysate contains dextrose in a concentration of 1.5%, 2.5%, or 4.25%, to promote an osmotic gradient for ultrafiltration. The selection of the dextrose concentration of the dialysate is based on individual requirements for fluid removal. For routine dialysis in animals, a standard dextrose concentration of 1.5% is used. This concentration exerts a mild osmotic force that counters the tendency for fluid absorption, facilitates fluid recovery, and prevents progressive fluid accumulation.

(1). For overhydrated patients, or to increase recovery of the dialysate transiently, more rapid ultrafiltration can be achieved by increasing the concentration of dextrose in the dialysate (usually to 4.5%). These solutions are used only on a short-term basis. Prolonged use causes excessive fluid removal and volume contraction.

(2). Solutions have been formulated with 2.5 or 3.5% dextrose to provide better control of ultrafiltration during the prolonged dwell times associated with chronic ambulatory peritoneal dialysis (CAPD), but such formulations may be used in patients that receive dialysate intermittently, to control fluid balance.

(3). The osmotic effects of dextrose in the dialysate dissipate as the dextrose diffuses into the extracellular fluid. The rate of ultrafiltration is maximal at the start of dwell, but diminishes thereafter until ultrafiltration stops, as dextrose comes into equilibrium. Intraperitoneal volume is maximal at ultrafiltration (dextrose) equilibrium, after which peritoneal fluid is reabsorbed and net fluid removal is decreased.

(4). Ultrafiltration depends, collectively, on the concentration of dextrose in the dialysate, the volume of dialysate instilled, and the rate of dextrose absorption across the peritoneum. For standard exchange procedures, however, the volume of ultrafiltrate produced is proportional to the osmolality of the dialysate.

3. Delivery techniques.

Three techniques for the delivery of peritoneal dialysis (manual peritoneal dialysis, cycler-assisted peritoneal dialysis, and chronic ambulatory peritoneal dialysis) have been described for animal patients.[33,36,41,42,46] The dialysis cycles for each procedure incorporate common infusion, dwell, and drain phases; however, each procedure differs in its clinical indications, methods of fluid transfer, and time allocated to each phase of the cycle.

a. Manual continuous peritoneal dialysis is the most commonly used form of peritoneal dialysis for acute and chronic renal failure in animals. It is performed with a short-term stylus catheter, a chronic Tenckhoff-type catheter, or column-disk catheter. Dialysate is infused from a reservoir bag through one limb of a Y connector and, following the dwell phase, is drained into an empty collection bag connected to the other limb. The inflow, dwell, and drain phases are adjusted to establish a cycle that is repeated sequentially to achieve the desired dialysis prescription. Short cycle times (approximately 60 minutes) are generally used to achieve rapid solute clearance and to maximize the efficiency of the dialysis sessions.

b. Cycler-assisted peritoneal dialysis is delivered with an automated mechanical device that repeatedly delivers programmed dialysis cycles. Infusion volume, dwell time, and drain volume are set for the dialysis session and are executed automatically, on fixed time intervals. Cyclers also warm the dialysate to the appropriate temperature and monitor the balance of fluid exchanges and ultrafiltration. Cycler techniques are appropriate for either continuous (24 hours per day) or intermittent (alternating periods of dialysis and no dialysis) delivery techniques. Cycler dialysis alleviates the considerable work load that manual techniques demand. Although the cost of automatic cyclers is moderate compared to that of hemodialysis delivery systems, the availability of the automatic devices is limited to specialty centers.

c. Continuous ambulatory peritoneal dialysis (CAPD) is a delivery technique most appropriate for patients who suffer chronic renal failure. Dialysis goes on continuously, throughout every day. Long dwell times of 4 to 8 hours are used to provide 6 to 8 cycles per day, permitting animals to be unrestrained and ambulatory throughout most of the daily sessions. CAPD is the most popular form of peritoneal dialysis for human patients, and it has been an attraction for animal patients with end-stage renal failure that cannot be managed effectively with conventional therapy.[42,46] The long dwell times associated with CAPD result in low-efficiency exchange cycles, but its continuous nature promotes effective cumulative weekly urea clearance.

C. Peritoneal dialysis prescription for acute renal failure.

The decision to institute peritoneal dialysis for acute uremia assumes that conventional attempts to initiate diuresis and to control the biochemical disturbances of uremia have failed. The goals of therapy are to stabilize the patient as quickly as possible and to control ongoing fluid, electrolyte, acid-base balance, and biochemical disorders. The BUN value should be reduced to less than 90 mg/dL, and serum potassium, bicarbonate, sodium, and phosphate should approximate reference ranges. To achieve these goals, the initial dialysis session is likely to extend beyond 48 hours, with continuous cycles throughout the session. At the end of each 12- to 24-hour period, the clinical and laboratory status of the patient should be reassessed and the dialysis prescription adjusted accordingly.

1. Catheter placement must be performed under strict aseptic conditions and in conjunction with a partial omentectomy. The column-disk catheter is preferable for most animals. Tenckhoff peritoneal dialysis catheters are also suitable, if they are placed carefully in the pelvic cavity after partial omentectomy. Trocar-type catheters commonly used for pleural lavage and drainage can be used in emergencies, but generally, they are inefficient and tend to leak.
2. A standard peritoneal dialysate containing 1.5% dextrose should be used unless greater ultrafiltration is required.
   a. When fluid removal is required in volume-overloaded patients, a dialysate with a higher dextrose concentration (usually 4.5%) should be prescribed for the initial cycles. Because fluid removal rates with these solutions can be quite rapid, close supervision of hydration and blood pressure is required.
   b. For initial cycles, potassium-free dialysate is appropriate; however, as the hyperkalemia is corrected, the dialysate solution should be modified to contain 2- to 4 mmol/L of potassium chloride.
   c. The dialysate must be warmed to 38 to 39° C, and it is delivered by gravity into the peritoneal cavity at 30 to 40 mL/kg.[23,33]
      (1). For the initial 10 to 12 cycles immediately following placement of the catheter, exchange volumes of 15 to 20 mL/kg may result in less leakage around the catheter and into subcutaneous tissues.
      (2). The exchange volume should be decreased if respiratory distress, abdominal discomfort, or pain develops.
      (3). Heparin, 100 to 500 U, can be added to each liter of dialysate during initial sessions, to prevent fibrin occlusions of the catheter.
3. Continuous delivery procedures with 60-minute cycle times are appropriate and effective for most patients.

a. Each cycle should encompass a 10-minute inflow time, 30 to 40 minutes of dwell time, and a 20- to 30-minute drain period. At the conclusion of each cycle, new cycles are initiated for the duration of the session.
b. The drained dialysate is collected in a sterile bag and inspected for cloudiness or abnormal color, and the recovered volume is determined.
c. Higher-efficiency dialysis sessions (greater urea clearance and fluid removal) can be achieved by shortening the dwell (10 to 20 minutes) and cycle (30 to 40 minutes) times. Although they are more effective for urea removal, these high-efficiency procedures are rarely necessary and require greater volumes of dialysate and extraordinary demands on technical staff.

4. A detailed record of exchange volumes and net fluid balance should be maintained for each cycle throughout the procedure. Body weight, hydration status, blood pressure, and central venous pressure should be assessed every 3 to 4 hours, to avert extremes of fluid balance.
   a. If fluid balance becomes excessively positive, dialysate with a higher dextrose concentration should be prescribed, to promote ultrafiltration and removal of additional fluid.
   b. If the fluid balance becomes negative, hyperosmotic dialysate should be discontinued, and appropriate measures should be taken to prevent hypotension and hypovolemia.
   c. Serum electrolytes, chemistry profile (BUN, creatinine, phosphate, calcium, total protein, and albumin), and acid-base parameters should be assessed every 12 to 24 hours, to monitor the efficacy of urea clearance and to help to formulate the dialysis prescription for the next session.
5. Following the initial 24 to 48 exchanges, the azotemia and clinical condition of the patient may warrant progressive increases in the dwell time, to extend the cycle length to 3 to 6 hours. Guidelines for these changes include BUN concentrations less than 90 mg/dL, normalization of electrolytes and acid-base status, and control of vomiting, diarrhea, seizures, and fluid volume. As excretory function is recovered, only three to four exchanges may be required each day to control the azotemia and clinical condition of the animal until the kidney damage is repaired.

D. Peritoneal dialysis prescription for chronic renal failure.

1. CAPD provides continuous dialysis with infrequent fluid exchanges during the day. It is indicated for animals with end-stage renal disease.[41,42,46] With the exception of the dialysis catheter, transfer tubing, and the dialysate solution containers, CAPD requires no specialized or costly equipment. The procedure is uncomplicated and seemingly within the capabilities of pet owners. To perform CAPD, dialysate is instilled by gravity into the peritoneal cavity and allowed to dwell for 4 to 8 hours before it is drained out. The abdomen is left filled overnight, so only four to six exchanges are needed during the day. Despite its lure, CAPD has never achieved clinical acceptance and is rarely considered as a therapeutic option. Nevertheless, it has merit for end-stage renal disease and it could be provided to animals with highly motivated owners. Although during each cycle urea clearance is low, the cumulative weekly effects of CAPD compare favorably with the results of more intensive forms of dialysis therapy, including hemodialysis.[30] CAPD provides more physiologic and sustained control of azotemia than does hemodialysis. As a goal, BUN should be maintained below 80 mg/dL, to control the clinical manifestations of uremia.
2. Peritoneal access is best achieved with a surgically placed column-disk or Tenckhoff peritoneal catheter.[4,46] Contemporaneously with catheter placement, partial omentectomy should be performed to improve catheter performance and longevity. The catheter is connected to a fluid transfer set that facilitates aseptic delivery and removal of dialysate from the peritoneal cavity.
   a. Currently, a variety of reusable and disposable transfer sets are available. The conventional transfer circuit incorporates a straight-spike design similar to intravenous fluid administration sets that use the spike repeatedly to access the port in the fluid bags. The transfer set should be treated with a povidone-iodine solution, to minimize bacterial contamination before it is removed from the empty bag and attachment to the new bag. One drawback to this technique is the fact that any bacterial contaminant in the transfer system is flushed into the abdomen along with the fresh dialysate.
   b. A more complicated delivery technique using a Y-transfer set appears to reduce the incidence of bacterial peritonitis.[28] The limbs of the Y-transfer tubing are flushed—either before or immediately after drainage of the peritoneum—into the drain bag with fresh dialysate, before it is instilled into the abdomen. The flushing effect eliminates the risk of bacterial contamination during removal and connection of the fluid bags. As a further modification, the limbs of the transfer circuit are filled with disinfectant during the dwell period. The disinfectant is flushed into the drain bag before fresh dialysate is introduced through the catheter.
   c. After dialysate has been introduced into the abdomen, the partially used or empty bag is secured to the patient, to permit free mobility during the dwell period. With standard transfer

circuits, the empty infusion bag is used for drainage. With the Y-transfer system, the entire transfer set can be disconnected from the dialysis catheter and the free ends can be sealed with disinfectant-containing caps. This arrangement is most appropriate for small animals that require multiple exchanges from a single set of solution and drain bags.

3. A dialysate with a standard composition and 1.5% dextrose is used as the base solution and is modified as appropriate to meet the needs of the patient.
   a. For maintenance CAPD in animals with chronic renal failure, the potassium concentration of the dialysate should be adjusted to 4 to 5 mmol/L with potassium chloride.
   b. A solution with 40 to 45 mmol/L of lactate better corrects metabolic acidosis.
   c. The addition of heparin, antibiotics, or other compounds should be considered on the basis of specific indications of peritonitis.
   d. Extensive ultrafiltration is rarely indicated in animal patients. If fluid retention is recognized, a dialysate with 2.5 or 4.5% dextrose can be substituted for the overnight exchanges.
4. For each exchange, the largest tolerated volume of dextrose should be administered. Initial exchange volumes of 15 to 20 mL/kg used during the initial 12 to 24 hours after catheter placement should be increased, as tolerated, to 30 to 40 mL/kg. Larger exchange volumes promote greater urea clearance and more effective dialysis. Three to four exchanges with 4- to 6-hour cycle times should be delivered during waking hours, and a final exchange should be provided before bedtime.

E. Complications of peritoneal dialysis.
Although the technical simplicity of peritoneal dialysis makes it an enticing therapy, complications associated with the peritoneal access (described previously), and with the technical and medical aspects of peritoneal dialysis, may prove formidable to clinicians, and fatal for patients.

1. Peritonitis is one of the most clinically significant consequences of peritoneal dialysis. In a recent review, 22% of patients treated with peritoneal dialysis for variable periods developed bacterial peritonitis,[11] and for animals treated for extended periods, the prevalence of infectious peritonitis is high.[11,33,23,43] Infectious peritonitis results from inadvertent contamination of the peritoneal cavity by the dialysate or the delivery apparatus. Sources of infection include contamination of the transfer set connections, owing to breaches of aseptic technique, periluminal infection of the catheter by bacteria on the skin along the subcutaneous tunnel, or transmural passage of bacteria from the bowel to the peritoneum.
   a. Infectious peritonitis is recognized by drainage fluid that looks cloudy or bloody, and/or by detection of organisms by cytology, Gram's stain, or culture of the dialysate, or by clinical signs of peritoneal inflammation (fever, anorexia, vomiting, diarrhea, abdominal tenderness). The diagnosis is confirmed by detection of inflammatory cells (>100/μL) in the dialysate and the identification of infectious organisms by cytology or culture.
   b. The peritoneal effluent should be examined and cultured at the first indications of peritonitis to determine what therapy is most appropriate. *Staphylococcus* organisms are cultured most often, but gram-negative bacteria, mixed cultures, and fungal isolates may be detected.
   c. Prevention by meticulous placement and care of the peritoneal access device and strict use of aseptic technique during fluid exchanges is, by far, the most effective approach to the potential complication of peritonitis.
      (1). In the event of a break in sterile technique, prophylactic administration of broad-spectrum antibiotics, such as cephalosporins or potentiated penicillins, is indicated. The transfer set should be replaced and the antimicrobial therapy maintained for 24 to 48 hours. Daily use of prophylactic saline–saline plus iodine rinses of the peritoneal cavity described in dogs have been shown to prevent peritonitis in the early stages of therapy or following a breach in aseptic technique without concurrent use of antibiotics.[41,43] These techniques may have value for both acute and chronic delivery techniques.
      (2). For confirmed infections, treatment should be initiated as soon as possible. The choice of antibiotics should be based on bacterial culture and on antimicrobial susceptibility testing. If the organism is gram positive, initial therapy with cephalosporins or potentiated penicillins, administered in the dialysate or systemically, is appropriate. Intraperitoneal administration of antibiotics in the dialysate is the traditional route for therapy.[15,43,45] For severe infections, a loading dose of antibiotic is given in the dialysate or intravenously, followed by maintenance doses. Guidelines for antimicrobial dosing have been established for human patients and have been extrapolated for animal schedules.[6,15,25,43,45] For cephalothin, a loading dose of 1000 mg/L and a maintenance dose of 250 mg/L of dialysate may be used.[25,43] Heparin, at 500 U/L, is added to the dialysate to prevent fibrin occlusion of the catheter. For gram-negative organ-

isms, initial treatment with aminoglycosides (4 mg/kg intramuscularly and 6 mg/L of dialysate, maintenance) is recommended.[43] For uncomplicated cases, therapy should be extended to 10 to 14 days. Mixed infections should be treated with combined cephalosporin and aminoglycoside therapy.

(3). If, after 96 hours of aggressive medical therapy no clinical improvement occurs, the peritoneal access should be removed. A new catheter should not be inserted until the peritonitis is resolved, which may necessitate alternative dialysis support to keep the patient alive.

(4). Tissue from exit site infections should be cultured and the pathogen addressed with appropriate systemic antibiotics, in addition to local wound care, including cleansing with antiseptics (povidone-iodine, hydrogen peroxide, or chlorohexadine solutions) and topical antimicrobials.

2. Hypoalbuminemia is a common complication of peritoneal dialysis, owing to the relative permeability to albumin of the peritoneal membrane.[11] The rate of albumin loss increases with peritonitis and may exacerbate the negative protein balance characteristic of uremic animals.
3. Pleural effusion has been described in dogs, coincident with delivery of peritoneal dialysis.[6] In the absence of anatomic defects in the diaphragm, the dialysate likely passes into the pleural cavity through subdiaphragmatic lymphatics, in response to pressure gradients across the diaphragm.[6] The pleural fluid may be sufficient to cause dyspnea, in which case thoracocentesis may be necessary.
4. Overhydration can develop as a result of ineffective removal of the exchange volume. This common outcome of drainage failure of the peritoneal catheter must be prevented.
5. Hypovolemia and dehydration can develop from excessive ultrafiltration associated with the prolonged use of dialysate containing 2.5 or 4.5% dextrose. These solutions are indicated to remove specific fluid loads—and *not* for routine dialysis. Fluid volume derangements are best prevented by accurate fluid balance records and routine weighing of the animal.

III. HEMODIALYSIS

A. Historical perspective.

Development of modern hemodialysis is punctuated by notable discoveries, technologic developments, and medical pioneers who seized these developments and applied them to this unique purpose.

1. The first prototype of the modern artificial kidney was developed by Able, Rowntree, and Turner in 1913.[1] Interestingly, their device contained many design characteristics that, today, are remotely visible in modern hollow-fiber artificial kidneys, and the design was employed experimentally and successfully in dogs, to usher in the development of therapeutic hemodialysis. The clinical application of dialysis techniques would not be realized for another decade because of the constraints of anticoagulation and the need for more suitable membranes and better vascular access.
2. The discovery and availability of purified heparin and a new membrane material named "cellophane" launched the beginnings of the dialysis era. In 1943, Wilhelm Kolff devised a "rotating drum artificial kidney," the surface of which was encoiled with cellophane tubing partially suspended in a batch dialysate. This was the first device suitable for human dialysis, and it was responsible for the first successful treatment of acute uremia with dialysis technology.
3. In 1960, Quinton, Dillard, and Scribner moved hemodialysis a quantum stride forward with the development of the Teflon/Silastic exteriorized arteriovenous shunt for repeated access to the vasculature.[35] From this point, the logistics of treating patients with end-stage renal failure by long-term maintenance hemodialysis was realized.
4. Since the realization that hemodialysis had a legitimate role in the management of all forms of renal failure, we have witnessed in the subsequent 3 decades exponential developments in dialysis delivery and technologic applications, including:
   a. Replacement of external arteriovenous shunts with surgically created internal arteriovenous fistulas and graphs.
   b. Development of new dialysis membranes with greater solute permeability and ultrafiltration characteristics and improved biocompatibility.
   c. Incorporation of these membranes into geometrically improved artificial kidney designs that optimize surface area–to–blood volume and dialysis efficiency.
   d. Technologic improvements in dialysis delivery systems that incorporate variable dialysate dilution, volumetric ultrafiltration control, electronic safety surveillance, microprocessor-controlled delivery systems, and high-efficiency dialysis techniques.
   e. Assessment and quantitation of dialysis delivery and adequacy of therapy.

B. Artificial kidneys (hemodialyzers), dialysate, and hemodialysis delivery systems.

1. Artificial kidneys (hemodialyzers)
   a. The artificial kidney, the heart of the hemodialysis process, simulates the excretory processes of natural kidneys. An ideal artificial kidney must possess many characteristics in common with biologic kidneys.

(1). It must have a high capacity to remove both small- and medium-molecular-weight waste products from the blood.

Conventional cellulosic hemodialyzers have good diffusive clearance rate for small-molecular-weight (<500 daltons) solutes, but poor dialyzability for solutes with higher molecular weights. The convective properties of high-flux synthetic hemodialyzers permit enhanced clearance of "middle molecules" (molecular weight 500 to 5000 daltons) and large molecules to approximately 12,000 daltons).

(2). It must selectively retain essential solutes, plasma proteins, and the cellular elements of blood. The pore size of all dialysis membranes prohibits filtration of the cellular components of blood and permits negligible flux of plasma proteins larger than albumin. The clearance of essential solutes like sodium and calcium is prevented by eliminating the transmembrane gradient required for diffusion.

(3). It must regulate water removal independently of solute flux. This feature is accomplished by the hydraulic permeability of the dialyzer through the process of ultrafiltration. Synthetic membrane dialyzers have greater hydraulic permeability than that of conventional dialyzers.

(4). Its blood compartment must be an efficient solute exchanger without disrupting or decompensating cardiovascular homeostasis.

(5). It must be sterile and nontoxic, and must not produce adverse biologic interactions with the patient.

b. The artificial kidney has evolved to approach these objectives more closely. Dialyzer design has incorporated innovations in membrane materials and manufacturing technology. Today, hemodialyzers are compact, disposable, efficient, reliable, relatively inexpensive, and tailored to the size, biologic incompatibilities, and excretory requirements of individual patients.

c. Hemodialyzers are classified as "parallel-plate" or "hollow-fiber," according to the physical characteristics and arrangement of the semipermeable membrane used in their construction. They may be categorized additionally by the composition of their membrane material into conventional (cellulosic) or high-flux (synthetic) dialyzers. The arrangement of closed compartments on each side of the membrane for the respective flow of blood and dialysate is common to each design. Compliance of the blood compartment, priming volume, blood flow resistance, and physical size distinguish each design.

(1). Parallel-plate dialyzers, initially proposed by Kiil, were among the first designs to be successfully employed for maintenance hemodialysis in human patients.[22] Plate dialyzers use flat sheets of semipermeable membrane sandwiched between plastic supports or mesh that disperse blood and dialysate over opposing sides of the membrane. This design has diminished in popularity since the late 1960s, but disposable, multilayer (stacked) parallel-plate designs are still in active use and are available with both cellulosic and synthetic membranes. Parallel-plate dialyzers are available with effective surface areas from 0.2 to 1.1 m^2. They have low blood flow resistance, but increased compliance of the blood compartment may cause fluctuations in extracorporeal volume, which is disadvantageous for small animals.

(2). The hollow-fiber artificial kidney was introduced in 1965 has become the standard for dialyzer design (Fig. 31–3). It is composed of a bundle of small-diameter cellulosic or synthetic capillary fibers encased

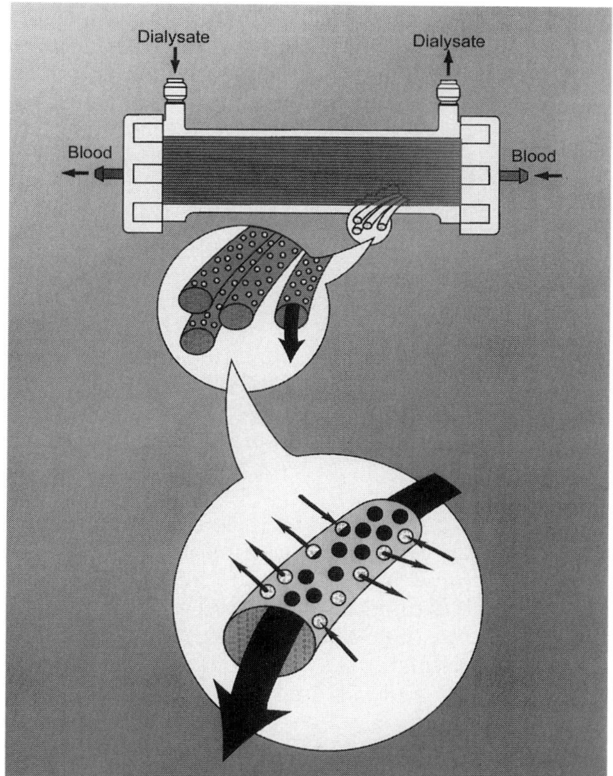

FIG. 31–3. Schematic illustration of a hollow-fiber dialyzer depicts the countercurrent flow of blood and dialysate. The expanded inserts portray the permeable nature of the fibers, the blood path (large arrow), and solute exchange (small arrows). (Burrows-Hudson S, Hudson MV. Module IV, hemodialysis devices. In:*Core Curriculum for the Dialysis Technician.* Thousand Oaks, California: Medical Media Publishing; 1992:14.)

in a plastic housing. This design provides a large surface area and low blood volume and blood flow resistance. Blood is channeled through the lumens of the fibers (approximately 200 μ in diameter) while the dialysate is distributed around the fiber bundle in a countercurrent direction. The thickness of the fiber wall (between 6 and 40 μ) allows efficient solute diffusion and sufficient rigidity to accommodate high transmembrane hydrostatic pressures for effective ultrafiltration. They are available with effective surface areas between 0.22 and 2.5 m^2. Pediatric hollow-fiber dialyzers have blood compartment volumes between 18 and 60 mL, making them well suited for small animal hemodialysis.

(3). Synthetic membrane (polysulfone and polyacrylonitrile) hollow-fiber dialyzers have high diffusion, ultrafiltration, and biocompatibility characteristics that permit high-efficiency hemodialysis therapy with shorter treatment intervals and better fluid, solute, and middle molecule removal. High-efficiency therapies require high blood and dialysate flow to exploit the increased diffusive and convective transfer rates and dialysis delivery systems capable of precise regulation, monitoring, and adjustment of these parameters.

2. Vascular access.
   a. Ready and repeatable access to the animal's vasculature to deliver blood to the dialyzer and to return the dialyzed blood to the animal is fundamental to hemodialysis.
   b. In 1960, the development of the exteriorized arteriovenous shunt facilitated the delivery of both acute and chronic hemodialysis to human patients.[35] Use of arteriovenous shunts has been largely replaced by alternative angioaccess in human patients, but until recently shunts were the mainstay in veterinary hemodialysis.[7,8,14,44] The arteriovenous shunt is composed of two exteriorized Silastic tubes connected to Teflon vessel cannulas inserted surgically in a peripheral artery and vein. For hemodialysis treatments, the arterial limb of the shunt supplies blood to the dialyzer; the dialyzed blood is returned to the patient via the venous limb. During nondialysis periods, the free ends of the silicone tubes are connected, to establish a free-flowing arteriovenous circuit (shunt). The low thrombogenicity of the shunt materials and the rapid flow of blood through the access maintain its patency until the next dialysis treatment, without the need for systemic anticoagulation.

      (1). Arteriovenous shunts are generally placed between the femoral artery and vein or the carotid artery and the external jugular vein.[8,44] Once in place, they are available for immediate use and therefore are suitable for acute dialysis treatments.

      (2). Arteriovenous shunts require meticulous surgical placement, impose the risks of arterial catheterization, are prone to clotting, and are ill-suited for ambulatory animals.
   c. More recently, transcutaneous, double-lumen venous catheters have been developed for temporary angioaccess in human patients. These catheters are a more desirable choice for either short-term or long-term use in animals and have generally replaced arteriovenous shunts.[10]

      (1). Transcutaneous catheters are made of polyurethane or silicone and are manufactured in a variety of diameters and lumen configurations, to accommodate either dogs or cats. The catheters may be placed with percutaneous techniques that do not require extensive surgery or prolonged anesthesia. For critical patients, temporary polyurethane catheters* can be inserted quickly with only local analgesia. Silastic catheters placed under general anesthesia are preferable for animals that require prolonged access. In dogs, the catheters† are inserted percutaneously into the external jugular vein, using guidewires and dilators, and are advanced down the vein until the vascular portals are located in the right atrium or cranial vena cava (Fig. 31–4). The extravascular portion of the catheter is tunneled subcutaneously to exit the skin in the cranial area of the neck. A subcutaneous Dacron cuff on the catheter stabilizes it in position, prevents accidental displacement from the vessel, and impairs extension of local infections. The external jugular vein of cats is too small to accommodate the percutaneous placement sheaths, but No. 8 French pediatric dialysis catheters‡ can be inserted through a transverse venotomy following surgical isolation of the external jugular vein.

      (2). Between dialysis treatments, both lumens of the catheter are filled with heparin to prevent clotting, the cutaneous exit site is treated with povidone-iodine ointment,

*Quinton Mahurkar Dual Lumen Catheters, Quinton Instrument Co., Seattle, Washington 98121-2791.

†Permcath Dual Lumen Catheters, Quinton Instrument Co., Seattle, Washington 98121-2791.

‡Pediatric Hemo-Cath (diameter, 18 cm; length, 18 cm) MEDCOMP, INC, Harleysville, Pennsylvania 19438.

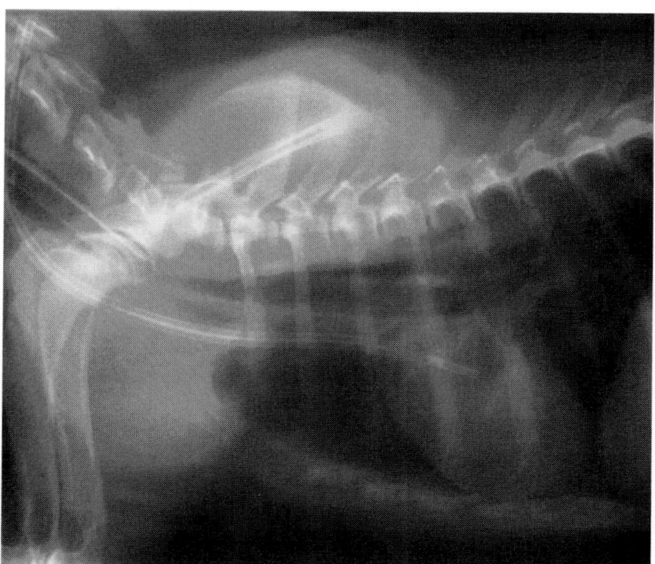

FIG. 31–4. Lateral thoracic radiograph illustrates a transcutaneous dual-lumen dialysis catheter in the external jugular vein of a dog. Note the tip of the catheter in the right atrium.

and the entire catheter is protected in a bandage. Long-term administration of small doses of aspirin, 1 to 5 mg/kg/d (dogs) or every 48 hours (cats), helps to prevent luminal thrombosis.

(3). Properly maintained, transcutaneous venous catheters remain patent and serviceable for many months. Catheters have to be replaced if they become physically damaged, nonpatent, or infected. In most cases, the catheter should be replaced in the opposite jugular vein. The less flexible polyurethane catheters used for acute temporary vascular access are prone to kinking and physical damage, but can often be replaced with a permanent catheter without additional surgery by using a wire guide.

d. Surgically constructed arteriovenous fistulas or grafts are the access of choice for humans with chronic renal failure. They are subcutaneous anastomoses created from native vessels (fistula) or synthetic (polytetrafluoroethylene) vessel material (graph) that directly interconnect a major peripheral artery (usually the radial artery) with a peripheral vein (the cephalic vein). Once created and matured, the fistula develops in a large-diameter completely subcutaneous vascular channel with a natural endothelial lining and fast blood flow. During dialysis sessions, blood is withdrawn with needles from the arterial end of the fistula and returned downstream toward the venous end. Recirculation of dialyzed blood is minimized by the distance between the needles and the rapid flow of blood through the access.

(1). Arteriovenous fistulas or grafts have not been used to any extent in dogs and cats because of the limited availability of adequately sized vessels in sites that would accommodate needle cannulation. Fistulas require many weeks to heal and mature before they become serviceable, and therefore are not suitable for animals with acute renal failure that need immediate dialysis.

(2). Accessible fistulas probably would not afford the rapid blood flow rates required for high-efficiency dialysis techniques used in animals with chronic renal failure.

3. Dialysis delivery system.

The dialysis delivery system (the hemodialysis machine) is the apparatus that determines the amount of dialysate to be delivered from concentrates and continuously monitors the composition, temperature, and pH of the final fluid, controls and monitors extracorporeal flow of blood, regulates the rate of ultrafiltration, and maintains the delivery of anticoagulant to prevent clotting in the blood circuit. The design and sophistication of the delivery system determine what type of dialysis therapy can be provided and what supervision is required during the dialysis session.

a. The dialysate proportioning system mixes a concentrated solute solution termed concentrate with highly purified water to formulate the final dialysate solution.

(1). The proportioning system may produce a fixed-ratio dilution for which the dialysate composition is determined by the content of the preformulated concentrate solution.

(2). More sophisticated proportioning systems use variable-ratio dilution, which permits adjustment and programming (modeling) of dialysate composition throughout the treatment.

(3). The proportioning system also monitors the composition of the dialysate by measuring its conductivity and pH to ensure that it is within safe tolerances. The proportioned dialysate is finally heated to body temperature, degassed, monitored for evidence of blood leaks, and pumped through the dialyzer at constant flow.

(4). If a bicarbonate-based dialysate is used, separate proportioning systems are required for bicarbonate concentrate and the other solutes. The interim solutions are mixed when appropriately diluted to prevent precipitation of calcium and magnesium with the bicarbonate.

(5). Internal alarms are activated if any alteration of conductivity (solute concentration), pH, or temperature occurs, or if a blood leak is detected, and the dialysate is diverted (bypassed) away from the dialyzer to protect the patient until the abnormality is corrected.

b. The extracorporeal circuit routes the patient's blood to and from the dialyzer via the vascular access. It includes the serial arrangement of the "arterial" blood line, an "arterial" drip chamber, the blood pump, the heparin infusion pump, the blood path through the dialyzer, a "venous" drip chamber, the "venous" blood line, an air-foam detector, and the venous line clamp (Fig. 31–5). Pressure and flow monitors detect any compromise to safe blood flow in the pathway.
   (1). If the vascular access is an external arteriovenous shunt, arterial blood is supplied by the arterial limb of the shunt and the dialyzed blood is returned to the venous circulation via the venous limb of the shunt.
   (2). With transcutaneous venous access catheters, "arterial" (to the dialyzer) blood is pumped from the right atrium and an equivalent volume (minus the amount of ultrafiltration) of "venous" (from the dialyzer) blood returns simultaneously to the right atrium.
   (3). Blood leaks, disconnected tubing, and kinks or clots in the blood circuit are detected by changes in pressure in the "arterial" or "venous" segments. They alarm the machine, halt blood flow, and place the system on standby until the alarm conditions are corrected.

c. The ultrafiltration control system regulates the rate and volume of ultrafiltration during the course of dialysis.
   (1). Older dialysis machines incorporate Venturi valves or vacuum pumps on the effluent side of the dialyzer to generate negative pressure in the dialysate compartment. The rate of ultrafiltration is regulated by adjusting the negative pressure in the dialysate compartment to achieve a transmembrane pressure appropriate for the desired fluid removal. Transmembrane pressure fluctuates as blood flow and dialysis conditions change. Therefore, they must be closely monitored on these systems to prevent excessive ultrafiltration and overt volume depletion in small animals.
   (2). More sophisticated delivery systems provide precise volumetric systems in which the desired volume or rate of fluid removal is selected at the start of the dialysis session and in which ultrafiltration controllers automatically and accurately regulate ultrafiltration throughout the treatment. Precision ultrafiltration controllers are preferable for dialysis in small animals to ensure that subtle or undetected fluctuations in transmembrane pressure do not cause serious volume depletion and hypotension.

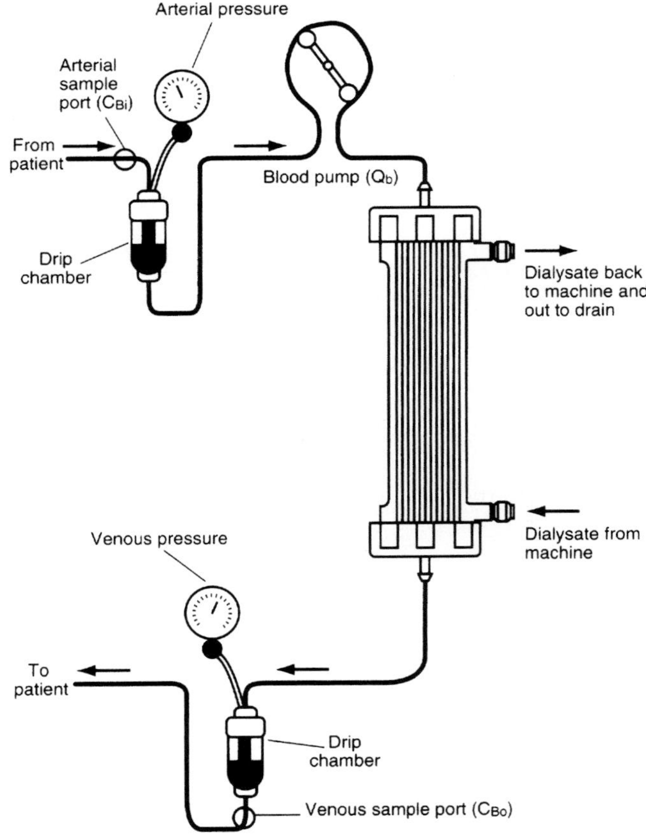

FIG. 31–5. Schematic representation of the typical extracorporeal blood path used for hemodialysis. (Burrows-Hudson S, Hudson MV. Module IV, hemodialysis devices. In: *Core Curriculum for the Dialysis Technician.* Thousand Oaks, California: Medical Media Publishing; 1992:34.)

4. Dialysate composition.
   a. The dialysate must be formulated to accomplish the diffusive and convective requirements of the dialysis prescription without adversely affecting normal solute composition, pH, and volume of body fluids. The composition of the dialysate approximates the composition of "normal" extracellular fluid, but it is frequently tailored to the particular needs of the patient or the type of dialysis being performed.
   b. The large and continuous volume of dialysate used in hemodialysis (approximately 500 mL/min) is produced by dilution of commercial salt concentrates; however, available concentrates

are formulated for human use and without modification are not necessarily suitable for dogs or cats. Dialysis delivery systems with fixed proportioning often require the addition of more solute to the concentrate to achieve the desired composition in the diluted dialysate. Delivery systems with flexible proportioning systems permit adjustment of the composition of the dialysate from a single concentrate and therefore are better able to match the needs of animals. When modifying the dialysate, one must calculate carefully the total amount of solute required to "spike" the concentrate to produce the desired adjustment in the diluted product.

(1). For example, 1 gallon (3.78 L) of concentrate may produce 35 gallons (132.3 L) of usable dialysate (1:35 fixed dilution). Adjustment of the sodium concentration of the dialysate from 135 mmol/L (a typical concentration for human dialysis) to 145 mmol/L (suitable for canine dialysis) requires the addition of 1323 mmol (10 mmol/L × 132.3 L) or 76.7 g of sodium chloride to the original gallon of concentrate. Whenever supplements are added to the concentrate, the composition of the diluted dialysate should be measured to determine if it matches the calculated expectation.

(2). Sodium is the major solute in the dialysate. Recommendations for its concentration have been revised in recent years. Dialysates with a sodium concentration lower than that of plasma (130 to 135 mmol/L) were advocated to facilitate fluid and sodium removal for hypertension control. Hyponatremic dialysate, however, causes exaggerated transcellular osmotic gradients, as both urea and sodium are rapidly removed from extracellular fluid, thereby promoting nausea, vomiting, muscle cramps, extracellular fluid volume contraction, and hypotension.[2,39] With modern hemodialyzers and high-efficiency delivery systems, the requirements for sodium and fluid removal can be accomplished readily with ultrafiltration. The current convention of using physiologic concentrations of sodium in the dialysate has minimized signs of osmotic shift disequilibrium and hypotension and permitted faster ultrafiltration.[2,27,34,38]

(a). Some delivery systems support sodium modeling, which allows delivery of variable dialysate sodium concentrations throughout the dialysis session. With sodium modeling, the sodium concentration of the dialysate is set high during the early phases of dialysis to counter the transcellular urea gradient when the potential for osmotic shift complications is greatest. Dialysate sodium is reduced later in the session, so the patient ends the treatment with a normal serum sodium concentration without the risk of hypernatremia and hypertonicity.[29,32]

(b). The relatively large extracorporeal volume and profound azotemia frequently seen with acute uremia predispose animal patients to hypotension and osmotic shift complications at the start of dialysis. Many animals are also volume depleted and hypotensive from protracted vomiting, diarrhea, and reduced consumption of water. We have found that modeling dialysate sodium remarkably improves the hemodynamic stability of these animals throughout the dialysis session and reduces the frequency of disequilibrium signs.

(1′). We routinely model the dialysate sodium to produce a programmed continuous reduction in sodium from 155 to 145 mmol/L in dogs, and from 160 to 150 mmol/L in cats.

(2′). If sodium modeling is not available, a dialysate sodium concentration within the physiologic range (145 mmol/L for dogs, 150 mmol/L for cats) is appropriate. Most commercial dialysate concentrates do not proportion to these concentrations unless the delivery system has a variable sodium option and is supplemented with sodium chloride.

(3). Commercial concentrates can be obtained with a variety of predefined potassium concentrations to meet the requirements of the dialysis session. Animals with acute oliguric renal failure, sepsis, or severe catabolism may be hyperkalemic and require rapid correction of serum potassium with a low-potassium dialysate (0 to 3 mmol/L). Later in the course of the therapy, but before the patient is eating and vomiting or diarrhea is controlled, the potassium in the dialysate may need to be adjusted to more physiologic values (3 to 4 mmol/L) to minimize the potential for potassium depletion. A dialysate concentrate formulated to yield a final potassium concentration of 3 mmol/L is generally satisfactory for both acute and maintenance hemodialysis. If hypokalemia is a persistent concern, a concentrate formulated for a higher potassium concentration should be prescribed, or the existing concentrate can be "spiked" to produce a more appropriate concentration.

(4). Selecting acetate or bicarbonate as the buffer replacement in the dialysate may significantly influence the tolerance of the animal for dialysis. The instability of bicarbonate in solution, and the difficulty of formulating a bicarbonate-based dialysate that would not precipitate calcium and magnesium, prompted industry-wide utilization of acetate for base-generating equivalents in commercial dialysate. For most human patients receiving conventional dialysis, the accumulated acetate load is readily converted to bicarbonate and adequately corrects the bicarbonate deficit. However, many elderly, diabetic, or critically ill humans undergoing conventional dialysis are unable to metabolize acetate to bicarbonate effectively, and thus become acetate intolerant as a result of its accumulation.[20,24,26] The current widespread use of highly permeable dialyzers and development of high-efficiency dialysis techniques exposed the consequences of excessive acetate accumulation and acetate intolerance, the uncompensated clearance of bicarbonate, and the negative base balance that developed during acetate-based dialysis in otherwise stable chronic dialysis patients.[19,24,31]

(a). Low acetate concentrations in the dialysate or its ineffective conversion to bicarbonate may not provide sufficient buffer to balance net acid production rates and replenish existing bicarbonate deficits. Consequently, bone buffer reserves are consumed to maintain hydrogen ion balance.[18,48]

(b). Large acetate loads produce peripheral vasodilation and reduce myocardial contractility and myocardial energetics, resulting in systemic hypotension and hemodynamic instability.[24,49]

(c). Acetate-based dialysis induces hypoxemia because of decreased metabolic production and gradient-dependent losses of carbon dioxide, which produce hypoventilation.

(d). Acetate dialysis is also associated with higher prevalences of nausea, vomiting, headache, and fatigue in human patients.

(e). Acetate-based dialysis is well tolerated by stable patients undergoing conventional hemodialysis; however, for patients with cardiovascular or hemodynamic instability, intermediary metabolic defects, such as diabetes or malnutrition, or sepsis, bicarbonate-based dialysis is preferable.

(f). Complications associated with acetate and the thrust for more efficient dialysis treatments promoted development of dialysis delivery systems with separate proportioning pathways for bicarbonate concentrates. Bicarbonate-based dialysis has now become widely accepted and preferred. It physiologically corrects the acidosis, promotes hemodynamic stability, facilitates rapid rates of fluid removal and solute transfer, obviates the symptoms of acetate intolerance, and improves patient comfort during the dialysis session.

(1′). No available data document the superiority of bicarbonate over acetate dialysis in animals; however, our experience using bicarbonate-based dialysis during the past 4 years confirms improvements in intradialysis hypotension, vomiting, fatigue, and hypoxemia, as compared with acetate dialysis. Also, acetate-based dialysis would be unlikely to permit the intensive hemodialysis prescriptions we currently use for intermittent maintenance dialysis in dogs.

(2′). Our dialysis experience in cats has been entirely with bicarbonate dialysates; however, the small blood volume of cats relative to the extracorporeal volume could easily exacerbate the hemodynamic effects of acetate and predispose cats to acetate intolerance.

(g). Owing to the nearly universal conversion to bicarbonate-based dialysis in human nephrology, more surplus acetate-based delivery systems will be available. Whether these systems will be as acceptable, effective, or safe for animal dialysis as are the newer bicarbonate-based delivery systems is unlikely.

(5). The most abundant component of dialysate is water. During a single dialysis session, the animal is exposed to approximately 150 L of water. The magnitude of this exposure demands that the water used for the dialysate be chemically pure. Minute traces of routine impurities, water treatment chemicals (fluorine, chloramine), herbicides, bacteria, viruses, or endotoxins (which are perfectly safe and tolerated in drinking water) constitute a formidable toxic and health risk for dialysis patients. To ensure that water quality meets these exacting standards, supply water must be processed sequentially with 1) filters to remove particulate materials, 2) carbon filters to absorb organic solutes, 3) water softeners to reduce excessive amounts of calcium and magnesium, and 4) deionization to remove inorganic cations and anions. Reverse osmosis is used as a final "polishing" treatment to remove approximately 99% of the contaminants. The supply plumbing must also be maintained free from bacterial and chemical contamination, so that the purified water is not tainted en route to the dialysis delivery system.

C. Hemodialysis prescription.

1. The prescription for hemodialysis is formulated to the specific needs of the patient and is influenced by the available facilities, the medical condition, and the species of the patient. The following guidelines reflect my current experience using a bicarbonate-based, volumetrically controlled dialysis delivery system.*
2. Acute hemodialysis.
   a. Dialyzer (hollow-fiber design) with a surface area between 0.6 and 1.0 m^2 and a priming volume of approximately 50 mL is appropriate for dogs larger than 5 kg body weight.† There have been no clinical comparisons of cellulosic and synthetic membrane dialyzers, but anecdotal experience has shown Hemophan to be less thrombogenic and better tolerated than Cuprophane materials. For cats, a dialyzer with a surface area between 0.2 and 0.3 m^2 and a priming volume of less than 20 mL is used.‡
   b. Blood flow rates should be restricted to 3 to 5 mL/kg/min for the first few treatments to prevent dialysis disequilibrium. In later sessions, blood flow can be increased to 10 to 15 mL/kg/min for more intensive treatments.
   c. Dialysis time for the initial 1 to 3 sessions, when the risk for dialysis disequilibrium is highest, should be limited to approximately 120 minutes. The combination of blood flow rate and the length of the dialysis session largely determines the intensity of the dialysis treatment. These parameters should be selected to achieve a postdialysis-predialysis BUN ratio no greater than 0.5. When the predialysis BUN is less than 100 mg/dL, subsequent treatments can be extended to 180 to 300 minutes and faster blood flow rates can be incorporated to achieve maximal reduction of azotemia.
   d. Dialysate composition should be formulated for each patient, but a standardized solution with the following composition is usually appropriate: sodium, 145 mmol/L (dogs) or 155 mmol/L (cats); potassium, 3.0 mmol/L; bicarbonate, 35 mmol/L; chloride, 107 mmol/L (dogs) or 117 mmol/L (cats); calcium, 3.0 mmol/L; magnesium, 1.0 mmol/L; dextrose 200 mg/dL. Dialysate flow is conventionally 500 mL/min.
      (1). If the delivery system permits variable proportioning, a modeled dialysate with sodium concentrations of 155 mmol/L for the initial 20% of the session, 150 mmol/L for the next 40% of the session, and 145 mmol/L for the remainder of the session have been effective in dogs to minimize dialysis disequilibrium and hypotension. For cats, the respective sodium concentrations are 165 mmol/L, 160 mmol/L, and 155 mmol/L.
      (2). A dialysate potassium value of 3.0 to 3.5 mmol/L corrects hyperkalemia in most animals and eliminates the need to stock concentrate with no potassium.
      (3). For bicarbonate-based delivery systems, the bicarbonate concentration should be 25 to 35 mmol/L for the initial treatments. The lower value is chosen for patients with severe metabolic acidosis, as rapid correction of the bicarbonate deficit might exacerbate dialysis disequilibrium or paradoxic cerebral acidosis. A lower bicarbonate concentration should be selected for animals with pre-existing alkalemia. If a dialysate containing acetate is used, the acetate concentration should be approximately 35 mmol/L for animals that are hemodynamically stable and not alkalemic.
   e. Ultrafiltration is prescribed, according to the condition of the patient. Initially most animals with acute uremia are volume depleted and require no ultrafiltration; however, aggressive fluid therapy to induce diuresis usually causes fluid overload in animals admitted for hemodialysis. An ultrafiltration rate is selected to lessen the fluid burden, correct pulmonary edema and congestive heart failure, and facilitate ongoing fluid therapies like parenteral nutrition. Elimination of the entire fluid load during the first dialysis session is usually unnecessary and unsafe, but 20 to 50 mL/kg of

*Centrysystem 3 Dialysis Delivery Systems, Cobe Laboratories, Inc., Lakewood, Colorado 80228.

†Cobe Centrysystem 200 HG, COBE Laboratories, Inc., Lakewood, Colorado 80228.

‡Cobe Centrysystem 100 HG, COBE Laboratories, Inc., Lakewood, Colorado 80228.

ultrafiltration can be prescribed at successive sessions in the early stages of therapy, to achieve a suitable dry weight.

3. Chronic intermittent hemodialysis.
   a. The application of intermittent dialysis therapy for supportive management of animals with end-stage renal disease is a new and provocative direction in veterinary therapeutics. The objective of dialysis therapy in human patients with end-stage renal disease is to provide excretory replacement for the failing kidneys. In contrast, the objective in animal patients is to provide merely an "excretory boost," which lessens the persistent azotemia and urea exposure. How much hemodialysis is necessary to control uremia *adequately* is a topic of considerable interest and controversy in human nephrology. At present, adequacy of the hemodialysis prescription is predicated on kinetic modeling of urea removal, which corresponds to clinical predictors of patient well-being.[5,12,17]
   b. Because of economic and logistic issues, attainment of similar adequacy standards in animals is unlikely. As an alternative, intensive intermittent hemodialysis can be provided every 3 to 7 days to supplement the residual excretory capacity of the diseased kidneys. The dialysis prescription is formulated to maximally reduce the azotemia during these intermittent sessions.
      (1). Animals with end-stage renal disease or decompensated chronic renal failure should be treated initially with an acute dialysis prescription until the predialysis BUN is less than 100 mg/dL. This usually requires 2 to 3 dialysis sessions, after which the animal can go to a more intensive maintenance dialysis schedule. The goals for maintenance dialysis are to reduce clinical signs of uremia, minimize the degree of azotemia, and facilitate conservative medical therapies. The dialysis prescription should promote a predialysis BUN value of less than 90 mg/dL and a time-averaged BUN of 60 mg/dL or less over the interdialysis interval. The time-averaged BUN concentration is a kinetically modeled value that reflects the effective urea exposure or total body burden of urea over the dialysis cycle (Fig. 31–6).
      (2). The choice of dialyzer and dialysate composition is generally the same as that for acute dialysis. The dialysate bicarbonate concentration is generally 25 to 35 mmol/L to maintain adequate buffer reserves in the interdialysis interval.
      (3). Blood flow and dialysis time are the major variables that change with maintenance dialysis. After initial dialysis sessions, the risks of dialysis disequilibrium are small. Therefore, more intensive prescriptions can be provided for maximum efficacy. Blood flow rates between 8 and 12 mL/kg/min are well tolerated, but a bicarbonate-based dialysate is probably required for blood flow rates greater than 5 mL/kg/min. For "high-efficiency" dialysis, blood flow can be cautiously increased to

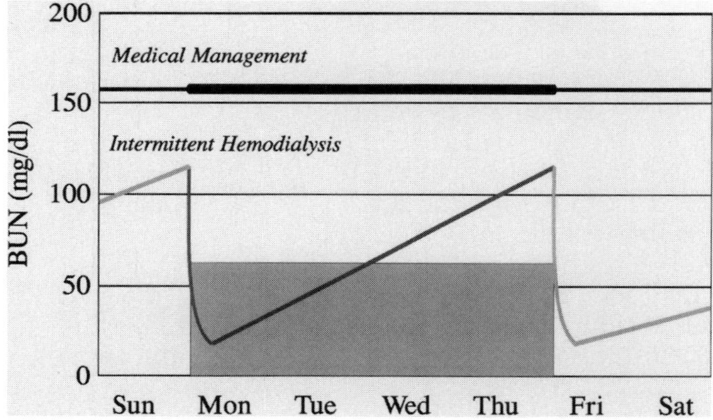

FIG. 31–6 Conceptualized daily changes in BUN before (Medical Management) and following (Intermittent Hemodialysis) the initiation of hemodialysis treatments in animals with end-stage renal disease. The darkened segment on the lower curve reflects the change in BUN during sequential hemodialysis treatments and the intervening interdialysis period. The shaded insert on this curve depicts the "time-averaged" urea concentration (see text) during the dialysis cycle. The expanded segment on the upper curve depicts the corresponding urea exposure in the animals before hemodialysis treatments. The data reflect the mean values from 12 dogs with chronic renal failure in response to 85 hemodialysis treatments. Reproduced with permission from Cowgill LD. Veterinary applications of hemodialysis: an update. In Bonagura JD, ed. Kirk's Current Veterinary Therapy XII. Philadelphia: WB Saunders; 1994.

15 to 20 mL/kg/min. At these faster flow rates, blood pressure and pulse rate must be carefully monitored to ensure that the animal remains hemodynamically stable. Dialysis time is extended to 240 to 300 minutes to maximize urea removal. The session can be shorter if the patient has reasonable residual renal function, if a high-efficiency dialyzer is used, or if the frequency of dialysis is increased to three times per week.

(4). The amount of residual renal function dictates the intensity of the dialysis schedule that must be maintained for an adequate dialysis prescription. Three treatments per week is traditional for human patients and is used as an intermediate schedule for animals with acute renal failure. The inconvenience, expense, and client commitment of thrice weekly dialysis is impractical for animals that require maintenance dialysis indefinitely. Consequently, a less frequent but more intensive dialysis regimen must be utilized. The frequency is determined by the residual renal function, dietary protein intake, and catabolic status of the patient.

(a). Our initial goal is to provide dialysis once weekly for as long as it is possible to maintain the predialysis BUN less than 90 mg/dL and the weekly time-averaged BUN less than 60 mg/dL. This regimen is effective for animals with a serum creatinine value that is approximately 6 to 8 mg/dL.

(b). As serum creatinine increases to 8 to 10 mg/dL, the schedule is increased to every 5 days.

(c). Animals with a serum creatinine value greater than 10 mg/dL require a twice weekly schedule to be dialyzed adequately. Fig. 31–7 illustrates the effect of different weekly dialysis schedules on BUN and time-averaged BUN in a dog receiving high-efficiency hemodialysis treatments. Despite the efficiency of the individual dialysis session, a once weekly schedule is clearly inadequate for animals with advanced uremia.

(d). Each dialysis session for animals with advanced renal failure must achieve a urea reduction rate approaching 85 to 90% (see Table 31–3). This requires blood flow rates approaching 20 mL/kg/min and a dialyzer with a high urea clearance.

D. Complications of hemodialysis.

1. Complications associated with hemodialysis result from both the technical complexities of the procedure and the clinical compromise of the dialysis patient. The prevalence of specific complications is different in the intradialysis and the interdialysis periods and for acute and chronic hemodialysis treatments. Elimination of all risks associated with hemodialysis is clearly impossible, but meticulous patient supervision and improvements in dialysis delivery minimize many of these hazards.
2. During the intradialysis period, the most common complications include transient hypotension,

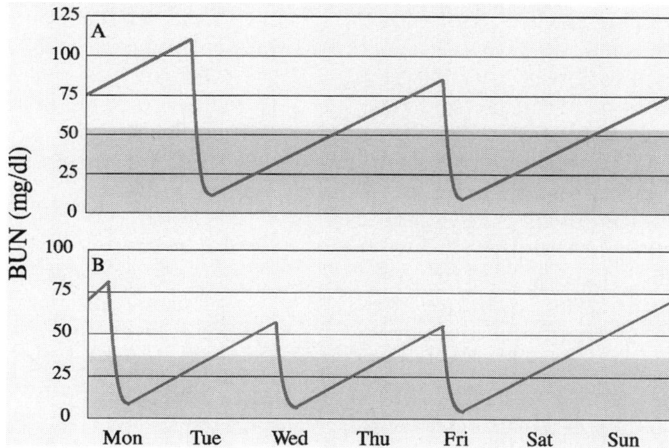

FIG. 31–7. Kinetically modeled effect of hemodialysis schedule on BUN and time-averaged BUN (shaded blocks) in a 25-kg dog with no residual renal function receiving 5 hours of intensive hemodialysis therapy (Kt/V = 2.59) twice (A, upper panel) or three (B, lower panel) times weekly. For the twice weekly (Tuesday, Friday) schedule, the average predialysis BUN is 98 mg/dL and the time-averaged BUN is 54 mg/dL. Thrice weekly (Monday, Wednesday, Friday) dialysis decreases the average predialysis BUN to 64 mg/dL and the time-averaged BUN to 36 mg/dL.

vomiting, tremors, seizures, clotting in the extracorporeal circuit, and blood loss.

a. Hypotensive episodes usually arise from aggressive ultrafiltration, excessive blood flow rates, or use of acetate-based dialysate, and they are readily resolved with modification of the dialysis prescription and fluid supplementation. Use of pediatric and neonatal extracorporeal blood sets, bicarbonate-based dialysate, ultrafiltration controllers, sodium modeling, and priming of the extracorporeal circuit with dextran solutions (in animals that weigh less than 6 kg) improves the hemodynamic stability of animals during dialysis.

b. Vomiting frequently occurs at the start of the dialysis session and may be caused by the dialysis procedure itself or by uremia. The association of vomiting with the initiation of dialysis indicates that it is caused by some aspect of the extracorporeal circulation, hypotension, or bioincompatibility reactions. Initiating the extracorporeal flow gradually and using bicarbonate-based dialysate reduce the incidence of vomiting. Protracted vomiting during the dialysis session is usually caused by uremia and should be treated with local and central-acting antiemetics.

c. During rapid dialysis of severely azotemic animals, the rate of solute removal from the extracellular space can exceed its redistribution from intracellular pools, causing transcellular osmotic gradients. Dialysis disequilibrium occurs as fluid shifts along the gradient into the intracellular compartment, causing an increase in brain water content. The signs of disequilibrium syndrome include restlessness, tremors, vocalization, and seizures and may develop during initial dialysis sessions in animals with severe azotemia. Dialysis disequilibrium is managed by decreasing the intensity and duration of the dialysis session, slowing changes in blood pH by lowering the dialysate bicarbonate concentration, and administering hypertonic mannitol to reduce the transcellular osmotic pressure. Seizures are treated symptomatically with diazepam. Sodium-modeling techniques and adherence to conservative dialysis prescriptions for severely azotemic animals minimize the tendency toward—and severity of—these episodes.

d. Clotting in the dialyzer or extracorporeal circuit can occur during acute or chronic dialysis sessions. It is more common in initial dialysis treatments, when blood flow is slower and the heparin requirement of the patient is not yet established. Clotting impairs the efficiency of the dialysis treatment and constitutes blood loss that cannot be returned at the end of the session. Clotting can be minimized by carefully regulating the heparin infusion, monitoring coagulation times, and using fast blood flow rates and substituted cellulosic or synthetic dialyzer.

e. Bleeding from the site of vascular access, venipuncture, a surgical incision, or renal biopsy or from gastrointestinal ulcers or intraocular hemorrhages may occur in excessively anticoagulated animals during or following hemodialysis treatments. Bleeding is more common in animals with acute renal failure. Whenever possible, access placement should be performed with the least invasive technique and as long as possible before the dialysis session. Anticoagulation prescriptions should be minimized and closely monitored with serial coagulation measurements during the dialysis session. Heparin requirements can be reduced by use of faster blood flow rates and cellulose or synthetic membrane dialyzers that are less thrombogenic. Animals with prolonged or severe bleeding and those at risk of intracranial, intraocular, or gastric hemorrhage should be treated with protamine sulfate at the end of the dialysis session, to neutralize the residual heparin and normalize coagulation time. Inadvertent chronic blood loss is a predictable consequence of hemodialysis that promotes or exacerbates anemia in animals with compromised ability to regenerate the losses. Blood loss occurs from blood sampling for laboratory procedures and anticoagulation monitoring, removal of the heparin lock, clotting in the dialyzer, and incomplete rinseback of extracorporeal blood at the end of the dialysis session. Cumulatively, these blood losses become significant and require regular transfusion or administration of recombinant human erythropoietin to replete red blood cell mass.[9] (See Chapter 29, Medical Management of the Anemia of Chronic Renal Failure.)

3. Major complications in the interdialysis period include clotting of the vascular access device, sepsis, bleeding, thromboembolism, and inadequate dialysis.

a. Clotting of the vascular access port is less common with transcutaneous venous catheters than with exteriorized arteriovenous shunts, but it can be anticipated in most patients as dialysis therapy extends beyond 2 weeks. Positioning of the catheter tip, the shape and composition of the catheter, and intrinsic characteristics of the patient influence the development of access clots. In most instances, repositioning of the access and careful dislodgement and aspiration of the clot are sufficient to restore patency. In some cases, instillation of fibrinolytic agents or replacement of the catheter is required. Catheter patency is prolonged by carefully maintained heparin locks in the interdialysis period and

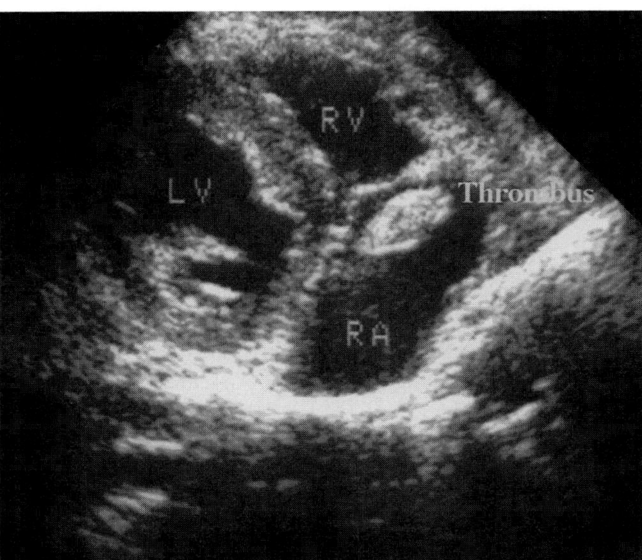

FIG. 31–8. Right parasternal cardiac ultrasound image demonstrating a thrombus in the right atrium (RA) of a cat with a transcutaneous venous hemodialysis catheter. RV, right ventricle; LV, left ventricle.

administration of small doses of aspirin (1 to 3 mg/kg/d for dogs and 1 to 3 mg/kg every 48 hours for cats).

b. Subcutaneous or exit site infection of the vascular access port and systemic infection are severe complications of hemodialysis. The potential for infection is high in uremic animals, and it is exacerbated by the exposure imposed with the vascular access and extracorporeal circulation. Every effort must be taken to minimize these risks by strict use of aseptic technique during the dialysis procedure and by active surveillance and treatment of infections.

c. Bleeding may occur in the interdialysis period if the caps and clamps on the vascular access port become disconnected, the catheter is cut or damaged inadvertently, or invasive procedures are performed after the dialysis session while the animal is still anticoagulated. Heparin appears to diffuse from the open portals of the catheter in the interdialysis period. If the concentration of heparin in the catheter lock is too high, the load of heparin may be sufficient to anticoagulate small animals, causing prolonged bleeding time or active hemorrhage. For cats and dogs that weigh less than 5 kg, we use heparin, 500 U/mL, as a lock solution in the catheter. For dogs between 5 and 15 kg, we use 1000 U/mL heparin locks. For dogs that weigh more than 15 kg, 1000 to 3000 U/mL heparin is used.

d. Venous thrombosis leading to pulmonary thromboembolism is a serious complication associated with transcutaneous venous catheters. Tachypnea is the most common clinical manifestation, but spontaneous pneumothorax and pulmonary infarction may also develop. The emboli arise from thrombus formation at the tip of the catheter, in the right atrium, or along the cranial vena cava (Fig. 31–8). Whether catheter design or materials, placement techniques, or host interactions predispose to thrombus formation in animals is not known. Venous thrombosis is an infrequent complication of transcutaneous dialysis catheters in human patients, suggesting its prevalence in dogs and cats may result from unique interactions between the catheters and their respective coagulation mechanisms.[47] We routinely monitor animals undergoing prolonged hemodialysis with cardiac ultrasound, to identify development of subclinical venous thrombi.

e. Inadequate dialysis and failure to control the manifestations of uremia occur if the dialysis schedule or the intensity of dialysis treatments for acute or chronic renal failure is insufficient to control the azotemia. Clearly, as residue renal function approaches zero, once weekly dialysis is inadequate for patients with chronic renal failure, regardless of the intensity of the dialysis delivered (see Fig. 31–7). Similarly, three sessions per week may be required to control uremia in animals with acute renal failure that are severely catabolic. Anorexia, nausea, weight loss, and vomiting may be difficult to correct with twice weekly dialysis, despite adequate control of the time-average BUN.

E. Future of dialysis therapy.

1. By the very nature of its complexity, and the specificity of the clinical conditions for which it is targeted, dialysis therapy is unlikely to become a staple of veterinary practice. Nevertheless, for a large population of companion dogs and cats with acute and chronic uremia, no alternative exists except renal transplantation or euthanasia.
2. For these animals, dialysis therapy is a technical reality. Increased awareness and acceptance of dialysis by primary care veterinarians, the increased sophistication of specialty veterinary practice and academic centers able to support these services, increased training of veterinary internists with an interest in nephrology, and the increased demand by pet owners for these services are sufficient reasons to foster expansion of veterinary dialysis on a regional basis. In my opinion, hemodialysis is the most versatile, uniformly effective, and promising form of dialysis therapy for animals; however, technical improvements will continue to improve the efficiency and safety of both peritoneal dialysis and hemodialysis in the future.
3. Chronic ambulatory peritoneal dialysis has never gained acceptance as a therapy for end-stage renal disease, but it should be re-evaluated as a home-management alternative for the supportive management of chronic renal failure in animals.

REFERENCES

1. Abel JJ, Rowntree LC, Turner BB. On the removal of diffusible substances from the circulating blood by means of dialysis. *Trans Assoc Am Physiol.* 1913; 28:41.
2. Acchiardo SR, Hayden AJ. Is Na^+ modeling necessary in high flux dialysis. *Trans Am Soc Artif Intern Organs.* 1991; 37:M135–M137.
3. Ash SR, Johnson H, Hartman J, et al. The column-disc peritoneal catheter. A peritoneal access device with improved drainage. *Trans Am Soc Artif Intern Organs.* 1980; 3:109.
4. Birchard SJ, Chew DJ, Crisp MS, Fossum TW. Modified technique for placement of a column disc peritoneal dialysis catheter. *J Am Anim Hosp Assoc.* 1988; 24:663–666.
5. Bosch JP. Prescribing high-efficiency treatments. *Cont Issues Nephrol.* 1993; 27:135–149.
6. Carter LJ, Wingfield WE, Allen TA. Clinical experience with peritoneal dialysis in small animals. *Comp Contin Educ.* 1989; 11:1335–1343.
7. Cowgill LD, Bovee KC. Current status of hemodialysis and renal transplantation. In: Kirk RW, ed. *Current Veterinary Therapy. Small Animal Practice.* 5th ed. Philadelphia, Pennsylvania: WB Saunders; 1977.
8. Cowgill LD. Current status of veterinary hemodialysis. In: Kirk RW, ed. *Current Veterinary Therapy. Small Animal Practice.* 7th ed. Philadelphia, Pennsylvania: WB Saunders; 1980.
9. Cowgill LD. Use of recombinant human erythropoietin: An update. In: Kirk RW, Bonagura JD, eds. *Kirk's Current Veterinary Therapy.* 12th ed. Philadelphia, Pennsylvania: WB Saunders; 1994.
10. Cowgill LD, Maretzki CH. Veterinary applications of hemodialysis: an update. In: Kirk RW, Bonagura JD, eds. *Kirk's Current Veterinary Therapy.* 12th ed. Philadelphia, Pennsylvania: WB Saunders; 1994.
11. Crisp MS, Chew DJ, DiBartola SP, Bichard SJ. Peritoneal dialysis in dogs and cats: 27 cases (1976–1987). *J Am Vet Med Assoc.* 1989; 195:1262–1266.
12. Depner TA. Urea modeling: Introduction. In: Depner TA, ed. *Prescribing Hemodialysis: A Guide to Urea Modeling.* Boston, Massachusetts: Kluwer Academic Publishers; 1991.
13. Depner TA. Measuring dialysis: How much is enough? In: Depner TA, ed. *Prescribing Hemodialysis: A Guide to Urea Modeling.* Boston, Massachusetts: Kluwer Academic Publishers; 1991.
14. Dhein CRM. Hemodialysis in the dog. *Comp Contin Educ.* 1981; 3:1031–1045.
15. Everett ED. Peritonitis: Risk assessment and management. *Contemp Issues Nephrol.* 1990; 22:145–165.
16. Excerpts from United States Renal Data System 1991 Annual Data Report. *Am J Kidney Dis.* 1993; 28:1–127.
17. Gotch FA, Sargent JA. A mechanistic analysis of the national cooperative dialysis study (NCDS). *Kidney Int.* 1985; 28:526–534.
18. Gotch FA, Sargent JA, Keen ML. Hydrogen ion balance in dialysis therapy. *Artif Organs.* 1982; 6:388–395.
19. Hakim RM, Pontzer MA, Tilton D, et al. Effects of acetate and bicarbonate dialysate in stable chronic dialysis patients. *Kidney Int.* 1985; 28:535–540.
20. Huyghebaert MF, Dhainaut J-F, Monsallier JF, Schlemmer B. Bicarbonate hemodialysis of patients with acute renal failure and severe sepsis. *Crit Care Med.* 1985; 13:840.
21. Khanna R. Peritoneal dialysis access. *Contemp Issues Nephrol.* 1990; 22:101–126.
22. Kiil F. Development of a parallel flow artificial kidney in plastics. *Acta Chir Scand.* 1960; 253(Suppl):142–150.
23. Lane IF, Carter LJ, Lappin MR. Peritoneal dialysis: An update on methods and usefulness. In: Kirk RW, ed. *Current Veterinary Therapy. Small Animal Practice.* Philadelphia, Pennsylvania: WB Saunders; 1992.
24. Ledebo I. Bicarbonate in high-efficiency hemodialysis. *Contin Issues Nephrol.* 1993; 27:9–25.
25. Leehey DJ, Gandhi VC, Daugirdas JT. Peritonitis. In: Daugirdas JT, Ing TS, eds. *Handbook of Dialysis.* Boston, Massachusetts: Little, Brown; 1988.
26. Leunissen KML, Hoorntje SJ, Fiers HA, et al. Acetate versus bicarbonate hemodialysis in critically ill patients. *Nephron.* 1986; 42:146–151.
27. Levine T, Falk B, Henriquez M, et al. Effects of varying dialysate sodium using large surface area dialyzers. *Trans Am Soc Artif Intern Organs.* 1978; 24:139–141.
28. Maiorca R, Cancarini GC. Experiences with the Y-system. *Contemp Issues Nephrol.* 1990; 22:167–186.
29. Muriassco A, France G, Leblond G, et al. Sequential sodium therapy allows correction of sodium volume balance and reduces morbidity. *Clin Nephrol.* 1985; 24:201–208.
30. Nolph KD. Peritoneal Dialysis. In: Brenner BM, Rector FC, eds. *The Kidney.* 4th ed. Vol. 2. Philadelphia, Pennsylvania: WB Saunders, 1991.
31. Novello A, Kelsch RC, Easterling RE. Acetate intolerance during hemodialysis. *Clin Nephrol.* 1976; 5:29.
32. Ogden DA. A double-blind cross-over comparison of high and low sodium dialysis. *Proc Dial Transplant Form.* 1978; 8: 157–165.
33. Parker HR. Peritoneal dialysis and hemofiltration. In: Bovee KC, ed. *Canine Nephrology.* Media, Pennsylvania: Harwal Publishing Co, 1984.
34. Port FK, Johnson WJ, Klass DW. Prevention of dialysis disequilibrium syndrome by use of high sodium concentration in the dialysate. *Kidney Int.* 1973; 3:327–333.
35. Quinton W, Dillard D, Scribner BH. Cannulation of blood vessels for prolonged hemodialysis. *Trans Am Soc Artif Intern Organs.* 1960; 6:104–113.
36. Rubin J, Quintus J, Quillen E, Bower JD. A model of long-term peritoneal dialysis in the dog. *Nephron.* 1983; 35:259–263.
37. Sargent JA, Gotch FA. Principles and biophysics of dialysis. In: Maher JF, ed. *Replacement of Renal Function by Dialysis.* 3rd ed. Dordrecht, Holland: Kluwer Academic Publishers; 1989.
38. Stewart WK, Fleming LW. Blood pressure control during maintenance heamodialysis with isonatric (high sodium) dialysate. *Postgrad Med J.* 1974; 50:260–264.
39. Stewart WK. The composition of dialysis fluid. In: Maher JF, ed. *Replacement of Renal Function by Dialysis.* 3rd ed. Dordrecht, Holland: Kluwer Academic Publishers; 1989.
40. Thornhill JA, Ash SR, Dhein CR, et al. Peritoneal dialysis with the purdue column-disc catheter. *Minn Vet.* 1980; 20:27–30.
41. Thornhill JA. Peritoneal dialysis in the dog and cat: An update. *Comp Contin Educ.* 1981; 3:20–32.
42. Thornhill JA, Hartman J, Boon GD, et al. Support of an anephric dog for 54 days with ambulatory peritoneal dialysis and a newly designed peritoneal catheter. *Am J Vet Res.* 1984; 45:1156–1161.
43. Thornhill JA. Peritonitis associated with peritoneal dialysis: diagnosis and treatment. *JAVMA.* 1983; 182:721–724.
44. Thornhill JA. Hemodialysis. In: Bovee KC, ed. *Canine Nephrology.* Media, Pennsylvania: Harwal Publishing Co; 1984.
45. Thornhill JA. Therapeutic strategies involving antimicrobial treatment of small animals with peritonitis. *J Am Vet Med Assoc.* 1984; 185:1181–1184.
46. Thornhill JA. Continuous ambulatory peritoneal dialysis. In: Kirk RW, ed. *Current Veterinary Therapy. Small Animal Practice.* 11th ed. Philadelphia, Pennsylvania: WB Saunders; 1983.
47. Vathada M, Neiberger RE, Pena DR, et al. Complications of hemodialysis catheters in children. *Dial Transplant.* 1994; 23: 240–247.
48. Ward RA, Wathen RL. Utilization of bicarbonate for base repletion in hemodialysis. *Artif Organs.* 1982; 6:396–403.
49. Ward RA. Acid-base homeostasis in dialysis patients. In: AR Nissenson, RN Fine, DE Gentile, eds. *Clinical Dialysis.* 2nd ed. Norwalk, Connecticut: Appelton & Lange; 1990.

CHAPTER 32

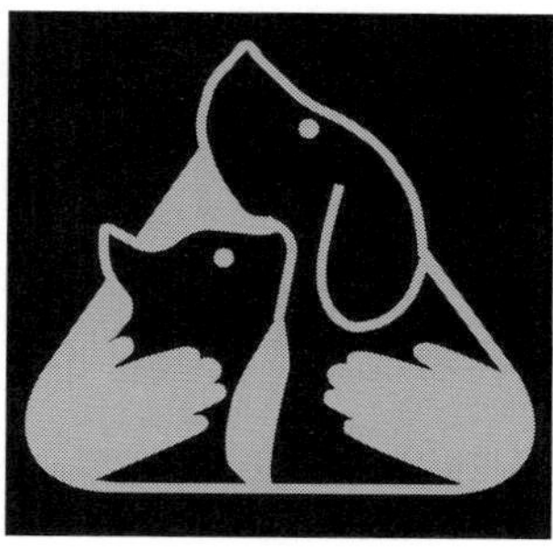

Clinical Renal Transplantation

CLARE R. GREGORY

I. INTRODUCTION

A. Definitions.

1. Tissue or organ from an unrelated donor of the same species. An allograft is unmatched if the cell surface antigens of the organ differ from those of the recipient. A matched allograft shares many of the same cell surface antigens with the donor.
2. Acute rejection.[11]
   a. Inflammatory response is initiated by T cells against the cells of the transplanted organ.
   b. T cells recognize foreign antigens on the surface of the cells of the allograft.
   c. T cells kill the cells of the allograft, or recruit other cells to kill the cells of the allograft or to form antibodies against the cells of the allograft.
   d. An acute rejection response destroys the function of a transplanted renal allograft in 5 to 10 days.

B. History.[14]

1. First kidney transplants in animals.
   a. Austria, Dr. Emerich Ulmann, 1902.
   b. United States, Dr. Alexis Carrel, 1905.
2. Recognition of acute allograft rejection, Mayo Clinic, Dr. Carl Williamson, 1923.
3. First kidney transplant between identical twins, Brigham Hospital, 1954.
4. First kidney transplants using unrelated donors.
   a. 1960s, owing to the development of azathioprine for immunosuppression.
   b. 1980s, increased early survival owing to the development of cyclosporine.
5. First successful clinical transplant in veterinary medicine.
   a. 1984.[3]
   b. Persian cat, 6 years old, female.
   c. Survived 2 years.

C. Clinical renal transplantation in feline veterinary medicine.[3–7]

1. Accepted treatment for patient in end-stage renal failure.
2. Provides good to excellent quality of life.
3. Transplantation is only a treatment, not a cure.
4. A transplanted feline kidney can function for 4 years or longer.
5. Retransplantation is an option if an allograft fails.
6. Cats rarely suffer acute allograft rejection.
7. The rarity of acute rejection episodes simplifies the management of feline patients and makes renal transplantation possible in clinical practice.

D. Clinical renal transplantation in canine veterinary medicine.[7]

1. Canine recipients of allografts from unrelated donors are subject to frequent and severe acute rejection episodes.
2. Immunosuppressive protocols require multiple agents.
3. Owing to the frequency of acute rejection episodes, intensive clinical management is often required.

4. Clinical renal transplantation in dogs is still under investigation.

II. DONOR SELECTION

A. Feline donor.

1. Healthy adult.
2. Free of feline leukemia and feline immunodeficiency virus.
3. Need not be related.
4. Blood must be crossmatch compatible with that of the recipient.
   a. The antigens on red blood cells are present on the endothelium of the allograft blood vessels.
   b. Preformed antibodies to these antigens cause clotting in the allograft vessels and infarcts in the organ at the time of surgery.
5. Donor should have no evidence of renal insufficiency based on clinical pathologic testing (complete blood count, serum chemistry panel, urinalysis).
6. Excretory urography is performed to ensure that the donor has two normally shaped, well-vascularized kidneys.

B. Canine donor.

1. Diagnostic testing as for feline donor.
2. If multiple related canine donors are available, they should be "tissue typed," to determine if they match the recipient. Antigen matching can be performed at many schools of veterinary medicine.

III. PREOPERATIVE MANAGEMENT

A. Diuresis using parenteral administration of balanced electrolyte solutions at rate of 75 to 100 mL/kg/24 h.

1. Monitor and correct severe acid-base and electrolyte imbalances.
2. Be careful not to overload patient with fluid.

B. Restrict protein intake. Placement of a gastrostomy (peg) tube greatly enhances nutritional management.

C. Correct anemia.

1. Packed cell volume (PCV) should be 30% or higher before surgery.
2. Erythropoietin.
   a. If used, it should be started 4 to 6 weeks before surgery.
   b. Concurrent administration of cyclosporine may prevent antibody formation to recombinant human erythropoietin.
   c. Greatly reduces perioperative need for whole blood.
3. Blood transfusions.
   a. Must be carefully cross-matched.
   b. Several blood donors must be available, as 180 to 250 mL of whole blood may be needed to attain a PCV of 30% in feline patients.

D. Evacuate the colon (warm-water enema or glycerin suppository) before surgery, to facilitate placement of the allograft in the iliac fossa.

IV. IMMUNOSUPPRESSION

A. Cyclosporine.[10]

1. First agent to specifically inhibit T cells.
2. Extremely effective as a single agent in cats; must be used in combination with other immunosuppressants in dogs.
3. Initial dose for cats: 7.5 mg/kg/12 h orally, administered in gelatin capsules.
4. Owing to extreme variability in absorption following oral administration; 12-hour trough levels of cyclosporine must be measured.
5. Target blood levels.
   a. For first 30 days postoperatively, 500 ng/mL of whole blood.
   b. Thereafter for life, 250 ng/mL of whole blood.
6. Clients and veterinarians must have access to the intravenous form of cyclosporine for periods when the patient cannot tolerate oral administration because of severe gastroenteritis.

B. Prednisolone.

1. Synergistic with cyclosporine.[13]
2. Dose: 0.25 mg/kg/12 h for the first 30 days postoperatively; 0.25 mg/kg/24 h thereafter, for life.

V. ANESTHESIA AND SURGERY[1,2,5,14]

A. Anesthesia for felines.

1. Medicate with atropine (0.03 mg/kg) and oxymorphone (0.05 mg/kg) before induction.
2. Induce anesthesia with isoflurane and oxygen.
3. Administer blood or balanced electrolyte solutions intravenously.
4. Administer dopamine (3 to 5 μg/kg/min) intravenously.
5. Monitor systemic arterial pressure.
   a. Doppler ultrasonography: maintain systolic pressure at ≥90 mm Hg.
   b. Direct arterial catheterization: maintain mean pressure at ≥60 mm Hg.
6. Assess arterial or venous blood gases and electrolytes periodically; correct imbalances as necessary.
7. As abdominal closure is begun, administer butorphenol or oxymorphone, to reduce postoperative pain and provide a quieter recovery.

B. Surgery.

1. For feline transplantation, loupes or a microscope providing 3.5× to 10× magnification (depending on the experience of the surgeon) is necessary.
2. The donor kidney is placed in the iliac fossa of the recipient.
   a. End-to-end anastomosis of the renal artery to the external iliac artery is performed.
   b. End-to-side anastomosis of the renal vein to the external iliac vein is performed.
3. Following completion of the vascular anastomoses, ureteroneocystostomy is performed.
4. Warm ischemia time of the transplanted kidney should not exceed 60 minutes.
5. The native kidneys are left *in situ,* to act as a reserve if the donor kidney fails to function or if function is delayed. Native kidneys can be removed after normal renal function is attained, if necessary.
6. Most transplanted kidneys function well by 72 hours after surgery.

VI. POSTOPERATIVE CARE

A. The recipient is given balanced electrolyte solutions until water and food are accepted.

B. PCV, total plasma protein (TPP), serum creatinine (SC), and trough whole blood levels of cyclosporine are determined at 2- to 4-day intervals.

C. Voided urine is collected daily to assess urine specific gravity.

D. Recipient is discharged from the hospital when it has good appetite, good attitude, decreased or normal SC, and urine specific gravity indicating concentrating ability.

E. Weekly examinations are performed by the primary care veterinarian for 4 weeks and gradually are extended to 4- to 6-week intervals.

1. PCV, TPP, SC, cyclosporine blood level, and urinalysis are performed at each examination period.
2. Complete blood count and serum chemistry panel are performed every 4 months.

VII. COMPLICATIONS OF RENAL TRANSPLANTATION

A. Acute allograft rejection.

1. Characterized by malaise, vomiting, and depression.
2. Rare in feline patients with adequate blood levels of cyclosporine.
3. Elevated SC or blood urea nitrogen occurs only late in the rejection process; if rejection is suspected by the clinical signs, treatment must begin immediately.
4. Treatment.
   a. Cyclosporine: intravenous form, 6 mg/kg/24 h in 5% dextrose or 0.9% NaCl over 4 to 6 hours.
   b. Corticosteroids: intravenous prednisolone, 5 to 10 mg/kg/12 h.
5. Oral administration of cyclosporine and prednisolone is reinstated when the signs of rejection subside and the recipient accepts water and food.

B. Ureteral obstruction.

1. Occurs 5 to 10 days after surgery.
2. Usually produced by granuloma formation at the new stoma.
3. Characterized by a rising SC and decreasing urine specific gravity.
4. Must not be confused with a rejection episode.
5. Diagnosis is made by ultrasonographic examination of the transplanted ureter and kidney.
6. Corrected by surgically excising the granuloma and reimplanting the ureter in the bladder.

C. Infections.

1. Fungal infections are associated with high blood levels of cyclosporine.
   a. Maximal blood levels should not exceed 500 ng/mL over long periods of time.
   b. Cyclosporine requirements decrease over time, as the drug becomes more bioavailable to the recipient.
2. Urinary tract infections (UTI) are the most common post-transplant infection.
   a. Treat UTI according to results of antibiotic sensitivity testing.
   b. Aminoglycoside antibiotics and trimethoprim are nephrotoxic when used in combination with cyclosporine.
   c. Cephalosporins and fluoroquinolone antibiotics are safe and effective.
3. Viral upper respiratory infections.
   a. If the recipient becomes severely affected, supplementation with balanced electrolyte solutions and nasogastric feedings may be necessary.
   b. With supportive therapy, most episodes are controlled in 7 to 10 days.

D. Complications in individual patients.

1. Lymphosarcoma developed following treatment of inflammatory bowel disease with large doses of prednisolone.[8]
2. Pulmonary toxoplasmosis developed in an asymptomatic carrier 3 months after transplantation.
3. Oxalate nephrosis, not associated with ethylene glycol intoxication, caused the loss of two allografts in one cat.[9]

VIII. PROGNOSIS FOLLOWING RENAL TRANSPLANTATION

A. Survival time increases as patient selection becomes more stringent.

1. Most postoperative deaths and complications are secondary to malnutrition and multiple organ failure that results in severe hypothermia, hypotension, and irreversible shock.
2. Pre-existing conditions, such as cardiac disease, continue to progress following transplantation.

B. Current survival time for cats that survive the procedure and leave the hospital with improved to normal renal function ranges from 2 to more than 4 years.

IX. SUMMARY

A. Renal transplantation offers a unique method for treating renal failure in veterinary medicine.

1. Many questions and problems have yet to be answered, particularly for perioperative management of critically ill patients.
2. If transplantation is performed and complications arise in the perioperative period, the patient will likely die from multiple organ failure.

B. Clients must be dedicated to lifelong attention to their pet.

1. They must medicate the pet two times daily for life.
2. They must return to the primary care veterinarian for periodic examinations of their pet. If an emergency arises, they must identify a 24-hour veterinary service where intravenous cyclosporine is available to the patient at all times.

C. No specific limitations are placed on the activity of the patient. Travel represents little or no problem, but boarding kennels should be avoided.

REFERENCES

1. Gourley IM, Gregory CR. Renal transplantation. In: *Atlas of Small Animal Surgery.* New York, New York: Gower; 1992:19.27–19.30.
2. Gourley IM, Gregory CR. Ureter. In: *Atlas of Small Animal Surgery.* New York, New York: Gower; 1992:19.7–19.12.
3. Gregory CR, Gourley IM, Broaddus TW, et al. Long-term survival of a cat receiving a renal allograft from an unrelated donor. *J Vet Intern Med.* 1990; 1:1–3.
4. Gregory CR. Status of renal transplantation in the 90's. *Semin Vet Med Surg (Small Anim).* 1992; 7:183–186.
5. Gregory CR, Gourley IM. Organ transplantation in clinical veterinary medicine. In: Slatter DH, ed. *Textbook of Small Animal Surgery.* 2nd ed. Philadelphia, Pennsylvania: WB Saunders, 1993.
6. Gregory CR, Gourley IM, Kochin EJ, et al. Renal transplantation for treatment of end-stage renal failure in cats. *J Am Vet Med Assoc.* 1992; 201:285–291.
7. Gregory CR, Gourley IM, Taylor NJ, et al. Preliminary results of clinical renal allograft transplantation in the dog and cat. *J Vet Intern Med.* 1987; 1:53–60.
8. Gregory CR, Madewell BR, Griffey SM, et al. Feline leukemia virus–associated lymphosarcoma following renal transplantation in a cat. *Transplantation.* 1991; 52:1097–1099.
9. Gregory CR, Olander HJ, Gourley IM, et al. Oxalate nephrosis and hypertensive renal sclerosis following renal transplantation in the cat. *Vet Surg.* (in press).
10. Gregory CR, Hietala SK, Pedersen NC, et al. Cyclosporine pharmacokinetics in cats following topical ocular administration. *Transplantation.* 1989; 47:516–519.
11. Gregory CR, Gourley IM, Ferriera H, et al. Pathologic studies of acute rejection of mismatched feline musculocutaneous flaps. *Transplantation.* 1991; 51:1170–1175.
12. Kochin EJ, Gregory CR, Gourley IM. Evaluation of a new method of ureteroneocystostomy in cats. *J Am Vet Med Assoc.* 1993; 202:257–260.
13. Manfro RC, Pohanka S, Tomlanovich S, et al. Cyclosporin A and prednisolone: an additive inhibitory effect of cell proliferation and interleukin-2 production. *Transplant Proc.* 1989; 21:1457–1459.
14. Morris PJ. Preface to the first edition. In: Morris PJ, ed. *Kidney Transplantation Principles and Practice.* 2nd ed. San Diego, California: Grune and Stratton; 1984:9–12.

P A R T 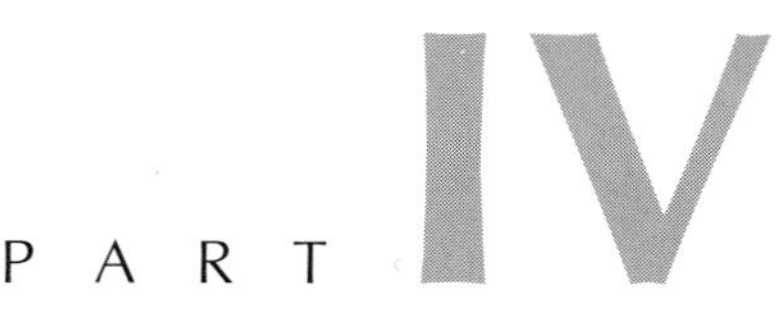

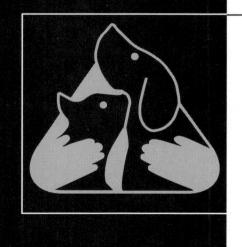

DISEASES OF THE URETERS

33

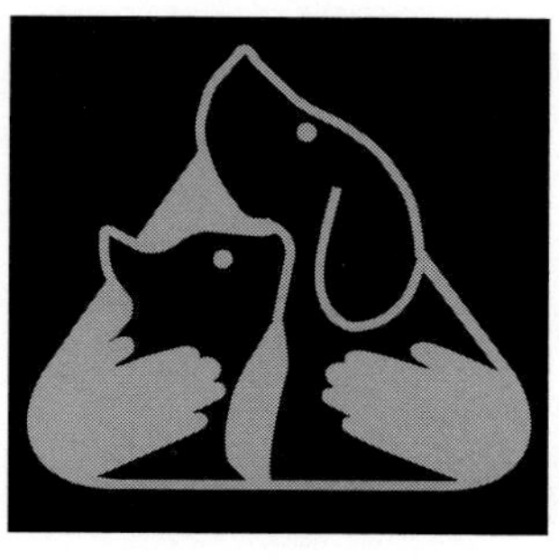

Vesicoureteral Reflux

CARL A. OSBORNE
DANIEL A. FEENEY

I. DEFINITION AND CLASSIFICATION

A. Vesicoureteral reflux is regurgitation or retrograde flow of urine from the urinary bladder into the ureters and renal pelves.

B. On the basis of pathogenesis, vesicoureteral reflux has been called primary or secondary.

1. The term primary vesicoureteral reflux denotes an intrinsic maldevelopment of the ureterovesical junction.
2. The term secondary vesicoureteral reflux implies an acquired disorder of the ureterovesical junction.

II. SIGNIFICANCE

A. The unidirectional flow of urine from the ureters into the bladder and the ureterovesical flap valve protect the kidneys from contamination by bladder urine.

B. If the ureterovesical junction becomes abnormal, or if intraluminal bladder pressure becomes excessive, vesicoureteral reflux occurs as soon as intraluminal bladder pressure exceeds intraluminal ureteral pressure.

1. If the refluxed urine contains pathogenic microbes, infection of the upper urinary tract (reflux nephropathy) may occur.
2. Renal parenchymal damage may also be associated with the escape of antigenic proteins derived from the excretory pathway into the renal interstitium. A correlation exists between the severity of vesicoureteral reflux and the risk of renal damage.[25]
3. If reflux is severe and associated with marked ureterectasis, voiding pressure may be transmitted to the renal pelvis. Intermittent elevation of intrapelvic pressure has been suggested to act as a water hammer predisposing the kidney to parenchymal damage.[11]
4. In addition to reflux nephropathy, vesicoureteral reflux may perpetuate lower urinary tract infection (UTI).
   a. Even if the bladder is capable of completely eliminating all urine from its lumen, it will be recontaminated with infected refluxed urine returning from the ureter.
   b. This phenomenon may increase the susceptibility of patients to persistent or recurrent UTI.

C. Hypertension is a well-known long-term complication of vesicoureteral reflux and renal scarring encountered in humans.

III. ETIOPATHOGENESIS

A. Many factors affect the functional competence of the ureterovesical valve.

1. The length of the submucosal (intravesical) segment of the ureter.
2. The diameter of the intravesical ureter.
3. The ratio of the length of the intravesical ureter to its width.
4. The pliability of the roof of the intravesical portion

of the distal ureter that functions as a flap valve.
5. The integrity of the detrusor muscle, which underlies and supports the intravesical portion of the ureter.[11,12]
6. Ureteral peristalsis.[16]
7. Intraluminal pressures in the ureters and urinary bladder.

B. The length of the intravesical portion of the ureter has an important role in the pathogenesis of vesicoureteral reflux. The longer it is, the less likely is reflux; ureters with relatively short intravesical portions are more likely to permit reflux.

C. Self-limiting primary vesicoureteral reflux commonly occurs in young dogs (7 to 12 weeks old) that have an otherwise normal urinary tract (Figs. 33–1, 33–2).[1–3]

1. Its presence is thought to be related to the fact that early development of the intravesical portion of the ureter is associated with a disproportionate increase in diameter as compared with length.
2. As growth proceeds, however, the submucosal portion of the distal ureter elongates, bringing about regression of reflux.
3. Vesicoureteral reflux in puppies has also been associated with development of adrenergic fibers.[13] The incidence of vesicoureteral reflux in puppies decreased dramatically as adrenergic fibers began to appear.
4. Primary vesicoureteral reflux has been reported to occur in fewer than 10% of adult dogs.[2] It is more frequent in female dogs than in male dogs and is more often bilateral than unilateral.

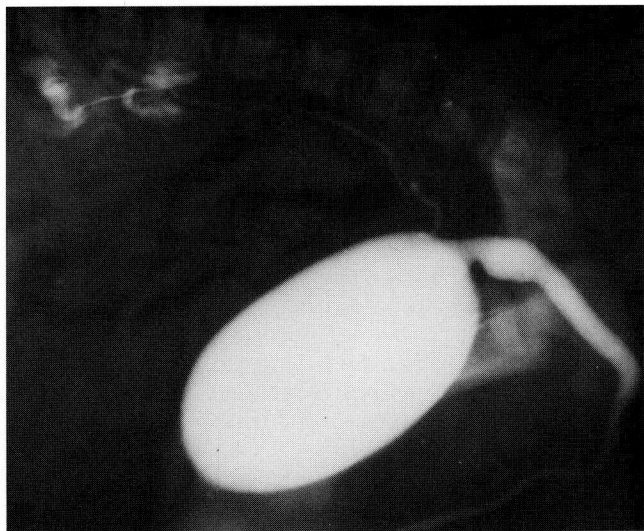

FIG. 33–1. Lateral view of a positive contrast retrograde urethrocystogram of a normal 8-week–old male beagle illustrates vesicoureteral reflux. (From Johnston GR, Feeney DA, Osborne CA. Radiographic findings in urinary tract infection. *Vet Clin North Am.* 1979;9:749–774.)

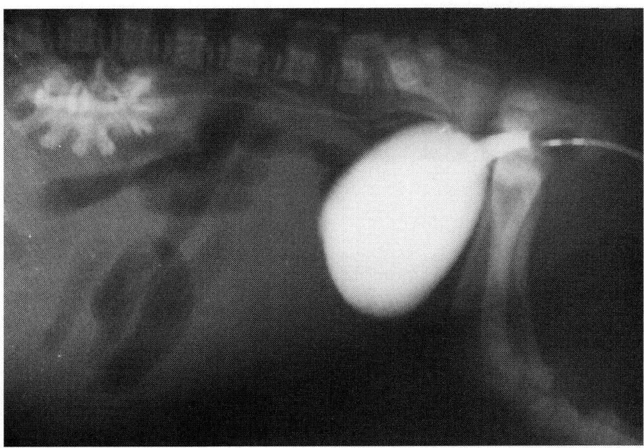

FIG. 33–2. Lateral view of a positive contrast retrograde urethrocytogram of a normal 8-week–old female beagle. Vesicoureteral reflux is associated with filling of the ureteral and pelvic lumens with contrast medium. (From Johnston GR, Feeney DA, Osborne CA. Radiographic findings in urinary tract infection. *Vet Clin North Am.* 1979;9:749–774.)

D. Secondary vesicoureteral reflux may be associated with inflammation of the vesicoureteral junction, surgical damage to the trigone, mechanical or functional obstruction below the bladder neck, neurogenic disease of the urinary bladder, and surgical techniques used for urine diversion.[3,15,17,19,22,23] Ureteral reflux may also occur in association with ectopic ureters. Although the consensus is that reflux may be a sequela to infection, one experimental study in dogs found that bladder infection *per se* was not significant in causing vesicoureteral reflux.[10] In another experimental study, however, reflux occurred in 4 of 8 dogs infected with *Escherichia coli* bacteria and in 16 of 17 dogs infected with *Proteus* species.[21]

1. When the ureterovesical flap valve is damaged by one or more of these disorders, vesicoureteral reflux occurs as soon as intraluminal bladder pressure exceeds intraluminal ureteral pressure.
   a. If infection becomes established in the urinary bladder, vesicoureteral reflux allows bacteria to ascend to the kidneys.[20] In one study of dogs, natural and surgically induced vesicoureteral reflux without concomitant persistent bladder infection was not associated with radiographic, gross, or microscopic changes in the kidneys or ureters.[18] When persistent infection of the urinary bladder was induced by implanting a foreign body in the bladder lumen, however, pyelonephritis and renal dysfunction developed.

b. Similar results of experimental studies in dogs have been reported by other investigators, although they concluded that impaired ureteral peristalsis was also an important factor.[24]

c. The fact that refluxed urine must contain bacteria to establish an infection of the kidneys has also been observed in experimental studies in rats.[8]

2. Studies in normal male and female dogs and cats have revealed that attempts to induce micturition by manual compression of the urinary bladder may cause vesicoureteral reflux (Figs. 33–3, 33–4).[6]

   a. Application of digital pressure to the urinary bladder for a prolonged period to initiate voiding of urine was associated with a greater prevalence of reflux than was the application of digital pressure for a short time.

   b. Vesicoureteral reflux associated with compression-induced micturition probably occurs as a result of lack of coordinated relaxation of the smooth muscle of the internal ureteral sphincter mechanism and striated muscle of the external urethral sphincter, which normally occurs during the voiding phase of spontaneous micturition.

IV. DIAGNOSTIC CONSIDERATIONS

A. A diagnosis of vesicoureteral reflux must be based on appropriate radiographic studies.

1. Due caution must be used because vesicoureteral reflux may be induced in normal patients as a result of the type of anesthetic agent used, the depth of anesthesia, patient positioning, and the degree of distention of the urinary bladder (Figs. 33–5, 33–6).

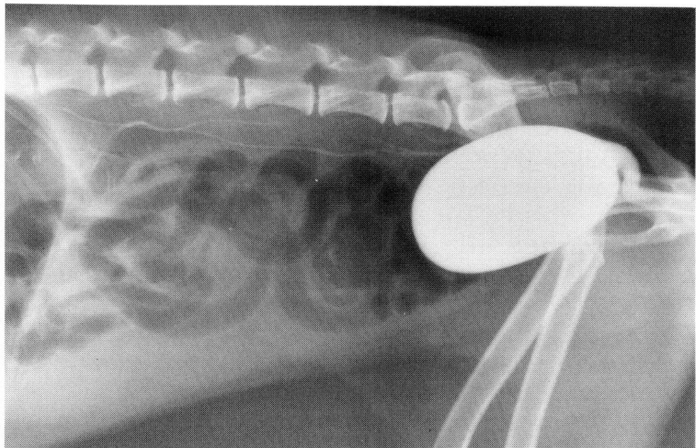

FIG. 33–3. Lateral view of the abdomen of an adult female poodle following distention of the urinary bladder with contrast medium. Increased abdominal pressure has resulted in caudad displacement of the urinary bladder and kinking of the urethra. Contrast medium has refluxed into the ureters.

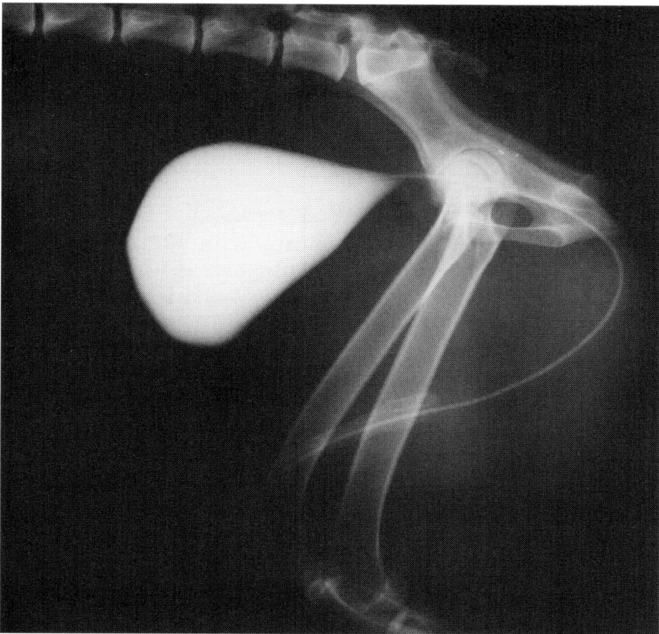

FIG. 33–4. Lateral view of the abdomen of an adult male mixed–breed dog obtained following positive contrast cystography. Vesicoureteral reflux is not evident. Arrows outline urinary catheter.

2. Too often, these variables are ignored in the evaluation of vesicoureteral reflux.

B. Radiographic techniques used to identify vesicoureteral reflux include voiding cystourethrography, retrograde urethrocystography, maximum distention cystourethrography, and compression cystourethrography.

1. Our current recommendation is to use either voiding or maximum distention retrograde urethrocystography.
2. Voiding cystourethrography has been the technique most often used in canine studies to demonstrate vesicoureteral reflux, but it is technically cumbersome.[3]

C. Vesicoureteral reflux can occur during bladder filling, voiding, or both (see Figs. 33–1 through 33–6).

1. In adult dogs, reflux occurs near the time of maximal bladder distention; in puppies it tends to occur earlier in the course of bladder filling.
2. Although unilateral reflux has been reported in dogs, it is usually bilateral.
3. Contrast medium generally reaches the renal pelves. Depending on the cause of reflux, other radiographic abnormalities may also be noted.

D. Retrograde urethrocystography is performed by infusing an iodinated radiocontrast agent into the urinary bladder after catheterization of the membranous or prostatic urethra. Reflux is observed more often if the urinary bladder is

distended to the point of trigone urethral dilatation before the urethral injection.[7]

1. This modified technique, termed maximum distention urethrocystography, was associated with a 50% incidence of reflux in adult male beagle dogs in studies performed at the University of Minnesota.
2. Care should be taken to prevent urinary bladder rupture, especially if balloon catheters are used to prevent spontaneous voiding.

E. Compression cystourethrography is performed with the dog or cat in a light plane of anesthesia.

1. The patient's urinary bladder is filled with an iodinated radiocontrast agent.
2. After the patient is placed in a lateral recumbent position, external pressure is applied to the bladder in an attempt to express urine.
3. When urine flow is observed, an abdominal radiograph is exposed or the vesicoureteral junction is observed fluoroscopically.

F. Reflux may be detected by cystoscopy by filling the urinary bladder with a solution containing a colored dye, such as methylene blue or indigo carmine, and then observing the efflux from each ureteral orifice after the bladder is emptied and filled with clear saline.[11]

G. Radionuclide cystography may be used to detect vesicoureteral reflux.[11]

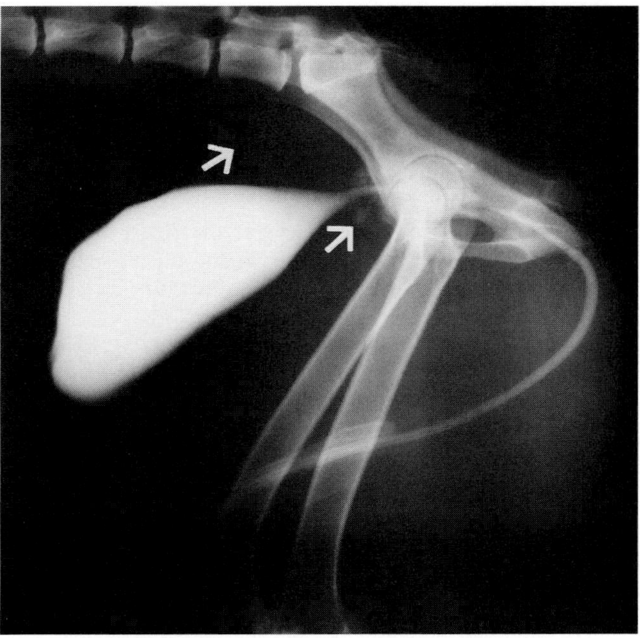

FIG. 33–5. Lateral view of the abdomen of the dog described in Figure 33–4 following removal of the urinary catheter and manual compression to the urinary bladder to induce voiding. Contrast medium has passed into the urethra but has also refluxed into a ureter (arrows) and the prostate gland (arrows).

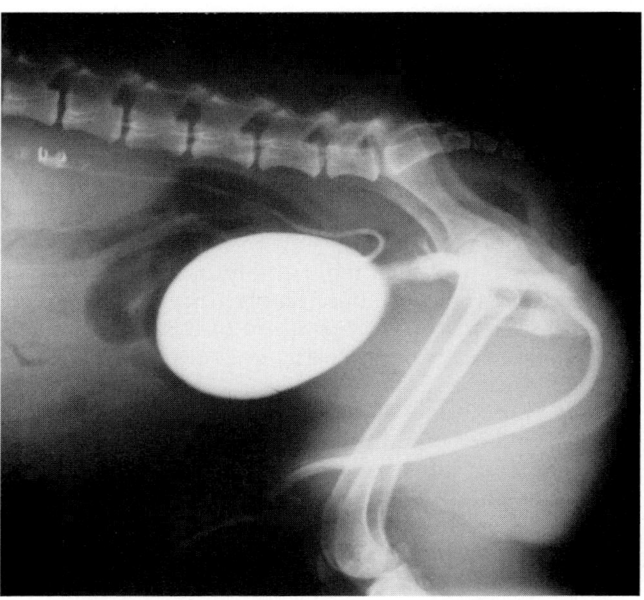

FIG. 33–6. Retrograde positive contrast urethrocystogram with vesicoureteral and urethroprostatic reflux of contrast medium.

V. MANAGEMENT

A. Therapeutic approaches to vesicoureteral reflux include medical therapy to eradicate the UTI and surgical therapy to correct an abnormal vesicoureteral junction.[11]

B. Because primary vesicoureteral reflux is common in young dogs, and because reflux usually ceases as the dogs mature, therapy is not indicated for young dogs with reflux without UTI.

C. If UTI and reflux coexist, antibiotics should be administered to sterilize the urine to prevent pyelonephritis. Urine must remain sterile as long as urethral reflux persists. Quantitative urine cultures should be obtained to ensure that infection has been eradicated. Techniques other than manual expression should be used to collect urine.

D. Surgical procedures have been developed to correct primary reflux in humans.[4,5,11,16] **An endoscopic procedure has been used to correct experimentally induced vesicoureteral reflux in dogs**[14] **and humans.**[11] **If reflux occurs secondary to some other urologic abnormality, therapy should be directed at the underlying problem. The urine should be kept sterile by appropriate antibiotic therapy.**

E. To prevent iatrogenic infection of the upper urinary tract, appropriate caution should also be used when performing manual compression to empty the urinary bladder of a patient with UTI before exploratory celiotomy.

1. If voiding cannot be induced with minimal digital pressure while the patient is anesthetized, the

need to empty the bladder before celiotomy should be re-evaluated.

2. If the bladder is distended to such a degree that iatrogenic damage during incision of the abdominal wall is a concern, alternative methods to reduce its size should be considered.

F. Appropriate caution is recommended to prevent damage to the ureters at the time other disorders of the lower urinary tract or genital tract are being corrected by surgery. Experimental studies performed in normal dogs revealed that superficial and total trigonectomy did not impair ureterovesical valve formation in 29 of 30 ureters evaluated by contrast radiography and light microscopy.[9]

REFERENCES

1. Christie BA. The ureterovesical junction in dogs. *Invest Urol.* 1971;9:10–15.
2. Christie BA. Incidence and etiology of vesicoureteral reflux in apparently normal dogs. *Invest Urol.* 1971;9:184–194.
3. Christie BA. Vesicoureteral reflux in dogs. *J Am Vet Med Assoc.* 1973;162:772.
4. Ehrlich RM. Vesicoureteral reflux: a surgeon's perspective. *Pediatr Clin North Am.* 1982;29:827–834.
5. Elo J, Tallgren LG, Alfthan O, et al. Character of urinary tract infections and pyelonephritis renal scarring after antireflux surgery. *J Urol.* 1983;129:343–346.
6. Feeney DA, Osborne CA, Johnston GR. Vesicoureteral reflux induced by manual compression of the urinary bladder of dogs and cats. *J Am Vet Med Assoc.* 1983;182:795–797.
7. Feeney DA, Johnston GR, Osborne CA, et al. Maximum distension retrograde urethrocystography in normal male dogs. II. Occurrence of vesicoureteral reflux. *Am J Vet Res.* 1984;45: 953–954.
8. Freeman RB, Murphy TE, Dickstein CD. Experimental renal infection. Acute and chronic studies of histology and function. *Kidney Int.* 1978;13:129.
9. Hannan QHA, Stephens D. The influence of trigomectomy on vesicoureteral reflux in dogs. *Invest Urol.* 1973;10:469–472.
10. Harrison L, Cass A, Cox C, et al. Role of bladder infection in the etiology of vesicoureteral reflux in dogs. *Invest Urol.* 1974; 12:123.
11. King LR. Vesicoureteral reflux, megaureter, and ureteral reimplantation. In: Walsh PC, Retik AB, Stamey TA, Vaughn ED, eds. *Campbell's Urology.* 6th ed. Philadelphia, Pennsylvania: WB Saunders; 1992;1689–1742.
12. Kind LR, Kazmi SO, Belman AB. Natural history of vesicoureteral reflux. Outcome of the trial nonoperative therapy. *Urol Clin North Am.* 1974;1:441.
13. Kiruluta HG, Fraser K, Owen L. The significance of the adrenergic nerves in the etiology of vesicoureteral reflux. *J Urol.* 1986;136:232–235.
14. Kohri K, Kataoka K, Akyama T, et al. Treatment of vesicoureteral reflux by endoscopic injection of blood. *Urol Int.* 1988;43: 324–326.
15. Levers PE, Ramage HC, Metcalfe JO. Vesicoureteral reflux, urethral resistance, and age. *Can J Surg.* 1964;7:196.
16. Levitt SB, Duckett J, Spitzer A, et al. Medical versus surgical treatment of primary vesicoureteral reflux: a prospective international reflux study in children. *J Urol.* 1981;125:277–283.
17. Montgomerie JZ, Guze L. The renal response to infection. In: Brenner BM, Rector FC, eds. *The Kidney.* Vol 2. Philadelphia, Pennsylvania: WB Saunders; 1976.
18. Newman L, Bucy JG, McAlister WH. Experimental production of reflux in the presence and absence of infected urine. *Radiology.* 1974;111:591.
19. Radzinski C, McGuire EJ, Smith D, et al. Creation of a feline model of obstructive uropathy. *J Urol.* 1991;145:859–863.
20. Ransley PG. Vesicoureteral reflux: continuing surgical dilemma. *Urology.* 1978;12:246.
21. Sommer JL, Roberts JA. Ureteral reflux resulting from chronic urinary infections in dogs: long-term studies. *J Urol.* 1966; 95:502.
22. St Clair SR, Hixson CJ, Ritchey ML. Enterocystoplasty and reflux nephropathy in the canine model. *J Urol.* 1992;148:728–732.
23. Tanagho EA, Hutch JA. Primary reflux. *J Urol.* 1965;93:158.
24. Tsuchida S, Sugawara H, Arai S. Ascending pyelonephritis in dogs induced by ureteral dysfunction. *Invest Urol.* 1973;10:450.
25. Weiss RA. Vesicoureteral reflux in children. *The Kidney.* 1993; 25:1–6.

CHAPTER 34

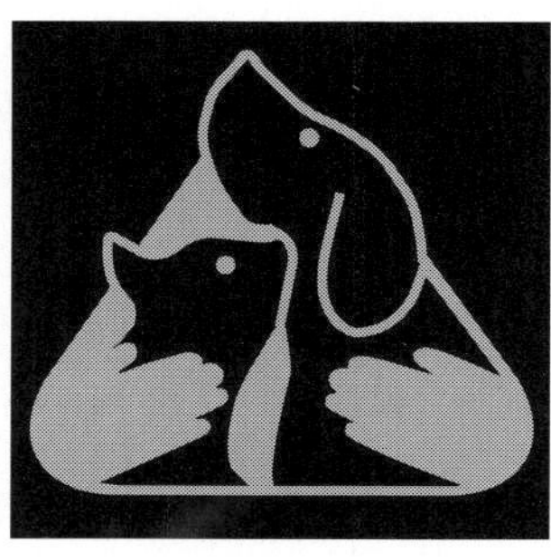

Ectopic Ureters and Ureteroceles

CARL A. OSBORNE
GARY R. JOHNSTON
JOHN M. KRUGER

I. ECTOPIC URETERS

A. Applied embryology and etiology.

1. Ureteral ectopia is a congenital anomaly of one or both ureters, which do not terminate normally in the trigone of the urinary bladder.
   a. The embryonic pathogenesis of ectopic ureters is related to abnormal origin or migration of the metanephric ducts, which become the ureters.[1,43]
   b. Ureters may terminate anywhere along the lower urinary or reproductive tract that originates from the mesonephrons.
   c. Ectopic ureters may bypass the urinary bladder completely (extramural ectopic ureter), or they may enter the serosal surface of the urinary bladder at the normal site and tunnel through the bladder wall, past the trigone, to terminate at an ectopic site (intramural ectopic ureter).
   d. Because of the close relationship of the mesonephros and the metanephros and development of other urogenital organs, ureteral ectopia may be associated with other anomalies, such as renal ectopia, renal hypoplasia, renal aplasia, ureterocele, urachal remnants, agenesis or hypoplasia of the urinary bladder, urethral agenesis or ectopia, phimosis, vulvovaginal strictures, and persistent hymen.
2. Although the underlying cause of ureteral ectopia in dogs and cats is unknown, its tendency to occur in certain canine breeds and the observation of Siberian husky littermates with ectopic ureters suggest a familial tendency.[9,26] A familial tendency has also been reported in golden retrievers.[23,27]
3. Rats fed a vitamin A-deficient diet have a high incidence of congenital urinary tract defects, including ureteral ectopia.[60] The anomalies were prevented by administration of vitamin A to pregnant rats at the appropriate time during gestation.[61]; however, no data link nutritional factors to development of ectopic ureters in dogs or cats.
4. Two cases of urinary incontinence in female cats caused by an acquired communication between the ureters and the vagina have been reported.[1a]

B. Diagnostic considerations.

1. Gender and breed.
   a. Dogs.
      (1). Ureteral ectopia is a common cause of urinary incontinence in young female dogs. Recognition of this clinical manifestation has been established to be 20 times greater in female than in male dogs,[19] perhaps because urinary incontinence is

less frequently associated with ectopic ureters in males.

(2). Breeds at high risk for ureteral ectopia in females include the Siberian husky, Newfoundland, English bulldog, Labrador retriever, collie, West Highland white terrier, fox terrier, Skye terrier, and miniature and toy poodle.[19,20,23,26,55]

(3). Although the majority of cases reported in male dogs have been in mixed breeds, Labrador retrievers, Welsh corgis, and fox terriers have been reported to be affected more frequently than other breeds.[38,55]

b. Cats.

(1). Eleven clinical cases of ureteral ectopia have been reported in cats.[3,6,13,14,28,31,50,54]

(2). Eight were females and three were males.

2. Age.

a. Dogs.

(1). Because ureteral ectopia is a congenital anomaly, the associated urinary incontinence is usually recognized in young animals.

(2). In the majority of female dogs, the anomaly is detected before they are 1 year old; in many it is diagnosed when they are 6 to 16 weeks old.

(3). Urinary incontinence caused by ureteral ectopia has been recognized in adult female dogs. However, if it occurs following ovariohysterectomy, the possibility that acquired fistulas developed following surgery should be considered.[8,16]

(4). In male dogs, urinary incontinence caused by ectopic ureters is usually recognized when the dogs are immature, but cases have been encountered in which the diagnosis was not established until the patients were 3 years old.[29,30]

b. Cats.

(1). Ectopic ureters were recognized in 8 of 11 cats when they were 3 to 6 months old.[3,6,13,14,28,31,50,54]

(2). In 3 cats, the diagnosis was established when they were at least 2 years old.

3. Sites of ectopic ureters.

a. Types of ectopic ureters.[52]

(1). Normal ureters enter the dorsolateral caudal surface of the serosal surface of the bladder, traverse the bladder wall, and terminate at the trigone (see Fig. 1–1).

(2). Intramural ectopic ureters contact and enter the bladder wall at the normal site but continue through the bladder musculature and submucosa, past the trigone, to terminate in the urethra or the vagina. They are associated with urinary incontinence (Fig. 34–1).

(3). Intramural ectopic ureters may not have a terminal orifice. They are associated with hydroureter and hydronephrosis.

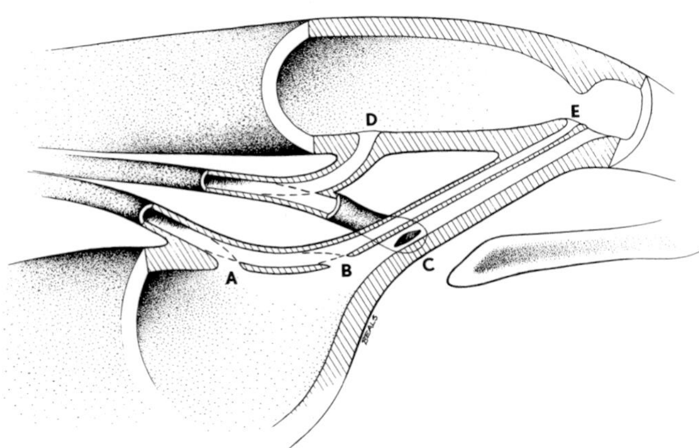

FIG. 34–1. Schematic illustration of sites of termination of ectopic ureters: A, normal site of termination of ureter in the urinary bladder; B, intramural ectopic ureter terminating in the proximal urethra; C, extramural ectopic ureter terminating in the urethra; D, extramural ectopic ureter terminating in the vagina; E, intramural ectopic ureter terminating in the vagina.

(4). Intramural ectopic ureters may open at the trigone in a normal fashion and then continue submucosally to a second, more distal opening (so-called ureteral branching).[9,10,33,52] They are associated with urinary incontinence.

(5). Ureteral troughs have been defined as ureters that pass through the serosa and bladder musculature normally, and may open into the bladder lumen in a normal or more distal location[52,52a]; however, the anomalous ureter continues as an incomplete structure, called a trough, beyond the trigone into the proximal urethral sphincter. They are associated with urinary incontinence.

(6). Extramural ectopic ureters totally bypass the urinary bladder, terminating in the urethra, vagina, or uterus (Fig. 34–1). They are associated with urinary incontinence.

(7). Intramural ectopic ureters are more common in dogs; extramural ectopic ureters are more common in cats.

b. Dogs.

(1). In female dogs, ectopic ureters were reported to terminate in the vagina (70%), urethra (20%), neck of the bladder (8%), or uterus (3%).[43] Results of other surveys suggest that the urethra is the most common site of ectopic ureters in females.[33]

(2). In males, ectopic ureters are most commonly recognized when they terminate in the cranial portion of the pelvic urethra (Fig. 34–2).

(3). Most investigators report that unilateral ectopic ureters are more common than bilateral ectopic ureters in female dogs; distribution between right and left ureters has been approximately equal.

(4). In male dogs, almost equal distribution of unilateral and bilateral ectopic ureters has been recognized. The left ureter more frequently has been ectopic in unilateral cases.

c. Cats.

(1). In 11 cats with ectopic ureters, both ureters were ectopic in 5 cases (Fig. 34–3); the left ureter was ectopic in 4 cats, and the right ureter was ectopic in 2 cats.[3,6,13,14,28,31,50,54]

(2). In six cats, the ectopic ureters terminated in the urethra (Fig. 34–3), whereas in four they terminated in the vagina. In one cat, the ectopic site of termination was not determined.

4. Clinical signs.

a. Clinical signs of ureteral ectopia depend on the site of termination of the ectopic ureter(s) and on the presence of other congenital or acquired abnormalities.

b. Constant or intermittent urinary incontinence during the storage phase of micturition is the most common clinical sign and is often associated with a normal voiding phase of micturition. Other causes of urinary incontinence (neurogenic disorders, hormone imbalance, neoplasia, cystitis, urethritis, psychologic dribbling, or other congenital abnormalities) should be considered (Table 34–1).

c. Females.

(1). In affected females, continuous or intermittent involuntary dribbling of urine may be noted by the client at the time of birth of the kitten or puppy, but the anomaly usually is not recognized until the animal is weaned.

(2). The severity of incontinence may vary from continuous dribbling from the vulva to intermittent incontinence that is associated with vaginal pooling of urine that gravitates out of the vulva when the body position is changed.

(3). Incontinent patients with unilateral ureteral ectopia usually micturate normally because urine continues to pass into the urinary bladder through the unaffected ureter.

(4). Although patients with bilateral ureteral ectopia may not micturate normally, reflux of a sufficient quantity of urine from the urethra into the bladder may allow normal micturition if the ureters terminate in the urethra.

(5). Persistent dribbling of urine that accumulates around the perivulvar area and caudal thighs may produce discoloration of the hair in this area, especially if it is white or light colored. Severe or prolonged incontinence may lead to urine-scald dermatitis.

d. Males.

(1). As in females, intermittent or continuous involuntary dribbling of urine detected

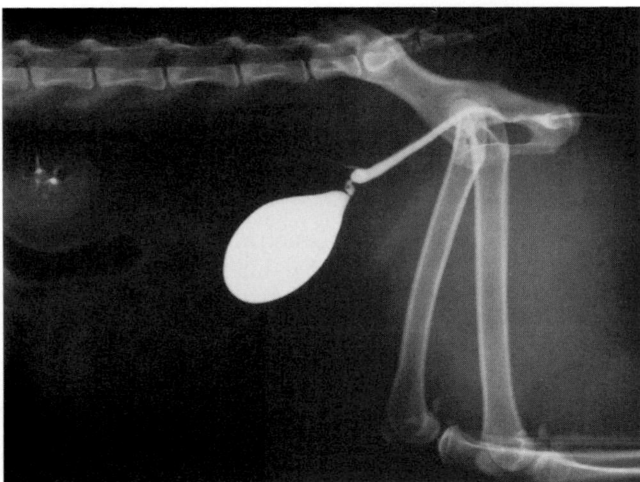

FIG. 34–3. Retrograde contrast urethrocystogram of a 5–year–old spayed female domestic shorthair cat with dysuria and hematuria. Note reflux of contrast medium into both ureters, which terminate in the proximal urethra. Bilateral extramural ureteral ectopia was not associated with dilation of the lumens of the ureters. Note also the constrictions of the proximal urethra craniad to the sites of ureteral ectopia. The cat had normal ability to concentrate urine and was not azotemic.

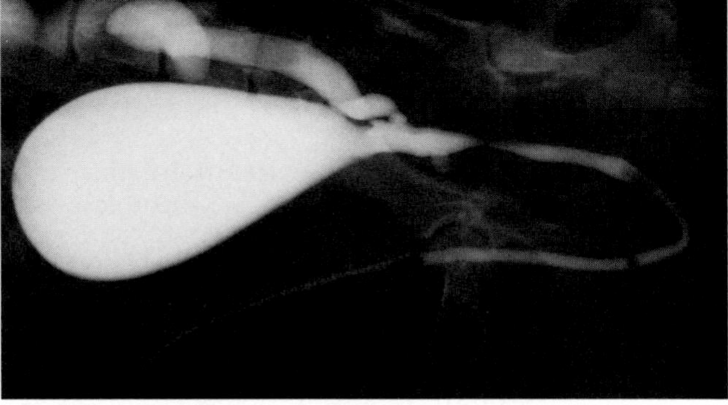

FIG. 34–2. Retrograde contrast urethrocystogram of an incontinent 7–year–old male Newfoundland with an ectopic dilated left ureter terminating in the proximal urethra. Air bubbles are in the urethral lumen.

when the animal is young is the sign most commonly associated with ureteral ectopia. In males, the longer urethra and strong external urethral sphincter may explain why urinary incontinence is intermittent or does not occur.[36,41] On occasion, the ectopic ureter has no distal orifice, and hydroureter and hydronephrosis result.

(2). Additional clinical findings observed in male cats include a constricted preputial opening (phimosis) with dilation of the sheath owing to accumulation of urine, urine staining of the perineum and hind limbs, and inflammation of the perineal skin.

(3). As in females, unilateral ureteral ectopia in males is usually associated with sufficient filling of the urinary bladder to initiate normal micturition.

(4). In male patients with bilateral ectopia, insufficient urinary bladder filling, which is associated with reduced size of the urinary bladder, may prevent normal micturition; however, reflux of urine from the urethra into the bladder may permit distention of the urinary bladder and normal micturition in addition to incontinence.[38,55]

e. Defects in urethral continence mechanisms may be associated with ectopic termination of ureters into the urethra. They may be associated with reduced intraurethral pressure when evaluated by urethral pressure profilometry. When present, this abnormality may result in persistent incontinence following surgical correction of the ectopic ureter(s).[48]

f. Bacterial urinary tract infections are commonly associated with ectopic ureters and may be associated with the following risk factors:

(1). Loss of the normal vesicoureteral valve that prevents vesicoureteral reflux of urine.

(2). Impaired ureteral peristalsis.

(3). Ureteroectasia.

(4). Stasis of urine in the lower genitourinary tract or in the ectopic ureter.

g. Progressive destruction of renal parenchyma of the associated kidney as a result of ascending bacteriuria and pyelonephritis may be associated with a progressive decrease in the severity of urinary incontinence. In one female dog with a unilateral ectopic ureter, complete destruction of the associated kidney resulted in remission of incontinence.[10]

h. If bilateral generalized renal infections develop, signs of renal failure or sepsis may develop.

5. Endoscopic findings.

a. Vaginoscopy.

(1). Examination of the vagina with a speculum may permit the identification of an ectopic ureteral orifice if the anomalous ureter enters the vagina; however, radiographic examination is usually more rewarding than is endoscopy.

(2). Unless two ureteral openings can be found, a definitive diagnosis of bilateral ureteral ectopia cannot be made by vaginal endoscopy.

(3). Satisfactory visualization of the entire mucosal surface of the vagina depends on the use of a vaginoscope that eliminates mucosal infoldings by distending the vaginal wall. We prefer to use glass (Pyrex) test tubes from which the bottoms have been removed and the ends fire polished, pediatric proctoscopes, disposable plastic syringe cases (Monoject) from which a large rectangular section has been removed from the wall, or fiberoptic endoscopes.* Otoscopic cones and nasal specula are less satisfactory alternatives.

(4). Injection of air into the vaginal lumen during endoscopy may enhance the visualization of the mucosa by causing distention of the vaginal wall.

(5). Many female dogs with ectopic ureters have a persistent hymen. Visual inspection of the vagina of such patients revealed a fleshy piece of tissue that was attached to

TABLE 34–1
PROBLEM-SPECIFIC DATABASE FOR URINARY INCONTINENCE

Medical history
- Age, sex, breed
- Owner's definition of incontinence
- Age of onset and duration of incontinence

Physical examination
- Observe micturition
- Evaluate bladder size before and after micturition
- Verify incontinence
- Perform vaginal examination
- Perform neurologic examination

Quantitative urine culture

Serum biochemistry (including at least serum urea nitrogen and creatinine)

Options to consider
- Survey abdominal radiographs
- Excretory urography, fluoroscopy
- Contrast urethrography or vaginography
- Endoscopy (vaginoscopy, urethroscopy, cystoscopy)
- Urethral pressure profilometry

*Available from Sherwood Medical Industries, Inc., 1831 Olive Street, St. Louis, Missouri 63101.

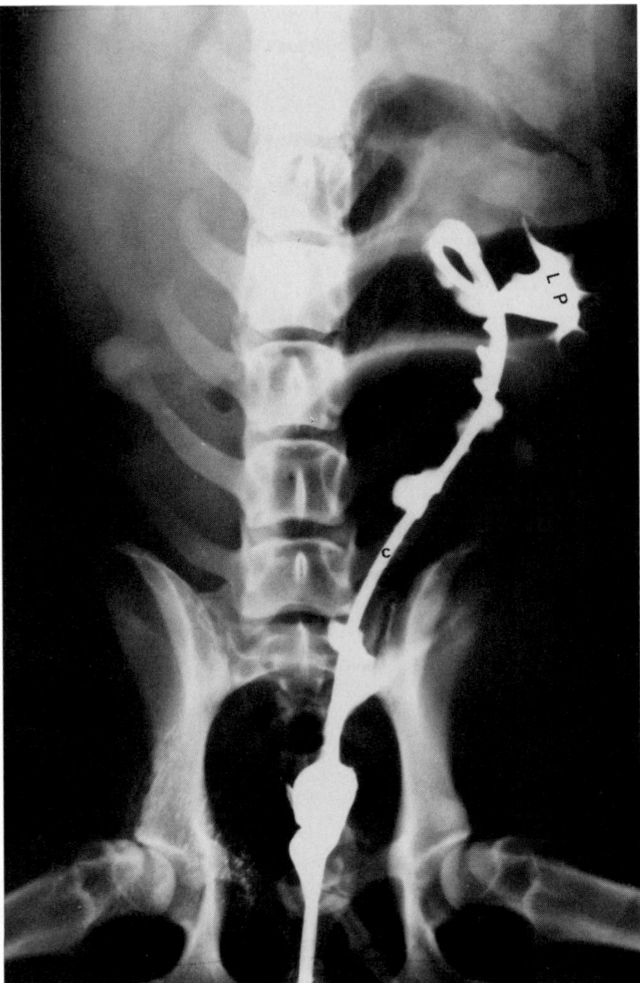

FIG. 34–4. Retrograde catheterization of the left ureter via ectopic ureteral orifice of a 21-month-old nonspayed female English bulldog. LP = left kidney pelvis; C = radiopaque fiber catheter.

the dorsal and ventral walls of the vagina. The lateral aspects of the structure often formed slitlike openings with the vaginal wall. Care must be used to avoid mistaking such openings for ectopic ureteral openings.

(6). When an abnormal orifice is detected by endoscopic examination, catheterization of the orifice with a radiopaque catheter followed by retrograde ureteropyelography may be performed (Fig. 34–4).[39] This technique should not be used as a substitute for intravenous urography, because it does not permit evaluation of other portions of the urinary system for concomitant abnormalities and may prevent recognition of bilateral ureteral ectopia.

b. Cystoscopy and urethroscopy.[34]

(1). Cystoscopy and urethroscopy may reveal the sites of termination of ectopic ureters.

(2). Urethral deformities associated with ectopic ureters may also be evaluated.

6. Urethral pressure profilometry.[17,18,22,24,48]

a. Defects in urethral continence mechanisms associated with ectopic termination of ureters into the urethra may be detected by urethral pressure profilometry.

b. The causes of abnormalities in urethral pressure are not well established, but they may be associated with segments of the ectopic ureter in the urethral wall, in addition to primary urethral abnormalities. Therefore, corrective surgery should be considered even if an abnormal urethral pressure profile is obtained. If urinary incontinence caused by primary urethral dysfunction persists after surgery, it may be controlled by administration of alpha-adrenergic agonists (such as phenylpropanolamine).

7. Radiographic findings.

a. Knowledge of the exact site or sites of termination of ectopic ureters has prognostic and therapeutic significance.

b. Retrograde contrast urethrography and vaginography are both excellent techniques for confirming ectopic ureters and for locating the site of termination (see Figs. 34–2, 34–3, and 34-5).[23,25,37] Either pediatric Foley catheters* or Swan-Ganz flow-directed balloon catheters† may be used.

(1). Care must be taken to avoid occluding the openings of ectopic ureteral orifices with the inflated balloons of these catheters, especially when ureters terminate in the distal urethra.

(2). In addition, the catheters should be filled with contrast medium before being inserted into the patient; this precaution prevents the formation of air bubbles in the urinary tract.

c. A standard technique and normal findings of excretory urography have been described.[5,11,12]

(1). Excretory urograms may permit confirmation of a diagnosis of ectopic ureter(s) (Figs. 34–6 through 34–8). The position, size, and shape of the kidneys, the size and shape of the renal pelvis, the size of the ureters, the site of termination of the ureters, and the position, shape, and size of the urinary bladder may also be evaluated. For best results, high-dose urography is recommended.[40]

*Available from Rusch Inc., 2450 Meadowbrook Parkway, Duluth, Georgia 30136.

†Available from Baxter-Edwards Laboratories, PO Box 11150, Santa Ana, California 92711.

(2). Unfortunately, localization of the exact site of termination of ectopic ureters is sometimes difficult with excretory urography (see Figs. 34–6 and 34–9).

(a). Poor visualization may occur if the ectopic ureter tunnels through the bladder wall (intramural ectopic ureter) for several centimeters before opening into the urethra. In addition, the ectopic orifice may be obscured by accumulation of contrast material

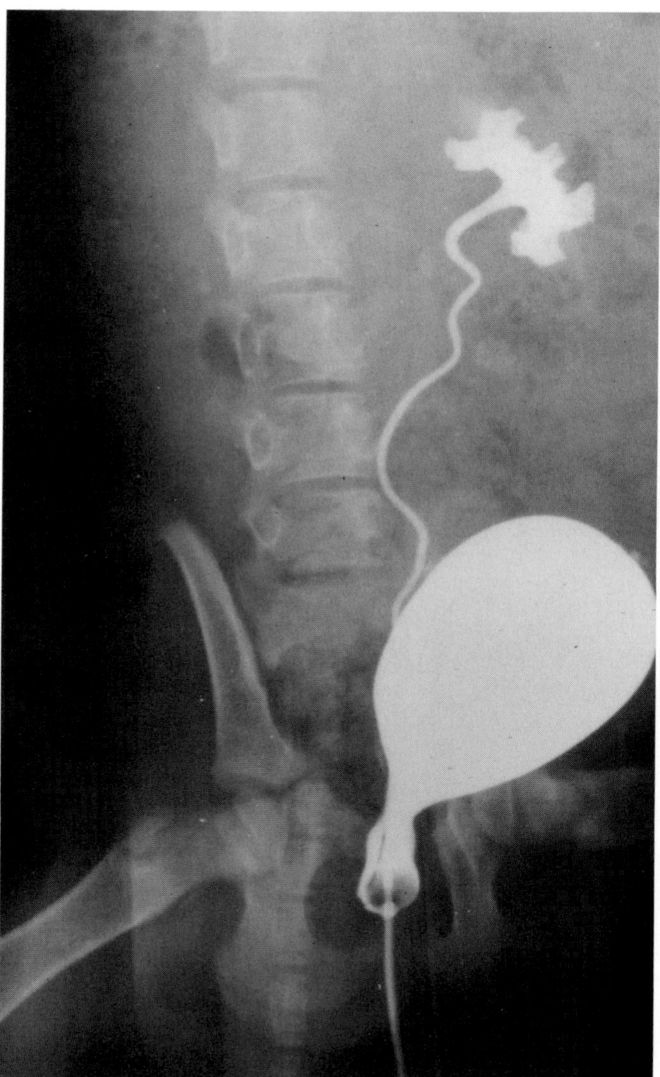

FIG. 34–5. Dorsoventral oblique view of a retrograde urethrocystogram of an incontinent immature female Siberian husky with unilateral left ectopic ureter. The distal end of the ectopic ureter entered the urethra (arrow). (Osborne CA, et al. The urinary system: Pathophysiology, diagnosis, treatment. In: Gourley IM, Vasseur PB, eds. *General Small Animal Surgery.* Philadelphia, Pennsylvania: JB Lippincott; 1985.)

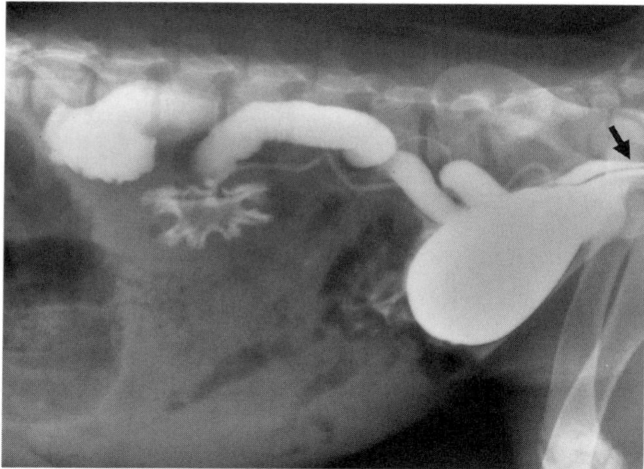

FIG. 34–6. Lateral view of the abdomen of a 10–week–old female black Labrador retriever following intravenous urography and retrograde urethrocystography. Note the dilated right renal pelvis and right ureter. The termination of the ectopic right ureter in the urethra can be identified (arrow). Note the normal termination of the left ureter in the urinary bladder. Overdistention of the urinary bladder with contrast medium resulted in self–limiting perivesical leakage of contrast medium into the peritoneal cavity.

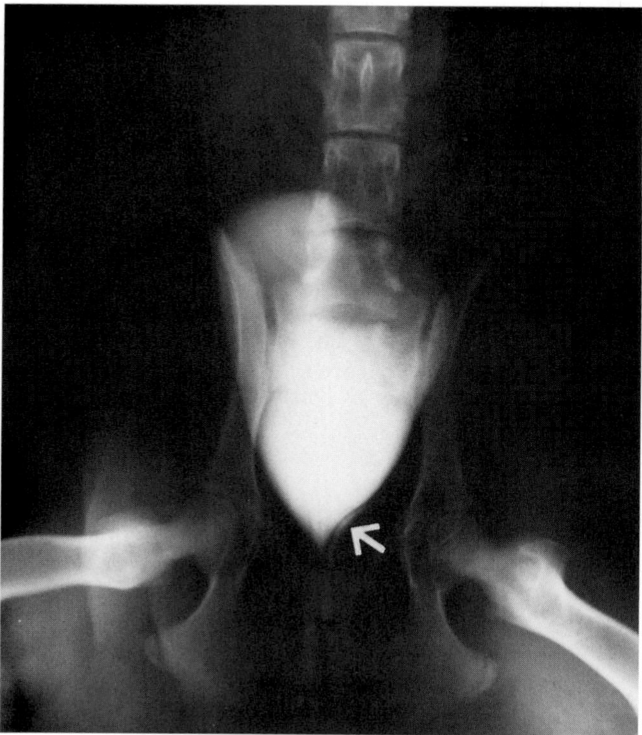

FIG. 34–7. Intravenous urogram of an incontinent 4–year–old spayed female golden retriever illustrates termination of the left ureter in the urethra (arrow). Left ureteral ectopia was not associated with dilation of the ureter or renal pelvis.

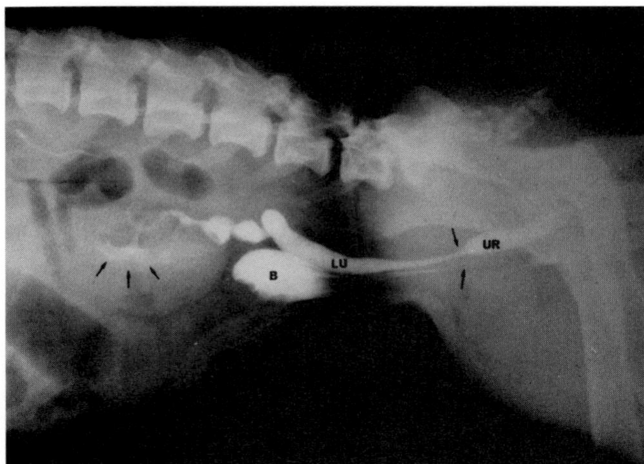

FIG. 34–8. Retrograde urogram shows termination of left ureter into the urethra (arrows) of a 21-month-old nonspayed female English bulldog. LV = left ureter; B = bladder; UR = urethra (arrows outline renal pelvis).

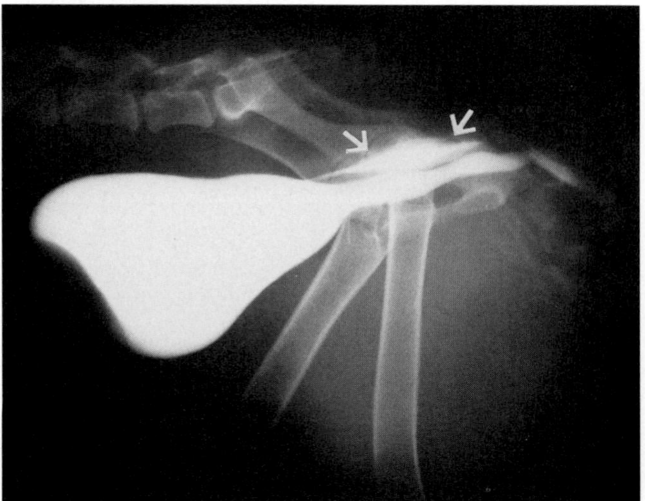

FIG. 34–9. Intravenous urogram of a 2–year–old spayed female soft–coated Wheaten terrier with bilateral ectopic ureters (not shown). Note the pooling of contrast medium in the vaginal lumen (arrows).

in the bladder lumen. However, an increase in intravesicular pressure caused by a full bladder may enhance shunting of urine through ectopic urethral branches of ureters that have openings at the trigone and the urethra.[9]

(b). Poor visualization of the ureter may result from reduced excretion of contrast medium in poorly concentrated urine formed by pyelonephritic kidneys.

(c). Interference with visualization of the distal portion of ectopic ureters caused by accumulation of contrast medium within the bladder lumen may be minimized by exposing films before the bladder becomes distended with contrast material, by fluoroscopy, by combining pneumocystography with intravenous urography, or by taking oblique radiographic views in addition to lateral, ventrodorsal, and dorsoventral views. In one study, ureteral structure was correctly identified by a combination of excretory urography and pneumocystography in six of seven dogs with ectopic ureters.[33] By comparison, ureteral structure was correctly predicted in only one of eight dogs evaluated by excretory urography alone.

(3). Megaureter (ureteroectasia), characterized by dilation of the ureteral lumen and abnormal peristalsis, is a common, but not consistent, finding in dogs with ectopic

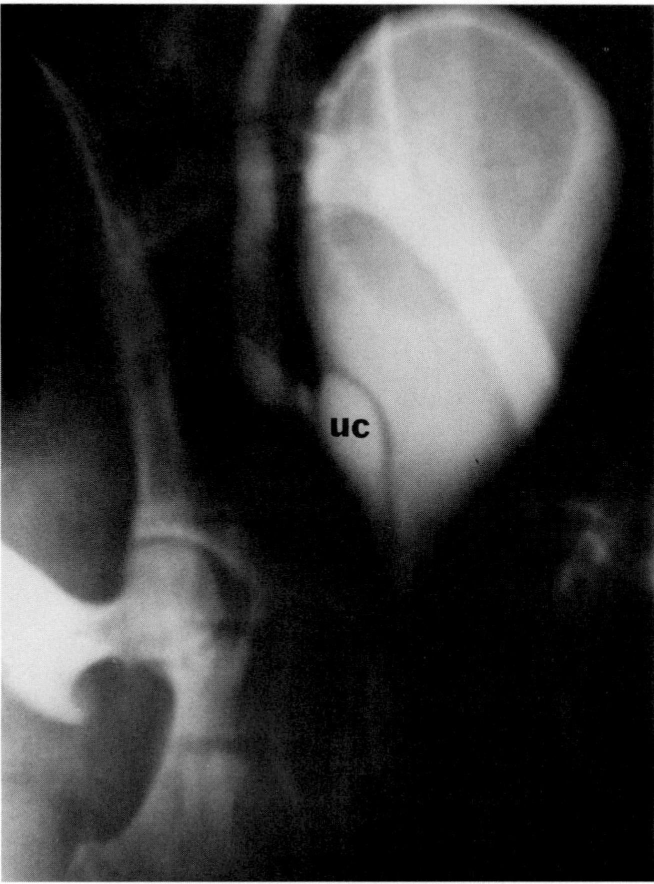

FIG. 34–10. Intravenous urogram of an incontinent 1–year–old intact female with a left ectopic ureterocele (uc) that terminated in the proximal urethra. A large bubble of air is in the bladder lumen (see Table 34–2).

ureters (see Figs. 34–2, 34–4 through 34–6, 34–8, and 34–10). This abnormality has not been observed as consistently in cats with urethral ectopia.

(a). Although the cause(s) of megaureter in dogs and cats have not been established, developmental abnormalities of the distal portion of the ureter have been cited as a cause in humans.[4]

(b). Because the distal end of an ectopic ureter has no functional valve, the pathogenesis of megaureter might be related to vesicoureteral or urethroureteral reflux.

(c). Increased resistance to urine flow through the distal ureters caused by submucosal tunneling of ectopic ureters through the bladder and urethra may also contribute to dilation of proximal portions.

(d). Urinary tract infection caused by bacteria (*Escherichia coli* and *Pseudomonas* species) known to impair ureteral peristalsis by releasing bacterial toxins or by stimulating biologically active substances produced by the host may also be contributing factors to megaureter.[7]

(4). The configuration of the ureterovesical junction, visualized by excretory urography, may arouse suspicion of an ectopic ureter. In a study, 20 of 23 ectopic ureters were identified by the observation that the ureterovesical junction had a straight rather than a normal J-shaped configuration.[33]

(5). Dilation and irregular margins of the renal pelvis (pyelectasis), accompanied by shortened or blunted renal pelvic diverticula, are characteristics of chronic pyelonephritis, which often occurs in dogs with ectopic ureter(s).

(6). Progressive reduction in renal size also commonly occurs in patients with ureteral ectopia.

(a). The abnormal focus of termination of the distal end of ectopic ureters and/or abnormal ureteral function are conducive to ascending bacterial infection of the kidneys.

(b). In our experience, contracted kidneys of patients with ectopic ureters typically have gross, microscopic, and bacteriologic findings typical of chronic generalized pyelonephritis.

(7). In summary, excretory urographic findings that may be associated with ectopic ureters include:

(a). Distal ureters that bypass the bladder trigone (see Figs. 34–1 through 34–3 and 34–5 through 34–8).

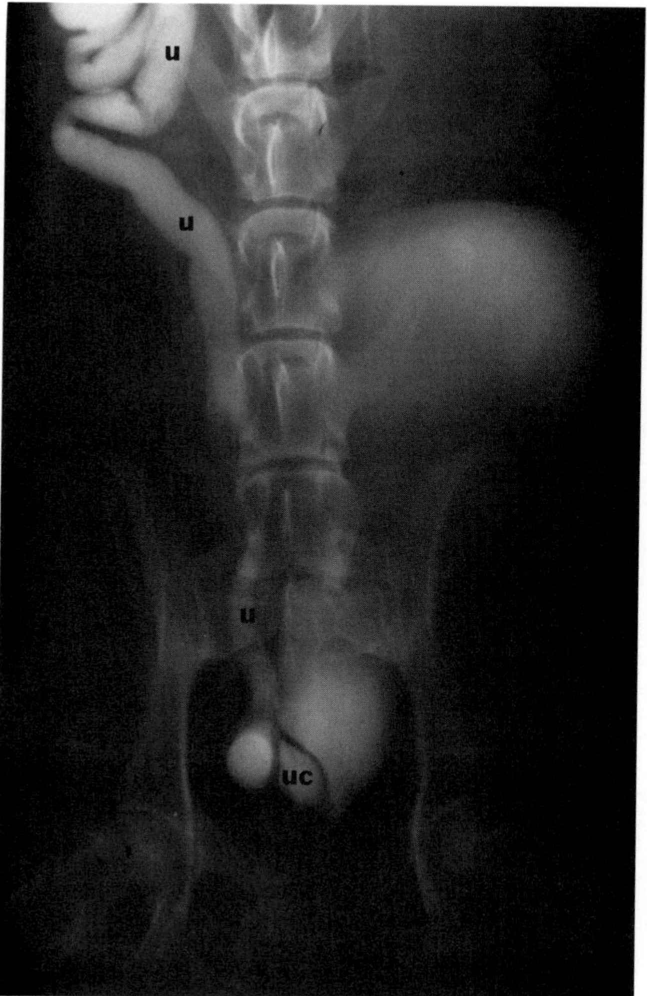

FIG. 34–11. Intravenous urogram of a 33-month-old intact female Newfoundland with a left ectopic ureterocele (uc) and associated dilation of the ureter (u) and renal pelvis. Incontinence decreased following neoureterocystotomy (see Table 34–2).

(b). Ectasia of the ureter and renal pelvis, and abnormalities or renal pelvic diverticula (Figs. 34–4 through 34–6, 34–8, 34–9, and 34–11).

(c). Decreased renal size.

(d). Appearance of radiographic contrast medium in the urethra or vagina during the storage phase of micturition (see Fig. 34–9).

(e). A straight ureterovesical junction.

d. Positive or negative contrast cystography (or cystometrography) is required to confirm abnormal reduction in the size and distensibility of the urinary bladder. Although this finding has been associated with embryonic cystic hypoplasia, it is most likely to occur in patients with bilateral ureteral ectopia as a consequence of disuse.

C. Management.

1. No effective primary medical management is available for urinary incontinence caused by an ectopic ureter; surgical correction is the only viable alternative. Urinary incontinence during the storage phase of micturition that persists following surgical correction of ectopic ureters may respond to administration of alpha-adrenergic agonists, such as phenylpropanolamine or ephedrine. This may be combined with small dosages of estrogen, which are thought to increase the sensitivity of alpha-adrenergic receptors.
2. Surgical management.
   a. The choice of surgical technique depends on the number of ectopic ureters, their termination sites, the functional status of the ureters and kidneys, and the presence of concomitant abnormalities. Reconstructive surgery designed to direct urine flow from the ectopic ureter into the urinary bladder should be seriously considered when function of the kidney drained by the ectopic ureter(s) is normal, extravesical termination of both ureters exists, or functional capacity of both kidneys is reduced. If generalized renal disease is present, removing an ectopic ureter and the associated kidney may reduce renal function enough to precipitate renal failure.
   b. Preoperative considerations.
      (1). A physical examination and evaluation by hemogram and urinalysis to assess the general health of the animal, and radiographic evaluation (excretory urography, urethrocystography) to detect concomitant congenital abnormalities and to localize the termination site(s) of the ectopic ureter(s), are essential.
      (2). The serum concentration of urea nitrogen or creatinine should be determined, to assess glomerular filtration rate.
      (3). Since persistent urinary tract infection (UTI) is common, bacterial culture of urine and determination of the antimicrobial susceptibility of pathogens are recommended. If significant bacteriuria is present, appropriate antimicrobial therapy should be instituted before surgery.
   c. Neostoma *in situ* (Fig. 34–12).
      (1). Creation of a neostoma *in situ* without transection of the ureter may be considered for intramural ectopic ureters.[9a,42,52,52a] The segment of ureter distal to the neostoma must be ligated, to prevent continued loss of urine through the ectopic ureteral opening.
      (2). The advantages of this technique are that the ureter is not transected, damage to the ureteral blood and nerve supply is minimal, the likelihood of postsurgical outflow obstruction is minimized, and the likelihood of postsurgical vesicoureteral reflux is minimized.

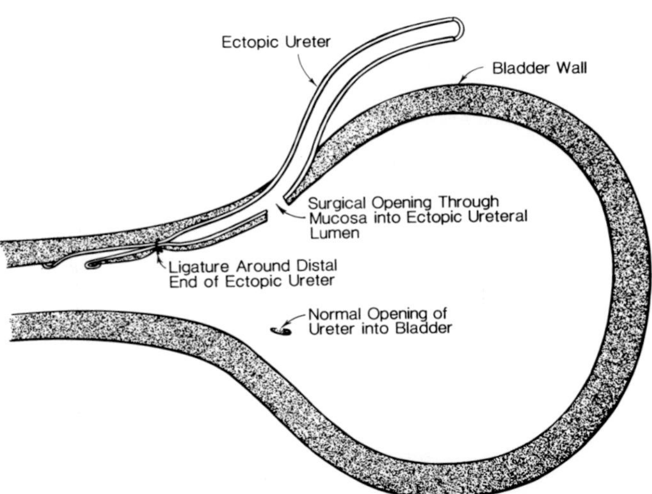

FIG. 34–12. Schematic illustration of a technique of ureterovesicular anastomosis in which the ectopic ureter is not transected. Urine is prevented from passing from the ureter into the urethra by ligating the distal portion of the ectopic ureter. Urine from the ectopic ureter is diverted into the bladder lumen by placing an opening between the transmural section of the ureteral and bladder mucosa. (Faulkner RT, Osborne CA, Feeney DA. Canine and feline ureteral ectopia. In: Kirk RW, ed. *Current Veterinary Therapy VIII.* Philadelphia, Pennsylvania: WB Saunders; 1983.)

   d. Ureterovesical anastomosis (ureteroneocystostomy) (Fig. 34–13).
      (1). Ureterovesicular anastomosis should be considered to correct urinary incontinence caused by extramural ectopic ureters.
      (2). The most widely accepted method of ureterovesicular anastomosis involves transecting the abnormal ureters near the bladder, spatulating their ends, and reimplanting them into the urinary bladder through a submucosal antireflux tunnel formed in the bladder wall.[15,44,46,52,57–59]
         (a). Transecting the ureter has the disadvantage of interrupting its vascular and nerve supply.
         (b). This technique may also be associated with formation of strictures at the site of anastomosis.
   e. When the ectopic ureter opens normally at the trigone, and at a site distal to the trigone (branching), the ureteral segment distal to the normal site of termination should be ligated.
   f. Ureteral troughs may be surgically corrected by closing them with a simple continuous suture pattern.[52,52a]
   g. Suture material allowed to remain in contact

with the lumen of the urinary tract should be absorbable. Nonabsorbable sutures that are exposed to urine predispose the patient to bacterial urinary tract infections and urolith formation.

h. Nephrectomy and ureterectomy.
   (1). Nephrectomy and removal of as much of the ectopic ureter as possible should be performed in patients with a unilateral ectopic ureter attached to a kidney affected by generalized and severe disease.
   (2). Nephrectomy and ureterectomy may be considered only if the contralateral kidney has function adequate to sustain renal function.
   (3). The ectopic ureter should be transected as close as possible to its site of termination, to minimize problems associated with infection of the distal ureteral stump.
i. Ligation of the renal artery and ureter.
   (1). Ligation of the renal artery and left ureter eliminated urinary incontinence in a 2-year-old female Burmese cat with an ectopic left ureter terminating in the vagina.[13] Ureteral transplantation was considered unwise. Nephrectomy and ureterectomy were not possible because the cat was in renal failure.
   (2). The goal was to increase compensatory function in the right kidney, based on results of studies in sheep indicating that renal infarction is a greater stimulus to compensatory renal function than is renal ablation.
j. Postsurgical recommendations.
   (1). Some degree of temporary occlusion of the ureteral lumen at the site of anastomosis is common and is caused by inflammatory swelling of tissues following surgery. It may persist several weeks (Fig. 34–14).
      (a). This finding does not necessarily indicate a poor surgical result.
      (b). If complete obstruction of the ureteral lumen is not corrected within 1 week after it occurs, irreversible damage to the associated kidney is likely.
      (c). An excretory urogram should be performed approximately 5 to 7 days after surgery, to assess patency of the ureter.
      (d). Evaluation of an excretory urogram 4 to 6 weeks after surgery may be necessary to reassess the functional status of the ureter.
      (e). Surgeons disagree about whether a ureteral stent should be used after ureterovesical anastomosis. The logic is to minimize occlusion of small ureters caused by postsurgical inflammation.
   (2). Every effort should be made to avoid the use of catheters for collecting urine samples or for obtaining retrograde radiographic studies, because postsurgical patients are predisposed to UTI. Samples for urinalysis and urine culture should be collected by cystocentesis. Urinalysis should be performed at appropriate intervals after surgery, to monitor the patient for UTI.
   (3). For bacterial UTI, antimicrobial therapy selected on the basis of urine culture and antimicrobial susceptibility tests should be

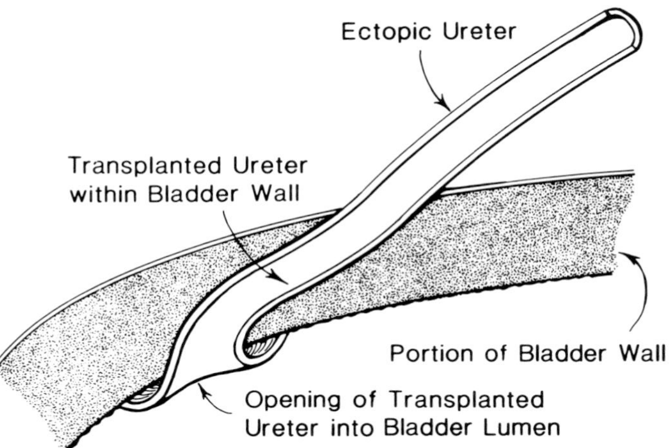

FIG. 34–13. Schematic diagram of ureterovesicular anastomosis illustrates a submucosal reflux tunnel. Distention of the bladder lumen with urine compresses the portion of the ureteral lumen located within the bladder wall and thus minimizes the reflux of urine from the bladder into the ureter. (Faulkner RT, Osborne CA, Feeney DA. Canine and feline ureteral ectopia. In: Kirk RK, ed. *Current Veterinary Therapy VIII.* Philadelphia, Pennsylvania: WB Saunders; 1983.)

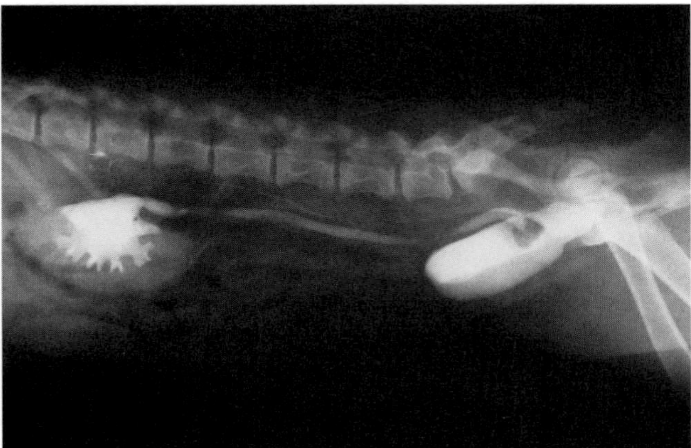

FIG. 34–14. Intravenous urogram of a 5–month–old female mixed–breed dog obtained 2 weeks following surgical correction of an ectopic left ureter by ureterovesical anastomosis with a submucosal reflux tunnel. Note the filling defect in the dorsal region of the bladder at the site of ureteral transplantation, and dilation of the left renal pelvis and ureter caused by partial outflow obstruction. Postsurgical distal ureteral outflow obstruction resolved spontaneously.

continued until clinical signs of infection subside, results of urinalysis are normal, and the urine is sterile.

k. Postsurgical complications may include the following.
   (1). Dehisence of the anastomosis may be caused by extensive tension at the transplantation site.
   (2). Permanent stenosis caused by excessive handling or suturing may result in hydroureter and hydronephrosis.
   (3). Uroliths may form around suture material that remains exposed to the excretory pathway.
   (4). Formation in the bladder wall of a ureteral tunnel that is too short may predispose to vesicoureteral reflux and upper urinary tract infections.
   (5). Recanalization of the distal ureter after closure of the distal segment of a branching ureter, or after neostoma formation, may result in recurrence of urinary incontinence.

l. Prognosis.
   (1). Surgical correction of ectopic ureters is often associated with immediate cessation of urinary incontinence; however, estimates show that some degree of incontinence during the storage phase of micturition (positional, exertional, nocturnal, etc.) may occur in 50% of dogs after surgery.[9,52a] Patients with ureters that terminate in the vagina or uterus are more likely to gain urinary continence. Surgical correction of ectopic ureters that terminated in the urethra has been associated with a higher rate of continence in males than in females.
   (2). Postoperative incontinence may be related to:
      (a). Persistent patency of the distal ureteral segment.
      (b). Failure to identify bilateral ectopic ureters.
      (c). Vaginal pooling of urine.
      (d). Reduced urinary bladder capacity.
      (e). Concomitant abnormalities of the urethra.
      (f). Damage to the sphincter mechanism as a result of surgery.
   (3). Female dogs with unilateral or bilateral ectopic ureters that terminate in the urethra may continue to have some degree of urinary incontinence following surgery. This may be related to concomitant abnormalities of the urethra.[48] Persistent postsurgical incontinence in these patients may be controlled by daily administration of phenylpropanolamine (0.5 to 1.0 mg/kg/d, divided into 2 or 3 subdoses), an alpha-adrenergic agonist.[47] This drug may be combined with small dosages of estrogens, given with the goal of increasing the sensitivity of alpha-adrenergic receptors to stimulation. Response to therapy may be monitored by urethral pressure profilometry. Pharmacologic stimulation of alpha-adrenergic receptors located in the bladder neck and proximal urethra may increase resting urethral pressure sufficiently to correct the problem.
   (4). The reimplantation of dilated ureters into the urinary bladder may be associated with varying degrees of vesicoureteral reflux. This phenomenon is clinically significant because it predisposes the patient to ascending infection of the kidney.
   (5). Even though a better long-term result may be obtained when the ureters have some degree of peristalsis and are not extremely dilated, we have obtained satisfactory long-term results in several dogs in which markedly dilated ectopic ureters were reimplanted into the urinary bladder. In some patients, ureteroectasia and pyeloectasia present prior to surgery subsided following surgery.[33,39,49] Reduction in the size of the ureters and renal pelves has been detected by postoperative excretory urography; however, excretory urography is not a definitive method for assessing ureteral structure because the degree of filling and of radiodensity of the renal pelves and ureters varies with the type, dosage, and rate of intravenous injection

TABLE 34–2
CLINICAL FEATURES OF FIVE FEMALE DOGS WITH ECTOPIC URETEROCELES DIAGNOSED AT THE UNIVERSITY OF MINNESOTA VETERINARY TEACHING HOSPITAL BETWEEN 1976 AND 1991

Age (mo)	Breed	Clinical Signs	Radiographic Findings	Clinical Outcome
2	Siberian husky	Urinary incontinence	Dilated right renal pelvis and ureter with ectopic right ureterocele terminating in vagina[1]	Vaginal ectopic ureter was transplanted (neoureterocystotomy) into the bladder; however, the incontinence did not resolve following surgery.*
33	Newfoundland	Urinary incontinence since birth	Left hydroureter and dilated left renal pelvis with ectopic left ureterocele terminating in the urethra 5-week postop intravenous urography (IVU) revealed reduced size of the left renal pelvis and ureter when compared to preop IVU	Left ureteral transplantation (neoureterocystotomy) into the bladder; incontinence was improved 5 weeks postoperatively.
11	Miniature poodle	Urinary incontinence since birth	Left hydroureter and dilated left renal pelvis with ectopic left ureterocele terminating in urethra	Transplanted left ectopic ureter into the bladder (neoureterocystotomy); incontinence resolved following surgery.
3	Brittany spaniel	Incontinence, stranguria, and nocturia	Left-sided hydroureter, hydronephrosis, and an ectopic ureterocele terminating in the urethra. The ureterocele obstructed the bladder neck. Follow up IVUs at 3 weeks, 5 months, 1 year, and 2 years post endoscopy revealed a gradual reduction in hydroureter and hydronephrosis.	Endoscopy revealed that the ureterocele entered into the urethra. By endoscopy, it was incised and catheterized. The incontinence resolved after endoscopic surgery but recurred following ovariohysterectomy. Treatment with phenylpropanolamine was unsuccessful.
48	Pekingese-poodle cross	Urinary incontinence after normal voiding and while sleeping noticed for 2 years following ovariohysterectomy. Treatment with stilbestrol for 2 years was initially satisfactory; however, increased dosages did not prevent recurrence of incontinence.	Dilated distal left hydroureter terminating in the urethra. A ureterocele was noted.‡	Urinary incontinence resolved following surgical transplantation of left ectopic ureter (neoureterocystotomy) into the bladder.

*Data from Johnston GR, Osborne CA, Wilson JW, Yano BL. Familial ureteral ectopia in the dog. *J Am Anim Hosp Assoc.* 1977;13:168–170.
‡Data from Johnston GR, Feeney DA. Radiographic evaluation of the urinary tract in dogs and cats. *Contemp Issues Small Anim Pract (Nephrol Urol).* 1986;4:203–273.

of contrast medium and with the rate of urine production.

II. URETEROCELES

A. Applied embryology and etiology.

1. A ureterocele is a cystic dilation of the terminal submucosal segment of the intravesicular ureter.
2. In humans, ureteroceles are classified according to location, structure, and other concurrent anatomic abnormalities.[2]
   a. Orthotopic (simple) ureteroceles are located at the trigone of the urinary bladder; the distal ureteral orifice is in normal position.
   b. Ureteroceles accompanying ectopic ureters are called ectopic ureteroceles.
3. Postulated causes of ureteroceles in humans.[1]
   a. Late rupture of the double epithelial layer between the lumen of the ureter and the lumen of the urogenital sinus.
   b. Ureteral dilation secondary to ureteral obstruction caused by stenosis of the ureteral orifice.
   c. Delayed ureteral migration such that the normal dilation occurs, but is not incorporated into the urogenital sinus and thus is retained as a dilated distal ureteral segment.
   d. Segmental embryonal arrest of the distal ureter resulting in a lack of superficial musculature in the distal ureteral segment.
4. Development of an acquired ureterocele in a 17-month-old male Labrador retriever was reported secondary to surgical correction of an ectopic ureter.[32]

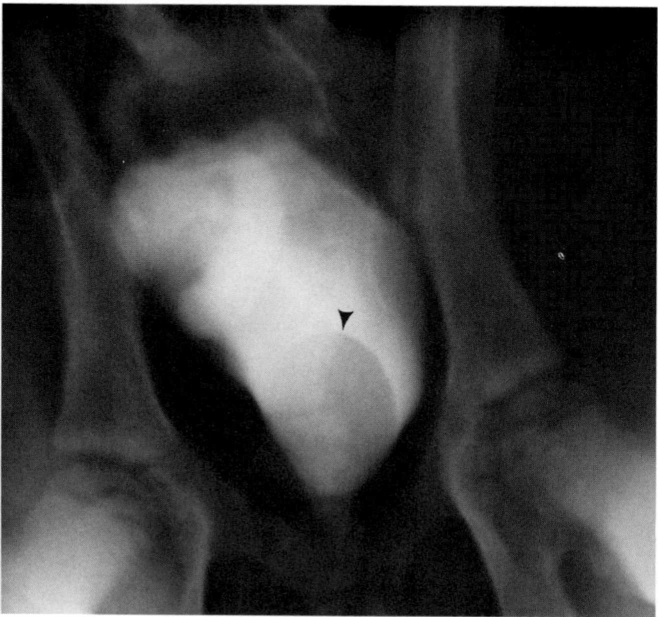

FIG. 34–15. Intravenous urogram of a 3–month–old Brittany spaniel with a left ectopic ureterocele (arrow) partially obstructing the neck of the urinary bladder (see Table 34–2).

5. Too few cases of canine ureterocele have been reported to determine breed predispositions. Most, but not all, ureteroceles have been detected in female dogs (Table 34–2).[1,21,35,51,53,56] Apparently they have not been reported in cats.

B. Diagnostic considerations.

1. As with ectopic ureters, clinical signs are usually, but not invariably, observed in young animals. Clinical signs depend on the location and size of the ureterocele and on the presence of concomitant abnormalities.
   a. Although dogs with orthotopic ureteroceles may be asymptomatic, the ureterocele may not be static. Continued enlargement of the ureterocele may cause partial outflow obstruction in the region of the bladder neck, leading to urine stasis, dysuria, and urinary tract infection. Obstruction of the ureter may result in hydroureter and hydronephrosis.
   b. Dogs with ectopic ureteroceles usually have urinary incontinence. Ipsilateral hydroureter and hydronephrosis are common, and may be complicated by bacterial UTI.
2. Excretory urography, especially when combined with pneumocystography, may reveal a "cobra head" dilation of the ureter within the bladder or urethra (see Figs. 34–10 and 34–11). Hydroureter and hydronephrosis may also be detected (see Table 34–2).
3. Intravenous urography or retrograde urethrocystography may reveal a filling defect in the bladder or urethra (Fig. 34–15). Contrast medium may reflux into an ectopic ureter.
4. Ultrasonography may reveal findings consistent with a cystic structure in the bladder or urethra.

C. Treatment (Table 34–2).

1. In general, treatment of ectopic ureteroceles should be directed at controlling associated clinical signs, preserving or improving renal function, and eliminating or preventing urinary tract infection.
2. Obstructive ureteroceles may be treated initially by cystoscopy and incision of the ureterocele.
3. Ureterocelectomy and ureteral transplantation should be considered if the ipsilateral kidney is functional.[35]
4. Ureteronephrectomy should be considered if severe hydroureter and hydronephrosis is present, provided adequate renal function can be sustained by the contralateral kidney.

REFERENCES

1. Alexander LG. Ectopic ureter and ureterocele. In: Bojrab MJ, ed. *Disease Mechanisms in Small Animal Surgery.* 2nd ed. Philadelphia, Pennsylvania: Lea & Febiger; 1993:513–519.

1a. Allen WE, Webbom PM. Two cases of urinary incontinence in cats associated with acquired vaginoureteral fistulas. *J Small Anim Pract.* 1980;21:367–371.

2. Bauer SB, Perlmutter AD, Retik AB. Anomalies of the upper urinary tract. In: Walsh PC, Retik AB, Stamey TA, et al., eds.

Campbell's Urology. 6th ed. Philadelphia, Pennsylvania: WB Saunders; 1992:1359–1442.

3. Bebko RL, Prier JE, Biery DN. Ectopic ureters in a male cat. *J Am Vet Med Assoc.* 1977;171:738–740.
4. Belman AB. Megaureter: classification, etiology, and management. *Urol Clin North Am.* 1974;1:497–513.
5. Biery DN. Radiographic evaluation of the kidneys. In: Bovee KC, ed. *Canine Nephrology.* Media, Pennsylvania: Harwal; 1984: 275–313.
6. Biewenga WJ, Rothuizen J, Voorhout G. Ectopic ureters in the cat: A report of two cases. *J Small Anim Pract.* 1978;19:531–537.
7. Boyarsky S, et al. *Urodynamics: Hydrodynamics of the Ureter and Renal Pelvis.* New York, New York: Academic Press; 1971.
8. Brodeur GY. Diagnosis of ectopic ureter. *Canine Pract.* 1977; 4:25–28.
9. Dean PW, Constantinescu GM. Canine ectopic ureter. *Comp Contin Ed.* 1988;10:146–157.

9a. Dingwall JS, Eger CE, Owen RR. Clinical experience with the combined technique of ureterovesical anastomosis for treatment of ectopic ureters. *J Am Anim Hosp Assoc.* 1976;12:406–410.

10. Faulkner RT, Osborne CA, Feeney DA. Canine and feline ureteral ectopia. In: Kirk RW, ed. *Current Veterinary Therapy VIII.* Philadelphia, Pennsylvania: WB Saunders; 1983:1043–1048.
11. Feeney DA, Barber DL, Osborne CA. Advances in excretory urography. In: *Proceedings of the 30th Gaines Veterinary Symposium.* White Plains, New York: Gaines Professional Services; 1981: 8–22.
12. Feeney DA, et al. Normal canine excretory urogram: Effects of dose, time, and individual dog variation. *Am J Vet Res.* 1979;40: 1596–1604.
13. Filippich LJ, et al. Ectopic ureter in a cat—A case report. *Aust Vet Pract.* 1985;15:7–9.
14. Grauer GF, Freeman LF, Nelson AW. Urinary incontinence associated with an ectopic ureter in a female cat. *J Am Vet Med Assoc.* 1983;182:707–710.
15. Greene RW, Greiner TP. The ureter: Repair of longitudinal defects and reimplantation. In: Bojrab MJ, ed. *Current Techniques in Small Animal Surgery.* Philadelphia, Pennsylvania: Lea & Febiger; 1975.
16. Greene JA, Thornhill JA, Blevins WE. Hydronephrosis and hydroureter associated with a unilateral ectopic ureter in a spayed bitch. *J Am Anim Hosp Assoc.* 1978;14:708–713.
17. Gregory CR, Willits NH. Electromyographic and urethral pressure evaluations: Assessment of urethral function in female and ovariohysterectomized female cats. *Am J Vet Res.* 1986;47:1472–1475.
18. Gregory SP, Holt PE. Comparison of stressed simultaneous urethral pressure profiles between anesthetized continent and incontinent bitches with urethral sphincter mechanism incompetence. *Am J Vet Res.* 1993;54:216–222.
19. Hayes HM. Ectopic ureter in dogs. Epidemiological features. *Teratology.* 1974;10:129–132.
20. Hayes HM. Breed associations of canine ectopic ureter: A study of 217 female cases. *J Small Anim Pract.* 1984;25:501–504.
21. Hoffman S, Ferguson HR. Ureterocele in a dog: Case study. *J Am Anim Hosp Assoc.* 1991;27:93–95.
22. Holt PE. Simultaneous urethral pressure profilometry: Comparisons between continent and incontinent bitches. *J Small Anim Pract.* 1988;29:761–769.
23. Holt PE, Gibbs C, Pearson H. Canine ectopic ureter: A review of twenty-nine cases. *J Small Anim Pract.* 1982;23:195–208.
24. Holt PE, Gregory SP. Resting urethral pressure profilometry in bitches: Artifact or reality? *Comp Contin Ed.* 1993;15:1207–1215.
25. Johnston GR, Jessen CR, Osborne CA. Retrograde contrast urethrography. In: Kirk RW, ed. *Current Veterinary Therapy VI.* Philadelphia, Pennsylvania: WB Saunders; 1977.
26. Johnston GR, et al. Familial ureteral ectopia in the dog. *J Am Anim Hosp Assoc.* 1977;13:168–170.
27. Jones BR. Diseases of the ureters. In: Ettinger SJ, ed. *Textbook of Veterinary Internal Medicine.* 2nd ed. Vol 2. Philadelphia, Pennsylvania: WB Saunders; 1983.
28. Kuzma AB, Holmberg DL. Ectopic ureter in a cat. *Can Vet J.* 1988;29:59–61.
29. Lane LG. Canine ectopic ureter: Two further case reports. *J Small Anim Pract.* 1973;14:555–560.
30. Lennox JS. A case report of unilateral ectopic ureter in a male Siberian husky. *J Am Anim Hosp Assoc.* 1978;14:331–336.
31. Lulich JP, et al. Urologic disorders of immature cats. *Vet Clin North Am.* 1987;17:663–696.
32. Martin RA, Harvey HJ, Flanders JA. Bilateral ectopic ureters in a male dog: A case report. *J Am Anim Hosp Assoc.* 1985;21:80–84.
33. Mason LK, et al. Surgery of ectopic ureters: Pre- and postoperative radiographic morphology. *J Am Anim Hosp Assoc.* 1990;26: 73–79.
34. McCarthy TC, McDermaid SL. Cystoscopy. *Vet Clin North Am.* 1990;20:1315–1338.
35. McLoughlin MA, Hauptman JG, Spaulding K. Canine ureteroceles: A case report and literature review. *J Am Anim Hosp Assoc.* 1989;25:699–706.
36. Osborne CA, Dietrich HF, Hanlon GF, Anderson LD. Urinary incontinence due to ectopic ureter in a male dog. *J Am Vet Med Assoc.* 1975;166:911–914.
37. Osborne CA, Low DG, Finco DR. *Canine and Feline Urology.* Philadelphia, Pennsylvania: WB Saunders; 1972.
38. Osborne CA, Finco DR, Low DG. Diseases of the ureters. In: Ettinger SJ, ed. *Textbook of Veterinary Internal Medicine.* Vol 2. Philadelphia, Pennsylvania: WB Saunders; 1975.
39. Osborne CA, Hanlon GF. Canine congenital ureteral ectopia: Case report and review of literature. *J Am Anim Hosp Assoc.* 1967;3:111–122.
40. Osborne CA, Oliver JE. Non-neurogenic urinary incontinence. In: Kirk RW, ed. *Current Veterinary Therapy VI.* Philadelphia, Pennsylvania: WB Saunders; 1977.
41. Osborne CA, Perman V. Ectopic ureter in a male dog. *J Am Vet Med Assoc.* 1969;154:273–278.
42. Osborne CA, Polzin DJ, Feeney DA, Caywood DD. The urinary system: Pathophysiology, diagnosis & treatment. In: IM Gourley, PB Vasseur, eds. *General Small Animal Surgery.* Philadelphia, Pennsylvania: JB Lippincott; 1985:479–658.
43. Owen RR. Canine ureteral ectopia: A review. I. Embryology and etiology. *J Small Anim Pract.* 1973;14:407–417.
44. Owen RR. Canine ureteral ectopia: A review. II. Incidence, diagnosis and treatment. *J Small Anim Pract.* 1973;14:419–427.
45. Pearson H, Gibbs C. Urinary tract abnormalities in the dog. *J Small Anim Pract.* 1971;12:67–84.
46. Rawlings CA. Repair of ectopic ureter. In: Bojrab MJ, ed. *Current Techniques in Small Animal Surgery.* 2nd ed. Philadelphia, Pennsylvania: Lea & Febiger; 1983.
47. Rigg DL, Zenoble RD, Riedesel EA. Neoureterostomy and phenylpropanolamine therapy for incontinence due to ectopic ureter in a dog. *J Am Anim Hosp Assoc.* 1983;19:237–241.
48. Rosin AE, Barsanti JA. Diagnosis of urinary incontinence in dogs: Role of urethral pressure profile. *J Am Vet Med Assoc.* 1981;178:814–822.
49. Ross LA, Lamb CR. Reduction of hydronephrosis and hydroureter associated with ectopic ureters in two dogs after ureterovesical anastomosis. *J Am Vet Med Assoc.* 1990;196:1497–1499.
50. Rutgers C, Chew DJ, Burt JK. Bilateral ectopic ureters in female

cats with urinary incontinence. *J Am Vet Med Assoc.* 1984;184: 1394–1395.

51. Scott RC, Greene RW, Patnaik AK. Unilateral ureterocele associated with hydronephrosis in a dog. *J Am Anim Hosp Assoc.* 1974;10:126–131.
52. Stone EA, Barsanti JA. *Urologic Surgery of the Dog and Cat.* Philadelphia, Pennsylvania: Lea & Febiger, 1992.

52a. Stone EA, Mason LK. Surgery of ectopic ureters: Types, method of correction, and postoperative results. *J Am Anim Hosp Assoc.* 1990;26:81–88.

53. Stowater JL, Springer AL. Ureterocele in a dog. *Vet Med Small Anim Clin.* 1979;74:1753–1756.
54. Smith CW, Burke TJ, Froehlich P. Bilateral ureteral ectopia in a male cat with urinary incontinence. *J Am Vet Med Assoc.* 1983; 182:172–173.
55. Smith CW, Stowater JL, Kneller SH. Bilateral ectopic ureter in a male dog with urinary incontinence. *J Am Vet Med Assoc.* 1980; 177:1022–1024.
56. Smith CW, Stowater JL, Kneller SK. Ectopic ureter in the dog—A review of cases. *J Am Anim Hosp Assoc.* 1981;17:245–248.
57. Tarvin GB. Surgical treatment of ectopic ureters. *Vet Clin North Am.* 1979;9:277–284.
58. Waldron DR. Ectopic ureter surgery and its problems. *Prob Vet Med.* 1989;1:85–92.
59. Waldron DR, et al. Ureteroneocystostomy: A comparison of the submucosal tunnel and transverse pull through techniques. *J Am Anim Hosp Assoc.* 1987;23:285–290.
60. Wilson JG, Warkang J. Malformations in the genitourinary tract induced by maternal vitamin A deficiency in the rat. *Am J Anat.* 1948;83:357–407.
61. Wilson JG, Roth CB, Warkang J. An analysis of the syndrome of malformations induced by maternal vitamin A deficiency. Effects of restoration of vitamin A at various times during gestation. *Am J Anat.* 1953;92:189–217.

PART V

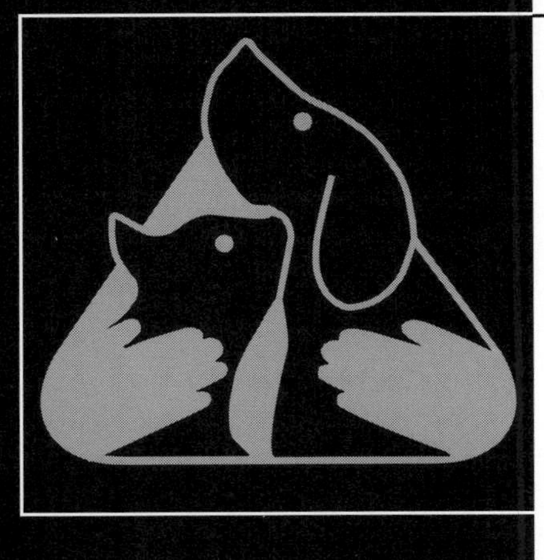

DISEASES OF THE LOWER URINARY TRACT

CHAPTER 35

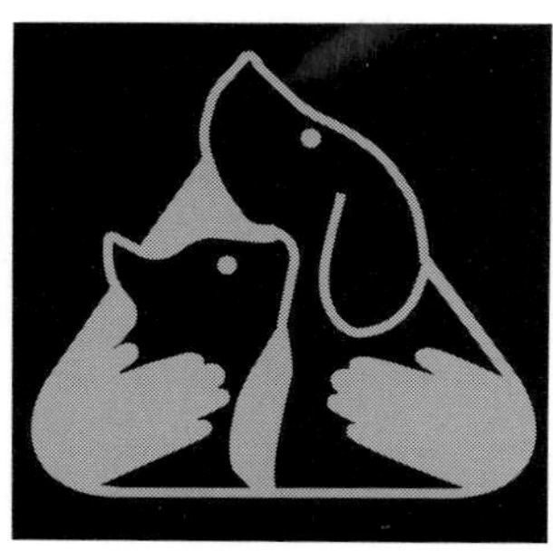

Disorders of the Feline Lower Urinary Tract

CARL A. OSBORNE
JOHN M. KRUGER
JODY P. LULICH
DAVID J. POLZIN

I. DEFINITION OF TERMS AND CONCEPTS

A. The terms feline urologic syndrome and FUS are being used less by the veterinary profession as diagnostic terms to describe disorders of domestic cats characterized by hematuria, dysuria, pollakiuria, and partial or complete urethral obstruction because various combinations of these signs may be associated with any cause of feline lower urinary tract disease (LUTD) (Table 35–1). The similarity of clinical signs caused by diverse causes is not surprising because the feline urinary tract responds to various diseases in a limited and predictable fashion. "FUS" should be redefined as feline urologic *signs*. In this context, FUS is no more a diagnosis than vomiting or pruritus is diagnosis.

B. A heterogeneous group of LUTDs of cats may result from fundamentally different causes. The causes may be single, multiple and interacting, or unrelated (see Table 35–1).[69]

1. Results of diagnostic procedures are required to localize and redefine causes of diseases that result in feline LUTD (Table 35–2).
2. When possible, refined diagnoses of LUTD should encompass descriptive terms pertaining to site (e.g., urethra, bladder), pathophysiologic mechanisms (e.g., obstructive uropathy, reflex dyssynergia), morphologic changes (e.g., inflammation, neoplasia), and causes (e.g., anomalies, urolithiasis, bacteria, fungi).

II. EPIDEMIOLOGIC STUDIES

A. Overview.

1. Several dozen epidemiologic studies of FUS have been published.[4,76] Although many contain useful data, almost all have utilized the nonspecific concept of FUS as the common denominator to group affected cats.
2. Few populations selected for study were defined on the basis of standard or contemporary clinical diagnostic procedures. Thus, results of most of these studies must be interpreted in the context of a combination of all types of feline LUTDs, rather than as specific disorders.

B. Incidence and proportional morbidity.

1. The incidence of a disease is defined as the annual rate of appearance of new cases of disease among the entire population of individuals at risk for the disease.[92] Although there have apparently been no recent studies, the incidence of hematuria, dysuria, and/or urethral obstruction in domestic cats in the United States and Great Britain was

TABLE 35–1
EXAMPLES OF CONFIRMED CAUSES OF LOWER URINARY TRACT DISEASE IN DOMESTIC CATS*

Metabolic disorders (including nutritional)
- Uroliths (see Table 35-5)
- Urethral plugs (see Table 35-6)

Inflammatory disorders
- Infectious agents
  - Viruses? (see Table 35-7)
  - Bacteria (see Table 35-7)
  - Mycoplasmas/ureaplasmas? (see Table 35-7)
  - Fungi (see Table 35-7)
  - Parasites (see Table 35-7)
  - Others
- Noninfectious
  - Immune-mediated?
  - Others?

Trauma

Neurogenic disorders
- Reflex dyssynergia
- Urethral spasm
- Hypotonic or atonic bladder (primary or secondary)
- Others

Iatrogenic disorders
- Reverse flushing solutions
- Urethral catheters (reverse flushing)
- Indwelling urethral catheters, especially open systems
- Postsurgical urethral catheters
- Urethrostomy complications

Anatomic abnormalities
- Congenital
  - Urachal anomalies
  - Persistent uterus masculinus
  - Urethrorectal fistula
  - Phimosis
  - Others?
- Acquired
  - Urethral strictures
  - Others?

Neoplastic
- Benign
  - Cystadenoma (bladder)
  - Fibroma (bladder)
  - Leiomyoma (bladder)
  - Papilloma (bladder)
  - Hemangioma (bladder)
  - Transitional cell carcinoma (bladder and urethra)
  - Squamous cell carcinoma (bladder)
  - Adenocarcinoma (bladder)
  - Unclassified carcinoma (bladder)
  - Hemangiosarcoma (bladder)
  - Lymphosarcoma (primary and metastatic in bladder)
  - Myxosarcoma (bladder)
  - Prostatic adenocarcinoma (urethra)
  - Rhabdomyosarcoma (bladder)
  - Endometrial adenocarcinoma (extraurinary invading and compressing urethra)

Idiopathic

*Except where noted with a question mark, all these causes have been identified in cats with naturally occurring urinary disorders.

previously reported to be approximately 0.5 to 1.0% per year.[44,76,92]

2. The incidence of naturally occurring hematuria, dysuria, and/or urethral obstruction in domestic cats should not be confused with the frequency with which such cats are seen in veterinary hospitals (so-called proportional morbidity ratios).[92]
   a. Although the proportional morbidity ratio of cats with LUTDs has been reported to be as high as 10%, the frequency most commonly reported is 1 to 6%.[76,92]
   b. Data from 23 colleges of veterinary medicine in North America compiled by workers at the Veterinary Data Base, Purdue University, indicated that, from 1980 to 1990, LUTD was diagnosed in 13,511 of 184,983 hospital admissions (7.3%).
   c. Proportional morbidity ratios for FUS are not a reliable index of its incidence, because they can be affected by such factors as local population economics, geography, season, type of veterinary practice, and the interest and training of veterinarians.[92]
3. In a prospective clinical study performed at the University of Minnesota, 143 untreated cats with hematuria, dysuria, urethral obstruction, or combinations of these signs were evaluated by contemporary diagnostic methods. The cats had no concomitant disease of other body systems. Specific diagnoses were established in 66 of 153 (46%) (Tables 35–3 and 35–4).[41,26]

C. Risk factors.

1. Many risk factors for FUS have been identified, some of which appeared to be synergistic.[4] This led to the hypothesis that FUS was a multifactorial disorder (Table 35–5). In fact, an "FUS profile" was identified. Based on older epidemiologic data, the typical FUS cat was depicted as a 2- to 4-year-old overweight neutered male that lived indoors and consumed primarily dry food.[76]
2. When considered in light of the design and population characteristics of many older epidemiologic studies, the hypothesis that FUS was a multifactorial disease is not surprising. Likewise, difficulty in identifying the specific mode(s) of interaction of identified risk factors is predictable. Resolution of these difficulties depends on contemporary controlled epidemiologic studies designed to evaluate subsets of cats with LUTDs defined on the basis of specific diagnostic criteria. (See sections about specific diseases for additional information about risk factors.)

III. INTERRELATIONSHIP BETWEEN UROPATHOGENS, CRYSTALLURIA, AND URINARY TRACT DEFENSE MECHANISMS: A UNIFYING HYPOTHESIS

A. Overview.

1. In a prospective diagnostic study of feline LUTD performed at the University of Minnesota, we

TABLE 35–2
DIAGNOSTIC PLAN FOR FELINE DYSURIC HEMATURIA

	With Urethral Obstruction		Without Urethral Obstruction	
Factor	**First or infrequent episodes**	**Frequent or persistent episodes**	**First or infrequent episodes**	**Frequent or persistent episodes**
Defined history	+++++	+++++	+++++	+++++
Defined physical exam	+++++	+++++	+++++	+++++
Urinalysis (with sediment)*	+++++	+++++	+++++	+++++
Screening, quantitative urine culture*	+++	++++	+++	++++
Serum chemistry profile (esp. SUN, creatinine, K^+, and T-CO_2)	+++++	+++++	+	++
Assess lesion(s), site(s), and cause(s)				
Palpation	+++++	+++++	+++++	+++++
Survey radiography	+++	+++++	+++	+++++
Contrast radiography (retrograde urethrocystography or antegrade cystourethrography)	+	+++++	+	++++
Analysis of urethral plug or urolith†	+++++	+++++	+++++	+++++
Urine urease activity	+	++	+	++
Complete blood count	+	+++	+	+++
Surgical biopsy	±	±	±	±
Urine electrolytes	±	±	±	±

*Urine sample, preferably collected by cystocentesis.
†If available, submit for quantitative analysis.
+ = estimate of recommended frequency; ± = sometimes.

TABLE 35–3
TYPE OF DISORDERS IN 143 CATS WITH HEMATURIA AND DYSURIA

Disorder	Number of Cats	%
Idiopathic conditions	77	53.8
Urethral plugs	32	22.4
Uroliths	30	21.0
Urolith and bacterial urinary tract infections	2	1.4
Bacterial urinary tract infections	2	1.4
Total	143	100

TABLE 35–4
RADIOGRAPHIC FINDINGS IN 143 CATS WITH NATURALLY OCCURRING HEMATURIA AND DYSURIA

Finding	Number of Cats	%
No abnormalities	14	9.8
Radiodense urethral plug*	5	3.5
Uroliths (31) and sand (1)†	32	21.7
Vesicourachal diverticula	33	23.1
Irregular mucosa	64	44.8
Vesicoureteral reflux	32	22.4

*Detected by survey radiography.
†Excludes material identified by double-contrast cystography that could not be distinguished from blood clots or sand.

interpreted our data to suggest that the clinical signs of hematuria, dysuria, pollakiuria, and/or urethral obstruction were most commonly related to various forms of urolithiasis and urinary tract infection LUTD.[41,76]

2. We have hypothesized that various combinations of these two etiologic events may lead to three different, but common, clinical manifestations of naturally occurring feline LUTD (Fig. 35–1).[80] Our hypothesis does not encompass all potential causes of feline LUTD (see Table 35–1).

B. Nonobstructive hematuria and dysuria.

1. UTIs with viruses, and occasionally with bacteria or fungal pathogens, lead to production of mucoprotein and inflammatory reactants and to the clinical signs of hematuria and dysuria (see Fig. 35–1).
2. Urethral obstruction is an uncommon clinical

TABLE 35–5
SOME RISK FACTORS REPORTED IN CATS WITH LOWER URINARY TRACT DISEASE

Factor	Comment
Age	Uncommon in cats younger than 1 year. Most common between age 1 and 10 years, with peak between 2 and 6 years.
Sex	Urethral obstruction occurs most commonly in males. Males and females have a similar risk for nonobstructive forms of the disease.
Neutering	Increased risk of disease in neutered males and females, regardless of age of neutering.
Diet	Consumption of an increased proportion of dry food in the daily ration is associated with increased risk of disease.
Feeding frequency	Increased frequency of feeding associated with increased risk of disease, regardless of diet.
Excessive weight	Obesity associated with increased risk of disease.
Water consumption	Decreased daily water consumption associated with increased risk for disease.
Sedentary life style	Lazy cats at increased risk for disease.
Spring or winter season	Seasonal variation has been implicated as a risk factor by some investigators, but not by others.
Indoor lifestyle	Cats using indoor litter boxes for micturition and defecation have increased risk for disease.

feature of this form of LUTD, because a noncrystalline gel of mucoprotein and inflammatory reactants can be passed through the urethra of female and male cats.

C. Urolithiasis.

1. The initial step in formation of a urine crystal is formation of the nidus, or crystal embryo. This phase of initiation of urolith formation, called nucleation, depends on supersaturation of urine with calculogenic crystalloids. The degree of urine supersaturation may be influenced by the magnitude of renal excretion of the crystalloid, urine pH, and/or factors that inhibit crystal formation or crystal aggregation. Noncrystalline proteinaceous matrix substances also play a role in nucleation in some instances.
2. Further growth of the crystal nidus depends on these variables:
   a. Its ability to remain in the lumen of the excretory pathway of the urinary system.
   b. The degree and duration of supersaturation of urine with crystalloids identical to or different from crystals in the nidus.
   c. Physical characteristics of the crystal nidus. If the nidus crystals are compatible with other crystalloids, epitaxial growth with different crystalloids may occur.
3. The presence of factors that promote crystal formation and growth in urine, in the absence of concomitant UTIs that cause production of large quantities of mucoprotein and inflammatory reactants, leads to formation of classic uroliths (Figs. 35–1 and 35–2, Table 35–6).
   a. Because struvite uroliths contain relatively small quantities of matrix, formation of large quantities of crystalline material is unlikely to stimulate production of matrix substances by tissues lining the lower urinary tract.
   b. Urolithiasis affecting the lower urinary tract is typically characterized by hematuria and dysuria. Urethral obstruction may occur if small uroliths become lodged in the urethra.

D. Obstruction with matrix-crystalline urethral plugs.

1. The concomitant occurrence of UTI (Fig. 35–1, I) and crystalluria (Fig. 35–1, III) may lead to formation of matrix-crystalline plugs (Fig. 35–1, II) that obstruct various portions of the urethra, especially in male cats (Figs. 35–1 through 35–3).[7]
   a. The same type of phenomenon is known to occur during formation of casts in renal tubular lumens.
   b. Tamm-Horsfall mucoprotein may form a gel in tubular lumens that traps intact cells (cellular casts), disintegrating cells (granular casts), or lipid droplets (fatty casts).
   c. This process of formation of matrix-crystalline urethral plugs could also be compared to preparation of fruited Jell-O; the matrix (comparable to gelatin) traps various types of crystals (comparable to fruit). In addition to various types of crystals, the matrix may also trap red cells, white cells, epithelial cells, bacteria, and cells containing viruses.
   d. This hypothesis provides a plausible explanation of the observed association of virus particles or bacteria in matrix-crystalline plug containing crystals of different mineral composition (Table 35–7).
2. Crystalluria per se is an unlikely cause of the production of large quantities of matrix, because classic uroliths, which are composed of at least 90% crystalline material, contain relatively little matrix.

IV. DIAGNOSIS AND TREATMENT OF ANATOMIC ABNORMALITIES

A. Overview.

1. As with other species, congenital and acquired abnormalities of the lower urinary tract may be associated with hematuria, dysuria, urinary in-

continence, and/or urethral obstruction (Table 35–1).

2. Vesicourachal diverticula, observed in approximately one of four cats with LUTD, are worthy of further review.

B. Vesicourachal diverticula.

1. Function and dysfunction of the urachus (Fig. 35–4).
   a. The urachus is a fetal conduit that provides communication between the developing urinary bladder and the allantoic sac (a portion of the placenta).
      (1). This structure allows varying quantities of fetal urine to pass from the urinary bladder through the urachus to the placenta, where unwanted metabolites are absorbed by maternal circulation and subsequently excreted in the mother's urine.
      (2). During later stages of fetal development, the function of the urachus as a conduit for urine apparently declines, whereas that of the urethra increases.
      (3). At birth, the urachus is nonfunctional. Thus, all urine that accumulates in the urinary bladder during the storage phase of micturition flows through the urethra during the voiding phase.
   b. Studies of feline urinary bladders obtained from a variety of sources have revealed microscopic evidence of urachal remnants located in the vertex of the urinary bladder (Fig. 35–5).[75]
      (1). From a two-dimensional light microscopic perspective, the abnormality is characterized by islands of transitional epithelium of varying size that occasionally contain microscopic lumens.
      (2). We assume that the three-dimensional appearance of these structures would be tubular.
      (3). These microscopic structures, thought to be remnants of the urachus, sometimes persist at the bladder vertex from the level of the submucosa to the subserosa.
   c. Although the nonfunctional status of the ura-

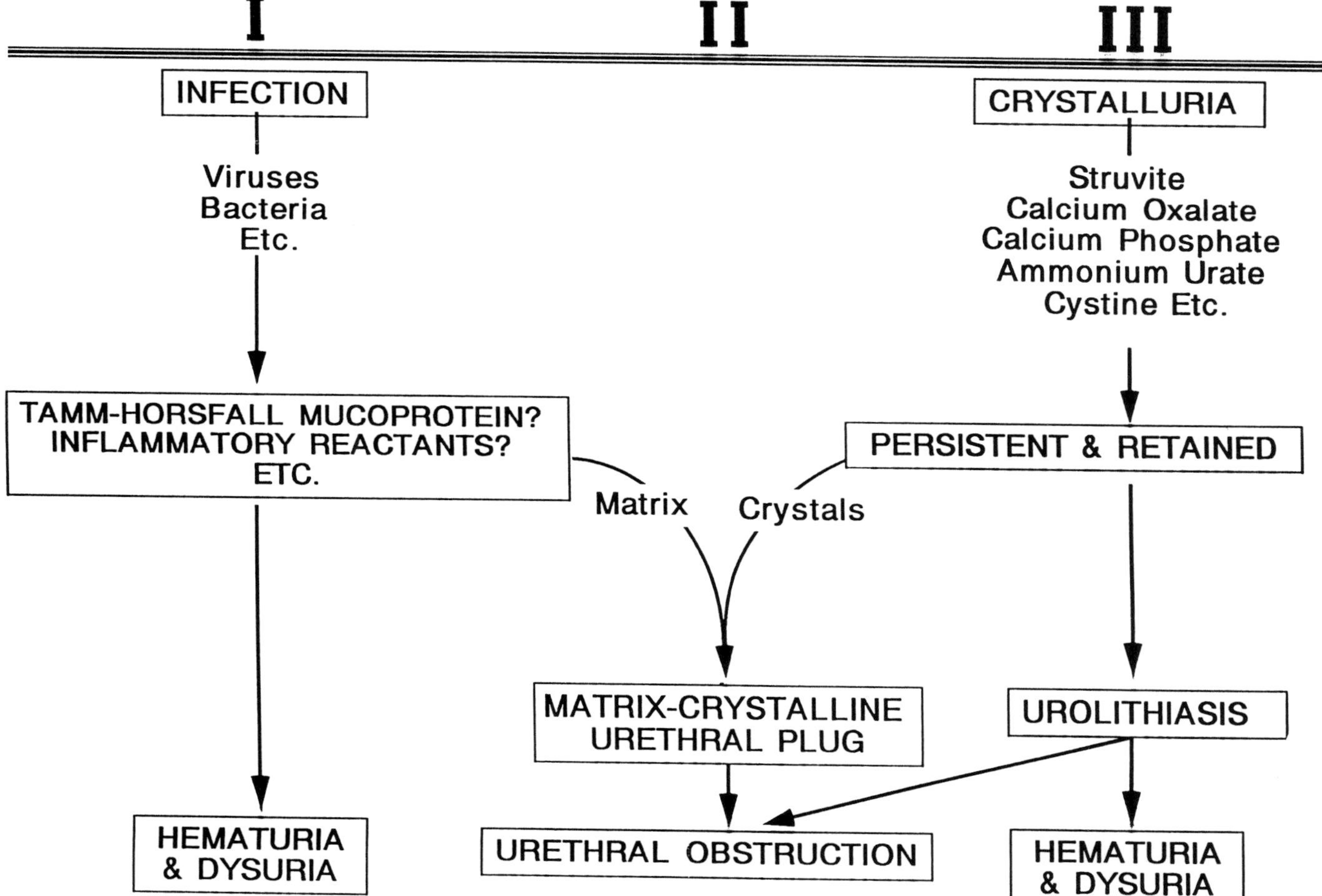

FIG. 35–1. Schematic illustration of different manifestations of feline LUTD associated with single or interacting underlying causes. (Modified from Osborne CA, et al. Feline matrix-crystalline urethral plugs: A unifying hypothesis of causes. *J Small Anim Pract.* 1992; 33:172–177.)

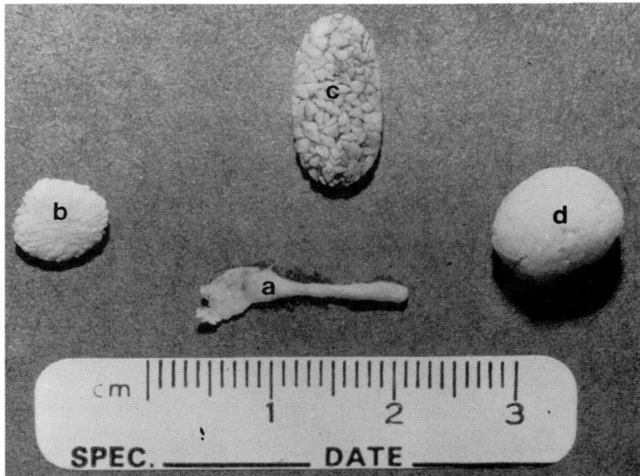

FIG. 35–2. a, Sterile struvite urethral plug removed from an adult male cat with urethral obstruction. One end of the plug was crushed with an index finger to illustrate its friable nature. **b** and **c,** Two wafer-shaped sterile struvite feline urocystoliths. **d,** An infected struvite urocystolith removed from an adult male cat. (From Osborne CA, et al. Redefinition of the feline urologic syndrome: Feline lower urinary tract disease with heterogeneous causes. *Vet Clin North Am.* 1984; 14:409–438.)

chus at birth is well established, the mechanism(s) responsible for atrophy of the urachus apparently have not been identified.

(1). Part of the atrophy may be associated with disuse.

(2). Because the mechanism(s) of physiologic atrophy are unknown to us, events that lead to persistence of microscopic urachal remnants in the bladder vertex are also unknown.

d. Microscopic urachal remnants that persist in the vertex of the urinary bladder following birth represent a risk factor for development of macroscopic diverticula of the urinary bladder in adult cats.[75] Abnormal and/or sustained increase of bladder intraluminal pressure associated with feline LUTDs may cause enlargement and/or tearing of microscopic diverticula, leading to development of self-limiting macroscopic diverticula of varying size.

2. Congenital and acquired vesicourachal diverticula.

a. In one study, radiographically detectable diverticula affecting the vertex of the urinary bladder wall were detected in almost one of four adult cats with hematuria, dysuria, and/or urethral obstruction (see Table 35–4).[75,76]

(1). They occurred twice as often in male (27%) as in female (14%) cats.[75]

(2). No breed predisposition was detected.

(3). The mean age of affected cats was 3.7 years (range, 1 to 11 years); clinical signs were not observed when the cats were younger than 1 year of age. The probable explanation of the higher frequency of occurrence in males is that they are more likely to develop urethral outflow obstruction caused by intraluminal precipitates and/or swelling or spasm of the urethral wall.

b. Two etiologically distinct forms of macroscopic vesicourachal diverticula are known.

(1). Congenital macroscopic vesicourachal diverticula, presumed to be caused by impaired urine outflow, probably develop before birth or soon after and may persist for an indefinite period. In our experience, they have been uncommon.

(a). The most likely explanation of persistence of that portion of the urachal canal adjacent to the bladder wall in immature cats is pressure in the bladder lumen that is abnormally high and/or sustained.

(b). Possibilities include anatomic or functional (reflex dyssynergia) outflow obstruction of the lower urinary tract, disorders associated with detrusor hyperactivity, and/or abnormal production of a large volume of urine. Further studies are required to investigate these possibilities (Fig. 35–6).

(c). Persistent congenital macroscopic diverticula may predispose to UTIs. If infections are caused by urease-producing calculogenic microbes (especially staphylococci), infection-induced struvite uroliths may develop.

(2). In the second (and most common) form, microscopic remnants of the urachus located at the bladder vertex of cats remain clinically silent until LUTD associated with increased bladder lumen pressure develops. Our clinical studies suggest that radiographically detectable acquired vesicourachal diverticula may develop at the bladder vertex of cats with microscopic vesicourachal remnants following onset of acquired diseases associated with increased intraluminal pressure caused by urethral obstruction and/or detrusor hyperactivity induced by inflammation (Figs. 35–7 through 35–10).

3. Diagnosis of vesicourachal diverticula.

a. Feline vesicourachal diverticula are best identified by radiographic studies, although extramural diverticula may be identified at celiotomy. On occasion, large extramural diverticula cause prominent pointed deformities of the bladder vertex that can be detected by survey radiography. In addition, the urinary bladder of affected patients may have an elliptic shape when incompletely distended, and the bladder vertex may be impaired from its normal movement toward the bony pelvis in the partially distended or undistended state.

b. Antemortem confirmation of vesicourachal diverticula requires some form of contrast cystography.

(1). In our opinion, positive antegrade cystourethrography and retrograde positive-contrast urethrocystography are the procedures of choice (Figs. 35–6 through 35–11).[76]

TABLE 35–6
MINERAL COMPOSITION OF 6335 FELINE UROLITHS EVALUATED BY QUANTITATIVE METHODS*

Predominant Mineral Type	% Mineral Composition	Uroliths (No.)	Prevalence (%)
Magnesium ammonium phosphate hexahydrate		3,413	53.9
	100	(2,904)	(45.8)
	70–99†	(509)	(8.0)
Magnesium hydrogen phosphate trihydrate		16	0.3
	70–99†	(16)	(0.3)
Calcium oxalate		2,037	37.2
Calcium oxalate monohydrate			
	100	(738)	(11.6)
	70–99†	(704)	(11.1)
Calcium oxalate dihydrate			
	100	(69)	(1.2)
	70–99†	(234)	(3.7)
Calcium oxalate monohydrate and dihydrate			
	100	(269)	(4.2)
	70–99†	(231)	(0.4)
Calcium phosphate		68	1.1
Calcium phosphate			
	100	(23)	(0.3)
	70–99†	(29)	(0.5)
Calcium hydrogen phosphate hexahydrate			
	100	(5)	(0.1)
	70–99†	(9)	(0.2)
Tricalcium phosphate			
	100	(1)	(<0.1)
	70–99†	(1)	(<0.1)
Uric acid and urates		432	6.8
Ammonium acid urate			
	100	(327)	(5.2)
	70–99†	(97)	(1.5)
Sodium urate			
	70–99†	(1)	(<0.1)
Uric acid			
	100	(4)	(0.1)
	70–99†	(3)	(<0.1)
Cystine		22	0.3
Xanthine		9	0.1
Silica		0	0
Mixed‡		118	1.9
Compound§		115	1.8
Matrix		106	2.0
	Total	6,335	100%

*Uroliths analyzed by polarized light microscopy and x-ray diffraction methods.
†Uroliths composed of 70–99% of mineral type listed; no nucleus or shell detected.
‡Uroliths did not contain at least 70% of mineral type listed; no nucleus or shell detected.
§Uroliths contained an identifiable nucleus and one or more surrounding layers of a different mineral type.

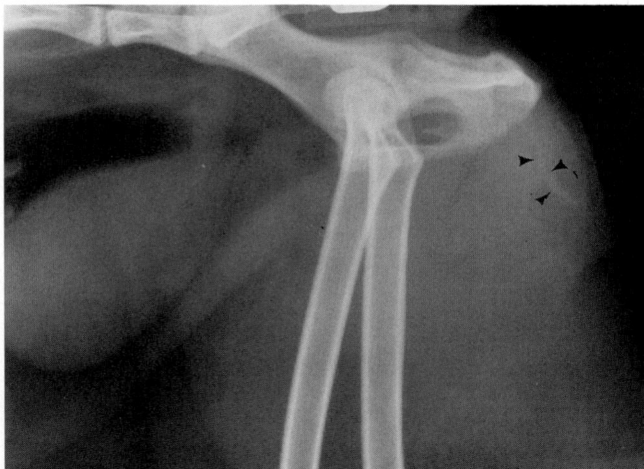

FIG. 35–3. Survey radiograph of the lateral aspect of the urethra of a 2-year-old male domestic shorthair cat with urethral obstruction. Note the radiodense structure in the location normally occupied by the penile urethra (arrows). A struvite urethral plug was expelled from the external urethral orifice by inducing micturition with the aid of manual compression of the urinary bladder. (From Osborne CA, et al. Feline urologic syndrome: A heterogeneous phenomenon? *J Am Anim Hosp Assoc.* 1984; 20:17–32.)

(2). Double-contrast cystography or intravenous urography may also be utilized.

(3). Pneumocystography has not been as consistently reliable as positive-contrast cystography, in our experience.

c. Complete distention of the lumen of the urinary bladder with contrast medium is usually recommended, to allow meaningful interpretation of the thickness of the bladder wall.

(1). However, maximum distention of the lumen of the urinary bladder with contrast medium may obscure small vesicourachal diverticula as a result of stretching of the vertex of the bladder.

(2). To minimize this problem, a series of radiographs (at least two) may be obtained with the bladder completely and then partially distended with contrast medium.

d. The radiographic appearance of extramural vesicourachal diverticula is often characterized by a convex or triangular protrusion from the bladder vertex (Figs. 35–6 through 35–12 and Fig. 35–16). Intramural diverticula may appear as cylindric duct-like structures or sac-like abnormalities with a narrow neck that allows communication with the bladder lumen.

4. Treatment of vesicourachal diverticula.

a. Introduction.

(1). Urachal diverticula are an uncommon primary factor in development of feline LUTD. Our studies suggest that most macroscopic diverticula of the bladder vertex are a sequela of lower urinary tract dysfunction.

(2). At least some, and probably most, macroscopic diverticula may be self-limiting if the urinary bladder and urethra return to a normal state of function.[75] We have observed spontaneous resolution of acquired macroscopic diverticula in 15 of 15 adult male cats evaluated by serial radiography.[77] Initially the diverticula were identified at radiographic evaluation of these patients for the underlying cause of hematuria, dysuria, and/or urethral obstruction. Subsequently, these clinical signs resolved spontaneously or in conjunction with some form of therapy. Acquired diverticula probably heal within 2 to 3 weeks following elimination of the underlying cause of increased intraluminal pressure (Figs. 35–12 through 35–14).[77]

b. Cats with bacterial urinary tract infection.

(1). Bacterial UTI confirmed by quantitative culture of urine samples properly collected from a cat with a diverticulum of the bladder vertex should be treated with appropriate antimicrobials. Any causes of unrelated diseases associated with increased bladder intraluminal pressure also should be eliminated or controlled. If the bladder diverticulum is self-limiting, eradication of the UTI eliminate the LUTD.

(2). If bacterial UTI persists or recurs despite proper antimicrobial therapy, the status of the diverticulum should be re-evaluated by contrast radiography. If a macroscopic diverticulum of the bladder vertex persists (longer than 4 to 8 weeks?) in a patient with persistent or recurrent UTI, diverticulectomy should be considered.

c. Abacteriuric cats scheduled for urethral surgery.

(1). If a diverticulum of the bladder vertex is detected by contrast radiography in an abacteriuric male cat being evaluated for perineal urethrostomy, the client should be informed that removal of the penile urethra (which contributes to local host defenses) combined with the diverticulum (an abnormality of local host defenses) may result in bacterial UTI. If the infection is caused by urease-producing bacteria, such as staphylococci, infection-induced struvite uroliths may develop.

(a). Rather than recommend perineal urethrostomy and/or diverticulectomy, one should re-evaluate the indications for urethral surgery and serially evaluate the size of the diverticulum.

(b). If the diverticulum subsides but a confirmed abnormality of the penile urethra that predisposes to urethral obstruction persists, the risk of postsurgical UTI is reduced (but not eliminated).

(c). If the diverticulum persists and an abnormality of the penile urethra that predisposes to an unacceptable recurrence of urethral obstruction persists, a perineal urethrostomy may be considered.

(2). If urethral surgery is performed in a patient with a persistent bladder diverticulum, the cat should be monitored periodically for bacterial UTI. If frequently recurrent or persistent UTI occurs after perineal urethrostomy, diverticulectomy should then be considered.

d. Abacteriuric cats with hematuria and dysuria (Figs. 35–12 through 35–14).

(1). The concomitant occurrence of hematuria, dysuria, and urethral obstruction with a diverticulum of the bladder vertex is not an immediate indication for diverticulectomy.

(2). Contrast radiography performed 2 to 3 weeks after the clinical signs subside may reveal varying degrees of resolution of the diverticulum.

TABLE 35–7
MINERAL COMPOSITION OF 820 FELINE URETHRAL PLUGS ANALYZED BY QUANTITATIVE METHODS*

Predominant Mineral Type	% Mineral Composition	Uroliths (No.)	Uroliths Prevalence (%)
Magnesium ammonium phosphate hexahydrate		636	77.6
	100	(540)	(65.9)
	70–99†	(96)	(11.7)
Newberyite		3	0.4
	100	(1)	(0.1)
	77–99†	(2)	(0.3)
Calcium oxalate		14	1.7
Calcium oxalate monohydrate			
	100	(4)	(0.5)
	70–99†	(5)	(0.6)
Calcium oxalate dihydrate			
	100	(2)	(0.2)
	70–99†	(2)	(0.2)
Calcium oxalate monohydrate and dihydrate			
		(1)	(0.1)
Calcium phosphate		21	2.6
Calcium phosphate			
	100	(11)	(1.3)
	70–99†	(7)	(0.9)
Calcium hydrogen phosphate hexahydrate			
	100	(2)	(0.3)
	70–99†	(1)	(0.1)
Ammonium acid urate		6	0.7
	100	(6)	(0.7)
Xanthine		1	0.1
Sulfadiazine		1	0.1
Mixed‡		27	3.3
Matrix		113	13.4
Total		820	100%

*Urethral plugs examined by polarizing light microscopy and x-ray diffraction methods.
†Uroliths composed of 70–99% of mineral type listed; no nucleus and shell detected.
‡Uroliths did not contain at least 70% of mineral type listed; no nucleus or shell detected.

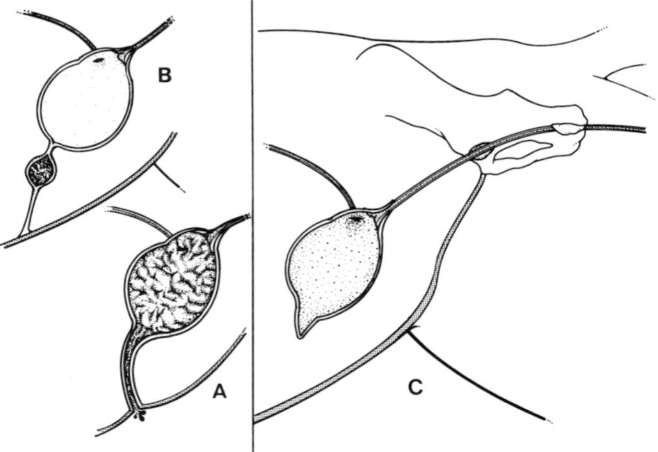

FIG. 35–4. Some congenital urachal anomalies. **A,** Persistent urachus. **B,** Urachal cyst. **C,** Vesicourachal diverticulum. (Osborne CA, Kruger JM, Johnston GR. Etiopathogenesis and biological behavior of feline vesicourachal diverticula. *Vet Clin North Am.* 1987; 17:700.)

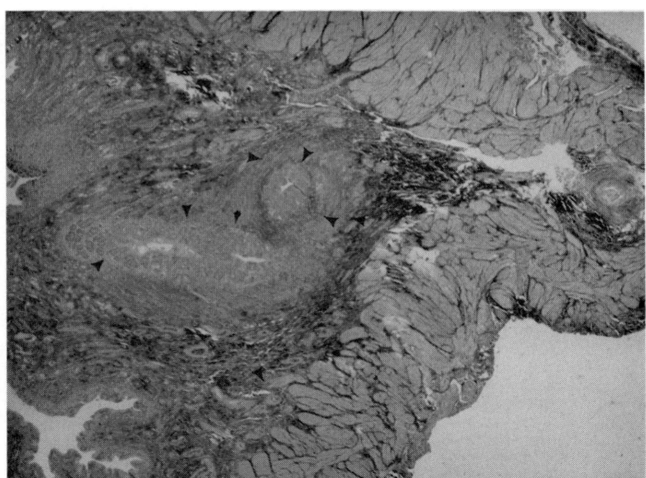

FIG. 35–5. Photomicrograph of a microscopic urachal remnant (arrows) located in the bladder vertex of an intact adult female domestic shorthair pound cat. Lack of connection between submucosal and subserosal urachal segments has probably been caused by the degree of distention of the bladder at the time of fixation with formalin and the plane of transection of the specimen. (Trichrome stain; original magnification, 4×.) (From Osborne CA, et al. Etiopathogenesis and biologic behavior of feline vesicourachal diverticula. *Vet Clin North Am.* 1987; 17: 697–732.)

(a). The major focus of effort should be directed at detection and elimination of the underlying cause of the lower urinary tract inflammation and the increased pressure within the bladder lumen.

(b). If an underlying cause (e.g., metabolic uroliths, urethral plugs, UTI, infection-induced struvite uroliths) cannot be identified, resolution of the hematuria, dysuria, and bladder di-

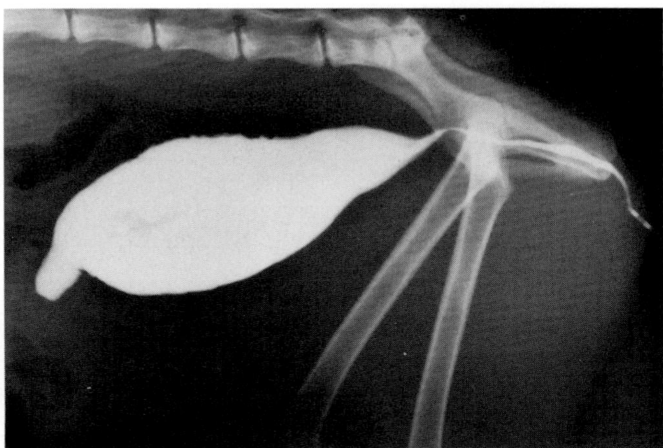

FIG. 35–6. Lateral view of a retrograde contrast urethrocystogram of an 8-month-old male Manx cat with histologically confirmed myelodysplasia. The cat had a history of dysuria. Note the narrowing of the prostatic urethra, dilation of the preprostatic urethra, and large diverticulum protruding from the bladder vertex. The diverticulum did not change in size during a 1-month period. Failure of resolution of the diverticulum may have been related to persistent partial outflow obstruction at the level of the prostatic urethra. (From Osborne CA, et al. Etiopathogenesis and biologic behavior of feline vesicourachal diverticula. *Vet Clin North Am.* 1987; 17:697–732.)

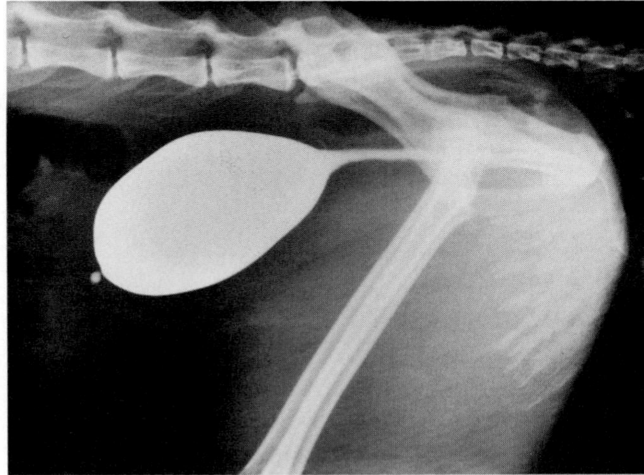

FIG. 35–7. Lateral view of a positive-contrast retrograde urethrocystogram of a 2-year-old castrated male domestic shorthair cat. The cat had nonobstructive hematuria and dysuria. Note the intramural diverticula of the bladder vertex. (From Osborne CA, et al. Etiopathogenesis and biologic behavior of feline vesicourachal diverticula. *Vet Clin North Am.* 1987; 17:697–732.)

verticulum may occur with or without symptomatic therapy.

e. Cats with urocystoliths.

(1). Cats with acquired diverticula of the bladder vertex and sterile struvite or infection-induced struvite urocystoliths may be successfully managed by medical therapy (Figs. 35–15 through 35–19).[75,78]

(2). Because effective protocols to induce medical dissolution of feline calcium oxalate, calcium phosphate, ammonium urate, uric acid, and cystine urocystoliths have not yet been developed, surgery

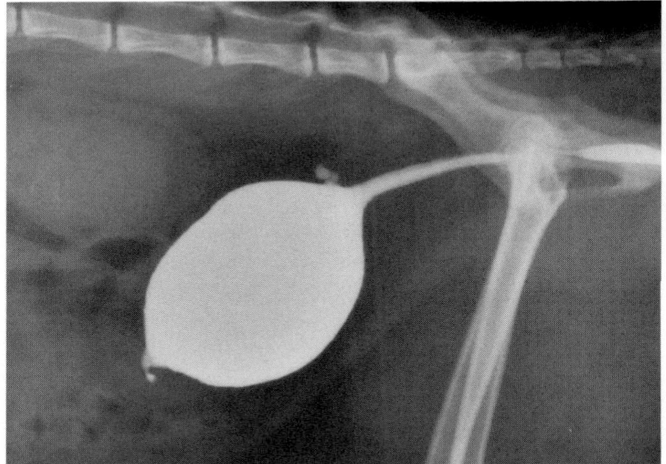

FIG. 35–8. Positive-contrast retrograde urethrocystogram of a 1-year-old male domestic shorthair cat illustrates an extramural diverticulum of the bladder vertex, and vesicoureteral reflux. The cat had an obstructed urethra caused by a urethral plug. (From Osborne CA, et al. Etiopathogenesis and biologic behavior of feline vesicourachal diverticula. *Vet Clin North Am.* 1987; 17:697–732.)

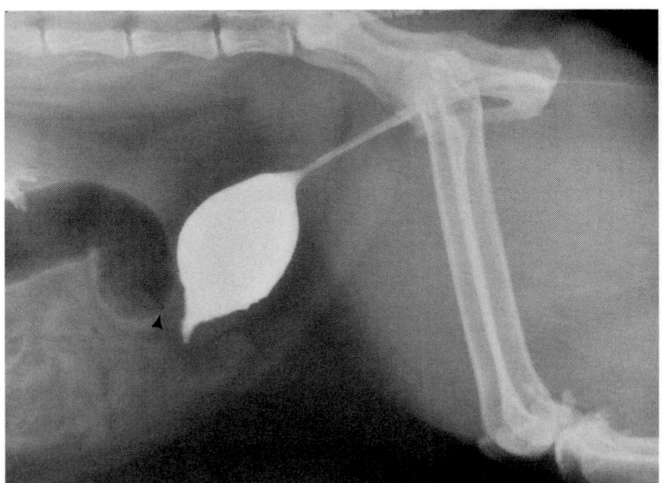

FIG. 35–9. Lateral view of a positive-contrast retrograde urethrocystogram of a 3-year-old castrated domestic shorthair cat obtained after correction of intraluminal urethral obstruction. Note the large diverticulum protruding from the vertex of the bladder. The lumen of the penile urethra is reduced in diameter. (From Osborne CA, et al. Etiopathogenesis and biologic behavior of feline vesicourachal diverticula. *Vet Clin North Am.* 1987; 17:697–732.)

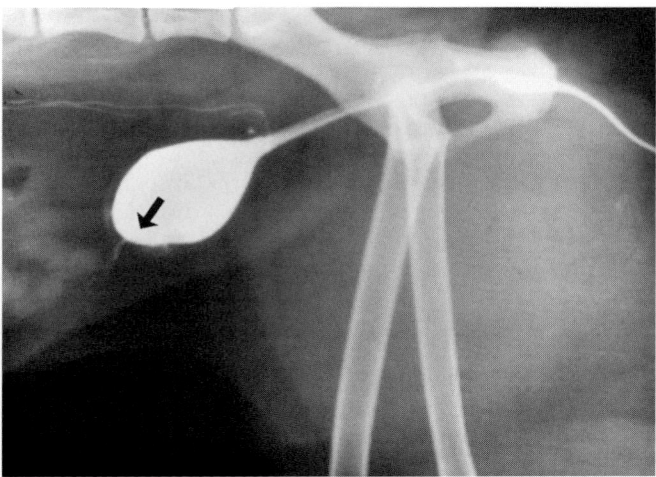

FIG. 35–10. Lateral view of a positive-contrast retrograde urethrocystogram of a 5-year-old castrated male domestic shorthair cat with nonobstructive hematuria and dysuria. Note the narrow intramural diverticulum protruding into the thickened wall of the bladder vertex (arrow) and ulcerations of the cranioventral surface of the bladder mucosa. (From Osborne CA, et al. Etiopathogenesis and biologic behavior of feline vesicourachal diverticula. *Vet Clin North Am.* 1987; 17:697–732.)

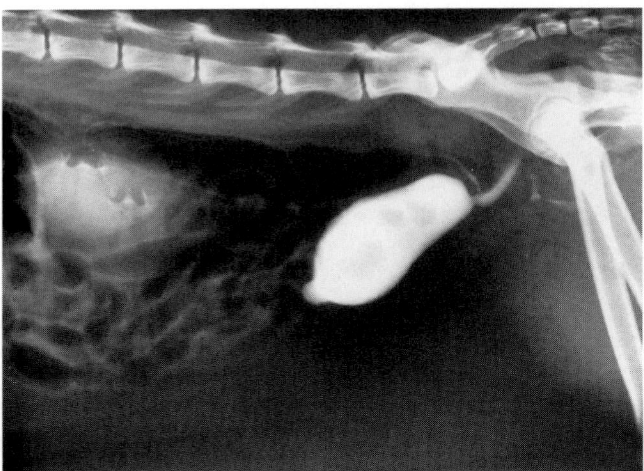

FIG. 35–11. Lateral view of an intravenous urogram of a 7-year-old domestic shorthair cat with struvite urocystoliths. The uroliths appear less dense than the contrast medium in the bladder lumen. A urachal diverticulum is at the vertex of the bladder wall. (From Osborne CA, et al. Feline urologic syndrome: A heterogeneous phenomenon? *J Am Anim Hosp Assoc.* 1984; 20:21.)

remains the most reliable method of treating patients with metabolic urolithiasis and diverticula of the vertex of the urinary bladder.

C. Urethral strictures.

1. Although in young cats we have encountered urethral strictures that are presumed to be of congenital origin, they are uncommon.
2. Urethral strictures usually occur as a sequela to:
   a. Catheter trauma induced at the time of treatment of urethral plugs or urethroliths.
   b. Use of indwelling transurethral catheters, especially those constructed of material that stimulates a foreign body response.
   c. Self-trauma.[13,76,89]
3. Formation of urethral strictures may be minimized by proper patient restraint during urethral catheterization, avoiding an indwelling urethral catheter when possible, and restraint devices to minimize self-trauma. If urethral strictures predispose to clinical signs, corrective surgery should be considered, but not before the lower urinary tract has been evaluated by antegrade cystourethrography or retrograde urethrocystography.[13,73]

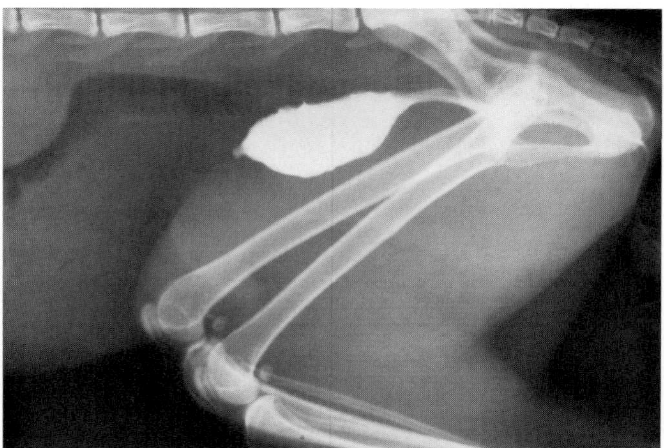

FIG. 35–12. Positive-contrast retrograde urethrocystogram of a 2-year-old male domestic shorthair cat illustrates a diverticulum protruding from the vertex of the urinary bladder. The cat had a urinary outflow obstruction caused by a urethral plug.

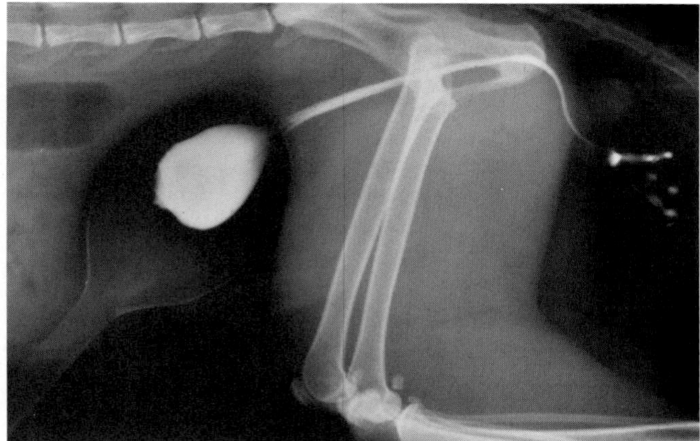

FIG. 35–13. Positive-contrast retrograde urethrocystogram of the cat described in Figure 35–12. This study was performed 9 days later. Note reduction in size of the diverticulum.

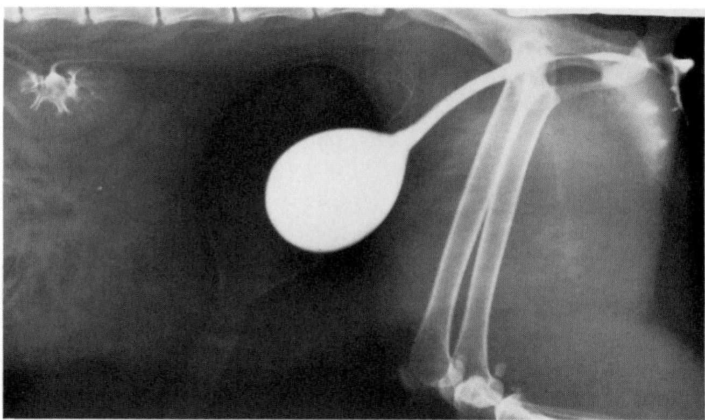

FIG. 35–14. Positive-contrast retrograde urethrocystogram of the cat described in Figures 35–12 and 35–13. This study was performed 19 days after initial evaluation. A perineal urethrostomy was performed on day 15. There is no evidence of the bladder diverticulum. Note the vesicoureteral reflux.

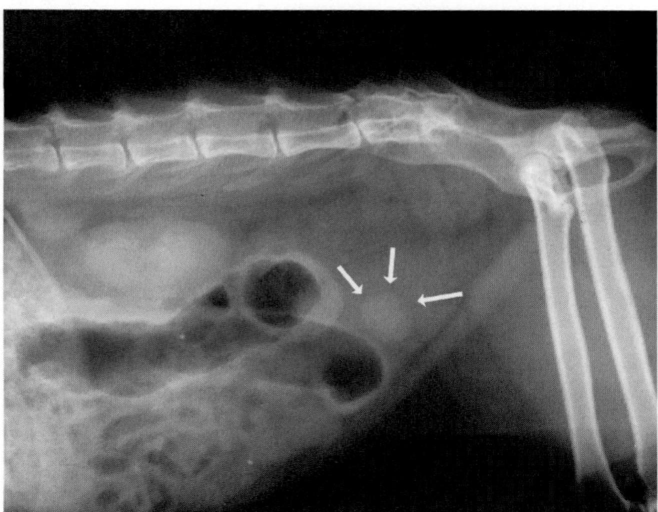

FIG. 35–15. Survey abdominal radiograph of a 3-year-old castrated male cat illustrates a radiodense urocystolith (arrows).

D. Compression of the urethral lumen.

1. Congenital or acquired disorders of the urethral wall, and space-occupying lesions located adjacent to the urethra, may compress the urethral lumen and induce clinical signs (Fig. 35–20).
2. We encountered a persistent cystic uterus masculinus in a dysuric 6-year-old castrated male domestic longhair cat that caused partial occlusion of the bladder neck and proximal urethra.[67] We also encountered a prostate adenocarcinoma in a

dysuric 6-year-old male domestic longhair that caused partial obstruction of the prostatic urethra (Fig. 35–21).[68]

3. Also, we have encountered a uterine adenocarcinoma that invaded and partially occluded the urethra of a dysuric adult female cat.

V. DIAGNOSIS AND TREATMENT OF INFECTIOUS AGENTS

A. Viral urinary tract infection.

1. Overview.
   a. Several hypotheses have been advanced about possible causes of idiopathic hematuria, dysuria, and/or matrix-crystalline urethral plug formation in male and female cats with LUTD.[42,69]
   b. One attractive hypothesis implicates viruses as causative agents of some forms of naturally occurring feline LUTD (Table 35–8).[21,42]
      (1). This hypothesis was supported by the isolation of cell-associated herpesvirus (CAHV), feline calicivirus (FCV), and syncytia-forming virus (SFV) from urine and tissues obtained from cats affected with naturally occurring LUTD.[21,42,63]
      (2). It is noteworthy that polyomavirus, adenovirus type 2, herpes simplex virus, and herpes zoster have been implicated as causes of hemorrhagic cystitis in humans.[1,17,42]

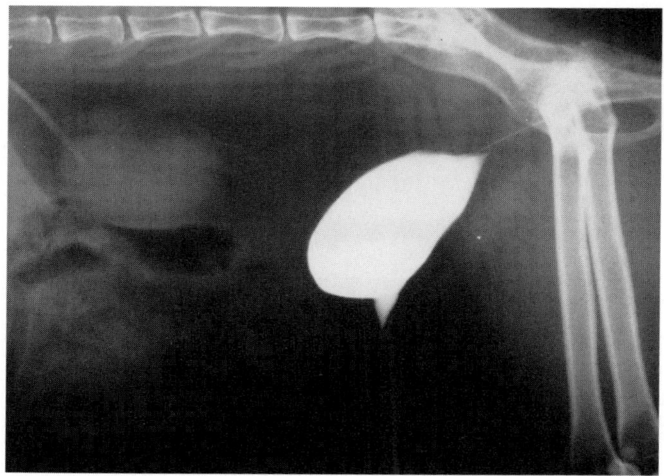

FIG. 35–16. Positive-contrast urethrocystogram of the cat described in Figure 35–15. Note the vesicourachal diverticulum.

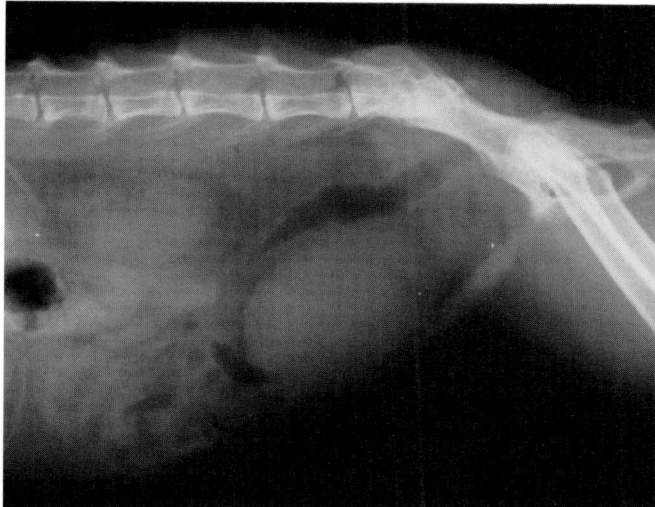

FIG. 35–17. Survey abdominal radiograph of the cat described in Figure 35–15 obtained 7 weeks after initiation of therapy with a diet designed to dissolve struvite uroliths. No radiodense stones are in the urinary tract.

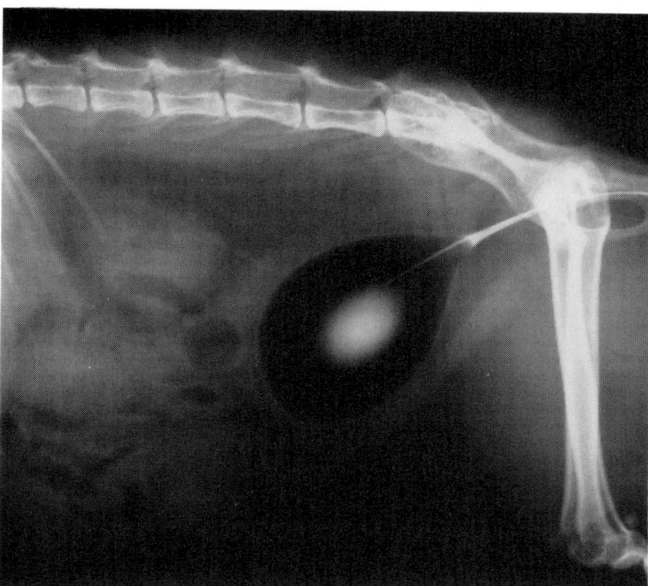

FIG. 35–18. Double-contrast cystogram of the cat described in Figure 35–17. There is no evidence of urocystoliths (see Fig. 35–16).

2. Etiopathogenesis.
   a. Calicivirus.
      (1). The first indirect evidence to support the hypothesis of a viral cause of feline LUTD was reported in 1969, when investigators at Cornell University produced urethral obstruction in male cats by inoculating the urinary bladder with centrifuged bacteriologically sterile urine obtained from male cats with naturally occurring urethral obstruction.[21]
      (2). Subsequent isolation of an FCV from a Manx cat with spontaneous urethral obstruction, and experimental induction of obstructive uropathy in conventionally reared cats by urinary bladder inoculation with this virus, directly supported the concept of a viral cause of feline LUTD.[21]

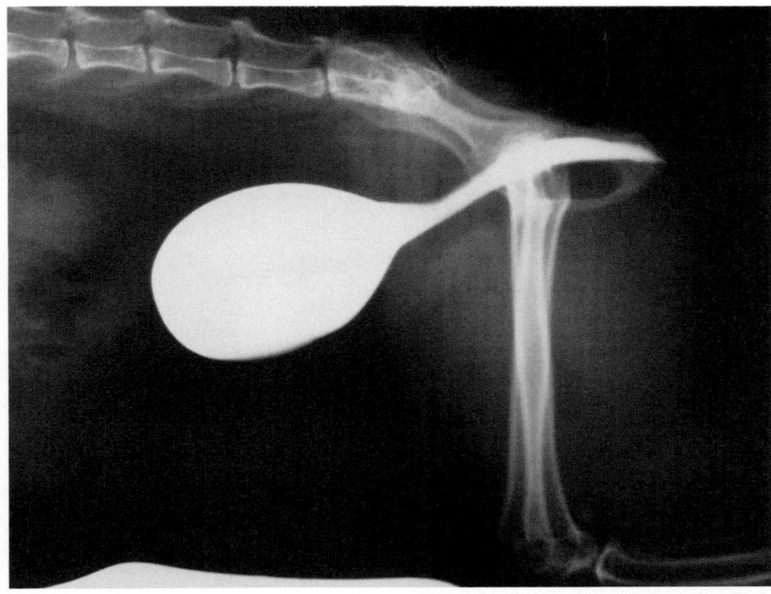

FIG. 35–19. Positive-contrast retrograde urethrocystogram of the cat described in Figure 35–17. The vesicourachal diverticulum has healed (see Fig. 35–16).

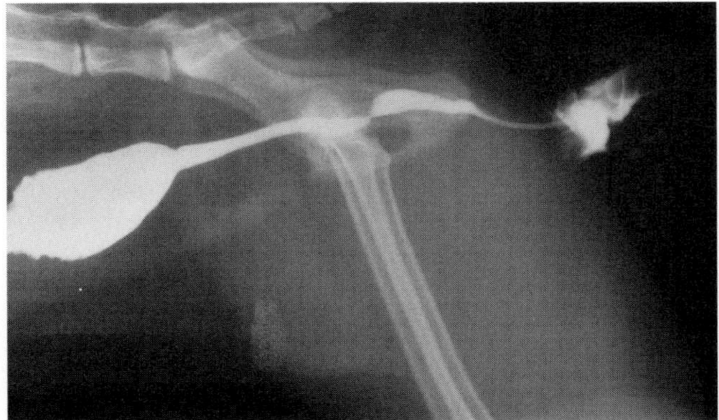

FIG. 35–20. Antegrade contrast cystourethrogram of a 3-year-old neutered male domestic shorthair cat illustrates partial outflow obstruction of the postprostatic urethra.

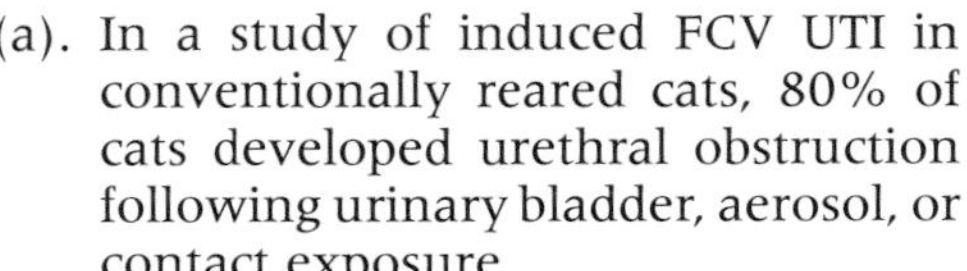

(a). In a study of induced FCV UTI in conventionally reared cats, 80% of cats developed urethral obstruction following urinary bladder, aerosol, or contact exposure.

(b). Despite these encouraging results, failure to reisolate FCV from urine past the fourth day after infection, lack of a significant serum neutralizing antibody response, and isolation of an additional virus (SFV) from all obstructed experimental cats prompted investigators to hypothesize that FCV was not a primary causative agent.[21]

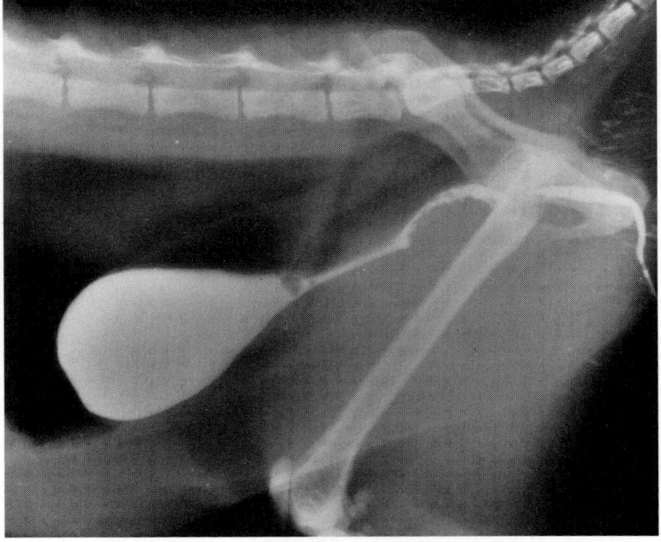

FIG. 35–21. Positive-contrast urethrocystogram of the lateral abdomen of a 6-year-old male domestic longhair cat with urethral obstruction. Note dorsal deviation of the section of urethra immediately craniad to the bony pelvis. The urethral lesion was caused by a carcinoma of the prostate gland. The radiolucent structures at the junction of the bladder with the urethra are air bubbles. (From Osborne CA, et al. Feline urologic syndrome: A heterogeneous phenomenon? *J Am Anim Hosp Assoc.* 1984; 20:17–32.)

(c). The notion was advanced that this virus incited other latent viruses present in the urinary tract to induce urethral obstruction.

(3). Results of a subsequent study comparing the effects of induced UTI with FCV alone or in combination with cell-associated herpesvirus appeared to support the concept that FCV played only a secondary role in the pathogenesis of feline LUTD.[21]

(4). The causative role of FCV was confounded by inability of other investigators to isolate FCV from urine obtained from cats with spontaneous forms of feline LUTD.

(a). Virus isolation by standard cell culture inoculation methods has been attempted in many cats with naturally occurring forms of feline LUTD[42,43]; however, FCV has been isolated only once from the urinary tract of an affected cat. Although these findings raise serious questions about the role of FCV, increasing evidence shows that FCV may be more prevalent in cats with feline LUTD than was previously believed.

(b). Transmission electron microscopic examination of urethral matrix-crystalline plugs obtained from male cats with urethral obstruction revealed virus-like particles similar in size (approximately 25 to 30 nm) and structure to caliciviruses (Figs. 35–22

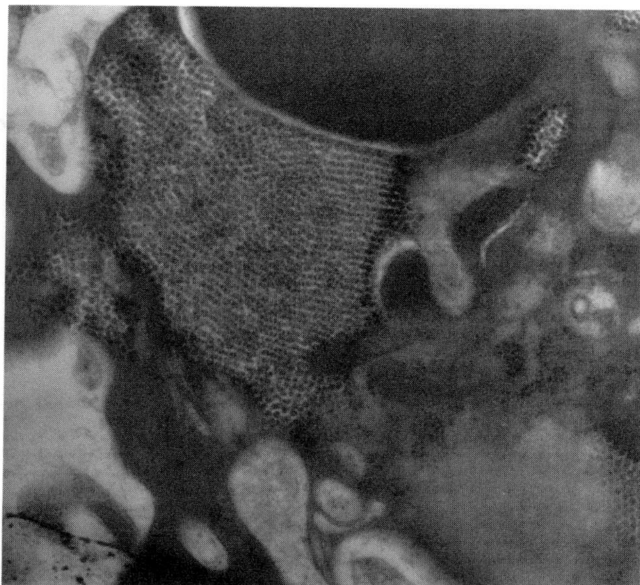

FIG. 35–22. Transmission electron micrograph of a section of matrix-crystalline urethral plug removed from a 12-year-old neutered male domestic shorthair cat. The crystals were composed of struvite. Note virus-like particles contained within an unidentified cell. Compare Figures 35–22 and 35–23. (Original magnification, 50,000×.)

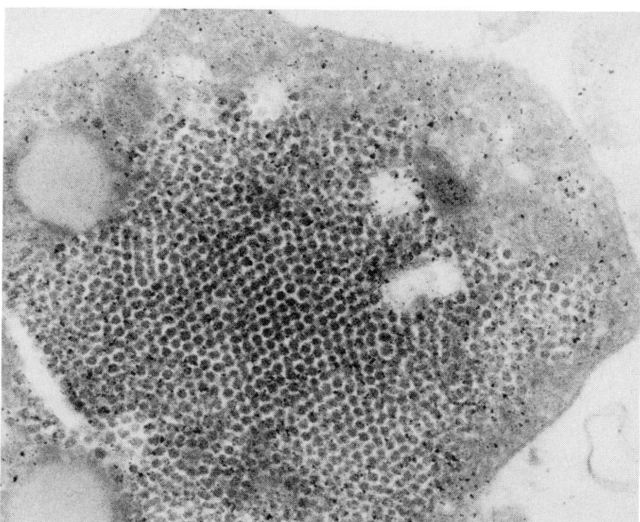

FIG. 35–23. Transmission electron micrograph of a section of urethral plug obtained from a 3-year-old domestic longhair cat. Note virus-like particles contained within an unidentified cell. Compare Figures 35–22 and 35–24. (Original magnification, 80,000×.) (From Osborne CA, et al. Feline matrix-crystalline urethral plugs: A unifying hypothesis of causes. *J Small Anim Pract.* 1992; 33:172–177.)

TABLE 35–8
FELINE UROPATHOGENS

Bacteria
Escherichia coli
Staphylococcus spp.
Streptococcus spp.
Pasteurella spp.
Proteus spp.
Pseudomonas spp.
Klebsiella spp.
Enterobachter spp.
Others
Fungi
Candida spp.
Aspergillus spp.
Trichosporon spp.
Cephalosporium spp.
Parasites
Capillaria feliscati
Potential pathogens
Viruses
Feline calicivirus
Feline syncytia-forming virus
Bovine herpesvirus-4
Mycoplasmas and ureaplasmas
Mycoplasma felis
Mycoplasma gateae
Ureaplasma spp.

through 35–24).[7,21] Studies are currently in progress to verify the viral origin of these structures.

b. Syncytia-forming virus (SFV).
   (1). Shortly after isolation of FCV, an SFV was isolated from eight cats with spontaneous LUTD.[21]
   (2). Unfortunately, studies investigating the etiopathogenic role of SFV in feline LUTD are limited.[43]
      (a). In one study, FCV-induced urethral obstruction in conventionally reared cats was consistently associated with isolation of SFV.[43]
      (b). In other studies, clinical signs of LUTD were not observed in a few cats following intravenous, intraperitoneal, intramuscular, intraarticular, or subcutaneous inoculation of SFV.[43]
   (3). In contrast to FCV, SFV has been isolated from urine, urinary tract tissues, and other tissues obtained from many cats affected with naturally occurring forms of LUTD.[21,42,63] In addition, SFV antibodies have been detected in serum samples obtained from cats affected with naturally occurring LUTD.[42]
      (a). In a colony of cats with a high incidence of LUTD, SFV antibodies were detected by agar gel immunodiffusion in 90% of serum specimens collected from male cats with urethral obstruction; SFV antibodies were also detected in all specimens obtained from clinically normal male cats.[43] Interestingly, signs of recurrent episodes of upper respiratory tract infection were observed in the same cats before the development of urethral obstruction. Unfortunately, a specific cause was not established for the recurrent upper respiratory tract disease; however, concurrent FCV or feline rhinotracheitis virus infection was suspected.
      (b). The relative ease and frequency with which SFV has been isolated from cats with LUTD, and the prevalence of SFV antibodies, suggests a potential role in the pathogenesis of the disease. However, the relative importance of SFV is difficult to assess on the basis of available experimental and clinical studies. Further investigations are necessary to determine the role of this virus in feline LUTD.

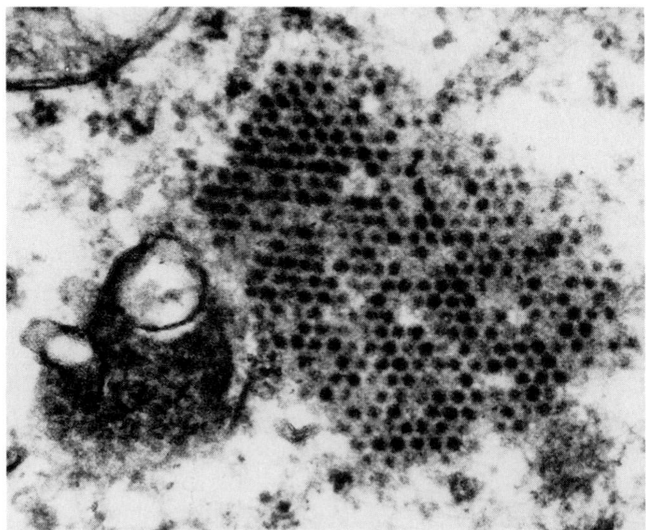

FIG. 35–24. Transmission electron micrograph of Crandell-Rees feline kidney cells grown *in vitro* and infected with feline calcivirus. Note the similarity of calcivirus structure to virus-like particles illustrated in Figures 35–22 and 35–23. (Original magnification, 60,000×). (From Osborne CA, et al.: *Consultations in Feline Medicine* 2. Philadelphia, Pennsylvania: WB Saunders; 1994.)

c. Herpesviruses (Fig. 35–25).
   (1). In addition to FCV and SFV, investigators at Cornell University isolated a strongly cell-associated herpesvirus (CAHV) from pooled kidney organ explants obtained from a litter of normal kittens, a kitten with upper respiratory tract disease, and a kitten with concurrent upper respiratory tract disease and urethral obstructions (Fig. 35–25).[21] Results of experimental studies designed to induce urethral obstruction in specific pathogen–free (SPF) cats with urinary bladder inoculation of FCV alone, CAHV alone, or CAHV in combination with FCV led to the hypothesis that CAHV was a primary causative agent in the etiopathogenesis of naturally occurring feline LUTD.[21,43]
   (2). Results of antigenic and genomic analyses have indicated that CAHV is related to a group of gamma herpesviruses collectively referred to as bovine herpesvirus-4 (BHV-4).[39]
      (a). Serologic cross-reactivity was demonstrated between the antigens of CAHV and those of BHV-4 (reference strain DN-599) by direct and indirect immunofluorescence.
      (b). Restriction endonuclease cleavage patterns (so-called viral DNA fingerprinting) of CAHV DNA were nearly identical to the DNA cleavage patterns of other BHV-4 isolates.
      (c). In addition, results of dot blot and Southern blot analyses performed in

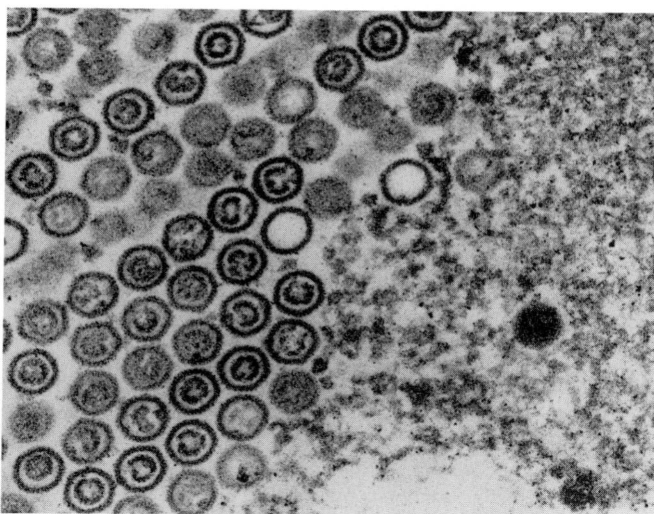

FIG. 35–25. Transmission electron micrograph of feline cell–associated herpesvirus particles isolated from primary tissue cultures established from the urinary bladder of a cat with an induced feline cell–associated herpesvirus UTI. (Original magnification, 50,000×.) (From Kruger JM, Osborne CA. The role of viruses in feline lower urinary tract disease. *J Vet Intern Med.* 1990; 4:71–78.)

our laboratory have demonstrated cross-hybridization between CAHV DNA and a BHV-4 (strain DN-599) DNA probe.[43]

(d). Based on antigenic and genetic analyses, CAHV appears to be a unique strain of BHV-4.

(3). The obvious question arises as to the origin of the CAHV strain of BHV-4.

(a). The BHV-4 group is composed of several related viruses, antigenically and genetically distinct from other bovine herpesviruses and feline herpesvirus type 1 (feline rhinotracheitis virus).[43]

(b). Strains of BHV-4 were originally isolated from cattle, where they typically established latent infections of mononuclear cells and lymphoid and nerve tissues, with or without clinical signs.[43]

(c). The fact that members of the BHV-4 group of herpesviruses have a unique ability to replicate in a variety of mammalian hosts (cattle, sheep, bison, buffalo, rabbits, owl monkeys, lions, and domestic cats) suggested that BVH-4 may be a pathogen of domestic cats.[43]

(4). In an effort to substantiate Cornell's studies, and to further characterize the clinicopathologic manifestations of herpesvirus-induced LUTD, BHV-4 (strain CAHV) was inoculated into the urinary bladder of 18 SPF male and female cats.[40]

(a). Results of these studies indicated that BHV-4 (strain CAHV) was capable of establishing persistent low-grade or latent UTIs in male and female SPF cats.

(b). However, in contrast to previous studies,[21] clinical signs of LUTD were uncommonly associated with persistent herpesvirus UTIs. Reasons for discrepancies between these results and those of others are unknown, but they may be related to differences in virus virulence or host susceptibility.

(5). Although initial virus isolations and experimental studies at Cornell were encouraging, subsequent clinical studies by other investigators yielded conflicting results about the causative role of BHV-4 in naturally occurring feline BHV-4 from spontaneous forms of feline LUTD. Attempts by other investigators have been uniformly unsuccessful in demonstrating LUTD using standard virus isolation techniques.[41,42,63]

(a). Although these findings raise serious questions about the role of BHV-4 in naturally occurring forms of LUTD, they may also reflect inappropriate or inconsistent selection of representative cases, failure to obtain suitable samples of tissues or fluids, or limited use of organ explanation techniques.

(b). Like other herpesviruses, BHV-4 produces persistent infections that exist as low-grade chronic infections or as latent infections.[43] Latent BHV-4 infections are difficult to detect by conventional virus isolation techniques.

(c). Isolation of herpesviruses from latent BHV-4 infections of cattle and rabbits required tissue explanation and cocultivation techniques. Likewise, tissue explanation techniques were necessary to identify viral persistence or latency in chronic BHV-4 (CAHV strain) infections of cats.[21,40]

(6). Serologic methods have also been used to evaluate the role of BHV-4 in naturally occurring feline LUTD.

(a). More than 250 serum samples collected from normal cats and cats with naturally occurring forms of LUTD have been evaluated for BHV-4 antibody by serum-neutralization assay.[41,43] BHV-4 serum-neutralizing antibodies were not detected in any of the serum specimens evaluated.

(b). However, results of other studies indicate that neutralization assays have limited usefulness in evaluating BHV-4 antibody responses.[39] Cats with experimentally induced BHV-4 UTI produced low or undetectable concentrations of BHV-4 serum-neutralizing antibodies; high concentrations of BHV-4 antibodies were detected when serum samples were evaluated with an indirect fluorescent antibody test (IFAT).[21,39]

(c). In a prospective study of feline LUTD, 167 serum specimens obtained from 26 normal cats and from 141 cats affected with naturally occurring LUTD were evaluated with the BHV-4 IFAT.[41] Antibodies against BHV-4 were detected by the IFAT in specimens obtained from 31% of cats affected with LUTD and from 23% of normal control cats. However, significant associations between positive BHV-4 IFAT results did not appear to be significantly associated with clinical signs, specific diagnosis, or abnormal laboratory findings.

(7). Detection of antibodies in clinically normal cats and in cats with LUTD indicates natural BHV-4 exposure.

(a). These results are consistent with previous experimental findings that demonstrate that BHV-4 (CAHV strain) readily establishes persistent low-grade or latent infections, which may or may not be associated with clinical signs.[21,40]

(b). However, the pathogenic role of BHV-4 in cats remains unresolved. Detection of BHV-4 antibody in clinically normal cats and lack of association of positive BHV-4 IFAT results with a clinical diagnosis of LUTD preclude assigning BHV-4 a primary role in naturally acquired LUTD.

(c). Concomitant isolation of BHV-4 and other viral or bacterial agents from cattle with systemic illness, and localization of BHV-4 in lymph nodes, spleen, and blood mononuclear cells of cattle with induced infections, has led to the hypothesis that BHV-4 has a potential immunomodulating role in some dual infections.[43] A similar phenomenon of infection in cats with LUTD or other disorders is suggested by recent detection of virus particles with ultrastructural characteristics of calicivirus in naturally forming urethral plugs.[26,80] The fact that BHV-4 was originally isolated from a cat with concurrent naturally acquired LUTD and calicivirus-induced upper respiratory tract disease lends further support to this hypothesis.[21]

(d). Additional studies are necessary to define the etiopathogenic role of BHV-4 infections in cats with naturally acquired LUTD or other disorders.

3. Diagnosis.

a. Identification and localization of viruses within the urinary tract are essential prerequisites to establishing a cause-and-effect relationship between viruses and various forms of feline LUTD.

(1). Clinical signs, clinical laboratory data, and microscopic evaluation of tissues stained from routine light microscopy cannot reliably distinguish virus-induced disease from other causes of LUTD.[40,43] Furthermore, not all cats with LUTD are likely to have viral infections.

(2). Exclusion of other known causes of hematuria, dysuria, and urethral obstruction should precede attempts to establish a diagnosis of viral UTI.

(3). In general, diagnostic criteria for viral infections include:

(a). Isolation and identification of viral agents.

(b). Direct demonstration of virus particles, viral antigens, or viral nucleic acids in tissues or body fluids.

(c). Detection and quantification of specific viral antibodies.[22]

b. Virus isolation is often a sensitive and specific means of establishing a viral diagnosis; however, use of standard cell culture inoculation techniques to isolate viral pathogens from urine of cats with experimentally induced and naturally occurring LUTD have been unrewarding.[21,41,43]

(1). Negative findings may be related to the highly cell-associated nature of some viruses, or to their propensity to establish low-grade or latent infections, or to the virucidal characteristics of feline urine.[42] In studies of induced BHV-4 (strain CAHV) UTI, herpesviruses could not be isolated from urine of infected cats, even though BHV-4 (strain CAHV) was consistently isolated from their urinary bladders by tissue explantation techniques.[40]

(2). Similarly, SFV was recovered only rarely from the urine of cats from whom SFV had been isolated by explanation of urinary tract tissues.[43]

c. Although virus isolation has historically been the primary method of establishing a specific diagnosis of viral infection, in some instances, expense, time, special sample requirements, and unusual biologic characteristics of viruses limit the diagnostic utility of virus isolation.
   (1). For example, isolation of BHV-4 by explanation requires a viable tissue sample obtained surgically or at necropsy, followed by a 4- to 6-week tissue culture incubation.[40]
   (2). Techniques designed to directly identify virus particles, viral antigens, or viral nucleic acids in tissues or body fluids are alternative means of virus identification and localization. Electron microscopy, immunofluorescence, immunohistochemistry, radioimmunoassay, enzyme-linked immunosorbent assay, DNA or RNA hybridization, and DNA amplification by the polymerase chain reaction (PCR) are procedures currently utilized for viral diagnosis.[16,22]

d. DNA or RNA hybridization using radioactively and nonradioactively labeled probes has proved to be an extremely sensitive, specific, and rapid method of identifying viral nucleic acids in cells or tissue (hybridization *in situ*), or in DNA extracts prepared from blood leukocytes, urine, exudates, or tissues.[16]
   (1). This technique exploits the ability of an appropriately labeled DNA probe to form a highly specific hybrid between itself and its complementary viral DNA or RNA sequence.
   (2). Recently, hybridization probes specific for BHV-4 DNA have been developed in our laboratory and elsewhere.[43]
   (3). In a study of induced BHV-4 infections of rabbits, dot blot DNA hybridization was found to be more sensitive for identifying sites of latent BHV-4 infections than was tissue explanation.[43]

e. Polymerase chain reaction methods have proved superior to conventional virus isolation and identification methods.[16]
   (1). Polymerase chain reaction logarithmically amplifies specific viral DNA sequences and allows detection of minute quantities of viral nucleic acid in a wide range of tissue or body fluids.
   (2). Its advantages—speed, specificity, and exquisite sensitivity—are rapidly making PCR the gold standard for viral diagnosis.
   (3). In our experience, PCR is more sensitive than either slot-blot DNA hybridization or tissue explanation for detecting latent BHV-4 infection in experimentally exposed cats.[43]

f. Detection and quantification of specific viral antibodies provide an indirect method of identifying viral infections.[8,22]
   (1). Ideally, paired serum samples obtained during the acute and convalescent phase of the disease should be evaluated for a rise in specific antibody titer.
   (2). In some cases, a single serum sample may be adequate if viral pathogens cause persistent or lifelong infections.
   (3). Because of the persistent—and often asymptomatic—nature of FCV, SFV, and BHV-4 infections in cats, and because of widespread use of calicivirus vaccines, caution must be used in establishing a cause-and-effect relationship between viruses and LUTD on the basis of serologic evidence alone.[43]
   (4). Choice of serologic methods to detect and quantitate viral antibodies should be based on test sensitivity and specificity. Whereas the IFAT appears to be a sensitive test for BHV-4 exposure in cats, standard serum neutralization assays have been unreliable.[39,21,43]

g. Because of the uncertainty surrounding the role of viral uropathogens in feline LUTD, future studies of viral causes of naturally occurring feline LUTD should encompass specialized sampling, cultivation, and identification techniques suitable for each individual uropathogen when attempting to establish a diagnosis of viral UTI.

4. Treatment.
   a. Interest in antiviral chemotherapeutic and biologic agents has grown considerably in recent years; however, antiviral agents available for clinical use are relatively few and of limited specificity.[31] Antiviral agents have not been evaluated in cats with LUTD.
   b. In cats, management of LUTD suspected to be caused by viral agents has been limited to supportive and symptomatic care given during the course of clinical signs. It is noteworthy that clinical signs of hematuria and dysuria in many nonobstructed cats with the idiopathic form of LUTD spontaneously subsided approximately 7 to 10 days after diagnosis.[41,76] Regardless of whether viruses have causative roles in idiopathic LUTD, these observations emphasize the unpredictability with which signs of feline LUTD undergo remission and exacerbation and illustrate the need for controlled studies evaluating the safety and efficacy of therapeutic and prophylactic regimens.[69]

B. Bacterial urinary tract infection.

1. Etiopathogenesis.
   a. Bacterial UTIs are common causes of LUTD in dogs. In contrast, results of several clinical studies indicate that initial episodes of feline LUTD usually occur in the absence of signifi-

cant numbers of detectable bacteria.[41,46,76] In a prospective diagnostic study of male and female obstructed and nonobstructed cats, bacterial UTIs were identified in fewer than 3% of patients (see Table 35–3).[41,76] The infrequency with which bacteria have been isolated from urine of cats during the initial phases of LUTD may be related to highly effective local host defense mechanisms in this species.[76]

(1). As with other species, unimpeded, frequent, and complete urination, urethral structure and function, and the intrinsic antibacterial properties of urinary mucosa are important local host defenses against bacterial colonization of the feline urinary tract.

(2). In addition, feline urine is apparently a less hospitable medium for bacterial growth than is the urine of other species.

(a). Physiochemical properties of urine that inhibit bacterial growth include low or high pH, high osmolality, high concentration of urea, and weak organic acids and uromucoid (Tamm-Horsfall mucoprotein).[5,80]

(b). The infrequency of primary bacterial UTIs in cats has been hypothesized to be related to their ability to produce highly concentrated urine (specific gravity up to 1.80) and their consumption of comparatively high-protein diets. High-protein diets promote formation of acid urine that is high in concentrations of urea and weak organic acids.[66,76]

b. When bacterial UTI has been detected in cats (see Table 35–8), it frequently was a secondary or complicating factor rather than a primary etiologic factor.[46,66,76] Local urinary tract defenses against bacterial infection are frequently compromised in cats with various forms of naturally occurring nonbacterial LUTD, especially if the episode is associated with urethral obstruction (see Table 35–1).

c. Indwelling transurethral catheters are associated with a high prevalence of secondary or complicating bacterial UTI.

(1). In studies of normal cats, catheter-induced bacteriuria was detected in 33% of cats after 1 day of catheterization, and in 50 to 83% of cats after 5 days of indwelling catheterization.[43,66]

(2). Similarly, in cats, bacterial UTIs are common sequelae of perineal urethrostomy. In a controlled prospective study of cats with naturally occurring LUTD, episodes of bacterial UTI occurred in 17% of cats treated with perineal urethrostomy, 10% of cats treated with perineal urethrostomy and diet, and none of the cats treated with dietary therapy alone.[79]

(3). Results of these studies emphasize the importance of the distal urethra in defending the urinary tract from bacterial colonization.

2. Diagnosis.

a. A diagnosis of bacterial UTI in cats with LUTD should be based on urinalysis and quantitative urine culture.

(1). Although urinalysis findings of hematuria, pyuria, and proteinuria are consistent with bacterial infection, a diagnosis of bacterial UTI should not be based on these findings alone. The constellation of hematuria, pyuria, and proteinuria is nonspecific and indicates urinary tract inflammation, which may result from infectious or noninfectious causes of LUTD.

(2). In a prospective study of cats with naturally occurring LUTD, hematuria and pyuria were detected in 20% of cats with idiopathic disease, 57% of cats with urethral matrix-crystalline plugs, and 60% of cats with urolithiasis.[41] Conversely, clinical and experimental studies in cats have demonstrated that pyuria may not be observed in urinalysis of cats with confirmed bacterial UTIs.[43]

b. Detection of bacteria in urine sediment is suggestive, but not conclusive, evidence of bacterial UTI because urine may be contaminated during collection and storage. The commensual population of bacteria that normally inhabits mucosal surfaces of the distal urinary tract commonly contaminates voided urine samples, and may contaminate samples collected by catheterization.

c. Quantitative urine culture provides the most definitive means of confirming and characterizing bacterial UTIs. Because of the innate antibacterial properties of cat urine as compared to dog urine, however, lower concentrations of bacteria are more likely to be clinically significant in cats.[46,66,76]

(1). Detection of more than 1000 colony-forming units per milliliter of urine collected by cystocentesis or catheterization is considered to be significant bacteriuria in cats.

(2). In urine samples collected by voluntary micturition or manual compression of the urinary bladder, detection of greater than 10,000 colony-forming units per milliliter is considered significant.

(a). Results of quantitative cultures performed on voided urine samples must be interpreted with caution.

(b). Studies in normal cats have shown that contamination of voided urine samples may result in colony counts greater than 100,000 per milliliter.[47]

d. Considering that bacterial UTIs are uncommon causes of initial episodes of feline LUTD and that most patients with significant bacteriuria have secondary or complicating UTIs, efforts should be made to identify factors that predispose to bacterial UTI. Additional diagnostic procedures that may be considered include survey and contrast radiography, ultrasonography, exfoliative cytology of urine sediment, serology, virus isolation, and biopsy.

3. Treatment.
   a. Antimicrobial agents remain the cornerstone of therapy for feline bacterial UTI; however, they should not be given indiscriminately or without clinical follow-up.
      (1). The infrequency with which bacterial uropathogens are isolated from cats with LUTD emphasizes that routine use of antimicrobial agents in treating LUTD is unnecessary.[41,66,76]
      (2). In a prospective study designed to evaluate the efficacy of chloramphenicol as compared with a placebo for treatment of male and female cats with LUTD, clinical signs resolved in the majority of cats within 5 days, regardless of treatment.[43]
   b. Once bacterial UTI has been confirmed, antimicrobial drugs should be selected on the basis of susceptibility tests. Urine should be recultured 3 to 5 days after initiation of therapy to confirm sterilization of urine. Antibiotic therapy should be continued until clinical and laboratory evidence shows response as determined by clinical signs, urinalysis, and bacterial culture.
   c. Prevention of recurrent bacterial UTI may depend on correction or control of abnormalities in host defenses (Table 35–9).

TABLE 35–9
SUMMARY OF OBJECTIVES FOR TREATMENT OF URINARY TRACT INFECTIONS

1. The predisposing or complicating causes of the UTI should be identified and eliminated.
2. Causative pathogens are identified by qualitative and quantitative culture, and antimicrobials are selected on the basis of antimicrobial susceptibility tests. Ideally, the agent chosen should have the narrowest possible spectrum of antimicrobial activity.
3. Aggressive treatment with appropriate dosages of antimicrobials is indicated.
4. Although usually unnecessary, urine pH can be altered to enhance antimicrobial activity.
5. Urine should be recultured 3 to 5 days after initiation of therapy, to check the efficacy of the antimicrobial agent in sterilizing the urine.
6. Antimicrobial therapy is continued until clinical and laboratory evidence of response is attained. The patient's response is monitored by bacterial culture and urinalysis.
7. Because symptomatic or asymptomatic recurrences may be associated with progressive and potentially irreversible disease, they should be anticipated, prevented, and, if necessary, treated.

C. Mycoplasma and ureaplasma urinary tract infections.

1. Unlike other bacteria, mycoplasmas and ureaplasmas are characterized by lack of a rigid cell wall, small size (0.2 to 0.3 μm), and limited biosynthetic abilities.[87]
   a. They are the smallest known self-replicating prokaryotic bacteria.
   b. Ureaplasmas differ from mycoplasmas in that they possess urease and are capable of hydrolyzing urea for energy.
   c. Mycoplasmas and ureaplasmas have been associated with naturally occurring or experimentally induced LUTD in humans and in dogs, sheep, and rats.[43,53,72,90]
   d. Although mycoplasmas and ureaplasmas have been isolated from the genitourinary tract of cats, their role as agents of feline LUTD is uncertain (Table 35–8).[6,43]
2. Efforts to isolate *Mycoplasma* and *Ureaplasma* organisms from urine of more than 141 cats with naturally occurring LUTD were unsuccessful.[41] Other investigators have reported similar findings.[63]
   a. Although these results raise questions about the causative role of mycoplasmas and ureaplasmas in feline LUTD, they may also reflect unsuitable culture factors (e.g., inappropriate or poor-quality media) or the presence of inhibitory host factors that limit recovery of mycoplasmas or ureaplasmas.[43]
   b. Host factors that may limit mycoplasma growth *in vivo* include high urine pH and osmolality, high ammonia concentration, and/or the presence of inhibitory antibiotics or enzymes.[6,72]
   c. *In vitro* studies using synthetic urine suggest that ureaplasmas, but not mycoplasmas, are capable of surviving osmotic conditions of normal feline urine.[6] These results were consistent with the isolation of *Ureaplasma* species, but not *Mycoplasma* species, from the urine of a limited number of cats.
3. Establishing an etiopathologic role for ureaplasmas or mycoplasmas in feline LUTD requires isolating the organisms from suitable urine or tissue samples and demonstrating a host cellular response.[51]
   a. Mycoplasmas and ureaplasmas are fragile and

fastidious organisms with exacting growth requirements, which vary considerably among *Mycoplasma* species.

b. Successful recovery and identification of these organisms require careful collection and transport of specimens and use of appropriate growth media and specific cultivation methods.[6,43]

c. Because many laboratories are not prepared to culture mycoplasmas and ureaplasmas, one should consult with laboratory staff for specific recommendations before collecting samples for submission.

4. Detection of mycoplasmas in host tissues and characterization of host responses to infection depend on use of specialized methods.

a. Because of their small size and amorphous shape, standard light microscopic techniques cannot reliably detect mycoplasmas in urine sediment or tissues.

b. Electron microscopy is usually required to visualize individual organisms and to demonstrate their interaction with host cells or tissue.[43]

D. Fungal urinary tract infections.

1. Although uncommon, fungal UTIs have been reported in cats (see Table 35–8).[19,27,58,76]

a. In humans, dogs, and cats, factors that predispose to fungal UTI include prolonged antibiotic and/or glucocorticoid therapy, aciduria (optimal pH for fungal growth is 5.1 to 6.4), indwelling transurethral catheters, and/or local urinary tract or systemic disorders that compromise host urinary tract defenses.[58]

b. Many cats with fungal UTIs have been given symptomatic treatment for clinical signs of LUTD.[19,27,76]

c. Many forms of therapy currently in vogue for empiric treatment of LUTD represent significant predisposing factors for fungal UTI.

2. Fungi detected in properly collected urine samples are abnormal.

a. A tentative diagnosis of fungal UTI may be established by identifying yeasts or mycelia in urine sediment.[58] Candida organisms typically appear as budding unicellular yeasts of approximately 3 to 7 μm. They may also appear as branching filamentous pseudohyphae as long as 600 μm.

b. Definitive diagnosis of fungiuria is based on culture or organisms on Sabouraud's dextrose agar or cycloheximide-free blood agar.[58]

(1). Quantitative fungal urine cultures appear to have little value in establishing a diagnosis of fungal UTI.

(2). Isolation of fungal organisms from two serial urine samples collected by cystocentesis should be considered significant, regardless of colony count.

(3). However, confirmation of fungal UTI requires demonstration of fungal organisms in urinary tract tissues.

3. Experience with treatment of fungal UTIs in cats is limited.

a. In patients with asymptomatic fungal UTI, correction of identifiable predisposing factors and alkalinization of urine to a pH greater than 7.5 may be sufficient.[58] We have not been successful in eradicating fungal UTIs with alkalinization of urine alone.

b. Patients that have concurrent clinical signs of LUTD or that have other debilitating or complicating disorders may require additional specific antifungal therapy to eliminate the organism. Flucytosine, amphotericin B, ketoconazole, itraconazole, and fluconazole have been used to treat *Candida* species UTIs in humans[41]; however, as yet no studies confirm the safety or efficacy of these agents against fungal UTIs of cats.

c. Response to treatment should be monitored by serial urine fungal culture. Treatment should be continued until 2 successive negative cultures are obtained at 1- to 2-week intervals.

E. Parasitic urinary tract infections.

1. Although parasitic UTIs are quite prevalent in certain regions of the world, parasites are rarely recognized as causes of feline LUTD in North America.[7]

2. To date, the nematode *Capillaria feliscati* is the only parasite that has been associated with clinical signs of feline LUTD (see Table 35–8).[7]

a. Most *C. feliscati* UTIs appear to be asymptomatic. Absence of clinical signs associated with these nematodes most likely reflects their small quantities and their superficial attachment to bladder mucosa.

b. Diagnosis of *C. feliscati* is based on identification of characteristic ova in urine sediment or visualization of adult worms in the urinary bladder. Ova of *C. feliscati* are bipolar, measuring 50 to 68 μm in length and 22 to 32 μm in width. Adults are small, thread-like worms 13 to 45 mm in length.[42]

c. Treatment is indicated when clinical signs of LUTD accompany *C. feliscati* UTI. In those instances, fenbendazole, 25 mg/kg every 12 hours for 3 to 10 days, has been suggested.[7]

VI. DIAGNOSIS, TREATMENT, AND PREVENTION OF UROLITHS AND URETHRAL PLUGS

A. Terminology.

1. Physical (see Fig. 35–2) and probably etiopathogenic differences exist between feline uroliths and urethral plugs (Tables 35–10 through 35–12). These terms should not be used interchangeably.

a. Uroliths are polycrystalline concretions composed primarily of minerals (organic and inor-

TABLE 35–10
COMMON CHARACTERISTICS OF FELINE STRUVITE UROLITHS

Chemical name: Magnesium ammonium phosphate hexahydrate. Crystal name: Struvite.
Formula: $MgNH_4PO_4 \cdot 6H_2O$
Variations in mineral composition
- Struvite only (especially sterile struvite)
- Struvite mixed with lesser quantities of calcium apatite and/or ammonium acid urate (especially infection-induced struvite)
- Nucleus of a different mineral surrounded by variable layers composed primarily of struvite.
  - Small quantities of calcium apatite and/or ammonium acid urate also may be present.

Physical characteristics
- Color: Struvite uroliths usually are white, cream, or light brown. The surface of uroliths commonly is red because of concomitant hematuria.
- Shape: Sterile struvite uroliths obtained from the urinary bladder of cats commonly have a wafer or disc shape; they are thicker at their center than at the periphery. Sterile struvite uroliths also may have a rough, jagged, quartz-like appearance. Infection-induced feline struvite urocystoliths often are larger than sterile struvite uroliths and tend to be more egg shaped. They also contain more matrix than do sterile struvite uroliths.
- Nuclei and laminations: Uncommon in sterile struvite uroliths. Infection-induced struvite may surround sterile struvite.
- Matrix: Sterile struvite uroliths contain little matrix and characteristically are dense and brittle. Infection-induced struvite uroliths are somewhat softer because they contain more matrix.
- Density: Struvite is radiodense compared with nonskeletal tissue on survey radiographs.
- Location: Most occur in the urinary bladder; some may lodge in the urethra, especially of male cats. Struvite uroliths may affect the kidneys, but this location has been uncommon.
- Number: Single or multiple.
- Size: Subvisual to a size limited by the capacity of structure (kidney and urinary bladder) in which they form.

Predisposing factors.
- Sterile struvite.
  - Tendency to form in alkaline or less acidic urine.
  - Supersaturation of urine with magnesium, ammonium, and/or phosphate.
  - Excessive consumption of magnesium and, perhaps, other minerals.
  - Formation of concentrated urine.
  - Retention of urine.
  - Unidentified factors.
- Infection-induced struvite.
  - UTI with urease-producing microbes, especially staphylococci.
  - Excretion of large quantities of urea in urine.

Characteristics of affected patients.
- May be detected at any age, but usually between 1 and 10 years of age.
- When uroliths occur in immature cats, they usually have infection-induced struvite.
- Somewhat more common in females than males.
- Obesity reflects excessive food consumption. Excessive calories are stored as fat. Minerals consumed with excessive food are excreted in urine and may predispose to urolith formation.

ganic crystalloids) and smaller quantities of matrix.

b. Feline urethral plugs commonly are composed of large quantities of matrix mixed with minerals,[72] although some are composed primarily of matrix, some consist of sloughed tissue, blood, and/or inflammatory reactants, and a few are composed primarily of aggregates of crystalline minerals.

2. A variety of different minerals have been identified in uroliths (see Table 35–6) and urethral plugs (see Table 35–7) of cats. The mineral composition of uroliths and urethral plugs should be used to describe them, because most therapeutic regimens have been based on their mineral composition.

B. Epidemiology of uroliths and urethral plugs.

1. As of mid 1994, the mineral composition of approximately 54% of the naturally occurring uroliths submitted to the University of Minnesota by veterinarians in the United States and Canada were primarily struvite (see Table 35–6). The 54% frequency of naturally occurring struvite uroliths observed in 1993 represents approximately a 26% decrease from the series we reported in 1989,[76] and a 36% decrease from the series we reported in 1984. (Please note that uroliths tabulated in 1994 include those analyzed in the 1989 and 1984 reports.)[70] In contrast, the frequency of feline uroliths composed of calcium oxalate rose from approximately 2% in 1984, and 5.6% in 1989, to approximately 37% in 1994 (see Table 35–5).[70,76]

2. As of mid 1993, the mineral composition of approximately 78% of the naturally occurring urethral plugs submitted to the University of Minnesota were primarily struvite (see Table 35–7). The 78% frequency of naturally occurring struvite urethral plugs observed in 1993 represents approximately a 12% decrease from the series we reported in 1987,[2] and a 16% decrease from the series we reported in 1984.[70]
3. The decline in appearance of naturally occurring struvite uroliths and urethral plugs during the past decade may be explained in part by the widespread use of a calculolytic diet designed to dissolve them, and by modification of maintenance and prevention diets designed to minimize struvite crystalluria.
   a. However, information submitted to our urolith laboratory indicates that diets known to be effective in dissolving and preventing struvite uroliths and struvite crystalluria are being used inappropriately in attempts to manage other types of uroliths.
   b. Likewise, once a protocol for dietary management is selected, follow-up evaluation of efficacy by urinalysis is performed too infrequently.

C. Biologic behavior of uroliths and urethral plugs.

1. Urolith activity.
   a. Uroliths may undergo spontaneous dissolution, remain active (growth occurs), or become inactive (no growth occurs).
      (1). Surgical activity has been defined as urolithiasis with colic, obstruction to urine outflow, or infection requiring surgical intervention.[82]
      (2). Metabolic activity occurs when one or more of the following are present:
         (a). Radiographic or ultrasonographic evidence of stone growth within the past year.
         (b). Radiographic or ultrasonographic evidence of a new stone within the past year.
         (c). Documented voiding of uroliths within the past year.
      (3). Intermediate activity is a term used to designate situations in which radiographs or ultrasonograms are not available or are inadequate to evaluate the status of urolithiasis during the past year. In a study of 101 consecutive human patients with

TABLE 35–11
COMMON CHARACTERISTICS OF FELINE CALCIUM OXALATE UROLITHS

Chemical name; Formula; Crystal name:
- Calcium oxalate monohydrate; $CaC_2O_4 \cdot H_2O$; Whewellite
- Calcium oxalate dihydrate; $CaC_2O_4 \cdot 2H_2O$; Whewellite

Variations in composition
- Calcium oxalate monohydrate only
- Calcium oxalate dihydrate only
- Combinations of calcium oxalate monohydrate and dihydrate.
- Calcium oxalate (monohydrate and/or dihydrate) mixed with variable quantities of calcium phosphate. Variable quantities of struvite or ammonium acid urate may also be present.
- Calcium oxalate (monohydrate and/or dihydrate) nucleus surrounded by other minerals, especially infection-induced struvite.

Physical characteristics
- Color: Calcium oxalate monohydrate uroliths are usually tan or brown. Calcium oxalate dihydrate uroliths are usually white or cream colored. The surface may be red to black if they are coated with blood.
- Shape: Variable. Calcium oxalate monohydrate uroliths are usually round or elliptic and have a smooth, polished surface. On occasion, they may develop a jackstone or mulberry shape. Calcium oxalate dihydrate uroliths and mixed calcium oxalate monohydrate–calcium oxalate dihydrate uroliths are usually round to ovoid and have an irregular surface caused by protrusion of sharp-edged crystals. On occasion, they may develop a jackstone shape.
- Nuclei: Nuclei, radial striations, and concentric laminations may occur.
- Density: Very dense and brittle. Survey radiographs reveal that they are radiodense compared with soft tissue.
- Number: Single or multiple.
- Location: May be located in renal pelves, ureters, urinary bladder (most common), and/or urethra.
- Size: Subvisual to several centimeters.

Prevalence
- Represent 45 to 50% of uroliths
- May be recurrent

Characteristics of affected cats
- More common in males (56%) than in females (44%).
- Mean age of diagnosis is about 7 years (range, <1 to >20).
- Most commonly observed in Burmese, Himalayan, and Persian breeds.

TABLE 35–12
CHARACTERISTICS OF FELINE STRUVITE URETHRAL PLUGS*

Chemical name: Magnesium ammonium phosphate hexahydrate; Crystal name: Struvite
Formula: $MgNH_4PO_4 \cdot 6H_2O$
Variations in composition
- Struvite only
- Struvite mixed with relatively small quantities of calcium apatite

Physical characteristics
- Color: Typically white, cream, or light brown
- Shape: Often have a cylindric shape; sometimes form a shapeless gelatinous mass
- Nuclei and laminations: None grossly visible
- Matrix: Contain large quantities of matrix and therefore are fragile
- Density: Soft and easily compressible
- Number: Usually single; occasionally multiple
- Size: Diameter conforms to diameter of urethra. Length varies from a few millimeters to several centimeters, and may be interrupted along length of urethra.

Predisposing factors
- Reduced diameter for the penile urethra
- Locally produced matrix?
- Factors affecting struvite crystalluria?

Characteristics of affected patients
- Mean age, 4 years (range, <1 to >12 years)
- No obvious breed disposition
- Consistently (if not invariably) in males

*With the exception of crystal composition, similar characteristics have been observed in urethral plugs containing calcium phosphate, calcium oxalate, ammonium acid urate, and xanthine.

uroliths of intermediate activity, 64 (63%) were found to have inactive urolithiasis and 37 (37%) were found to have active urolithiasis.[82] Similar studies have not been performed in cats with uroliths.

b. The concept of metabolic activity is of prognostic and therapeutic relevance, especially if urolith treatment is likely to be associated with complications. Detection of a urolith is not always justification for medical surgical management.
   (1). In cats, small uroliths may remain asymptomatic in the urinary tract (especially the renal pelvis and urinary bladder) for months or years. However, the underlying cause(s) of uroliths and their sequelae (partial or total obstruction, UTI) remain potential hazards.
   (2). When uroliths are detected fortuitously in asymptomatic patients without significant bacteriuria, the option of monitoring urolith activity by appropriate procedures is an accepted alternative to surgery.
   (3). If the urolith(s) remain inactive, therapy designed to dissolve or remove them is not mandatory.
   (4). If the urolith(s) become active, appropriate medical and/or surgical therapy is recommended.

2. Biologic behavior of uroliths.
   a. Few studies of the natural course of urolithiasis in cats have been performed.
      (1). Although empiric observations suggest that most uroliths that cause clinical signs persist or increase in number and size, we have observed spontaneous dissolution of naturally occurring bladder uroliths presumed to be sterile struvite in two adult cats.
      (2). In 1 cat, a 5-year-old female domestic shorthair, uroliths presumed to be composed of sterile struvite spontaneously dissolved 18 days following their radiographic detection. Radiographic evidence of uroliths was not detected during 7 monthly follow-up examinations; however at the eighth month, multiple urocystoliths were detected. Subsequently they dissolved spontaneously during the next 3½ months.
      (3). In 2 retrospective studies of uroliths, recurrence rates of 19 and 37% were reported.[32,82] Unfortunately, the type of minerals in the recurrent uroliths was not specified.
      (4). In our experience, sterile and infection-induced struvite uroliths have recurred within weeks to several months after elimination.

(5). Cystine urocystoliths also typically recur within a few weeks to several months following removal.

(6). Calcium oxalate, calcium phosphate (brushite), and ammonium urate uroliths also have an unpredictable tendency to recur, typically within months, rather than weeks, following removal.

b. Small uroliths that form in the urinary bladder may pass into the urethra of male or female cats (Fig. 35–26). Likewise, small renoliths may pass into the ureters. Because of the tendency of uroliths to change size and position, radiographic evaluation of the urinary system should be repeated if there has been a significant interval between diagnosis and scheduling of surgery to remove them.

c. Because many feline uroliths are small, complete surgical removal of all uroliths may be difficult. In a retrospective clinical study performed at the University of Minnesota, uroliths were detected by radiographs taken within 14 days following cystotomy in 20% of the patients.[59] Results of this study emphasize the importance of postsurgical radiography to assess urolith status before evaluating recurrence or therapeutic efficacy.

3. Biologic behavior of urethral plugs.

a. The biologic behavior of any disorder is influenced by its cause. Future studies of the biologic behavior of obstructive uropathy in male cats must encompass efforts to detect and specify the nature of the obstruction (Table 35–13).

b. Of the various manifestations of feline LUTD, the consequence of urethral obstruction and postrenal azotemia have received the greatest emphasis. Obstruction to urine outflow produces predictable clinical and biochemical abnormalities that vary with the duration and degree of obstruction. However, systemic abnormalities in fluid, acid-base, and electrolyte balance caused by urethral obstruction probably occur, regardless of the specific cause (e.g., uroliths, plugs, strictures, regardless). Feline urethral plugs are associated with a frequent but unpredictable tendency to recur. However, this generality appears to be an overstatement, because most investigators have considered urethral obstruction in male cats and struvite urethral plugs to be identical. Recent clinical studies, however, indicate that urethral obstruction in male cats may be initiated and maintained at one or more sites by one or a combination of primary, secondary, and/or iatrogenic causes (see Tables 35–1 and 35–13). Even when recurrent obstruction is caused by urethral plugs, no studies have been designed specifically to evaluate comparisons of the nature and composition of first-occurrence plugs and recurrent obstructing material.

D. Diagnosis.

1. Uroliths.

a. Information obtained from the Purdue University Veterinary Medical Data Base suggests that uroliths may be overlooked in cats with LUTD. From 1980 to 1990, uroliths from the bladder and urethra were detected in 7.1% of 13,511 cats with LUTD admitted to 23 veterinary teaching hospitals in North America. In contrast, in a prospective diagnostic study of feline LUTD performed at the University of Minnesota, uroliths were detected by survey and

TABLE 35–13
POSSIBLE CAUSES OF URETHRAL OBSTRUCTION IN MALE CATS

Primary Causes	Perpetuating Causes	Iatrogenic Causes
Intraluminal	Intraluminal	Tissue Damage
Urethral plugs (matrix and/or crystals)	Increased production of mucoprotein, red and white blood cells, and fibrin	Reverse flushing solutions
Urethroliths	Sloughed tissue	Catheter trauma
Tissue sloughed from urinary bladder or urethra	Mural	Catheter-induced foreign body reaction
Mural or extramural	Inflammatory swelling	Catheter-induced infection
Strictures	Muscular spasm (reflex dyssynergia?)	Postsurgical dysfunction
Prostatic lesions	Strictures	
Urethral neoplasms		
Anomalies		
Reflex dyssynergia		
Combinations	Combinations	
Others?	Others?	

TABLE 35–14
CHECKLIST OF FACTORS THAT SUGGEST PROBABLE MINERAL COMPOSITION OF FELINE UROLITHS

Urine pH
- Struvite and calcium apatite uroliths, usually alkaline. Sterile struvite uroliths may be observed with urine pH 6.5 or higher.
- Ammonium urate uroliths, acid to neutral*
- Cystine uroliths, acid*
- Calcium oxalate, often acid to neutral*

Identification of crystals in uncontaminated fresh urine sediment, preferably at body temperature

Type of bacteria, if any, isolated from urine
- Urease from bacteria, especially staphylococci and less frequently *Proteus* spp., may be associated with struvite uroliths.
- UTIs often are absent in patients with calcium oxalate, cystine, or ammonium urate.
- Calcium oxalate, cystine, or ammonium urate uroliths may predispose to UTI; if infections are caused by urease-producing bacteria, struvite may precipitate around metabolic uroliths.

Radiographic density and physical characteristics of uroliths

Serum chemistry evaluation
- Hypercalcemia may be associated with calcium-containing uroliths.
- Hyperuricemia may be associated with uric acid or urate uroliths.
- Hyperchloremia, hypokalemia, and acidemia may be associated with distal renal tubular acidosis and calcium phosphate or struvite uroliths.

Urine chemistry evaluation
- Patient should be consuming a standard diagnostic diet or the diet consumed when uroliths formed.
- Excessive quantities of one or more minerals contained in the urolith are expected. The concentration of crystallization inhibitors may be decreased.

Breed of cat and history of uroliths in patient's ancestors or littermates.

Drugs
- Corticosteroids and furosemide predispose to hypercalciuria.
- Allopurinol predispose to xanthine.
- Drugs containing sulfadiazine predispose to formation of uroliths containing varying quantities of sulfadiazine.

Quantitative analysis of uroliths passed during micturition or collected via catheter technique.

*Concomitant infection with urease-producing microbes may result in formation of alkaline urine.

contrast radiography in more than 20% of the patients (see Tables 35–3 and 35–4).

b. Most uroliths in cats cannot be detected by abdominal palpation.
   (1). For example, in a study of 30 urocystoliths in cats, stones were detected by palpation in only 3 patients.[78]
   (2). Likewise, uroliths located in the renal pelves cannot be detected by palpation through the abdominal wall.
      (a). Therefore, radiographic and/or ultrasonographic evaluation of the urinary tract is required to consistently detect feline uroliths (Figs. 35–11 and 35–15).
      (b). Double-contrast cystography is usually required to detect urocystoliths smaller than 3 mm in diameter, especially those of low radiodensity.
   (3). From a diagnostic yield perspective, radiography of the abdomen of previously untreated cats with hematuria, dysuria, and/or urethral obstruction is more likely to yield positive information (>20%) than are quantitative urine cultures (±3%).

c. Medical dissolution of uroliths poses the problem of formulating therapy without the availability of surgically removed uroliths for analysis.
   (1). To overcome this problem, we follow a checklist that facilitates "guesstimates" of urolith composition (Table 35–14); however, quantitative mineral analysis of representative portions of uroliths by polarizing light microscopy, infrared spectroscopy, x-ray defractometry, or energy-dispersive x-ray spectroscopy remains the diagnostic gold standard. Small uroliths located in the urinary bladder are commonly voided during micturition.
   (2). Small urocystoliths may also be retrieved for analysis by aspirating them through a catheter into a syringe while an assistant vigorously and repeatedly moves the patient's abdomen in an up-and-down direction.[57,81]
      (a). This maneuver causes uroliths located in the dependent portion of the bladder to disperse throughout fluid in the bladder lumen.
      (b). Small uroliths in the vicinity of the catheter tip may then be sucked into

the catheter along with urine (or saline previously injected into the bladder lumen).

2. Urethral plugs.
   a. In addition to an appropriate history and physical examination, survey abdominal radiographs should be obtained of the lower urinary tract before therapy designed to re-establish urethral patency (see Table 35–2, Fig. 35–3, and Treatment and Prevention of Urethral Plugs). Localization of the site(s) and cause(s) of urethral obstruction is especially important if urethrostomy is being considered.
   b. A complete urinalysis, with special emphasis on evaluation of urine sediment unadulterated with reverse flushing solution, is especially valuable.
   c. Pretreatment urine samples may be obtained during decompressive cystocentesis.
   d. Quantitative analysis of the mineral components of plugs removed from the urethra should be done routinely.

E. Ammonium urate uroliths.

1. Etiopathogenesis.
   a. In our feline urolith series, ammonium urate and uric acid, collectively called purines, comprised approximately 6.8% of the total (see Table 35–6).
      (1). The urinary bladder was the most common site of purine uroliths (253), whereas the urethra (23), bladder and urethra (11), and ureter (1) were less common sites (the site of 17 purine uroliths was not recorded).
      (2). Purine uroliths were not found in the kidneys in our series; however, ammonium urate and uric acid uroliths have been found by others in the kidneys of cats.[76]
      (3). In our series, males (151) were affected as often as females (153). Neutered males (133) and neutered females (134) were affected more frequently than intact males (18) and intact females (19) (in 10 affected cats, the gender was not specified).
      (4). The mean age of affected cats was 5.8 ± 2.9 years (range, 5 months to 15 years).
   b. Isolated case reports of uric acid and ammonium urate uroliths in cats have appeared during the past 20 years.[76]
      (1). Although a renal tubular reabsorptive defect and portovascular anomalies have been implicated as causes in a few cases, the cause of formation of most feline urate uroliths has not been established.
      (2). We have not been able to determine precisely the cause of feline urate uroliths in our stone series. This problem has been compounded by the difficulty of reproducibly measuring the concentration of uric acid in serum and urine by methods commonly used in clinical laboratories.
      (3). Nonetheless, formation of highly acidic, and highly concentrated, urine associated with consumption of diets high in purine precursors (especially liver) appear to be risk factors in some cases.
   c. We have encountered xanthine uroliths in the bladder of two cats that were not given allopurinol.
      (1). One patient was a 15-month-old neutered male domestic longhair cat. A urolith surgically removed from the urinary bladder was composed of 95% xanthine and 5% uric acid.
      (2). The other patient was a 9-month-old neutered male domestic shorthair cat with uroliths in the bladder and the urethra.
         (a). Many crystals resembling uric acid were observed in the urine sediment.
         (b). Evaluation of a hemogram and serum biochemical profile revealed no abnormalities.
         (c). Quantitative analysis revealed that the uroliths were composed of 100% xanthine.
         (d). Evaluation of a urine sample by high-pressure liquid chromatography revealed that the uric acid concentration was 3.4 mg/dL whereas the xanthine concentration was 54 mg/dL.
2. Treatment and prevention.
   a. Medical protocols that consistently promote dissolution of ammonium urate uroliths in cats have not yet been developed.
   b. Urocystoliths small enough to pass through the urethra may be removed with the aid of a urinary catheter or by voiding urohydropropulsion.[56,57,81]
   c. Surgery remains the most reliable method for removing larger, inactive uroliths from the urinary tract.
   d. Prevention should encompass consumption of a diet low in purine precursors (e.g., low in liver), and that promotes formation of less acidic urine (pH ± 7) that is not highly concentrated.
   e. Induced dissolution of an ammonium urate urocystolith affecting a 3-year-old male castrated domestic shorthair cat was associated with a combination of allopurinol, 30 mg/kg/d divided into 2 equal doses, and a diet relatively low in purine precursors. Although allopurinol may be considered to reduce formation of uric acid, additional studies of the efficacy and potential toxicity of allopurinol in cats are required before meaningful generalities can be

established. Of particular concern is the potential of inducing xanthine uroliths.

F. Calcium oxalate uroliths.

1. Etiopathogenesis.
   a. In our most recent series, calcium oxalate uroliths comprised approximately 37% of the total (see Tables 35–6 and 35–11).
      (1). They were detected in the kidneys (39), ureter (22), kidney and ureter (7), kidney and bladder (8), ureter and bladder (5), ureter, bladder, and urethra (1), ureter and urethra (1), urinary bladder (884), urethra (100), urinary bladder and urethra (108), and kidney, ureter, bladder, and urethra (1; Fig. 35–26). Fifty-two calcium oxalate uroliths were voided. The location of 50 calcium oxalate stones was not recorded.
      (2). In our series, male cats (707) were affected more often than females (543). Neutered males (649) and neutered females (494) were affected more often than intact males (58) and intact females (49) (for 28 affected cats, the gender was not recorded).
      (3). The mean age of affected cats was 7.2 ± 3.5 years (range, 3 months to 22 years).
      (4). Case control epidemiologic studies performed at the University of Minnesota indicate a higher prevalence of calcium oxalate uroliths in Burmese, Himalayan, and Persian breeds.

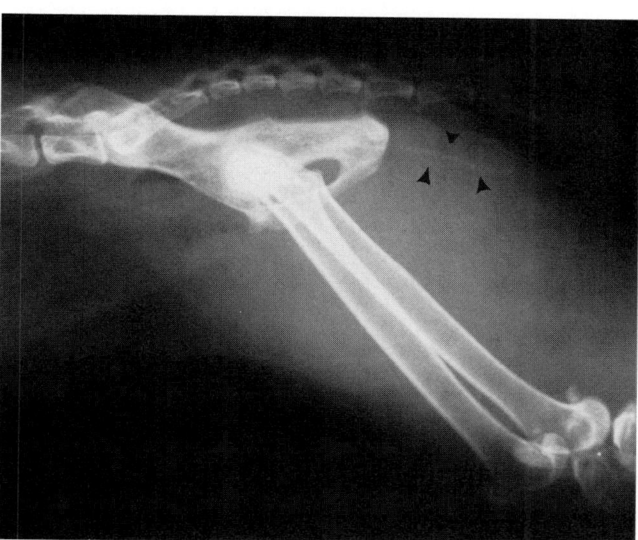

FIG. 35–26. Survey radiograph of the lateral aspect of the urethra of an 11-year-old neutered male Siamese cat with urethral obstruction. Note the radiodense structures in the site normally occupied by the penile urethra (arrows). Following return of the structures to the urinary bladder by urohydropulsion, numerous small uroliths composed of calcium oxalate were removed by cystotomy.

   b. In most cats with calcium oxalate uroliths, serum concentrations of minerals, including calcium, have been normal.
      (1). Mild hypercalcemia (11.1 to 13.5 mg/dL) has been observed with sufficient frequency to warrant routine evaluation of serum calcium concentration in affected patients.
      (2). Hypercalcemia promotes urinary calcium excretion and may result in precipitation of calcium oxalate crystals.
      (3). Although primary hyperparathyroidism has been recognized as a cause of hypercalcemia and calcium oxalate uroliths in cats, the underlying cause of hypercalcemia in most cats with calcium oxalate uroliths has not been detected.
      (4). The relationship between hypercalcemia, parathyroid hormone secretion, vitamin D homeostasis, and calcium oxalate urolith formation deserves further study.
   c. Cats with calcium oxalate urolithiasis typically have concentrated (mean pretreatment urine specific gravity of about 1.040) and acidic (urine pH of 6.3 to 6.7) urine. Pretreatment blood pH is often reduced (pH = 7.3).
      (1). The association between aciduria, acidemia, and calcium oxalate urolithiasis may be that acidemia promotes mobilization of carbonate and phosphorus from bones to buffer hydrogen ions.[2,15,23]
      (2). Concomitant mobilization of bone calcium may result in hypercalciuria.
   d. Although hyperoxaluria and nephrocalcinosis have been observed in kittens that consumed diets deficient in vitamin B_6, a naturally occurring form of this syndrome has not been observed.[2]
      (1). Urinary oxalic acid excretion in kittens that consumed diets oversupplemented with vitamin B_6 was similar to urinary oxalic acid excretion by kittens that consumed diets with adequate vitamin B_6.[2]
      (2). Hyperoxaluria has been encountered in related cats with deficient quantities of hepatic D-glycerate dehydrogenase, an enzyme required for metabolism of oxalic acid precursors[65]; however, to date, the clinical manifestations of this metabolic disorder have been related primarily to weakness and acute onset of renal failure in young cats.
   e. Magnesium has been reported to be a calcium oxalate inhibitor in rats and humans.[74] For this reason, orally administered magnesium sometimes is recommended to prevent recurrence of calcium oxalate uroliths.
      (1). Use of urine acidifiers and/or supplemen-

tal sodium (usually sodium chloride) has been associated with hypercalciuria in some species.

(2). Because therapy for feline struvite uroliths often encompasses restriction of magnesium, sodium chloride–induced diuresis, and acidification of urine, the relationship of these factors to feline calcium oxalate uroliths deserves further study.

2. Treatment and prevention.
 a. Overview.
  (1). Medical protocols that promote dissolution of calcium oxalate uroliths in cats are not yet available.
   (a). Urocystoliths small enough to pass through the urethra may be removed by voiding urohydropropulsion.[56]
   (b). Very small urocystoliths may be retrieved with the aid of a urinary catheter.[57,81]
   (c). Surgery is the only practical alternative for removal of larger active calcium oxalate uroliths; however, some calcium oxalate uroliths, especially those in the kidneys, may remain clinically silent for months to years. Because of the unavoidable destruction of nephrons during nephrotomy, this procedure is not recommended unless it can be established that the stones are a cause of clinically significant disease. Serial urinalysis, renal function tests, serum electrolyte evaluations, and/or radiographic studies may be indicated to evaluate the clinical activity of calcium oxalate uroliths.
  (2). Following urolith removal, medical protocols should be considered to minimize urolith recurrence or to prevent further growth of the uroliths that remain in the urinary tract.
   (a). In general, medical therapy should be formulated in a stepwise fashion, with the initial goal of reducing urine concentration of calculogenic substances. Medications that have the potential to induce a sustained alteration in body composition of metabolites, in addition to urine concentration of metabolites, should be reserved for patients with active or frequently recurrent calcium oxalate uroliths. Caution must be used so that side effects of treatment are not more detrimental than the effects of uroliths.
   (b). In cats with hypercalcemia, the cause of hypercalcemia (e.g., primary hyperparathyroidism) should be corrected. Whether calcium oxalate uroliths remaining in the patient following appropriate therapy subsequently dissolve is not known; however, growth or recurrence of calcium oxalate uroliths is less likely.
   (c). In patients with a normal serum calcium concentration, an attempt should be made to identify risk factors for urolith formation. Amelioration or control of the consequences of risk factors should minimize urolith growth and recurrence.
 b. Dietary considerations.
  (1). Although reduction of urine calcium and oxalic acid concentrations by reduction of dietary calcium and oxalic acid appears to be a logical therapeutic goal, it is not necessarily a harmless maneuver.
   (a). Reducing consumption of only one of these constituents (e.g., calcium) may increase the availability of the other (e.g., oxalic acid) for intestinal absorption and subsequent urinary excretion.
   (b). In general, reduction of dietary calcium should be accompanied by an appropriate reduction of dietary oxalic acid.
  (2). Humans with calcium oxalate uroliths are often advised to avoid milk and milk products because the carbohydrate component (lactose) of these products may augment intestinal absorption of calcium from any dietary source.[55] Likewise, they are often discouraged from consuming foods containing relatively large quantities of oxalic acid (chocolate, nuts, beans, sweet potatoes, wheat germ, spinach, and rhubarb).
  (3). Consumption of much sodium may augment renal excretion of calcium.
   (a). Twenty-four–hour urinary calcium excretion of normal dogs consuming diets with 0.8% sodium (dry weight analysis) was comparable to calcium excretion in dogs with naturally occurring calcium oxalate uroliths.[55]
   (b). If similar results occur in cats, moderate dietary restriction of sodium would be a logical recommendation for cats that form active calcium oxalate uroliths.
  (4). Dietary phosphorus should not be restricted for patients with calcium oxalate urolithiasis because reduction in dietary phosphorus may be associated with activation of vitamin D, which in turn promotes intestinal calcium absorption and

subsequent urinary calcium excretion. In addition, pyrophosphate is an inhibitor of calcium oxalate urolith formation.

(a). If calcium oxalate urolithiasis is associated with hypophosphatemia and normal serum calcium concentration, oral phosphorus supplementation may be considered (Neutra-Phos, Willen Drug Company, Baltimore, Maryland.)

(b). Caution must be used, however, because excessive dietary phosphorus may predispose to formation of calcium phosphate uroliths.

(5). Increased urine magnesium concentration reduces formation of calcium oxalate crystals *in vitro*. For this reason, supplemental magnesium has been used to minimize recurrence of calcium oxalate uroliths in humans.

(a). However, supplemental dietary magnesium may contribute to formation of magnesium ammonium phosphate uroliths and to hypercalciuria.

(b). Pending further studies, we do *not* recommend dietary magnesium restriction or supplementation for treatment of calcium oxalate uroliths in cats.

(6). Ingestion of foods that contain large quantities of animal protein may contribute to calcium oxalate urolithiasis by increasing urinary calcium and oxalic acid excretion, and by decreasing urinary citric acid excretion. Some of these consequences result from obligatory acid excretion associated with protein metabolism.

(7). A diet with reduced quantities of protein, calcium, and sodium and one that does not promote formation of acidic urine (e.g., Prescription Diet Feline k/d, Hill's, Topeka, Kansas) should be considered to help to minimize recurrence of active calcium oxalate uroliths in cats. We have had success in reducing mild hypercalcemia in some cats that form calcium oxalate uroliths by feeding them a high-fiber reducing diet (Prescription Diet Feline w/d, Hill's, Topeka, Kansas).

(a). Ideally, diets should not be restricted or supplemented with phosphorus or magnesium.

(b). Excessive levels of vitamin D (which promote intestinal absorption of calcium) and ascorbic acid (a precursor of oxalate) should also be avoided.

(c). The diet should be adequately fortified with vitamin B_6, because vitamin B_6 deficiency promotes endogenous production, and subsequent urinary excretion, of oxalic acid.

(d). Moist foods may prove more beneficial than dry foods if they are associated with compensatory diuresis.

c. Citrate.

(1). Citric acid inhibits calcium oxalate crystal formation because of its ability to form soluble salts with calcium. This may explain why some humans with abnormally small quantities of urine citric acid are at risk for development of calcium oxalate uroliths.[55]

(2). Oral administration of potassium citrate (approximately 90 mg/kg/d) to human patients has been associated with marked increases in urinary citric acid excretion.[83]

(3). Potassium citrate also may be beneficial in the management of calcium oxalate because of its alkalinizing effects. In dogs, chronic metabolic acidosis inhibits renal tubular reabsorption of calcium, whereas metabolic alkalosis enhances tubular reabsorption of calcium.[83]

(4). Potassium citrate (Urocit-K, Mission Pharmaceuticals, San Antonio, Texas) is preferred to sodium bicarbonate, an alkalinizing agent, because oral administration of sodium may enhance urinary calcium excretion. We currently recommend a total of 80 to 120 mg/kg/d (divided into 2 or 3 doses.

d. Vitamin B_6.

(1). Vitamin B_6 increases the transamination of glyoxylate, an important precursor of oxalic acid, to glycine.

(2). Although experimentally induced vitamin B_6 deficiency resulted in renal precipitation of calcium oxalate and hyperoxaluria in kittens, a naturally occurring form of this syndrome has not been observed.

(3). Although additional vitamin B_6 was associated with decreased oxalic acid excretion in cats that consumed a diet deficient in vitamin B_6, the ability of supplemental vitamin B_6 to reduce urinary oxalic acid excretion in cats with calcium oxalate uroliths that were fed a diet with an adequate quantity of vitamin B_6 is unknown.

(4). In our hospital, administration of vitamin B_6 (10 mg/kg/d) to a normal cat for 10 days was not associated with decreased urine oxalic acid concentration (1.13 ± 0.11 mmol/L before vitamin B_6 supplementation as compared with 1.39 ± 0.19 mmol/L during vitamin B_6 administration).[60]

e. Thiazide diuretics.
 (1). Thiazide diuretics have been recommended to reduce recurrence of calcium-containing uroliths in humans because of their ability to reduce urine calcium excretion. The exact mechanism(s) by which thiazide diuretics reduce urinary calcium excretion are unknown; however, several factors appear to be involved.[55]
  (a). For instance, studies in rats reveal that thiazide diuretics directly stimulated distal renal tubular resorption of calcium.
  (b). Although results of studies in humans suggest that thiazide diuretics potentiate the action of parathyroid hormone, effects of thiazide diuretics on urinary excretion were not altered in parathyroidectomized rats or dogs.[55]
  (c). Because the hypocalciuric response to thiazide diuretics was blocked when volume depletion was prevented by sodium chloride administration in humans, thiazide diuretics were hypothesized to promote mild extracellular volume contraction and, thus, proximal tubular reabsorption of several solutes, including sodium and calcium.[55]
 (2). Although hydrochlorothiazide diuretics may be beneficial in minimizing urinary calcium excretion in humans and dogs, no data have been provided to indicate their efficacy in cats with calcium oxalate uroliths. Because thiazide diuretics can be associated with adverse effects (dehydration, hypokalemia, hypercalcemia), we cannot yet recommend their routine use, pending further evaluation.

f. Other agents.
 (1). A variety of other agents has been suggested for management of calcium oxalate uroliths in humans. They include allopurinol, to minimize heterogenous nucleation of calcium oxalate on uric acid crystals; sodium cellulose phosphate, to bind intestinal calcium; and orthophosphates, to minimize calcium excretion.
 (2). We have not used these agents in cats. Consult references for further details about applications to veterinary medicine.[28,74]

G. Calcium phosphate uroliths.

1. Etiopathogenesis.
 a. In our current series, calcium phosphate accounted for approximately 1% of the naturally occurring feline uroliths (Table 35–6).
  (1). They were located in the kidneys (17), ureters (3), urinary bladder (27), urethra and bladder (3), and urethra (1). Two calcium phosphate uroliths were voided (the location of six uroliths was not recorded).
  (2). Calcium phosphate uroliths occurred more commonly in females (31) than in males (23).
  (3). The mean age of affected cats was 8 ± 5 years (range, 5 months to 19 years).
 b. We have documented nephroliths composed of blood clots mineralized with calcium phosphate.
  (1). Contrary to one theory, they are not composed of bile metabolites.
  (2). Such mineralized blood clots may be found in renal pelvic diverticula in addition to the renal pelvis.
   (a). Formation of highly concentrated urine in patients with gross hematuria may favor formation of blood clots.
   (b). In a persistently hematuric patient, such nephroliths remained inactive (i.e., did not increase in quantity or size or cause outflow obstruction or predispose to bacterial UTI) over a 3-year period of evaluation.
 c. Calcium phosphate uroliths may occur in association with primary hyperparathyroidism in humans and dogs,[37] and this association has also been made in cats. One 3-year-old male castrated domestic shorthair cat with multiple calcium hydrogen phosphate (brushite) urocystoliths and urethroliths consumed large quantities of spinach, according to the owner. Spinach contains large quantities of oxalate salts.
2. Treatment and prevention.
 a. Protocols designed to dissolve or prevent calcium phosphate uroliths in cats have not been studied.
 b. Urocystoliths small enough to pass through the urethra may be removed with the aid of a urinary catheter, or by voiding urohydropropulsion.[56,57,81]
 c. Surgery remains the most reliable way to remove larger active uroliths from the urinary tract. We emphasize that surgery may be unnecessary for clinically inactive calcium phosphate uroliths.
 d. Studies in other species suggest that avoiding excessive dietary protein and sodium may minimize hypercalciuria.

H. Cystine uroliths.

1. Cystine urocystoliths occur with equal frequency in male and female cats (Table 35–6).
2. The mean age at diagnosis of cats with cystine uroliths in our series was 4.1 years (range, 10 months to 11 years).
3. All affected cats, with the exception of a Korat, were of the domestic shorthair breed.
4. Evaluation of urine amino acid profiles of three

affected cats revealed increased concentrations of arginine, lysine, and ornithine in addition to cystine. A similar pattern of amino aciduria was reported in a 10-month-old male Siamese cat with cystine urocystoliths.[18]

I. Struvite uroliths.

1. Etiopathogenesis.
   a. Overview. Results of our clinical and experimental studies indicate that three distinct etiologic mechanisms may be responsible for development of clinically significant urinary tract precipitates containing large quantities of struvite.[22,76]
      (1). Formation of sterile struvite uroliths (perhaps in association with dietary risk factors) is one type.
      (2). Formation of "infected" or "urease" struvite uroliths as a sequela to UTI with urease-producing bacteria is a second type. A combination of a sterile struvite nidus that predisposes to UTI plus urease-producing microbes may result in formation of an outer layer of infection-induced struvite.
      (3). Formation of urethral plugs containing a large quantity of matrix, in addition to varying quantities of struvite, is a third form.
   b. Experimental studies of sterile struvite uroliths.
      (1). Results of experimental studies of cats indicate that sterile struvite uroliths may be initiated by altering the composition of the diet.
         (a). Several groups of investigators have reported convincing data concerning experimental production of magnesium phosphate and magnesium ammonium phosphate uroliths in previously normal cats that consumed calculogenic diets containing 0.15 to 1.0% dry weight magnesium.[9,26,72,76] However, we emphasize that the percentage of magnesium in experimental diets (and in commercial diets) may be a misleading indication of dietary magnesium intake because of differences in calorie density, palatability, and digestibility.[26,45]
         (b). Calcium, phosphorus, and other dietary minerals may also influence the calculogenic potential of various diets containing magnesium.
         (c). Although consumption, absorption, and urinary excretion of comparatively large quantities of magnesium have been often implicated as important features of calculogenic diets, recent studies indicate that other factors may also play a role.[26]
      (2). Uroliths experimentally produced in cats by one group of investigators[91] were similar in gross appearance and mineral composition to naturally occurring sterile struvite uroliths commonly encountered in male and female cats.[72]
         (a). However, in all experimental studies of feline struvite calculogenesis reported to date, none have resulted in production of urethral plugs containing substantial quantities of matrix in addition to struvite crystals.
         (b). When urethral obstruction has occurred, aggregates of crystalline material with little, if any, matrix have been observed.
         (c). These observations suggest that the aforementioned dietary models of struvite urolithiasis are not analagous to the naturally occurring form of feline urethral obstruction associated with matrix struvite plugs (see Table 35–12).
      (3). Uroliths produced during early experimental studies were composed of magnesium phosphate,[2] whereas those produced in subsequent studies were found to contain magnesium, ammonium, and phosphate.[9,26] Results of further studies indicate that the precise mineral composition of uroliths induced by excess dietary magnesium may be influenced by urine pH.[9,10,25]
         (a). Administration of a sufficient quantity of magnesium oxide alkalinizes urine produced by cats. Uroliths formed in this situation often contain magnesium hydrogen phosphate trihydrate (newberyite).[72] They are nearly devoid of ammonium ion.
         (b). However, if the composition of the diet is modified so that urine of neutral or slightly acidic pH is produced, uroliths composed of magnesium ammonium phosphate may be induced.[25,26]
         (c). Subsequent studies further emphasized the importance of urine pH on the calculogenic potential of magnesium-supplemented diets. Consumption of diets supplemented with magnesium oxide may produce struvite uroliths in cats; however, consumption of diets with a similar quantity of magnesium in the form of magnesium chloride (a urine-acidifying agent) did not result in struvite urolith formation because urine acidification was sufficient to prevent oversaturation of urine with struvite.[9]
         (d). Addition of a sufficient quantity of

acidifier (ammonium chloride) to diets supplemented with potentially calculogenic quantities of magnesium oxide inhibited struvite urolith formation.[91]

(4). The association of alkaline urine with formation of sterile struvite uroliths needs further study.

(a). Magnesium hydrogen phosphate (newberyite) was produced in cats consuming canned food supplemented with as much as 1% magnesium in the form of magnesium oxide.[72,76] Presumably, reduction of the need of the renal tubules to produce ammonia buffer because of formation of alkaline urine reduced the quantity of ammonium available to combine with magnesium and phosphate.

(b). In a clinical study of 20 cats with naturally occurring struvite urocystoliths and no detectable UTI, the mean urine pH at the time of diagnosis was 6.9 ± 0.4. The urine of affected cats was not persistently alkaline. This point is clinically significant when attempting to modify urine pH to dissolve or prevent sterile struvite uroliths.

(c). Based on available data, one should strive to achieve a pH value of approximately 6.0 to 6.3, in an attempt to dissolve or prevent struvite uroliths.

(5). The relationship of water content of the diet and formation of uroliths in cats has also been studied by several investigators.

(a). Factors involved include dietary moisture, drinking behavior, digestibility of food and its relationship to fecal water loss, and the quantity of sodium chloride in the diet.

(b). Because of numerous variables, a cause-and-effect relationship between dietary moisture, urine volume, and urolithiasis has not been clearly established.

(c). Pending further studies, consideration of highly digestible, high-moisture diets is recommended to minimize recurrence of uroliths.

(6). In conclusion, data derived from cats with induced sterile struvite uroliths indicate that several dietary factors play a role in the etiopathogenesis of naturally occurring sterile struvite uroliths. Of these, factors affecting urine magnesium concentration and urine pH have major therapeutic importance.

c. Naturally occurring sterile struvite uroliths.

(1). As described in the preceding section on experimental study of sterile struvite uroliths, the mineral composition and physical characteristics of some experimentally induced and naturally occurring sterile struvite uroliths are almost identical (see Tables 35–6 and 35–10).

(a). At this time, less than 50% of the naturally occurring uroliths removed from cats contain primarily struvite (Table 35–6).

(b). Although the exact percentage of sterile versus infection-induced struvite uroliths in our series could not be precisely determined, we estimate that at least 90 to 95% were composed of sterile struvite.

(c). Sterile struvite uroliths contain less matrix than do infection-induced struvite uroliths and have other characteristic features (see Table 35–10).

(d). Bacteria cannot be detected in the matrix of sterile struvite uroliths by culture, light microscopy, or electron microscopy, as they can in infection-induced struvite uroliths.

(2). Of the 2867 struvite uroliths, 1510 occurred in females and 1225 were encountered in males.

(a). Neutered males (1016) and neutered females (1290) were affected more commonly than were intact males (209) and intact females (220) (for 132 affected cats, gender was not recorded). In a study performed at the University of California, males younger than 2 years predominated 2/1 over females, whereas females older than 2 years predominated 3/1 over males.[52]

(b). A case-control comparison performed at the University of Minnesota revealed no breed prevalence for struvite urolithiasis.

(c). The mean age of affected cats was 7.2 ± 3.5 years (range, 3 months to 22 years).

(d). The urinary bladder was the most common site of struvite uroliths (2201); the urethra (238), bladder and urethra (136), voided urine (131), kidney (4), ureters (3), kidney and ureters (1), ureters and bladder (1), and kidney, ureters, and bladder (1) were less common sites (the site of 151 struvite uroliths was not recorded) (see Figs. 35–2 and 35–15).

(3). Additional case-control epidemiologic studies of cats known to have naturally occurring sterile struvite uroliths are needed. Based on currently available information, several associations can be predicted.

(a). For example, a decrease in urine volume and increase in urine specific gravity secondary to decreased water consumption would be a logical risk factor for urolith formation.

(b). Likewise, excessive consumption of food (perhaps associated with *ad libitum* feeding) would be expected to result in obesity and excretion of excess minerals (some of which could be calculogenic) in urine. Cats have been reported to maintain magnesium homeostasis by excreting excessive dietary magnesium in their urine.[26] Rather than link obesity as a risk factor for FUS, both obesity and urolithiasis may be linked logically to excessive food consumption.

(c). Finally, the infrequency with which immature cats develop sterile struvite uroliths may be associated with their tendency to form more acidic urine than that of adults. The capacity to form significantly alkaline urine does not develop until cats are approximately 1 year of age[86]; however, this factor does not protect immature cats from infection-induced struvite uroliths. In our experience, most uroliths encountered in immature male and female cats have been infection-induced struvite secondary to abnormalities in local host defense mechanisms.

d. Naturally occurring infection-induced struvite uroliths.

(1). Infection of the feline urinary tract with urease-producing microbes (especially staphylococci) may result in rapid production of magnesium ammonium phosphate uroliths in a fashion identical to that in dogs (Figs. 35–2 and 35–11).[72] Rather than being linked to urinary excretion of excessive quantities of dietary minerals, the etiopathogenesis of infection-induced struvite is linked to microbial urease that hydrolyzes urea. The result is alkalinization of urine associated with large quantities of ammonia and phosphate ion. The difference in etiopathogenesis of infection-induced and sterile struvite uroliths is of great therapeutic significance.

(2). Because cats are innately resistant to bacterial UTI, infection-induced struvite uroliths are encountered far less commonly than are sterile struvite uroliths. However, when encountered, they usually affect cats in which local host defenses have been altered by persistent diseases (e.g., congenital anomalies, neoplasia, perineal urethrostomy, or indwelling urinary catheters).[69,72,76]

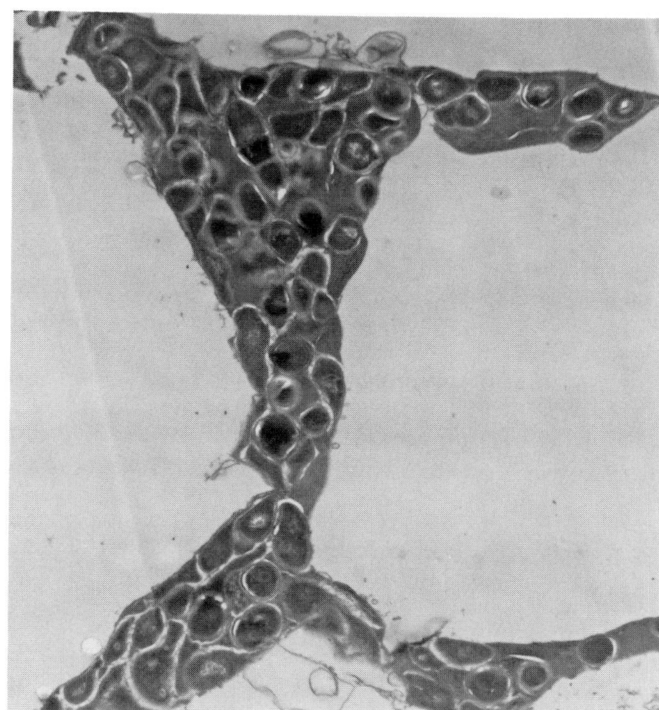

FIG. 35–27. Transmission electron micrograph of a section of an infection-induced struvite urolith removed from the urinary bladder of a 1-year-old neutered Manx cat. Note the spaces previously occupied by struvite crystals surrounded by matrix containing staphylococci. (Original magnification, 6,300×.)

(3). Infection-induced struvite often contains more matrix than does sterile struvite, presumably as a result of increased production of inflammatory reactants (Table 35–10).[72] They also tend to grow more rapidly and frequently are larger. Urease-producing microbes can readily be cultured from their inner portions and can be detected by light and electron microscopy (Fig. 35–27).

2. Treatment.

a. Sterile struvite uroliths.

(1). Experimental and clinical studies of feline sterile struvite uroliths have confirmed the feasibility of inducing their dissolution by medical therapy (see Figs. 35–15 through 35–19).

(2). Probable risk factors for formation of sterile struvite uroliths include mineral composition, energy content, moisture content, and urine-alkalinizing metabolites in the diet, quantity of food consumed, *ad libitum* versus controlled feeding schedule, formation of concentrated urine, and retention of urine.

(3). Key components in inducing dissolution of most struvite uroliths in cats appear to be:
   (a). Reduction of urine pH to approximately 6.0 to 6.3.
   (b). Reduction of urine magnesium by feeding a magnesium-restricted diet (Table 35–15).

(4). In a clinical study of 22 (11 male and 11 female) cats, uroliths presumed to be composed of sterile struvite dissolved in 20 cats in a mean period of 36.2 ± 26.6 days (range, 14 to 141 days) (see Figs. 35–15 to 35–19).[78] The cats were fed a high-moisture (canned), high-energy (640 kilocalories metabolizable energy per 15 ounces), caculolytic diet (Prescription Diet Feline s/d, Hill's, Topeka, Kansas) containing 41/4% dry weight protein.
   (a). The diet was formulated to contain reduced quantities of magnesium (0.058% dry weight) and to promote formation of acidic urine (pH ± 6.0).
   (b). The diet was also supplemented with sodium chloride (0.79% of dry weight sodium), to stimulate thirst and promote diuresis.
   (c). Because the feline struvitolytic diet is supplemented with sodium chloride, and because it is formulated to produce aciduria, neither sodium chloride nor urine acidifiers should be given with it.
   (d). It should not be given to immature cats because they may develop metabolic acidosis, anorexia, and dehydration.
   (e). Likewise, this diet should not be given to cats that are acidemic (e.g., owing to postrenal azotemia, primary renal dysfunction) or to cats with positive fluid balance (e.g., secondary to cardiac dysfunction, hypertension).
   (f). Consumption of the struvitolytic diet by cats with struvite uroliths of the lower urinary tract is typically associated with remission of dysuria and pollakiuria within 2 to 3 weeks.[78] Reduction in the magnitude of hematuria and pyuria coincides with remission of clinical signs. Reduction in urine pH and reduction or elimination of struvite crystalluria also occurs. At the time abdominal radi-

TABLE 35–15
SUMMARY OF RECOMMENDATIONS FOR MEDICAL DISSOLUTION OF FELINE STRUVITE UROLITHS

Perform appropriate diagnostic studies, including complete urinalysis, quantitative urine culture, and diagnostic radiography. "Guesstimate" urolith composition by evaluation of appropriate clinical data.

Institute dietary management designed to reduce the urine concentration of magnesium and create a pH of approximately 6.0 to 6.3. No other food should be fed to patients consuming calculolytic diets. Monitor urine pH 4 to 8 hours after eating. Urine that is acidic at this time is likely to be acidic throughout the day.

Although attempts may be made to stimulate thirst-induced diuresis by addition of sodium chloride to the diet, this step is not essential. Thirst-induced diuresis may benefit patients with slowly dissolving uroliths.

Antimicrobial therapy

Sterile struvite: Attempt to eradicate or control secondary UTIs with antimicrobial agents. Although control of secondary UTI is not essential to induce sterile struvite urolith dissolution, it is warranted to prevent damage of tissues of the urinary tract by bacteria and their metabolites.

Infection-induced struvite: Initiate antimicrobial therapy to eradicate or control urease-positive UTIs. Maintain therapy as long as uroliths can be detected by radiography.

Periodically (2- to 4-week intervals) monitor the size of uroliths by survey radiography. Survey radiography is preferable to retrograde contrast radiography to monitor urolith dissolution because use of catheters during retrograde radiographic studies may result in iatrogenic UTI. Alternatively, intravenous urography may be considered.

Periodic evaluation of urine sediment for crystalluria may be considered. *In vivo* struvite crystals should not form if therapy has been effective in promoting formation of urine that is undersaturated with magnesium ammonium phosphate.

Continue calculolytic diet therapy for at least 1 month following radiographic disappearance of uroliths. The rationale is to provide therapy of adequate duration to dissolve small uroliths that cannot be detected by survey radiography.

If uroliths increase in size during dietary management or do not begin to shrink after approximately 4 to 8 weeks of appropriate medical management, alternative methods should be considered. Difficulty in inducing complete dissolution of uroliths by creating urine that is undersaturated with the suspected calculogenic crystalloid should prompt consideration that 1) the wrong mineral component was identified (see Table 35–14); 2) the nucleus of the urolith is of different mineral composition than other portions of the urolith; and 3) the owner of the patient is not complying with medical recommendations.

ography indicates urolith dissolution, urinalysis findings are typically normal.

(5). Empiric clinical studies performed at the University of Minnesota indicate that acidification of urine to a pH of approximately 6.0 to 6.3 and consumption of a low-magnesium diet are effective in preventing recurrence of naturally occurring sterile struvite urocystoliths in male and female cats. No attempt was made to determine whether acidification of urine and/or a low-magnesium diet were the major factor(s) responsible for the beneficial results. If diets designed to promote formation of acidic urine are used, additional urine acidifiers should not be routinely used. Excessive consumption of acidifiers may result in metabolic acidosis, which, if prolonged, can result in bone demineralization and increase blood ionized calcium concentration.[15,20,23,86]

(6). If nonacidifying diets are used, such acidifiers as methionine may be mixed with them. Alternatively, acidifiers in tablet form may be given at mealtime.

(a). The goal is to reduce postprandial alkalinization of urine. Therefore, the dosage of urine acidifiers should be monitored by evaluation of 4- to 6-hour postprandial urine pH values.

(b). Adequate acidification to prevent sterile struvite uroliths has been achieved with methionine (approximately 1000 mg/cat/d) or ammonium chloride (approximately 800 mg/cat/d).[24,45,54,76,88,91] We prefer methionine, because ammonium chloride occasionally causes gastrointestinal signs.

(c). Caution should be used to avoid toxic doses of methionine, because it has been reported to cause anorexia, ataxia, cyanosis, methemoglobinemia, and Heinz body anemia in cats.[61]

b. Infection-induced struvite uroliths.

(1). Probable risk factors for infection-induced struvite urolithiasis include infections with urease-producing microbial pathogens, abnormalities (including perineal urethrostomies) in local host defenses of the urinary tract that allow bacterial infections, and the quantity of urea (the substrate of urease) excreted in urine.

(2). Because of different etiopathogenic mechanisms involved in formation of sterile and infection-induced struvite uroliths, some important differences in dissolution protocols exist.

(a). In addition to dietary therapy, antimicrobials must be used as long as infection-induced struvite uroliths can be detected radiographically. The reason is that viable calculogenic microbes tend to persist in inner portions of the uroliths and may cause a relapse of infection (see Table 35–15; Fig. 35–27) (See Chapter 40, Bacterial Infections of the Canine and Feline Urinary Tract.) Control of urease-positive infection in cats with infection-induced struvite uroliths is especially important because the calculolytic diet (Prescription Diet Feline s/d, Hill's, Topeka, Kansas) is not protein restricted. Protein restriction has been avoided because cats normally have a relatively high protein requirement.

(b). We emphasize that the protein-restricted struvitolytic diet designed for use in dogs (Prescription Diet Canine s/d, Hill's, Topeka, Kansas) is contraindicated for cats.

(3). Differences in the causes and treatment of feline sterile uroliths and infection-induced struvite uroliths are associated with differences in their dissolution. In a prospective clinical trial performed at the University of Minnesota, the time required to dissolve staphylococcus-induced struvite uroliths in 3 cats was 79 days (range, 64 to 92 days).[78]

(4). Prevention of infection-induced struvite uroliths in cats should be based on the same principles described for dogs (see Chapter 41, Canine and Feline Urolithiases: Relationship of Etiopathogenesis to Treatment and Prevention). The key to preventing recurrence is eradication or control of infection.

J. Miscellaneous uroliths.

1. Compound uroliths (nucleus composed of one mineral type and shells of a different mineral type) accounted for approximately 2% of uroliths analyzed in our series (Table 35–6).

   a. Examples include 1) a nucleus of 100% calcium oxalate monohydrate surrounded by a shell of 80% magnesium ammonium phosphate and 20% calcium phosphate and 2) a nucleus composed of 95% magnesium ammonium phosphate and 5% calcium phosphate surrounded by a shell of 95% ammonium acid rate and 5% magnesium ammonium phosphate.

   b. Sulfadiazine comprised 30% of the shell of a compound urocystolith removed from a 7-year-old female domestic shorthair cat.

2. Because risk factors that predispose to precip-

itation (nucleation) of different minerals vary, the occurrence of compound uroliths poses a unique challenge, in terms of preventing recurrence.

a. In the absence of clinical evidence to the contrary, the logically recommended management protocols are designed principally to minimize recurrence of nucleation of minerals comprising the nucleus (rather than those in shells) of compound uroliths.
b. Followup studies designed to evaluate the efficacy of preventive protocols should include complete urinalysis, radiography, and, if available, evaluation of the urine concentration of calculogenic metabolites.

K. Urethral plugs.

1. Etiopathogenesis.
   a. Mineral composition.
      (1). Urethral plugs contain varying quantities of minerals in proportion to large quantities of matrix (see Table 35–12).
      (2). Various different minerals have been identified in urethral plugs of cats, suggesting that multiple factors are involved in their formation (see Table 35–7).
         (a). Risk factors associated with the formation of ammonium urate, calcium oxalate, calcium phosphate, and magnesium ammonium phosphate crystals found in urethral plugs are probably similar to those associated with mineral formation in classic uroliths.
         (b). The mineral composition of urethral plugs should be used to describe them, at least in part, because therapeutic regimens are often influenced by knowledge of their mineral composition.

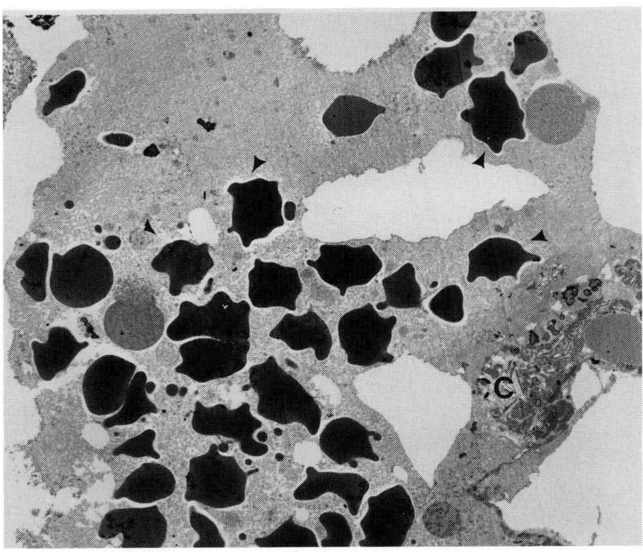

FIG. 35–29. Transmission electron micrograph of a section of matrix-crystalline urethral plug removed from a 3-year-old male neutered Himalayan cat. Note spaces previously occupied by struvite crystals surrounded by matrix containing red blood cells (arrows) and an unidentified cell (c). (Original magnification, 2,070×.)

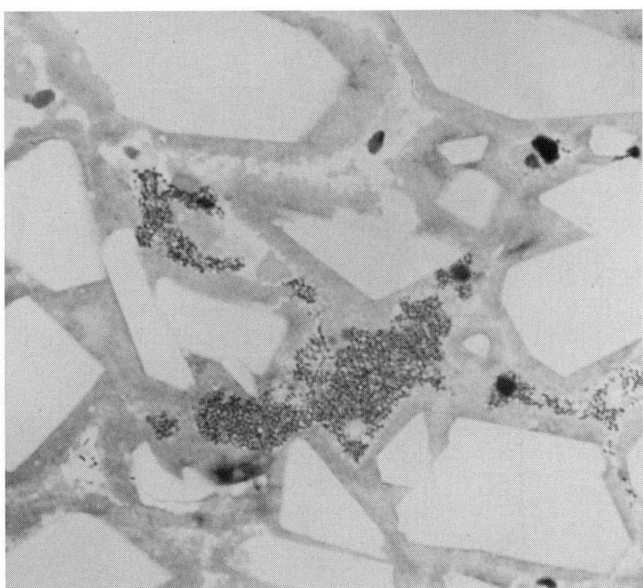

FIG. 35–28. Photomicrograph of a urethral plug removed from an adult male cat with obstructive urethropathy. Note spaces previously occupied by struvite crystals surrounded by matrix containing bacterial cocci. (Hematoxylin and eosin stain; original magnification, 450×.)

   b. Matrix composition.
      (1). Compared to uroliths, urethral plugs contain large quantities of matrix (Figs. 35–2, 35–28 through 35–34).
         (a). The question about specific composition of urethral plug matrix has not yet been answered.
         (b). The observation that the urine concentration of Tamm-Horsfall mucoprotein is increased in cats with LUTD prompts the hypothesis that a major component of plug matrix is this type of mucoprotein.[85] Tamm-Horsfall mucoprotein has been identified in human and ovine uroliths.[7,44] Preliminary results suggest that feline urethral plugs also contain Tamm-Horsfall mucoprotein. The ultrastructure of purified Tamm-Horsfall protein obtained from feline

urine resembles some matrix components identified by transmission electron microscopy in some matrix-crystalline urethral plugs. Tamm-Horsfall mucoprotein has been hy-

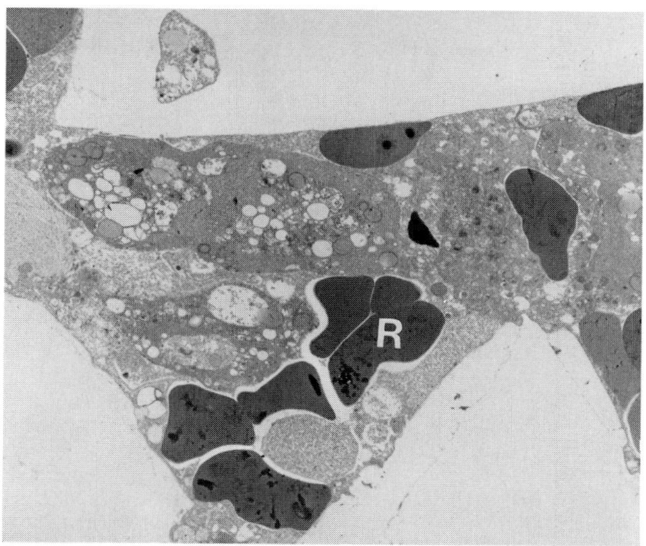

FIG. 35–30. Transmission electron micrograph of a urethral plug removed from an adult male cat with obstructive urethropathy. The clear spaces were previously occupied by struvite crystals. The matrix contains red blood cells (R), cellular debris, and other unidentified substances.

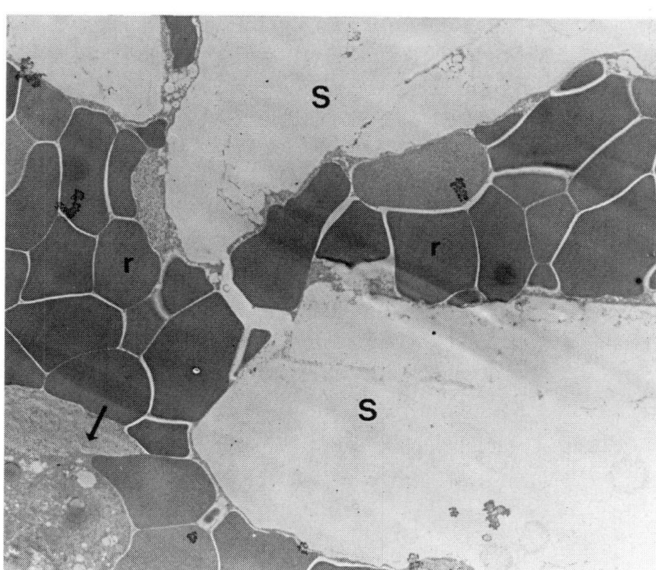

FIG. 35–31. Transmission electron micrograph of a urethral plug removed from a 4½-year-old neutered male Siamese cat. Note clear spaces previously occupied by struvite crystals (s), red blood cells (r), and unidentified disintegrated cell (arrow) surrounded by matrix. (Original magnification, 2,070×.)

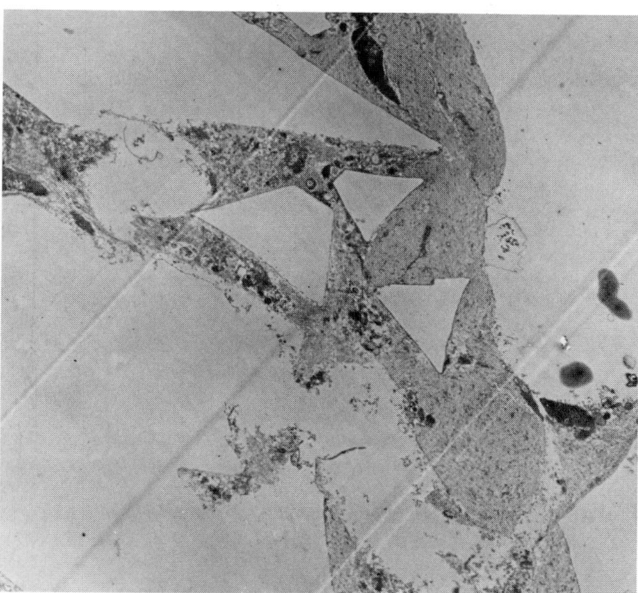

FIG. 35–32. Transmission electron micrograph of a section of matrix crystalline urethral plug removed from the urethra of a 1-year-old male neutered domestic shorthair cat. Note the clear spaces previously occupied by struvite crystals surrounded by amorphous matrix. (Original magnification, 3,300×.)

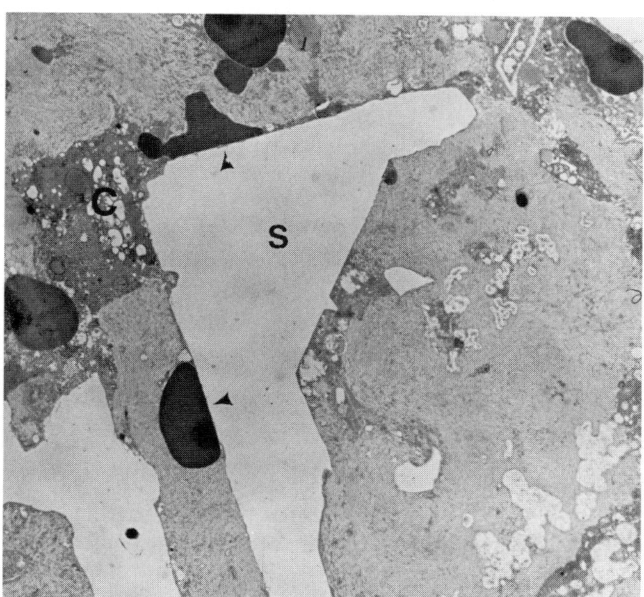

FIG. 35–33. Electron micrograph of a section of urethral plug removed from an 11-month-old male Siamese cat. Note the struvite crystal(s), red blood cells (arrows), unidentified cell (c), and cell fragments trapped in proteinaceous matrix. (Original magnification, 3,300×.) (From Osborne CA, et al. Feline matrix-crystalline urethral plugs: A unifying hypothesis of causes. *J Small Anim Pract.* 1992; 33:172–177.)

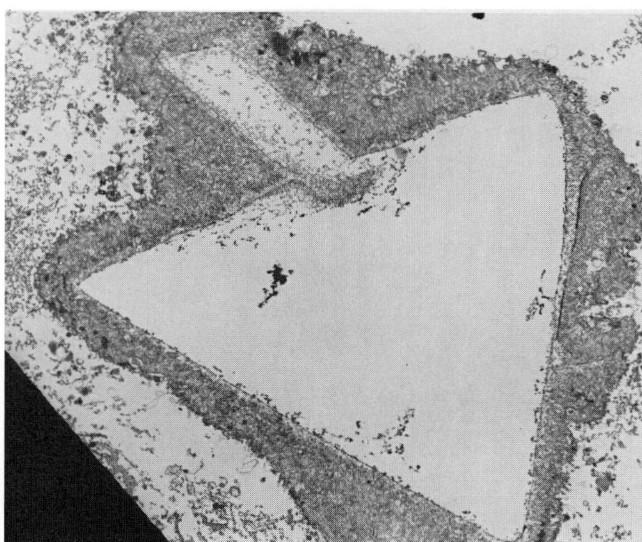

FIG. 35–34. Transmission electron micrograph of a section of urethral plug removed from a 3-year-old neutered male domestic shorthair cat. Note the triangular and rectangular struvite crystals surrounded by amorphous matrix. (Original magnification, 3,300×.)

pothesized to be a local host defense mechanism against viral and bacterial UTIs.[5]

(2). Light and transmission electron microscopic evaluation of naturally occurring feline urethral plugs have revealed that noncrystalline components of plugs also include red blood cells, white cells, epithelial cells, spermatozoa, virus-like particles, and bacteria surrounded by amorphous material (Figs. 35–21, 35–22, and 35–28 through 35–35).[76,80,82] These structures apparently have been trapped by the amorphous matrix.

(3). Some urethral plugs do not contain crystalline components (Figs. 35–36 through 35–38).

c. Relationship of minerals and matrix.

(1). As outlined earlier in this chapter, we hypothesize that formation of matrix by an infectious or inflammatory agent in a cat with concomitant crystalluria may lead to the formation of matrix-crystalline urethral plugs (Fig. 35–1).[80]

(2). We emphasize that obstructive urethropathy in male cats may also be caused by one or more intraluminal, mural, or extramural abnormalities located at one or more sites (see Table 35–13). Formation of matrix-crystalline plugs appears to be the most common, but not the only, cause of urethral obstruction (Fig. 35–12).

2. Treatment of urethral plugs.

a. Medical treatment.

(1). Whatever the cause of urethral obstruction, predictable clinical and biochemical abnormalities subsequently develop.

(a). They are characterized by systemic deficits and/or excesses in fluid (dehydration), electrolyte (e.g., hypercalcemia, hyperphosphatemia), and acid-base (metabolic acidosis) balance, and retention of metabolic

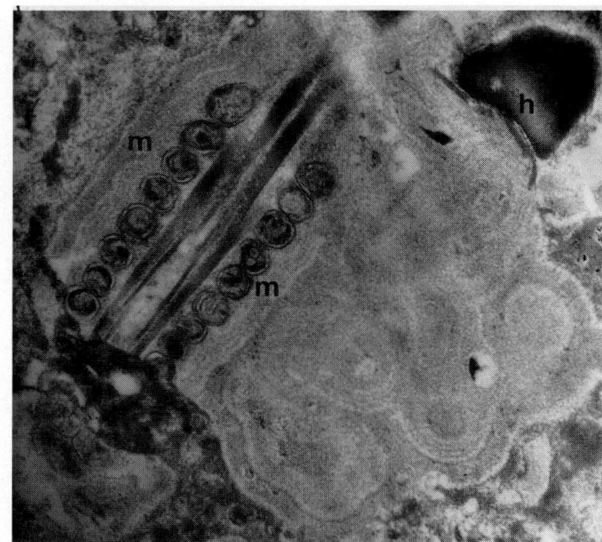

FIG. 35–35. Transmission electron micrograph of a section of matrix crystalline urethral plug removed from the urethra of the cat described in Figure 35–34. Note head (h) and midpiece (m) of a sperm trapped in matrix. (Original magnification, 20,000×.)

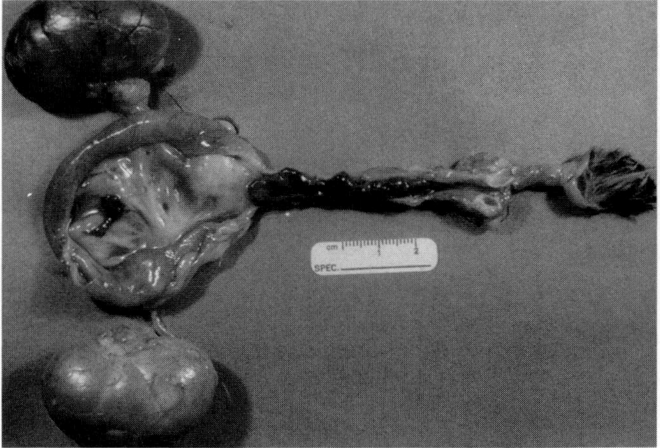

FIG. 35–36. Noncrystalline matrix plug in the preprostatic, prostatic, and postprostatic urethra of an adult male cat found dead by the owner. The plug consists of necrotic tissue, red blood cells, inflammatory cells, and fibrin-like material.

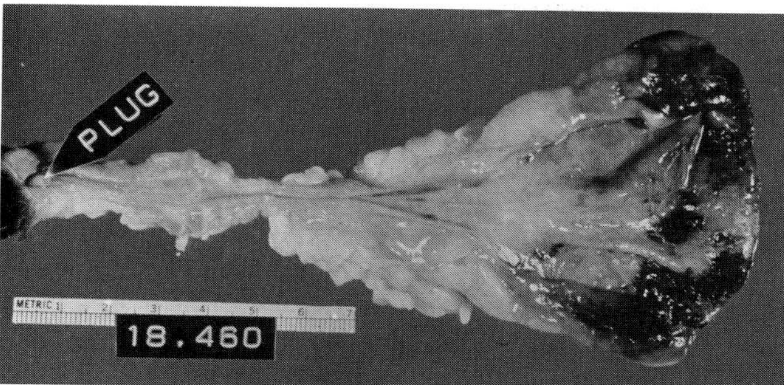

FIG. 35–37. Photograph of the lower urinary tract of a 3-year-old male domestic shorthair cat with a transitional cell carcinoma of the urinary bladder. A portion of sloughed neoplasm originating in the urinary bladder has occluded the penile urethra. (Courtesy of Dr. T.P. O'Leary.)

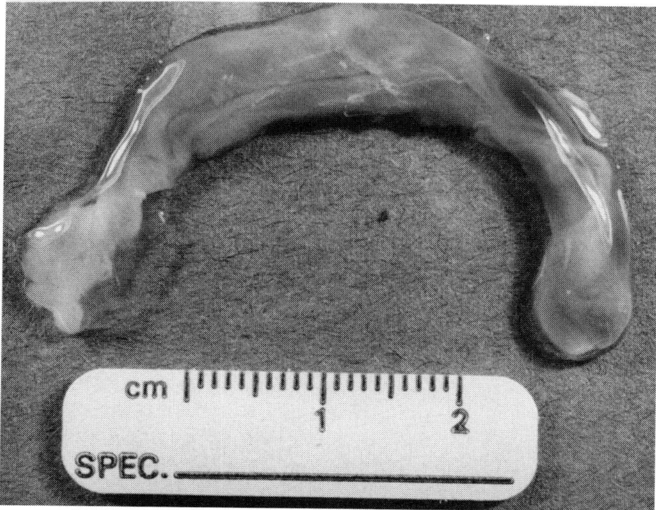

FIG. 35–38. Matrix plug voided through the urethra of a 1-year-old neutered Siamese cat. The plug did not contain crystals but was composed of inflammatory cells, necrotic tissue, fibrin, and bacteria.

wastes (creatinine, urea, other protein catabolites). The magnitude of these systemic abnormalities varies with the degree and duration of obstruction.

(b). Obstructive uropathy that persists longer than about 24 hours usually results in postrenal uremia. This occurs because increased back-pressure induced by obstruction to outflow impairs glomerular filtration, renal blood flow, and tubular function. In normal cats obstruction of the urethra results in death in 3 to 6 days. Damage to the mucosal surface of the urinary bladder may shorten survival time. Despite the potentially catastrophic outcome of urethral obstruction, the biochemical consequences of this disorder are potentially reversible, provided appropriate supportive and symptomatic parenteral therapy is given (See chapters in Part III). In severe cases, supportive therapy to correct hyperkalemia, metabolic acidosis, and volume depletion should be instituted immediately after decompression of the excretory pathway by cystocentesis. (See the following section, Re-establishment of Urethral Patency, for details.)

(2). The immediate need to remove urethral plugs within hours of their discovery precludes attempts to dissolve them over a period of days or weeks; however, urethral plugs can often be repulsed into the bladder lumen. Thus, the question arises, can such plugs be dissolved by medical therapy?

(a). As previously described, urethral plugs contain a substantially greater quantity of matrix than do classic uroliths. Although medical protocols effective in inducing sterile struvite urolith dissolution probably would also be effective in dissolving the struvite crystalline component of urethral plugs located in the bladder lumen, such therapy may not result in dissolution of plug matrix.

(b). Calcium oxalate and ammonium urate crystals have been identified in a few naturally occurring feline urethral plugs (Table 35–7). These factors may account for lack of expected response to therapy in some patients.

(3). No attempt should be made to dissolve struvite crystals with urine acidifiers or diets designed to promote acidic urine if a cat has postrenal azotemia. The metabolic sequelae of urethral obstruction, particularly severe metabolic acidosis, must be corrected before a diet designed to acidify urine is utilized.

b. Re-establishment of urethral patency.

(1). Obstructive urethropathy may be caused by one or more intraluminal, mural, or extramural abnormalities at one or more sites (Table 35–13; Figs. 35–3, 35–20, 35–21, 35–26, 35–39, 35–40).

(a). Thus, reverse flushing solutions may be effective in dissolving urethral plugs but might not have an effect on obstructive lesions in the urethral wall or periurethral tissue.

(b). Inability to restore the patency by flushing the urethral lumen with a solution should arouse suspicion of a mural or periurethral lesion in addition to, or instead of, a firmly lodged urethral plug or urethrolith.

(2). Physical restraint alone, or in combination with topical anesthesia, may be sufficient for obstructed patients that are particularly docile or severely depressed.

(a). Wrapping the cat in a bath towel may help to protect the patient and the assistant.

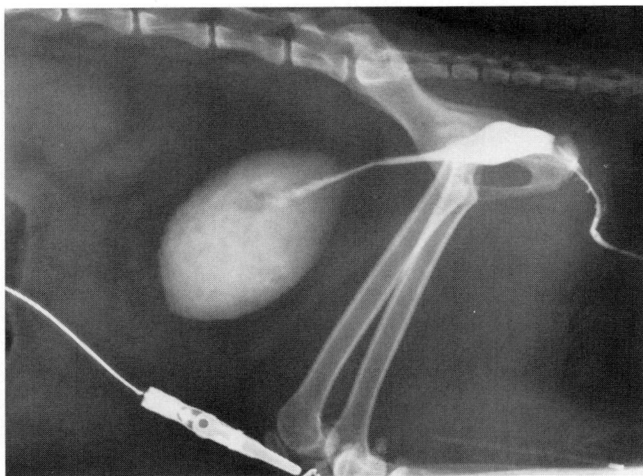

FIG. 35–39. Positive-contrast urethrocystogram of a 12-year-old neutered male Persian cat illustrates almost complete obstruction of the postprostatic urethra (arrow) by a transitional cell carcinoma.

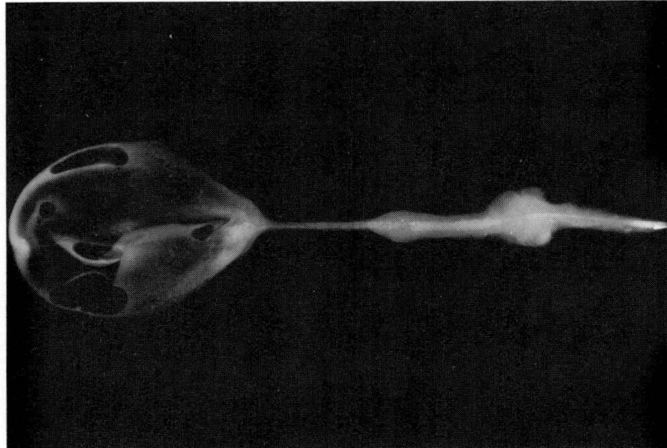

FIG. 35–40. Survey radiograph of the lower urinary tract of a neutered adult male cat at necropsy. Note the varied diameter and interrupted continuity of the matrix crystalline plug in the penile, postprostatic, and prostatic urethra. Radiodense crystalline material is apparent in the bladder lumen. The crystals in the urethral plug and urinary bladder were composed of struvite.

(b). If local anesthetics are used to anesthetize the urethral mucosa, they should be administered only in a quantity sufficient to accomplish this goal. We do not recommend use of local anesthetic agents as primary reverse flushing solutions, because they may induce systemic toxicity if absorbed in sufficient quantity. Absorption may be enhanced by damage to the urothelium, and their toxic potential may be enhanced by postrenal uremia.

(3). Because of an increased risk of adverse drug reactions associated with obstructive uropathy, pharmacologic restraint should be avoided when feasible. However, the risk of adverse drug reactions must be weighed against the possibility of iatrogenic trauma to the urethra of an uncooperative patient.

(a). If the disposition of the patient is such that attempts to dislodge the urethral obstruction are likely to be associated with additional damage to the urethra, or if the patient has a high risk of iatrogenic UTI, some form of pharmacologic restraint should be considered.

(b). Short-acting barbiturates that are metabolized by the liver (thiamylal), propofol, and/or inhalant anesthetics may be considered if general anesthesia is required. Anesthetics must be given cautiously, because dosages smaller than those recommended for patients with normal renal function are required for patients with postrenal azotemia.

(c). If ketamine hydrochloride is administered, similar caution must be used, because it is excreted in active form by the kidneys. Small doses (1 to 2 mg/kg given intravenously) have been used successfully by many clinicians; however, if difficulty is encountered in relieving outflow obstruction, administration of additional quantities of ketamine is inadvisable.

(4). We recommend a step-by-step approach when attempting to restore urethral patency to an obstructed male cat (Table 35–16).[71] In order of priority, these steps are 1) massage of the distal urethra, 2) attempts to induce voiding by gentle palpation of the urinary bladder, 3) cystocen-

TABLE 35–16
GENERAL GUIDELINES FOR REVERSE FLUSHING THE MALE FELINE URETHRA OBSTRUCTED WITH INTRALUMINAL MATERIAL (SEE FIGS. 35-44 TO 35-48)

1. Make every effort to protect the patient from iatrogenic complications associated with catheterization of the urethra (especially trauma and bacterial UTI).
2. Strive to use meticulous aseptic "feather-touch" technique.
3. Use only sterile catheters.
4. Cleanse the penis and prepuce with warm water prior to catheterization.
5. Select the shortest Minnesota olive-tipped feline urethral catheter* for initial catheterization of the urethra, and attach it to a flexible IV connection set and a syringe.
6. Coat the olive tip with sterile aqueous lubricant.
7. Prior to insertion of the catheter into the external urethral orifice, the extended penis should be displaced dorsally until the long axis of the urethra is approximately parallel to the vertebral column.
8. Carefully advance the catheter to the site of obstruction. If necessary, replace the short olive-tipped Minnesota needle with a longer one. Record the site of suspected obstruction, because this information may be of value when considering use of muscle relaxants and/or when considering urethral surgery to prevent recurrent obstruction. CAUTION: Do not mistake resistance induced by curvature of the feline male urethra for a site of obstruction. In addition, never use excessive force when advancing the catheter.
9. Next, a large quantity of physiologic saline or lactated Ringer's solution (as much as several hundred milliliters) should be flushed into the urethral lumen and allowed to reflux out the external urethral orifice. When possible, the catheter may be advanced toward the bladder. As a result of this maneuver, the obstructed urethral plugs may be gradually dislodged and flushed around the catheter and out of the urethral lumen. Application of steady but gentle digital pressure to the bladder wall after the urethra has been flushed with physiologic saline or lactated Ringer's solution may result in expulsion of a urethral plug or urolith from the urethral lumen. Excessive pressure should not be used because it may result in: 1) trauma to the bladder, 2) reflux of potentially infected urine into the ureters and renal pelvis, and/or 3) rupture of the bladder wall.
10. If the technique outlined in Step 9 is unsuccessful, it may be necessary to attempt repulsion of suspected urethral plugs or uroliths back into the bladder lumen by occluding the distal end of the urethra around the olive tip of the catheter before injecting fluid into the urethra. By preventing reflux of solutions out of the external urethral orifice, this maneuver tends to dilate the urethral lumen. If the obstruction persists, an attempt may be made to gently advance the suspected plug or urolith toward the bladder. *Excessive force should not be used.*
11. On occasion, it is advantageous to allow the reverse flushing solution to soften the obstructing urethral plugs (this technique is ineffective for most uroliths) before attempting to propel them back into the bladder. Allowing lapse of several hours between attempts to remove firmly lodged plugs by reverse flushing has been effective.

*Minnesota feline olive-tipped urethral catheters are available from EJAY International, Inc, P.O. Box 1835, Glendora, California 91740.

tesis, 4) retrograde urethral flushing, 5) combinations of steps 1 to 4, 6) diagnostic radiography to determine if the urethral obstruction is intraluminal, mural, or extramural, and 7) surgical procedures.

(a). Gentle massage of the penis between the thumb and fingers may help to dislodge plugs in the penile urethra (Figs. 35–41 and 35–42). If necessary, the penis may be manipulated while it is retracted within the prepuce. Plugs located in the preprostatic (abdominal) or membranous (pelvic) urethra may occasionally be dislodged by massaging the urethra per rectum. Although these methods are often ineffective, their simplicity and occasional success make them worth trying before considering cystocentesis or catheterization. In addition, they may disrupt material in urethral plugs confined to the penile urethra to such a degree that subsequent palpation of the urinary bladder may dislodge them.

(b). Inability of a cat to void urine spontaneously indicates that increasing intraurethral pressure by digitally compressing the urinary bladder is unlikely to be effective. However, if this technique is utilized *following* urethral massage, sufficient intraluminal pressure may be generated to dislodge fragments of urethral precipitates. Appropriate caution should be used to prevent iatrogenic damage to the urinary bladder. If UTI is likely, the consequence of inducing vesicoureteral reflux of urine during palpation should be considered, as microbes could be forced into the upper urinary tract.

(c). In general, *cystocentesis* should be performed if the aforementioned tech-

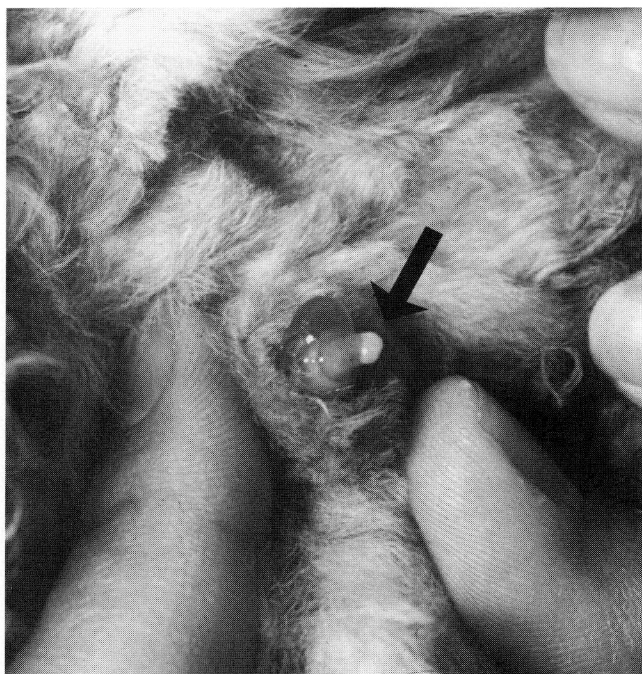

FIG. 35–41. Photograph of a 3-year-old male domestic shorthair cat with urethral obstruction. Note the matrix-crystalline plug at the external urethral orifice (arrow).

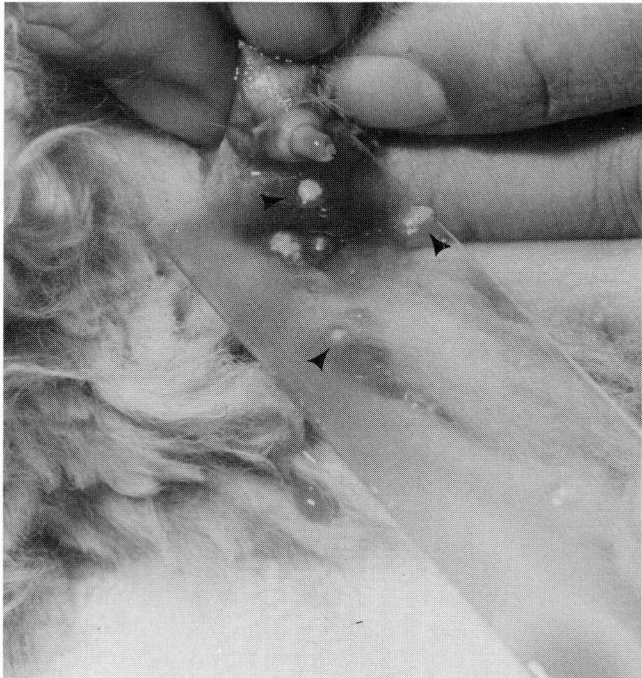

FIG. 35–42. Photograph of the cat described in Figure 35–41 after digital manipulation of the distal urethra and manual compression of the urinary bladder. Fragments of urethral plug are visible on the microscope slide (arrows).

niques are ineffective in reestablishing urethral patency (Fig. 35–43).[71]

(1′). The advantages of performing decompressive cystocentesis before flushing the urethral lumen via a catheter are:

(a′). A urine sample suitable for analysis and culture is obtained.

(b′). Decompression of an overdistended urinary bladder by removing most (but not all) of the urine provides a mechanism to temporarily halt the continued adverse effects of obstructive urethropathy, whatever the cause.

(c′). Decompression of an overdistended urinary bladder and proximal urethra may facilitate repulsion of a urethral plug or urolith into the bladder lumen.

(d′). The gross character of aspirated urine may provide valuable clues about the nature of the obstructive disorder (intraluminal precipitates of matrix and crystalline material versus ex-

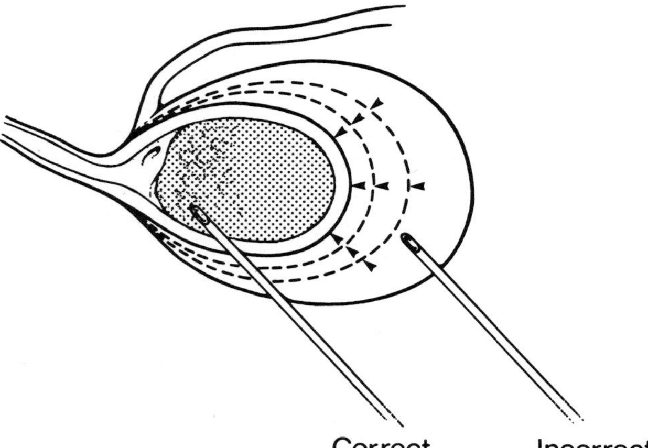

FIG. 35–43. Schematic drawing illustrates correct and incorrect sites of insertion of a needle into the bladder for the purpose of evacuating urine. The needle should be inserted in the ventral or ventrolateral surface of the wall a short distance craniad to the junction of the bladder with the urethra rather than at the vertex of the bladder. This position permits removal of urine and decompression of the bladder without need for reinsertion of the needle into the bladder lumen. (Medical illustrations by Michael P. Schenk, College of Veterinary Medicine, University of Minnesota.)

traluminal compression). Urine that contains large quantities of visible precipitates suggests a greater likelihood of reobstruction following subsequent flushing of the urethral lumen.

(2′). The potential disadvantages of performing decompressive cystocentesis are:

(a′). It may result in extravasation of urine into the bladder wall and/or peritoneal cavity.

(b′). It may injure the bladder wall or surrounding structures.

(c′). Although these complications could be severe in patients with a devitalized bladder wall, in our experience this has been the exception rather than the rule if most, but not all, of the urine is removed from the bladder. Loss of a small quantity of urine into the peritoneal cavity is usually of little consequence, especially if it does not contain pathogens. The potential of trauma to the bladder and adjacent structures can be avoided by proper technique.

(3′). We are not advocating an "always or never" recommendation regarding compressive cystocentesis. Clinical judgment is required in every case. However, decompression of the urinary bladder by cystocentesis (saving an aliquot for appropriate diagnostic tests) prior to use of reverse flushing procedures is preferable in patients:

(a′). That are likely to have adequate integrity of the bladder wall.

(b′). In which immediate overdistention of the bladder lumen is not allowed to recur.

(4′). We recommend that a 22-gauge needle be attached to a flexible intravenous extension set, which in turn is attached to a large-capacity syringe.

(a′). One individual should immobilize the urinary bladder and 22-gauge needle, while another aspirates urine from the bladder lumen.

(b′). Gentle agitation of the bladder with an up-and-down motion before cystocentesis may disperse particulate matter or crystals throughout the urine and thus facilitate its aspiration into the collection system.

(c′). The bladder should be emptied as completely as is consistent with atraumatic technique.

(d′). An attempt at complete evacuation of the bladder lumen is undesirable, because doing so allows the sharp point of the needle to damage the bladder wall. We recommend that 15 to 20 mL of urine be allowed to remain in the bladder.

(5′). In the event that patency of the urethra is not established before the bladder fills with urine again, decompressive cystocentesis should be repeated. On occasion, we have performed serial decompressive cystocentesis over a span of several days until urethral patency was reestablished.

(6′). The need for prophylactic antibacterial therapy following cystocentesis must be determined on the basis of the status of the patient and on retrospective evaluation of technique. If subsequent restoration of urethral patency requires intermittent or indwelling catheterization, preventive antimicrobial therapy should be considered.

(d). Flushing the urethral lumen with sterilized solutions following urethral catheterization may dislodge urethral plugs and uroliths. However, urethral obstruction may be caused by a combination of intraluminal precipitates (uroliths or urethral plugs), swelling of the urethral wall, and/or spasm of urethral musculature (see Tables 35–1 and 35–13).

(1′). Reverse flushing solutions should be selected cautiously because accumulation and absorption of large quantities of acid or anesthetic solutions from an inflamed urinary bladder may cause systemic toxicity. In addition, they may damage the coating of glycosaminoglycans that lines the surface of the urothelium. Glycosaminoglycans normally minimize adherence of crystals and microbes to the urethral mucosa.[35,66]

(a′). Adherence of crystals to the urothelium is most likely to occur if acidic solutions utilized to dissolve struvite crystals are used.

(b′). Pending results of further studies, we prefer physiologic saline or lactated Ringer's solution, because both are readily available, sterilized, nontoxic, nonirritating, and economical.

(2′). The general guidelines to be followed when reverse flushing feline urethras to re-establish patency are outlined in Table 35–16. Use of proper restraint, atraumatic urethral catheters (Figs. 35–44 through 35–48), and nonirritating flushing solutions greatly minimizes damage to the urethral mucosa and surrounding structures.

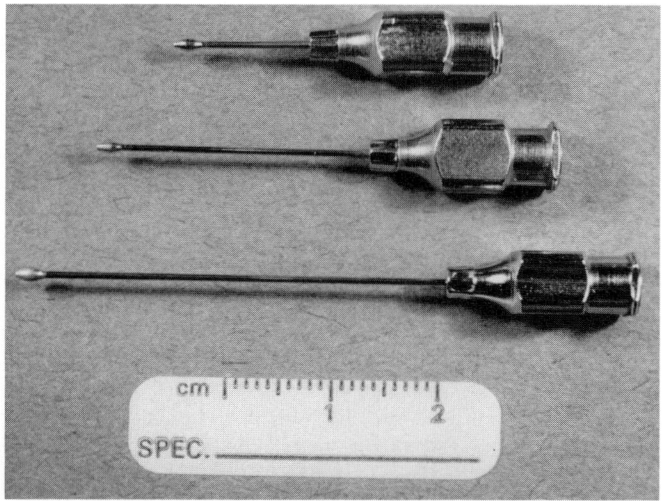

FIG. 35–44. Photograph of Minnesota olive-tipped urethral catheters. The catheters are 1/2, 1, and 1 1/2 inches long. (Available from EJAY International, P.O. Box 1385, Glendora, California 91740.)

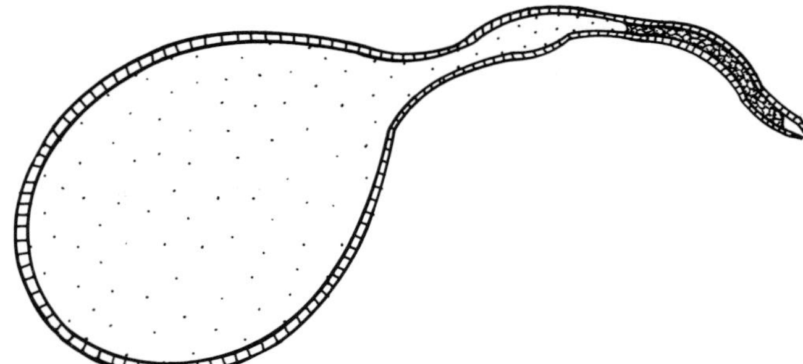

FIG. 35–45. Schematic illustration of a matrix-crystalline plug obstructing the urethral lumen of a male cat (see Figs. 35–46 to 35–48).

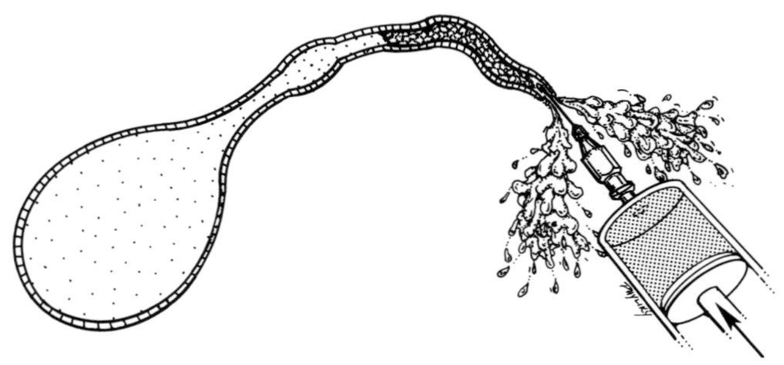

FIG. 35–46. Schematic illustration of flushing feline urethra obstructed with a urethral plug. After insertion of a Minnesota olive-tipped feline urethral catheter, a large quantity of saline is injected into the urethral lumen and allowed to reflux out of the distal urethra. Some 50 to 200 mL of saline may be required to flush away all the obstructing material (see Figs. 35–47 and 35–48).

(e). Inability to establish adequate urethral patency by use of catheters and reverse flushing should arouse a high index of suspicion that the underlying cause is not a urethral plug (see Table 35–13; Figs. 35–20, 35–21, 35–39).

(1′). Appropriate diagnostic procedures should be considered (see Table 35–2).[34]

(2′). Overdistention of the bladder lumen may be prevented by serial decompressive cystocentesis.

(3′). We do not recommend surgical intervention to correct obstructive urethropathy in uremic cats unless no reasonable alternative is available.

c. Immediate aftercare.

(1). After urine flow has been re-established by nonsurgical techniques, most of the urine should be removed from the bladder lumen. Removal of all the urine from the lumen is unnecessary and inadvisable because trauma associated with such efforts may aggravate the severity of bladder lesions.

(a). Manual compression may be used, provided it does not require substantial pressure to induce voiding. Manual compression of the bladder is not necessarily the procedure of choice if an overdistended bladder has been recently decompressed by cystocentesis, because extravasation of urine into the bladder wall or peritoneal cavity may result.

(b). Alternative methods include use of a catheter and syringe and cystocentesis.

(c). Each of these procedures has advantages or disadvantages that must be considered in light of the status of the urinary bladder and urethra of each patient.

(d). If the gross appearance of voided or aspirated urine suggests that reobstruction as a result of intraluminal debris is likely, removal of this material with saline or lactated Ringer's solution flushes of the bladder lumen may be of value in minimizing reobstruction. Particulate material located in the dependent portion of the bladder may be dispersed throughout the bladder lumen by digitally moving the bladder in an up-and-down fashion, which may in turn facilitate aspiration of crystals, inflammatory reactants, and blood clots into the catheter and syringe.

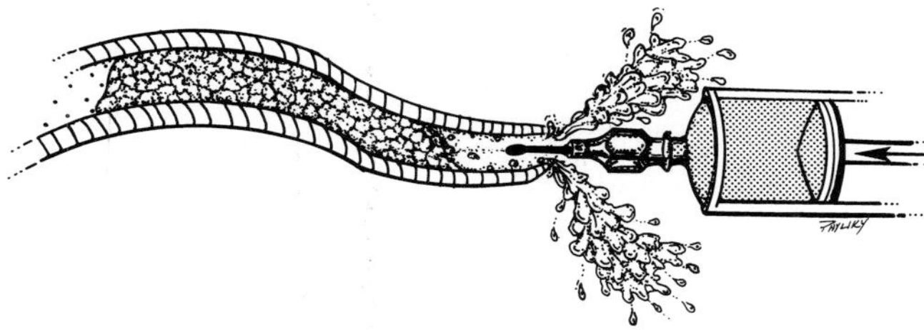

FIG. 35–47. Schematic illustration of the beneficial effects of flushing without occlusion of the urethra and the catheter. A portion of the matrix-crystalline plug has been flushed out the external urethral orifice.

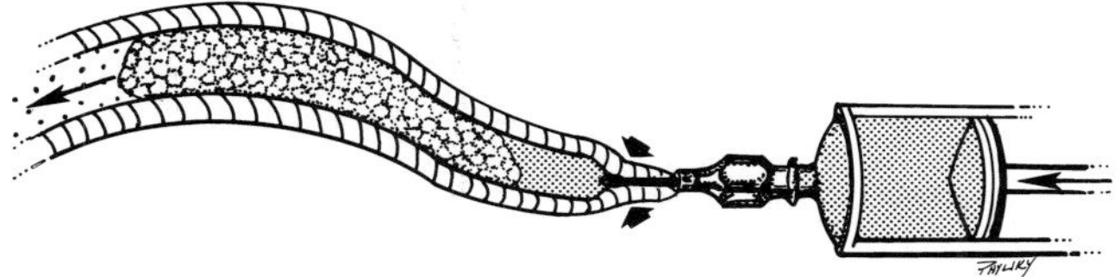

FIG. 35–48. Schematic illustration of technique of reverse flushing the urethra following compression of the distal urethra around the Minnesota olive-tipped catheter.

(e). Local instillation of antimicrobial agents into the bladder lumen in attempts to prevent or treat UTI has no proven value. Unless the bladder wall is hypotonic or atonic, the antimicrobial agent is likely to be voided soon after it is instilled. If circumstances dictate the need for antimicrobial agents, they should be given orally or parenterally, to maximize their effectiveness.

(2). The urinary bladder should be evaluated periodically following restoration of adequate urethral patency, to ensure that urethral obstruction has not recurred or that the detrusor muscle is not hypotonic. Micturition induced by gentle digital compression of the bladder may facilitate evaluation of urethral patency.

(3). Caution must be used when selecting various drugs for azotemic cats.

(a). Although glucocorticoid therapy has been advocated to minimize inflammatory swelling of the urethra, glucocorticoids may aggravate the severity of potentially life-threatening anemia by inducing protein catabolism (via gluconeogenesis).

(b). Likewise, administration of acidifying agents to azotemic cats may exacerbate existing metabolic acidosis.

(c). Indiscriminate use of any drug in patients with renal dysfunction must be avoided because of potential adverse drug reactions associated with the uremic state.

(4). Following relief of urethral obstruction, transitory obligatory postobstructive diuresis may develop. Even though polyuric cats may consume some water, the quantity consumed is often insufficient to maintain proper fluid balance. Thus, supplementation of water intake may be necessary with parenteral administration of rehydrating or maintenance fluids.

d. Indwelling transurethral catheters

(1). We do not recommend routine use of indwelling urinary catheters in cats following relief of urethral obstruction because they may induce further damage to the urinary tract.[80]

(a). Disruption of the glycosaminoglycan coating of the urothelium as a result of indwelling urethral catheters may promote adherence of microbes and UTI.

(b). Disruption of the glycosaminoglycan coating may also facilitate adherence of crystals to the urothelium, facilitating their growth or aggregation.[35]

(2). Indwelling urinary catheters may be indicated following relief of urethral obstruction to:

(a). Facilitate measurement of urine formation rate during intensive care of critically ill cats.

(b). Promote recovery of detrusor atony by maintaining an empty bladder.

(c). Prevent recurrence of urethral obstruction caused by urine precipitates or mural abnormalities in high-risk patients (Table 35–13).

(3). The likelihood of whether or not a cat will voluntarily resume micturition may be assessed by evaluation of:

(a). The caliber of the urine stream during the voiding phase of micturition.

(b). The abundance of material in urine with the potential to occlude the urethral lumen.

(c). The adequacy of detrusor tone immediately following relief of urethral obstruction.

(4). When use of indwelling urinary catheters is deemed to be beneficial, several precautions minimize catheter-induced complications.[50]

(a). Sterilized catheters composed of soft, pliable material are preferred because they are less likely to cause trauma to the urinary tract.

(b). Catheters constructed of relatively inert material minimize toxicity to adjacent tissues.

(c). To minimize injury to proximal portions of the urethra, and especially to the urinary bladder, one should avoid insertion of an excessive length of catheter. If the wall of the urinary bladder is not hypotonic, use of an open-ended catheter that extends only a short distance into the bladder lumen is recommended.

(d). To minimize ascending UTI, the urethral catheter should be connected to a closed sterilized drainage system when possible.[50]

(e). Administration of a broad-spectrum antimicrobial agent, such as ampicillin, may be considered.

(1′). However, because UTI by resistant microbes develops in some patients during antimicrobial therapy, follow-up urine culture and susceptibility tests are essential to determine the need for, and the type of, additional antimicrobial therapy.

(2′). An alternative is to consider administration of antibiotics during indwelling transurethral catheterization only if evidence of infection is detected. This minimizes the likelihood of infection caused by bacteria that are resistant to antimicrobial agents. If catheter-induced bacterial infection develops and remains asymptomatic, it may be treated with antibiotics following removal of the catheter.

(f). Urethral catheters should be removed as soon as possible (12 to 36 hours?) to minimize catheter-induced iatrogenic disease. The cat should then be observed for signs of recurrent obstruction during a 12- to 24-hour period before being discharged from the hospital.

(g). In one study of cats with induced cystitis and indwelling transurethral catheters attached to a closed collection system, glucocorticoids increased the susceptibility of the cats to bacterial UTI without decreasing urinary tract inflammation.[81] Intravesicular injection of dimethyl sulfoxide (DMSO) did not decrease the incidence of bacterial UTI or the severity of inflammation.[81]

e. Hypotonic urinary bladder and reflex dyssynergia.

(1). Severe or prolonged distention of the urinary bladder caused by obstruction to urine outflow may cause the detrusor muscle to become hypotonic. The underlying cause is thought to be related to disruption of specialized portions of bladder smooth muscle cells (so-called tight junctions) that normally transmit neurogenic impulses from smooth muscle pacemaker cells.

(a). Once urethral patency has been reestablished, therapy designed to maintain relatively low pressure within the bladder lumen often restores the normal micturition reflex.

(1′). One alternative consists of trial therapy with bethanecol, a parasympathomimetic agent. The recommended oral dose for cats is 1.25 to 2.5 mg every 8 hours.[49,76] Bethanecol may be given in conjunction with phenoxybenzamine, an alpha-adrenergic antagonist, to facilitate relaxation of smooth muscle in the proximal urethra (oral dose, 2.5 to 10 mg given once per day).[49,62]

(2′). Alternatively, an indwelling catheter with its tip located within the bladder lumen may be utilized.

(3′). Periodic attempts to induce voiding by manual compression of the urinary bladder may also be considered, provided they do not markedly increase intraluminal pressure.

(b). If an indwelling urinary catheter is utilized to minimize accumulation of urine in the bladder, the previously described precautions designed to prevent catheter-induced injury should be considered. In addition to orally administered antimicrobial agents, irrigation of the bladder lumen with antimicrobial solutions may be considered, provided a sufficient quantity of the agent remains in the bladder long enough to have a beneficial effect. Only sterile solutions should be injected in volumes sufficient to allow contact with all portions of the bladder mucosa.

(2). Reflex dyssynergia may be a cause or a complication of urethral outflow obstruction in male cats and may coexist with a hypotonic detrusor muscle (see Table 35–1).[49,69]

(a). This disorder is characterized by failure of the urethral sphincter to relax during the voiding phase of micturition.

(b). The suggested treatment of this complex of neuromuscular dysfunction is administration of an alpha-adrenergic blocking agent (phenoxybenzamine) for dyssynergia of the internal urethral smooth muscle sphincter.

(c). If dyssynergia of the external urethral skeletal muscle sphincter is present, a skeletal muscle relaxant may be given.

(d). Simultaneously, the hypotonic detrusor muscle may be treated with bethanecol in the dosage previously described.

3. Prevention of urethral plugs.

a. Overview.

(1). We emphasize that obstructive urethropathy may occur at different sites, owing to different causes (see Tables 35–1 and 35–13). Therefore, the need for, and the type of, prophylactic therapy should be based on appropriate diagnostic information (Table 35–2). The following review pertains to obstructive urethropathy associated with matrix-crystalline urethral plugs.

(2). A significant but unpredictable potential exists for recurrence of urethral obstruction caused by matrix-crystalline plugs. Because of associated morbidity and mortality, many medical and surgical protocols have been advocated to deal with this problem. Unfortunately, lack of understanding of the diverse cause(s) of this disorder has resulted in recommendations of a variety of therapeutic maneuvers based on personal opinion and empiric clinical evidence rather than on studies of relevant experimental models and controlled clinical trials.[1,85]

b. Medical protocols.

(1). Because insoluble crystals appear to be an integral component of many matrix-crystalline urethral plugs, use of medical protocols to prevent crystal formation in affected patients is logical. Struvite has been the primary mineral component of most naturally occurring urethral plugs, although other mineral types have been encountered (see Table 35–7). Successful prevention of recurrent urethral obstruction utilizing diets designed to reduce urine pH and urine magnesium and phosphorus concentration has been reported.[31]

(2). See the preceding sections on medical prevention of various types of feline urethral stones for details.

c. Surgical protocols.

(1). Perineal urethrostomy is an effective method for minimizing recurrent obstruction of the penile urethra of patients that do not respond to nonsurgical therapeutic and prophylactic management. However, contrast antegrade cystourethrography or retrograde urethrocystography should be performed to localize the site(s) of urethral obstruction before considering this technique (Figs. 35–20, 35–21, 35–26, and 35–39).[34]

(2). We emphasize that perineal urethrostomy may be associated with significant short-term and long-term complications.

(a). They include bacterial UTIs,[30,79] abnormal urethral pressure profiles,[29,30] and urethral strictures.[76]

(b). If staphylococcal UTI develops as a

result of surgical removal of the penile urethra and associated local host defense mechanisms, infection-induced struvite urocystoliths may subsequently develop.[79]

VII. IDIOPATHIC LOWER URINARY TRACT DISEASE

A. Current status of etiopathogenesis.

1. The cause(s) of hematuria, dysuria, and urethral obstruction cannot be detected in a substantial number of patients.
2. In a prospective clinical study designed to detect causes of hematuria, dysuria, and urethral obstruction in 143 untreated male and female cats with naturally occurring disease, a causative agent (e.g., infectious agents, uroliths, neoplasms) could not be detected in 77 cases (53%) (see Table 35–3).[41,76]
   a. Although we were unable to identify viruses in urine of affected patients, no attempt was made to explant tissues for virus isolation. This fact is noteworthy in light of our ability to identify herpesvirus from explanted tissue, but not urine, of cats with induced cell-associated herpesvirus infection.[80,82]
   b. The subsequent course of clinical signs in many of these 77 cats was consistent with a viral cause (Fig. 35–1). Clinical signs of gross hematuria, dysuria, and pollakiuria resolved spontaneously without treatment.

B. Interstitial cystitis.

1. Interstitial cystitis is a nonmalignant inflammatory disorder of humans of unknown cause.[64] The disease is characterized by dysuria, pain above the pubic region that is relieved by voiding, urinalysis which typically is normal, and distinctive mucosal lesions detected by cystoscopy (Table 35–17).[33,64]
   a. Although interstitial cystitis has affected humans of all ages and both sexes, it is most common in middle-aged white women.
   b. The pathology and etiopathogenesis of human interstitial cystitis have not been clearly defined. Proposed causes include viral infections, autoimmunity, mast cell–mediated disease, lymphatic or vascular obstruction, neurogenic disease, endocrinopathies, and defects in the GAG coating of the mucosal surface of the bladder.[64]
   c. A reliable and effective treatment of human interstitial cystitis currently is unavailable.
      (1). A variety of pharmacologic agents have

TABLE 35–17
CLINICAL FEATURES OF FELINE IDIOPATHIC LOWER URINARY TRACT DISEASE AND HUMAN INTERSTITIAL CYSTITIS

	Idiopathic LUTD	Interstitial Cystitis
Signalment	Young animal Male or female	Middle-aged Predominantly female
Signs	Dysuria Pollakiuria Hematuria Urethral obstruction	Pollakiuria Nocturia Pelvic pain
Clinical course	Episodic Self-limiting	Chronic Persistent
Urinalysis	Hematuria Proteinuria ±Pyuria Decreased GAGs?	Usually normal ±Pyuria Decreased GAGs?
Urine culture	Sterile	Sterile
Radiography	Irregular mucosa	Unremarkable
Cystography	Glomerulations?	Glomerulations Reduced bladder capacity Hunner's ulcers
Light microscopy	Ulceration Hemorrhage Mononuclear cell infiltrate Increased mast cells?	Ulceration Hemorrhage Mononuclear cell infiltrate Increased mast cells? Granulation tissue Vasculitis Perineural inflammatory infiltrate

GAGs = glycosaminoglycans

been used, including intravesicular administration of DMSO or silver nitrate and chlorpactin.

(2). Oral agents that have been used include antihistamines, nonsteroidal anti-inflammatory agents, cimetidine, doxepin (a histamine H_1, H_2 antagonist), amitriptyline, and sodium pentosan polysulfate.[64]

(3). In approximately 10% of the patients, surgery is used to reconstruct a small contracted or ulcerated bladder.

(4). Although symptomatic treatment may be associated with a decrease in the severity of clinical signs, complete and permanent remission of interstitial cystitis has been rare.[64]

2. Some cats with feline LUTD have findings similar to those observed in humans with interstitial cystitis. They include decreased urine concentrations of glycosaminoglycans, and similar gross and light microscopic changes (see Table 35–17).[11,12] These similarities have prompted the hypothesis that some forms of feline LUTD are an analog of human interstitial cystitis; however, further studies are essential to prove or disprove this hypothesis.

C. Treatment.

1. The clinical signs of hematuria and dysuria in many untreated nonobstructed male and female cats with idiopathic LUTD frequently subside within approximately 1 week.[69,76] These signs may recur after a variable period and again subside without treatment.
   a. In this situation, any form of therapy might appear to be beneficial, as long as it is not harmful.
   b. The self-limiting nature of some forms of idiopathic feline LUTD underscores the need for controlled clinical trials to prove efficacy of various forms of therapy.
2. Antibacterial agents.
   a. The infrequency with which bacteria have been identified at the onset of clinical signs of LUTD has been well established.[41,48,63]

      (1). The uselessness of antimicrobial agents in the treatment of abacteriuric cats with LUTD has also been documented.[3,76]

      (2). Indiscriminate use of antimicrobial agents has undoubtedly been responsible, at least in part, for the emergence of the resistant strains of microbes that populate veterinary hospitals.

   b. Cats with perineal urethrostomies may develop recurrent bacterial UTIs.[30,79] (See Chapter 40, Bacterial Infections of the Canine and Feline Urinary Tract, for recommendations about management of recurrent bacterial UTI caused by relapses and reinfections.)
3. Urinary tract antiseptics.
   a. Urinary tract antiseptics are sometimes used as adjunctive agents in the treatment, control, and prevention of UTI in humans. Although their use is frequently acknowledged in treatment of bacterial UTI in dogs, and is occasionally mentioned for treatment of LUTD in cats, no studies have substantiated their effectiveness in these species.
   b. Methenamine is a cyclic hydrocarbon. In an acid environment (pH < 6.0), methenamine hydrolyzes to form formaldehyde, an essential component of its antimicrobial activity.

      (1). Because of the necessity of acidic urine for formation of formaldehyde, methenamine is usually given in combination with acidifiers, such as mandelic acid (methenamine mandelate) or hippuric acid (methenamine hippurate). Methenamine must remain in the urinary tract for a sufficient period to allow generation of effective concentrations of formaldehyde.

      (2). Once generated in sufficient concentration, formaldehyde is capable of killing microbes at any urine pH.

      (3). In light of the hypothesis that some forms of LUTD in cats are caused by viruses, the unproven suggestion that methenamine may have viricidal action in urine is of interest.

         (a). However, the intracellular location of viruses poses the problem of access of formaldehyde to them.

         (b). Lack of definitive proof that viruses are a cause of naturally occurring LUTD in cats and lack of studies of the efficacy of methenamine in such patients are additional problems.

         (c). At this time, use of methenamine to treat feline urinary tract disorders represents no more than an idea.

   c. Methylene blue (tetramethylthionine chloride) is a weak antiseptic agent that at one time was popularly used in combination products designed to treat lower urinary tract symptoms. Medications containing methylene blue are contraindicated for cats because methylene blue has the potential to cause Heinz bodies and severe anemia (Fig. 35–49).[76]
4. Urinary tract analgesics.
   a. Phenazopyridine is an azo dye that is commonly used as a urinary tract analgesic in humans.
   b. Its use, alone or in combination with sulfa drugs, is contraindicated for cats because it has the potential to cause methemoglobinemia and irreversible oxidative changes in hemoglobin, resulting in formation of Heinz bodies and anemia. Cats have been susceptible to dose-related toxicity of this agent.[76]

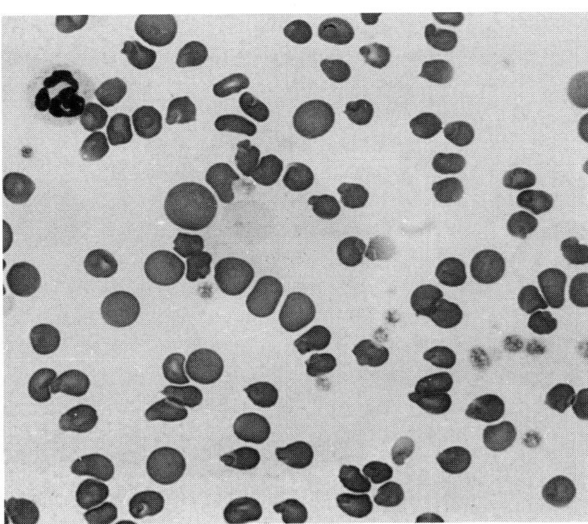

FIG. 35–49. Photomicrograph of a blood smear obtained from an anemic adult male cat that had been receiving a urinary antiseptic containing methylene blue. Many red cells contain Heinz bodies. Immature red cells indicate that the Heinz body anemia is regenerative. (Wright's stain; original magnification, 256×.) (Courtesy of Dr. Victor Perman, College of Veterinary Medicine, University of Minnesota, St. Paul).

5. Smooth muscle antispasmodics.
   a. Many cats with inflammation of the lower urinary tract develop urge incontinence, which is an uncontrollable desire to void that results in involuntary loss of urine. Incontinence occurs soon after the sensation of bladder fullness.
      (1). It is characterized by inability to control micturition between the time of urge to micturate and the actual time of voiding.
      (2). Micturition usually occurs at a low volume of bladder filling.
      (3). Apparently, the urethral sphincter mechanisms are not damaged, because continuous loss of urine is not observed.
   b. Because the exact mechanism of urge incontinence is unknown, details about specific therapy are unavailable.
      (1). The use of smooth muscle antispasmodics for symptomatic treatment of urge incontinence is logical.
      (2). Combination preparations designed to treat signs of LUTD frequently contain atropine, hyoscyamine, and/or scopolamine. The efficacy, if any, of these agents in cats with dysuria has not been established by properly controlled clinical trials.
   c. Propantheline minimizes the force and frequency of uncontrolled detrusor contractions, but has negligible effect on urethral sphincter pressure.
      (1). In a controlled clinical study of the efficacy of propantheline (7.5 mg given orally on 1 occasion) for treatment of naturally occurring hematuria and dysuria in nonobstructed male and female cats, no difference in rate of recovery was observed between cats treated with propantheline and control groups.[4] This finding is not unexpected, because propantheline represents a symptomatic form of therapy.
      (2). Propantheline may be considered to reduce the severity and frequency of urge incontinence in nonobstructed male and female cats.
         (a). It has a rapid onset of action; however, care must be used to prevent urine retention as a result of excessive dosages.
         (b). Because the smallest tablet is 7.5 mg, the suggested dose is 7.5 mg given orally approximately every 72 hours.
         (c). Further studies utilizing appropriate dosages and maintenance intervals are required to substantiate a beneficial symptomatic effect of propantheline in cats with urge incontinence.
6. Anti-inflammatory agents.
   a. Overview.
      (1). One can reasonably assume that most cats with hematuria and dysuria have an inflammatory lesion of the lower urinary tract. Hematuria is indicative (but not pathognomonic) of inflammation; dysuria indicates involvement of the lower urinary tract. The cause of the inflammation in many cats is unknown. For many patients, however, it can be established what the cause is not.
      (2). Lack of specific therapy for abacteriuric cats with hematuria and dysuria has stimulated many to question the value of anti-inflammatory agents to reduce the severity of clinical signs.
         (a). Success in minimizing the frequency of voiding not only would be beneficial to affected cats, but would eliminate owner frustration associated with the socially unacceptable problem of frequent voiding on floors, carpets, and furniture.
         (b). Unfortunately, few controlled clinical trials have studied the short- and long-term effectiveness of anti-inflammatory agents in the symptomatic treatment of dysuria and hematuria in cats. We emphasize that hematuria and dysuria in abacteri-

uric cats without uroliths is often self-limiting.

b. Glucocorticoids.
   (1). Consideration of glucocorticoids to minimize persistent signs associated with inflammation in cats with idiopathic dysuria and hematuria is logical. To test this logic, we conducted a double-blind, controlled therapeutic trial utilizing adult male and female cats with previously untreated idiopathic hematuria and dysuria.
      (a). Six symptomatic cats selected randomly were given 1.0 mg/kg of prednisolone orally, twice each day; 6 symptomatic cats were given a placebo.
      (b). In both groups, clinical signs subsided in a mean of 1 to 2 days, and in both groups, hematuria and pyuria subsided in approximately 2 to 5 days.
      (c). In one cat with recurrent idiopathic dysuria and hematuria, treatment with prednisolone and the placebo were given at different times. No difference in response to the two different forms of management was detectable.
   (2). Because of their catabolic effect, glucocorticoids are generally contraindicated in cats with urethral obstruction and postrenal azotemia.
      (a). They should not be considered in such patients until deficits and excesses in fluid, electrolyte, and acid-base balance have been corrected.
      (b). Likewise, glucocorticoids are contraindicated in cats with bacterial UTI. Use of glucocorticoids in cats with indwelling catheters is especially apt to be hazardous.[3]

c. Dimethyl sulfoxide
   (1). DMSO is an analgesic anti-inflammatory agent with weak antibacterial, antifungal, and antiviral activity.
      (a). It has been reported to be effective in the treatment of a variety of genitourinary disorders of humans, including interstitial cystitis, radiation cystitis, chronic prostatitis, and female chronic trigonitis.
      (b). Retrograde infusion of 50% solutions of pyrogen-free DMSO into the bladder lumens of humans with interstitial cystitis has been reported to minimize associated clinical signs in some patients.[64]
   (2). DMSO has been used to treat FUS in cats, presumably because of its reported efficacy in humans with interstitial cystitis.
      (a). Whether any type of LUTD in cats is morphologically similar to interstitial cystitis in humans is not known. All forms of LUTD in cats are not similar to interstitial cystitis in humans, however.
      (b). Appropriately controlled clinical trials that are designed to evaluate the effectiveness of local instillation of DMSO into the urinary bladder of cats with signs of LUTD have not been reported. In a controlled study of cats with induced cystitis, intravesicular administration of 45% DMSO for 3 days was of no detectable benefit in minimizing bacterial infection or inflammation.[3]
      (c). Dosages and frequency of administration of DMSO has been entirely empiric.
         (1′). Local instillation of varying quantities (as much as 25 ml) of solutions containing 25 to 50% DMSO into the urinary bladders of dogs weighing 15 to 40 kg every other week for as long as 6 months revealed no detectable side effects. Use of solutions containing 100% DMSO caused mucosal edema and hemorrhage. Licensed products available to veterinarians contain 90% DMSO and are not pyrogen free; licensed products available to physicians contain 50% DMSO and are pyrogen free.
         (2′). Side effects of DMSO in cats apparently have not been evaluated. Pending further studies, we discourage its use to treat idiopathic feline LUTD.

d. Other agents.
   (1). A variety of other agents have been advocated by various authors to treat and prevent feline LUTD. None has been evaluated by appropriate selection of patients for study, nor by controlled clinical trials.
   (2). Recommendations for testosterone, castor oil, progesterone, vitamin A, hyaluronidase, and various homeopathic preparations appear to be based on supposition rather than fact. We do not recommend them.

e. Urothelial Debridement.
   (1). Cystotomy to lavage and debride the blad-

der mucosa has been recommended by some to treat cystitis, urethritis, and/or urethral obstruction.

(2). Although this procedure is still used by some veterinarians, no controlled experimental or clinical studies indicate efficacy for the procedure. In fact, reports of clinical experiences suggest that the technique is of little benefit.

(a). This is not surprising, because the urethra and urinary bladder are affected in many cats with dysuria, hematuria, and pollakiuria. If one assumes (and we do not) that debridement of the urothelium has some therapeutic benefit, removal of the bladder mucosa would have no obvious beneficial effect on the urethra.

(b). We do not recommend this procedure.

REFERENCES

1. Arthur RR, et al. Association of BK viruria with hemorrhagic cystitis in recipients of bone marrow transplants. *N Engl J Med.* 1986; 315:230.
2. Bai SC, et al. Vitamin B_6 requirement of growing kittens. *J Nutr.* 1989; 119:1020–1027.
3. Barsanti JA, et al. Effect of therapy on susceptibility of urinary tract infection in male cats with indwelling urethral catheters. *J Vet Intern Med.* 1992; 6:64–70.
4. Barsanti JA, Finco DR. Feline urologic syndrome. In: Breitschwerdt EB, ed. *Contemporary Issues in Small Animal Practice–Nephrology and Urology.* Vol. 4. New York, New York: Churchill Livingstone; 1986.
5. Bjugn R, Flood RR. Scanning electron microscopy of human urine and purified Tamm-Horsfall's glycoprotein. *Scand J Nephrol Urol.* 1988; 22:313.
6. Brown MR, et al. Survival of mycoplasmas in urine. *J Clin Microbiol.* 1991; 29:1078.
7. Brown SA, Prestwood AK. Parasites of the urinary tract. In: Kirk RW, ed. *Current Veterinary Therapy IX.* Philadelphia, Pennsylvania: WB Saunders; 1986:1153.
8. Bryan A. The serological diagnosis of viral infection. *Arch Pathol Lab Med.* 1987; 111:1015.
9. Buffington CA, et al. Feline struvite urolithiasis: Magnesium effect depends on urinary pH. *Feline Pract.* 1985; 15:29.
10. Buffington CA, et al. Effect of diet on struvite activity product in feline urine. *Am J Vet Res.* 1990; 151:2025–2030.
11. Buffington CA, et al. Decreased urine glycosaminoglycan (GAG) in cats with idiopathic lower urinary tract disease. *J Vet Intern Med.* 1993; 7:126.
12. Buffington CA, Chew DJ. Presence of mast cells in submucosa and detrusor of cats with idiopathic lower urinary tract disease. *J Vet Intern Med.* 1993; 7:126.
13. Caywood DD, Raffe MR. Perspectives on surgical management of feline urethral obstruction. *Vet Clin North Am.* 1984; 14:677.
14. Ching SV, et al. The effect of chronic dietary acidification using ammonium chloride on acid-base and mineral metabolism in the adult cat. *J Nutr.* 1989; 119:902–915.
15. Ching S, et al. Trabecular bone remodeling and bone mineral density in the adult cat during chronic dietary acidification with ammonium chloride. *J Bone Mineral Res.* 1990; 5:547–556.
16. Clabough DL. Molecular biology and diagnosis of viral infection. In: *Proceedings of the 9th ACVIM Forum.* New Orleans, Louisiana: 1991:375.
17. Deltertogh DA, Brettman LR. Hemorrhagic cystitis due to herpes simplex virus as a marker of disseminated herpes infection. *Am J Med.* 1988; 84:632.
18. Di Bartola SP, et al. Cystinuria in a cat. *J Am Vet Med Assoc.* 1991; 198:102–104.
19. Doster AR, et al. Trichosporonosis in two cats. *J Am Vet Med Assoc.* 1987; 190:1184.
20. Dow SW, et al. Effects of dietary acidification and potassium depletion on acid-base balance, mineral metabolism, and renal function in adult cats. *J Nutr.* 1990; 120:509–518.
21. Fabricant CG. The feline urologic syndrome induced by infection with a cell-associated herpesvirus. *Vet Clin North Am.* 1984; 14:493.
22. Fenner F, et al. *Veterinary Virology.* New York, New York: Academic Press; 1987:237.
23. Fettman MJ, et al. Effect of dietary phosphoric acid supplementation on acid-base balance and mineral and bone metabolism in adult cats. *Am J Vet Res.* 1992; 53:2125–2135.
24. Finco DR, et al. Ammonium chloride as a urinary acidifier in cats. *Mod Vet Pract.* 1986; 67:537.
25. Finco DR, Barsanti JA. Diet-induced feline urethral obstruction. *Vet Clin North Am.* 1984; 14:529.
26. Finco DR, et al. Characteristics of magnesium-induced urinary disease in the cat and comparison with feline urologic syndrome. *Am J Vet Res.* 1985; 46:391.
27. Fulton RB, Walker RD. *Candida albicans* urocystitis in a cat. *J Am Vet Med Assoc.* 1992; 200:524.
28. Goldfarb S. Dietary factors in the pathogenesis and prophylaxis of calcium nephrolithiasis. *Kidney Int.* 1988; 34:544–555.
29. Gregory CR, Vasseur PB. Electromyographic and urethral pressure profilometry: Long-term assessment of urethral function after perineal urethrostomy. *Am J Vet Res.* 1984; 45:1318–1321.
30. Griffin DW, Gregory CR. Prevalence of bacterial urinary tract infection after perineal urethrostomy in cats. *J Am Vet Med Assoc.* 1992; 200:681–684.
31. Gustafson DP. Antiviral therapy. *Vet Clin North Am.* 1986; 16:1181.
32. Hesse A, et al. Analysis of urinary stones using infrared spectroscopy and scanning electron microscopy. *Scan Electron Microscop.* 1986; 4:1705.
33. Johansson SL, Fall M. Clinical features and spectrum of light microscopic changes in interstitial cystitis. *J Urol.* 1990; 143:1118–1124.
34. Johnston GR, Feeney DA. Localization of feline urethral obstruction. *Vet Clin North Am.* 1984; 14:555.
35. Khan SR, et al. Crystal retention by injured urothelium of the rat urinary bladder. *J Urol.* 1984; 132:153.
36. King JM. Pigment calculi. *Vet Med.* 1990; 85:1179.
37. Klausner JS, Osborne CA. Canine calcium phosphate uroliths. *Vet Clin North Am.* 1986; 16:171.
38. Koziol JA, et al. The natural history of interstitial cystitis: A survey of 374 patients. *J Urol.* 1993; 149:465–469.
39. Kruger JM, et al. Genetic and serologic analysis of cell-associated herpesvirus infection of the urinary tract in conventionally reared cats. *Am J Vet Res.* 1989; 50:2023.
40. Kruger JM, et al. Clinicopathologic analysis of herpesvirus-induced urinary tract infection in specific pathogen–free cats given methylprednisolone. *Am J Vet Res.* 1990; 51:878.
41. Kruger JM, et al. Clinical evaluation of cats with lower urinary tract disease. *J Am Vet Med Assoc.* 1991; 199:211–216.
42. Kruger JM, Osborne CA. The role of viruses in feline lower urinary tract disease. *J Vet Intern Med.* 1990; 4:71–78.

43. Kruger JM, Osborne CA. The role of uropathogens in feline lower urinary tract disease. *Vet Clin North Am.* 1993; 23:101–123.
44. Lawler DF, et al. Incidence rates of feline lower urinary tract disease in the United States. *Feline Pract.* 1985; 15:13.
45. Lewis LD, Morris ML, Hand MS. *Small Animal Clinical Nutrition.* 3rd ed. Topeka, Kansas: Mark Morris Associates; 1987.
46. Lees GE. Epidemiology of naturally occurring feline bacterial urinary tract infections. *Vet Clin North Am.* 1984; 14:471.
47. Lees GE, et al. Results of analyses and bacterial culture of urine specimens obtained from clinically normal cats by three methods. *J Am Vet Med Assoc.* 1984; 184:449.
48. Lees GE, et al. Diseases of the lower urinary tract. In: Sherding RG, ed. *The Cat: Diseases and Clinical Management.* New York, New York: Churchill Livingstone; 1989:1397–1454.
49. Lees GE, Moreau PM. Management of hypotonic and atonic urinary bladders in cats. *Vet Clin North Am.* 1984; 14:641.
50. Lees GE, Osborne CA. Use and misuse of indwelling urinary catheters in cats. *Vet Clin North Am.* 1984; 14:599.
51. Lichtenberg F. Infectious disease. In: Cotran RS, Kumar V, Robbins SL, eds. *Pathologic Basis of Disease.* 4th ed. Philadelphia, Pennsylvania: WB Saunders; 1989:307.
52. Ling GV, et al. Epizootiologic evaluation and quantitative analysis of urinary calculi from 150 cats. *J Am Vet Med Assoc.* 1990; 196:1459–1462.
53. Livingston CW, et al. Effect of experimental infections with ovine ureaplasma upon the development of uroliths in feedlot lambs. *Isr J Med.* 1984; 20:958.
54. Lloyd WE, Sullivan DJ. Effects of orally administered ammonium chloride and methionine on feline urinary acidity. *Vet Med.* 1984; 79:773.
55. Lulich JP. Calcium oxalate urolithiasis: Etiology, pathophysiology, and therapy. PhD Thesis. University of Minnesota; 1991: 123–133.
56. Lulich JP, et al. Nonsurgical removal of urocystoliths in dogs and cats by voiding urohydropropulsion. *J Am Vet Med Assoc.* 1993; 203:660–663.
57. Lulich JP, Osborne CA. Catheter assisted retrieval of urocystoliths from dogs and cats. *J Am Vet Med Assoc.* 1992; 201: 111–113.
58. Lulich JP, Osborne CA. Fungal urinary tract infection. In: Kirk RW, ed. *Current Veterinary Therapy XI.* Philadelphia, Pennsylvania: WB Saunders; 1992:914.
59. Lulich JP, et al. Incomplete removal of canine and feline urocystoliths by cystotomy. In: *Proceedings 11th ACVIM Forum.* Washington DC; 1993:397.
60. Lulich JP, et al. Feline calcium oxalate urolithiasis: Cause, detection, control. In: August JR, ed. *Consultations in Feline Internal Medicine 2.* Philadelphia, Pennsylvania: WB Saunders; 1994:343–349.
61. Maede Y, et al. Methionine toxicosis in cats. *Am J Vet Res.* 1987; 48:289.
62. Marks SL, et al. The effects of phenoxybenzamine and acepromazine maleate on urethral pressure profiles of anesthetized healthy male cats. In: *Proceedings 11th ACVIM Forum.* Washington DC; 1993:935.
63. Martens JG, et al. The role of infectious agents in naturally occurring feline urologic syndrome. *Vet Clin North Am.* 1984; 14:503.
64. Messing EM. Interstitial cystitis and related syndromes. In: Walsh PC, et al, eds. *Campbell's Urology.* 6th ed. Philadelphia, Pennsylvania: WB Saunders; 1992:982–1005.
65. McKerrell RE, et al. Primary hyperoxaluria (L-glyceric aciduria) in the cat: A newly recognized inherited disease. *Vet Res.* 1989;125:31–34.
66. Osborne CA. Bacterial infections of the canine and feline urinary tract: Cause, cure and control. In: Bojrab MJ, ed. *Disease Mechanisms in Small Animal Surgery.* 2nd ed. Philadelphia, Pennsylvania: Lea & Febiger; 1993:426–463.
67. Osborne CA, et al. Etiology of feline urologic syndrome: Hypothesis of heterogeneous causes. In: *Proceedings 7th Kal Kan Symposium.* Vernon, California: 1983:107–124.
68. Osborne CA, et al. Feline urologic syndrome: A heterogeneous phenomenon? *J Am Anim Hosp Assoc.* 1984; 20:17–32.
69. Osborne CA, et al. Redefinition of the feline urologic syndrome: Feline lower urinary tract disease with heterogeneous causes. *Vet Clin North Am.* 1984; 14:409.
70. Osborne CA, et al. Epidemiology of naturally occurring feline uroliths and urethral plugs. *Vet Clin North Am.* 1984; 14:481.
71. Osborne CA, et al. Immediate relief of feline urethral obstruction. *Vet Clin North Am.* 1984; 14:585.
72. Osborne CA, et al. Struvite urolithiasis in animals and man: Formation, detection, and dissolution. *Adv Vet Sci Comp Med.* 1985; 29:1.
73. Osborne CA, et al. The urinary system: Pathophysiology, diagnosis and treatment. In: Gourley IM, Vasseur PB, eds. *General Small Animal Surgery.* Philadelphia, Pennsylvania: JB Lippincott; 1985:622–624.
74. Osborne CA, et al. Etiopathogenesis, clinical manifestations, and management of canine calcium oxalate urolithiasis. *Vet Clin North Am.* 1986; 16:133–170.
75. Osborne CA, et al. Etiopathogenesis and biological behavior of feline vesicourachal diverticula. *Vet Clin North Am.* 1987; 17:697.
76. Osborne CA, et al. Feline lower urinary tract disorders. In: Ettinger SJ, ed. *Textbook of Veterinary Internal Medicine.* 3rd ed. Vol. 2. Philadelphia, Pennsylvania: WB Saunders; 1989:2057–2082.
77. Osborne CA, et al. Medical management of vesicourachal diverticula in 15 cats with lower urinary tract disease. *J Small Anim Pract.* 1989; 30:608–612.
78. Osborne CA, et al. Medical dissolution of feline struvite urocystoliths. *J Am Vet Med Assoc.* 1990; 196:1053–1063.
79. Osborne CA, et al. Perineal urethrostomy versus dietary management in prevention of recurrent lower urinary tract disease. *J Small Anim Pract.* 1991; 32:296.
80. Osborne CA, et al. Feline matrix-crystalline urethral plugs: A unifying hypothesis of causes. *J Small Anim Pract.* 1992; 33:172–177.
81. Osborne CA, et al. Nonsurgical retrieval of uroliths for mineral analysis. In: Kirk RW, Bonagura JD, eds. *Current Veterinary Therapy XI.* Philadelphia, Pennsylvania: WB Saunders; 1992: 886–889.
82. Osborne CA, et al. Feline lower urinary tract disease: Relationships between crystalluria, urinary tract infections, and host factors. In: August JR, ed. *Consultations in Feline Internal Medicine 2.* Philadelphia, Pennsylvania: WB Saunders; 1994:351–363.
83. Pak CYC, et al. Augmentation of renal citrate excretion by oral potassium citrate administration: Time course, dose frequency schedule, and dose-response relationship. *J Clin Pharmacol.* 1984; 24:19–26.
84. Polzin DJ, Osborne CA. Medical prophylaxis of feline lower urinary tract disorders. *Vet Clin North Am.* 1984; 14:661.
85. Rhodes DCJ, et al. Urinary Tamm-Horsfall glycoprotein concentrations in normal and urolithiasis-affected male cats determined by an ELISA. *J Vet Med A.* 1992; 39:621–634.
86. Rogers QR. Unpublished data. Department of Physiology, School of Veterinary Medicine, University of California, Davis, California, 1987.
87. Rozin S. Characteristics of the mycoplasmas as a group. In: Rozin S, Tully JG, eds. *Methods in Mycoplasmology.* Vol. I. New York, New York: Academic Press; 1983:3.

88. Senior DF, et al. Testing the effects of ammonium chloride and *dl*-methionine on the urinary pH of cats. *Vet Med.* 1986; 81:88.
89. Smith CW. Surgical diseases of the urethra. In: Slatter DH, ed. *Textbook of Small Animal Surgery.* Vol. 2. Philadelphia, Pennsylvania: WB Saunders; 1985:1803–1806.
90. Takebe S, et al. Stone formation by *Ureaplasma urealyticum* in human urine and its prevention by urease inhibitors. *J Clin Microbiol.* 1984; 20:859.
91. Taton GF, et al. Urinary acidification in the prevention and treatment of feline struvite urolithiasis. *J Am Vet Med Assoc.* 1984; 184:437.
92. Willeberg P. Epidemiology of naturally occurring feline urologic syndrome. *Vet Clin North Am.* 1984; 14:455.

CHAPTER 36

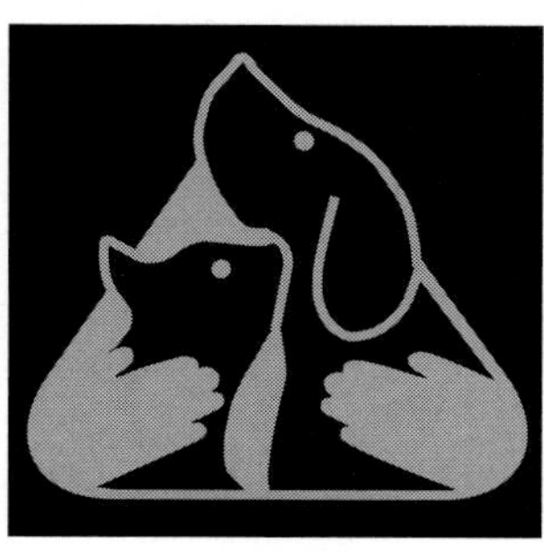

Inherited and Congenital Disease of the Lower Urinary Tract

JOHN M. KRUGER
CARL A. OSBORNE
JODY P. LULICH

I. OVERVIEW

A. Urinary tract disorders of young animals may result from heritable (genetic) or acquired disease processes that affect differentiation and growth of the developing urinary tract, or from similar processes that eventually affect the structure or function of the mature urinary system.

B. As with animals of all ages, successful management of pediatric urinary tract disorders depends on familiarity with the structure and functions of the kidneys, ureters, urinary bladder, and urethra. In addition, a conceptual understanding of the unique anatomic features and physiologic limitations that accompany urinary tract embryogenesis and maturation is essential for developing effective strategies for diagnosis, treatment, and prevention of urinary tract diseases in young dogs and cats.

II. APPLIED EMBRYOLOGY

A. Formation of the urinary system depends on sequential and coordinated development and interaction of multiple embryonic tissues.[37,41]

B. The urinary bladder and urethra are formed by subdivision of the cloaca, the caudal portion of the embryonic hindgut. Formation of the urorectal septum divides the cloaca into the rectum dorsally and the urogenital sinus ventrally.

C. The urogenital sinus communicates caudally with the amniotic cavity via the urogenital orifice and cranially with the allantois (a portion of the placenta) via the urachus and allantoic stalk. The urinary bladder eventually develops from the proximal urachus and the cranial portion of the urogenital sinus. The caudal portion of the urogenital sinus differentiates into the urethra, whereas the remainder of the urachus narrows and is functionally closed by birth.

D. As the embryo grows, the mesonephric ducts and the embryonic ureters (ureteral buds) establish separate openings in the caudal portion of the urogenital sinus. Initially, the ureteral orifice is located caudal to the opening of the mesonephric duct, but as the bladder develops, positions of the embryonic ureter and the mesonephric ducts are transposed, so that the ureter opens cranially in the neck of the bladder and the mesonephric duct opens in the cranial urethra. In male dogs and cats, the mesonephric ducts differentiate into components of the male reproductive system. In females, the mesonephric ducts contribute to formation of the vagina.

III. DEVELOPMENTAL PHYSIOLOGY

A. Although the mesonephros and metanephros produce urine, maintenance of fetal homeosta-

sis is primarily the responsibility of the placenta. Varying quantities of urine formed by the fetal kidneys pass from the developing urinary bladder through the urachus to the placenta, where unwanted waste products are absorbed by the maternal circulation and subsequently excreted in the mother's urine.[40]

B. Fetal urine also passes through the urethra into the amniotic cavity, where urine forms one of the major constituents of amniotic fluid.[40]

C. Normal patterns of urine storage and bladder emptying are evident during the later part of gestation in human and ovine fetuses.[37]

D. Most newborn puppies and kittens void urine shortly after birth; however, micturition is rarely observed in most canine and feline neonates because of maternal hygiene.

IV. CONGENITAL AND HEREDITARY ANOMALIES OF THE UROCYST

A. Urinary bladder agenesis and hypoplasia.

1. Complete agenesis of the urinary bladder is extremely rare but has been reported in a 4-month-old mixed-breed female dog with a lifelong history of urinary incontinence.[54]
2. Hypoplasia of the urinary bladder has been reported more frequently in dogs and cats and typically has been associated with bilateral and, occasionally, unilateral ectopic ureters.[21,52]
3. Although hypoplastic bladders are often implicated as being the result of embryonic maldevelopment, studies in rats and dogs indicate that defunctionalization of the urinary bladder may be associated with potentially reversible reductions in bladder capacity.[14,58] Small urinary bladder capacity may contribute to the urinary incontinence occasionally observed after surgical correction of ectopic ureters; however, bladder capacity may increase substantially over a period of several months following correction of ureteral ectopia.[3]
4. The incidence of urinary bladder hypoplasia resulting from embryonic maldevelopment is unknown.

B. Exstrophy.

1. The term exstrophy encompasses several congenital anomalies characterized by ventral midline defects in the ventral abdominal wall, urinary bladder, intestines, and external genitalia.
2. They are rare disorders in dogs and cats and the cause is uncertain.
3. Lifelong urinary incontinence, ascending urinary tract infection (UTI), and pyelonephritis were the predominant clinical features of exstrophy of the urinary bladder and ventral abdominal wall in an 8-month-old female English bulldog.[20]
4. Physical examination often differentiates exstrophy from other causes of urinary incontinence in young dogs and cats (Tables 36–1 and 36–2).
5. Correction of exstrophy requires reconstructive surgery, and success depends on the severity of the

TABLE 36–1
CAUSES OF URINARY INCONTINENCE IN IMMATURE DOGS AND CATS

- Neurogenic
  - Spinal dysraphism
  - Spinal trauma
  - Dysautonomia
  - Others
- Nonneurogenic
  - Anatomic anomalies
    - Ectopic ureter
    - Ureterocele
    - Ureteral ectasia
    - Ureteral valves
    - Urinary bladder agenesis/hypoplasia
    - Urinary bladder duplication
    - Exstrophy
    - Ectopic uterine horns
    - Colorurocystic fistula
    - Persistently patent urachus
    - Urethral agenesis
    - Urethral hypoplasia
    - Pseudohermaphroditism/intersex
    - Epispadias/hypospadias
  - Obstructive (paradoxical) incontinence
    - Urolithiasis
    - Ureterocele
    - Urethral stricture
    - Neoplasia
    - Periurethral mass lesion
  - Urge incontinence
  - Inappropriate (submissive) micturition

TABLE 36–2
PROBLEM-SPECIFIC DATA BASE FOR URINARY INCONTINENCE IN IMMATURE DOGS AND CATS

- Medical history
  - Note age, sex, and breed
  - Note owner's definition of incontinence
  - Note age of onset and duration of incontinence
- Physical examination
  - Observe micturition
  - Evaluate bladder size before and after micturition
  - Verify incontinence
  - Examine vagina
  - Examine neurologic status
- Quantitative urine culture
- Serum biochemistry (at least serum urea nitrogen and creatinine)
- Consider
  - Survey abdominal radiographs
  - Excretory urography
  - Contrast urethrography or vaginography
  - Endoscopy (vaginoscopy, urethroscopy, cystoscopy)

defect and the presence of other urinary tract abnormalities.

C. Anomalies of the urachus.

1. Overview.
   a. Anomalies of the urachus are relatively common congenital disorders of the urinary bladder.
   b. The urachus is a fetal conduit that allows urine to pass from the developing urinary bladder to the placenta.[40] It usually undergoes complete atrophy and is nonfunctional at birth. The atrophied urachus is typically seen as a fibrous connective tissue remnant at the bladder vertex. If, however, the urachus fails to undergo complete atrophy, macroscopic or microscopic remnants may remain and result in persistent urachal patency or formation of urachal cysts or diverticula.[44]
   c. Factors responsible for incomplete closure and atrophy of the urachus have not been defined.
2. Persistent urachus.
   a. A persistent (or patent) urachus exists when the entire urachal canal remains functionally patent between the bladder and the umbilicus (Fig. 36–1).
   b. It has been observed in immature dogs and cats and is characterized by inappropriate loss of urine through the umbilicus.[15,49,53] A persistent urachus is often accompanied by omphalitis, ventral dermatitis, and UTI. Rarely, a persistent urachus may terminate in the abdominal cavity, resulting in uroabdomen.[17]
3. Urachal cysts.
   a. Urachal cysts may develop if secreting urachal epithelium persists in isolated segments of a persistent urachus (see Fig. 36–1).
   b. These anomalies are rare in dogs and have not, as yet, been reported in cats.[3,44]
4. Vesicourachal diverticula.
   a. When the portion of urachus located at the bladder vertex fails to close, the result is a blind diverticulum of variable size that protrudes from the bladder vertex (see Fig. 36–1).
   b. Congenital *microscopic* urachal diverticula are characterized by microscopic lumens lined by transitional epithelium that may persist at the bladder vertex from the level of the submucosa to the subserosa.[44]
      (1). In a study of 80 feline urinary bladders, more than 40% had microscopic urachal diverticula.[68]
      (2). Microscopic remnants persisting in the urinary bladder vertex after birth are usually clinically silent; however, recent studies suggest that *macroscopic* diverticula may develop at the bladder vertex of cats and dogs with microscopic urachal remnants following the onset of concurrent but unrelated acquired diseases of the lower urinary tract (e.g., bacterial cystitis, urolithiasis, crystalline-matrix urethral plugs, idiopathic disease).[35,45]
      (3). Presumably, urethral obstruction and/or detrusor hyperactivity induced by inflammation results in increased intraluminal pressure and subsequent enlargement of microscopic diverticula.[44] This hypothesis is supported by the observation that many macroscopic diverticula in cats appear to be self-limiting within 2 to 3 weeks following amelioration of clinical signs of lower urinary tract disease.[45,46]
   c. Congenital *macroscopic* vesicourachal diverticula, presumed to be caused by impaired urine outflow, probably develop before or soon after birth and may persist indefinitely.[44]
      (1). The incidence of congenital macroscopic vesicourachal diverticula in dogs and cats is unknown.
      (2). Persistent congenital macroscopic vesicourachal diverticula in young animals are potential risk factors in the pathogenesis of recurrent bacterial UTI.[44,69]
      (3). Although macroscopic diverticula in abacteriuric animals are usually clinically silent, diverticula with concurrent UTI may be associated with signs of lower urinary tract inflammation (e.g., hematuria, pyuria, dysuria, and pollakiuria).
   d. Vesicourachal diverticula are best identified by positive- or double-contrast cystography or by excretory urography.[44] Survey abdominal ra-

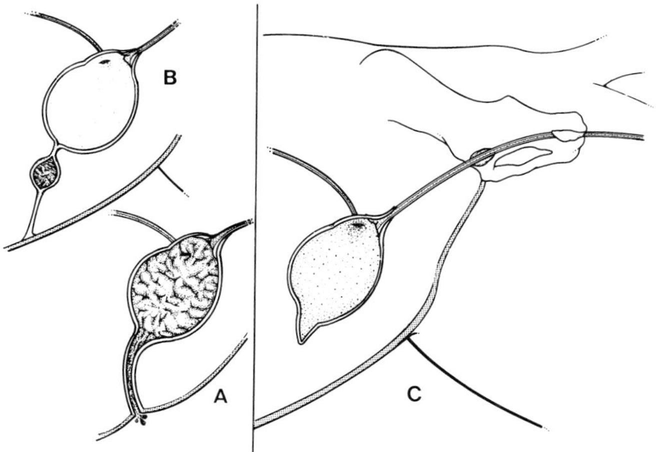

FIG. 36–1. Congenital urachal anomalies. **A,** Persistent urachus; **B,** urachal cyst; **C,** vesicourachal diverticulum. (From Osborne CA, et al. Etiopathogenesis and biological behavior of feline vesicourachal diverticula. *Vet Clin North Am Small Anim Pract.* 1987;17:697–733.)

diographs and pneumocystography have been inconsistent in identifying diverticula.

e. In the past, therapeutic recommendations for any macroscopic vesicourachal diverticula associated with recurrent UTI have consisted of partial cystectomy/diverticulectomy and appropriate antimicrobial therapy.[69] The observation that many macroscopic diverticula of cats (and sometimes dogs) are acquired and self-limiting suggests that therapeutic efforts should be directed toward eliminating underlying causes of lower urinary tract disease.[35,45] If bacterial UTI persists or recurs despite appropriate therapy, the urinary bladder should be re-evaluated by contrast radiography. If a macroscopic diverticulum persists because of persistence of the predisposing cause, and if the patient has persistent or recurrent UTI, diverticulectomy should be considered.

D. Urinary bladder duplication.

1. Complete and partial duplication of the urinary bladder, with or without concomitant duplication of the urethra, are rare congenital disorders of dogs.[23,34] Similar anomalies have not been reported in cats.
2. Urinary bladder duplication may result from any pathologic process that alters the normal morphogenesis of the cloaca or its subdivision into the urogenital sinus and rectum.[1]
3. Clinical signs, which usually develop early in life, include dysuria, urinary incontinence, and abdominal distention.
4. Diagnosis is based on physical examination and identification of a duplicated urinary bladder by contrast radiography, cystoscopy, or exploratory celiotomy (Tables 36–1 and 36–2).[1,23,34]
5. Anomalies involving duplication of the urinary bladder are amenable to surgical correction; however, prognosis is guarded and depends on the degree of malformation and the presence of other concurrent anomalies.

E. Colourocystic fistula.

1. Communication between the urinary bladder and colon is a rare congenital defect that has been observed in a 5-week-old male domestic shorthair cat.[31]
2. This anomaly may result from incomplete division of the cloaca during embryogenesis or it may be acquired after birth.
3. Colourocystic fistulas potentially predispose animals to UTI and urinary incontinence.
4. Surgery design to obliterate the fistula without compromising the urinary bladder and colonic function would be of potential benefit.

F. Ectopic uterine horns entering the urinary bladder.

1. Although the close association between development of the urinary and genital systems might be expected to result in anomalies shared by the two systems; such anomalies are rare.
2. One case of a 9-month-old female domestic shorthair cat with both uterine horns terminating in the urinary bladder has been reported.[27] Clinical signs relating to this anomaly included dysuria, hematuria, and urinary incontinence.

G. Primary urinary bladder neoplasia.

1. In general, neoplasms of the urinary bladder are rare in immature dogs and cats.[10] However, botryoid rhabdomyosarcomas are commonly seen in large-breed dogs younger than 18 months of age.[29]
2. Botryoid rhabdomyosarcomas are embryonic mesenchymal tumors believed to arise from pleuripotent stem cells originating from primitive urogenital ridge remnants.[60]
3. Grossly, these neoplasms are infiltrating tumors that arise from the trigone and project into the bladder lumen as botryoid (resembling a cluster of grapes) masses.[29]
4. Botryoid rhabdomyosarcomas are characterized by clinical signs of hematuria, dysuria, and stranguria. They may also be associated with a complete or partial urethral obstruction, ureterectasis, hydronephrosis, and hypertrophic osteoarthropathy.[16,29] In dogs, botryoid rhabdomyosarcomas are locally invasive; however, distant metastases appear to be uncommon.[29]
5. Unfortunately, little is known about the biologic behavior of botryoid rhabdomyosarcomas and their response to various therapeutic approaches.
   a. Surgical resection alone has been reported to result only in short-term remissions of 3 months or less.[29,61] We observed long-term (greater than 1 year) remission in an 8-month-old male golden retriever following radical surgical excision and ureteral transplantation.
   b. A partial response to combination chemotherapy utilizing doxorubicin, cyclophosphamide, and vincristine sulfate was observed in a female Doberman pinscher with local recurrence and distant metastases following surgical excision.[65]
   c. Combinations of surgery, chemotherapy, and radiation therapy are routinely used to manage botryoid rhabdomyosarcomas of children.[60]
6. Until further studies are performed, the prognosis for botryoid rhabdomyosarcoma in dogs following treatment remains unpredictable.

H. Urocystoliths.

1. Overview.
   a. Formation of urocystoliths and their sequelae is a common manifestation of congenital disorders associated with excess urinary excretion of calculogenic crystalloids.[5,48]
      (1). Cystine uroliths are observed exclusively in patients with congenital renal tubular transport defects resulting in cystinuria.
      (2). Uroliths composed predominantly of urates are often associated with congenital metabolic or morphologic anomalies characterized by decreased biodegrada-

tion and increased urinary excretion of uric acid.

b. Surprisingly, cystine and urate uroliths often are not recognized until affected dogs and cats reach maturity (Tables 36–3 and 36–4). At the University of Minnesota Urolith Center, struvite was the most common urolith type identified in dogs and cats younger than 1 year of age, comprising approximately 65% of all uroliths in both species (see Tables 36–3 and 36–4). In our experience, most struvite uroliths encountered in pediatric patients have been induced by bacterial UTI with urease-producing microorganisms.

c. Cystine and urate uroliths may be found anywhere in the urinary tract, but they are usually detected in the urinary bladder or urethra of affected dogs and cats.[8,9,48,50]

2. Cystine uroliths.

a. Cystine urocystoliths and urethroliths are the most frequent manifestation of hereditary cystinuria in dogs and cats, but the exact mechanisms of cystine urolith formation are unknown. Because not all cystinuric dogs and cats form uroliths, cystinuria is a predisposing cause of cystine urolith formation rather than the primary cause.[48]

(1). Cystinuria results from a heritable defect in renal tubular transport of cystine and other dibasic amino acids.[5]

(2). Cystinuria has been observed in more than 60 breeds of dogs, and occasionally in cats.[8,46,66]

(3). In the United States, a high prevalence of cystinuria and cystine urolithiasis has been observed in mastiffs, Australian cattle dogs, English bulldogs, Chihuahuas, bull mastiffs, Newfoundlands, dachshunds, basenjis, Australian shepherd dogs, Scottish deerhounds, Staffordshire terriers, miniature pinschers, pitbull terriers, Welsh corgis, silky terriers, and Bichon Frises.[8]

(4). Analysis of pedigrees of several breeds with hereditary cystinuria suggests an autosomal recessive or X-linked recessive mode of inheritance.[5,7,63]

b. This disorder has been observed primarily in male dogs, but cystinuria and cystine uroliths have been detected in cats and female dogs.[5,8,46,48] Cystine uroliths appear to occur with equal frequency in both male and female cats.[46]

c. Although cystinuria is detectable at birth, cystine uroliths are uncommon in affected dogs and cats younger than 6 months of age (see Tables 36–3 and 36–4). Most cystine uroliths are observed in somewhat older dogs (mean age 4.5 years) and cats (mean age 4.1 years).[8,46]

d. For additional information on pathogenesis, clinical signs, diagnosis, treatment, and prevention of cystine uroliths, consult Chapter 41, Canine and Feline Urolithiases: Relationship of Etiopathogenesis to Treatment and Prevention.

3. Urate uroliths.

a. Uroliths composed of uric acid, ammonium urate, and sodium urate account for approximately 6% of all canine and feline uroliths.[46,48] Ammonium urate is the major mineral constituent of more than 90% of urate uroliths in both dogs and cats.

b. Urate urolithiasis has been associated with congenital and acquired disease processes resulting in decreased metabolism and/or increased urinary excretion of uric acid.[30]

c. Hyperuricuria is recognized as a major predisposing factor in the formation of urate uroliths; however, the observation that not all dogs and cats with hyperuricuria develop urate urolithiasis suggests that additional factors must be involved in promoting or inhibiting urate lithogenesis.[30]

d. Dalmation dogs are recognized as being uniquely predisposed to urate uroliths, owing to excretion of comparatively large amounts of uric acid in urine.

(1). Etiopathogenic factors responsible for hyperuricuria in this breed appear to involve impaired hepatic conversion of uric acid to allantoin by the enzyme uricase and enhanced renal tubular secretion of uric acid.[13,55]

(2). Hyperuricuria in dalmation dogs is transmitted by a recessive nonsex-linked mode of inheritance.[28]

(3). Although hyperuricuria is present at birth, urate uroliths are uncommon in dalmations younger than 6 months of age. They are most frequently detected in middle-aged dogs (mean age 5.0 years).[9]

e. English bulldogs are also predisposed to formation of ammonium urate uroliths.[4]

(1). The odds that uroliths submitted to the University of Minnesota Urolith Center for analysis were urate was 17 times greater for English bulldogs than for other breeds (95% confidence interval = 11 to 25).

(2). Urate uroliths were retrieved more frequently from male English bulldogs (89%) than from females (11%).

(3). A familial predisposition is suspected.

f. A high prevalence of ammonium urate uroliths has been observed in immature dogs with portal vascular anomalies.[38,57]

(1). Direct communication between the portal vasculature and systemic veins allows blood to bypass the liver, resulting in hepatic atrophy, diminished hepatic func-

TABLE 36–3
AGE DISTRIBUTION OF UROLITHS IN 391 IMMATURE DOGS

Age (mo)	Mineral Type*															
	Struvite	Calcium Oxalate	Calcium Apatite	Calcium Carb-Apat	Tricalcium Phosphate	Brushite	Uric Acid	Ammonium Urate	Sodium Urate	Xanthine	Cystine	Silica	Mixed†	Compound‡	Other	Total
≤1	15		1	2		1	1	1					1	1	1	24
1<age≤2	76	4	2	2	1		3	4					7	6		105
2<age≤3	40		1					4					1	4		50
3<age≤4	20		2					3					2	1		28
4<age≤5	10							6					1	2		19
5<age≤6	20							8	1		2			2		33
6<age≤7	12							3					2	1		18
7<age≤8	18	1	1					9			1		3			33
8<age≤9	11							10			1					22
9<age≤10	20	2						10					2	2		36
10<age≤11	13							9			1					23
Total	255	7	7	4	1	1	4	67	1	0	5	0	19	19	1	391

Carb-Apat = carbonate-apatite
*Urolith composed of 70–99% of mineral type listed.
†Urolith contained less than 70% of predominant mineral; no nucleus or shell was detected.
‡Urolith contained an identifiable nucleus and one or more surrounding layers of a different mineral.
(Data from the University of Minnesota Urolith Center. Analyses performed by optical crystallography and x-ray diffraction.)

TABLE 36–4
AGE DISTRIBUTION OF 64 IMMATURE CATS WITH UROLITHS

	Mineral Type*														
Age (mo)	**Struvite**	**Cal-cium Oxalate**	**Cal-cium Apatite**	**Cal-cium Carb-Apat**	**Trical-cium Phos-phate**	**Brush-ite**	**Uric Acid**	**Ammo-nium Urate**	**Sodium Urate**	**Xan-thine**	**Cys-tine**	**Silica**	**Mixed†**	**Com-pound‡**	**Other**	**Total**
≤1	1															1
1<age≤2	4															4
2<age≤3	8	1											1			10
3<age≤4	7															7
4<age≤5	4	1		1				2			1					9
5<age≤6	4							1								5
6<age≤7	6		1					1								8
7<age≤8	3		1											1	2	7
8<age≤9	3							4		1						8
9<age≤10								1							1	2
10<age≤11	2														1	3
Total	42	2	2	1	0	0	0	9	0	1	1	0	1	1	4	64

Carb-Apat = carbonate-apatite
*Urolith composed of 70–99% of mineral type listed.
†Urolith contained less than 70% of predominant mineral; no nucleus or shell was detected.
‡Urolith contained an identifiable nucleus and one or more surrounding layers of a different mineral.
(Data from the University of Minnesota Urolith Center. Analyses performed by optical crystallography and x-ray diffraction.)

tion, and reduced conversion of uric acid to allantoin and of ammonia to urea.[30]

(2). Extrahepatic shunts, composed of a single anomalous vessel connecting the portal vasculature to systemic veins, are most frequently observed in small-breed dogs, such as Yorkshire terriers, miniature schnauzers, dachshunds, Shih Tzus, Malteses, and pugs.[67]

(3). Intrahepatic shunts (e.g., patent ductus venosus) are found predominantly in large-breed dogs, such as golden retrievers, Labrador retrievers, and Irish wolfhounds.[67]

(4). Etiopathogenic factors involved in formation of congenital portal vascular anomalies have not been defined; however, the predisposition of certain breeds of dogs to portal vascular anomalies and subsequent formation of urate uroliths suggests that hereditary factors may be involved. Confirmation of this hypothesis requires further investigation.

g. Congenital renal tubular reabsorptive defects and portal vascular anomalies have been incriminated as causes in a few cases of urate urolithiasis in cats. The cause of formation of most feline urate uroliths has not been established.

h. For additional information regarding pathogenesis, clinical signs, diagnosis, treatment, and prevention of urate uroliths, consult Chapter 41, Canine and Feline Urolithiases: Relationship of Etiopathogenesis to Treatment and Prevention.

V. CONGENITAL AND HEREDITARY ANOMALIES OF THE URETHRA

A. Urethral aplasia and hypoplasia.

1. Urethral aplasia is a rare congenital anomaly characterized by complete absence of a patent urethra. Urethral aplasia and urinary bladder aplasia have been reported in a 4-month-old female mixed-breed dog with a lifelong history of urinary incontinence.[53] In this case, both ureters were ectopic and terminated on the floor of the vagina.
2. Urethral hypoplasia resulting in urinary incontinence has been described in nine immature female cats.[21] With one exception, all affected cats were domestic shorthairs; no familial tendency was evident.
   a. Early in life, cats with urethral hypoplasia typically develop severe urinary incontinence, which is most pronounced when the animal is recumbent or sleeping.
   b. Diagnosis is based on clinical signs and retrograde contrast vaginourethrography (see Tables 36–1 and 36–2). Radiographic features include marked urethral shortening and vaginal aplasia.
   c. Urethral hypoplasia may be accompanied by other urogenital anomalies (urinary bladder hypoplasia, renal and ureteral aplasia, vaginal aplasia) and is frequently complicated by a secondary UTI.
   d. Clinical signs resolved completely in two cats and improved in four cats following surgical reconstruction of the bladder neck.

B. Urethrorectal fistula.

1. Fistulas connecting the lumens of the urethra and large bowel may be congenital anomalies or may be acquired secondary to traumatic, inflammatory, or neoplastic processes.[42]
2. Most urethrorectal fistulas in dogs and cats appear to be congenital.[42,64]
3. One investigator has hypothesized that congenital ureterorectal fistulas develop as a result of incomplete division of the cloaca into a ventral urethrovesical segment and a dorsal rectal segment; precise etiopathogenic factors in dogs and cats are unknown.[32]
4. Male dogs appear to be affected more frequently than females, and an apparent breed predilection exists for English bulldogs.[42] Breed or sex predispositions have not been reported in cats.
5. Abnormal urination patterns, usually observed early in life, are characterized by simultaneous passage of urine from the anus and the penis (male) or vulva (female) during micturition. Additional clinical signs may include diarrhea, perianal dermatitis, and signs associated with secondary UTI. In two cases, urethrorectal fistulas were associated with infection-induced struvite urolith formation.[39,51]
6. Diagnosis is based on clinical signs and identification of a urethrorectal fistula by antegrade or retrograde contrast urethrography or retrograde colonography.
7. Clinical signs are usually controlled by fistulectomy and eradication of the secondary UTI.

C. Urethrogenital malformations.

1. Urinary incontinence is a common clinical manifestation of urethrogenital malformations associated with diseases of intersexuality, especially pseudohermaphroditism.[22]
2. Pseudohermaphrodites have the gonads of one sex and external genitalia resembling those of the opposite sex.[24] It occurs in both males and females as a result of simultaneous development of Müllerian duct derivatives (oviduct, uterus, and portions of the vagina) and masculinization of the urogenital sinus. The phenotypic appearance of the animal depends on the degree of masculinization of the urogenital sinus.

3. The precise etiopathogenesis of pseudohermaphroditism is incompletely understood; however, a familial tendency has been reported in some canine cases.[18,57] This disorder has not been observed in cats.
4. Incontinence develops early in life and may, on occasion, be accompanied by signs of dysuria and hematuria caused by secondary bacterial UTI. Urinary incontinence related to pseudohermaphroditism most likely results from retention of urine in anomalous communications between the urethra and the genital tract and subsequent passive leakage of urine to the exterior.[25]
5. Diagnosis is based on history, physical examination, and contrast radiography (retrograde contrast urethrography and excretory urography) (see Tables 36–1 and 36–2).
6. Urinary incontinence and pseudohermaphroditism may be reversible following surgical correction of urethrovaginal malformations.[22]

D. Epispadias and hypospadias.

1. Epispadias is a rare congenital anomaly characterized by variably sized defects in the dorsal aspect of the distal urethra.
   a. In humans, both males and females may be affected.
   b. Epispadias associated with exstrophy of the urinary bladder has been reported in an 8-month-old female English bulldog.[20]
2. Hypospadias, a more common anomaly, affects predominantly male dogs and is characterized by ventral malposition of the urethral meatus.[19]
   a. In affected male dogs, an abnormal ventral urethral meatus may be located anywhere along the shaft of the penis, scrotum, or perineum. It is usually associated with malformation of the prepuce and penis.[2]
   b. This anomaly has also been described in female dogs, most of which have concurrent disorders of intersexuality. Hypospadias has not yet been reported in cats.
   c. Embryonically, hypospadias results from incomplete fusion of the urogenital fold.
      (1). Studies in other species suggest that hypospadias may be caused by genetic defects, hormonal teratogens (DES, progesterone), or nonhormonal factors (hypovitaminosis A, anticonvulsant drugs, viruses).[62]
      (2). Precise etiologic factors in dogs with hypospadias are unknown; however, the high prevalence of hypospadias in Boston terriers may suggest a genetic basis for some cases.[19]
   d. Affected dogs are of various ages and may be asymptomatic or develop clinical signs of urinary incontinence, periurethral dermatitis, or recurrent secondary bacterial UTI.[2]
   e. Diagnosis is often based on physical examination.
   f. The presence of an os penis in male dogs precludes surgical reconstruction in most cases. Scrotal or perineal urethrostomy, combined with castration and removal of vestigial preputial and penile tissues, may be of cosmetic value.

E. Urethral duplication.

1. Duplication of the urethra is an uncommon congenital anomaly that has been encountered in immature dogs, but not cats.[26,34,71]
2. Because of the close association between embryonic development of the urogenital and gastrointestinal systems, urethral duplication is almost invariably accompanied by other duplication anomalies. These anomalies are believed to result from abnormal sagittal midline division and subsequent parallel development of the embryonic hindgut, cloaca, rectum, or urogenital sinus.[1] The spectrum of anomalies that accompany urethral duplication depends on the stage at which dysmorphogenesis occurs.
3. Complete urethral duplication, observed in both male and female dogs, may be associated with concurrent duplication of descending colon, rectum, urinary bladder, vagina and vulva in females, and penis in males, and with other urogenital anomalies (unilateral renal hypoplasia, bilateral cryptorchidism).[26,34]
4. Examination of affected dogs may reveal gross anatomic abnormalities, urinary incontinence, or clinical signs of secondary UTI.
5. Diagnosis is based on physical examination, contrast radiography, and exploratory celiotomy.
6. Anomalies of urethral duplication may, in some cases, be amenable to surgical extirpation of the duplicated structure. However, surgical reconstruction has rarely been attempted in cases involving extensive duplication.

F. Ectopic urethra.

1. Urethral ectopia is a rare congenital anomaly characterized by abnormal position of the external urethral orifice.
2. Embryonically, urethral ectopia may result from anomalous morphogenesis of the urogenital sinus, paramesonephric ducts (Müllerian ducts), or mesonephric ducts.[41]
3. Clinical signs depend on the site of termination of the abnormal urethra and other concomitant urogenital anomalies.
   a. Lifelong urinary incontinence was the predominant clinical feature in a 21-month-old female English bulldog with unilateral ureteral ectopia and an ectopic urethra terminating in the cranial vagina.[43]

b. In contrast, a 2-month-old female domestic shorthair cat with an ectopic urethra terminating in the ventral rectum did not have urinary incontinence, but voided urine through the anus.[36]

G. Urethral prolapse.

1. Prolapse of the mucosal lining of the distal portion of the urethra through the external urethral orifice occurs primarily in male dogs 4 months to 5 years of age.[50]
2. An apparent predilection exists for brachycephalic breeds, especially English bulldogs and Boston terriers.[50,59]
3. The exact cause is unknown; however, we have hypothesized that the predilection of brachycephalic dogs to urethral prolapse may be related to abnormal development of the urethra with superimposed increased intra-abdominal pressure as a consequence of labored breathing, dysuria, and/or sexual activity.[50]
4. Diagnosis of urethral prolapse is based on characteristic historical and physical examination findings.[50]
   a. Affected dogs are usually recognized because of bleeding from the prolapsed urethra independent of micturition and because of intermittent or persistent licking of the penis.
   b. Physical examination usually reveals a red to purple, pea-sized, doughnut-shaped mass protruding from the distal end of the penis.
   c. Signs related to UTI or to uroliths affecting the lower urinary tract may also be present.
   d. Results of urinalysis, quantitative urine culture, survey abdominal radiography, and contrast urethrocystography may be of value for identification and characterization of predisposing urinary tract abnormalities.
5. Treatment of urethral prolapse has traditionally involved surgery[59]; however, clinical observations suggest that, in some cases, urethral prolapse may be associated with only minor clinical signs, or may be asymptomatic.[50] In these situations, specific therapy may not be required.
6. If the urethral prolapse is small and further therapy is deemed necessary, manual reduction should be considered.
7. Surgery should be considered for patients with excessive bleeding, pain, or extensive ulceration or necrosis of the prolapsed tissue. Urethral prolapse recurred in 4 of 5 bulldogs 1 week to 18 months following surgical resection.[50]

H. Urethral stricture.

1. Urethral strictures, presumed to be congenital, have been encountered occasionally in young dogs and cats.[6,47]
2. Clinical signs are usually related to partial or complete urethral obstruction. If obstruction is of sufficient magnitude and duration, increased pressure proximal to the stricture site may cause bladder distention, overflow incontinence, ureterectasia, and hydronephrosis.
3. Urinary incontinence, bilateral hydronephrosis, and hydronephrosis were observed in an 8-month-old male German shepherd with a congenital midurethral stricture.[6]
4. Congenital strictures must be differentiated from acquired lesions secondary to trauma, inflammation, or iatrogenic causes.
5. Treatment depends on location and size of the stricture. Extrapelvic strictures may be managed by urethrostomy, whereas intrapelvic strictures may require urethral resection and anastomosis.

I. Urethroliths.

1. Urocystoliths, urethroliths, and partial or complete urethral obstruction are common manifestations of congenital disorders associated with cystinuria or hyperuricuria (see section on urocystoliths).[5,9,48,66]
2. Most urethroliths composed of cystine or urate are detected in male dogs and cats. This finding may be related to gender-specific differences in the etiopathogenesis of cystine and urate uroliths, although cystinuria, hyperuricuria, and uroliths composed of cystine and urate have been observed in female dogs and cats.[5,8,9,46,48] These observations suggest that failure to detect urethroliths in females may be related to passage of small uroliths through their relatively short, wide, and distensible urethra.[48]
3. For additional information on clinical signs, diagnosis, treatment, and prevention of cystine and urate urethroliths, consult Chapter 41, Canine and Feline Urolithiases: Relationship of Etiopathogenesis to Treatment and Prevention.

J. Spinal dysraphism.

1. The term spinal dysraphism collectively refers to cleft-like malformations of the spine and spinal cord resulting from incomplete closure of the neural tube.
2. Clinically, spinal dysraphism is revealed by urinary and fecal incontinence and locomotor disturbances of the hindlimbs.[33,70]
   a. Most dysraphic lesions affect the caudal lumbar, sacral, and coccygeal cord segments and are characterized by hydromyelia, syringomyelia, meningocele formation, demyelination, neuronal necrosis, and defective closure or development of adjacent vertebral arches (spinal bifida and sacrococcygeal vertebral agenesis).[11,70]
   b. Malformation of the sacral spinal cord segments disrupts nerve pathways responsible for micturition, resulting in loss of detrusor responsiveness and urethral sphincter control.
   c. Lack of a normal micturition reflex may result

in abnormal intraluminal pressure and bladder overdistention.

3. Spinal malformations are genetically transmitted as an autosomal dominant trait in Manx cats.[11,33] Spinal dysraphism has been reported in other breeds of cats and dogs.[12,70] English bulldogs appear to have an unusually high incidence of spinal malformations as compared with other breeds.[70]
4. Affected animals often develop urinary incontinence early in life.[11,33,70] Pyuria and bacteriuria are frequent urinalysis findings indicative of secondary UTI. Extraurinary tract signs may include perivulvar or periprepucial dermatitis, fecal incontinence, constipation, plantigrade stance, and a hopping gait.
5. A tentative diagnosis of spinal dysraphism is based on age, breed, and clinical signs (see Tables 36–1 and 36–2). Survey radiographs may confirm vertebral abnormalities of the caudal spine; identification of meningoceles requires contrast myelography.[33,70]
6. Therapy should be directed at relieving urinary incontinence and eliminating or preventing secondary UTI. For patients without excessive urethral sphincter tone, manual compression may be utilized to minimize bladder overdistention and subsequent overflow incontinence.

REFERENCES

1. Abrahamson J. Double bladder and related anomalies: Clinical and embryological aspects and a case report. *Br J Urol.* 1961;33: 195–214.
2. Ader PL, Hobson HP. Hypospadias: A review of the veterinary literature and a report of three cases in the dog. *J Am Anim Hosp Assoc.* 1978;14:721–727.
3. Archibald J, Owen RR. Urinary system. In: Archibald J, ed. *Canine Surgery.* Santa Barbara, California, American Veterinary Publications; 1974:627–701.
4. Bartges JW, et al. Prevalence of cystine and urate uroliths in English bulldogs and urate uroliths in dalmations. *J Am Vet Med Assoc.* 1994;204:914–918.
5. Bovée KC. Genetic and metabolic diseases of the kidney. In: Bovée KC, ed. *Canine Nephrology.* Philadelphia, Pennsylvania: Harwal; 1984:339–354.
6. Breitschwerdt EB, et al. Bilateral hydronephrosis and hydroureter in a dog associated with congenital urethral stricture. *J Am Anim Hosp Assoc.* 1982;18:799–803.
7. Casal ML, et al. Inherited cystinuria in the Newfoundland dog. *J Vet Intern Med.* 1993;7:124.
8. Case LC, et al. Cystine-containing urinary calculi in dogs: 102 cases (1981–1989). *J Am Vet Med Assoc.* 1992;201:127–133.
9. Case LC, et al. Urolithiasis in dalmations: 275 cases (1981–1990). *J Am Vet Med Assoc.* 1993; 203:96–100.
10. Caywood DD, Osborne CA, Johnston GR. Neoplasia of the canine and feline urinary tracts. In: Kirk RW, ed. *Current Veterinary Therapy VII.* Philadelphia, Pennsylvania: WB Saunders; 1980:1203–1212.
11. Deforest ME, Basrur PK. Malformation and the Manx syndrome in cats. *Can Vet J.* 1979;20:304–314.
12. Frye FL. Spina bifida occulta with sacrococcygeal agenesis in a cat. *Anim Hosp.* 1967;3:238–242.
13. Giesecke D, Tiemeyer W. Defect of uric acid uptake in dalmation dog liver. *Experientia.* 1984;40:1415–1416.
14. Goss RJ, Singleton SD. Disuse atrophy of the bladder after bilateral nephrectomy. *Pract Soc Exp Biol Med.* 1971;138:861–884.
15. Greene RW, Bohning RH. Patent persistent urachus associated with urolithiasis in a cat. *J Am Vet Med Assoc.* 1971;158:489–491.
16. Halliwell WH, Ackerman N. Botryoid rhabdomyosarcoma of the urinary bladder and hypertrophic osteoarthropathy in a young dog. *J Am Vet Med Assoc.* 1974;165:911–913.
17. Hanson JS. Patent urachus in a cat. *Vet Med Small Anim Clin.* 1972;67:379–381.
18. Hare WCD, McFeely RA, Kelly DF. Familial 78XX male pseudohermaphroditism in three dogs. *J Reprod Fertil.* 1974;36: 207–210.
19. Hayes HM, Wilson GP. Hospital incidence of hypospadias in dogs in North America. *Vet Rec.* 1986;118:605–607.
20. Hobson HP, Ader PL. Exstrophy of the bladder in a dog. *J Am Anim Hosp Assoc.* 1979;15:103–107.
21. Holt PE, Gibbs C. Congenital urinary incontinence in cats: A review of 19 cases. *Vet Rec.* 1992;130:437–442.
22. Holt PE, Long SE, Gibbs C. Disorders of urination associated with canine intersexuality. *J Small Anim Pract.* 1983;24:475–487.
23. Hoskins JD, Abdelbaki YZ, Rost CR. Urinary bladder duplication in a dog. *J Am Vet Med Assoc.* 1982;181:603–604.
24. Jackson DA. Pseudohermaphroditism. In: Kirk RW, ed. *Current Veterinary Therapy VII.* Philadelphia, Pennsylvania: WB Saunders; 1980:1241–1243.
25. Jackson DA, et al. Nonneurogenic urinary incontinence in a canine female pseudohermaphrodite. *J Am Vet Med Assoc.* 1978; 172:926–930.
26. Johnston SD, Bailie NC, Hayden DW, et al. Diphallia in a mixed-breed dog with multiple anomalies. *Theriogenology.* 1989; 31:1253–1260.
27. Jones AK. Unusual case of feline incontinence. *Vet Rec.* 1983; 112:555.
28. Keeler CE. The inheritance of predisposition of renal calculi in the dalmation. *J Am Vet Med Assoc.* 1940;96:507–510.
29. Kelly DF. Rhabdomyosarcoma of the urinary bladder in dogs. *Vet Pathol.* 1973;10:375–384.
30. Kruger JM, Osborne CA. Etiopathogenesis of uric acid and ammonium urate uroliths in non-dalmation dogs. *Vet Clin North Am Small Anim Pract.* 1986;16:87–126.
31. Lawler DV, Monti KL. Morbidity and mortality in neonatal kittens. *Am J Vet Res.* 1984;45:1455–1459.
32. LeDuc E. Congenital rectourethral fistula: Report of a case without rectal anomaly. *J Urol.* 1965;93:272–275.
33. Leipold HW, et al. Congenital defects of the caudal vertebral column and spinal cord in Manx cats. *J Am Vet Med Assoc.* 1974;164:520–523.
34. Longhofer SL, Jackson RK, Cooley AJ. Hindgut and bladder duplications in a dog. *J Am Anim Hosp Assoc.* 1991;27:97–100.
35. Lulich JP, Osborne CA, Johnson GR. Non-surgical correction of infection-induced struvite uroliths and a vesicourachal diverticulum in an immature dog. *J Small Anim Pract.* 1989; 30:613–617.
36. Lulich JP, Osborne CA, Lawler DF, et al. Urologic disorders of immature cats. *Vet Clin North Am Small Anim Pract.* 1987;17: 663–696.
37. Maizels M. Normal development of the urinary tract. In: Walsh PC, Retik AB, Stamey TA, et al., eds. *Campbell's Urology.* 6th ed. Philadelphia, Pennsylvania: WB Saunders; 1992: 1301–1343.
38. Marretta SM, et al. Urinary calculi associated with portosystemic shunts in six dogs. *J Am Vet Med Assoc.* 1981;178:133–137.

39. Miller CF. Urethrorectal fistula with concurrent urolithiasis in the dog. *Vet Med Small Anim Clin.* 1980;75:73–76.
40. Noden DM, de Lahunta A. *The Embryology of Domestic Animals.* Baltimore, Maryland: Williams & Wilkins; 1985:47–69.
41. Noden DM, de Lahunta A. *The Embryology of Domestic Animals.* Baltimore, Maryland: Williams & Wilkins; 1985:312–320.
42. Osborne CA. Urethrorectal fistulas. In: Kirk RW, ed. *Current Veterinary Therapy VI.* Philadelphia, Pennsylvania: WB Saunders; 1977:985–986.
43. Osborne CA, Hanlon GF. Canine congenital ureteral ectopia: Case report and review of literature. *Anim Hosp.* 1967; 3:111–122.
44. Osborne CA, et al. Etiopathogenesis and biological behavior of feline vesicourachal diverticula. *Vet Clin North Am Small Anim Pract.* 1987;17:697–733.
45. Osborne CA, et al. Medical management of vesicourachal diverticula in 15 cats with lower urinary tract disease. *J Small Anim Pract.* 1989;30:608–612.
46. Osborne CA, et al. Feline lower urinary tract diseases. In: Ettinger SJ, Feldman EC, eds. *Textbook of Veterinary Internal Medicine.* 4th ed. Philadelphia, Pennsylvania: WB Saunders; 1995:1805–1832.
47. Osborne CA, et al. The urinary system: Pathophysiology, diagnosis, treatment. In: Gourley IR, Vasseur PB, eds. *General Small Animal Surgery.* Philadelphia, Pennsylvania: JB Lippincott; 1985: 510–511.
48. Osborne CA, et al. Canine urolithiasis. In: Ettinger SJ, ed. *Textbook of Veterinary Internal Medicine.* 3rd ed. Philadelphia, Pennsylvania: WB Saunders; 1989:2083–2107.
49. Osborne CA, Rhoades JD, Hanlon GR. Patent urachus in the dog. *J Am Anim Hosp Assoc.* 1966;2:245–250.
50. Osborne CA, Sanderson SL. Medical management of urethral prolapse in male dogs. In: Bonagura JD, Kirk RW, eds. *Current Veterinary Therapy XII.* Philadelphia, Pennsylvania: WB Saunders; (in press).
51. Osuna DJ, Stone EA, Metcalf MR. A urethrorectal fistula with concurrent urolithiasis in a dog. *J Am Anim Hosp Assoc.* 1989;25: 35–39.
52. Owen RR. Canine ureteral ectopia—a review. 1. Embryology and aetiology. *J Small Anim Pract.* 1973;14:407–417.
53. Pearson H, Gibbs C. Urinary tract abnormalities in the dog. *J Small Anim Pract.* 1971;12:67–84.
54. Pearson H, Gibbs C, Hillson JM. Some abnormalities of the canine urinary tract. *Vet Rec.* 1965;77:775–780.
55. Roch-Ramel F, Wong NLM, Dirks JH. Renal excretion of urate in mongrel and dalmation dogs: A micropuncture study. *Am J Physiol.* 1976;231:326–331.
56. Rothuizen J, et al. Congenital porto-systemic shunts in sixteen dogs and three cats. *J Small Anim Pract.* 1982;23:67–81.
57. Rothuizen J, et al. Urovagina associated with female pseudohermaphroditism in four bitches from one litter. *Tijdschr Diergeneeskd.* 1978;103:1109–1113.
58. Schmaelzle JF, Cass AS, Hinman F. Effect of disuse and restoration of function on vesical capacity. *J Urol.* 1969;101:700–705.
59. Sinibaldi KR, Green RW. Surgical corrections of prolapse of the male urethra in three English bulldogs. *J Am Anim Hosp Assoc.* 1973;9:450–453.
60. Snyder HM, et al. Pediatric oncology. In: Walsh PC, Retik AB, Stamey TA, et al, eds. *Campbell's Urology.* 6th ed. Philadelphia, Pennsylvania: WB Saunders; 1992:1967–2014.
61. Stamps P, Harris DL. Botryoid rhabdomyosarcoma of the urinary bladder of a dog. *J Am Vet Med Assoc.* 1968;153:1064–1068.
62. Sweet RA, et al. Study of the incidence of hypospadias in Rochester, Minnesota, 1940–1970, and a case-control comparison of possible etiologic factors. *Mayo Clinic Proc.* 1974;49:52–58.
63. Tsan MF, et al. Canine cystinuria: Its urinary amino acid pattern and genetic analysis. *Am J Vet Res.* 1972;33:2455–2461.
64. Van Den Broek AHM, Else RW, Hunter MS. Atresia ani and urethrorectal fistula in a kitten. *J Small Anim Pract.* 1988; 29:91–94.
65. Van Vechten M, Goldschmidt MH, Wortman JA. Embryonal rhabdomyosarcoma of the urinary bladder in dogs. *Comp Cont Ed Pract Vet.* 1990;12:783–793.
66. Wallerstöm BI, Wågberg TI, Lagergren CH. Cystine calculi in the dog: An epidemiological retrospective study. *J Small Anim Pract.* 1992;33:78–84.
67. Whiting PG, Peterson SL. Portosystemic shunts. In: Slatter D, ed. *Textbook of Small Animal Surgery.* 2nd ed. Philadelphia, Pennsylvania: WB Saunders; 1993:660–677.
68. Wilson GP, Dill LS, Goodman RZ. The relationship of urachal defects in the feline urinary bladder to feline urological syndrome. In: *Proceedings 7th Kal Kan Symposium.* Vernon, California: Kal Kan Foods; 1983:125–129.
69. Wilson JW, et al. Canine vesicourachal diverticula. *Vet Surg.* 1979;8:63–67.
70. Wilson JW, et al. Spina bifida in the dog. *Vet Pathol.* 1979;16: 165–179.
71. Wolff A, Radecky M. Anomaly in a poodle puppy. *Vet Med Small Anim Clin.* 1973;68:732–733.

CHAPTER 37

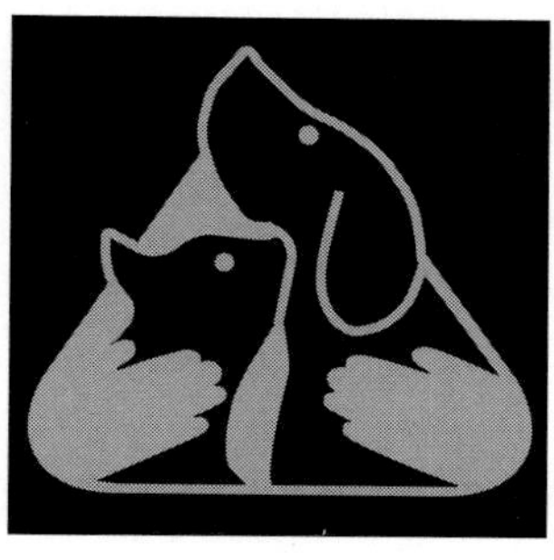

Disorders of Micturition

INDIA F. LANE

I. INTRODUCTION

A. Normal micturition and urinary continence requires a combination of neurologic, anatomic, and muscular coordination.

1. Micturition encompasses both a storage phase, during which the bladder is relaxed and fills against an appropriate degree of outlet resistance in the bladder neck and urethra, and an emptying phase, during which the urinary bladder contracts and the outlet relaxes until voiding is complete.
2. Disturbances in either phase may create dysfunction, or loss of voluntary, coordinated, and complete micturition.
3. Disorders of storage result in pollakiuria, nocturia, and urinary incontinence.
4. Disorders of emptying result in urine retention, incomplete voiding, and overflow urinary incontinence.

B. Disorders of micturition are best approached with a careful history, physical examination, neurologic examination, urinalysis, and selected ancillary diagnostic procedures designed to characterize urinary bladder and urethral function.

C. Disorders of micturition are classified according to the phase of micturition affected (disorders of voiding, disorders of storage), pathophysiology (neurogenic, nonneurogenic disorders), frequency (continuous, intermittent), and residual urine volume (distended urinary bladder, nondistended urinary bladder).

D. Diagnosis and management of nonneurogenic disorders of micturition are enhanced by the characterization of bladder and urethral activity contributing to the disorder.

E. Management of disorders of micturition is similar for neurogenic and nonneurogenic disorders and may include urinary bladder management, pharmacologic manipulation, or surgical procedures.

F. If clinical improvement is not observed following an appropriate evaluation and management, re-evaluation of the pharmacologic agent, dosage, contributing factors, and diagnosis is recommended (Table 37–1).

II. NORMAL PHYSIOLOGY

A. Anatomy and neurophysiology.

1. In the normal animal, micturition requires the coordinated effects of various anatomic, central nervous system, and local neuromuscular components affecting the lower urinary tract.
2. Anatomic components include the ureterovesicular junctions, the detrusor muscle of the urinary bladder, the smooth muscle of the bladder neck and urethra (internal urethral sphincter), and the striated muscle of the external urethral sphincter.
   a. The urinary bladder is functionally divided into a bladder body and bladder neck (or base).
   b. The detrusor muscle is composed of an inter-

TABLE 37–1
POSSIBLE CAUSES OF POOR RESPONSE TO THERAPY OF DISORDERS OF MICTURITION

Inadequate dosage, frequency, or duration of pharmacologic therapy
Inadequate ancillary management (e.g., bladder management)
Poor client compliance
Inappropriate diagnosis, inappropriate pharmacologic agent
Untreated urinary tract infection
Uncorrected polyuria
Mixed disorder of micturition present
Underlying neurologic impairment
Underlying anatomic abnormality
Refractory functional disorder

woven network of smooth muscle bundles in varying orientation and layers. Tight cellular junctions between smooth muscle cells allow rapid transmission of neuromuscular impulses.[1]

c. The smooth muscle of the urethra is an extension of detrusor smooth muscle with both longitudinal and circular or spirally arranged fibers.
d. In dogs, a striated muscle zone is located primarily in the prostatic urethra in males and the midurethra in females.
e. In cats, the striated muscle zone is located primarily in the postprostatic urethra in males and the distal urethra in females.[35]

3. Local neuromuscular responsiveness, intact peripheral nerves and spinal pathways, and input from higher centers in the cerebral cortex, midbrain, and cerebellum are required for voluntary, coordinated micturition.
   a. The pelvic nerve originates from sacral spinal cord segments (S-1 to S-3), and projects parasympathetic impulses to ganglia in the urinary bladder wall and cholinergic (muscarinic) receptors in the urinary bladder.[39,98,117] Acetylcholine is the primary neurotransmitter at the terminal receptors; other neurotransmitters, such as adenosine triphosphate (ATP), vasoactive intestinal peptide, histamine, and serotonin, may also be involved.[7,27,39,40,139]
   b. The hypogastric nerve originates from the lumbar spinal cord (L-1 to L-4 in dogs, L-2 to L-5 in cats), synapses in the caudal mesenteric ganglion, and supplies sympathetic input to adrenergic receptors in the urinary bladder and urethra.[98,106]
      (1). Norepinephrine is the primary neurotransmitter at postganglionic adrenergic receptors; however, ATP and neuropeptide Y may also be involved.[27]
      (2). Beta-adrenergic receptors are distributed primarily in the urinary bladder.
      (3). Alpha-adrenergic receptors are concentrated in the bladder neck and urethra.
   c. The pudendal nerve also originates from sacral spinal cord segments and provides somatic innervation to the striated muscle of the external urethral sphincter.
   d. Although micturition is essentially a spinal reflex, supraspinal organization appears increasingly important for voluntary, coordinated, and complete micturition.[24,38]
      (1). A micturition center located in the pons is responsible for modulating the storage-voiding cycle and for coordinating bladder and urethral activity during voiding.
      (2). Cerebral cortical input is important for voluntary initiation, inhibition, and interruption of voiding.
      (3). Additional modulatory input, primarily inhibitory, is received from the cerebellum, basal ganglia, and hypothalamus.
   e. Afferent (sensory) information from stretch receptors in the urinary bladder and from additional nerve endings in the bladder submucosa, which respond to extreme distention and pain, is relayed via the pelvic and the hypogastric nerve, respectively. Afferent information from the urethra, including perception of urine flow, urethral distention, and pain, is transmitted to the spinal cord and higher centers via the pudendal nerve.[40,106]

B. Storage phase.

1. The storage phase of micturition is characterized by sympathetic dominance.
2. Slow filling of the urinary bladder is characterized by minimal change in intravesicular pressure until critical threshold volumes are reached. Inhibition of bladder contractility during filling involves characteristics of the detrusor muscle, sympathetic input, and the influence of higher centers.
   a. Activation of beta receptors in the urinary bladder facilitates relaxation of the detrusor muscle.
   b. Inhibitory neurotransmitters in the central nervous system probably include enkephalins, gamma aminobutyric acid (GABA), and serotonin.[38]
3. Activation of alpha receptors in the urethra facilitates smooth muscle contraction and urethral closure.
   a. During bladder filling, outlet resistance is provided by the mechanical factors of urethral diameter and wall tension, and by basal tonic activity in the striated and smooth muscle of the urethra.[79]
   b. Later in the filling phase, as trigonal distention occurs, alpha-mediated increases in urethral resistance preserve continence.[79]

4. Additional urethral resistance is provided by the striated muscle of the external urethral sphincter, which reflexively contracts if intra-abdominal pressure is increased. This sphincter may also be voluntarily controlled.[39,98]
5. Alpha-adrenergic activity also plays a role in the inhibition of parasympathetic transmission during bladder filling, probably via direct interactions with parasympathetic components at bladder surface ganglia.[40,106]

C. Voiding phase.

1. As distention of the urinary bladder increases, afferent impulses from stretch receptors in the bladder wall are transmitted to the brain stem and cerebral sensory areas via the pelvic nerve and spinal pathways. With severe overdistention and pain, additional sensory information is transmitted via the hypogastric nerve and sympathetic system as well.
2. Micturition occurs as a pure reflex in infants and neonates; however, the reflex is modulated in adults, and voluntary release of inhibition is required for initiation of voiding at an appropriate time and place.[40,47]
3. Parasympathetic motor impulses are transmitted from the micturition center via reticulospinal pathways and the pelvic nerve to initiate bladder contraction. Spread of contraction in the detrusor muscle is facilitated by the tight junctions between smooth muscle fibers.
4. Relaxation and opening of the urethral outlet is a function of mechanical and neurogenic factors.
   a. Contraction of the bladder may alter the orientation of muscles occluding the bladder neck and help to pull the outlet open.[15,97]
   b. Sympathetic and striated muscle input is reflexively inhibited to facilitate urethral opening. This is mainly a function of the micturition center and spinal responses.
   c. In cats, urethral activity during voiding is characterized by the synergistic relaxation of circular muscle fibers and contraction of longitudinal muscle fibers, resulting in dilation and shortening of the urethra.[2]
   d. In rats and dogs, electrical activity is detectable in the muscle of the external urethral sphincter (EUS) during voiding, suggesting some influence of urethral activity in promoting urine flow.[38]
   e. Electrodiagnostic studies in cats have also demonstrated increased EUS activity associated with pulsatile urine flow during voiding, particularly toward the end of emptying, indicating that an active urethral process aids urine flow.[127]
5. Secondary reflexes reinforce voiding responses and favor complete emptying of the urinary bladder.
   a. Afferent information from the bladder and urethra (particularly urine flow and urethral distention) is organized within the sacral spinal cord to facilitate inhibition of the external urethral sphincter.[40]
   b. Input from ganglia on the urinary bladder surface helps to sustain contraction.[40]
   c. Influence of the micturition center in the pons is required for sustained contraction, sustained inhibition of outlet sphincters, and complete emptying.[38]
6. Following complete voiding, sympathetic dominance resumes, and the system is "reset" for urine storage.

III. CLASSIFICATION OF DISORDERS OF MICTURITION

A. Micturition disorders may be classified according to origin (neurogenic versus nonneurogenic), frequency (intermittent versus continuous), or residual volume (distended bladder versus nondistended bladder) (Table 37–2).[15,99]

B. The most useful classification of urinary incontinence is based on the functional status of the urine "pump" (urinary bladder) and outlet (bladder neck and urethra).

1. Hypocontractile bladder (detrusor atony, detrusor hyporeflexia, hypercompliance): Animals with poor contractile function of the urinary bladder are unable to generate sufficient intravesicular pressure to initiate or to complete voiding.
2. Hypercontractile bladder (hypoaccomodation): Normal filling and storage of urine in the urinary bladder is lost owing to inappropriate neurologic signals, changes in urinary bladder compliance or capacity, or idiopathic causes. Detrusor reflexes are triggered at low urinary bladder volumes or pressures. Detrusor hyperreflexia, detrusor instability, and urge incontinence are terms used to describe variations of this condition and its symptoms.
3. Hypotonic urethra (urethral incompetence): Poor outlet resistance during urine storage is a common cause of urinary incontinence in small animals.
4. Increased outlet resistance caused by physical obstruction or functional hypertonicity of urethral sphincters may disrupt or prevent complete voiding.

IV. NEUROGENIC DISORDERS OF MICTURITION

A. Lesions of local neuroreceptors, peripheral nerves, spinal pathways, or higher centers may disrupt urine storage or voiding. The term neurogenic is usually reserved for overt lesions of peripheral nerves or central nervous system components, however.

B. Lesions of the sacral spinal cord (lower motor neuron deficits).

1. Examples include congenital malformation of the sacral spinal column, cauda equina compression, lumbosacral disc disease, sacral or sacrococcygeal

TABLE 37–2
MAJOR TYPES OF MICTURITION DISORDERS OF SMALL ANIMALS

Disorder	Characteristics
Neurogenic disorders of micturition	
Sacral spinal cord/peripheral nerve lesions	Distended, flaccid urinary bladder, easily expressed; depressed genitoanal reflexes; weak or absent voiding efforts
Suprasacral spinal cord lesions	Distended, often firm urinary bladder, not easily expressed; weak or incomplete voiding efforts with time; proprioceptive deficits
Brain stem lesions	Distended urinary bladder; interrupted voiding pattern; cranial nerve or gait deficits
Cerebellar lesions	Inappropriate voluntary voiding; pollakiuria, nocturia; ataxia, intention tremors
Nonneurogenic disorders of micturition	
Congenital or anatomic abnormalities	
Ectopic ureter(s)	Continuous or severe intermittent incontinence since birth
Patent urachus	Urine dribbling from umbilicus
Acquired disorders characterized by increased residual volumes	
Urinary bladder dysfunction (hypocontractility) due to acute or chronic overdistention	Distended urinary bladder, intermittent overflow incontinence; absent or incomplete voiding
Urethral dysfunction (increased outlet resistance)	
Physical obstruction	Distended urinary bladder; dysuria with little or no urine voided; intermittent overflow incontinence if partial obstruction
Functional urethral obstruction	Same as physical obstruction
Detrusor-urethral dyssynergia	Distended urinary bladder, dysuric or interrupted voiding pattern
Acquired disorders characterized by normal residual volumes	
Urinary bladder dysfunction (hypercontractility) due to urinary tract infection, neoplastic infiltration or mass, or idiopathic causes	Small urinary bladder; intermittent urine leakage; may leak urine when active; possible urinary tract infection or feline leukemia virus infection
Urethral dysfunction (hypotonicity)	Small urinary bladder; voiding pattern normal; intermittent urinary incontinence, often when animal is recumbent
Reproductive hormone responsive	
Congenital	
Urinary tract infection	
Prostatic disease	

fractures, and traumatic or degenerative lesions of peripheral nerves supplying the bladder and urethra.

2. Loss of most afferent and all efferent input to the bladder and urethral sphincters results in loss of bladder sensory responses, voluntary control of micturition, and spinal micturition reflexes.[42,43,98,106]
3. Clinical signs associated with lower motor neuron disorders may include paraparesis or paralysis, decreased anal tone and perineal reflexes, depressed bulbocavernosus reflexes, fecal incontinence, and tail pain or loss of tail tone.
4. The bladder is usually distended but flaccid; high residual volumes exacerbate detrusor muscle damage and atony.
5. Typically, outlet resistance is low and urine is easily expressed from the bladder because direct innervation to outlet sphincters is abolished. However, the urethral outlet may instead become "fixed" and provide passive outlet obstruction.[1,106]
6. Overflow incontinence may be observed when pressure within the distended urinary bladder exceeds urethral pressure.
7. Management of lower motor neuron disorders includes correction of the primary lesion, if pos-

sible, and pharmacologic or physical manipulation to facilitate urinary bladder emptying.

C. Lesions of the suprasacral spinal cord (upper motor neuron deficits).

1. Thoracolumbar disc disease, fractures, and other lesions of the suprasacral spinal cord produce upper motor neuron deficits to the urinary bladder and urethra.
2. Clinical signs include proprioceptive deficits, paraparesis or tetraparesis, ataxia, and hyperreflexia.
3. Sensory and motor pathways to the urinary bladder are interrupted; bladder function is lost, but sphincter tone usually remains. Uninhibited pudendal nerve activity may create a hypertonic striated muscle sphincter and excessive outlet resistance.[1,98,106]
4. Initially, upper motor neuron disorders are characterized by a distended, firm urinary bladder that is difficult to express.
5. Over time, some urinary bladder contractile function may return with emergence of a purely sacral reflex. Voiding is usually uninhibited, incomplete, and poorly coordinated. Frequent, involuntary voiding of small volumes may be observed.
6. If contractile function returns while sphincter tone remains hyperactive, the urinary bladder may contract against inappropriate outlet resistance (detrusor-urethral dyssynergia). Dysuria, interrupted urination, and large residual volumes are observed.[29,98,110]
7. Management of upper motor neuron disorders includes correction of the primary lesion and pharmacologic manipulation to reduce outlet resistance and improve urinary bladder emptying.

D. Lesions of higher centers.

1. Brain stem lesions at or below the level of the micturition center in the pons affect micturition in a fashion similar to that of suprasacral spinal lesions. Coordination of the micturition cycle is affected, and a distended bladder with exaggerated or dyssynergic urethral sphincter activity is observed. Other brain stem signs include disturbances of mental status, gait, and posture; cranial nerve deficits may be apparent.
2. With central nervous system lesions above the level of the pons, voluntary control of micturition is primarily affected, and inhibitory input is lost. Unconscious urination, nocturia, and urination in inappropriate places are common. Urination of small volumes, similar to a hypercontractile urinary bladder, may be observed as well.[15,38,106]
3. Some loss of inhibition is also observed with cerebellar disease; urination is again inappropriate. Other signs of cerebellar disease, such as ataxia and intention tremor, may be apparent.

E. Mixed and incomplete or undifferentiated disorders of micturition are observed following spinal injury in humans and probably are encountered in small animals as well.[98]

V. Nonneurogenic disorders of micturition.

A. When overt neurologic disease is not apparent, disorders of micturition are characterized by determining the functional status of the urinary bladder and the urethra. Historical information, physical examination findings, and observation are the most valuable tools in this determination.

B. Disorders of micturition characterized by a distended urinary bladder or increased residual volume are usually caused by hypocontractility of the urinary bladder or physical or functional obstruction of the urethra.[15,99,87]

1. Physical obstruction of the urethra may be characterized by marked urinary bladder distention, large residual urine volumes following voiding, dysuria, stranguria, or an attenuated urine stream.
   a. If the obstruction is partial, paradoxic urinary incontinence may be observed as the urinary bladder fills and pressure within the bladder eventually exceeds urethral resistance and allows overflow of urine.
   b. Causes of urethral obstruction include urethroliths, bladder neck or urethral neoplasia, urethral strictures, prostate disease, and mucoprotein-crystalline plugs in cats.
   c. Physical obstruction is diagnosed by attempting urethral catheterization and may be confirmed by contrast radiography.
2. If physical obstruction is eliminated as a possible cause of incomplete voiding or urinary incontinence with increased residual volume, detrusor atony (bladder hypocontractility) or functional urethral obstruction is likely. These two disorders may be more difficult to differentiate.
   a. Gentle attempts to express urine manually from the bladder may trigger detrusor activity and allow subjective assessment of urethral resistance.
   b. If the animal initiates voiding, but the urine stream is rapidly interrupted, functional obstruction or detrusor-urethral dyssynergia should be considered.
   c. Functional urethral obstruction, owing to increased urethral resistance or muscular urethral spasm, may follow neurologic injury, urethral or pelvic surgery, urethral obstruction, or urethral inflammatory disease, and often appears clinically identical to mechanical urethral obstruction.
   d. Detrusor-urethral dyssynergia is a lack of coordination between urinary bladder contraction and urethral relaxation. Shortly following detrusor contraction, urethral smooth muscle, striated muscle, or both contract to prevent complete voiding.
      (1). Dyssynergia may be a consequence of neurologic lesions or metabolic, local, or idiopathic causes.[40]

(2). Confirmation of dyssynergia requires urodynamic studies that simultaneously provide information on urinary bladder activity and urine flow.

e. Detrusor atony is usually characterized by a distended, flaccid bladder that is fairly easy to express. Clinically, the animal may posture to urinate or apply an abdominal press, and fail to produce an adequate stream. Some make little if any attempt to urinate voluntarily.

(1). Urinary bladder atony is usually secondary to neurologic disorders or acute or chronic overdistention of the urinary bladder. Detrusor atony and functional urethral obstruction are common sequelae to urethral obstruction, particularly in male cats.[87]

(2). Clinical signs of dysautonomia, a disturbance of autonomic ganglia primarily observed in cats in Great Britain and also described in dogs in the United States, may include detrusor atony and overflow incontinence. However, other clinical signs usually predominate, including mydriasis, prolapsed third eyelids, constipation or diarrhea, regurgitation or vomiting, xerostomia, and anorexia.[122]

(3). Electrolyte disturbances, acid-base disorders, and circulatory disturbances associated with generalized muscle weakness may also affect detrusor muscle contractile function.[87]

f. Management of detrusor atony may include maintaining small bladder volumes to facilitate smooth muscle recovery and pharmacologic manipulation to increase detrusor contractile function and minimize urethral resistance.

C. Urinary incontinence with normal residual volume reflects failure of urine storage. Anatomic abnormalities that disrupt or bypass storage structures, an inappropriate urinary bladder filling phase, or reduced urethral resistance are causes of storage dysfunction.

1. Anatomic urinary incontinence.

a. Congenital abnormalities.

(1). Ectopic ureters, in which the termination of one or both ureters bypasses the normal reservoir function of the urinary bladder, typically create continuous urinary incontinence observed at birth or at a very early age. Intermittent or positional incontinence has also been described with ectopic ureters, and additional concurrent anatomic anomalies are frequently observed.[36,84,92,95,108,114,115,131,132]

(2). A urachal remnant that remains patent allows urine to flow from the urinary bladder through the structure. Urine dribbles from the umbilicus of the affected animal.

(3). Vaginal anomalies, including vestibulovaginal constrictions and vaginal bands, have been variably associated with urinary incontinence.[66,73,141] Urinary incontinence has been attributed to pooling of urine in the cranial vagina, with intermittent leakage; however, many dogs with urinary incontinence and vestibulovaginal anomalies likely have functional abnormalities that create incontinence.

(4). Pseudohermaphroditism, exstrophy of the urinary bladder, ureteroceles, urethral diverticula, and urethral fistulas are other anatomic anomalies that have been associated with urinary incontinence.[47,72,74,100]

(5). The urethra in animals with congenital urethral dysfunction may or may not be grossly abnormal.

b. Acquired anatomic abnormalities.

(1). The development of ureterovaginal fistulas is an uncommon complication of ovariohysterectomy.[5,116] Urinary incontinence is observed shortly after surgery. Vesicovaginal fistulas have also been described following ovariohysterectomy in dogs.[45,61]

(2). Narrowing of the vestibule, creating urovagina and positional urinary incontinence, was described as a complication of vaginal surgery in a dog.[9]

(3). Other acquired anomalies may be expected in individual animals following surgical procedures or trauma.

2. Urinary bladder storage dysfunction is characterized by poor accommodation during the filling phase or urinary bladder hypercontractility.

a. Accommodation, or compliance of the urinary bladder, may be affected by chronic inflammatory processes, infiltrative masses, or radiation injury.

b. Congenital urinary bladder hypoplasia has been reported in dogs,[138] and reduced bladder storage function has been suspected to accompany other congenital abnormalities, such as ectopic ureters.[33,84]

c. Hypercontractility of the urinary bladder, in which detrusor contractions are triggered at low bladder volumes and pressures, has been described in small animals.[21,60,86]

(1). Inflammatory or neoplastic disease of the urinary bladder may create involuntary hypercontractility (sensory hyperreflexia) with urinary incontinence, pollakiuria, or both.[8,80,86]

(2). Neuropathic hypercontractility (detrusor hyperreflexia), may be observed following upper motor neuron lesions and the subsequent evolution of local reflex pathways with involuntary and incomplete detrusor activity. Neuropathic hyperreflexia is also associated with other neurologic disorders in humans, including cerebrovascular diseases, demyelinating diseases, and Parkinson's disease.[8,139]

(3). Idiopathic hypercontractility (detrusor instability) is a common type of urge incontinence in women and is described in dogs and cats. Instability was documented in one cat with urinary incontinence associated with feline leukemia virus.[86]

(4). Other causes of instability include chronic partial obstruction and prostate disease.[21,80]

d. A syndrome of reduced bladder storage, in which urinary bladder capacity and accommodation are reduced but involuntary contractions are not observed, may be an additional clinical entity.[14]

e. Clinically, disorders of bladder storage are characterized by urinary incontinence and pollakiuria. Urinary incontinence may appear similar to the resting intermittent incontinence observed with urethral dysfunction or may be associated with positional change, standing, barking, or jumping.[86]

f. Management of urinary bladder storage dysfunction may include elimination of urinary tract inflammation, correction of neurologic disorders, or pharmacologic manipulation designed to reduce detrusor muscle contractile responses. Therapy may be less successful in the urinary bladder with fibrotic change.[120]

3. Urethral incompetence.

a. Weakened closure responses of the smooth or striated muscle of the urethra allow urine leakage during storage. The problem has a variety of underlying causes and may be observed in males or females. Urethral incompetence occurs most frequently in neutered females and is characterized by intermittent leakage of small amounts of urine, often while the animal is sleeping or relaxed.

b. Urethral incompetence is the most common cause of urinary incontinence in adult dogs.[64]

c. Congenital urethral dysfunction has been described in young, intact animals.

(1). Urethral incompetence may be observed alone or in addition to other congenital urogenital anomalies, such as ectopic ureters, vaginal anomalies, or upper urinary tract malformations.[69,71,73,84,95,120,133,137]

(2). In cats, congenital urethral incompetence is rare and frequently appears to be associated with vaginal aplasia.[69]

(3). Urethral structure may be normal or the urethra may be dilated or grossly shortened.[70,88]

(4). Some authors have reported reduction or resolution of urinary incontinence following the first estrous period in affected animals.

(5). Response of severely affected animals to pharmacologic manipulation often is poor.

d. Reproductive hormone–responsive (acquired) urethral incompetence.

(1). Varied reports of the incidence of acquired urethral incompetence in spayed females range from 4.5%,[136] to 18%,[75] to 20%.[13]

(a). Medium-sized to large breed dogs are most commonly affected. Breeds that commonly develop urinary incontinence caused by urethral sphincter incompetence include the German shepherd, boxer, dachshund, poodle, spaniel, Old English sheepdog, Doberman pinscher, collie, and Irish setter.[13,64]

(b). An overall incidence of 20.1% was reported in a large review of 412 spayed female dogs completed in Switzerland. The incidence reached 30.9% in dogs of more than 20 kg body weight in this series.[13] Anatomic and functional urethral length has been correlated to body weight in dogs[10,19]; however, urethral closure pressure[10] and response to therapy[85] did not appear to be related to body weight.

(2). The pathophysiology of acquired urethral sphincter incompetence remains unclear. Many factors probably contribute to the development of urethral incompetence in neutered animals (Table 37–3).[11,62]

(a). An early theory suggested that the

TABLE 37–3
FACTORS THAT MAY CONTRIBUTE TO URETHRAL SPHINCTER INCOMPETENCE IN ADULT DOGS

Body weight, body size
Obesity
Reproductive status
Reproductive hormone sensitivity
Effects of aging on urethral function
Bladder neck position
Urethral length
Urethral or vaginal conformation
Vaginal abnormalities
Cystourethritis

uterine stump remaining following ovariohysterectomy created interference at the level of the bladder neck or proximal urethra. Investigators suggested that adhesions between the stump and bladder neck altered the position and function of urethral sphincter mechanisms.[46]

(b). Because many neutered dogs with sphincter incompetence respond to reproductive hormone administration, hormone deficiency was considered a likely factor in the development of incontinence. However, serum hormone alterations have not been detected in incontinent dogs,[119] and many neutered animals do not become incontinent. Furthermore, some incontinent animals do not respond to hormone supplementation.

(c). Reduced urethral closure pressures documented by urethral pressure profilometry have confirmed poor urethral contractile tone in many incontinent animals.[67,119,124]

(d). The effects of aging on urethral musculature are questionable. Urethral pressure profile measurements change with age in women[126] and in older, multiparous dogs[123]; however, in a larger group of adult dogs, urethral closure pressures did not seem to be affected by increasing age.[11]

(e). Lower urinary tract conformation may play a role in urethral incompetence.

- (1′). The urethra of incontinent female dogs was found by retrograde vaginourethrography to be shorter than that in continent female dogs in a series of 60 dogs.[66] Functional urethral lengths determined by urethral pressure profilometry may also be short in incontinent animals; however, functional urethral length does vary with body size, and comparisons may be difficult.
- (2′). In a series of female dogs evaluated radiographically, incontinent dogs were more likely to have a urethral conformation in which the proximal urethra deviated dorsally relative to the pubis; continent dogs typically had a urethral conformation in which the urethral axis remained parallel to the pubis.[57]
- (3′). Bladder neck position may play a role in urinary incontinence. Caudal displacement of the bladder neck has been observed in incontinent females, and clinicians theorize that this finding may be associated with a short urethra and poor urethral tone, or an abnormal response to abdominal pressure changes. If the bladder neck is intrapelvic, increases in intra-abdominal pressure may be transmitted to the bladder body and not to the bladder neck, increasing intravesicular pressure and causing urine leakage.
  - (a′). In a retrospective series of contrast radiographic findings, 10 of 17 dogs with a pelvic location of the bladder neck were incontinent. Of 57 dogs with urinary incontinence, 18 had a pelvic bladder.[4]
  - (b′). A subsequent experimental study demonstrated that bladder neck position varied with bladder distention in dogs and questioned the significance of pelvic bladder location in the incontinent animal.[77,89,90]
  - (c′). Measurement of bladder neck position in relation to the cranial brim of the pubis was completed in a series of 60 female dogs evaluated by retrograde vaginourethrography. Mean bladder neck position was caudad to the cranial brim of the pubis in incontinent females, whereas mean bladder neck position was 1.5 cm craniad to the brim in continent females.[66]
- (4′). Urinary incontinence has been an inconsistent finding in dogs with vaginal anomalies.
  - (a′). Urinary incontinence was observed in 12 of 22 dogs with vestibulovaginal stenoses in 1 series[73]; incontinence was not ob-

served in another series of 13 dogs undergoing surgical correction of vaginal anomalies.[141]

(b′). A similar frequency of vestibulovaginal stenoses was observed in a group of dogs with urinary incontinence attributed to urethral incompetence and a group of continent females.[66]

(c′). Urinary incontinence associated with vaginal anomalies has been attributed to pooling of urine craniad to vaginal strictures, persistent urinary tract infection, and concurrent urethral dysfunction.

(d′). Vaginal anomalies were observed in 12 of 33 dogs with urethral incompetence documented by urethral pressure profilometry and subsequently managed with phenylpropanolamine. Dogs with vaginal anomalies in this group tended to develop incontinence at a younger age and at a shorter interval after ovariohysterectomy than did dogs without vaginal anomalies. Response to therapy was also somewhat less favorable in dogs with vaginal anomalies.[85]

(f). Other causes of urethral dysfunction include cystourethritis and infiltrative diseases of the urethra.

(g). Management of urethral incompetence may include elimination of urinary tract inflammation and pharmacologic or surgical manipulation to increase urethral contractile tone.

4. Mixed disorders of micturition are common in humans[14] and probably occur in small animals. Reduced urinary bladder storage function may be observed in addition to urethral incompetence; functional disorders may be observed along with anatomic abnormalities or mechanical obstruction.

5. Miscellaneous disorders.

a. Prostate disorders are the most common cause of urinary incontinence in adult male dogs.[60,64]

(1). Urinary incontinence has been associated with suppurative inflammation, cystic hyperplasia, squamous metaplasia, and neoplasia of the prostate gland in dogs. Clinical experience suggests that urinary incontinence may be more likely in dogs with prostatic neoplasia, probably because of partial obstruction or severe interference with the prostatic urethra.

(2). Prostatic disease may contribute to many different types of disorders of micturition, including inflammatory cystitis or urethritis, urethral incompetence, detrusor instability, urethral spasm, or partial obstruction with overflow incontinence and detrusor atony.[21,51]

(3). In an experimental group of healthy male dogs, mildly reduced urethral closure pressures were observed following total prostatectomy; however, clinical incontinence was not observed.[22]

(4). A high incidence (93%) of urinary incontinence was observed in a prospective series of 14 dogs undergoing prostate surgery. Urethral incompetence and detrusor instability were documented by urodynamic measurements. Response to alpha-agonist administration in dogs with urethral incompetence was poor.[21]

(5). In another series of 11 dogs with clinical prostate disease, only 3 exhibited incontinence following prostatectomy, 2 of which were incontinent prior to prostatectomy.[51]

b. Urinary incontinence associated with feline leukemia virus.

(1). Idiopathic urinary incontinence in cats, characterized by intermittent urine leakage and small residual urine volumes, has been associated with feline leukemia virus infection.[16,18,86]

(2). In a review of 11 cats with urinary incontinence of undetermined origin, 9 of 9 cats tested positive for feline leukemia virus. Other signs of illness were reported in many of the cats, including anorexia, weight loss, vomiting, ptyalism, polydipsia, infertility, abortion, and neonatal kitten death.[16]

(3). Anisocoria, a possible indication of multifocal autonomic dysfunction, was a common physical finding.[16]

(4). Detrusor instability was identified by cystometrographic measurements in one feline leukemia–positive cat with urinary incontinence. This cat exhibited urinary incontinence when walking, and responded well to anticholinergic therapy.[86]

However, cystometrographic findings in another cat with feline leukemia virus were normal.[16]

(5). Whether or not urinary dysfunction may develop in association with other potentially neurotropic viral infections, such as feline immunodeficiency virus, is not known at this time.

VI. APPROACH TO DIAGNOSIS

A. The diagnosis of micturition disorders relies primarily on the clinical skills of history, physical examination, and observation. Specific points to be addressed during the clinical evaluation and the use of ancillary diagnostic procedures are given in this section and Table 37–4.

B. Signalment.

1. Young animals are more likely to have congenital anatomic or neurologic abnormalities; older animals may be more likely to have acquired dysfunction or underlying urologic or systemic disease.
2. Neutered animals may be more likely to have urethral incompetence responsive to reproductive hormone, particularly if urinary incontinence is observed within 2 to 3 years following neutering.
3. Disorders of micturition in intact males are frequently a result of prostate disease.
4. In cats, neurologic injuries or congenital anatomic abnormalities are the most common causes of urinary incontinence, but functional abnormalities are encountered.

C. Points to address in a problem-specific history.

1. Reproductive status and time of neutering.
2. Characterization of any previous urinary problems.
3. Characterization of voiding, including frequency, posture, urine stream, and urine volume.
4. Characterization of urine, including color, smell, presence of blood.
5. Pattern of urinary incontinence, if present.
   a. Continuous or intermittent?
   b. Small volumes or large?
   c. Normal urine or abnormal?
   d. During resting or during activity or movement?
   e. Positional?
6. Previous traumatic injuries to spine, pelvis, tail, limbs?
7. Difficulties walking, standing, defecating?
8. Previous medical problems and medications administered?
9. Estimated daily water consumption, if possible.

D. Physical examination of the animal with urinary incontinence.

1. General appearance, including attitude, mental status, ambulation, gait, and conformation.
2. Examination of external genitalia for conformational abnormalities, lesions, masses, urine staining.
3. Abdominal palpation focusing on urinary bladder size and degree of tone or firmness, presence of pelvic masses, pain.
4. Digital rectal palpation to assess anal tone, prostate and prostatic urethra in males, pelvic canal, urethra, and bladder neck in females.
5. Digital vaginal examination should be performed in females to evaluate conformation and to detect vaginal bands, strictures, masses.

E. Neurologic assessment.

1. Because neurologic disruption accounts for many disorders of micturition, an assessment of spinal and peripheral nerve integrity is imperative in the initial evaluation of animals with micturition disorders.
2. A brief assessment of the caudal spine and innervation to the hindquarters can be made in animals without obvious evidence of neurologic dysfunction.
   a. Pudendal nerve integrity and sacral spinal cord reflex arcs can be assessed indirectly by assessing anal tone, perineal sensation, and bulbospongiosus reflexes. Pressure or a quick squeeze on the bulbis glandis in the male, or the

TABLE 37–4
STEPS IN THE DIAGNOSTIC EVALUATION OF DISORDERS OF MICTURITION IN SMALL ANIMALS

Signalment
History
  Characterization of voiding urine
  Pattern of incontinence
  Previous injuries, neurologic or urinary problems
  Medications administered
Physical examination
  Urinary bladder size, expressibility
  Vaginal/preputial conformation
  Rectal/vaginal examination
Neurologic evaluation
  Mental status
  Hindlimb function
  Tail tone, function
  Anal tone, genitoanal reflexes
  Lumbosacral palpation
Observation of micturition, including estimate or measure of residual urine volume
±Urethral catheterization (if dysuric voiding pattern is observed)
Urinalysis and urine sediment examination
Feline leukemia testing (cats)
±Complete blood count, biochemical panel
±Diagnostic workup for polyuria
±Radiographic procedures
  Plain: Further evaluation of bladder, prostate gland
  Contrast: Continuous incontinence, juvenile animals, postoperative incontinence
±Urodynamic procedures
Pharmacologic trials

vulva in the female, should elicit a visible contraction of the anal sphincter.

b. The sacral spinal cord can be further assessed by evaluating the tone and carriage of the tail and by palpating for lumbosacral pain. This is particularly important in animals known to have a high incidence of lumbosacral disc disease or degenerative disorders of the spinal cord associated with voiding difficulties.

c. The thoracolumbar spinal cord should be evaluated by palpation, proprioception and placing responses of the hindlimbs, and postural reactions if indicated.

3. Recall that disorders of higher centers, including the cerebrum, cerebellum, and midbrain, may also influence micturition.
4. If any subtle neurologic deficits are detected, a complete neurologic examination is indicated, to localize the lesion and plan further diagnostic procedures.

F. Observation.

1. Micturition should be observed, if possible. The urinary bladder should be palpated before voiding. Gentle attempts to express urine manually may be made.
2. The animal should be allowed to void independently; then the bladder should be palpated or catheterized, to determine residual volume. Normal residual volume in the dog is 0.2 to 0.4 mL/kg.[98]

G. Urinalysis.

1. A complete urinalysis should be performed to identify infection or inflammation of the lower urinary tract.
2. Specific gravity of randomly collected urine samples also gives some indication of urine-concentrating ability. If concentration is suboptimal, repeated specimens or further evaluation should be considered.
3. Culture and antibiotic susceptibility testing of urine should be completed if any inflammatory changes are noted or if clinical signs suggest urinary tract infection.

H. Other laboratory data, including a complete blood count and serum biochemical analyses, may be necessary if these findings indicate an underlying medical problem, polyuria, or renal insufficiency.

I. Testing for feline leukemia virus and feline immunodeficiency virus infection should be completed in all cats with urinary incontinence.

J. Radiography.

1. Survey radiography is of limited value in evaluation of most disorders of micturition; however, urinary bladder size, position, prostatic contour, and pelvic conformation may be evaluated. Radiodense urocystoliths or urethroliths may be identified on survey radiographs as well.
2. Contrast radiography may be more helpful if specific information is required about urinary tract or reproductive anatomy, urinary bladder conformation, wall thickness, and urethral characteristics.
3. Contrast radiography is recommended for diagnostic evaluation of the following conditions:
   a. Urinary incontinence or other abnormalities of micturition in juvenile animals.
   b. Continuous urinary incontinence or urine leakage from abnormal anatomic sites.
   c. Urinary incontinence in breeds with an increased incidence of anatomic abnormalities (e.g., ectopic ureters).
   d. Urinary incontinence or dysuria observed shortly after ovariohysterectomy or other surgical procedures.
4. Contrast radiographic techniques.
   a. Excretory urography may be utilized to evaluate the kidneys, ureters, ureteral terminations, and urinary bladder.
      (1). This technique is valuable in the identification of ectopic ureters and ureterovaginal or vesicovaginal fistulas and allows qualitative estimations of upper urinary tract function.
      (2). With fluoroscopy, or combined with negative contrast cystography, the technique usually reliably detects ectopic ureteral terminations; however, the excretory urogram may not be as sensitive as retrograde studies in some animals.
   b. Cystourethrography allows visualization of the urinary bladder, bladder neck, and proximal urethra. Filling defects in the urinary bladder or bladder neck, as well as uroliths, urachal diverticula, and abnormalities of the bladder wall, may be identified.
   c. Retrograde vaginourethrography is an additional easily performed technique that has been particularly valuable in evaluation of dogs with urinary incontinence. The technique is also valuable in evaluation of the lower urinary tract when urethral catheterization is impossible or hazardous.[61,70,89,138]
      (1). Contrast material is infused into the vagina via a urinary catheter positioned in the vestibule. Once the vagina is filled, contrast material enters the urethra and urinary bladder.
      (2). Retrograde studies provide visualization of vaginal anomalies, urethral length, and urinary bladder neck position and allow detection of urethral mucosal lesions, urethral rupture, and urethral or bladder neck masses.
      (3). Retrograde filling of ectopic ureters, vesicovaginal fistulas , and ureterovaginal fistulas may also be observed.

TABLE 37–5
FEATURES OF URODYNAMIC PROCEDURES EMPLOYED IN SMALL ANIMALS

Procedure	Function Assessed	Indications	Limitations
Cystometrography	Urinary bladder storage and contractile function	Urinary incontinence Suspected detrusor instability Detrusor atony Neurogenic disorders Disorders affecting bladder capacity	Relies on artificial filling Detrusor function affected by outlet resistance Detrusor reflex may be in small animals
Urethral pressure profilometry	Urethral storage function	Urinary incontinence Urinary obstruction Dysuria, urethral spasm Preoperative evaluation of ectopic ureters	Assess storage phase only Affected by sedation Much variability in results in normal animals
Electromyography	Activity of striated muscle of urethra	Urinary incontinence Neurogenic disorders Perioperative evaluations Dysuria, suspected dyssynergia	Subject to artifact Affected by sedation
Uroflowmetry	Urine flow characteristics, outlet resistance	Dysuria Urinary incontinence Detrusor atony Suspected dyssynergia	Flow measurement cumbersome Interpretation relies on other urodynamic results
Evoked potentials, electromyelography	Neurologic integrity of micturition, sacral reflexes	Neurogenic disorders Refractory detrusor atony or urinary incontinence	Availability limited Sophisticated equipment required

(4). An alternative method of retrograde identification of ectopic ureters involves catheterization of the urinary bladder and injection of contrast material as the catheter is slowly withdrawn through the urethra. If the ureter empties into the urethra, contrast material may fill the ureter as the catheter passes the urethral termination.

VII. URODYNAMIC PROCEDURES

A. General information and indications.

1. Urodynamic procedures are specialized diagnostic studies that objectively measure various facets of micturition. They may be used to help to characterize dysfunction (Table 37–5).[3,81,118,135]
2. Urodynamic evaluation is available at many veterinary teaching hospitals and is indicated in animals with disorders of micturition when the diagnosis is in doubt, multiple abnormalities are suspected, or an animal does not respond to appropriate trial medical management.
3. Urodynamic procedures are also valuable in the evaluation of urinary bladder and urethral function when anatomic abnormalities, such as ectopic ureters or vaginal anomalies, are present.[84,118]
4. Urodynamic procedures applied in the evaluation of animals with micturition disorders include cystometrography (CMG), urethral pressure profilometry (UPP), electromyography (EMG), and urine flow studies (uroflowmetry).[109]
5. General limitations of urodynamic procedures include the need for specialized recording instruments and personnel familiar with performance of the procedures.
6. Many clinical and investigational applications of urodynamic procedures have contributed to the understanding of lower urinary tract disorders in veterinary medicine.

B. Cystometrography (CMG).

1. Urinary bladder capacity, elasticity, and contractile function can be objectively evaluated by CMG. CMG may also be combined with urine flow measurements.[96,111,118]
2. The cystometrogram is completed by recording the pressure within the urinary bladder as the bladder is slowly distended with air, carbon dioxide, saline, or water. A graph of intravesicular pressure versus volume infused provides a curve depicting the filling and contractile phases of micturition.[3,96,111]
3. In normal dogs and cats, intravesicular pressure rises slowly until a threshold volume and pressure are reached. At this point, the slope of the filling phase may increase just before the sharp peak of a detrusor contraction.[111]
4. Variables identified on a standard cystometrogram include: (Fig. 37–1).[112]

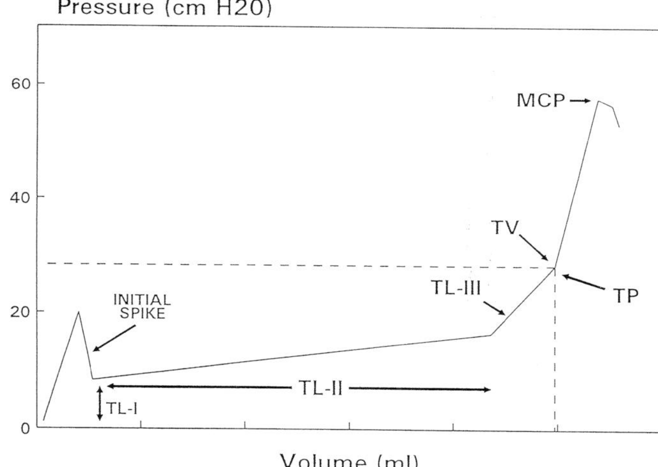

FIG. 37-1. Schematic representation of a typical cystometrographic recording. TL-I = Tonus limb I, initial intravesicular pressure; TL-II = tonus limb II; TL T-III = tonus limb III; TV = threshold volume; TP = threshold pressure; MCP = maximum contractile pressure. (From Lane IF, Barsanti JA. Urinary incontinence. In: August JR, ed. *Consultations in Feline Internal Medicine*. 2nd ed. Philadelphia, Pennsylvania: WB Saunders; 1994:377).

a. Tonus limb I (TL-I or T-I); the initial intravesicular pressure measured following initiation of infusion.
b. Tonus limb II (TL-II or T-II); the slope of the filling phase from T-I to threshold, expressed as change in pressure per 100 ml infused.
c. Tonus limb III (TL-III or T-III); the sharp change in slope observed in some cystometrographic recordings just prior to the contractile peak.
d. Threshold volume (TV) and threshold pressure (TP); volume infused and pressure recorded at which T-III is observed or a detrusor reflex is initiated.
e. Maximum contractile pressure (MCP); maximum pressure observed during the sharp, sustained pressure peak of a detrusor contraction.

5. Large filling volumes and the lack of a sustained contractile peak are evidence of a hypocontractile (or hypercompliant) urinary bladder or of detrusor atony.
6. Reduced threshold volumes and threshold pressures may represent reduced urinary bladder elasticity or detrusor instability.
7. Indications for cystometrography in small animals include:
   a. Neurogenic disorders of micturition in which contractile function is in question.
   b. Suspected bladder atony.
   c. Refractory urinary incontinence.
   d. Assessment of functional storage capacity in animals with multiple disorders, urinary bladder damage, or ectopic ureters.
8. Interpretation.
   a. The primary advantages of CMG are its abilities to evaluate detrusor reflex function during storage and to rule out detrusor instability.[105]
   b. Overinterpretation of detrusor function or lack thereof must be avoided, because detrusor contraction is a function of both bladder contractile strength and outflow resistance.[101]
   c. Women and female dogs often produce urine flow without significant changes in intravesicular pressure; detrusor contractile strength may erroneously appear absent or reduced.[101]
9. Disadvantages and potential pitfalls of CMG.[44,81,101,107,111,129]
   a. The requirement for controlled filling rates and sophisticated recording equipment limits availability.
   b. Urinary catheters, whether transurethral or percutaneous, may interfere with the study.
   c. Filling of the urinary bladder during CMG is artificial and may not exactly mimic natural filling. The rate of filling of the urinary bladder also may affect CMG measurements, and urinary bladder capacity is often underestimated.
   d. Sedation is usually required and may affect results.[19,76,112]
   e. Sensation of filling and voluntary control of detrusor contractions are difficult to assess in animals.
   f. Detrusor contractions are frequently inhibited in animals, despite sedation.
   g. Intra-abdominal pressures influence recorded intravesicular pressure. Ideally, intra-abdominal pressures are recorded simultaneously via rectal or vaginal transducers and subtracted.
10. Since adaptation of the technique for small animals,[112] CMG has been applied to the evaluation of urinary bladder physiology and dysfunction.
   a. Results of transurethral air cystometry in dogs with several different sedative regimens were reported; xylazine with atropine was considered optimal.[76] Reasonable results were also observed with use of oxymorphone/acepromazine for sedation.[19]
   b. Cystometrographic measurements obtained via percutaneously placed transabdominal catheters were combined with urine flow measurements to provide more complete micturition studies in dogs.[101-103]
   c. Transabdominal cystometrographic measurements combined with EMG recordings of external urethral sphincter muscles in cats provided characterization of sphincter activity during filling and voiding in normal cats.[127]
   d. Cystometrographic measurements were utilized to characterize idiopathic detrusor insta-

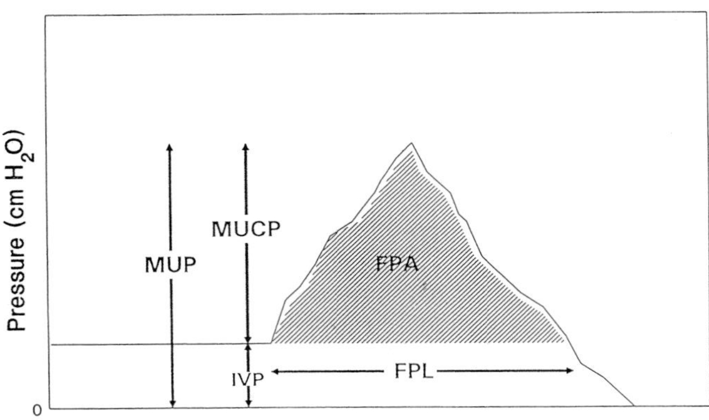

FIG. 37-2. Schematic representation of a typical urethral pressure profile in a female dog. IVP = intravesicular pressure; MUP = maximal urethral pressure; MUCP = maximal urethral closure pressure; FPL = functional profile length. (Modified from Lane IF, et al. Evaluation of results of preoperative urodynamic measurements in dogs with ectopic ureters: nine cases (1990-1992). *J Am Vet Med Assoc.* (In press.)

bility in two dogs and a cat with urinary incontinence.[86]

e. Cystometrographic measurements were also used to confirm optimal urinary bladder filling in an evaluation of cystographic technique in dogs.[89]

11. Additional potential applications of CMG in small animals include evaluation of pharmacologic agents affecting bladder storage capacity or detrusor contractility, and assessment of detrusor function and filling in other lower urinary tract disorders, such as inflammatory diseases.

C. Urethral pressure profilometry (UPP).

1. Objective measurements of urethral resistance may be obtained by UPP.[26,41,54,56,118,123,124]
2. Intraurethral pressure measurements are made by recording resistance to infusion of fluid through a urinary catheter or via catheter-mounted transducers.
3. The profile is completed by plotting pressures measured along the length of the urethra.
4. With a controlled rate of catheter withdrawal, a plot of pressure versus length is made, and measurement of functional urethral length, as well as of maximal urethral pressures, is possible.
5. Variables identified from standard UPP (Fig. 37–2).[3,123]
   a. Intravesicular pressure (IVP), defined as the initial resting pressure measured with the catheter tip remaining in the urinary bladder.
   b. Maximum urethral pressure (MUP), defined as the maximum pressure observed along the urethral pressure profile.
   c. Maximum urethral closure pressure (MUCP), defined as the maximum pressure gradient observed above resting bladder pressure, i.e., MUP minus IVP.
   d. Functional profile length (FPL) or functional urethral length (FUL), defined as the length of profile in which urethral pressure exceeds initial IVP.
   e. Additional variables that may be measured include functional profile area (FPA), the area under the curve generated by the urethral closure pressure, and location of the peak closure pressure (proximal urethra, distal urethra).
6. Indications for UPP in small animals.
   a. Diagnostic evaluation of urinary incontinence.
   b. Localization of urethral obstructions.
   c. Identification of increased urethral resistance or urethral spasm.
   d. Assessment of urethral responses to pharmacologic agents.
   e. Evaluation of urethral function in dogs with anatomic abnormalities, such as ectopic ureters and vaginal anomalies.
   f. Preoperative and postoperative evaluation of surgical procedures that manipulate urethral function or length.
7. The primary advantages of UPP are its simplicity and its ability to provide a graphic image of urethral characteristics.
8. Disadvantages or potential pitfalls of UPP.[44,81,108,123,135]
   a. Pressure recording capabilities and, ideally, a mechanized withdrawal device are required.
   b. The procedure assesses the urethra in the storage phase only.
   c. Urethral resistance may be affected by sedation, infection, inflammation, or bladder disease.
   d. The recording urinary catheter may interfere with urethral dynamics and recordings.
   e. Urethral measurements may vary considerably in normal and abnormal individuals.
   f. Many sources of error may affect measurements, including filling of the bladder, the rate of saline perfusion, catheter size, and position and orientation of catheter sensors.
9. Many varied applications of UPP have been described in small animals.
   a. The saline perfusion technique for UPP was described and reference measurements for healthy dogs under xylazine sedation were given by Rosin and co-workers in 1980.[123]
   b. Clinical application of UPP, including documentation of urethral incompetence and urethral obstruction in dogs, was described later.[124]
   c. Nonsedated UPP was compared to xylazine-sedated UPP in dogs. Significant reductions in MUP, MUCP, FPL, and EMG activity were noted following xylazine administration.[120]
   d. Nonsedated UPP was completed in 19 dogs

with urethral incompetence, and the clinical and UPP response to phenylpropanolamine administration was reported.[119]

e. Double-sensor microtip pressure transducer catheters were used to record simultaneous urinary bladder and urethral pressures in 50 continent and 50 incontinent female dogs. Urethral incompetence was defined by a drop in urethral pressure below bladder pressure during all or part of the profile.[67]

f. MUCPs recorded in 46 spayed female dogs with incontinence were generally lower than those of 44 healthy intact female dogs examined under general anesthesia.[11]

g. UPP findings in healthy intact male cats and intact and ovariohysterectomized cats have been described.[54,56]

h. UPP has been valuable in the critical evaluation of perineal urethrostomy in cats.[52-55,58,128]

  (1). Significant reductions in MUCP, localization of MUCP, and striated muscle activity were observed in healthy male cats 1 and 3 weeks following perineal urethrostomy.[54] Long-term follow-up of other cats was also reported, in which partial recovery of external urethral sphincter (EUS) activity was apparent over time.[55]

  (2). Urethral function following alternative dissection techniques in perineal urethrostomy have been compared. Preservation of the dorsal pudendal nerve branches was considered critical for preservation of urethral function in one study,[58] but not in another.[128] Effects of sedative agents on the UPP procedure may have affected the results of both studies, however.

  (3). UPP has been applied to clinically affected perineal urethrostomy cats with urinary incontinence for documentation of urethral dysfunction.[53]

i. The effect of pharmacologic agents on UPP in cats has been investigated in several studies, to define the autonomic responsiveness of the feline urethra and direct therapy of feline urethral disorders.[49,93,94,134]

j. UPP has been applied to the study of the effect of prostate disease and surgical manipulations of the prostate gland on urethral dynamics.

  (1). In an experimental group of normal dogs undergoing complete prostatectomy, minimal change in postoperative MUCP was observed.[22]

  (2). In the evaluation of a series of dogs with clinical prostate disease and postprocedural urinary incontinence, marked urodynamic alterations were often observed.[21]

k. UPP has been applied to the evaluation of urinary incontinence in dogs with ectopic ureters.[84,124] Preoperative UPP characteristics were used to predict the likelihood of postoperative continence or the need for additional medical management in a small series of dogs with ectopic ureters.[84]

l. Urethral pressure measurements were utilized to adjust placement and tightness of urethral prosthetic devices in three dogs with refractory urinary incontinence.[37]

D. Electromyography (EMG).

1. Activity in the striated muscle of the external urethral sphincter may be measured by standard EMG techniques.
2. Recording electrodes are inserted percutaneously or mounted on a urinary catheter used for other urodynamic procedures.[20,54,56,119,127] Skin patch pads, anal plug electrodes, and rectal catheter electrode methods have been described in humans.[3,107]
3. A qualitative assessment of the contribution of the EUS to the UPP can thus be identified and may be particularly valuable in the assessment of neurogenic innervation to the EUS.[6]
4. EMG of the EUS recorded during filling and voiding is also valuable in the evaluation of voiding dysfunction and detrusor-striated urethral dyssynergia.[3]
5. Indications for EMG in the urodynamic evaluation of small animals include neurogenic disorders of urethral function, incomplete or interrupted voiding with suspected dyssynergia, and urinary incontinence.
6. Applications of EMG in the urodynamic evaluation of small animals.
   a. Catheter-mounted electrodes have been used with UPP measurements in dogs[21,119,120] and cats,[54,56] and the effect of xylazine sedation on EMG activity has been described.[120]
   b. Percutaneous placement of needle electrodes for EMG recording of the EUS has been described in cats; EMG activity during filling and voiding in healthy cats was characterized.[127]
   c. Measurement of EMG activity of the EUS has been applied to the evaluation of perineal urethrostomy techniques to evaluate postoperative pudendal nerve function.[58,128]

E. Uroflowmetry.

1. Simple measurements of urine flow (uroflowmetry) are particularly valuable in the evaluation of humans, in whom progressive urinary obstructive disorders are common. The measurement of urine flow in small animals is more difficult, owing to the difficulty of "commanding" urine flow and collecting urine in an appropriate reservoir.
   a. Methods of recording urine flow include weight recording, electromagnetic fields, air displacement, rotating trays, acoustic methods, droplet dispersal analysis, and radionuclide techniques.[23,30,59]
   b. Variables identified in urine flow studies in-

clude peak flow rate, voiding time, time to peak flow, average urine flow, and voided volume.[3]

2. When IVP is measured along with urine flow, a more complete assessment of filling and voiding is possible. Premature leakage of urine, interrupted voiding, and dyssynergia may be detected.
3. Micturition studies incorporating IVP measurement and urine flow recording are described in dogs.[101,102] The technique has been used clinically to characterize urethral incompetence and outflow obstruction.[103]
4. Urine flow measurements are affected by position, abdominal straining, catheterization, and volume of fluid or urine voided; variations for age and gender are described in humans.
5. Indications for urine flow measurements in small animals include:
   a. Dysuria or obstructed voiding pattern.
   b. Urethral incompetence.
   c. Urinary bladder dysfunction or incomplete voiding.
   d. Neurogenic disturbances of micturition.
   e. Perioperative evaluation of surgical procedures affecting the lower urinary tract.

F. Other electrodiagnostic techniques may be applied at some institutions for the evaluation of neurologic innervation of the lower urinary tract.

1. Results of stimulation of urinary bladder or urethral receptors may be measured in recordings of pudendal nerve activity (electromyelography), to assess integrity of the sacral reflex arc.[25]
2. Evoked potentials or evoked responses may be measured from the anal sphincter muscle in response to local stimuli, such as stimulation of the perineal area, penis, or clitoris.[31,32,130] Scalp-derived cortical evoked responses are also described in humans.[50]
3. Evoked genitoanal reflexes have been performed clinically in cats with sacral injury, to help predict recovery of neurologic function.[31]

G. The potential applications of urodynamic procedures to small animals are unlimited. Areas of study may include the evaluation of new pharmacologic agents, surgical procedures, and mixed urinary disorders.

VIII. MANAGEMENT OF MICTURITION DISORDERS

A. General principles.

1. Potentially life-threatening abnormalities such as urine retention, azotemia, and fluid or electrolyte imbalances should be addressed immediately.
2. Primary neuromuscular, anatomic, or obstructive disorders should be identified and corrected if possible.
3. UTI or inflammation should be identified and appropriately managed before further pharmacologic manipulations are undertaken.

B. Pharmacologic manipulation of micturition (see Table 37–6).

1. Pharmacologic intervention is chosen when the disorder is solely functional or when supplemental manipulation is required for treatment of primary neurologic or muscular dysfunction. Ideally, pharmacologic agents are used for the minimum time necessary.
2. The choice of pharmacologic agents is based on the urinary bladder and urethral classifications described.
3. Since pharmacologic activity is directed at the end-organ (postganglionic receptors in the urinary bladder or urethra), pharmacologic agents are applied similarly for neurogenic and non-neurogenic disorders of micturition.
4. As most pharmacologic agents affect the lower urinary tract, initial doses should be at the low end of effective dose ranges and be gradually increased for the desired effect. Animals should be monitored carefully for adverse effects, as these agents rarely affect the urinary system alone.

C. Management of urinary bladder dysfunction.

1. Management of the atonic urinary bladder is designed to increase detrusor muscle contractile function and facilitate urinary bladder emptying.
   a. The urinary bladder should be kept as small as possible during therapy, to maximize recovery of the tight neuromuscular junctions between smooth muscle cells. Frequent manual expression, intermittent urinary catheterization, or a temporary indwelling urinary catheter may be required.
   b. Parasympathomimetic (cholinergic) agents are frequently employed to increase parasympathetic input and stimulate contraction.
      (1). Bethanechol chloride is administered in doses of 5 to 25 mg orally every 8 to 12 hours (dogs) or 1.25 to 7.5 mg orally every 8 to 24 hours (cats).[15,83,99]
      (2). Starting doses of 2.5 mg (cats), 5 mg (small dogs), and 10 mg (larger dogs) are recommended, and the dosage may be slowly increased in 2.5- to 5-mg increments until the desired effect is seen or adverse effects are noted.
      (3). Parenteral administration in doses of 2.5 to 10.0 mg subcutaneously (every 8 hours) have been recommended for dogs[83,125] and may be more effective than bethanechol administered orally. However, caution is advised because the possibility of adverse effects is markedly increased with this route of administration.
   c. Potential adverse effects of parasympathomimetic agents include ptyalism, lacrimation, abdominal cramping, vomiting, and diarrhea.[100]
   d. Parasympathomimetic agents are contraindicated in the presence of urinary or gastrointestinal obstruction and should be used with caution in animals with bronchial disease or ulcerative disease. Urethral resistance must be

TABLE 37–6
PHARMACOLOGIC AGENTS USED IN THE MANAGEMENT OF DISORDERS OF MICTURITION IN SMALL ANIMALS

Agent	Mechanism of Action	Recommended Dosage	Adverse Effects	Contraindications, Comments
Agents used to increase urinary bladder contractility				
Bethanechol	Parasympathomimetic; direct cholinergic activity	5–25 mg PO q8h (dogs)[15,83] 5–15 mg PO q8h (dogs)[99] 2.5–7.5 mg PO q8h (cats)[15] 1.25–5.0 mg PO q8h (cats)[99]	Nausea, vomiting, abdominal cramping, salivation	Urethral obstruction Gastrointestinal obstruction Pregnancy Phenoxybenzamine often used concurrently
Agents used to decrease urinary bladder contractility				
Propantheline	Parasympatholytic; acetylcholine blockade	7.5–15 mg PO q8h (dogs)[15] 15–30 mg PO q8h (dogs)[125] 5–7.5 mg PO q8h (cats)[99] 7.5 mg PO q72h (cats)[113]	Nausea, vomiting, constipation, increased ocular pressure, sedation	Glaucoma Tachycardia
Oxybutynin	Parasympatholytic, antispasmodic; detrusor smooth muscle relaxation	1.25–3.75 mg PO q8–12h (dogs) 5 mg PO q8–12 h (dogs)[83,125] 0.5–1.25 mg PO q8–12h (cats) 0.5 mg PO q12h (cats)[86]	Nausea, vomiting, urine retention, diarrhea, sedation	As for propantheline
Imipramine	Tricyclic antidepressant with anticholinergic, alpha- and beta-agonist effects; detrusor smooth muscle relaxation and urethral muscle contraction	5–15 mg PO q12h (dogs)[99] 2.5–5 mg PO q12h (cats)[99]	Seizures, tremors, tachycardia, hyperexcitability	Onset of action may be delayed

*See text for details on prescribing information
†Dosage from investigational application

Continued

minimized before initiating therapy. Administration of an alpha antagonist, striated muscle relaxant, or both may be required prior to initiating bethanechol therapy.[15,88,99,125]

e. The clinical efficacy of bethanechol in small animals remains questionable. Parasympathomimetic agents are most likely to be effective in conditions in which some neurologic input is preserved, such as partial neurologic lesions or acute overdistention of the urinary bladder.[15,42,43,48]

f. Alternative pharmacologic agents utilized to improve urinary bladder contractile function include cholinesterase inhibitors, beta antago-

TABLE 37–6 CONT'D
PHARMACOLOGIC AGENTS USED IN THE MANAGEMENT OF DISORDERS OF MICTURITION IN SMALL ANIMALS

Agent	Mechanism of Action	Recommended Dosage	Adverse Effects	Contraindications, Comments
Agents used to increase urethral resistance				
Diethylstilbestrol or stilbestrol	Reproductive hormone; may increase sensitivity or urethral alpha receptors	0.1–1.0 mg PO q24h for 5 d (approximately 0.2 mg/kg), followed by 0.1–1.0 mg PO q7d* (female dogs)[99,83] 0.04–0.06 mg PO q24h for 7 d, reduce dosage to 0.01 mg PO q4h (female dogs)[4,10]	Signs of estrus, bone marrow suppression	
Testosterone propionate	Reproductive hormone	2.2 mg /kg SC or IM q2–3d (male dogs)[83] 5–10 mg IM as needed (male cats)[18]	Aggression, prostatic disease, aggravation or perianal adenoma, perineal hernia	Prostatic disorders
Testosterone cypionate		2.2 mg/kg IM q30d (male dogs)[99] 200 mg IM q30d (male dogs)[83,17]		
Phenylpropanolamine	Alpha-agonists; urethral smooth muscle contraction	1.5 mg/kg PO q8h (dogs & cats)[99] 12.5–5.0 mg PO q8h (dog)[125] 12.5 mg PO q8h (cat)[83]	Anxiety, cardiac arrhythmias, anorexia, hypertension	Cardiac disease Hypertensive disease
Ephedrine	Alpha-agonist; urethral smooth muscle contraction	1.2 mg/kg PO q8h (dog)[99] 5–15 mg PO q8h (dog)[83] 2–4 mg/kg PO q8–12h (cat)[99] 2–4 mg PO q8h (cat)[83]	Anxiety, cardiac arrhythmias, hypertension	Same as phenylpropanolamine
Agents used to decrease urethral resistance				
Phenoxybenzamine	Alpha-antagonist; urethral smooth muscle relaxation	0.25 mg/kg PO q12h (dogs and cats)[15,99] 5–15 mg PO q12h (dogs) 2.5–10 mg PO q24h (cats)[18,87]	Hypotension Tachycardia Vomiting/diarrhea Increased intraocular pressure	Use with caution in cardiac patients

Continued

nists, dopamine antagonists, and selected prostaglandins.[99] None of these agents has received much attention in small animals.

2. Management of the hypercontractile urinary bladder, conversely, is designed to reduce contractile activity and improve urinary bladder accommodation.
   a. Sensory or neurogenic disorders that contribute to the dysfunction should be identified and addressed, if possible.
   b. Parasympatholytic (anticholinergic) agents are administered to alleviate clinical signs of urinary incontinence or pollakiuria.
      (1). Propantheline is a readily available anticholinergic agent. Recommended doses range from 5.0 to 7.5 mg as needed for cats (frequency required varies from every 8 hours to every 2 to 3 days) and 7.5 to 30 mg every 12 hours for dogs. Starting doses of 7.5 to 15 mg are recommended for dogs.[86,99,113]
      (2). Oxybutynin is an anticholinergic agent with the added properties of antispasmodic and smooth muscle relaxant actions. Doses of approximately 0.2 mg/kg orally appear effective in dogs and cats. Total doses of 0.5 to 1 mg every 8 to 12 hours are recommended for cats and small dogs; 1.25 to 5 mg every 8 to 12 hours is usually effective for larger dogs.[86]
   c. Potential adverse effects of anticholinergic agents include drowsiness, ileus, vomiting, constipation, and urine retention and often are dose related. Glaucoma is an absolute contraindication to the use of anticholinergic agents.[83,99]
   d. Tricyclic antidepressants, with their varied pharmacologic actions, are recommended for women with both urge and stress incontinence.
      (1). These agents possess anticholinergic, antihistaminic, sedative, and neurotransmitter effects.[91]
      (2). Both the anticholinergic effects and mild

TABLE 37–6 CONT'D
PHARMACOLOGIC AGENTS USED IN THE MANAGEMENT OF DISORDERS OF MICTURITION IN SMALL ANIMALS

Agent	Mechanism of Action	Recommended Dosage	Adverse Effects	Contraindications, Comments
Agents used to decrease urethral resistance				
Diazepam	Striated muscle relaxation; central nervous system depressive effect	0.2 mg/kg PO q8h (dogs)[99] 2–10 mg PO q8h (dogs)[83,125] 2.5–5.0 mg PO q8h or prn (cats)[18,87] 0.5 mg/kg IV† (cats)[94]	Sedation Vertigo Paradoxic excitement	Short duration of activity
Aminopromazine	Smooth muscle relaxation	2.2 mg/kg PO q12h (both)[100]		
Acepromazine	Urethral muscle relaxation by neuroleptic effect; alpha antagonism	0.1 mg/kg IV† (cats)[93] 1.1–2.2 mg/kg PO (cats)	Sedation Hypotension Seizures	Seizure disorders Cardiac patients
Dantrolene	Striated muscle relaxation; direct action	3–15 mg/kg PO q24h divided (dogs)[126] 0.5–1.0 mg/kg PO q8h (dogs)[100] 0.5–1.0 mg/kg PO q12h (cats)[100]	Weakness Hepatotoxicity	
Nicergoline	Alpha-antagonism; urethral smooth muscle relaxation	1–5 mg PO q8h (both)[99]		

stimulatory effects on lower urinary tract alpha and beta receptors facilitate urine storage.

(3). In small animals, imipramine is recommended in doses of 5 to 15 mg orally every 12 hours (dogs) and 2.5 to 5 mg orally every 12 hours (cats). Clinical effects of imipramine may not be observed for 5 to 7 days.[99]

(4). Imipramine has been particularly useful in humans with a fibrotic, poorly compliant urinary bladder.[139]

e. Alternative agents utilized to reduce urinary bladder contractility include beta agonists, calcium channel antagonists, and other smooth muscle relaxants.[99,139] These agents have been variably successful in humans with urge incontinence.

f. Long-term therapy is usually required for idiopathic detrusor instability.

D. Management of urethral dysfunction.

1. Management of excessive urethral resistance or detrusor-urethral dyssynergia.

a. Urethral resistance is a function of both smooth muscle and striated muscle. Both components may be manipulated pharmacologically to reduce urethral tone.

b. Smooth muscle relaxation is best achieved by administration of alpha antagonists.

(1). Phenoxybenzamine has been the most reliable agent for this purpose and is administered in doses of approximately 0.25 mg/kg[99] (2.5 to 5 mg orally every 12 to 24 hours in cats and 5 to 20 mg orally every 12 hours in dogs).

(2). Potential adverse effects of alpha antagonists include hypotension, reflex tachycardia, and gastrointestinal irritation. Phenoxybenzamine and other adrenergic agents should be avoided or used cautiously in animals with cardiovascular disease.[99]

c. Striated muscle relaxants, such as diazepam, may be used in addition to alpha antagonists and may be indicated for patients with upper motor neuron lesions in which striated muscle activity is likely to be uninhibited.

(1). Diazepam has a short duration of action and is therefore administered several times daily. It is primarily used to facilitate voluntary bladder emptying or manual expression of the bladder.

(2). Approximate dosages of oral diazepam are 2.5 to 5.0 mg orally every 6 to 8 hours (cats)[87] and 2 to 10 mg orally every 6 to 8 hours (dogs).[83,125]

(3). The major side effect of diazepam is sedation, although vertigo and paradoxic excitement occasionally are observed.[99]

(4). Other skeletal muscle relaxants that may reduce urethral resistance include baclofen, dantrolene, and calcium channel inhibitors. Use of these agents in small animals has been limited.[95,99,134]

d. The alpha-blockade and tranquilizing effects of the phenothiazine acepromazine have led some clinicians to use this agent for relaxation of the urethra, particularly following urethral obstruction in cats. Intravenously administered acepromazine was effective in reducing preprostatic and prostatic urethral pressures in anesthetized male cats in one experimental study.[93] If sedation and cardiovascular effects are minimal, this drug may be valuable in the short-term management of functional urethral obstruction or spasm.

e. Although long preferred as a sedative for urodynamic studies in animals, the sedative xylazine appears to consistently reduce urethral pressures measured in dogs and cats. Although xylazine is a peripheral alpha agonist, its central alpha$_2$-agonist properties probably account for this urethral response. The sedative and cardiovascular effects of xylazine limit its therapeutic applications.[21,94,120]

f. Urethral pressure profilometry has been used to help to delineate the actions of pharmacologic agents on the urethra of male cats.

(1). Antagonism of alpha receptors with the intravenous administration of prazocin, phenoxybenzamine, and acepromazine results in some reduction in preprostatic urethral pressures.[49,94]

(2). The skeletal muscle relaxant diazepam may reduce prostatic urethral pressures[93]; diazepam had no effect on urethral pressure of cats in another study.[134] Dantrolene, a direct-acting skeletal muscle relaxant, more effectively reduced prostatic, postprostatic, and penile urethral pressures.[134]

2. Management of urethral incompetence.

a. General principles.

(1). Urinary tract infections (UTI) should be identified and treated appropriately before initiation of therapy with pharmacologic agents.

(2). Polyuria, if present, should be evaluated. Reversible disorders should be corrected, if possible.

(3). Weight reduction should be recommended for obese animals.

(4). If incontinence is severe, general cleansing and clipping of hair should be encouraged to improve hygiene.

b. Pharmacologic manipulation.

(1). Reproductive hormone administration.

(a). Estrogens affect the urethra in several

ways, including enhancement of mucosal characteristics, urethral collagen content, and vascularity. Estrogen administration also appears to increase the density and sensitivity of alpha receptors in the bladder neck and urethra.

(b). Diethylstilbestrol (DES) and stilbestrol are effective and reasonably safe choices for female dogs with urethral incompetence.

(1′). DES is administered in doses of 0.1 to 1.0 mg orally daily for 5 to 7 days, followed by a similar dose every 5 to 14 days. The dosage is adjusted to be the minimum required for acceptable continence and client compliance. Cumulative doses greater than 1 mg per week are avoided.[99]

(2′). Daily estrogen therapy, using minimal dosages of DES or stilbestrol, also has been recommended. The protocol includes starting doses of 0.04 to 0.06 mg orally administered daily for 1 week then reduced at weekly intervals to 0.01 mg per day. After 4 weeks, the treatment is discontinued; a residual effect may be observed. If urinary incontinence recurs rapidly, 0.01 to 0.02 mg per day may be administered indefinitely.[10]

(3′). Potential side effects of estrogen administration include bone marrow suppression, alopecia, behavior changes, and signs of estrus.[99] Estrogen supplementation also may be dangerous for animals with immune-mediated diseases.

(4′). Although the risk of bone marrow suppression with these protocols is minimal, intermittent monitoring of a complete blood count is recommended for animals receiving estrogen therapy.

(5′). Administration of estrogen to cats is not recommended.[99]

(c). Testosterone may be administered to males with acquired urethral incompetence.

(1′). Testosterone propionate may be administered for short-term effects. Injections may be required every 2 to 3 days. Longer-lasting activity may be obtained with repository preparations, such as testosterone cypionate or testosterone enanate; followup injections are administered every 30 to 60 days, as required.

(2′). Doses of 2.2 mg/kg intramuscularly are recommended.[99] Doses up to 200 mg intramuscularly may be required in some cases.[17]

(3′). In neutered male cats, 5 to 10 mg testosterone propionate has been administered, with variable success.[16]

(4′). Significant potential adverse effects include behavior changes, aggression, prostate disease, perianal adenomas, and perineal hernias.[99]

(5′). Because of the potential for abuse in humans, testosterone compounds currently are controlled substances in the United States.

(2). Alpha-adrenergic agonists act at urethral alpha receptors to stimulate urethral smooth muscle contractile tone.

(a). Effective doses of phenylpropanolamine in dogs range from 1 to 2 mg/kg orally every 8 to 12 hours.[99,119] Ephedrine or pseudoephedrine is administered in doses of 5 to 15 mg orally every 8 hours[83] or 1 to 2 mg/kg every 12 hours.[10]

(b). Alpha agonists, like estrogens, can be slowly reduced to the minimum amount and frequency of administration required. Young animals with congenital urethral incompetence initially may require doses as large as 3 mg/kg.[84]

(c). Potential side effects of alpha agonists include anxiety, hyperactivity, anorexia, tachycardia, hypertension, and gastrointestinal upset.[99]

(d). Alpha-adrenergic agonists are contraindicated in animals with cardiac disease, hyperthyroidism, and other hypertensive disorders, such as renal failure, diabetes mellitus, or hyperadrenocorticism.

(3). Combination therapy.

(a). A synergistic effect on urethral tone may be observed when alpha agonist administration is combined with reproductive hormone administration.[34] Starting regimens are similar to those described for each agent; the doses of each agent required for long-term maintenance frequently are smaller than those required if either drug were used alone.

(b). In some animals, poor urinary bladder storage function may contribute to the urinary incontinence observed with urethral incompetence. The combination of an anticholinergic agent with alpha agonist or reproductive hormone therapy may be valuable in these cases.

(c). Prophylactic or long-term antimicrobial administration may be required in some animals with recurrent or persistent UTI and refractory urinary incontinence.

c. Response to medical management in dogs with acquired urethral incompetence generally is good.[13,104,119,140]

(1). Resolution of incontinence was observed in close to 90% in several small groups of dogs treated with alpha agonists.[119,140]

(2). In another series of 57 dogs, good responses were reported in 73.7% of female dogs managed with alpha agonists and 64.7% of dogs managed with estrogens.[13]

(3). In a prospective group of 33 female dogs treated with phenylpropanolamine, dogs that responded best (complete continence) tended to develop incontinence at a later age and at a longer interval after ovariohysterectomy than did dogs that had incomplete or poor responses.[85]

(4). If urinary incontinence does not resolve with seemingly appropriate therapy, a thorough evaluation for exacerbating problems, such as UTI, polyuria, or subtle neurologic deficits, and re-evaluation of the diagnosis are in order.

d. If urinary incontinence that is attributed to urethral incompetence does not improve sufficiently following appropriate medical therapy, surgical management may be considered.

(1). The goals of surgical treatment of urethral incompetence are to increase urethral resistance by repositioning the urethra, increasing urethral pressure, or increasing urethral length.[65]

(2). A seromuscular urethral sling, fashioned from excessive tissue in the proximal urethra, was constructed to increase resistance in an adult dog with urethral dilation and urinary incontinence.[28]

(3). Artificial mesh "sphincters" encircling the urethra were implanted in three female dogs with refractory urethral incompetence; acceptable results were observed in two dogs.[37]

(4). Polytetrafluoroethylene (Teflon) deposits have been injected into the proximal urethral submucosa in dogs with refractory urinary incontinence. Of 22 dogs in which the procedure was performed, 36% became continent following 1 injection. An additional 41% became continent following a second injection, for an overall success rate of 77%.[12]

(5). Other endoscopic procedures have been described for the correction of stress incontinence in women.[82]

(6). Colposuspension techniques, which are designed to reposition the intrapelvic bladder neck into a more intra-abdominal position, have been performed in dogs.

(a). The procedure involves pulling the vagina craniad and anchoring the vaginal wall to the prepubic tendon at the level of the proximal urethra. Cranial movement of the vagina and urethra results in cranial displacement of the urinary bladder neck.[63,65] An excellent outcome following colposuspension was observed in approximately 50% of dogs in a large series, and some improvement was observed in close to 90%.[63]

(b). Cystourethropexy, a similar technique for repositioning the bladder neck and proximal urethra, has also been described.

(7). Other bladder neck reconstructive techniques designed to elongate and "tighten" congenitally short and dilated urethras have provided improvement or resolution of urinary incontinence in cats and dogs.[68]

REFERENCES

1. Abdel-Azim M, Sullivan M, Yalla SV. Disorders of bladder function in spinal cord disease. *Neurol Clin.* 1991;9:727–740.
2. Abdel-Rahman M, Galeano C, LaMarche J, Elhilali M. A new approach to the study of the voiding cycle in the cat. *Invest Urol.* 1981;18:475–478.
3. Abrams P, Feneley R, Torrens M. *Urodynamics.* Berlin: Springer-Verlag; 1983.
4. Adams WM, DiBartola SP. Radiographic and clinical features of pelvic bladder in the dog. *J Am Vet Med Assoc.* 1983;182:1212–1217.
5. Allen WE, Webbon PM. Two cases of urinary incontinence in cats associated with acquired vagino-ureteral fistulas. *J Small Anim Pract.* 1980;21:367–371.
6. Andersen JT, Bradley WE. Urethral pressure profilometry: Assessment of urethral function by combined intraurethral pressure and electromyographic recording. *J Urol.* 1977;118:423–427.
7. Andersson PO, Bloom SR, Mattiasson A, Uvelius B. Bladder vasodilation and release of vasoactive intestinal polypeptide

from urinary bladder of the cat in response to pelvic nerve stimulation. *J Urol.* 1987;138:671–673.

8. Anon. Standardization of terminology of lower urinary tract function. Fourth report: Neuromuscular dysfunction. *Urology.* 1981;17:618–620.
9. Appledoorn A, Lemmens P, Schrauwen E. Urinary incontinence due to urovagina. *Vet Rec.* 1990;126:121.
10. Arnold S. Diagnosis and treatment of urinary incontinence. *Nephrology and Urology Proceedings of the 16th Waltham/OSU Symposium.* Columbus, Ohio: 1992;75–79.
11. Arnold S. Relationship of incontinence to neutering. In: Kirk RW, ed. *Current Veterinary Therapy XI: Small Animal Practice.* Philadelphia, Pennsylvania: WB Saunders; 1992:875–877.
12. Arnold S, et al. Treatment of urinary incontinence in dogs by endoscopic injection of Teflon. *J Am Vet Med Assoc.* 1989;195: 1369–1374.
13. Arnold S, Arnold P, Hubler M, et al. Incontinentia urinae bei der kastriertem Hunden: Haufigkeit und Rassedisposition. *Schweiz Arch Tierheilkd.* 1989;131:259–263.
14. Awad SA, Gajewski JB, Katz NO, Acker-roy K. Final diagnosis and therapeutic implications of mixed symptoms of urinary incontinence in women. *Urology.* 1992;39:352–357.
15. Barsanti JA. Urinary incontinence. In: Lorenz MD, Cornelius LM, eds. *Small Animal Medical Diagnosis.* Philadelphia, Pennsylvania: JB Lippincott; 1987:343–355.
16. Barsanti JA, Downey R. Urinary incontinence in cats. *J Am Anim Hosp Assoc.* 1984;20:979–982.
17. Barsanti JA, Edwards PD, Losonsky J. Testosterone responsive urinary incontinence in a castrated male dog. *J Am Anim Hosp Assoc.* 1981;17:117–119.
18. Barsanti JA, Finco DR. Feline urinary incontinence. In: Kirk RW, ed. *Current Veterinary Therapy IX: Small Animal Practice.* Philadelphia, Pennsylvania: WB Saunders; 1987:1159–1163.
19. Barsanti JA, Finco DR, Brown J. Effect of atropine on cystometry and urethral pressure profilometry in the dog. *Am J Vet Res.* 1988;49:112–114.
20. Barsanti JA, Mahaffey MB, Crowell WA, Barber DL. Cystometry in dogs under oxymorphone and acepromazine restraint. *Am J Vet Res.* 1984;45:2152–2153.
21. Basinger RR, Rawlings CA, Barsanti JA, Oliver JE. Urodynamic alterations associated with clinical prostatic diseases and prostatic surgery. *J Am Anim Hosp Assoc.* 1989;25:385–392.
22. Basinger RR, et al. Urodynamic alterations after prostatectomy in dogs without clinical prostatic disease. *Vet Surg.* 1987;16: 405–410.
23. Bloom DA, Foster WD, McLeod DG. Cost effective uroflowmetry in men. *J Urol.* 1985;133:421–424.
24. Bradley WE, Timm GW. Physiology of micturition. *Vet Clin North Am.* 1974;4:487–499.
25. Bradley WE, Timm GW, Rockswold GL, Scott FB. Detrusor and urethral electromyelography. *J Urol.* 1975;114:891–894.
26. Brown M, Wickham JEA. The urethral pressure profile. *Br J Urol.* 1969;41:211–217.
27. Burnstock G. Innervation of bladder and bowel. *Neurobiology of Incontinence.* (Ciba Foundation Symposium 151.) New York, New York: John Wiley; 1990:2–26.
28. Bushby PA, Hankes GH. Sling urethroplasty for the correction of urethral dilatation and urinary incontinence. *J Am Anim Hosp Assoc.* 1980;16:115–118.
29. Chancellor MB, Kaplan SA, Blaivas JG. Detrusor-external sphincter dyssynergia. *Neurobiology of Incontinence.* (Ciba Foundation Symposium.) New York, New York: John Wiley; 1990: 195–213.
30. Chaudhuri TK, Fink S, Netto ICV, Palmer JDK. Correlation of radionuclide urodynamometric and clinical data in 20 men with urinary symptoms. *Urology.* 1991;38:43–46.
31. Cook JR, Oliver JE, Purinton PT. Measurement of anal and genitoanal reflexes in cats. *Am J Vet Res.* 1991;52:29–33.
32. Cook JR Jr, Oliver JE Jr, Purinton PT. Comparison of genitoanal and bulbospongiosus reflexes and measurement of penile nerve conduction velocity in cats. *Am J Vet Res.* 1992;52:24–28.
33. Cotard JP, Collas G, Leclere C. L'ectopie ureterale chez le chien a propos d'onze cas. *Rec Med Vet.* 1984;160:731–744.
34. Creed KE. Effect of hormones on urethral sensitivity to phenylephrine in normal and incontinent dogs. *Res Vet Sci.* 1983;34: 177–181.
35. Cullen WC, Fletcher TF, Bradley WF. Morphometry of the female feline urethra. *J Urol.* 1983;129:190–192.
36. Day DG, et al. Postoperative evaluation of renal function after surgical correction of a ureterovaginal fistula in a cat. *J Am Vet Med Assoc.* 1993;202:104–106.
37. Dean PW, Novotny MJ, O'Brien DP. Prosthetic sphincter for urinary incontinence: Results in three cases. *J Am Anim Hosp Assoc.* 1989;25:447–454.
38. deGroat WC. Central neural control of the lower urinary tract. *Neurobiol Incontinence.* 1990;151:27–56.
39. deGroat WC. Nervous control of the urinary bladder of the cat. *Brain Res.* 1975;87:201–211.
40. deGroat WC, Booth AM. Physiology of the bladder and urethra. *Ann Intern Med.* 1980;92:312–315.
41. Edwards L, Malvern J. The urethral pressure profile: Theoretical considerations and clinical application. *Br J Urol.* 1974;46: 325–336.
42. El-Salmy S, Downie JW, Awad SA. Bladder and urethral function and sensitivity to subcutaneously administered bethanechol in cats with chronic cauda equina lesions. *J Urol.* 1985;134:1011–1018.
43. El-Salmy S, Downie JW, Awad SA. Effect of acute selective sacral rhizotomy in cats on bladder and urethral function and the response to bethanechol chloride. *J Urol.* 1985;134: 795–799.
44. Evans AT, Felker JR, Shank A III, Sugarman SR. Pitfalls of urodynamics. *J Urol.* 1992;122:220–222.
45. Ewers RS, Holt PE. Urological complications following ovariohysterectomy in a bitch. *J Small Anim Pract.* 1992;33: 236–238.
46. Finco DR, Osborne CA, Lewis RE. Non-neurogenic causes of abnormal micturition in the dog and cat. *Vet Clin North Am (Small Anim Pract).* 1974;4:501–516.
47. Firlit FC, Smey P, King LR. Micturition urodynamic flow studies in children. *J Urol.* 1978;119:250–253.
48. Finkbeiner AE. Is bethanechol chloride clinically effective in promoting bladder emptying? *J Urol.* 1985;134:443–449.
49. Frenier SL, et al. Urethral response to alpha-adrenergic agonist and antagonist drugs in anesthetized male cats. *Am J Vet Res.* 1992;53:1161–1165.
50. Ganzer H, Madersbacher H, Rumpl E. Cortical evoked potentials by stimulation of the vesicourethral junction: Clinical values and neurophysiological considerations. *J Urol.* 1991; 146:118–123.
51. Goldsmid SE, Bellenger CR. Urinary incontinence after prostatectomy in dogs. *Vet Surg.* 1991;20:253–256.
52. Gregory CR. The effects of perineal urethrostomy on urethral function in male cats. *Compend Contin Ed Pract Vet.* 1987;9:895–899.
53. Gregory CR. Electromyography and urethral pressure profilometry; clinical application in male cats. *Vet Clin North Am.* 1984;14:567–574.
54. Gregory CR, et al. Electromyographic and urethral pressure profilometry: Assessment of urethral function before and after

perineal urethrostomy in cats. *Am J Vet Res.* 1984;45:2062–2065.

55. Gregory CR, Vasseur PB. Electromyographic and urethral pressure profilometry: Long-term assessment of urethral function after perineal urethrostomy in cats. *Am J Vet Res.* 1984;45:1318–1321.
56. Gregory CR, Willits NH. Electromyographic and urethral pressure evaluations: Assessment of urethral function in female and ovariohysterectomized female cats. *Am J Vet Res.* 1986;47:1472–1475.
57. Gregory SP, Parkinson TJ, Holt PE. Urethral conformation and positioning in relation to urinary incontinence in the bitch. *Vet Rec.* 1992;131:167–170.
58. Griffin DW, Gregory CR, Kitchell RL. Preservation of striated—muscle urethral sphincter function with use of a surgical technique for perineal urethrostomy in cats. *J Am Vet Med Assoc.* 1984;194:1057–1060.
59. Groshar D, et al. Radionuclide assessment of bladder outlet obstruction; a noninvasive method for measurement of voiding time, urinary flow rates and residual urine. *J Urol.* 1988;139:266–269.
60. Holt PE. Urinary incontinence in dogs and cats. *Vet Rec.* 1990;127:347–350.
61. Holt PE. Positive-contrast vaginourethrography for diagnosis of lower urinary tract disease. In: Kirk RW, ed. *Current Veterinary Therapy X; Small Animal Practice.* Philadelphia, Pennsylvania: WB Saunders; 1989:1142–1145.
62. Holt PE. Pathophysiology and treatment of urethral sphincter mechanism incompetence in the incontinent bitch. *Vet Internat.* 1992;3:15–26.
63. Holt PE. Long-term evaluation of colposuspension in the treatment of urinary incontinence due to incompetence of the urethral sphincter mechanism in the bitch. *Vet Rec.* 1990;127:537–542.
64. Holt PE. Urinary incontinence in the bitch due to sphincter mechanism incompetence; prevalence in referred dogs and retrospective analysis of sixty cases. *J Small Anim Pract.* 1986; 26:181–180.
65. Holt PE. Urinary incontinence in the bitch due to sphincter mechanism incompetence: Surgical treatment. *J Small Anim Pract.* 1985;26:237–246.
66. Holt PE. Importance of urethral length, bladder neck position and vestibulovaginal stenosis in sphincter mechanism incompetence in the incontinent bitch. *Res Vet Sci.* 1985;39:364–372.
67. Holt PE. Simultaneous urethral pressure profilometry: Comparisons between continent and incontinent bitches. *J Small Anim Pract.* 1988;29:761–769.
68. Holt PE. Surgical management of congenital urethral sphincter mechanism incompetence in eight female cats and a bitch. *Vet Surg.* 1993;22:98–104.
69. Holt PE, Gibbs C. Congenital urinary incontinence in cats: A review of 19 cases. *Vet Rec.* 1992;130:437–442.
70. Holt PE, Gibbs C, Latham J. An evaluation of positive contrast vaginourethrography as a diagnostic aid in the bitch. *J Small Anim Pract.* 1984;25:531–549.
71. Holt PE, Gibbs C, Pearson H. Canine ectopic ureter; a review of twenty-nine cases. *J Small Anim Pract.* 1982;23:195–208.
72. Holt PG, Long SE, Gibbs C. Disorders of urination associated with canine intersexuality. *J Small Anim Pract.* 1993;24:475–487.
73. Holt PE, Sayle B. Congenital vestibulo-vaginal stenosis in the bitch. *J Small Anim Pract.* 1981;22:67–75.
74. Jackson DA, Osborne CA, Brasmer TH, Jessen CR. Nonneurogenic urinary incontinence in a canine female pseudohermaphrodite. *J Am Vet Med Assoc.* 1978;172:926–929.
75. Janssens LAA, Janssens GHRR. Bilateral flank ovariectomy in the dog—surgical technique and sequelae in 72 animals. *J Small Anim Pract.* 1991;32:249–252.
76. Johnson CA, et al. Effects of various sedatives on air cystometry in dogs. *Am J Vet Res.* 1988;49:1525–1528.
77. Johnston GR, Osborne CA, Jessen CR, Feeney DA. Effects of urinary bladder distention on location of the urinary bladder and urethra of healthy dogs and cats. *Am J Vet Res.* 1986;47:404–415.
78. Kinn A, Lindskog M. Estrogens and phenylpropanolamine in combination for stress urinary incontinence in postmenopausal women. *Urology.* 1988;32:273–279.
79. Kiruluta HG, Downie JW, Awad SA. The continence mechanisms: The effect of bladder filling on the urethra. *Invest Urol.* 1981;18:460–465.
80. Klein LA. Urge incontinence can be a disease of bladder sensors. *J Urol.* 1988;139:1010–1014.
81. Kondo A. Status and tasks of today's urodynamics. *Urol Internat.* 1991;47:16–18.
82. Kursh ED, Ahgell AH, Resnicj MI. Evolution of endoscopic urethropexy: Seven-year experience with various techniques. *Urology.* 1991;37:428–431.
83. Labato MA. Disorders of micturition. In: Morgan R, ed. *Handbook of Small Animal Medicine.* 2nd ed. New York, New York: Churchill Livingstone; 1992:611–618.
84. Lane IF, Lappin MR, Seim HB. Predictive value of urodynamic measurements in the management of dogs with ectopic ureters (abstr). *J Vet Intern Med.* 1992;6:119.
85. Lane IF, Lappin MR. Unpublished data, 1994.
86. Lappin MR, Barsanti JA. Urinary incontinence secondary to idiopathic detrusor instability; cystometrographic diagnosis and pharmacologic management in 2 dogs and a cat. *J Am Vet Med Assoc.* 1987;191:1439–1442.
87. Lees GE, Moreau PM. Management of hypotonic and atonic bladders in cats. *Vet Clin North Am.* 1984;14:641–647.
88. Leveille R, Atilola MAO. Retrograde vaginocystography: A contrast study for evaluation of bitches with urinary incontinence. *Comp Contin Ed Pract Vet.* 1991;13:934–943.
89. Mahaffey MB, Barber DL, Bassanti JA, Crowell WA. Simultaneous double-contrast cystography and cystometry in dogs. *Vet Radiol.* 1984;25:254–259.
90. Mahaffey MB, Barsanti JA, Barber DL, Crowell WA. Pelvic bladder in dogs without urinary incontinence. *J Am Vet Med Assoc.* 1984;184:1477–1479.
91. Malkowicz SB, Wein AJ, Ruggieri MR, Levin RM. Comparison of calcium antagonist properties of antispasmodic agents. *J Urol.* 1987;138:667–670.
92. Mason LK, et al. Surgery of ectopic ureters: Pre- and postoperative radiographic morphology. *J Am Anim Hosp Assoc.* 1990; 26:73–79.
93. Marks SL, et al. The effects of phenoxy benzene and acepromazine maleate on urethral pressure profiles of anesthetized healthy male cats (abstr). *J Vet Intern Med.* 1993;7:122.
94. Mawby DI, Meric SM, Crichlow EC, Papich MG. Pharmacologic relaxation of the urethra in male cats; a study of the effects of phenoxybenzamine, diazepam, nifedipine and xylazine. *Can J Vet Res.* 1990;55:28–32.
95. McLaughlin R, Miller CW. Urinary incontinence after surgical repair of ureteral ectopia in dogs. *Vet Surg.* 1991;20:100–103.
96. Merrill DC, Bradley WE, Markland C. Air cystometry. I. Technique and definitions of terms. *J Urol.* 1971;106:678–681.
97. Michell AR. Ins and outs of bladder function. *J Small Anim Pract.* 1984;25:237–247.
98. Moreau PM. Neurogenic disorders of micturition in the dog and cat. *Comp Contin Ed Pract Vet.* 1982;4:12–22.

99. Moreau PM, Lappin MR. Pharmacologic manipulation of micturition. In: Kirk RW, ed. *Current Veterinary Therapy X; Small Animal Practice.* Philadelphia, Pennsylvania: WB Saunders; 1989:1214–1222.
100. Moreau PM, Lees GE. Incontinence, enuresis and nocturia. In Ettinger SJ, ed. *Textbook of Veterinary Internal Medicine.* 3rd ed. Philadelphia, Pennsylvania: WB Saunders; 1989;148–154.
101. Moreau PM, Lees GE, Gross DR. Simultaneous cystometry and uroflowmetry (micturition study) for evaluation of the caudal part of the urinary tract in dogs: Studies of the technique. *Am J Vet Res.* 1983;44:1769–1773.
102. Moreau PM, Lees GE, Gross DR. Simultaneous cystometry and uroflowmetry (micturition study) for evaluation of the caudal part of the urinary tract in dogs: Reference values for healthy animals sedated with xylazine. *Am J Vet Res.* 1983;44:1774–1781.
103. Moreau PM, Lees GE, Hobson HP. Simultaneous cystometry and uroflowmetry for evaluation of micturition in two dogs. *J Am Vet Med Assoc.* 1983;183:1084–1088.
104. Nendick PA, Clark WT. Medical therapy of urinary incontinence in ovariectomized bitches: A comparison of the effectiveness of diethylstolboestrol and pseudoephedrine. *Aust Vet J.* 1987;64:117–118.
105. Nordling J. Functional assessment of the bladder. In: *Neurobiology of Incontinence* (Ciba Foundation Symposium 151). New York, New York: John Wiley; 1990:139–155.
106. O'Brien DP. Disorders of the urogenital system. *Semin Vet Med Surg.* 1990;5:57–66.
107. O'Donnell PD. Pitfalls of urodynamic testing. *Urol Clin North Am.* 1991;18:257–267.
108. O'Handley P, Carrig CB, Walshaw R. Renal and ureteral duplication in a dog. *J Am Vet Med Assoc.* 1979;174:484–487.
109. Oliver JE. Urodynamic assessment. In: Oliver JE, Hoerlein BF, Mayhew IG, eds. *Veterinary Neurology.* Philadelphia, Pennsylvania: WB Saunders; 1987:180–184.
110. Oliver JE. Dysuria caused by reflex dyssynergia. In: Kirk RW, ed. *Current Veterinary Therapy VIII (Small Animal Pract).* Philadelphia, Pennsylvania: WB Saunders; 1983:1088–1089.
111. Oliver JE, Young WO. Air cystometry in dogs under xylazine-induced restraint. *Am J Vet Res.* 1973;34:1433–1435.
112. Oliver E Jr, Young WO. Evaluation of pharmacologic agents for restraint in cystometry in the dog and cat. *Am J Vet Res.* 1973;34:665–668.
113. Osborne CA, et al. Medical management of male and female cats with nonobstructive lower urinary tract disease. *Vet Clin North Am.* 1984;14:617–640.
114. Owen RR. Three case reports of ectopic ureters in bitches. *Vet Rec.* 1973;93:2–10.
115. Owen RR. Canine ureteral ectopia; a review; 1. Embryology and aetiology. *J Small Anim Pract.* 1973;14:407–417.
116. Pearson H, Gibbs C. Urinary incontinence in the dog due to accidental vagino-ureteral fistulation during hysterectomy. *J Small Anim Pract.* 1980;21:287–291.
117. Purinton PT, Oliver JE Jr. Spinal cord origin of innervation to the bladder and urethra of the dog. *Exp Neurol.* 1979;65:422–434.
118. Richter KP. Use of urodynamics in micturition disorders in dogs and cats. In: Kirk RW, ed. *Current Veterinary Therapy X; Small Animal Practice.* Philadelphia, Pennsylvania: WB Saunders; 1989:1145–1150.
119. Richter KP, Ling GV. Clinical response and urethral pressure profile changes after phenylpropanolamine in dogs with primary sphincter incompetence. *J Am Vet Med Assoc.* 1985;187:605–610.
120. Richter KP, Ling GV. Effects of xylazine on the urethral pressure profile of healthy dogs. *Am J Vet Res.* 1985;46:1881–1886.
121. Rigg DL, Zenoble RD. Neoureterostomy and phenylpropanolamine therapy for incontinence due to ectopic ureter in a dog. *J Am Anim Hosp Assoc.* 1983;19:237–241.
122. Rochlitz I. Feline dysautonomia (the Key-Gaskell or dilated pupil syndrome); a preliminary review. *J Small Anim Pract.* 1984;25:587–598.
123. Rosin A, Rosin E, Oliver JE. Canine urethral pressure profile. *Am J Vet Res.* 1980;41:1113–1116.
124. Rosin AE, Barsanti JA. Diagnosis of urinary incontinence in dogs: Role of the urethral pressure profile. *J Am Vet Med Assoc.* 1981;178:814–822.
125. Rosin AH, Ross L. Diagnosis and pharmacological management of disorders of urinary continence in the dog. *Comp Contin Ed Pract Vet.* 1981;3:601–608.
126. Rud T. Urethral pressure profile in continent women from childhood to old age. *Acta Obstet Gynecol Scand.* 1980;59:331–335.
127. Sackman JE, Sims MH. Electromyographic evaluation of the external urethral sphincter during cystometry in male cats. *Am J Vet Res.* 1990;51:1237–1241.
128. Sackman JE, Sims MH, Krahwinkel DJ. Urodynamic evaluation of lower urinary tract function in cats after perineal urethrostomy with minimal and extensive dissection. *Vet Surg.* 1991;20:55–60.
129. Schmidt RA. Urodynamics simplified. *Urology.* 1991;37:449–454.
130. Schou J, Overgaard K, Vedel P, Nordling J. Evoked potentials in urology: A method to make an exact diagnosis? *Urol Internat.* 1991;47:153–155.
131. Seidenberg L, Knecht CD. Ectopic ureter in the dog. *J Am Vet Med Assoc.* 1971;159:876–877.
132. Smith CW, Stowater JL, Kneller SK. Ectopic ureter in the dog; a review of cases. *J Am Anim Hosp Assoc.* 1990;17:245–248.
133. Stone EA, Mason LK. Surgery of ectopic ureters: Types, method of correction, and postoperative results. *J Am Anim Hosp Assoc.* 1990;26:81–88.
134. Strater IM, Knowlen GG, Speth RC, Marks SL. The effect of succinylcholine, diazepam and dantrolene on the urethral pressure profile of the anesthetized, healthy intact male cat (abstr.). *Proceedings of the ACVIM Forum.* Washington DC; 1992:823.
135. Tanagho EA. Evolution of urodynamic studies. *Urol Internat.* 1991;47:5–8.
136. Thrusfield MV. Association between urinary incontinence and spaying in bitches. *Vet Rec.* 1985;116:695.
137. Waldron DR. Ectopic ureter surgery and its problems. *Probl Vet Med.* 1989;1:85–92.
138. Webbon PM. The radiological investigation of congenital urinary incontinence in the bitch. *Vet Ann.* 1982;22:199–206.
139. Wein AJ. Pharmacologic management of lower urinary tract storage failure. In: Finkbeiner AG, ed. *Pharmacology of the Lower Urinary Tract and Male Reproductive System.* New York, New York: Appleton-Century-Crofts; 1982:237–272.
140. White RAS, Pomeroy CJ. Phenylpropanolamine: An α-adrenergic agent for the management of urinary incontinence in the bitch associated with urethral sphincter mechanism incompetence. *Vet Rec.* 1989;125:478–480.
141. Wykes PM, Soderberg SF. Congenital abnormalities of the canine vagina and vulva. *J Am Anim Hosp Assoc.* 1983;19:995–1000.

CHAPTER 38

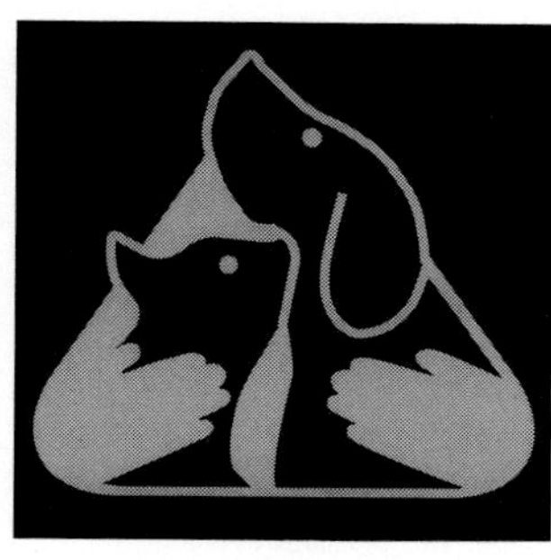

Urethral Diseases of Dogs and Cats

DONALD R. KRAWIEC

I. URETHRAL ANATOMY AND NEUROPHYSIOLOGY ARE COVERED IN DETAIL IN CHAPTER 1, APPLIED ANATOMY OF THE URINARY SYSTEM WITH CLINICOPATHOLOGIC CORRELATION

II. URETHRAL FUNCTION DURING MICTURITION

A. Effect of bladder filling on the urethra.

1. Effect of bladder filling on urethral length and position in the dog and cat.[1,2]
   a. In both dogs and cats, the urethra becomes uniformly longer as the bladder distends.
   b. The urethra tends to be closer to the floor of the pelvis in animals in lateral recumbency and tends to be displaced laterally in animals in ventrodorsal recumbency when the bladder is full.
2. Effect of bladder filling on urethral resistance.[3]
   a. Urethral wall tension must increase to maintain continence in the presence of increasing pressure as the bladder fills with urine. This increase in resistance occurs in two phases in cats. The initial phase appears to be mediated by both striated and smooth muscle. The late phase is secondary to alpha-adrenergic stimulation of smooth muscle and appears to be secondary to trigone distention.
   b. Canine urine has been hypothesized to induce the secretion of serotonin, which then increases urethral resistance.[4]
3. Effect of stress on the urethra.[5–7]
   a. Data from studies involving female dogs suggest that the urethral closure mechanism has three components. The first component is normal urethral tension. Proximal closure, the second mechanism, consists of the smooth muscle of the intrapelvic urethra. This smooth muscle is activated by passive transmission from abdominal pressure. The third component, the distal mechanism, involves active contraction of the external skeletal sphincter and pelvic floor muscles. This active contraction accounts for as much as 89% of the resistance required to maintain continence during abdominal stress.
   b. The active contraction of the third component of the urethral closure mechanism is mediated almost totally by periurethral striated sphincter muscles. Only 4% of the contraction is caused by intraurethral striated sphincter muscles.

B. The emptying phase of micturition in cats has two stages.[8]

1. The prevoiding (isovolumetric) stage results in increased urethral resistance, and occurs secondaryto relaxation of longitudinal and contraction of circular urethral muscles. This tightens the bladder neck.
2. Voiding in cats is accomplished during the second stage by the synergistic contraction of longitudinal and relaxation of circular urethral muscles.

3. This response does not require urine to flow and can be reproduced by filling the bladder with a balloon.

III. URETHRAL DISEASE

A. Congenital disorders.

1. Although no comprehensive retrospective studies have been reported, congenital urethral disorders appear to occur infrequently in dogs and rarely in cats. They are reported more frequently in male dogs than in female dogs.
2. Congenital disorders that have been reported include urethral agenesis, urethral duplication, hypospadias, diverticula, stricture, accessory meatus, urethral ectopia, hermaphroditism, and pseudohermaphroditism.[9–20]
   a. Hypospadias is an anomaly characterized by urethral openings caudal to the end of the penis. The urethra, penis, and prepuce anterior to the opening may be partially or completely open on the ventral aspect. This anomaly results from incomplete fusion of the urethral grooves.
      (1). Hypospadias may be classified anatomically according to the position of the urethral opening. The urethral meatus has been described as being normal, glandular, penile, scrotal, perineal, or anal.
      (2). Clinical signs usually refer to owner identification of an anatomic abnormality, urine scalding, urinary incontinence, or recurrent urinary tract infection. Animals with this condition may not require treatment or may require surgical amputation of the anterior penis and prepuce and/or repositioning of the urethral orifice.[9]
   b. Urethral ectopia has been reported in a female German shepherd, a female English bulldog, and a female Pekapoo. All dogs had urinary incontinence and had shortened urethras, with the urethral orifice in the anterior vagina. One dog also had ectopic ureters. No adequate therapy has been identified.[12,19,20]
   c. Congenital pelvic urethral stricture has been reported in a male German shepherd with urinary incontinence. The stricture was surgically corrected.[16]
   d. Urethrorectal fistulas seem to be the most common congenital fistula of dogs. They have been reported in male English bulldogs (three cases) and a female miniature poodle, and usually result in hematuria, dysuria, incontinence, and recurrent urinary tract infection.[14,15,17] Associated anomalies included ectopic ureters and pseudohermaphroditism.
      (1). Signs include urination from the anus as well as from the urethra, dysuria, and hematuria.
      (2). Bacterial urethrocystitis is a common complicating problem.
      (3). Treatment includes surgical correction and control of concomitant urinary tract infection.
   e. Hermaphroditism and pseudohermaphroditism are commonly associated with urinary incontinence and dysuria. The most common urethral abnormality associated with these conditions is vaginourethral communication. Other abnormalities include urethral rectal fistulas, duplicate urethral openings, and ventral opening of the urethra in the prepuce.

B. Inflammatory urethral disorders.[21–24]

1. Granulomatous urethritis is an idiopathic infiltrative disease of older female dogs. Signs include dysuria, hematuria, and urethral obstruction. The disease may mimic urethral neoplasia, but the histologic lesion consists primarily of mononuclear cell infiltration of the urethral mucosa and submucosa. The lesion may represent an immune-mediated reaction to infectious agents or other antigens. Whether the disorder is associated with chronic urinary tract infection is not known.
   a. Diagnosis is based on cytologic or histologic assessment of affected urethral tissue.
   b. Therapy is aimed at maintaining urethral patency with an indwelling urethral catheter, treating concomitant bacterial urinary tract infection with an appropriate antibiotic, and using anti-inflammatory agents (prednisolone and/or cyclophosphamide). Antibiotic therapy should be continued for the duration of anti-inflammatory therapy and for 3 weeks after such therapy is discontinued.
2. Bacterial urethritis is a common urethral abnormality usually associated with cystitis. Signs include dysuria, stranguria, urinary incontinence, and pollakiuria. Severe chronic urethritis may result in marked urethral swelling and obstruction.
   a. Culturing urethral discharges or urethral swabs may be helpful in making a diagnosis; however, the normal canine urethra is often colonized with a variety of microbes, including *Staphylococcus* spp, *Streptococcus* spp, and *Mycoplasma* spp, making interpretation of culture results difficult.
   b. Treatment of bacterial urethritis is similar to therapy for cystitis. Vaginal and urethral concentrations of trimethoprim, rosamicin, and, to some degree, erythromycin exceeded simultaneous plasma concentrations. Ampicillin concentrations are the same in urethral secretions and plasma. Trimethoprim, rosamicin, and erythromycin, therefore, may be better urinary antibiotics if the urethra is significantly involved.[25] Antibiotic therapy should be continued 2 to 3 weeks.
   c. Ancillary therapy using antispasmodic agents or prednisolone may be helpful for severe or

chronic urethritis. Prednisolone should be used only for short periods and should not be used unless the patient is also receiving an appropriate antibiotic.

3. Chlamydial urethritis has been produced in the cat utilizing the feline keratoconjunctivitis agent *Chlamydia psittaci*.[22] This organism has also been implicated as a cause of genital infections in catteries. Tetracyclines or chloramphenicol may be effective in treating this problem.

C. Noninflammatory urethral abnormalities.[10,11,26–32]

1. Urethral trauma may occur secondary to pelvic fracture, os penis fracture, urethral catheterization, or bite wounds. Urethral trauma may result in mild bruising or hemorrhage, which heal spontaneously without treatment, or may result in severe laceration and/or severance, causing urine leakage into the surrounding tissues or abdominal cavity. Urine leakage into tissues produces inflammation and necrosis, whereas urine leakage into the abdominal cavity may result in ascites, postrenal azotemia, and uremia.
   a. Partial rupture of the urethra may be treated conservatively with the aid of an indwelling urethral catheter until the urethra heals.
   b. Complete transection of the urethra must be treated by surgical anastomoses to allow healing to occur. A permanent urethrostomy may be produced using the proximal undamaged portion of the urethra if urethral anastomosis is not possible.
2. Urethral strictures may result from any severe traumatic insult or chronic inflammatory condition (urethral calculi or chronic urethritis). Signs include dysuria, stranguria, oliguria, and urinary incontinence. If severe, this condition may result in hydroureter, hydronephrosis, postrenal azotemia, and uremia. Therapy for severe urethral stenosis may be either surgical transection and anastomosis or urethrostomy proximal to the obstruction.
3. Urethral prolapse is an uncommon condition that occurs in young males of brachycephalic breeds (English bulldogs and Boston terriers). Predisposing conditions appear to be sexual excitement and urethritis. Signs include urethral mucosa protruding from the penis, along with dysuria, urinary incontinence, and hemorrhage from the urethral orifice.
   a. Amputation of the protruding tissue along with careful suturing of the urethra to the squamous epithelium of the penile tissue is usually curative. The animal must be prevented from damaging the penis by utilizing an Elizabethan collar or neck brace and sedation until healing has occurred.
   b. A more conservative therapeutic approach has been to catheterize the urethra, manually reduce the prolapse, place a string suture in the penile orifice, and then remove the catheter. The animal should be prevented from damaging the penis as previously described. This approach is less likely to be successful.
   c. Ancillary therapy may include antibiotics, antispasmodics, and anti-inflammatory agents to prevent the straining that occurs secondary to the infection and irritation.
4. Urethral catheters are irritating to urethral mucosa. Severe urethritis and stricture have been reported secondary to indwelling urethral catheterization. Silicone, Teflon-coated latex, and polyvinylchloride catheters seem to be less irritating to urethral mucosa than are latex catheters. Careful atraumatic placement, proper management of indwelling urethral catheters, and use for as short a period as possible minimize urethral irritation.

D. Urinary incontinence is a common sign of urethral disease.

1. Urethral incompetence is the most common cause of urinary incontinence in dogs.[33] It most often affects spayed females but can occur in either sex and in both neutered and intact animals.
   a. Bladder position has been implicated as a cause of urethral incompetence in spayed female dogs. Urinary incontinence has been identified radiographically in animals with bladders located within the pelvic canal (pelvic bladder).[34] This anatomic bladder site, however, can be observed in normal dogs.[35] One study reports a tendency of animals with urinary incontinence to have an intrapelvic bladder neck.[36]
   b. In a study of 47 continent and 57 incontinent dogs, a statistically significant degree of urethral shortening was observed in the incontinent animals.[36]
   c. Spayed female dogs with apparent urethral incompetence become continent when treated with oral diethylstilbestrol.[37] Male dogs with this problem may improve when treated with testosterone.[38] Urinary incontinence caused by urethral incompetence, therefore, is often referred to as "hormone-responsive urinary incontinence." Estrogen receptors have been identified in the urethra of both male and female dogs.[39] Estrogen receptors seem to be located only in the proximal smooth muscle portion of the urethra of both sexes. Stimulation of these estrogen receptors by diethylstilbestrol may ameliorate urinary incontinence in these animals.
2. Upper motor neuron lesions may cause urethral sphincter hypertonia and reflex dyssynergia. Lower motor neuron lesions may produce decreased urethral tone.[33]
3. Animals without physical obstruction may develop signs of urethral obstruction and paradoxic

incontinence. These animals may develop postrenal azotemia and uremia and a large bladder, and they attempt to urinate without success. They often have a history of chronic or intermittent bladder infections. Affected animals may be difficult to catheterize while awake but are easily catheterized without encountering resistance while asleep. The urethral obstruction is probably caused by spastic contraction and inflammation secondary to chronic urethritis. Utilizing indwelling urinary catheterization or cystotomy catheters to keep the bladder empty until the urethral irritation and inflammation subside is advisable. Specific therapy includes antibiotics and both smooth and skeletal muscle relaxants. Antispasmodics often are not employed because of their effect on bladder tone. Bladders of these animals usually are atonic owing to chronic overdistention.

E. Urethral obstruction.

1. Causes of urethral obstruction include urethral stricture, inflammatory stenosis, urethral calculi, and feline urethral lower urinary tract disease. These problems have been described in other portions of this chapter and in other chapters of this book.

F. Urethral neoplasia.[11,26]

1. Urethral neoplasia is uncommon in dogs and rare in cats.
2. The two most common types of urethral neoplasm are squamous cell carcinoma and transitional cell carcinoma. Other reported tumors include adenocarcinoma, rhabdomyosarcoma, and hemangiosarcoma. Bladder and prostate tumors may also extend into the urethra.
3. Urethral tumors are found mostly in older animals and are more common in females than in males. Female urethras are lined predominantly with squamous epithelium, whereas those of males are lined with transitional epithelium. This may play a role in the susceptibility of females.
4. Urethral tumors in males are located primarily in the prostatic urethra, whereas tumors in females are more common in the distal urethra.
5. Metastasis may occur to regional lymph nodes and lungs.
6. Signs include dysuria, hematuria, bloody urethral discharge, and/or urethral obstruction. Rectal or vaginal palpation may reveal an irregular urethra or a mass. Other diagnostic tests that help to localize the problem include contrast urethrography, cystoscopy, and vaginoscopy. Chest and abdominal radiography may help to identify metastasis.
7. Diagnosis is based on identification of neoplastic cells on cytologic or histologic evaluation of affected urethral tissue. Tissue for cytologic examination may be obtained from urine or urethral discharges, and tissue for histologic examination may be obtained by catheter biopsy, cystoscopy, or exploratory surgery.
8. Therapy is primarily supportive. Exploratory surgery and resection of the major tumor mass may be attempted; however, no studies are available concerning the success of this procedure. The success of medical therapy (radiation or chemotherapy) has not been described.
9. Recently, a technique involving photodynamic therapy using a cylindric fiber has been described.[40] This technique involves the use of a photosensitizing agent (dihematoporphyrin ether) that destroys tissue when interacted with absorbed light. The development of a 1-mm fused silica optical fiber with cylindric light distribution has allowed the application of this technique for use in the treatment of urethral carcinoma.

G. Urethral response to prostate disease.[41]

1. Prostate disease may result in inability to void or in urinary incontinence. Urethral discharge of prostatic fluid can be mistaken for urinary incontinence.
2. Intact and neutered male animals with urinary incontinence should be evaluated for prostate disease.

IV. DIAGNOSIS OF URETHRAL DISORDERS

A. Accurate diagnosis of urethral disorders requires interpretation of data obtained from the history, a thorough physical examination, and appropriate laboratory assays.

1. History.
   a. The history often suggests that the problem is in the lower urinary tract but rarely specifically localize the abnormality to the urethra.
   b. Information that should be obtained during the history is listed in Table 38–1.
2. Physical examination.
   a. A complete physical examination should be performed on all animals with suspected urethral disease.

TABLE 38–1.
INFORMATION THAT SHOULD BE OBTAINED FROM OWNERS OF DOGS AND CATS WITH SUSPECTED URETHRAL DISEASE

Description of the immediate problem
Severity and course of the current problem
Presence of urethral discharge or incontinence
Hematuria at the beginning, end, or throughout urination
Lower urinary tract signs
Signs referring to prostate disease
Water intake
Urine output
Previous illness or surgery
Current medications

TABLE 38–2.
PROCEDURES TO PERFORM DURING PHYSICAL EXAMINATION OF DOGS WITH SUSPECTED PROSTATE DISEASE

Complete general physical examination
Abdominal palpation to evaluate the prostate and bladder
Inspection of the external genitalia and perineal area for growths, trauma, or inflammation
Digital rectal examination to assess for urethral abnormalities and for prostatic abnormalities
Evaluation of the urine stream for duration, character, stranguria, dysuria, and hematuria
Evaluation for tenesmus and stool character

(1). Digital vaginal and rectal examinations should be performed on all females with signs of lower urinary tract disease. Digital rectal examination, as well as examination of the penis and prepuce, should be performed on male dogs.

(2). The entire urethra of female dogs should be palpated. The most distal portion can be palpated vaginally. The urethra can be palpated as it courses over the ischium both vaginally and externally in the perianal area. The intrapelvic urethra and proximal urethra can be palpated rectally on the floor of the pelvis. Most of the male urethra can also be palpated. The portion of the urethra that courses through the os penis, however, is inaccessible to physical examination.

b. Procedures that should be performed during physical examination are listed in Table 38–2.

3. Diagnostic assays. Several diagnostic assays can be performed to evaluate for urethral disease, including urethral discharge evaluation, urethrography, ultrasound evaluation of the prostate and urethra, electromyography, urethral pressure profiles, and urethroscopy.
   a. Urethral discharges should be evaluated by both cytology and culture. Cytologic evaluation may help to differentiate neoplasia from inflammation.
   b. If a palpable mass can be identified by physical examination, performance of a catheter biopsy may help to obtain a tissue sample. This technique is performed by placing a catheter in the urethra. The urethral mass and catheter are digitally palpated per rectum. The catheter should be advanced until it is in the abnormal area. A 12-mL syringe is placed on the end of the catheter, and negative pressure is applied. The catheter is then briskly pulled back while negative pressure is maintained by the syringe. Negative pressure forces tissue into the holes of the catheter. The tissue is torn loose by the pulling motion and can be removed from the area with the catheter while maintaining a minimal amount of negative pressure. Material may be ejected on a slide for cytologic evaluation. Occasionally, a large enough tissue sample is obtained to submit for histologic evaluation.
   c. Urethroscopy can also be utilized to identify urethral abnormalities in female dogs. Human pediatric cystoscopes or small bronchoscopes can be used for this purpose. The abnormal area then can be visualized directly and a biopsy performed.

B. Procedures for performing radiographic, ultrasonographic, and cystoscopic diagnostic procedures, as well as for lower urinary tract function tests, are described in detail in other chapters of this book.

V. TREATMENT OF URETHRAL DISORDERS

A. Surgical therapy.

1. Surgical therapy for urethral anomalies, feline urethral obstruction, urethral neoplasia, and urethral trauma is reviewed elsewhere in this book.
2. Surgical therapy for urethral incompetence.
   a. Numerous surgical procedures have been advocated for use in treating human female stress (urethral incompetence) incontinence.
   b. Recently, a procedure involving transurethral suspension of the neck of the bladder and urethra was described in the dog.[42] This procedure involves the use of an operative cystoscope to place three or four sutures from the anterior wall of the proximal urethra to the anterior fascia of the suprapubic region. Successful positioning of these sutures results in anterior and ventral displacement of the urethrovesical junction.
   c. To date, no information is available regarding the usefulness of surgical intervention in the treatment of canine urethral incompetence.
3. Surgical therapy for feline upper motor neuron disease.
   a. Recently, a surgical procedure was described that facilitated relaxation of the external urethral sphincter in cats with midthoracic level (T-5–T-6) spinal cord transection.[43]
   b. The procedure involves severing the pudendal nerve on one side, followed by maneuvering the hindlimbs to cause inhibition of reflex firing of the intact pudendal nerve.
   c. The limb ipsilateral to the intact pudendal nerve is maneuvered so that hip, knee, and ankle are in full flexion. This positioning stretches the major extensor muscles in the limb, which in turn inhibits ipsilateral motor neurons supplying the urethral sphincter. The limb contralateral to the intact pudendal nerve is then placed in full extension to inhibit im-

pulses from the contralateral pudendal nerve.

d. This procedure (unilateral pudendal nerve severing plus manipulation of the hindlimbs) resulted in relaxation of the urethral sphincter and urination in all animals with experimental paraplegia.

e. These results indicate that this procedure may have some use in clinical cases of paraplegia.

B. Medical management of urethral disorders.

1. Pharmacologic manipulation of urethral function.

a. Numerous pharmaceutic agents are available that affect urethral function. An incomplete list of such agents includes bethanechol chloride, bradykinin, dobutamine, dopamine, ephedrine, guanethidine, haloperidol, hexamethonium, imipramine, labetalol, nicergoline, phenoxybenzamine, phentolamine, phenylephrine, phenylpropanolamine, prazosin, prostaglandin E_2, prostaglandin $F_{2\alpha}$, salbutamol, sotalol, substance P, thymoxamine, verapamil, and yohimbine.[44–59]

(1). Pharmaceutic agents that decrease urethral resistance.

(a). Effective decrease in urethral tone may be accomplished with medications that relax both smooth and skeletal muscle sphincters.

(b). Alpha-adrenergic blocking agents decrease urethral smooth muscle tone. Phenoxybenzamine, nicergoline (not available in the United States), moxisylyte (not available in the United States), or prazosin (toxicity may make this medication less desirable) may be used for this purpose (Table 38-3).

(c). Relaxation of the skeletal urethral sphincter can be accomplished with diazepam or dantrolene (see Table 38–3).[50,59]

(d). Prostaglandin E_2 has been reported experimentally to induce both bladder contraction and urethral relaxation in dogs. This drug may prove useful in the future to treat neurologic lower urinary tract dysfunction.[45,49]

(2). Pharmaceutic agents that increase urethral tone.

(a). Urethral incompetence is one of the most common urethral problems requiring therapy.

(b). Alpha-adrenergic agents increase urethral tone. The most commonly used agents for this purpose are ephedrine and phenylpropanolamine (see Table 38–3).[33,59]

(c). Beta-adrenergic agents (propranolol) may help in cases refractory to alpha-adrenergic therapy alone. Cardiac and respiratory side effects make this drug less desirable.[59]

(d). Imipramine, a tricyclic antidepressant used to treat cataplexy in dogs

TABLE 38–3.
PHARMACOLOGIC AGENTS USED TO INCREASE AND DECREASE URETHRAL TONE[33,59]

	Medication	Canine Dose	Feline Dose	Side Effects or Signs of Overdose
Medications used to decrease urethral smooth muscle tone	Phenoxybenzamine	0.25 mg/kg PO q12h	0.25 mg/kg PO q12h	Hypotension, fainting, tachycardia, vomiting, lethargy, shock
Medications used to decrease urethral skeletal muscle tone	Diazepam	0.20 mg/kg PO q8h	2.5 to 5 mg PO q8h	Drowsiness, fatigue, ataxia
	Dantrolene	1 to 5 mg/kg PO q8h	None	Drowsiness, weakness, general malaise, fatigue, diarrhea
Medications used to increase urethral muscle tone	Ephedrine	25 to 50 mg PO q8 to 24h (no more than 4 mg/kg q8h)	2 to 4 mg/kg PO q8–24 h	Hyperactivity, tachycardia, hypertension
	Phenylpropanolamine	1.5 mg/kg PO q12h	1.5 mg/kg PO q12h	Hyperactivity, tachycardia, hypertension
	Imipramine	5 to 15 mg PO q12h	2.5–5 mg PO q12h	Hypotension, hypertension, tachycardia, anxiety, ataxia, nausea

and humans, has been reported to decrease bladder tone and increase urethral sphincter tone. It has been used with some success to treat canine urethral incompetence, especially if bladder hypertonia is a complicating problem.[44,59]

b. Therapeutic use of estrogens and testosterone for urethral incompetence is covered in another chapter of this book.

REFERENCES

1. Johnston GR, et al. Effects of urinary bladder distention on location of the urinary bladder and urethra of healthy dogs and cats. *Am J Vet Res.* 1986; 47:404.
2. Johnston GR, Osborne CA, Jessen CR. Effects of urinary bladder distention on the length of the dog and cat urethra. *Am J Vet Res.* 1985; 46:509.
3. Kiruluta HG, Downie JW, Awad SA. The continence mechanisms: The effect of bladder filling on the urethra. *Invest Urol.* 1981; 18:460.
4. Hanyu S, Iwanaga T, Kano K, Fujita T. Distribution of serotonin-immunoreactive paraneurons in the lower urinary tract of dogs. *Am J Anat.* 1987; 180:349.
5. Thuroff JW, Bazeed MA, Schmidt RA, Tanagho EA. Mechanisms of urinary continence: An animal model to study urethral responses to stress conditions. *J Urol.* 1982; 127:1202.
6. Thuroff JW, Heidler CH. Pelvic floor stress response: Reflex contraction with pressure transmission to the urethra. *Urol Int.* 1987; 42:185.
7. Heidler H, Casper F, Thuroff JW. Role of striated sphincter muscle in urethral closure under stress condition: An experimental study. *Urol Int.* 1987; 42:195.
8. Abdel-Rahman M, Galeano C, Lamarche J, Elhilali MM. A new approach to the study of the voiding cycle in the cat. *Invest Urol.* 1981; 18:175.
9. Ader PL, Hobson HP. Hypospadias: A review of the veterinary literature and a report of three cases in the dog. *J Am Anim Hosp Assoc.* 1978; 14:721.
10. Greene RW, Scott RC. Diseases of the bladder and urethra. *In:* Ettinger SJ, ed. *Textbook of Veterinary Internal Medicine.* 2nd ed. Philadelphia, Pennsylvania: WB Saunders; 1983.
11. Brown SA, Barsanti JA. Diseases of the bladder and urethra. *In:* Ettinger SJ, ed. *Textbook of Veterinary Internal Medicine.* 3rd ed. Philadelphia, Pennsylvania: WB Saunders; 1990.
12. Ladkin A. Urethral ectopia and anomalous cervix in a dog. *Vet Rec.* 1979; 104:555.
13. Holt PE, Long SE, Gibbs C. Disorders of urination associated with canine intersexuality. *J Small Anim Pract.* 1983; 24:475.
14. Goulden B, Bergman MM, Wyburn RS. Canine urethrorectal fistulae. *J Small Anim Pract.* 1973; 14:143.
15. Osborne CA, et al. Congenital urethrorectal fistula in two dogs. *J Am Vet Med Assoc.* 1975; 166:999.
16. Breitschwerdt EB, Olivier BB, King GK, Pavletic MM. Bilateral hydronephrosis and hydroureter in a dog associated with congenital urethral stricture. *J Am Anim Hosp Assoc.* 1982; 18:799.
17. Miller CF. Urethrorectal fistula with concurrent urolithiasis in a dog. *Vet Med/Small Anim. Clin.* 1980; 75:73.
18. Todoroff RJ. Congenital urological anomalies. *Compend Contin Educ Pract Vet.* 1979; 1:780.
19. Finco DR, Osborne CA, Lewis RE. Nonneurogenic causes of abnormal micturition in the dog and cat. *Vet Clin North Am Small Anim Pract.* 1974; 4:515.
20. Osborne CA, Hanlon GF. Canine congenital ureteral ectopia. Case report and review of literature. *Anim Hosp.* 1967; 3:111.
21. Matthiesen DT, Moroff SD. Infiltrative urethral diseases in the dog. *In:* Kirk RW, ed. *Current Veterinary Therapy X.* Philadelphia, Pennsylvania: WB Saunders; 1989.
22. Moller BR, Mardh P. Animal models for the study of chlamydial infections of the urogenital tract. *Scand J Infect Dis.* 1982; 32(Suppl):103.
23. Ling GV, Ruby AL. Aerobic bacterial flora of the prepuce, urethra, and vagina of normal adult dogs. *Am J Vet Res.* 1978; 39:695.
24. Polzin DJ, Jeraj K. Urethritis, cystitis, and ureteritis. *Vet Clin North Am Small Anim Pract.* 1979; 9:661.
25. Hoyme U, Baumueller A, Madsen PO. Antibiotics excretion in canine vaginal and urethral secretions. *Invest Urol.* 1978; 16:35.
26. Lipowitz AJ. Diseases of the canine urethra. *In:* Kirk RW, ed. *Current Veterinary Therapy VIII.* Philadelphia, Pennsylvania: WB Saunders; 1983.
27. Jones GH, Testerman WT, Howland TP, Bjerk TJ. Ruptured urethra caused by trauma in a dog. *Vet Med/Small Anim Clin.* 1981; 76:672.
28. Goodpasture JC, Cianci J, Zaneveld LJD. Long-term evaluation of the effect of catheter materials on urethral tissue in dogs. *Lab Anim Sci.* 1982; 32:180.
29. Nacey JN, Delahunt B, Tullock AGS. The assessment of catheter-induced urethritis using an experimental dog model. *J Urol.* 1985; 134:623.
30. Goldman AL, Beckman SL. Traumatic urethral avulsion at the preputial fornix in a cat. *J Am Vet Med Assoc.* 1989; 194:88.
31. Nacey JN, Horsfall DJ, Delahunt B, Marshall VR. The assessment of urinary catheter toxicity using cell cultures: Validation by comparison with an animal model. *J Urol.* 1986; 136:706.
32. Lees GE, Osborne CA, Stevens JB, Ward GE. Adverse effects caused by polypropylene and polyvinyl feline urinary catheters. *Am J Vet Res.* 1980; 41:1836.
33. Krawiec DR. Diagnosis and treatment of acquired canine urinary incontinence. *Companion Anim Pract.* 1989; 3:12.
34. DiBartola SP, Adams WM. Urinary incontinence associated with malposition of the urinary bladder. *In:* Kirk RW, ed. *Current Veterinary Therapy VIII.* Philadelphia, Pennsylvania: WB Saunders; 1983.
35. Mahaffey MB, Barsanti JA, Barber DL, Crowell WA. Pelvic bladder in dogs without urinary incontinence. *J Am Vet Med Assoc.* 1984; 184:1477.
36. Holt PE. Importance of urethral length, bladder neck position, and vestibulovaginal stenosis in sphincter mechanism incompetence in the incontinent bitch. *Res Vet Sci.* 1985; 39:364.
37. Barsanti JA, Finco DR. Hormonal responses to urinary incontinence. *In:* Kirk RW, ed. *Current Veterinary Therapy VIII.* Philadelphia, Pennsylvania: WB Saunders; 1983.
38. Barsanti JA, Edwards PD, Losonsky J. Testosterone-responsive urinary incontinence in a castrated male dog. *J Am Anim Hosp Assoc.* 1981; 17:117.
39. Schulze H, Barrack ER. Immunocytochemical localization of estrogen receptors in the normal male and female canine urinary tract and prostate. *Endocrinology.* 1987; 121:1773.
40. Manyak MJ, et al. Photodynamic therapy: Response of normal canine urethra using a cylindrical fiber. *Lasers Surg Med.* 1988; 8:301.
41. Basinger RR, Barsanti JA. Urodynamic abnormalities associated with canine prostatic diseases and therapeutic intervention. *In:* Kirk RW, ed. *Current Veterinary Therapy X.* Philadelphia, Pennsylvania: WB Saunders; 1989.
42. Lattanzi CA, Montague DK, Stowe NT. Endoscopic transurethral suspension of bladder neck and urethra. *Urology.* 1986; 27:243.

43. Jolesz FA, Ruenzel PW, Henneman E. Reflex inhibition of urethral sphincters to permit voiding in paraplegia. *Arch Neurol.* 1988; 45:38.
44. Creed KE, Tulloch GS. The action of imipramine on the lower urinary tract of the dog. *Br J Urol.* 1982; 54:5.
45. Kondo A, Kobayashi M, Takita T, Narita H. Effect of prostaglandin on urethral resistance and micturition. *Urol Res.* 1983; 11:19.
46. Abdel-Hakim A, et al. Response of urethral smooth muscles to pharmacological agents. II. Noncholinergic, nonadrenergic agonists and antagonists. *J Urol.* 1983; 130:988.
47. Nishizawa O, et al. Effect of verapamil on the lower urinary tract. *Tohoku J Exp Med.* 1983; 140:223.
48. Slack BE, Downie JW. Pharmacological analysis of the responses of the feline urethra to autonomic nerve stimulation. *J Auton Nerv Syst.* 1983; 8:141.
49. Mutoh S, et al. Effects of some prostaglandins on the urinary bladder and urethra isolated from the dog. *Urol Int.* 1983; 38:219.
50. Caine M, Mazouz B, Rossini BM. The effect of nicergoline on the lower urinary tract muscle. *Urol Res.* 1984; 12:287.
51. Sogbein SK, Downie JW, Awad SA. Urethral response during bladder contraction induced by subcutaneous bethanechol chloride: Elicitation of a sympathetic reflex urethral constriction. *J Urol.* 1984; 131:791.
52. Richter KP, Ling GV. Clinical response and urethral pressure profile changes after phenylpropanolamine in dogs with primary sphincter incompetence. *J Am Vet Med Assoc.* 1985; 187:605.
53. El-Salmy S, Downie JW, Awad SA. Effect of acute selective sacral rhizotomy in cats on bladder and urethral function and the response to bethanechol chloride. *J Urol.* 1985; 134:795.
54. Nishizawa O, et al. Effects of autonomic agonists on *in vivo* female canine urethral motility. *Urol Int.* 1985; 40:320.
55. Nishizawa O, et al. Effect of the autonomic antagonists on canine urethral responses to autonomic nerve stimulation. *Urol Int.* 1985; 40:314.
56. Moriya I, et al. Effects of dobutamine on the *in vivo* urethra in the female dog. *Tohoku J Exp Med.* 1985; 147:311.
57. Poirier M, Riffaud JP, Lacolle JY, Dupont C. Effects of five alpha-blockers on the hypogastric nerve stimulation of the canine lower urinary tract. *J Urol.* 1988; 140:165.
58. Harada T, et al. Effect of adrenergic agents on urethral pressure and urethral compliance measurements in the dog proximal urethra. *J Urol.* 1989; 142:189.
59. Moreau PM, Lappin MR. Pharmacologic management of urinary incontinence, *In:* Kirk RW, ed. *Current Veterinary Therapy X.* Philadelphia, Pennsylvania: WB Saunders, 1989.

CHAPTER 39

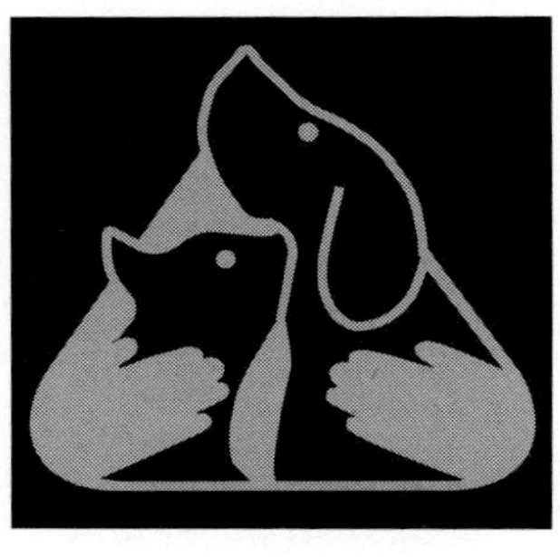

Diseases of the Prostate Gland

JEANNE A. BARSANTI

I. INTRODUCTION

A. Feline prostate gland.

1. The prostate gland of cats is located along the urethra. It is bilobed but covers the urethra only dorsally and laterally. The cat's urethra is proportionally longer, and the prostate gland is more caudal to the neck of the bladder than in the dog (Fig. 39–1). In addition, some prostatic lobules are disseminated within the urethral wall caudal to the prostate gland.[3,106]
2. Prostate disease is uncommon in cats. The feline prostate does not undergo spontaneous hyperplasia with age, and bacterial infections within the urinary tract are uncommon. A few cases of prostate neoplasia have been reported. Knowledge of the feline prostate gland is limited. In this chapter I refer only to dogs unless the cat is specifically mentioned.

B. Canine prostate gland.

1. Anatomy.
   a. The prostate gland, the only accessory sex gland in male dogs, is a bilobed organ with a median septum on the dorsal surface.[63,185] It is located predominantly in the retroperitoneal space, just caudal to the bladder in the area of the bladder neck and proximal urethra (Fig. 39–2; see Fig. 6–14). Only the craniodorsal side is covered by peritoneum. A variable amount of adipose tissue covers the gland ventrally. Dorsally, the prostate is attached to the rectum by a fibrous band.[139]
   b. The prostate encircles the proximal urethra at the neck of the bladder and its ducts enter the urethra throughout its circumference.[62] The urethra passes through the prostate slightly dorsal to the center of the gland.
   c. The position of the prostate in the caudal abdomen depends on age, bladder distention, and disease state.[95]
      (1). In neonates, the prostate is abdominal.
      (2). After loss of the urachal remnant (before age 2 months), the prostate resides within the pelvic inlet.[238]
      (3). With increasing age, the prostate again tends to become abdominal in location, so that in intact male dogs older than 5 years most of the prostate gland is abdominal.[95]
   d. The main arterial supply is from the urogenital artery, which divides into two or three prostatic branches, a prostatic vesical branch, and a prostatic urethral branch, all of which are on the dorsal and dorsolateral surfaces of the gland.[62,139] The veins course next to the arteries. Innervation is both sympathetic (hypogastric) and parasympathetic (pelvic nerve).[62,139]
2. Histology.
   a. The prostate gland is composed of glandular acini supported by a stroma of connective tissue and smooth muscle, enclosed by a thick fibromuscular capsule (Fig. 39–3).
   b. Columnar glandular epithelium changes to the

transitional type in the excretory ducts that open into the urethra.

c. The cells within the prostate gland are of two types, epithelial and stromal.[121]
   (1). Epithelial cells.
      (a). Tall columnar secretory epithelium.
      (b). Basal epithelium.
         (1′). Basal epithelial cells are located sporadically along the basement membrane.
         (2′). The role of the basal epithelial cells is unknown, but they may be precursors of the secretory epithelium.[121,173]

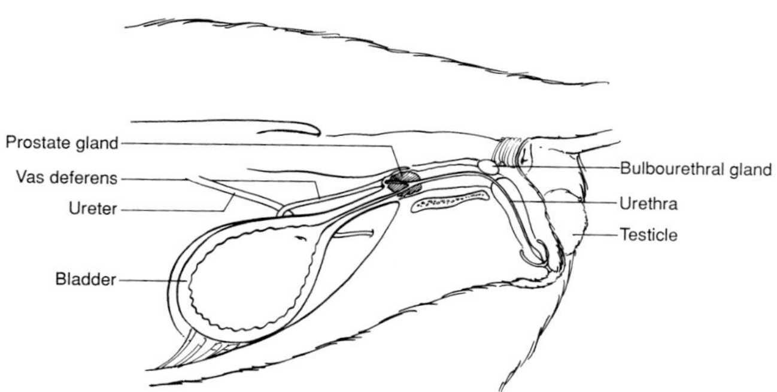

FIG. 39–1. The relationship of the prostate gland to other structures in the caudal abdomen of the male cat.

   (2). The stroma consists of fibroblastic and smooth muscle cells enmeshed in collagen with blood vessels and nerves.
      (a). The fibromuscular stroma is predominant prior to sexual maturity.[31,142] The histologic development of the prostate from immature to mature is most marked between 20 and 32 weeks of age, the time during which plasma testosterone levels increase.[134]
      (b). After this time, the epithelium is predominant.

3. Physiology.
   a. The purpose of the prostate gland is to produce prostatic fluid as a transport and support medium for sperm during ejaculation.
      (1). Formerly, parasympathetic stimulation was thought to increase the rate of fluid production just before ejaculation.[42] More recently, the sympathetic system was found to be more important in release of fluid produced.[258]
      (2). Under sympathetic stimulation, the prostate gland ejects the fluid during ejaculation.[42,258]
      (3). The hypogastric nerve (alpha-adrenergic fibers) is the main neuronal control of prostatic contraction.
   b. Basal secretion of small amounts (<1 ml/h) of

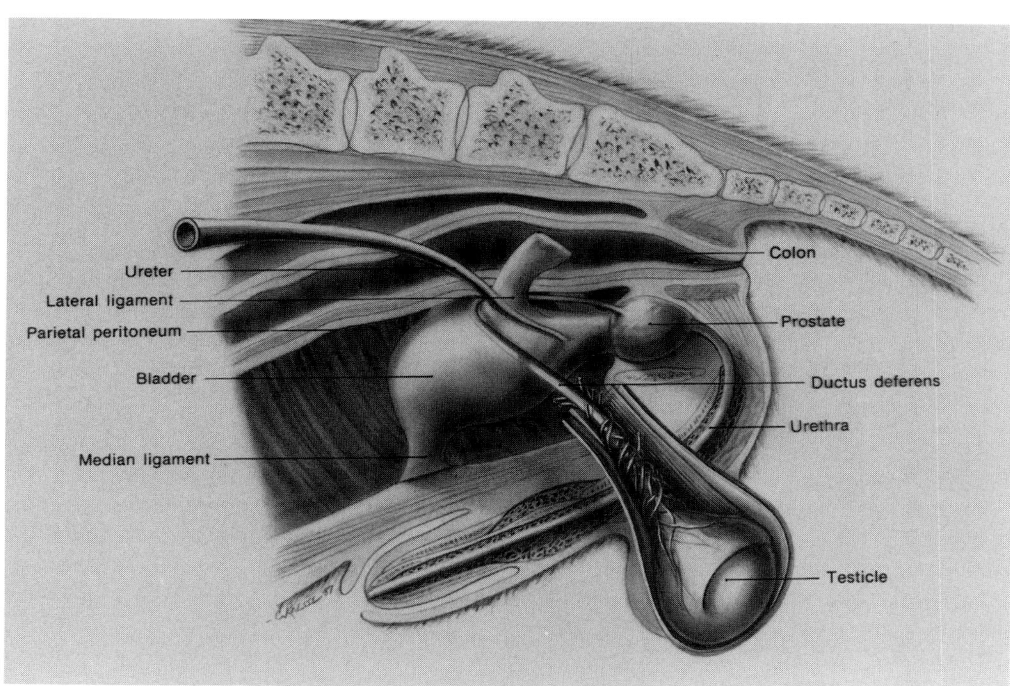

FIG. 39–2. The relationship of the prostate gland to other structures in the caudal abdomen of the male dog. (Barsanti JA. Canine prostatic disease. *In:* Ettinger SJ, ed. *Veterinary Internal Medicine.* Philadelphia, Pennsylvania: W.B. Saunders, 1989;1859.)

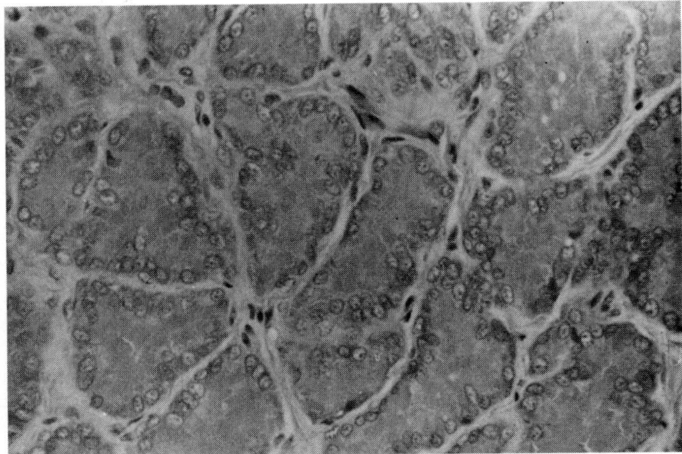

FIG. 39–3. Histologic slide of a normal canine prostate gland. Note that most of the gland is composed of acini, separated by small amounts of interstitial connective tissue. (Courtesy of Dr. W.A. Crowell, College of Veterinary Medicine, University of Georgia.)

prostatic fluid constantly flows into the prostatic excretory ducts and prostatic urethra normally.[73,258]

(1). When neither micturition nor ejaculation is occurring, urethral pressure moves this basally secreted fluid craniad into the bladder (prostatic fluid reflux).

(2). During micturition, urine enters the prostate gland in men (intraprostatic urinary reflux).[136] Whether this occurs in dogs is not known.

c. With age, the prostate gland increases in weight.[31,38,124]

(1). Between 4 and 16 months of age (for beagles), the prostate grows with a constant doubling time of 0.64 years.[120] This corresponds to the time when serum testosterone is rising to its normal adult level.[120]

(2). Once the prostate reaches its normal adult size (12 to 14 gs in beagles), growth stops until prostatic hyperplasia develops.

(3). Benign prostatic hyperplasia has been identified in 40% of beagles by 2.5 years of age, in more than 80% of beagles older than 6 years of age,[31,33,65] and in more than 95% of beagles older than 9 years of age.[33]

d. The prostate gland requires the presence of testosterone to grow and to maintain its size.

(1). There is apparently increased sensitivity of the growth of the prostate gland to testosterone with aging, because testosterone secretion and prostatic testosterone concentration decrease with aging.[31]

(2). If a dog is castrated before sexual maturity, normal prostatic growth is completely inhibited.[120]

(3). If a dog is castrated as an adult, involution shrinks the prostate to 20% of its normal adult size.[115]

e. Prostatic secretory function, as measured by ejaculate volume, reaches a peak at 4 years of age in beagles and then begins to decline.[31]

4. Microbiology. The prostate gland is normally sterile.

5. Prostate diseases are common in older male dogs. Although prostate disease occurs in all breeds of dogs, larger breeds, especially Doberman pinschers and German shepherds, have a higher than expected prevalence.[141] Whether the high incidence of von Willebrand's disease in Dobermans, which typically appears as urogenital bleeding,[40] is related to the higher rate of detection of prostate disease in Dobermans is not known. The most common signs of prostate disease are also those of lower urinary tract disease.[141] Other common signs are related to the gastrointestinal tract, systemic disease, and locomotor difficulty.[141]

a. Benign hyperplasia.

(1). With aging, the prostate gradually enlarges.

(2). Because of the glandular nature of the prostate, intraparenchymal prostate fluid cysts may develop in association with hyperplasia.

(3). Although all dogs develop histologic evidence of prostatic hyperplasia with aging, most are asymptomatic.[141]

b. Squamous metaplasia of the prostate gland develops in the presence of excess estrogens, either endogenous or exogenous.[10,180]

c. Infection.

(1). Most prostate infections are bacterial in origin.

(2). Bacterial infections of the prostate gland can be acute, or chronic and insidious, leading to abscessation.

(3). Decreased secretory function in the aging prostate may increase its susceptibility to infection.

(4). Chronic infection, with or without abscessation, was the most common prostatic disease observed in a teaching hospital.[141] This finding may reflect the fact that difficulty of diagnosis and treatment of such infections prompts referral or may reflect the incidence of such infections in symptomatic prostatic disease.

d. Paraprostatic cysts, which may or may not be of prostatic origin, are usually associated with the prostate and cause the same signs as those associated with prostatomegaly.

e. The aging prostate gland is also subject to neoplastic transformation, most commonly adenocarcinoma. Prostatic neoplasia is the only prostatic disease diagnosed in dogs that are neu utered before the onset of prostatic disease.[141]

f. Calculi may be found in canine prostate glands.[74]

g. Prostatic pain and a stilted gait have been observed in young dogs exposed to, but unable to breed, a bitch in estrus. Prostatomegaly that resolves within 24 hours was attributed to vascular engorgement.[139] This condition is rarely described in the literature, either because it is uncommon or because it resolves so rapidly without intervention.

6. The diagnostic plan for suspected prostatic disease always involves a thorough history, physical examination, and urinalysis and often includes a complete blood count, biochemical profile, evaluation of prostatic fluid and tissue, radiography, and ultrasonography.

a. History findings related to prostate diseases.

(1). Urinary tract problems: hematuria (common), urethral discharge (common), dysuria (less common, and usually associated with marked prostatomegaly), and polyuria (associated with abscessation).

(2). Gastrointestinal problems: rectal tenesmus (common), large bowel diarrhea (less common), vomiting (usually associated with acute infection or abscessation).

(3). Systemic problems: lethargy, anorexia, fever.

(4). Prostate pain.

(5). Locomotor problems: stilted gait.

(6). Reproductive problems.

(a). Prostatic disease is the most common cause of hematospermia.[192]

(b). Infertility.

(7). When taking a history of a patient with suspected prostate disease, one must ask about all the systems previously listed as certain signs are more common with certain diseases (Table 39–1).

b. Physical examination.

(1). The prostate gland is best examined with two hands, using digital rectal palpation and caudal abdominal palpation (Fig. 39–4). The hand palpating the caudal abdomen can gently push the prostate gland toward the pelvis, if necessary, so that it is more accessible per rectum. During rectal palpation, an attempt should be made to palpate the sublumbar lymph nodes.

(2). The normal prostate gland is smooth, symmetric, painfree, and movable. Size varies with age, but the normal gland does not compromise the rectal canal or push the bladder craniad.

(3). The rest of the urogenital system should also be examined carefully, as concomitant urinary tract, testicular, and epididymal abnormalities are not uncommon.

(4). The physical examination may also uncover related abnormalities in other systems, such as icterus in some cases of abscessation, heart murmurs associated with bacteremia,[192] or abnormal gait associated with spinal metastasis from neoplasia.

c. Urinalysis should be part of the minimum data base for all suspected cases of prostate disease because of the frequency of urinary tract abnormalities (see Table 39–1). Urine culture is also indicated in cases of suspected prostate infection.

d. A complete blood count and biochemical profile are useful in patients with systemic signs and with marked prostatomegaly (Table 39–2). Because most dogs with prostate disease are old, the complete blood count and biochemical profile are important in screening for other occult diseases of aged dogs.

e. Imaging techniques, such as survey and contrast radiography (especially retrograde urethrography) and ultrasonography are important parts of the evaluation for prostatomegaly (Table 39–3). (See Chapter 12, Canine and Feline Renal Biopsy.)

TABLE 39–1.
CLINICAL SIGNS ASSOCIATED WITH PROSTATIC DISEASES

Prostatic Diseases That Can Cause the Abnormal Sign				
Fecal Tenesmus	**Dysuria**	**Urethral Discharge**	**Systemic Signs***	**Urinary Tract Infection**
Hyperplasia Cyst Abscess Neoplasia	Cyst Abscess Neoplasia	Cyst Bacterial prostatitis Abscess Neoplasia	Acute bacterial prostatitis Abscess Cyst Neoplasia	Bacterial prostatitis

*Signs include fever, depression, pain, anorexia, lethargy.
(Adapted from Barsanti JA, Finco DR. Canine prostatic diseases. *In:* Morrow DA, ed. *Current Therapy in Theriogenology 2.* Philadelphia, Pennsylvania: WB Saunders; 1986.)

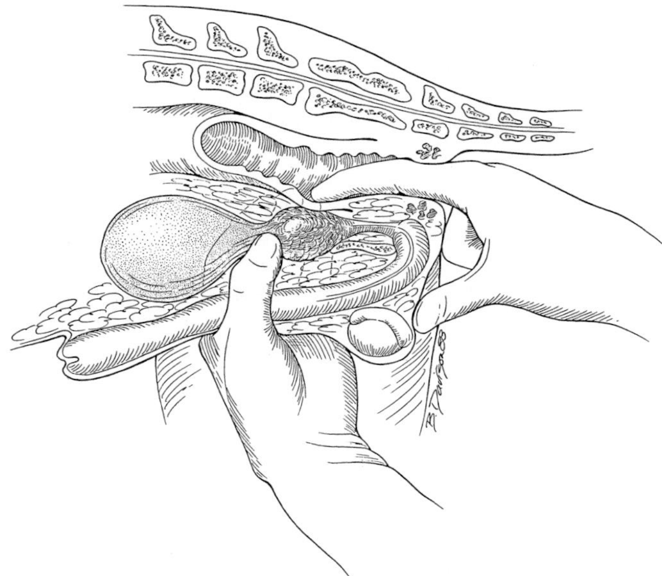

FIG. 39–4. Rectal palpation of the prostate gland in male dogs. One hand should apply pressure on the caudal abdomen while the other palpates rectally. The prostate gland, when enlarged, can be palpated in the caudal abdomen as well as per rectum. (Barsanti JA. Prostatomegaly. *In:* Stone EA, Barsanti JA, eds. *Urologic Surgery of the Dog and Cat.* Philadelphia, Pennsylvania: Lea & Febiger, 1992;30.)

f. A definitive diagnosis usually requires evaluation of prostatic fluid and/or tissue. (See Chapter 6, Collection and Analysis of Prostatic Fluid and Tissue.)

II. BENIGN HYPERPLASIA/CYSTIC HYPERPLASIA

A. Pathophysiology.

1. Benign prostatic hyperplasia (BHP) is an aging change that occurs in only two species, humans and dogs.[6,30–33,92,120,124]
   a. In dogs, hyperplasia is primarily uniform and epithelial,[38,120,271] although increased stromal volume has also been noted.[150,271]
   b. In men, hyperplasia is primarily stromal and nodular.[18,108,120,157,185]
   c. Despite the histologic differences, the natural course of hyperplasia is remarkably similar in both species.[30,92,122]
   d. Dogs show an increase in epithelial cell number (hyperplasia) and epithelial cell size (hypertrophy), but the increase in number is more marked.[271]
2. Hyperplasia is associated with an altered androgen/estrogen ratio,[38,148,196,272] and requires the presence of the testes.[223]
   a. To produce BPH in young castrated dogs, both androgens and estrogens must be administered.[10,120]

TABLE 39–2.
USUAL LABORATORY FINDINGS IN CYSTIC HYPERPLASIA, PARAPROSTATIC CYSTS, PROSTATITIS, AND PROSTATIC NEOPLASIA

	Laboratory Findings						
Prostatic Disease	**Leukocytosis**	**Hematuria**	**Pyuria**	**Bacteriuria**	**Hemorrhagic Prostatic Fluid**	**Purulent Prostatic Fluid**	**Bacteria in Prostatic Fluid**
Cystic Hyperplasia	No	Yes††	No	No	Yes††	No	No
Paraprostatic Cysts	No‡‡	No‡‡	No	No	No‡‡	No	No
Acute Prostatitis	Yes	Yes	Yes	Yes	NA	NA	NA
Chronic Prostatitis	No	Yes‡	Yes§	Yes‖	No#	Yes**	Yes
Prostatic Abscessation	Yes*	Yes	Yes	Yes	No#	Yes	Yes
Prostatic Neoplasia	No†	Yes	Yes	No	Yes	Yes	No

*60% of cases in 1 survey had a neutrophilic leukocytosis.[14]
†Only 20% of dogs with prostatic neoplasia had leukocytosis in 1 survey.[14]
‡60% of cases in 1 survey had hematuria.[14]
§72% of cases in 1 survey had pyuria.[14]
‖80% of cases in 1 survey had positive urine cultures.[14]
#33% of cases in 1 survey had hemorrhagic prostatic fluid.[14]
**75% of cases in 1 survey had purulent prostatic fluid.[14]
††75% of cases in 1 survey had bleeding.[14]
‡‡Leukocytosis and hematuria occasionally reported.
(From Barsanti JA, Finco DR. Canine prostatic diseases. *In:* Ettinger SJ, ed. *Textbook of Veterinary Internal Medicine.* Philadelphia, Pennsylvania: WB Saunders, 1986.)

b. The hyperplastic process is facilitated by estrogens, which may enhance androgen receptors.[61,215,248,257,268] In older dogs, despite declining androgen production, estrogen production (estrone and estradiol) increases.[38,148,268]

3. Dihydrotestosterone (DHT) within the gland probably serves as the main hormonal mediator of hyperplasia,[86,92,118,119,148,176,268] although some disagree.[64] The changes in DHT concentration with age are considered to be the most likely explanation for the development of prostatic hyperplasia.[86]
   a. DHT accumulates because of changes in catabolism and enhanced binding.[178,268]
   b. The concentration of enzyme that converts testosterone to DHT is higher in the prostatic epithelium than in the prostatic stroma of dogs.[251] The opposite is thought to be true in men, which may explain why hyperplasia is mainly epithelial in dogs and stromal in men.[251]
   c. Inhibitors of the final enzyme (5-alpha reductase) in the synthetic pathway for DHT may hold promise for treatment of BPH.[86,108]
4. Three other theories have been proposed to explain the development of BPH.[122]
   a. "Embryonic reawakening." The prostatic stroma responds to aging changes in androgens by regaining its embryonic induction properties, causing the prostatic epithelium to renew growth.
   b. "Stem cell hypothesis." An increase in the number of stem cells or in their ability to proliferate other cells; because a prostate that has involuted after castration can still be restored to normal size by androgen administration, the presence of two or more populations of prostate cells is assumed. One population is very androgen sensitive. The other, much smaller in quantity, is androgen insensitive as far as survival and is available to repopulate the prostate when androgens are administered (stem cells).
      (1). Stem cell development is androgen dependent early in life. When dogs were castrated at 14 months of age, normal prostate size could not be restored by androgen administration, whereas when beagles were castrated at 24 months of age, normal prostatic size was restored by androgen administration.[33,34]
      (2). One factor that may modify the amount of stem cell is stromal-epithelial interaction.
      (3). Because hyperplastic prostatic tissue is metabolically different from normal epithelium, the cells must be changed in type as well as amount.[122]
   c. Increased amounts of intraprostatic growth factors.[188]
5. Benign prostatic hyperplasia in dogs begins as glandular hyperplasia.[65] This begins as early as 2½ years of age in some dogs.[33,52,65]
6. After 4 years of age, a tendency to cystic hyperplasia begins.[33,65,150] This condition looks like a honeycomb in cross section (Fig. 39–5).
   a. Intraprostatic cystic hyperplasia is an extension of glandular hyperplasia.[52,115,116,142]
   b. Intraparenchymal cysts often communicate with the urethra and may be largest at the periphery of the gland.[115]
   c. The cysts vary in size and contour and contain a thin, clear to amber fluid.[142]
7. In an individual dog, BPH seems to develop rapidly (within 1 year).[33] Almost all men and sexually intact male dogs develop prostatic hy-

TABLE 39–3.
RADIOGRAPHIC AND ULTRASONOGRAPHIC FINDINGS ASSOCIATED WITH PROSTATIC DISEASES

Disease	Radiographic Findings	Ultrasonographic Findings
Benign Hyperplasia	Mild to moderate prostatomegaly	Diffusely hyperechoic, may contain focal hypoechoic areas (cysts)
Paraprostatic Cyst	Asymmetric prostatomegaly; caudal abdominal mass, may mineralize	Large hypoechoic or anechoic mass
Squamous Metaplasia	Mild to moderate prostatomegaly; accentuated colliculus seminalis	Diffusely hyperechoic
Acute Prostatitis	Normal to mild loss of detail in vicinity of prostate	Diffusely or focally hyperechoic
Chronic Prostatitis	Normal or granular mineralization	Focally or diffusely hypoechoic
Abscessation	Asymmetric prostatomegaly	Asymmetric; diffusely hyperechoic with focal anechoic areas
Neoplasia	Asymmetric prostatomegaly; may have granular mineralization; distortion of prostatic urethra	Multifocally hyperechoic; asymmetric

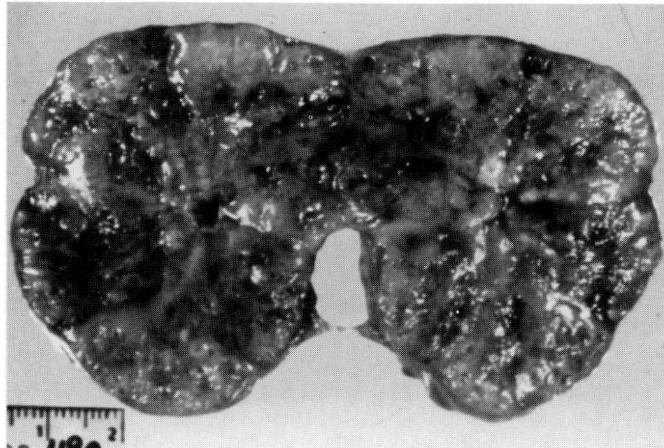

FIG. 39–5. A prostate gland involved with cystic hyperplasia; note the multifocal cystic areas and the mildly irregular "cobblestone" contour. (Courtesy of Drs. WA Crowell and LA Cowan, College of Veterinary Medicine, University of Georgia; from Barsanti JA, Diagnosis and medical therapy of prostatic disorders. *In:* Stone EA, Barsanti JA, eds. *Urologic Surgery of the Dog and Cat.* Philadelphia, Pennsylvania: Lea & Febiger, 1992;215.)

perplasia with age; however, most do not develop clinical signs.[122,150]

8. Although size increases with hyperplasia, prostatic secretory function decreases (decreased seminal volume).[38,115,263]
9. The vascularity of the prostate is increased with hyperplasia, and the gland has a tendency to bleed.[115]
10. Histologic evidence of mild chronic inflammation is common in dogs with hyperplasia.[38,124,150] Inflammation is primarily interstitial.[150]

B. Clinical signs.

1. History.
   a. Most dogs with prostatic hyperplasia have no signs.
   b. In some dogs, tenesmus associated with defecation may be present because of encroachment on the pelvic canal by the enlarged prostate.
   c. An intermittent hemorrhagic or clear, light yellow urethral discharge occurs in some dogs.
   d. Intermittent or persistent hematuria has also been associated with hyperplasia.
   e. Hyperplasia is not associated with any systemic signs of illness. Affected dogs are usually alert, active, and afebrile, although some reported cases have had anorexia, lethargy, and caudal abdominal pain.[141] However, this case review combined intraprostatic cysts with prostatic retention cysts, and prostatic retention cysts have been associated with more severe signs because of their larger size. I prefer to group prostatic retention cysts with paraprostatic cysts.
2. Physical examination.
   a. The prostate gland is not painful and is symmetrically enlarged. Consistency varies from normal to mild irregularity (cobblestone surface contour).
   b. In a study of 30 dogs with hyperplasia, the average size of the prostate was $5.5 \times 5.1 \times 3.1$ cm.[142]
3. Urine is normal or contains blood, either gross or microscopic.
4. Hematologic and serum biochemical parameters are unaffected by hyperplasia.
5. Prostatic fluid.
   a. If a urethral discharge is present, the discharge is hemorrhagic or clear but not purulent.[14]
   b. Semen and postprostatic massage samples may be normal or hemorrhagic (see Fig. 6–8).[14] Prostatic epithelial cells, when seen, appear normal.[246]
6. Imaging techniques. (See Chapter 11, Diagnostic Imaging of the Urinary Tract.)
   a. Survey abdominal radiographs confirm mild to moderate prostate enlargement with dorsal displacement of the colon and cranial displacement of the bladder. The prostate otherwise appears normal.[240]
   b. On distention retrograde urethrocystography, the prostatic urethra may be normal or may appear narrowed and undulant without distortion or destruction.[75] Urethroprostatic reflux may be greater than normal.
   c. On ultrasonography, the prostate is often normal, but it may also be diffusely hyperechoic with parenchymal cavities if intraparenchymal cysts have developed. The prostatic capsule is smooth and the gland is symmetrically enlarged.[202] The degree of enlargement is often mild.[128] The cavitary areas are typically well defined and smoothly marginated.[128]
7. Definitive diagnosis is possible only by biopsy.
   a. A presumptive diagnosis can be based on history and physical examination, with support from hematologic tests, urinalysis, and prostatic fluid analysis.
   b. I usually do not recommend biopsy for confirmation of the diagnosis if the clinical signs are typical.
   c. Response to castration can be used to help to confirm the diagnosis.

C. Treatment.

1. Treatment is required only if abnormal signs occur.
2. The most effective treatment is castration, which results in a 70% decrease in prostate size.[115,117,223]
   a. The prostate gland exhibits involution within days, and a palpable decrease in prostatic size is expected within 7 to 14 days.[36,130]
   b. Prostatic secretion becomes minimal 7 to 16 days after castration.[114,115]
   c. In both young and old dogs, prostatic weight declines most rapidly within the first month

after castration.[32] In dogs older than 6 years, prostatic weight continues to decline for 3 to 4 months.[32,115]

d. With cystic hyperplasia, small, irregular spaces may remain after castration.[115]

3. If castration is not feasible, small doses of estrogens can be used.
   a. Estrogens cause prostatic atrophy by reducing androgen concentrations. Estrogens reduce androgen levels by depressing gonadotropin secretion by the pituitary gland.
   b. Estrogens act primarily to decrease prostate size by decreasing cellular mass. There may be no effect on intraparenchymal cysts.[115]
   c. Diethylstilbestrol (DES) administered orally in doses of 0.2 to 1 mg per day for 5 days, or every few days for 3 weeks, has been recommended.[127]
      (1). Effective dosages of estrogens have not been determined.
      (2). In a study, 0.1 mg of injectable DES per day for 5 days markedly reduced prostatic secretory capability for 2 months.[180]
   d. The potential side effects of estrogens must be compared to their potential clinical benefit in each case before a decision is made to administer them.
      (1). With toxicity, an initial leukocytosis with a leftward shift is followed by severe bone marrow depression, with resultant anemia, thrombocytopenia, and leukopenia.
         (a). These effects have been noticed with overdosing, with repeated administration, and at the recommended dosage as an idiosyncratic reaction.[79,149,174,207,239]
         (b). Oral doses of 5 mg per day of DES usually resulted in death within 2 months, but doses of 1 mg per day were given for 9 months without development of anemia.[253] Single doses of estradiol cyclopentylpropionate (ECP) greater than 0.22 mg/kg given intramuscularly produced hematologic abnormalities; doses greater than 0.9 mg/kg consistently produced estrogen toxicity.[46] The dosage and duration of estrogen therapy that produce toxicity vary with the presence or absence of other factors (e.g., physical condition, parasitism) that modify bone marrow function.[50]
      (2). Although small doses of estrogens decrease prostate size, repeated administration and overdosing can also cause growth of the fibromuscular stroma of the prostate, metaplasia of prostatic glandular epithelium, and secretory stasis.[27,115] These changes can result in further prostatic enlargement and a predisposition to cyst formation, bacterial infection, and abscessation.

4. A drug that avoids the side effects of estrogens is the antiandrogen flutamide.[183]
   a. This drug specifically blocks DHT activity in the prostate by competing for DHT receptors. Thus, it has few effects on testicular function.[86] In men, flutamide shrinks the hyperplastic prostate without affecting libido, but benefits in clinical signs have been equivocal.[158,242] Mild gynecomastia and breast pain are the major side effects.[242]
   b. This drug was administered orally to research dogs in doses of 5 mg/kg/d for 1 year. Within 6 weeks of initiating treatment, prostatic size decreased dramatically. No changes were observed in libido, sperm production, or apparent fertility.[182] In another study, a significant decrease in prostate size, as detected by ultrasonography, was evident within 10 days.[44] Prostatic hyperplasia recurred within 2 months of drug discontinuation.[183]
   c. The drug is not approved for veterinary use, and it is expensive.[171]

5. Megestrol acetate also has antiandrogenic properties.[85,86,147,234]
   a. In men, megestrol reduces serum testosterone concentration, competitively inhibits binding of DHT to intracellular receptors, decreases DHT concentrations by inhibiting 5-alpha reductase, and decreases the number of androgen receptors in the prostate.[85,86,158,234] However, the degree of improvement in symptoms was little better in men treated with megestrol than in men treated with placebo.[86]
   b. Plasma concentrations of testosterone tend to rise again with continued therapy.[234]
   c. For dogs, a dose of 0.55 mg/kg/d for 4 weeks has been recommended.[192] This therapy resulted in no decrease in sperm numbers in 7 of 7 dogs (1 dog sired puppies[192]), and clinical signs of hyperplasia resolved in all 20 dogs.[192,224] This drug is not approved for use in male dogs nor for use for longer than 32 days in female dogs. Therefore, its principal application is for owners who want to maintain a short period of breeding soundness before neutering. A few owners who refused to have their dogs castrated allowed treatment at a dose of 0.55 mg/kg once a week, but effects of prolonged use have not been studied.[192] Prolonged use in cats has resulted in significant side effects, including diabetes mellitus, hypoadrenocorticism, and mammary gland hyperplasia.

6. The antifungal drug ketoconazole and gonadotropin-releasing hormone analogs (which block the release of luteinizing hormone) are antiandrogenic.[126,135,147,158,192,249,250] However, these drugs are essentially chemical castrators.[159]

Thus, they have no advantage over surgical castration in dogs.

7. Finasteride is a 5-alpha reductase inhibitor that was approved in 1992 for oral administration to men for prostatic hyperplasia. The drug caused a decrease of approximately 20 to 30% in prostate size in men within 6 to 12 months.[131] Although the drug had no effect on libido, it can cause fetal anomalies and is present in semen. If the same adverse effects occur in dogs, the drug would not be useful as an alternative to castration for owners who wish to maintain the breeding soundness of their dog.[170] Discontinuation of therapy results in return of hyperplasia.[131] Another 5-alpha reductase inhibitor (4-MA) was effective experimentally in the treatment of canine prostatic hyperplasia[39,262]; however, development for clinical use in humans was not pursued because the compound also affected other androgen receptors.[159]

III. SQUAMAOUS METAPLASIA

A. Pathophysiology.

1. Squamous metaplasia of prostatic columnar epithelium is secondary to exogenous or endogenous hyperestrogenism.[10,27,115,143,180,196,227,274]
   a. The mucosa and the submucosa of the prostatic urethra, the prostatic stroma, and the periurethral prostatic ductal epithelium contain estrogen receptors.[226]
   b. The glandular epithelium of normal dogs does not have estrogen receptors, but in dogs with BPH, epithelium in a few (<10%) glands exhibits estrogen receptors.[226]
   c. In dogs treated with estrogen, estrogen receptors become evident in all epithelium that develops squamous metaplasia.[226] Plasma cell infiltration was also noted, especially in the periurethral stroma. Short-term use of estrogens results in squamous metaplasia of the prostatic urethra and ducts only, whereas longer-term use of estrogens causes squamous metaplasia throughout the prostate. These findings fit well with the localization of estrogen receptors: those along the ducts are always present, whereas those in glandular epithelium require induction by exposure to higher levels of estrogen or to increases in the estrogen/androgen ratio in the prostate gland.
2. The major endogenous cause is a functional Sertoli cell tumor.
3. In addition to causing squamous metaplasia of the epithelial cells, estrogens also cause secretory stasis.
4. The epithelial change and secretory stasis predispose to cyst formation, infection, and abscessation.[109,116,123,127,145,198,235]

B. Clinical signs.

1. Physical examination.
   a. The prostate varies in size. Estrogens can result in prostatic atrophy secondary to inhibition of testosterone production; however, prolonged exposure to estrogens results in mild to moderate prostatic hypertrophy.[198] Secondary development of cysts or abscesses can be associated with marked prostatic enlargement.[198]
   b. With endogenous hyperestrogenism, the testicles may be palpably abnormal or one or both may be undescended. The opposite testicle is usually atrophic. With exogenous hyperestrogenism, both testicles may be atrophic.
   c. Other physical signs of hyperestrogenism, including alopecia, hyperpigmentation, gynecomastia, and pendulous prepuce, may be present.
2. Hematology/biochemical profile.
   a. Hematologic findings may reflect toxicity of estrogens.[227]
      (1). Nonregenerative anemia.
      (2). Thrombocytopenia.
      (3). Granulocytosis followed by granulocytopenia.
   b. Biochemical profile. Hyperestrogenism does not directly affect biochemical parameters unless the prostate gland becomes abscessed. (See Section VII of this chapter.)
3. Prostatic fluid. Increased quantities of squamous epithelial cells may be noted; inflammation may also be evident (see Fig. 6–4).[198,214,246]
4. Imaging.
   a. Survey radiographs usually indicate prostatomegaly.
   b. On retrograde urethrography, reflux of contrast material into cavities within the prostate gland and a persistent radiolucent filling defect in the prostatic urethra have been noted in some cases (Fig. 39–6).[123] The filling defect was

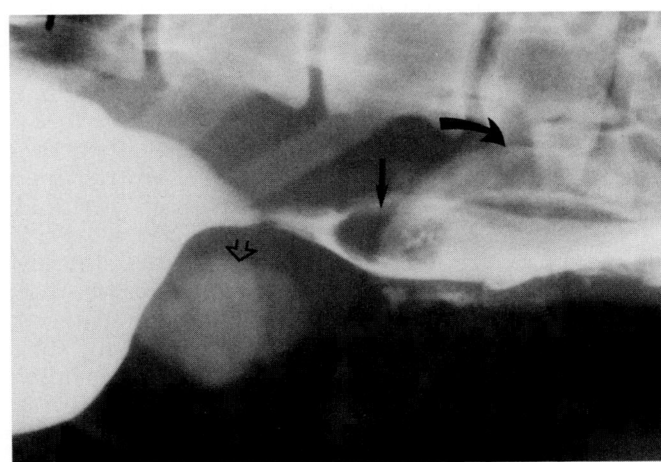

FIG. 39–6. Retrograde urethrogram in a dog with prostatomegaly, cryptorchidism, and gynecomastia. A large nipple is evident (open arrows), as are urethroprostatic reflux (curved arrow) and the colliculus seminalis (solid arrow). A Sertoli cell tumor of the testicle and squamous metaplasia of the prostate were identified in tissue specimens removed surgically. (Barsanti JA. Canine prostatic disease. *In:* Ettinger SJ, ed. *Veterinary Internal Medicine.* Philadelphia, Pennsylvania: W.B. Saunders, 1989;1859.)

an enlarged colliculus seminalis secondary to squamous metaplasia and edema.

c. Ultrasonography may also identify filling defects within the prostate gland. These can be either cysts or abscesses associated with squamous metaplasia.[123]

5. Prostatic tissue: The prostatic ducts and acini are lined by squamous rather than columnar epithelium.[198,214,246] The epithelium of the prostatic urethra and the uterus masculinus also become squamous in cell type.[198]

C. Treatment.

1. Treatment requires removing the source of estrogens.
   a. Castration in cases of endogenous hyperestrogenism.
   b. Discontinuation of estrogen therapy in cases of exogenous hyperestrogenism.
2. Squamous metaplasia of the epithelium is reversible.[115]

IV. INFLAMMATORY PROSTATIC DISEASES: AN OVERVIEW

A. Bacterial infection.

1. The most common inflammatory diseases of the canine prostate gland are associated with bacterial infection, either acute or chronic, with or without abscessation. Each is considered separately in depth.
   a. The prostate gland can be predisposed to infection by
      (1). Urethral diseases: Urolithiasis, trauma, strictures, neoplasia.
      (2). Urinary tract infection (UTI).
      (3). Prostatic diseases: Cysts, neoplasia, squamous metaplasia, neoplasia.
   b. Possible routes of infection.
      (1). The urethra (considered to be most common).
      (2). Infected urine.
      (3). The blood.
      (4). The vas deferens.
      (5). Direct extension or lymphatic transmission of rectal flora.
2. Bacteria usually involved[141]:
   a. *Escherichia coli* (most common)
   b. *Staphylococcus* spp.
   c. *Proteus* spp.
   d. *Klebsiella* spp.
   e. *Pseudomonas* spp.
   f. *Streptococcus* spp.
   g. *Brucella canis.* Signs of *B. canis* infection more often are related to orchiitis and scrotal dermatitis than to the prostate gland.[98]
   h. The role of anaerobes is unclear; anaerobes have been involved in some cases of abscessation.
   i. Note that the organisms commonly involved are the same as those that cause UTIs.

B. Infection with other organisms.

1. Infection by other organisms, fungi, or mycoplasmas[192,235] is rarely reported. Granulomatous chronic prostatitis has been noted in association with blastomycosis[13,141,230] and cryptococcosis.[255]
2. Although the controversy persists, most carefully performed studies in men indicate that ureaplasmas, mycoplasmas, and chlamydias are unlikely to be agents of chronic prostatitis.[28,54]

C. Noninfectious inflammation.

1. Noninfectious inflammatory disease is commonly described in humans, but the role of the inflammatory changes associated with hyperplasia in dogs is unknown.
2. In men, inflammatory prostatitis is 12 times as likely to be nonbacterial as it is to be bacterial.[168] This is in marked contrast to the case for dogs, in which most cases of clinically significant inflammation are associated with bacterial infection.

V. ACUTE BACTERIAL PROSTATITIS

A. Pathophysiology.

1. Bacterial prostatitis generally affects sexually mature male dogs.
2. Acute bacterial prostatitis can result in septicemia, which may be responsible for the severity of clinical signs in some patients.[168]

B. Clinical signs.

1. History.
   a. Signs of systemic illness, such as anorexia and lethargy, are usually noted.
   b. Vomiting is possible.
   c. A small percentage of affected dogs has a stiff, stilted gait.
   d. Fluid may drip from the prepuce.
2. Physical examination.
   a. Depression and fever are usually present.
   b. Caudal abdominal pain may be present, causing the dog to walk stiffly (Fig. 39–7). The pain can be localized by palpation to the prostate gland.
   c. In size, symmetry, and contour, the prostate gland is often normal, unless it is hyperplastic.
   d. Constant or intermittent urethral discharge may be present.
3. Urinalysis/urine culture.
   a. Urine usually contains blood, white blood cells (WBC), and bacteria.
   b. If urinalysis indicates UTI, a quantitative urine culture and sensitivity testing should be performed with a sample collected by cystocentesis or catheterization. The purpose of the culture is to identify the organism and its relative antibiotic sensitivity. This information is important for selecting an appropriate therapeutic agent and determining whether subsequent infections are relapses or new infections.
4. Hematology/blood chemistry. A neutrophilic leukocytosis, with or without a leftward shift, is often observed.
5. Prostatic fluid.
   a. In dogs, acute prostatitis is often so painful as to prevent ejaculation.

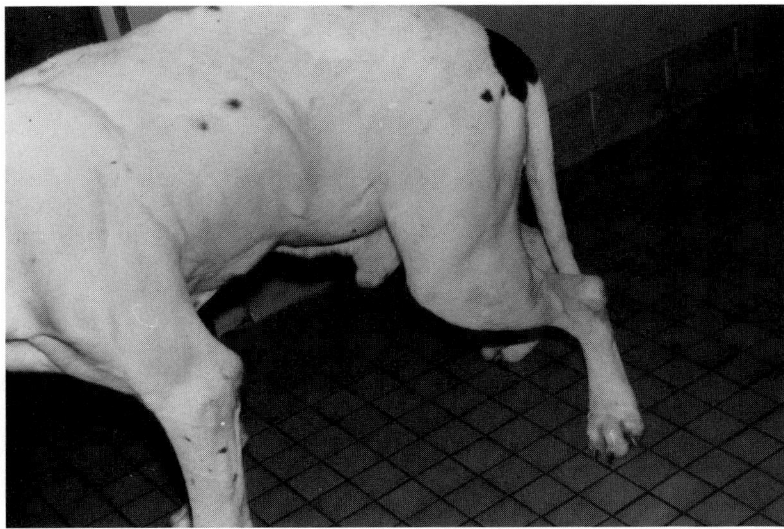

FIG. 39–7. A dog exhibiting pain in the rear limbs by standing on its toes and squatting slightly. In this dog, the source of the pain was localized to the prostate gland by rectal palpation. The concurrent presence of fever, leukocytosis, and urinary tract infection with only mild prostatomegaly in the young adult supported a presumptive diagnosis of acute bacterial prostatitis. (Barsanti JA. Diagnosis and medical therapy of prostatic disorders. *In:* Stone EA, Barsanti JA, eds. *Urologic Surgery of the Dog and Cat.* Philadelphia, Pennsylvania: Lea & Febiger, 1992.)

b. In human medicine, prostatic massage is contraindicated, for fear of inducing septicemia.[166,193]
   (1). We have not induced bacteremia with massage in dogs with experimental infections.
   (2). However, the results of prostatic massage in dogs with UTI are difficult (or impossible) to interpret. (See Chapter 6, Collection and Analysis of Prostatic Fluid and Tissue.)

6. Imaging.
   a. Survey abdominal radiographs may be normal or show a loss of detail at the margins of the prostate gland.
   b. With ultrasonography, echogenicity of the prostate gland may be focally to diffusely increased.

C. Treatment.

1. An antibiotic should be administered for at least 28 days.
   a. The choice of the antibiotic can be based on findings of urine culture and antibiotic sensitivity testing.
   b. With acute inflammation, the blood–prostatic fluid barrier is usually not intact, thus allowing a wide choice of antibiotics initially.[93,200]
   c. If the presenting signs are severe, the antibiotic initially should be given intravenously. Oral antimicrobials can be used once the condition of the dog improves.
   d. An oral antimicrobial with prostatic penetrance is preferred for the remainder of therapy. (See Section VI of this chapter.)[168]
2. Normal hydration should be sustained. If the dog exhibits vomiting or adipsia, intravenous fluid is needed. A balanced electrolyte solution, such as lactated Ringer's, with supplemental potassium (as needed) is generally the fluid of choice. The amount should be sufficient to meet maintenance fluid needs, correct gastrointestinal losses, and correct any evident dehydration.
3. Because acute infections may become chronic, the animal should be re-examined 3 to 7 days after antibiotic therapy is completed. The examination should include a physical examination, urinalysis, urine culture, and examination of prostatic fluid by cytology and culture. Acute bacterial prostatitis can also cause epididymitis or pyelonephritis.

VI. CHRONIC BACTERIAL PROSTATITIS

A. Pathophysiology.

1. Chronic prostatic infection may be a sequela to an acute infection, or it may develop insidiously, without a prior bout of a clinically evident acute infection.
2. In dogs, lower UTIs and prostatic infections are almost inseparable.
   a. Experimental infection of the bladder is difficult without infecting the prostate, and vice versa.[146]
   b. Any intact male dog with a UTI should be considered to have a prostate infection until it can be proved otherwise, even if clinical signs are absent.

3. The incidence of chronic prostate infections in dogs is unknown.
   a. Some 6 to 10% of male dogs have a UTI,[137] and an accompanying prostate infection would be expected.
   b. This percentage would be similar to the 5% prevalence reported for human males.[193] In men, prevalence increases with age—to 16% after age 80 years.[193] A higher prevalence of occult prostatic infection (21%) was reported when the diagnosis was based on cultures of prostate tissue at the time of prostatectomy.[96]
   c. Chronic prostatitis was the most common prostatic disease diagnosed in a series of patients seen at a veterinary teaching hospital.[141]
4. The prostate glands of normal male dogs and of men produce an antibacterial substance, referred to as "prostatic antibacterial factor" (PAF).[71]
   a. PAF is a heat-stable, water-soluble, low-molecular-weight, zinc-complexed polypeptide with wide antibacterial efficacy, especially against gram-negative enteric organisms.[71]
   b. PAF owes its antibacterial activity to its zinc content.[71]
      (1). Men with chronic bacterial prostatitis have a decreased zinc concentration in the prostatic fluid, but whether this finding is a cause or an effect is not known.[67,68,71,132,133,167,193]
      (2). Dietary supplementation with zinc had no effect on zinc concentrations in the prostate fluid.[68,133,193]
      (3). Dogs with chronic prostatitis have normal concentrations of zinc in their prostatic fluid and tissue.[21,38,48]
5. Men with acute or chronic prostatic infections have in their prostatic fluid increased concentrations of IgA antibodies against the specific bacteria involved.[79,80,151,228] Antibody concentrations in urine and prostatic fluid have been used to help to differentiate chronic bacterial prostatitis from nonbacterial prostatitis in men.[193,229]

B. Clinical signs.

1. History.
   a. Most often, no signs are directly referable to the prostate gland.
   b. The dog may appear for recurrent episodes of cystitis or for constant or intermittent urethral discharge or hematuria.
   c. Some dogs are lethargic.[141]
   d. Chronic prostatitis is a consideration in male dogs that appear for infertility.
      (1). Some investigators have reported an association of chronic prostatitis with infertility in men.[87]
      (2). No effects on sperm parameters were found in one study of experimentally induced chronic bacterial prostatitis in dogs.[15]
      (3). Chronic prostatitis in dogs seemed to be associated with infertility in one series of clinical cases.[141]
2. Physical examination.
   a. The prostate is not painful when palpated, and its size is variable, owing to the degree of hyperplasia and of fibrosis. Chronic infection, by itself, does not increase the size of the prostate.[12]
   b. The prostate gland may vary in symmetry and consistency, owing to formation of fibrous tissue secondary to chronic inflammation. Areas of fibrous tissue are more firm than areas of normal prostatic tissue. The areas of infection may be focal, multifocal, or diffuse.
3. Urinalysis/urine culture.
   a. Evidence of a UTI (pyuria, hematuria, and bacteriuria)[12] on urinalysis in an intact male dog should prompt consideration of chronic prostatitis.
      (1). Chronic bacterial prostatitis is the most common cause of recurrent UTI in men.[166]
      (2). Whether the same is true in dogs is not known.
4. Hematology/biochemical profile.
   a. WBC count is usually normal unless abscessation is present.[12,14]
   b. The rest of the hemogram and the biochemical profile is usually normal.
5. Prostatic fluid.
   a. Assessment of prostatic fluid is essential to the diagnosis of chronic prostatitis, but interpreting the results can be difficult.[57] (See Chapter 6, Collection and Analysis of Prostatic Fluid and Tissue.) Semen samples are preferred for evaluation because samples collected by prostatic massage usually contain urine, which, if infected, can invalidate the results (Fig. 39–8). To utilize prostatic massage to diagnose chronic

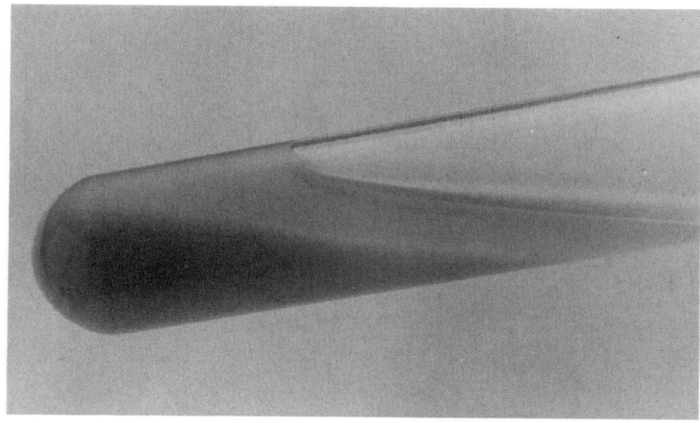

FIG. 39–8. Ejaculate from a dog with chronic bacterial prostatitis. The sediment contained many neutrophils. (Barsanti JA. Canine prostatic disease. *In:* Ettinger SJ, ed. *Veterinary Internal Medicine.* Philadelphia, Pennsylvania: W.B. Saunders, 1989; 1859.)

bacterial prostatitis, UTI must first be controlled.

b. Prostatic fluid collected by ejaculation or after prostatic massage contains inflammatory cells, and quantitative bacterial cultures usually grow one species of bacteria (see Fig. 6–5).[12]
   (1). The usual pathogen is *Escherichia coli.*
   (2). Dogs with experimental chronic bacterial prostatitis harbored more than 1000 organisms per milliliter.[12] Establishing a definitive number that separates infection from contamination is difficult, because chronic prostatitis is a multifocal disease and number of bacteria vary.[168] When interpreting the results of a culture, the clinician must consider all relevant findings: history, physical examination, urinalysis and urine culture, ultrasonography, and prostatic fluid cytology.
   (3). The finding of macrophages in ejaculates correlated with prostatic infection and inflammation.[12]
   (4). Although prostatic fluid from most dogs with prostatic infection is acidic,[12,21,22,37,163,192] the determination of prostatic fluid pH is useful for determining an appropriate course of therapy. (See the following section on treatment.)

6. Prostate imaging. (See Chapter 11, Diagnostic Imaging of the Urinary Tract.)
   a. No radiographic findings specifically suggest chronic bacterial prostatitis.
   b. With survey radiographs, granular parenchymal mineralization has been noted with chronic inflammation. Prostate size and contour are affected only if abscessation develops.
   c. Findings of distention retrograde urethrocystography usually are normal, except for greater than normal urethroprostatic reflux in some dogs.[74]
   d. By ultrasound, the prostate gland may be diffusely to multifocally hyperechoic.[76,128] Multifocal mineralization may also be seen, although mineralization is more common with neoplasia.[128] Hypoechoic areas suggest abscessation. Ultrasonography alone cannot differentiate chronic prostatitis from hyperplasia or neoplasia.

7. Prostatic tissue.
   a. Definitive diagnosis of chronic bacterial prostatitis is achieved by prostate tissue culture and histopathologic examination.
      (1). Culture of prostatic tissue may fail to grow bacteria even though infection is present.
         (a). A false-negative finding can result from missing a site of focal or multifocal infection.
         (b). A false-negative finding can also result from failure to retrieve the organism from the tissue (failure to macerate the tissue adequately or to use proper isolation methods for the pathogen at hand).
      (2). False-positive results are also possible if the sample is contaminated during collection.
   b. A presumptive diagnosis is reached by history, physical examination, hematologic studies, urinalysis, and prostatic fluid cytology and quantitative culture. In most cases, if these techniques are done carefully and assessed correctly, biopsy and culture of prostatic tissue are not needed to confirm the diagnosis.

C. Treatment.

1. The treatment of chronic bacterial prostatitis is antimicrobial therapy.
   a. Chronic bacterial prostatitis is difficult to treat effectively, because the blood–prostatic fluid barrier is intact (Fig. 39–9).[93,151,166]
      (1). The blood–prostatic fluid barrier results:
         (a). Partly from the differences in hydrogen ion concentrations in blood, prostatic interstitium, and prostatic fluid.
         (b). Partly from the characteristics of the prostatic acinar epithelium.
         (c). Partly from the protein-binding characteristics of antibiotics.[104,236,269]
      (2). The pH of blood and prostatic interstitium is 7.4. The pH of normal canine prostatic fluid is approximately 6.4.[12,16,37,73,116,216,269] Successful therapy correlates best with drug concentration of prostatic fluid, not of the prostatic interstitium.[168]
         (a). The presence of a pH gradient of at least 1.0 pH unit between compartments allows the phenomenon of ion trapping to occur (see Fig. 39–9).
         (b). The charged fraction of a drug is greater on one side of the system, depending on the pH.
         (c). Because the uncharged fraction of a lipid-soluble drug equilibrates, more total drug (charged plus uncharged) is on the side of greater ionization.
         (d). In contrast to humans, whose prostatic fluid becomes alkaline with infection,[7,69,70,204] most dogs with prostatic infection have acidic prostatic fluid.[12,21,22,37]
         (e). In acidic prostatic fluid, basic antibiotics with high pKa values, such as erythromycin, oleandromycin, clindamycin, and trimethoprim, ionize to a greater extent than in plasma (see Fig. 39–9). Prostatic fluid concentra-

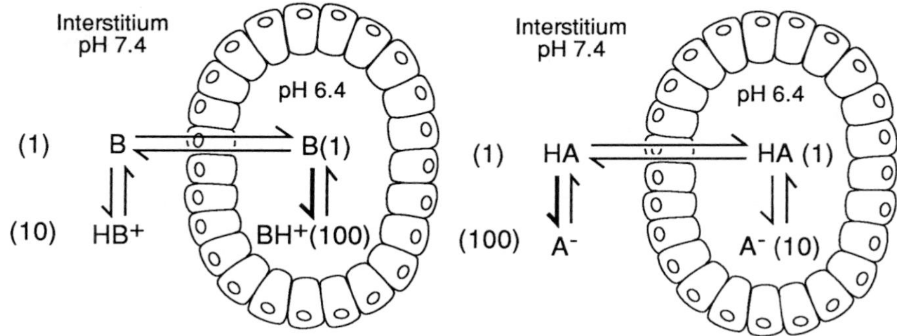

FIG. 39–9. Effect of the pH difference between the prostatic interstitium and prostatic fluid on ion trapping of antibiotics. Basic antibiotics are present in larger concentrations within prostatic acini **(A)** while acidic antibiotics do not enter the acini **(B).**

tion of trimethoprim can exceed plasma concentrations by two to ten times.[97,164,210,237]

(f). In alkaline prostatic fluid, acidic antibiotics, such as carbenicillin, are more effective.

(g). Distribution of nonionizable drugs, such as chloramphenicol, is not affected by pH differences.

(3). Lipid solubility is also an important factor in determining drug movement across prostatic epithelium.

(a). Drugs with low lipid solubility cannot cross into the prostatic acini. Many antibiotics, including penicillin, ampicillin, cephalosporins, oxytetracycline, and the aminoglycosides, are lipid insoluble.

(b). Chloramphenicol, the macrolide antibiotics, trimethoprim, the quinolones, and carbenicillin are examples of lipid-soluble drugs that can potentially enter prostatic fluid.

(4). Protein binding in plasma also determines the amount of drug available to enter prostatic fluid.

(a). Protein-bound drug is not available to diffuse. For highly protein-bound drugs, little free drug remains to enter prostatic epithelium.

(b). Protein binding factor is probably less important than lipid solubility or pKa, because biologic systems rarely reach equilibrium.

(c). Examples of drugs significantly bound by protein are clindamycin, chloramphenicol, and nalidixic acid.

b. In general, diffusion of tetracyclines into canine prostatic fluid is limited.

(1). Oxytetracycline does not enter prostatic fluid.

(2). If given intravenously, tetracycline may enter prostatic fluid.[107]

(3). Despite clinical studies in men that demonstrate efficacy for minocycline[199–201] and doxycycline,[84,213] penetration of these drugs into prostatic fluid of normal dogs was minimal.[23,166,167,209] The drugs may diffuse better into alkaline prostatic fluid,[167] and this possibility might explain the differences between the human and canine study findings.

c. Some newer quinolone antibiotics concentrate in human prostatic fluid.[49,169,181,193] They may be less efficacious in dogs, because their activity is enhanced in alkaline, not acidic, environments.[168]

(1). Norfloxacin is lipid soluble, a weak base with a high pKa, and poorly bound to proteins. It is concentrated in human prostate glands[29,34,35,80] and has been used to treat chronic UTIs and chronic prostatitis in men.[218,221] Norfloxacin was the first fluoroquinolone to be licensed for human use in the United States. Although norfloxacin has not been approved for use in dogs, its pharmacokinetics have been studied.[42] A dose of 20 mg/kg every 12 hours for 3 to 4 weeks was recommended for prostatic infection, although prostatic tissue levels were not studied.[42] An experimental study in dogs indicated that norfloxacin did not concentrate as well in canine prostatic fluid as in that of men.[55] In fact, in dogs, prostatic concentrations were slightly weaker than serum concentrations. The difference may be explained by the alkaline prostatic fluid in men, a condition that favors norfloxacin penetration.[55]

(2). Ciprofloxacin and ofloxacin also penetrate prostatic tissue.[1,2,169,247] Like norfloxacin, ciprofloxacin did not penetrate as well into canine prostatic fluid and tissue as into those of men. In fact, prostatic tissue levels in dogs were only 38% of prostatic tissue concentrations in men.[55] Prostatic ciprofloxacin concentrations were less than serum concentrations. The reasons for these findings are unclear because ciprofloxacin is a zwitterion: most is not ionized at pH 7.4. At higher and lower pH values, more should be ionized, and thus trapped.[1]

(3). Enrofloxacin is the first fluoroquinolone licensed for use in small animals.[254] The manufacturer reports prostatic penetrance in dogs. Enrofloxacin is not used in human medicine.

(4). Not all quinolones have prostatic penetrance. Rosoxacin is also a weak acid with a high pKa, but it is highly protein bound.[154] In dogs, rosoxacin and cinoxacin concentrations in prostatic fluid were only 10% of those in plasma.[55,154,155]

d. Most of the penicillins and cephalosporins do not diffuse into prostatic fluid because they are lipid insoluble and weak acids.[23,138,200,187,191]

(1). An exception is hetacillin, which is lipid soluble and cleaves to ampicillin within the prostatic acini.[138]

(2). Another exception is carbenicillin indanyl sodium.[222]

(a). In esterified form, carbenicillin is lipid soluble and uncharged, and its prostatic tissue concentrations are approximately 70% of plasma concentrations in dogs; however, prostatic fluid concentrations were not detectable.[187]

(b). In recent studies in humans, carbenicillin administered for 4 to 8 weeks resulted in a cure rate of about 70%, whereas trimethoprim sulfamethoxazole, given for 8 weeks, resulted in a 40% cure rate.[175,191]

(c). Prostatic fluid of men with chronic prostatitis is alkaline[7,69,70,204]; thus, an acidic antibiotic, such as carbenicillin, should be more successful than an alkaline antibiotic, such as trimethoprim.[93,222] The reverse may be the case in dogs, in which prostatic fluid is acidic.

e. Trimethoprim has excellent tissue penetrance into prostatic tissue of dogs.[97,164,209,210,237] Trimethoprim is a base that is able to diffuse into the more acidic canine prostatic fluid. Although it is less effective than quinolones for treatment of chronic prostatitis in men,[221,222] one would expect the opposite to be true in dogs because of the acidity of their prostatic fluid. The usual sulfa components of trimethoprim-sulfa combinations, sulfadiazine and sulfamethoxazole, do not diffuse well into normal canine prostatic fluid.[152,270]

f. Current recommendations for choosing an antimicrobial agent depend on whether a gram-positive or a gram-negative organism is the infective agent (Table 39–4).

(1). If the causative organism is gram positive, erythromycin, clindamycin, oleandromycin, chloramphenicol, or trimethoprim-sulfonamide can be chosen, depending on bacterial sensitivity.

(2). If the organism is gram negative, chloramphenicol, a quinolone, or trimethoprim-sulfonamide would be best.

TABLE 39–4.
USUAL ANTIBIOTIC DOSAGES FOR TREATING BACTERIAL PROSTATITIS

Drug	Dose (mg/kg)	Frequency	Route
Chloramphenicol	30-55	q 8 h	PO, IV
Ciprofloxacin	5-8	q 12 h	PO, IV
Clindamycin	11	q 12 h	PO, IV[43]
Enrofloxacin	2.5-11*	q 12 h	PO, IM
Norfloxacin	20	q 12 h	PO
Trimethoprim/sulfa	15	q 12 h	PO, SQ
Erythromycin	10	q 8 h	PO

*Higher dosages are required for infections caused by *Pseudomonas aeruginosa*.[256]
PO = oral; IV = intravenous; IM = intramuscular; SQ = subcutaneous.

(3). In difficult cases, measurement of prostatic fluid pH could help the clinician to choose a potentially effective drug.

g. Antibiotics should be continued at least 6 weeks. Treatment courses as long as 24 weeks are used in men.[45,168] Adverse effects are possible with long-term use of antimicrobial agents.

(1). Trimethoprim-sulfa has been associated with adverse effects.[51]

(a). Keratoconjunctivitis sicca.[177]

(b). Folate deficiency anemia when given longer than 6 weeks.

(c). Hepatopathy.[51,72,217]

(d). Bone marrow failure.[88]

(e). Arthropathy.[88,103,263]

(f). Wheals, skin rash, drug eruption.[51,88]

(g). The arthropathy, polymyositis, skin rash, and bone marrow failure were found to be associated with sulfadiazine rather than with trimethoprim.[88] All but one of the reported animals were receiving the veterinary product containing sulfadiazine rather than the human product containing sulfamethoxazole.[51] The animals reported to have hepatopathy were also receiving the veterinary, rather than the human, product.[51,217] Whether this experience reflects a difference in capacity of the two sulfonamides to produce such a reaction or merely the difference in use of the two products in dogs is not known. Cutaneous drug eruptions have been reported as frequently with combinations containing sulfamethoxazole as with those containing sulfadiazine.[172] Doberman pinschers have been reported to be most commonly affected with arthropathy, but arthropathy affects other breeds as well.[51] Other types of reactions have not been related to breed.

(h). Dose and duration of therapy are related to the development of keratoconjunctivitis sicca.[177] Whether dose is related to other toxicities is not clear, but several reports of this complication cite treatment at twice the recommended dose (30 mg/kg twice daily rather than 30 mg/kg once daily).[88,217,263] The larger dose was recently recommended for prostate disease.[266] No experimental evidence suggests that such a large dose is necessary; until such evidence is produced, the standard dose is recommended, at least for initial therapy.

(2). Chloramphenicol has been associated with anorexia, lethargy, and, when given to dogs longer than 6 weeks, nonregenerative anemia.

h. Urine and prostatic fluid should be recultured 3 to 7 days and 1 month after discontinuing antibiotics, to be sure the infection has been eliminated and not merely suppressed.

i. The prognosis for cure with antibiotic therapy alone, based on human medicine, is only 30 to 60%.[168,222,261] Cultures taken during and immediately after therapy may be negative, but a relapse within a few months after therapy is discontinued is common. Part of the difficulty in curing the infection is the possibility of abnormalities in host immune competence, as well as in the blood–prostatic fluid barrier.[162]

j. If initial therapy fails, a 3-month course of therapy should be used; therapy is discontinued only if drug side effects emerge.

(1). For such long-term therapy, trimethoprim-sulfa or a quinolone is currently the best choice.

(2). Trimethoprim-sulfa can induce keratoconjunctivitis sicca or mild anemia secondary to folate deficiency. We administer folic acid when a dog must take trimethoprim longer than 6 weeks at full dosage. Preformed folic acid cannot be utilized by bacteria; thus, giving it to the animal does not cancel the efficacy of the drug. We familiarize owners with the symptoms of keratoconjunctivitis sicca.

(3). The side effects of long-term use of quinolones in dogs are not well studied.

2. Castration may be beneficial as adjunctive therapy for chronic bacterial prostatitis.

a. In dogs, castration performed 2 weeks after induction of experimental chronic prostatitis hastened spontaneous resolution of the infection.[47]

b. This research suggested that castration may be beneficial in resolving prostatic infection in clinical cases, but the efficacy of this approach remains to be proved, because the interval between establishment of infection and castration may be important.

3. If oral antibiotics plus castration fail to cure the prostatic infection, only two options remain: low-dose antibiotic therapy and prostatectomy.

a. Low-dose antibiotic therapy can be instituted to suppress the UTI so that it will be asymptomatic.

(1). Trimethoprim, in 50% of the usual daily dose each night, is useful for this purpose.

(2). Other drugs that have been given in one nightly dose include nitrofurantoin, quinolones, and cephalosporins.

b. Prostatectomy eliminates infected prostatic tissue and can be used for dogs that are refractory to antibiotic therapy and to castration.

(1). The standard surgical procedure is difficult, and urinary incontinence is a frequent sequela in advanced cases of prostatic disease.[19,140]

(a). Urodynamic evaluation (cystometry and urethral pressure profilometry) should be performed before prostatectomy is undertaken, to discover pre-existing abnormalities.[19]

(b). If significant abnormalities are present, incontinence is likely sequela.[19]

(c). Several possible mechanisms of incontinence are associated with prostatic disease and prostatectomy.[19,94]

(1′). Decreased resting urethral pressure. Unfortunately, such alpha-adrenergic agonists as phenylpropanolamine, which are usually effective for primary sphincter incontinence, have been ineffective in most patients with postprostatectomy incontinence.[19]

(2′). Detrusor instability is less common than decreased urethral pressure, but it responds to therapy with oxybutynin. This diagnosis can be distinguished from urethral sphincter incompetence only with cystometry.

(3′). Overflow incontinence can be differentiated from urethral incompetence because of the high postvoiding residual volume with overflow incontinence.

(2). The development of newer techniques for prostatectomy in dogs may reduce the adverse effects so that in the future the technique becomes a more acceptable alternative.[208]

4. Outside the United States, direct injection of antimicrobial agents into the prostate gland has been used to treat chronic prostatic infections in men. Results were similar to those achieved with oral antibiotics. The number of injections varied from 1 to 10.[9,125,206] The route of injection was generally transperineal. The frequency of injections varied from weekly to every few months. Such therapy has not been evaluated in dogs.

VII. PROSTATIC ABSCESSATION

A. Pathophysiology.

1. Prostatic abscessation is a severe form of chronic bacterial prostatitis in which pockets of septic, purulent exudate develop within the parenchyma of the prostate gland (Fig. 39–10). Prostatic abscesses vary in size and number in any given dog.
2. Aerobic organisms similar to those that cause bacterial prostatitis are most often isolated in dogs (*E. coli* organisms 70% of the time).[179] Nevertheless, in 19% of cases no aerobic organisms were found.[179] This discovery may be related to prior antibiotic therapy or to infection with anaerobes or mycoplasmas. In human medicine, anaerobes have been associated with aerobic organisms in prostatic abscesses.[17]

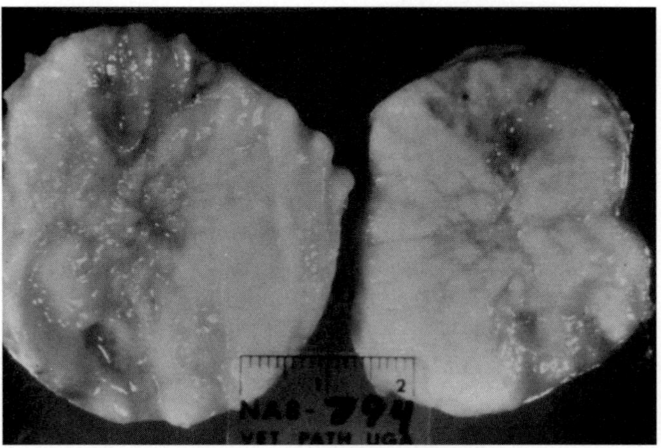

FIG. 39–10. A prostate gland with multifocal, abscessed areas. (Courtesy of Drs. WA Crowell and LA Cowan, College of Veterinary Medicine, University of Georgia; from Barsanti JA. Diagnosis and medical therapy of prostatic disorders. *In:* Stone EA, Barsanti JA, eds. *Urologic Surgery of the Dog and Cat.* Philadelphia, Pennsylvania: Lea & Febiger, 1992;215.)

B. Clinical signs.

1. History.
   a. The dog may appear for signs related either to prostatic enlargement or to infection.
   b. If the abscess, or abscesses, become large, the dog may appear for tenesmus from incursion on the colon or rectum or dysuria from incursion on the urethra. Incursion on the urethra can lead to partial urethral obstruction and, in turn, a chronically distended bladder, eventual detrusor dysfunction, and overflow urinary incontinence.
   c. Clinical signs related to infection include constant or intermittent urethral discharge, which may be hemorrhagic or purulent. If the abscess ruptures on the outer surface of the prostate gland, localized or generalized peritonitis results in lethargy, pain, and, possibly, vomiting. Such signs may also signal secondary septicemia.
   d. In one survey of cases,[179] the most common signs were depression and lethargy. Other findings in more than 50% of cases were stranguria, tenesmus, and hematuria. Signs observed in 10 to 35% of patients included vomiting, pain, polyuria and polydipsia, and dripping of blood from the prepuce. Uncom-

mon signs were dripping of pus from the prepuce and edema of the hind limbs, scrotum, or prepuce.

2. Physical examination.
   a. On palpation, the prostate gland is usually abnormal.
      (1). The prostate is usually enlarged, but the degree of enlargement depends on the size and location of the abscess pockets.[179]
      (2). The prostate gland is often asymmetric and its consistency may vary from one part to another, with firmer and softer areas. Occasionally, a fluctuant area may be palpated. The inability to palpate such an area does not rule out abscessation, because the abscess may lie deeper within the gland or have a firm, fibrous capsule.
      (3). Pain on palpation is more often related to localized peritonitis than to the abscess itself. Absence of pain does not rule out abscessation. Caudal abdominal pain was noted in 73% of cases in one large survey.[179]
   b. The dog may be systemically ill, with fever and depression. Evidence of shock (tachycardia, pale mucous membranes, delayed capillary refill, and weak pulses) were noted in about 10% of patients.[179] Peritonitis, with depression, abdominal pain, and pyrexia, occurred in about 20% of patients, owing to rupture of a prostatic abscess.[179]
   c. Icterus secondary to reactive hepatopathy may be present.[100] Reactive hepatopathy refers to abnormal findings in tests of liver function or of liver enzymes. Such findings relate not to primary liver disease but to the reaction of the liver to disease outside the hepatobiliary system.[78] Reactive hepatopathy is usually noted in association with sepsis or endotoxemia, fever, dehydration, and/or hypoxia.
3. Urinalysis/urine culture. A UTI is often present.
4. Complete blood count and biochemical profile.
   a. Hematology.
      (1). Neutrophilic leukocytosis, with or without a leftward shift, is common with abscessation, but the WBC count may also be normal.[179]
      (2). Neutrophilic leukocytosis with a leftward shift and toxic change are often seen with localized peritonitis secondary to prostatic abscessation.
      (3). Mild anemia (packed cell volume 30 to 35%) was found in 10% of cases.[179]
   b. Blood chemistry.
      (1). Serum bilirubin and liver enzyme concentrations (especially alkaline phosphatase) may be elevated.[100,179]
      (2). Even in the absence of icterus, findings of liver function tests, such as bromsulfthalein (BSP) retention or bile acids, may be abnormal.[20,100]
      (3). The pattern of abnormalities usually suggests cholestasis.[78]
      (4). Liver biopsy findings are minimally abnormal and thus consistent with reactive hepatopathy (as described under previous section entitled, Physical Examination).[78,100]
      (5). Biochemical evidence of liver disease resolves after successful therapy of abscessation.
      (6). Hypoglycemia was noted in 40% of cases.[179]
      (7). Approximately 10% have hyperglobulinemia and/or azotemia.[179] Hypokalemia, the most common electrolyte abnormality, was noted in only 2% of cases.[179] The cause of the azotemia was not determined, as urinalysis was not routinely performed in this study.
5. Prostatic fluid.
   a. Prostatic fluid, collected by ejaculation or post-prostatic massage, is usually purulent and septic. It may also be hemorrhagic. (See the section on diagnostic techniques for description of the difficulty of accurately assessing the results of prostatic massage when UTI is present).
   b. Quantitative culture of urine and prostatic fluid should yield significant numbers of the same organisms. Either aerobic or anaerobic bacteria may be involved in prostatic abscesses.
6. Imaging. (See Chapter 11, Diagnostic Imaging of the Urinary Tract.)
   a. Prostatic enlargement, which can be asymmetric or irregular in outline, may be evident on survey radiographs. Radiographic contrast of structures in the caudal abdomen can be poor.[179] The sublumbar lymph nodes may be enlarged.
   b. Reflux into the prostate gland may be noted on retrograde urethrography if the abscess communicates with the urethra. Periurethral asymmetry and narrowing of the prostatic urethra are observed on distention retrograde urethrocystography.[74] The prostatic urethral lumen may appear undulant, but it is neither distorted nor destroyed.[74]
   c. On ultrasound, the prostate gland is usually hyperechoic, with parenchymal cavities, irregular outline, and asymmetric shape.[76] The degree of asymmetry depends on the size of the abscess and its location relative to the capsule. The cavitary area(s) usually exhibit distal enhancement.[128] The internal margin of the cavity is often irregular, and the lumen may be septate.[128] Hematomas, hematocysts, and abscesses are indistinguishable.[128] The other major disease that must be considered is cystic hyperplasia.

7. Prostatic tissue.
   a. Although a presumptive diagnosis of abscessation can be based on findings of the history and physical examination and or studies of hematology, urinalysis, prostatic fluid cytology and culture, and imaging, the diagnosis should be confirmed by aspiration or exploratory celiotomy, because the current treatment of choice is surgical drainage.
   b. At surgery, the contents of the abscess should be collected for aerobic and anaerobic culture, and a tissue section should be obtained for microscopic examination and bacterial culture. The usual histologic finding is suppurative or chronic active prostatitis, although pyogranulomatous inflammation may also be noted.

C. Treatment.

1. Currently, surgical drainage is the treatment of choice.[99,127,140,232,241] Many methods can accomplish this goal, including needle aspiration, tube or Penrose drains, and marsupialization. Complications occur in almost every case.[100,179]
   a. Drainage through the abdomen often results in septic shock immediately after surgery because of absorption of bacteria and their toxins.[20,100,179] Intensive care is usually required for several days after surgery.[20,179]
   b. Drains placed around the prostate can sever the urethra, causing a urine fistula.[100]
   c. When drains are placed, ascending infection with antibiotic-resistant bacteria is possible.[100]
   d. Marsupialization leaves a chronic draining stoma in some dogs.[100] If the stoma closes too early, the abscess may reform.[100]
   e. Severe polyuria and polydipsia has been noted in a few dogs after surgical drainage of prostatic abscesses.[100] The polyuria and polydipsia resolved within 1 month of initiation of treatment.
   f. Failure to control prostatic infection and recurrent UTIs is common.[101] The prostatic abscess may recur.[179]
   g. Other common short-term complications are hypoproteinemia, edema of the scrotum, the prepuce, or the hind legs, anemia, hypokalemia, urine leakage from the drains, and urinary incontinence.[179]
   h. Other long-term complications include urinary incontinence and urethrocutaneous fistulas.[179] Urinary incontinence occurred in 46% of the cases.
2. For extensive prostate involvement, removal of the prostate may be considered[100,101]; however, serious complications are also associated with prostatectomy.
   a. Transurethral prostatectomy often results in incontinence in dogs with severe underlying prostatic disease.[100] Total prostatectomy is technically difficult, and the procedure takes a long time.
   b. Bladder and urethral function must be assessed before undertaking prostatectomy, because pre-existing abnormalities increase the likelihood of postoperative incontinence.[19]
   c. Subtotal prostatectomy was associated with a higher rate of intraoperative mortality than were drainage procedures in one small study in dogs. Death was attributed to sepsis.[101] This complication may have been the result of the severity of the illnesses of the dogs. Subtotal prostatectomy can be accomplished by standard surgical techniques,[241] by laser,[101] and by a Cavitron ultrasonic surgical aspirator.[208]
3. If prostatic enlargement has resulted in partial urethral obstruction, bladder and urethral function should be carefully assessed.
   a. Prolonged bladder distention may have resulted in bladder atony, so the dog may have overflow incontinence.[100] An indwelling urinary catheter may be necessary to let the detrusor muscle recover.
   b. If the bladder wall has been chronically distended and infected, it may be irreversibly damaged.
4. Castration is recommended as adjunctive therapy. Castration without abscess drainage leads to reduction of prostatic tissue but continuation of the abscess pocket(s).
5. Regardless of which surgical procedure is elected, affected dogs must receive antibiotic therapy.
   a. If the dog is systemically ill, intravenous antimicrobials should be used initially.
   b. Based on prostatic penetration, chloramphenicol, trimethoprim, or a quinolone is the initial drug of choice; however, the choice should be modified based on knowledge of the causative organism, its antibiotic sensitivity, and the presence or absence of bacteremia.
   c. After clinical signs improve, the dog should be managed in the same way as a dog with chronic bacterial prostatitis.
6. If the condition of an affected dog stabilizes on antibiotic therapy and the owners decline surgery, the dog can be managed with long-term suppressive antibiotic therapy, so long as the owners realize that the abscess will persist and could result in life-threatening infection.
7. In addition to antibiotic therapy, dogs with sepsis or peritonitis also require intensive fluid therapy.[179] Such therapy usually includes balanced electrolyte solutions administered intravenously at rates up to 90 mL/kg/h, depending on the severity of the signs and the response of the dog. Intravenous glucocorticoids are often given once, at the initiation of therapy, in doses used to treat shock. Dextrose also is often administered intra-

venously, to maintain normal blood glucose concentration.

8. Prostatic abscesses are difficult and expensive to treat.[20] The survival rate is approximately 50% after 1 year.[100,179] These facts underscore the importance of aggressive treatment of chronic prostatitis to try to halt progression to abscessation.

VIII. PARAPROSTATIC CYSTS

A. Pathophysiology.

1. Occasionally, one or more large cysts are found adjacent to the prostate (paraprostatic cyst) and attached to it via a stalk (patent or nonpatent) or adhesions.[127,260,266] The cyst also may be closely associated with the dorsal wall of the bladder[259] (see Fig. 6–13). The cyst may or may not communicate with the urethra. These are differentiated from the multiple small intraprostatic cysts often found in association with prostatic hyperplasia. (See Section II of this chapter.) Some paraprostatic cysts contain blood (hematocyst)[109]; whether this blood is similar to the bleeding occasionally associated with intraprostatic cysts is not known.
2. These large cysts may be remnants of the uterus masculinus or of prostatic origin.[4,214,259] In clinical cases, the origin of most large cysts is obscure. The terminology for these large cysts varies with different authors. The term paraprostatic cyst has been used as a general term for any large cyst largely outside of, but in the vicinity of, the prostate gland, regardless of whether or not there is a patent connection to the prostate gland. Others have reserved the term paraprostatic cyst for those without a patent connection and used the term prostatic retention cyst for those with a patent connection, especially if the cyst seems to arise from the parenchyma of the gland. Still others have reserved the term paraprostatic cyst for those that do not have an obvious patent connection to the prostate gland but that also do not have characteristics of a uterus masculinus and that seem histologically to be of prostatic origin.
   a. During development, the uterus masculinus is a bicornate structure with a stalk that opens on the dorsal wall of the urethra within the prostate gland. Normally, the structure degenerates within the prostate gland as the fetus develops masculine traits. Why this structure would become cystic is not known, but estrogen therapy, endogenous hyperestrogenism, and a congenital defect have been suggested.[8] Prostatic cysts have been associated with Sertoli cell tumors and hyperestrogenism in dogs.[109,235] With a cyst arising from the uterus masculinus, the origin should be on the dorsal midline of the prostate gland.[8,127] The prostate gland itself should be normal for the age of the dog (i.e., hyperplasia may be present). The epithelium lining the cyst should be the simple columnar type.[8] Evidence of hermaphroditism or pseudohermaphroditism may exist. A cystic uterus masculinus often communicates with the urethra.[8] Proven cases of paraprostatic cysts caused by uterus masculinus are rare.[8,205] Cases of cystic uterus masculinus have been reported in cats.[53,77,195,225]
   b. With a prostatic retention cyst and with paraprostatic cysts of apparently prostatic origin, the rest of the prostate gland is usually abnormal.
      (1). They may be in the abdomen, craniolateral to the prostate gland, or in the pelvis, caudal to the prostate, even extending to the perineum, lateral to the anus. Some are in both sites.[265]
      (2). They can have a thin or thick wall with a smooth lining or masses of calcified material.[127,212,231]
      (3). They may or may not communicate with the urethra. Most do not.[265]
      (4). The type of epithelium lining the cyst is usually transitional urothelium. Communication with prostatic ductule epithelium may be found.
   c. Identification of the cause of these cysts is largely irrelevant, for the clinical signs and treatment are the same.
   d. The first case of a cyst of apparently prostatic origin in a cat was reported recently.[186]

B. Clinical signs.

1. History.
   a. With large cysts, clinical signs may be related to their size, as encroachment on the urethra or colon results in dysuria or tenesmus, respectively.[8,259,265] Urinary incontinence has also been noted[265] and generally is associated with bladder overdistention and partial urethral obstruction.[8]
   b. If the cyst is sufficiently large, abdominal distention may be seen.[8,212,265]
   c. Alternatively, the cyst may extend into the perineal region and be noted as a swelling.[212,259,265]
   d. Hematuria or an intermittent hemorrhagic, serosanguineous, or yellow urethral discharge may be noted.
2. Physical examination. The cysts may be palpable in the caudal abdomen or the perineal area. If calcified, they may feel firm.[127,231,265]
3. Urinalysis/urine culture.
   a. Findings of urinalysis are usually normal, although hematuria is possible if hemorrhage occurs into the cyst and the cyst communicates with the urethra.
   b. A UTI is present in some cases.
4. Hematology/biochemical profile. Hematologic findings are usually normal, but neutrophilic leukocytosis was noted in about 30% of cases in 1 series.[259]

5. Prostatic fluid.
   a. If a urethral discharge appears to be the same color as the urine of the dog, the discharge should be examined cytologically to differentiate prostatic fluid from urine (urinary incontinence); "urinalysis" can be performed on both specimens for comparison. Cyst fluid usually has more protein than does urine from the same patient.[259]
   b. Prostatic fluid collected by ejaculation or postprostatic massage should be examined. Whether cyst fluid is obtained by ejaculation or prostate massage depends on whether the cyst communicates with the urethra. Alternatively, fluid from a prostatic cyst can be aspirated under ultrasound guidance.
   c. Prostatic cyst fluid is usually yellow to serosanguineous to brown, has few WBCs, variable amounts of red blood cells (RBC), variable amounts of epithelial cells, and is usually sterile (see Figs. 6–11 and 6–13).[127] If cyst fluid becomes infected, the cyst may be considered an abscess.
6. Imaging. (See Chapter 11, Diagnostic Imaging of the Urinary Tract.)
   a. On survey radiographs contrast between structures in the caudal abdomen may be poor, with asymmetric or irregular prostatic shape.[129] Paraprostatic cysts may mineralize to a density similar to that of egg shells (Fig. 39–11).[4,75,205,259] With large cysts, two "bladders" may be evident.

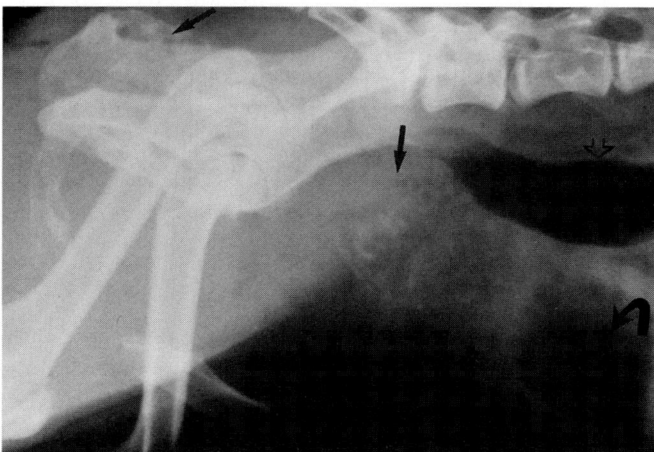

FIG. 39–11. Survey radiograph of the caudal abdomen shows a mineralized prostatic cyst (solid arrows). Note that the cyst extends from the caudal abdomen through the pelvic canal and into the perineal area. The colon is visible as the air-filled viscus dorsal to the cyst (open arrow), and the bladder is visible cranial to the cyst (curved arrow). (Barsanti JA. Canine prostatic disease. *In:* Ettinger SJ, ed. *Veterinary Internal Medicine.* Philadelphia, Pennsylvania: W.B. Saunders, 1989;1859.)

   b. A cystogram is often necessary to determine which structure is the bladder.
   c. On distention retrograde urethrocystography, the prostate may appear asymmetric around the urethra and the prostatic urethral lumen may be narrowed.[74] Urethroprostatic reflux may be greater than normal; however, contrast material often does not reflux into the large cyst.[259]
   d. Ultrasound can confirm that the mass is cystic by its hypoechoic to anechoic character and smooth internal margins.[76,128] Ultrasound can be used to direct fine-needle aspiration.

C. Treatment.

1. The recommended treatment for paraprostatic cysts is surgical drainage with excision or marsupialization.[99,109,127,231,232,235,241,259,265] One potential complication of marsupialization is chronic infection.[100]
2. Castration is also recommended.

IX. PROSTATIC NEOPLASIA

A. Pathophysiology.

1. The incidence of prostatic neoplasia appears to be low in dogs; about 5% of all dogs with prostatic disease had neoplasia.[197,260] In relation to prostatic diseases that prompted diagnostic evaluation at teaching hospitals, prostatic neoplasia represented about 15% of cases,[102,141] following chronic prostatitis (38%) and prostatic cystic disease (31%).[141] Prostatic neoplasia has been reported in cats.[105,111,113,194]
2. In contrast to most prostatic diseases, prostatic neoplasia can develop in both intact and neutered males.[25,59,63,102,110,113,141,189,201,272] In fact, prostatic neoplasia should be highest on the list of differential diagnoses in an old dog that was neutered when young and now appears with signs referable to prostatic disease or prostatic enlargement (Fig. 39–12).
3. All the common neoplasms that affect the prostate gland are malignant.
   a. The most common primary prostatic neoplasm of dogs, cats, and men is adenocarcinoma.[197]
      (1). This neoplasm tends to metastasize through the external and internal iliac lymph nodes to vertebral bodies and to the lungs.[60,143,272]
      (2). The tumor may grow into the neck of the bladder and obstruct the ureters.[143] The colonic and pelvic musculature may be invaded via direct extension through the prostatic capsule.[143]
      (3). The urethra may also become obstructed from neoplastic extension.[260]
      (4). Cysts, abscesses, and areas of hemorrhage can be found in association with neoplasia, making diagnosis difficult in some dogs.[195,197,260]
      (5). Prostatic adenocarcinoma arises in old

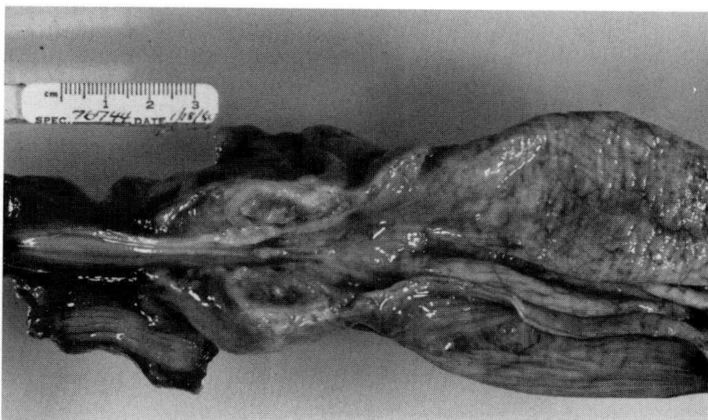

FIG. 39–12. Necropsy specimens of bladder and urethra opened on the midline from a castrated dog that appeared for overflow incontinence. Note the flaccid-looking bladder. The cause of the incontinence was urethral obstruction caused by prostatic adenocarcinoma. Note that the prostate is not grossly enlarged but is larger than expected for a dog neutered as a puppy. (Barsanti JA. Canine prostatic disease. *In:* Ettinger SJ, ed. *Veterinary Internal Medicine.* Philadelphia, Pennsylvania: W.B. Saunders, 1989; 1859.)

dogs (mean age 9 to 10 years).[25,102,141,143,260] Medium-sized to large breeds seem to be more commonly affected.[102,143,260]

b. The second most common neoplasm of the prostate gland is transitional cell carcinoma.[197]
   (1). Transitional cell carcinoma of the prostate can occur via direct extension from a bladder or urethral lesion or from neoplastic changes in the periurethral prostatic duct cells themselves.[219]
   (2). Clinical signs are often related to partial urethral obstruction.

c. Squamous cell carcinoma has been found in the prostate.[144]

d. Leiomyosarcomas and primary lymphoma have been reported but apparently are quite rare.[142,156]

e. The prostate gland may also be involved by a metastatic neoplasm from another site.
   (1). Any type of neoplasm may metastasize to the prostate gland.
   (2). Such neoplastic foci are often subclinical.
   (3). I have encountered a few cases of lymphosarcoma in dogs with clinical signs principally related to prostatomegaly. Prostatic lymphosarcoma was also noted in one dog in an early series of cases[196]; however, in this dog, the prostate was reported to be atrophied.

4. Benign tumors of the prostate are not reported; however, recently a case of nodular benign hyperplasia was reported in a dog.[90] In this case, a large nodule was localized to one lobe of the prostate gland and was surgically resectable. The only clinical signs were dyschezia, prostatomegaly, and microscopic hematuria. Surgical removal of the mass and castration were apparently curative. Although histologically this lesion was hyperplasia, the clinical evaluation suggested benign neoplasia. The distinction between hyperplasia and neoplasia is often difficult in men as well.

B. Clinical signs.

1. History.
   a. The owner's complaints are often related to increased prostatic size and include tenesmus and dysuria.[60,110,141,143,211,245,260] Hematuria was the sign observed in one cat,[113] whereas another was presented for urethral obstruction.[194]
   b. A hemorrhagic urethral discharge may be noted.[143]
   c. Rear limb weakness or stiffness and pain in the hindquarters is commonly reported, (prevalence, 40 to 50% of affected dogs).[60,110,143] More recent surveys found a much lower incidence of such signs.[25,141] These case surveys are retrospective, and the differences may be the result of differences in observing and/or reporting such signs. The pain may be related to necrosis and inflammation as the tumor outgrows its blood supply, or it may be caused by metastasis to lumbar vertebrae.[60]
   d. Chronic weight loss and anorexia are often present.[25,60,141,143,245,260]
2. Physical examination.
   a. With neoplasia, one or more firm, irregular nodules may be palpated before marked prostatic enlargement and clinical signs become evident.
   b. In most dogs with clinical signs, the prostate gland is enlarged, asymmetric, and unusually firm.[110,260] It may be painful on palpation and is often immovable.[25,143] In determining whether the prostate is enlarged, the examiner must consider the hormonal status of the dog. The prostate of a neutered dog exhibits involution to a small size. Thus, a prostate gland that would be normal in size for an intact dog is abnormal for a neutered dog.
   c. An attempt should be made to palpate the iliac lymph nodes rectally. Lymphadenopathy occurs with both infection and neoplasia.[74,143]
   d. Hypertrophic osteopathy affecting all four limbs was reported in a dog that had no evidence of lung metastasis.[211]
   e. Systemic signs may include depression, cachexia, and pyrexia.[25]
   f. Generalized bleeding noted in men with metastatic prostate carcinoma may be caused by disseminated intravascular coagulation.[243]
3. Urinalysis/urine culture.

a. Hematuria is the predominant abnormality on urinalysis.[14,25]
b. Pyuria may also be present, owing to prostatic necrosis and inflammation secondary to tumor growth.[11,14,25,143,201]
c. UTI and prostatic infection occasionally occur concomitantly with prostatic neoplasia.[25]
d. Atypical cells were found in the urine sediment of 17% of cases in a survey.[25]

4. Complete blood count/biochemical profile.
a. Hemogram.
(1). WBC count is usually normal, but neutrophilic leukocytosis, with or without a leftward shift, may be observed if sufficient necrosis and inflammation are associated with tumor growth.[14,25,143,201]
(2). Mild nonregenerative anemia was noted in 19% of cases, whereas regenerative anemia was noted in 7% of cases.[25]
(3). One case has been reported in which neoplastic cells were seen in the blood.[5]
(4). Thrombocytopenia may be associated with secondary development of disseminated intravascular coagulation.[243]
b. Biochemical profile.
(1). Azotemia.
(a). If the tumor obstructs both ureters, hydronephrosis and azotemia result.
(b). If the tumor causes partial urethral obstruction, loss of bladder function and azotemia may result.
(2). Hypercalcemia has been noted, although rarely, in association with prostate carcinoma in humans and dogs,[25,153] as has hypocalcemia.[25,243] In both men and dogs, hypocalcemia is more common than hypercalcemia. The reasons for these changes have not been explored.
(3). Approximately 50% of affected dogs had an increased serum alkaline phosphatase value.[25] Some of these dogs had bone or hepatic metastasis or had received glucocorticoids, but for others no obvious reason for the increase was determined.
(4). Plasma acid phosphatase, which is a useful tumor marker in men, is not increased in dogs[26,260] and has been reported not to be present in species other than human.[83] Prostate-specific antigen, a more specific prostatic tumor marker in men,[190] was not detectable in canine serum.[26] The concentration of canine prostatic secretory protease was different in normal dogs and dogs with prostatic disease, but the differences did not differentiate between types of prostatic disease and were not a useful tumor marker.[26] A study of canine adenocarcinomas found that few contained prostate-specific antigen or prostate-specific acid phosphatase, and only 25% contained canine prostatic secretory protease.[160] This finding was in contrast to normal and hyperplastic canine prostatic tissue, in which all three compounds were found.[160]

5. Prostatic fluid.
a. Semen samples are difficult to collect from dogs with advanced neoplasia.
b. Abnormal epithelial cells may be detected following postprostatic massage (see Fig. 6–10).[14,89]
(1). These cells are usually large, often appear in groups, and display anisocytosis and anisokaryosis.
(2). Irregular and variably sized nucleoli and, occasionally, abnormal mitotic figures may be present.
(3). Because epithelial cells in urine can normally vary in appearance, identification of such cells should be used as supportive, but not definitive, evidence for neoplasia.[246]

6. Imaging. (See Chapter 11, Diagnostic Imaging of the Urinary Tract.)
a. Asymmetric or irregular prostatic enlargement, which may be marked, may be evident on survey abdominal radiography.[240]
(1). Occasional prostatic carcinomas are associated with multifocal or granular ill-defined mineral densities.[75]
(2). The lumbar vertebral bodies and the pelvic bones always should be examined carefully for areas of lysis or proliferative changes suggestive of metastasis (Fig. 39–13).[56,143,238,260,273] Metastasis may also

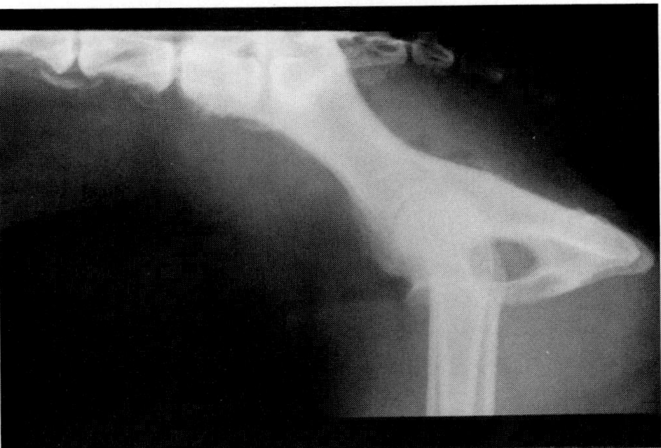

FIG. 39–13. Metastasis to the sixth and seventh lumbar vertebrae, sacrum, and medial aspect of the left ileum in a dog with prostatic adenocarcinoma. Also note the ventral deviation and compression of the colon by a soft tissue mass in the area of the sublumbar lymph nodes. The prostate gland is enlarged and irregular.

occur to long bones, scapula, ribs, and digits.[60,243]

(3). The degree of enlargement of the iliac lymph nodes should also be determined (see Fig. 39–13).

b. Thoracic radiographs are indicated to check for metastasis to the lungs. Metastasis may appear either as a generalized increase in nodular interstitial density or as single to multiple discrete nodules.[25] Even if thoracic radiographs show no evidence of metastasis, at least a 40% chance exists that metastases are present, indicating the relative insensitivity of thoracic radiographs for this purpose.[25]

c. Scintigraphic techniques can also be used to detect metastasis to bone.

d. With distention retrograde urethrocystography, periurethral asymmetry and narrowing, distortion, or destruction of the prostatic urethra may be detected.[74] Urethroprostatic reflux that is greater than normal is also common.[74] Spread of the neoplasm into the bladder is possible.

e. Ultrasound usually shows focal or multifocal hyperechoic parenchyma with asymmetry and irregular prostatic outline.[76] Echogenicity tends to be heterogeneous, with ill-defined hyperechoic foci that seem to coalesce.[129] Multifocal irregularly distributed mineralization may appear. Occasionally, cavitary lesions, which can represent infarction, necrosis, hemorrhage, or edema, may also be noted. Both intraparenchymal and paraprostatic cysts are occasionally associated with neoplasia.[128] The other major disease that can have similar hyperechoic foci with mineralization is chronic prostatitis.[128] Ultrasound may help to differentiate neoplasia originating from within the prostate gland from neoplasia originating from within the urethra (usually transitional cell carcinoma) by imaging the bladder neck, the prostatic urethra, and the hilar echo (where the prostatic ducts enter the prostatic urethra).[128]

7. Prostatic tissue.
   a. Unless metastatic disease is evident radiographically, the diagnosis of neoplasia should always be confirmed by aspiration or biopsy, because the prognosis is poor.
   b. Examination of a biopsy specimen or aspirate is necessary to determine the type of neoplasm. If a surgical biopsy is performed, a specimen should also be taken from the iliac lymph nodes.

C. Treatment for prostatic adenocarcinoma.

1. Before instituting therapy, the clinician should conduct a thorough search for metastasis, to allow a more accurate prognosis. Such a search should include, at least, thoracic radiographs and contrast radiographs of the lower urinary tract. A bone scan would also be advisable if available. At the advanced stage that most canine cases are currently diagnosed, metastases are usually present.[25]
2. Radiation therapy is the treatment of choice if metastatic disease is not evident.[252]
   a. Intraoperative orthovoltage therapy has been recommended.[252] Median and mean survival times for 10 dogs with radiotherapy were 114 and 196 days, respectively.[252] Three dogs with no evidence of metastatic disease appeared to be cured.
   b. External beam (cobalt) radiotherapy has been reported in two cases.[25] One dog had no response, and the other had an approximately 50% decrease in prostatic size initially, but was euthanized 4 months later for urinary obstruction. Androgen ablation therapy (castration and/or ketoconazole) was also used in these two dogs.
   c. The usual goal is temporary control of the tumor and amelioration of clinical signs. Cure is unlikely, because metastasis is likely to have occurred even if it is not clinically detectable.[25,252]
3. Prostatectomy is the alternative therapy, but the owner must be willing to accept the probable postsurgical development of urinary incontinence.[100,112,127] The longest reported postoperative survival for a dog with adenocarcinoma was 9 months.[100,203] One dog that survived 9 months had only small foci of neoplasia at the time of initial diagnosis.[100]
4. In advanced metastatic cases, euthanasia may be the most humane course because of lack of effective therapy at this time. Most patients are euthanized within 2 months of diagnosis because of progressive disease; however, one survived 19 months without therapy.[25] Therefore, the decision for euthanasia should be based on the physical condition of the animal and its quality of life, not only on the fact that it has prostate cancer.
5. Although androgen ablation is effective in some humans, castration has had no beneficial effect in dogs.[25,59,142,197,260,273] Prostatic adenocarcinoma has been reported in a dog with hyperestrogenism and in castrated dogs.[5,25,63,102,110,189,272,273] Lack of decrease in prostate size after castration may help to differentiate neoplasia from other prostatic diseases.
6. Chemotherapy has not been shown to improve survival in men.[91]

X. PROSTATIC CALCULI

A. Prostatic calculi are usually small and smoothly marginated.[75] They have been considered incidental findings that are not associated with clinical disease. (See Chapter 11, Diagnostic Imaging of the Urinary Tract.) Prostatic calculi are the least common cause of prostatic mineralization in dogs.[128]

B. In recent years in human medicine, prostatic calculi have been identified as the source of

chronic infection[66,165,193] or as a factor that makes elimination of infection more difficult.[222]

1. Human prostatic calculi are composed largely of urinary, not prostatic, constituents.[136,193]
2. Prostatic calculi are thought to be more common in men than in dogs.[128]

XI. MULTIPLE DISEASES

A. A prostate gland may be the focus of several disease processes. For example, it may be hyperplastic, abscessed, cystic, and/or neoplastic.[109,143,197,259]

B. The occurrence of multiple diseases is a limitation of all diagnostic tests. For markedly abnormal prostate glands, multiple biopsies may be indicated.

C. Clinicians should always keep an open mind should the disease course not fit the disease "diagnosed," even when a biopsy has been obtained.

REFERENCES

1. Aagaard J, Gasser T, Rhodes P, Madsen PO. MICs of ciprofloxacin and trimethoprim for *Escherichia coli:* Influence of pH, inoculum size, and various body fluids. *Infection.* 1991;19:s167.
2. Aagaard J, Knes J, Madsen PO. Prostatic tissue levels of ofloxacin. *Urology.* 1991;38:380.
3. Ackerman N. Radiology and ultrasonography of urogenital diseases in dogs and cats. Ames, Iowa: Iowa State University Press, 1991.
4. Akpavie SO, Sullivan M. Constipation associated with calcified cystic enlargement of the prostate in a dog. *Vet Rec.* 1986; 118:694.
5. Alsaker RD, Stevens JB. Neoplastic cells in the blood of a dog with prostatic adenocarcinoma. *J Am Anim Hosp Assoc.* 1977; 13:486.
6. Andersen JT, Bradley WF. Detrusor and urethral dysfunction in prostatic hypertrophy. *Br J Urol.* 1976;48:493.
7. Anderson RU, Fair WR. Physical and chemical determinations of prostatic secretion in benign hyperplasia, prostatitis and adenocarcinoma. *Invest Urol.* 1976;14:137.
8. Atilola MAO, Pennock PW. Cystic uterus masculinus in the dog. *Vet Radiol.* 1986;27:8.
9. Baert L, Leonard A. Chronic bacterial prostatitis: 10 years of experience with local antibiotics. *J Urol.* 1988;140:755.
10. Barrach ER, Berry SJ. DNA synthesis in the canine prostate: Effects of androgen and estrogen treatment. *Prostate.* 1987; 10:45.
11. Barsanti JA, et al. Evaluation of diagnostic techniques for canine prostatic diseases. *J Am Vet Med Assoc.* 1980;177:160.
12. Barsanti JA, et al. Evaluation of various techniques for diagnosis of chronic bacterial prostatitis in the dog. *J Am Vet Med Assoc.* 1983;183:219.
13. Barsanti JA. Blastomycosis. *In:* Greene CE, ed. *Clinical Microbiology and Infectious Diseases of the Dog and Cat.* Philadelphia, Pennsylvania: WB Saunders, 1984.
14. Barsanti JA, Finco DR. Evaluation of techniques for diagnosis of canine prostatic diseases. *J Am Vet Med Assoc.* 1984;185:198.
15. Barsanti JA, et al. Effect of induced prostatic infection on semen quality in the dog. *Am J Vet Res.* 1986;47:709.
16. Bartlett DJ. Studies in dog semen 1. Biochemical characteristics. *J Reprod Fertil.* 1962;3:190.
17. Bartlett JG, et al. Prostatic abscesses involving anaerobic bacteria. *Arch Intern Med.* 1978;138:1369.
18. Bartsch G, Rohr HP. Comparative light and electron microscopic study of the human, dog, and rat prostate. *Urol Int.* 1980;35:91.
19. Basinger RR, Rawlings CA, Barsanti JA, Oliver JE. Urodynamic alterations associated with clinical prostatic diseases and prostatic surgery. *J Am Anim Hosp Assoc.* 1989;25:38.
20. Bauer MS. Prostatic abscess rupture in three dogs. *J Am Vet Med Assoc.* 1986;188:735.
21. Baumueller A, Madsen PO. Experimental bacterial prostatitis in dogs. *Urol Res.* 1977;5:211.
22. Baumueller A, et al. Prostatic tissue and secretion concentration of rosamicin and erythromycin: Experimental studies in the dog. *Invest Urol.* 1977;15:158.
23. Baumueller A, Madsen PO. Secretion of various antimicrobial substances in dogs with experimental bacterial prostatitis. *Urol Res.* 1977;5:215.
24. Baumueller A, Madsen PO. Penicillanic acid derivatives in the canine prostate. *Prostate.* 1980;1:79.
25. Bell FW, et al. Clinical and pathologic features of prostatic adenocarcinomas in sexually intact and castrated dogs: 31 cases (1970–1987). *J Am Vet Med Assoc.* 1991;199:1623.
26. Bell FW, et al. Evaluation of prostatic acid phosphatase, prostate specific antigen, and canine prostatic secretory prostease measurements in the diagnosis of canine prostatic disorders. *Proc Vet Cancer Soc.* 1991;11:71.
27. Berg OA. Effect of stilbestrol on the prostate gland in normal puppies and adult dogs. *Acta Endocrinol.* 1958;27:155.
28. Berger RE, et al. Case-control study of men with chronic idiopathic prostatitis. *J Urol.* 1989;141:328.
29. Bergeron MG, et al. Norfloxacin penetration into human renal and prostatic tissues. *Antimicrobial Agents Chemother.* 1985; 28:349.
30. Berry SJ, et al. The development of human benign prostatic hyperplasia with age. *J Urol.* 1984;132:474.
31. Berry SJ, et al. Effects of aging on prostate growth in beagles. *Am J Physiol.* 1986;250:R1039.
32. Berry SJ, et al. Effect of age, castration and testosterone replacement on the development and restoration of canine benign hyperplasia. *Prostate.* 1986;9:295.
33. Berry SJ, et al. Development of canine benign prostatic hyperplasia with age. *Prostate.* 1986;9:363.
34. Bologna M, et al. Bactericidal intraprostatic concentrations of norfloxacin. *Lancet.* 1983;2:280.
35. Bologna M, et al. Norfloxacin in prostatitis: Correlation between HPLC tissue concentrations and clinical results. *Drugs Exper Clin Res.* 1985;11:95.
36. Borthwich R, Mackenzie CP. Signs and results of treatment of prostatic disease in dogs. *Vet Rec.* 1971;89:374.
37. Branam JE, et al. Selected physical and chemical characteristics of prostatic fluid collected by ejaculation from healthy dogs and from dogs with bacterial prostatitis. *Am J Vet Res.* 1984;45:825.
38. Brendler CB, et al. Spontaneous benign prostatic hyperplasia in the beagle. *J Clin Invest.* 1983;71:1114.
39. Brooks JR, et al. Effect of a new 5-alpha-reductase inhibitor on size, histological characteristics, and androgen concentrations of the canine prostate. *Prostate.* 1982;3:35.
40. Brooks M, Dodds WJ, Raymond SL. Epidemiologic features of von Willebrand's disease in Doberman pinschers, Scottish terriers, and Shetland sheepdogs: 260 cases (1984–1988). *J Am Vet Med Assoc.* 1992;200:1123.
41. Brown SA, et al. Pharmacokinetics of norfloxacin in dogs after single intravenous and single and multiple oral administrations of the drug. *Am J Vet Res.* 1990;51:1065.

42. Bruschini H, et al. Neurologic control of prostatic secretion in the dog. *Invest Urol.* 1978;15:288.
43. Budsberg SC, Kemp DT, Wolski N. Pharmacokinetics of clindamycin phosphate in dogs after single intravenous and intramuscular administrations. *Am J Vet Res.* 1992;53:2333.
44. Cartee RE, et al. Evaluation of drug-induced prostatic involution in dogs by transabdominal B-mode ultrasonography. *Am J Vet Res.* 1990;51:1773.
45. Childs SJ. Current concepts in the treatment of urinary tract infections and prostatitis. *Am J Med.* 1991;91:6A120s.
46. Chiu T. Studies on estrogen-induced proliferative disorders of hemopoietic tissue in dogs. Thesis, University of Minnesota, 1974.
47. Cowan LA, Barsanti JA, Crowell WA, Brown J. Effects of castration on chronic bacterial prostatitis in dogs. *J Am Vet Med Assoc.* 1991;199:346.
48. Cowan LA, et al. Effect of bacterial infection and castration on prostatic tissue zinc concentration in dogs. *Am J Vet Res.* 1991;52:1262-4.
49. Cox CE, Childs SJ. Treatment of chronic bacterial prostatitis with temafloxacin. *Am J Med.* 1991;91:6A134s.
50. Crafts RC. The effects of estrogens on the bone marrow of adult female dogs. *Blood.* 1948;3:276.
51. Cribb A. Idiosyncratic reactions to sulfonamides in dogs. *J Am Vet Med Assoc.* 1989;195:1612.
52. DeKlerk DP, et al. Comparison of spontaneous and experimentally induced canine prostatic hyperplasia. *J Clin Invest.* 1979; 64:842.
53. Diegmann FG, Loo BJ, Grom PA. Female pseudohermaphroditism in a cat. *Feline Pract.* 1978;8:45.
54. Doble A, et al. The role of chlamydia trachomatis in chronic abacterial prostatitis: A study using ultrasound guided biopsy. *J Urol.* 1989;141:332.
55. Dorflinger T, Larsen EH, Gasser TC, Madsen PO. The concentration of various quinolone derivatives in the dog prostate. *In: Therapy of Prostatitis.* Munich: W. Zuckschwerdt, 1986.
56. Douglas SW, Williamson HD. *Veterinary Radiological Interpretation.* Philadelphia, Pennsylvania: Lea & Febiger, 1970;260.
57. Drach GW. Problems in diagnosis of bacterial prostatitis: Gram-negative, gram-positive and mixed infections. *J Urol.* 1974; 111:630.
58. Dube JY, et al. Involution of spontaneous benign prostatic hyperplasia in the dog under the influence of chronic treatment with a LHRH agonist. *Prostate.* 1984;5:417.
59. Dube JY, et al. Single case report of prostate adenocarcinoma in a dog castrated 3 months previously. Morphological, biochemical and endocrine determinations. *Prostate.* 1984;5:495.
60. Durham SK, Dietze AE. Prostatic adenocarcinoma with and without metastasis to bone in dogs. *J Am Vet Med Assoc.* 1986;188:1432.
61. Ehrlichman RJ, Isaacs JT, Coffey DS. Differences in the effects of estradiol on dihydrotestosterone induced prostatic growth of the castrate dog and rat. *Invest Urol.* 1981;18:466.
62. Evans HE, Christensen GE. *Miller's Anatomy of the Dog.* 2nd ed. Philadelphia, Pennsylvania: WB Saunders, 1979;565.
63. Evans JE. Prostatic adenocarcinoma in a castrated dog. *J Am Vet Med Assoc.* 1985;186:78.
64. Ewing LL, et al. Dihydrotestosterone concentration of beagle prostatic tissue: Effect of age and hyperplasia. *Endocrinology.* 1983;113:2004.
65. Ewing LL, et al. Testicular androgen and estrogen secretion and benign hyperplasia in the beagle. *Endocrinology.* 1984;114: 1308.
66. Eykyn S, et al. Prostatic calculi as a source of recurrent bacteriuria in the male. *Br J Urol.* 1974;46:527.
67. Fair WR, et al. Prostatic antibacterial factor: Identity and significance. *Urology.* 1976;7:169.
68. Fair WR, Heston WDW. The relationship of bacterial prostatitis and zinc. *Progr Clin Biol Res.* 1977;14:129.
69. Fair WR, Cordonnier JJ. The pH of prostatic fluid: A re-appraisal and therapeutic implications. *J Urol.* 1978;120:695.
70. Fair WR, et al. A re-appraisal of treatment in chronic bacterial prostatitis. *J Urol.* 1979;121:437.
71. Fair WR, Parrish RF. Antibacterial substances in prostatic fluid. *Progr Clin Biol Res.* 1981;75:247.
72. Farrar ET. Severe trimethoprim-sulfonamide induced hepatopathy in a Bichon Frise dog. *Pulse.* 1991;33:17.
73. Farrell JI. The newer physiology of the prostate gland. *J Urol.* 1938;39:171.
74. Feeney DA, et al. Canine prostatic disease—comparison of radiographic appearance with morphologic and microbiologic findings: 30 cases (1981-1985). *J Am Vet Med Assoc.* 1987;190: 1018.
75. Feeney DA, Johnston GR. Urogenital imaging: A practical update. *Semin Vet Med Surg.* 1986;1:144.
76. Feeney DA, et al. Canine prostatic disease—comparison of ultrasonographic appearance with morphologic and microbiologic findings: 30 cases (1981-1985). *J Am Vet Med Assoc.* 1987;190:1027.
77. Felts JF, Randell MG, Greene RW, Scott RC. Hermaphroditism in a cat. *J Am Vet Med Assoc.* 1982;181:925.
78. Fenster LF. Reactive hepatopathy. *Postgrad Med.* 1984;76:62.
79. Fogle B. Iatrogenic oestrogen poisoning in a Maltese terrier. *Vet Rec.* 1981;109:201.
80. Forchetti C, et al. High-performance liquid chromatographic procedure for the quantitation of norfloxacin in urine, serum, and tissues. *J Chromatography.* 1984;309:177.
81. Fowler JE, et al. Immunologic response of the prostate to bacteriuria and bacterial prostatitis. *J Urol.* 1982;128:158.
82. Fowler JE, Mariano M. Immunologic response of the prostate to bacteriuria and bacterial prostatitis. *J Urol.* 1982;128:165.
83. Frenette G, et al. Radioimmunoassay in blood plasma of arginine esterase: The major secretory product of dog prostate. *Prostate.* 1987;10:145.
84. Garnes HA. Doxycycline levels in serum and prostatic tissue in man. *Urology.* 1973;1:205.
85. Geller J, et al. Effect of megestrol acetate on steroid metabolism and steroid-protein binding in the human prostate. *J Clin Endocrinol Metab.* 1976;43:1000.
86. Geller J. Overview of benign prostatic hypertrophy. *Urology.* 1989;34(Suppl):57.
87. Giamarellou H, et al. Infertility and chronic prostatitis. *Andrologia.* 1984;16(5):417.
88. Giger U, et al. Sulfadiazine-induced allergy in six Doberman pinschers. *J Am Vet Med Assoc.* 1985;186:479.
89. Gill CW. Prostatic adenocarcinoma with concurrent sertoli cell tumor in a dog. *Can Vet J.* 1981;22:230.
90. Gilson SD, Miller RT, Hardie EM, Spaulding KA. Unusual prostatic mass in a dog. *J Am Vet Med Assoc.* 1992;200:702.
91. Gittes RF. Carcinoma of the prostate. *N Engl J Med.* 1991; 324:236.
92. Gloyna RE, et al. Dihydrotestosterone in prostatic hypertrophy. *J Clin Invest.* 1970;49:1746.
93. Goldfarb M. Clinical efficacy of antibiotics in treatment of prostatitis. *Urology.* 1984;24(Suppl):1213.
94. Goldsmid SE, Bellenger CR. Urinary incontinence after prostatectomy in dogs. *Vet Surg.* 1991;20:253.
95. Gordon N. Position of the canine prostate gland. *Am J Vet Res.* 1961;22:142.
96. Gorelick JI, Senterfit LB, Vaughn ED. Quantitative bacterial

tissue cultures from 209 prostatectomy specimens: Findings and implications. *J Urol.* 1988;139:57.
97. Granato JJ, et al. Trimethoprim diffusion into prostatic and salivary secretions of the dog. *Invest Urol.* 1973;11:205.
98. Greene CE, George LW. Canine brucellosis. *In:* Greene CE, ed. *Clinical Microbiology and Infectious Diseases of the Dog and Cat.* Philadelphia, Pennsylvania: WB Saunders, 1984.
99. Greiner TP, Betts CW. Diseases of the prostate gland. *In:* Ettinger SJ, ed. *Veterinary Internal Medicine.* Philadelphia, Pennsylvania: WB Saunders, 1975.
100. Hardie EM, et al. Complications of prostatic surgery. *J Am Anim Hosp Assoc.* 1984;20:50.
101. Hardie EM, Stone EA, Spaulding KA, Cullen JM. Subtotal canine prostatectomy with the neodymium:yttrium-aluminum-garnet laser. *Vet Surg.* 1990;19:348.
102. Hargis AM, Miller LM. Prostatic carcinoma in dogs. *Comp Contin Ed Pract Vet.* 1983;5:647.
103. Harvey RG. Possible sulphadiazine-trimethoprim induced polyarthritis. *Vet Rec.* 1987;120:537.
104. Haveland H. Prostatic pharmacokinetics. In: Bernsteen LS, Salter AJ, eds. *Trimethoprim/Sulphamethoxazole in Bacterial Infections.* Int Sympos Sardinia. London: Churchill Livingstone; 1972.
105. Hawe RS. What is your diagnosis? *J Am Vet Med Assoc.* 1983; 182:1257.
106. Herron MA. Feline physiology of reproduction. *In:* Burke TJ, ed. *Small Animal Reproduction and Infertility.* Philadelphia, Pennsylvania: Lea & Febiger, 1986.
107. Hessl JM, Stamey TA. The passage of tetracycline across epithelial membranes with special reference to prostatic epithelium. *J Urol.* 1971;106:253.
108. Hieble JP, Caine M. Etiology of benign prostatic hyperplasia and approaches to its pharmacological management. *Fed Proc.* 1986;45:2601.
109. Hoffer RE, Dykes NL, Greiner TP. Marsupialization as a treatment for prostatic disease. *J Am Anim Hosp Assoc.* 1977;13:98.
110. Hornbuckle WE, et al. Prostatic disease in the dog. *Cornell Vet.* 1978;68:284.
111. Hornbuckle WE, Kleine LJ. Medical management of prostatic disease. *In:* Kirk RW, ed. *Current Veterinary Therapy VII.* Philadelphia, Pennsylvania: WB Saunders, 1980;1146.
112. Howard DR. The prostate gland. *In:* Bojrab MJ, ed. *Current Techniques in Small Animal Surgery.* Philadelphia, Pennsylvania: Lea & Febiger, 1975.
113. Hubbard BS, Vulgamott JC, Liska WD. Prostatic adenocarcinoma in a cat. *J Am Vet Med Assoc.* 1990;197:1493.
114. Huggins C, et al. Quantitative studies of prostatic secretion. *J Exp Med.* 1939;70:543.
115. Huggins C, Clark PG. Quantitative studies of prostatic secretion II. The effect of castration and of estrogen injection on the normal and on the hyperplastic prostate glands of dogs. *J Exp Med.* 1940;72:747.
116. Huggins C. The physiology of the prostate gland. *Physiol Rev.* 1945;25:281.
117. Huggins C. The etiology of benign prostatic hypertrophy. *Bull NY Acad Med.* 1947;23:696.
118. Isaacs JT. Common characteristics of human and canine benign prostatic hyperplasia. *Progr Clin Biol Res.* 1984;145:217.
119. Isaacs JT, Coffey DS. Changes in dihydrotestosterone metabolism associated with the development of canine benign prostatic hyperplasia. *Endocrinology.* 1981;108:445.
120. Isaacs JT. Changes in dihydrotestosterone metabolism and the development of benign prostatic hyperplasia in the aging beagle. *J Steroid Biochem.* 1983;18:749.
121. Isaacs JT. Structural and functional components in normal and hyperplastic canine prostates. *Progr Clin Biol Res.* 1984; 145:307.
122. Isaacs JT, Coffey DS. Etiology and disease process of benign prostatic hyperplasia. *Prostate.* 1989;2:33.
123. Jacobs G, Barsanti JA, Prasse K, Selcer B. Colliculus seminalis as a cause of a urethral filling defect in two dogs with Sertoli cell testicular neoplasms. *J Am Vet Med Assoc.* 1988;192:1748.
124. James RW, Heywood R. Age-related variations in the testes and prostate of beagle dogs. *Toxicology.* 1979;12:273.
125. Jimenez-Cruz JF, Tormo FB, Gomez JG. Treatment of chronic prostatitis: Intraprostatic antibiotic injections under echography control. *J Urol.* 1988;139:967.
126. Johnson DE, et al. Ketoconazole therapy for hormonally refractive metastatic prostate cancer. *Urology.* 1988;31:132.
127. Johnston DJ. The prostate. *In:* Slatter DH, ed. *Textbook of Small Animal Surgery.* Philadelphia, Pennsylvania: WB Saunders, 1985.
128. Johnston GR, Klausner JS, Bell FW. Canine prostatic ultrasonography—1989. *Semin Vet Med Surg.* 1989;4:44.
129. Johnston GR, et al. Diagnostic imaging of the male canine reproductive organs. *Vet Clin North Am (Small Anim Pract).* 1991;21:553.
130. Juniewicz PE, et al. Dose-dependent hormonal induction of benign prostatic hyperplasia (BPH) in castrated dogs. *The Prostate.* 1989;14:341.
131. Kane MM, Fields DW, Vaughn ED. Medical management of benign prostatic hyperplasia. *Urology.* 1990;36(Suppl):5.
132. Kavanagh JP, et al. The response of seven prostatic fluid components to prostatic disease. *Int J Androl.* 1982;5:487.
133. Kavanagh JP, et al. Zinc in post prostatic massage (VB3) urine samples: A marker of prostatic secretory function and indicator of bacterial infection. *Urol Res.* 1983;11:167.
134. Kawakami E, Tsutsui T, Ogasa A. Histological observations of the reproductive organs of the male dog from birth to sexual maturity. *J Vet Med Sci.* 1991;53:241.
135. Keane PF, et al. Response of the benign hypertrophied prostate to treatment with an LHRH analogue. *Br J Urol.* 1988;62:163.
136. Kirby RS, et al. Intra-prostatic urinary reflux: An aetiological factor in abacterial prostatitis. *Br J Urol.* 1982;54:729.
137. Kivisto AK, et al. Canine bacteriuria. *J Small Anim Pract.* 1977;18:707.
138. Kjaer T, Madsen PO. Prostatic fluid and tissue concentrations of ampicillin after administration of hetacillin ester. *Invest Urol.* 1976;14:57.
139. Knecht CD. Diseases of the canine prostate gland (Part I). *Compend Contin Ed Pract Vet.* 1979;1:385.
140. Knecht CD. Diseases of the canine prostate gland (part II: surgical techniques). *Comp Contin Ed Pract Vet.* 1979;1:426.
141. Krawiec DR, Helfin D. Study of prostatic disease in dogs: 177 cases (1981–1986). *J Am Vet Med Assoc.* 1992;200:1119.
142. Leav I, Cavazos LF. Some morphologic features of normal and pathologic canine prostate. *In:* Goland M, ed. *Normal and Abnormal Growth of the Prostate.* Springfield, Illinois: Charles C Thomas, 1975;69.
143. Leav I, Ling GV. Adenocarcinoma of the canine prostate. *Cancer.* 1968;22:1329.
144. Leib MS, et al. Squamous cell carcinoma of the prostate gland in a dog. *J Am Anim Hosp Assoc.* 1986;22:509.
145. Lindberg R, Jonsson OJ, Kasstrom H. Sertoli cell tumours associated with feminization, prostatitis, and squamous metaplasia of the renal tubular epithelium in a dog. *J Small Anim Pract.* 1976;17:451.
146. Ling GV, et al. Chronic urinary tract infection in dogs: Induction by inoculation with bacteria via percutaneous nephropyelostomy. *Am J Vet Res.* 1987;48:794.

147. Liu J, et al. Effects of androgen blockade with ketoconazole and megestrol acetate on human prostatic protein patterns. *Prostate.* 1986;9:199.
148. Lloyd JW, et al. Androgens and estrogens in the plasma and prostatic tissue of normal dogs and dogs with benign prostatic hypertrophy. *Invest Urol.* 1975;13:220.
149. Lowenstine LJ, Ling GV, Schalm OW. Exogenous estrogen toxicity in the dog. *California Vet.* 1972;26:14.
150. Lowseth LA, Gerlach RF, Gillett NA, Muggenburg BA. Age-related changes in the prostate and testes of the beagle. *Vet Pathol.* 1990;27:347.
151. Madsen PO, et al. Chronic bacterial prostatitis: Theoretical and experimental. *Urol Res.* 1983;11:1.
152. Madsen PO, et al. Experimental models for determination of antimicrobials in prostatic fluid, interstitial fluid and secretion. *Scand J Infect Dis.* 1978;14(Suppl):145.
153. Mahadevia PS, et al. Hypercalcemia in prostatic carcinoma. *Arch Intern Med.* 1983;143:1339.
154. Maigaard S, et al. Rosoxacin and cinoxacin distribution in prostate, vagina, and female urethra in dogs. *Invest Urol.* 1979;17:149.
155. Maigaard S, et al. Rosoxacin distribution in kidney and prostate: Experimental studies in dogs. *Urol Res.* 1980;8:113.
156. Mainwaring CJ. Primary lymphoma of the prostate in a dog. *J Small Anim Pract.* 1990;31:617.
157. Mariotti A, et al. Collagen and cellular proliferation in spontaneous canine prostatic hypertrophy. *J Urol.* 1982;127:795.
158. Matzkin H, Braf Z. Endocrine treatment of benign prostatic hypertrophy: Current concepts. *Urology.* 1991;37:1.
159. McConnell JD. Antiandrogen therapy for benign prostatic hyperplasia. *Monogr Urol.* 1990;11:7.
160. McEntee M, Isaacs W, Smith C. Adenocarcinoma of the canine prostate: Immunohistochemical examination for secretory antigens. *Prostate.* 1987;11:163.
161. McGuire EJ, Lytton B. Bacterial prostatitis. Treatment with trimethoprim-sulfamethoxazole. *Urology.* 1976;7:499.
162. McGuire EJ. Theoretical basis for treatment of prostatitis. *Urology.* 1984;24(Suppl):10.
163. Meares EM. Observations on activity of trimethoprim-sulfamethoxazole in the prostate. *J Infect Dis.* 1973;128:s679.
164. Meares EM. Observations on activity of trimethoprim-sulfamethoxazole in the prostate. *J Infect Dis.* 1973;128:s679.
165. Meares EM. Infection stones of prostate gland: Laboratory diagnosis and clinical management. *Urology.* 1974;4:560.
166. Meares EM. Prostatitis syndromes: New perspectives about old woes. *J Urol.* 1980;123:141.
167. Meares EM. Prostatitis. *Kidney Int.* 1981;20:289.
168. Meares EM. Prostatitis. *Med Clin North Am.* 1991;75:405.
169. Medical Letter. Ofloxacin. *Med Lett Drugs Ther.* 1991;33:71.
170. Medical Letter. Finasteride for benign prostatic hypertrophy. *Med Lett Drugs Ther.* 1992;34:83.
171. Medical Letter. Flutamide for prostatic cancer. *Med Lett Drugs Ther.* 1989;31:69.
172. Medleau L, Shanley KJ, Rakich PM, Goldschmidt MH. Trimethoprim-sulfonamide–associated drug eruptions in dogs. *J Am Anim Hosp Assoc.* 1990;26:305.
173. Merk FB, et al. Ultrastructural and biochemical expressions of divergent differentiation in prostates of castrated dogs treated with estrogen and androgen. *Lab Invest.* 1982;47:437.
174. Mills JN, Slatter DH. Stilbestrol toxicity in a dog. *Aust Vet J.* 1981;57:39.
175. Mobley DF. Bacterial prostatitis: Treatment with carbenicillin idanyl sodium. *Invest Urol.* 1981;19:31.
176. Moore RJ, et al. Concentration of dihydrotestosterone and 3-androstanediol in naturally occurring and androgen-induced prostatic hyperplasia in the dog. *J Clin Invest.* 1979;64:1003.
177. Morgan RV, Bacharach A. Keratoconjunctivitis sicca associated with sulfonamide therapy in dogs. *J Am Vet Med Assoc.* 1982;180:432.
178. Morimoto I, et al. Alteration in the metabolism of dihydrotestosterone in elderly men with prostate hyperplasia. *J Clin Invest.* 1980;66:612.
179. Mullen HS, Matthiesen DT, Scavelli TD. Results of surgery and postoperative complications in 92 dogs treated for prostatic abscessation by a multiple Penrose drain technique. *J Am Anim Hosp Assoc.* 1990;26:369.
180. Mulligan RM. Feminization in male dogs: A syndrome associated with carcinoma of the testes and mimicked by the administration of estrogen. *Am J Pathol.* 1944;20:865.
181. Naber KG. Use of quinolones in urinary tract infections and prostatitis. *Rev Infect Dis.* 1989;11:s1321.
182. Neri RO, Monahan M. Effects of a noval nonsteroidal antiandrogen on canine prostatic hyperplasia. *Invest Urol.* 1972;10:123.
183. Neri R. Pharmacology and pharmacokinetics of flutamide. *Urology.* 1989;34(suppl):19.
184. Netto NR, et al. Concentrations of norfloxacin in prostatic tissues following oral administration in patients with benign prostatic hyperplasia. *Int Urol Nephrol.* 1988;20:47.
185. Neumann F, et al. Male accessory sex glands: Experimental basis and animal models in prostatic tumor research. *In:* Serio M, Marteni L, eds. *Animal Models in Human Reproduction.* New York, New York: Raven 1980;249.
186. Newell SM, Mahaffey MB, Binhazim A, Greene CE. Paraprostatic cyst in a cat. *J Small Anim Pract.* 1992;33:399.
187. Nielsen OS, et al. Penicillamic acid derivatives in the canine prostate. *Prostate.* 1980;1:79.
188. Nishi N, et al. Comparative analysis of growth factors in normal and pathologic human prostates. *Prostate.* 1988;13:39.
189. Obradovich J, Walshaw R, Goullaud E. The influence of castration on the development of prostatic carcinoma in the dog. *J Vet Intern Med.* 1987;1:183.
190. Oesterling JE. Prostate specific antigen: A critical assessment of the most useful tumor marker for adenocarcinoma of the prostate. *J Urol.* 1991;145:907.
191. Oliveri RA, et al. Clinical experience with geocillin in the treatment of bacterial prostatitis. *Curr Ther Res.* 1979;25:415.
192. Olson PN, Wrigley RH, Thrall MA, Husted PW. Disorders of the canine prostate gland: Pathogenesis, diagnosis, and medical therapy. *Compend Contin Ed Pract Vet.* 1987;9:613.
193. Orland SM, et al. Prostatitis, prostatosis, and prostatodynia. *Urology.* 1985;25:439.
194. Osborne CA, et al. Feline urologic syndrome: A heterogeneous phenomenon? *J Am Anim Hosp Assoc.* 1984;20:17.
195. Osborne CA, et al. Redefinition of the feline urologic syndrome: Feline lower urinary tract disease with heterogeneous causes. *Vet Clin North Am.* 1984;14:409.
196. O'Shea JD. Studies of the canine prostate gland. I. Factors influencing its size and weight. *J Comp Pathol.* 1962;72:321.
197. O'Shea JD. Studies on the canine prostate gland. *J Comp Pathol.* 73:244-252, 1963.
198. O'Shea JD. Squamous metaplasia of the canine prostate gland. *Res Vet Sci.* 1963;4:431.
199. Paulson DF, White RD. Trimethoprim-sulfamethoxazole and minocycline hydrochloride in the treatment of culture-proved bacterial prostatitis. *J Urol.* 1978;120:184.
200. Paulson DF, et al. Treatment of bacterial prostatitis: Comparison of cephalexin and minocycline. *Urology.* 1986;27:379.
201. Penwick RC, Clark DM. Prostatic cyst and abscess with subse-

quent prostatic neoplasia in a Doberman pinscher. *J Am Anim Hosp Assoc.* 1990;26:489.
202. Peter AT, Jakovljevic S. Real-time ultrasonography of the small animal reproductive organs. *Compend Contin Ed Vet Med.* 1992; 14:739.
203. Pettit GD. A clinical evaluation of prostatectomy in the dog. *J Am Vet Med Assoc.* 1960;136:486.
204. Pfau A, et al. The pH of the prostatic fluid in health and diseases: Implications of treatment in chronic bacterial prostatitis. *J Urol.* 1978;119:384.
205. Pinegger H. Uterus masculinus in a male dog. *Kleintier-Praxis* 1975;20:231.
206. Plomp TA, Baert L, Maes RA. Treatment of recurrent chronic bacterial prostatitis by local injection of thiamphenicol into the prostate. *Urology.* 1980;15:542.
207. Pyle RL, Hill BL, Johnson JR. Estrogen toxicity in a dog. *Canine Pract.* 1976;August, 39-41.
208. Rawlings CA, Barsanti JA, Oliver JE, Crowell WA. Intracapsular subtotal prostatectomy in normal dogs: Use of an ultrasonic surgical aspirator. *Vet Surg.* 1994;23:182-189.
209. Reeves DS, et al. Twenty-three further studies on the secretion of antibiotics in the prostatic fluid of the dog. *In: Proceedings, 2nd International Symposium on Urinary Tract Infection.* London, 1972;197.
210. Reeves DS, Ghilchik M. Secretion of the antibacterial substance trimethoprim in the prostatic fluid of dogs. *Br J Urol.* 1980;42:66.
211. Rendano VT, Slauson DO. Hypertrophic osteopathy in a dog with prostatic adenocarcinoma and without thoracic metastasis. *J Am Anim Hosp Assoc.* 1982;18:905.
212. Rife J, Thornburg LP. Osteocollagenous prostatic retention cyst in the canine. *Canine Pract.* 1980;7:44.
213. Ristuccia AM, Cunha BA. Current concepts in antimicrobial therapy of prostatitis. *Urology.* 1982;20:338.
214. Rogers KS, et al. Diagnostic evaluation of the canine prostate. *Comp Contin Ed Pract Vet.* 1986;8:799.
215. Rohr HP, et al. The dog prostate under defined hormonal influences: An approach to experimentally induced prostatic growth. *Pathol Res Pract.* 1960;166:347.
216. Rosenkrantz H, et al. The chemical analysis of normal canine prostatic fluid. *Am J Vet Res.* 1961;22:1057.
217. Rowland PH, Center SA, Doughterty SA. Presumptive trimethoprim-sulfadiazine–related hepatotoxicosis in a dog. *J Am Vet Med Assoc.* 1992;200:348.
218. Sabbaj J, Hoagland VL, Cook T. Norfloxacin versus cotrimoxazole in the treatment of recurring urinary tract infections in men. *Scand J Infect Dis.* 1986;48(Suppl):48.
219. Sawczuk I, et al. Primary transitional cell carcinoma of prostatic periurethral ducts. *Urology.* 1985;25:339.
220. Schaeffer AJ. Pharmacokinetics of antibiotics used in treatment of prostatitis. *Urology.* 1984;24(Suppl):8.
221. Schaeffer AJ, Darras FS. The efficacy of norfloxacin in the treatment of chronic bacterial prostatitis refractory to trimethoprim-sulfamethoxazole and/or carbenicillin. *J Urol.* 1990;144:690.
222. Schaeffer AJ. Diagnosis and treatment of prostatic infections. *Urology.* 1990;36:13.
223. Schlotthauer CF. Observations on the prostate gland of the dog. *J Am Vet Med Assoc.* 1932;81:645.
224. Schuberth VBG, Weiger G. Zur Therapie der Prostatahypertrophie des Hundes mit Medroxyprogesteron. *KleintierPraxis.* 1978;23:331.
225. Schulman J, Levine SH. Pyometra involving uterus masculinus in a cat. *J Am Vet Med Assoc.* 1989;194:690.
226. Schulze H, Barack ER. Immunocytochemical localization of estrogen receptors in spontaneous and experimentally induced canine benign prostatic hyperplasia. *Prostate.* 1987;11:145.
227. Sherding RG, et al. Bone marrow hypoplasia in 8 dogs with Sertoli cell tumor. *J Am Vet Med Assoc.* 1981;178:497.
228. Shortliffe LMD, Wehner N, Stamey T. The detection of a local prostatic immunologic response to bacterial prostatitis. *J Urol.* 1981;125:509.
229. Shortliffe LMD, Elliott K, Sellers RG. Measurement of urinary antibodies to crude bacterial antigen in patients with chronic bacterial prostatitis. *J Urol.* 1989;141:632.
230. Shull RM, et al. Urogenital blastomycosis in a dog. *J Am Vet Med Assoc.* 1977;171:730.
231. Sisson DD, Hoffer RE. Osteocollagenous prostatic retention cyst: Report of a canine case. *J Am Anim Hosp Assoc.* 1977;13:61.
232. Smith CW. Marsupialization of the prostate gland. *In:* Bojrab MJ, ed. *Current Techniques in Small Animal Surgery.* Philadelphia, Pennsylvania: Lea & Febiger, 1975.
233. Smith JW. Recurrent urinary tract infections in men: Characteristics and response to therapy. *Ann Intern Med.* 1979;91:544.
234. Soloway MS. Treatment of prostatic cancer. *Postgrad Med.* 1986;80:249.
235. Spackman CJA, Roth L. Prostatic cyst and concurrent Sertoli cell tumor in a dog. *J Am Vet Med Assoc.* 1988;192:1096.
236. Stamey TA, et al. Chronic bacterial prostatitis and the diffusion of drugs into prostatic fluid. *J Urol.* 1970;103:187.
237. Stamey TA, et al. The concentration of trimethoprim in prostatic fluid: Nonionic diffusion or active transport? *J Infect Dis.* 1973;128(Suppl):S686.
238. Stead AC, Borthwich R. The canine urinary bladder and prostate. *J Small Anim Pract.* 1976;17:629.
239. Steinberg S. Aplastic anemia in a dog. *J Am Vet Med Assoc.* 1970;157:966.
240. Stone EA, et al. Radiographic interpretation of prostatic disease in the dog. *J Am Anim Hosp Assoc.* 1978;14:115.
241. Stone EA, Barsanti JA. *Urologic Surgery of the Dog and Cat.* Philadelphia, Pennsylvania: Lea & Febiger, 1992.
242. Stone NN. Flutamide in treatment of benign prostatic hypertrophy. *Urology.* 1989;34(Suppl):64.
243. Surya BV, Provet JA. Manifestations of advanced prostate cancer: Prognosis and treatment. *J Urol.* 1989;142:921.
244. Sutor DJ, Wooley SE. The crystalline composition of prostatic calculi. *Br J Urol.* 1974;46:533.
245. Taylor PA. Prostatic adenocarcinoma in a dog and a summary of 10 cases. *Can Vet J.* 1973;14:162.
246. Thrall MA, et al. Cytologic diagnosis of canine prostatic disease. *J Am Anim Hosp Assoc.* 1985;21:95.
247. Tolkoff-Rubin NE, Rubin RH. Ciprofloxacin in management of urinary tract infection. *Urology.* 1988;31:359.
248. Trachtenberg J, Hicks LL, Walsh PC. Androgen- and estrogen-receptor content in spontaneous and experimentally induced canine prostatic hyperplasia. *J Clin Invest.* 1980;65:1051.
249. Trachtenberg J. Effects of ketoconazole on testosterone production and normal and malignant androgen dependent tissues of the adult rat. *J Urol.* 1984;132:599.
250. Trachtenberg J. Ketoconazole therapy in advanced prostatic cancer. *J Urol.* 1984;132:61.
251. Tunn S, Hochstrate H, Habenicht UF, Krieg M. 5-Alpha-reductase activity of prostates from intact and castrated dogs treated with androstenedione, the aromatase inhibitor 1-methyl-1,4-androstadiene-3,17-dione, and cyproterone acetate. *Prostate.* 1988;12:243.
252. Turrel JM. Intraoperative radiotherapy of carcinoma of the prostate gland in 10 dogs. *J Am Vet Med Assoc.* 1987;190:48.
253. Tyslowitz R, Dingemanse E. Effect of large doses of estrogens on the blood picture of dogs. *Endocrinology.* 1941;29:817.

254. Vancutsem PM, Babish JG, Schwark WS. The fluoroquinolone antimicrobials: Structure, antimicrobial activity, pharmacokinetics, clinical use in domestic animals and toxicity. *Cornell Vet* 1990;80:173.
255. Walde I, Burtscher H. Retinal detachment as a result of cryptococcosis in a dog. *Kleintierpraxis.* 1980;25:251.
256. Walker RD, Stern GE, Hauptman JG, MacDonald KH. Pharmacokinetic evaluation of enrofloxacin administered orally to healthy dogs. *Am J Vet Res.* 1992;53:2315.
257. Walsh PC, Wilson JD. The induction of prostatic hypertrophy in the dog with androstanediol. *J Clin Invest.* 1976;57:1093.
258. Watanabe H, Shima M, Kojima M, Ohe H. Dynamic study of nervous control on prostatic contraction and fluid excretion in the dog. *J Urol.* 1988;140:1567.
259. Weaver AD. Discrete prostatic (paraprostatitic) cysts in the dog. *Vet Rec.* 1978;102:435.
260. Weaver AD. Fifteen cases of prostatic carcinoma in the dog. *Vet Rec.* 1981;109:71.
261. Weidner W, Schiefer HG, Dalhoff A. Treatment of chronic bacterial prostatitis with ciprofloxacin, results of a one-year follow-up study. *Am J Med.* 1987;82(Suppl 4A):280.
262. Wenderoth UK, George FW, Wilson JD. The effect of a 5-alpha-reductase inhibitor on androgen-mediated growth of the dog prostate. *Endocrinology.* 1983;113:569.
263. Werner LL, Bright JM. Drug-induced immune hypersensitivity disorders in two dogs treated with trimethoprim sulfadiazine: Case reports and drug challenge studies. *J Am Anim Hosp Assoc.* 1983;19:783.
264. Wheaton LG, et al. Relationship of seminal volume to size and disease of the prostate in the beagle. *Am J Vet Res.* 1979;40:1325.
265. White RAS, Herrtage ME, Dennis R. The diagnosis and management of paraprostatic and prostatic retention cysts in the dog. *J Small Anim Pract.* 1987;28:551.
266. Wilcke JR. Therapeutic application of sulfadiazine/trimethoprim in dogs and cats: A review. *Companion Anim Pract.* 1988;2:3.
267. Willard MD, et al. Ketoconazole-induced changes in selected canine hormone concentrations. *Am J Vet Res.* 1986;47:2504.
268. Wilson JD. The pathogenesis of benign hyperplasia. *Am J Med.* 1986;68:745.
269. Winningham DC, et al. Diffusion of antibiotics from plasma into prostatic fluid. *Nature.* 1968;219:139.
270. Winningham DG, Stamey TA. Diffusion of sulfonamides from plasma into prostatic fluid. *J Urol.* 1970;104:559.
271. Zirkin BR, Strandberg JD. Quantitative changes in the morphology of the aging canine prostate. *Anat Rec.* 1984;208:207.
272. Zontine WJ. The prostate gland. *Mod Vet Pract.* 1975;56:341.
273. Zontine WJ. Prostatic disease. *Mod Vet Pract.* 1975;56:485.
274. Zuckerman S, McKeoun T. The canine prostate in relation to normal and abnormal testicular changes. *J Pathol Bacteriol.* 1938;46:7.

PART VI

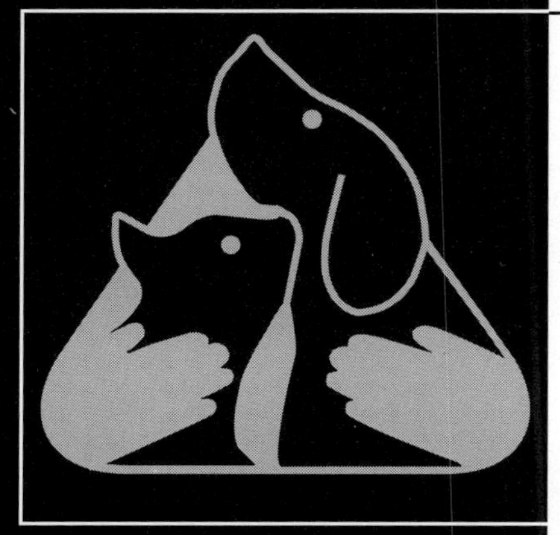

DISEASES OF THE UPPER AND LOWER URINARY TRACT

CHAPTER 40

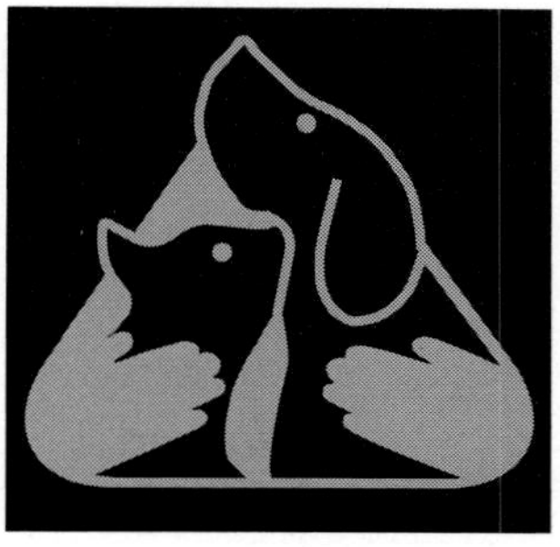

Bacterial Infections of the Canine and Feline Urinary Tract

CARL A. OSBORNE
GEORGE E. LEES

I. DEFINITION OF TERMS AND CONCEPTS[149]

A. Urinary tract infection (UTI).

1. Bacterial infection of the urinary tract encompasses a wide variety of clinical entities for which the common denominator is microbial invasion of any of its components.
   a. Infection may predominate at a single site, such as the kidney (pyelonephritis), ureter (ureteritis), bladder (cystitis), urethra (urethritis), or prostate gland (prostatitis), at two or more of these sites, or may be restricted to the urine (bacteriuria).
   b. Although such terms as pyelonephritis, cystitis, and urethritis are commonly used, they reflect localized expressions of UTI that have the potential of affecting the entire urinary tract.
   c. The important point is that the entire system is at risk of invasion once any of its parts becomes colonized with bacteria.
2. Because bacterial infections are unlikely to be confined to the urinary bladder without affecting the urethra, "lower urinary tract infection" or "urethrocystitis" is more appropriate than "cystitis." Likewise, because bacterial infections are unlikely to be confined to the renal parenchyma and renal pelvis without affecting portions of the ureters, of "upper urinary tract infection" is more appropriate than "pyelonephritis."
3. Although the pathogenesis of UTIs is still somewhat obscure, it is now known that it depends on the balance between uropathic infectious agents (analogous to seeds) and host resistance (analogous to soil).
   a. Evidence obtained in recent years indicates that growth of microbial "seeds" is enhanced if a suitable "soil," characterized by increased host susceptibility, is present.
   b. Although use of antimicrobial agents to eliminate uropathogens remains the cornerstone of therapy, the status of host defense mechanisms is also an important factor in the pathogenesis of UTIs. In other words, abnormalities in host defenses represent a major predisposing cause of UTIs that underlies microbial agents, the traditionally accepted cause.
4. A UTI is not a definitive diagnostic entity.
   a. Because bacterial UTI encompasses a spectrum of etiologic factors, diagnostic and therapeutic requirements vary from case to case.
   b. Conceptual understanding of the interaction of various host defense mechanisms with pathogenic microbes permits the development of a diagnostically and therapeutically significant classification of UTIs.
   c. The common denominator of this classification is the presence or absence of detectable abnormalities in host defense mechanisms, allowing

differentiation of complicated UTIs from uncomplicated (or simple) UTIs.

B. Significant bacteriuria.

1. Identification of bacteria in urine is not synonymous with UTI because the bacteria may represent contaminants or pathogens.
   a. Bacteria that normally inhabit the urethra and genitalia in the absence of UTI may appear in urine that is obtained by either spontaneous voiding or catheterization.
   b. Urine may also be contaminated with bacteria after it is voided.
2. Significant bacteriuria is a term coined to describe bacteriuria that represents UTI.
   a. A high bacterial count in a properly collected and cultured urine sample is indicative of UTI.
   b. Few bacteria obtained from untreated patients usually indicate contamination.
   c. Therefore, quantitative urine cultures aid differentiation between bacterial pathogens and contaminants.
3. Asymptomatic bacteriuria is defined as significant bacteriuria unaccompanied by signs referable to disease of the urinary tract.
   a. The term is used synonymously with covert bacteriuria.
   b. Asymptomatic or covert bacteriuria may be encountered in dogs given glucocorticoids or with hyperadrenocorticism. (See Section VB5, Impaired Immunocompetence, in this chapter.)
4. The concept of significant bacteriuria is based on probability. When interpreting quantitative bacterial cultures, several variables should be considered. (See Chapter 8, Diagnostic Urine Culture.)

C. Pyuria.

1. Pyuria is defined as the presence of white blood cells (WBC) in urine.
2. When WBCs are present in urine in significant numbers, they usually represent a normal response by the body to an irritant.
3. Pyuria and infection are not synonymous because pyuria may occur with inflammation that results from causes other than infection.
4. Although the normal range of WBCs (neutrophils) in urine sediment prepared from a 5-mL aliquot of urine has been reported to be 0 to 3 WBCs per high-power field (hpf) (450X) in samples collected by cystocentesis, and 0 to 8 WBCs per hpf in catheterized or midstream voided samples,[110] several variables should be considered when interpreting the numbers of WBCs in urine sediment (See Section VIII, Urinalysis, of this chapter.)

D. Inflammation versus infection.

1. Inflammation must be distinguished from infection as they relate to urinary tract disease.
   a. Many diverse disease processes, including bacterial infection, neoplasia, and urolithiasis, result in inflammatory lesions of the urinary tract characterized by exudation of red blood cells (RBCs), WBCs, and protein into urine. The resultant hematuria, pyuria, and proteinuria suggest inflammatory urinary tract disease, but do not indicate its cause or location within the urinary tract.
   b. Urine culture, renal function tests, radiographic and ultrasonographic studies, endoscopy, urodynamic studies, and biopsy procedures often provide the additional information necessary to localize the disease process and establish its cause.
2. Bacterial UTI is a common cause of urinary tract disease in dogs and is estimated to affect 14% of all dogs during their lifetime.[97] In contrast, results of several investigations of feline lower urinary tract disease indicate that the initial episode is associated with bacterial UTI in only 1 to 3% of the patients.[15,88,95,139,147]
   a. Detection of infection should be established by urine culture, because diagnosis based solely on recognition of inflammatory cells in urinalyses results in overdiagnosis of infection.
   b. Conversely, absence of hematuria, pyuria, and proteinuria does not rule out the existence of infection, because it may occur without stimulating detectable inflammatory response (asymptomatic or covert bacteriuria).
   c. Positive urine culture results indicate that bacterial infection is either the cause of the disease process or a secondary complication of another process, such as neoplasia, metabolic urolithiasis, or perhaps postsurgical sequelae.

II. NORMAL HOST DEFENSES

A. Overview.

1. The urinary tract communicates with an external environment laden with bacteria.
   a. Evidence that most UTIs result from ascending migration of pathogens has focused attention on the urethra and adjacent portions of the genital tract as immediate sources of bacteria.
   b. Numerous studies have revealed that a resident population of bacteria is normally present in the lower genital tract and urethra of animals and humans (Table 40–1).[16,28,66,67,102]
   c. Gram-positive bacteria appear to be especially common inhabitants of the canine urethra. *Mycoplasma* spp also are commonly present.
   d. The microflora of the lower genitourinary tract may be considered to be protective in the context that these microbes normally inhibit adherence of transient pathogenic microbes to adjacent mucosal cells and may also inhibit their growth. Seldom do these microbes cause UTI in normal dogs.
2. Although the urinary tract communicates with an environment loaded with bacteria and other potentially pathogenic agents, most of it is normally

TABLE 40–1.
BACTERIA DETECTED IN THE UROGENITAL TRACT OF NORMAL MALE AND FEMALE DOGS[16,66,67,102]

Genus	Distal Urethra (Males)	Prepuce	Vagina
Acinetobacter		+	+
Bacillus		+	+
Bacteroides			+
Citrobacter			+
Corynebacterium	+	+	+
Enterobacter			+
Enterococcus			+
Escherichia	+	+	+
Flavobacterium	+	+	+
Haemophilus	+	+	+
Klebsiella	+	+	+
Micrococcus			+
Moraxella		+	+
Mycoplasma	+	+	+
Neisseria			+
Pasteurella		+	+
Proteus		+	+
Pseudomonas			+
Staphylococcus	+	+	+
Streptococcus	+	+	+
Ureaplasma	+	+	+

sterile, and all of it is normally resistant to infection.

a. Experimental studies performed in dogs, rabbits, and humans revealed that large quantities of *Escherichia coli* inoculated into the lumina of their bladders were usually eliminated within 72 hours.[36,59,127]

b. Although one may logically assume that intact local host defenses may be inadequate to prevent infection by an overwhelming exposure to bacterial pathogens, continuous instillation of bacteria into intact urinary bladder lumina of dogs for 2 weeks to 3 months failed to establish infection.[59]

c. UTI can be experimentally induced by overwhelming normal host defenses with a massive inoculum of pathogenic bacteria; however, such a phenomenon is uncommon in naturally occurring cases.

d. Although systemic host defense mechanisms undoubtedly have an important role in preventing hematogenous spread of pathogens to and from the urinary tract, local host defense mechanisms appear to represent the initial line of defense in the prevention of ascending infection of the urinary tract (Table 40–2).[32]

3. Studies in animals have revealed some findings that, at first glance, appear to be paradoxic.
   a. By inducing an intense water diuresis, rats may be made resistant to attempts to induce pyelonephritis via intravenous injection of a large dose of certain bacteria (staphylococci and enterococci).[5-8]
   b. In contrast, dilution of urine increases the susceptibility of animals to urinary colonization with certain bacteria following their instillation into the urinary bladder.[49,78]
   c. As will be elucidated in subsequent sections of this chapter, these observations suggest differences in host defense mechanisms of the kidneys and urinary bladder.
4. Mechanisms of host resistance to bacterial UTIs may be divided into two basic categories:
   a. Natural resistance factors inherent to the urinary tract. Natural resistance factors include complete and frequent unidirectional voiding of urine, mucosal defense barriers, and the antimicrobic properties of urine (Table 40-2).

TABLE 40–2.
NATURAL AND ACQUIRED HOST DEFENSES OF THE URINARY TRACT

I. Normal Micturition
   A. Adequate urine volume
   B. Frequent voiding
   C. Complete voiding
II. Anatomic Structures
   A. Urethral high-pressure zones
   B. Surface characteristics of urethral urothelium
   C. Urethral peristalsis
   D. Prostatic secretions (antibacterial fraction and immunoglobulins)
   E. Length of urethra
   F. Ureterovesical flap valves
   G. Ureteral peristalsis
   H. Glomerular mesangial cells?
   I. Extensive renal blood supply and flow
   J. Others?
III. Mucosal Defense Barriers
   A. Antibody production
   B. Surface layer (glycosaminoglycans)
   C. Intrinsic mucosal antimicrobial properties
   D. Exfoliation of cells
   E. Bacterial interferences by commensal microbes of distal urethra and distal genital tract
   F. Others?
IV. Antimicrobial Properties of Urine
   A. Extremes (high or low) of urine pH
   B. Hyperosmolality
   C. High concentration of urea
   D. Organic acids
   E. Small molecular weight carbohydrates
   F. Tamm-Horsfall mucoprotein
   G. Others?
V. Systemic Immunocompetence
   A. Cell-mediated immunity
   B. Humoral-mediated immunity

b. Acquired or induced resistance factors that are activated only after infection with bacteria. Immune responses to bacterial infection are an example of acquired resistance (Table 40–2).
c. Both categories contribute to host resistance to bacterial UTI, but at least initially, natural local host defenses are thought to be the initial line of defense.

B. Normal micturition.

1. Because some bacteria can survive and multiply in urine, the hydrodynamics associated with unidirectional voiding of urine are thought to represent one of the most important natural defense mechanisms against infection of the urinary tract.[145]
   a. The fact that at least some bacteria may normally gain access to the urinary bladder is suggested by experimental studies in normal dogs in which radiolabeled colloidal particles the size of bacteria were detected in the lumen of the bladder following their placement in the urethra.[35] Likewise, spermatozoa are occasionally observed in urine collected from dogs and cats by cystocentesis, providing evidence that urine may reflux from the urethra into the bladder lumen.
   b. Mechanical washout induced by unimpeded, frequent, and complete voiding of urine inhibits bacterial colonization of the urinary tract by rapidly eliminating organisms that reach the lumen of the proximal urethra and urinary bladder.
      (1). Micturition also reduces the population of bacteria lining the urethral mucosa by flushing the urethral lumen with sterile urine.[171]
      (2). Washout of urethral bacteria may be aided by urethral distention, which obliterates mucosal folds and crevices in which bacteria may be lodged.[106]
      (3). Estimates suggest that the normal bladder clears 99.9% of the bacteria injected into it by the mechanical washout effect of voiding in combination with other defense mechanisms.[133,153]
2. Frequent voiding also eliminates toxic products produced by bacteria that may damage the urinary tract. Likewise, it permits accumulation of fresh urine with renewed quantities of antimicrobial metabolites.
3. The effectiveness of voiding depends on the rate of urine production and flow, the frequency of voiding, the completeness of emptying (the amount of residual urine), the virulence of bacteria, and the rate of bacterial multiplication in urine. The physiologic dilution of bacterial quantities that results from the constant inflow of sterile urine from the kidneys, and subsequent voiding stimulated by distention of the bladder wall, are significant. As will be reviewed, disorders that impair the frequency or volume of micturition, or that permit residual urine to remain in the urinary bladder following micturition, predispose the patients to infection.
   a. For example, the elimination of urine flow through the urethra of female dogs by surgical methods increased the number and distribution of bacteria in the urethra and urinary bladder.[116]
   b. Experimental reduction of the size of the distal urethra of female dogs also was associated with increased numbers of bacteria.[117]
   c. In contrast, dilation of the urethras of female dogs was associated with a decreased number of bacteria in the urethral lumen, presumably as a result of improved washout during micturition.[116]

C. Anatomic defense mechanisms.

1. Overview. A resident population of bacteria is normally present in progressively increasing amounts from the midportion of the urethra to the distal urethra (see Table 40–1). These organisms do not cause lesions in normal animals, a fact that may be related in part to the following anatomic features.
2. Urethral High-Pressure Zone
   a. A functional high-pressure zone in the midurethra of female dogs and humans has been hypothesized to inhibit the migration of bacteria from the distal urethra into the upper portions of the excretory pathway (urethrovesical reflux).[119,189]
   b. The urethral zone of high pressure corresponds to an area shown microscopically to consist of smooth and striated muscle.[65]
   c. This high-pressure zone might also have an important role in maintenance of urinary continence during the storage phase of micturition.
3. Surface Characteristics of Urethral Urothelium
   a. Scanning electron microscopy has revealed differences in the structure of the transitional epithelial cells that line the proximal and distal urethra of dogs.
      (1). Whereas the urothelium of the proximal urethra contains microplicae, the urothelium of the distal urethra contains microvilli.
      (2). Entrapment of bacteria that gain access to the proximal urethra by microplicae may hinder further migration and colonization.[134]
      (3). During the voiding phase of micturition, dilation of the urethral lumen is associated with flattening of the microplicae, allowing urine to flush bacteria to the exterior.
   b. The ability of bacteria to adhere to the surface of cells is an important factor in the colonization of mucosal surfaces.[38,48,138,194] The surface char-

acteristics of bacteria and mucosal cells are important factors influencing bacterial adherence to cells.[48,81]

(1). Recent studies in humans indicate that the ability of *E. coli* to adhere to vaginal mucosa is determined, at least in part, by the surface characteristics of the epithelial cells,[48] in addition to the adhesive property of bacteria.[73,85,187]

(2). Alteration of the surface characteristics of urothelial cells following infection and inflammation may reduce the effectiveness of bacterial washout by micturition.[107]

4. Urethral Peristalsis
   a. Intrinsic symmetric peristaltic contractions of the urethra have been identified in female dogs.[118] The peristaltic contractions begin in the proximal urethra and move to the distal urethra.
   b. Urethral peristalsis may aid unidirectional flow of urine and may assist in inhibiting the ascending migration of bacteria.
5. Prostatic Antibacterial Fraction
   a. Studies of prostatic fluid obtained from dogs, rats, and humans have revealed a substance(s) called prostatic antibacterial fraction (PAF) that is bactericidal to gram-positive and gram-negative organisms.[181]
      (1). Although the exact composition of PAF has not been determined, it is known to be a low-molecular-weight zinc compound, probably a zinc salt.[42]
      (2). Other factors, such as spermine and lysozyme, may be involved.[32]
      (3). Continuous, or at least frequent, exposure of the urethral mucosa to prostatic fluid may modify the ability of microbes to adhere to and colonize uroepithelial cells.
   b. Secretory cells have been identified in the urethra of female dogs and female humans, and investigators have speculated that their secretions may inhibit bacterial growth.[69]
   c. The vaginal fluid of women acts as an antimicrobial agent against some species of bacteria.[180]
6. Length of urethra. In humans and dogs, the incidence of cystitis is higher in females than in males.
   a. Uncontrolled clinical observations at the University of Minnesota and by other investigators revealed a similar pattern in dogs.[80]
   b. One popular but unproven hypothesis that has been advocated to explain this observation is that the shorter length of the female urethra provides less of a barrier to the ascending migration of bacteria than does the longer male urethra.
   c. The antimicrobial activity of PAF and spermine also may be involved.
   d. Of interest also is that urine from women supports bacterial growth better than does urine from men.[10]
7. Ureterovesical Flap Valves
   a. Although well-defined ureterovesical sphincters are not present, the oblique course of the ureters through the bladder wall and the specialized arrangement of the smooth muscle fibers in the distal ureter with the smooth muscle fibers of the bladder trigone form a one-way flap valve that normally prevents retrograde flow of urine from the bladder (so-called vesicoureteral reflux).[79,199]
   b. Unidirectional flow of urine from the ureters into the bladder protects the kidneys from contamination with infected bladder urine.
8. Ureteral Peristalsis
   a. The predominantly unidirectional movement of boluses of urine propelled by peristaltic waves in the ureters also may help to prevent ascending migration of bacteria.[169]
   b. The contraction of smooth muscle in the renal pelvis also promotes unidirectional movement of urine toward the urinary bladder.[205]

D. Renal medullary and cortical defenses.

1. Renal Medulla
   a. Results of studies of most experimental models of renal infection caused by ascending or hematogenous exposure to bacteria indicate that the renal cortex is much more resistant to infection than is the renal medulla.[5,7,50,51,85,123,163]
      (1). In a study in rats, fewer than 10 coliform bacilli injected into the medulla were required to initiate infection, whereas approximately 100,000 were required to infect the cortex.[51]
      (2). Experimental studies in rabbits indicate that the renal cortex is more susceptible to infections with *Candida* spp than is the renal medulla.[52]
   b. Vulnerability of the medulla to bacterial infection is not a consistent finding in all models of induced bacterial pyelonephritis, however. In some species, cortical and medullary lesions are observed simultaneously, and occasionally cortical lesions are observed initially.[165]
   c. Several factors have been associated with the increased susceptibility of the renal medulla to bacterial infection.[76,85] Comparatively slow blood flow through the renal medulla, an important feature of the countercurrent system and urine concentration, may be associated with a decrease in antibodies, complement factors, and leukocytes delivered to this area.
      (1). Although high osmolality tends to inhibit the survival and growth of bacteria in urine, the normal hyperosmolality of the renal medulla inhibits migration and phagocytosis of leukocytes.[5,9,31,86]

(2). The protective effect of water diuresis against infection of the renal medulla has been postulated to be associated with a reduction in medullary osmolality.[85]

(3). The hyperosmolality of the renal medulla also permits the survival of bacterial variants (L-forms) with cell wall deficiencies that are resistant to antibiotics (such as ampicillin) that impair bacterial cell wall synthesis.[3,86,192]

(a). These atypical forms are able to survive in a concentrated environment, but are lysed if osmotic pressure is reduced as a result of a decrease in the solute concentration.

(b). They may cause a relapse of infection if they revert to the parent form of bacteria after microbial therapy has been withdrawn.

d. The high concentration of ammonia in the renal medulla has been reported to enhance its susceptibility to infection by interfering with antigen-antibody reactions[165] and inhibiting the fourth component of complement.[28] This conclusion deserves further study, however, because studies in rats indicate that ammoniagenesis activates the alternate pathway of complement.[129] Once established, urease-producing bacteria may further contribute to the production of ammonia by degrading urea.

e. Because of the concept of reduced effectiveness of host defense mechanisms in the renal medulla, this region of the kidney has been likened to an "immunologic desert."[76]

2. Renal Cortex

a. Most investigators have focused on the susceptibility of the renal medulla to bacterial UTI rather than on the relative resistance of the renal cortex to UTI.

b. Inability of blood-borne bacterial microbes to reach the renal tubular lumens by filtering through normal glomerular capillary walls can be readily explained by the large size of the bacteria.

c. If bacteria gain access to a functional mesangium, the logical hypothesis is that they will become trapped and phagocytosed in this region before they initiate glomerular damage.

E. Mucosal defense barriers.

1. Overview

a. To promote infection and inflammation, bacteria must first attach themselves to urothelial receptors (adherence) and proliferate (colonization).

b. They must also penetrate the mucosal surface, which is separated from the underlying muscle layers by a thin layer called the lamina propria. The lamina propria is formed by loose, fibrous, and amorphous connective tissue containing blood vessels, nerve fibers, and occasional reticuloendothelial cells.

c. Numerous clinical and experimental studies indicate that intrinsic mucosal defense mechanisms have an important role in limiting bacterial colonization of the proximal urethra and urinary bladder and in preventing ascending migration of bacteria.

2. Surface Mucoprotein Layer.

a. Studies in humans, rabbits, and rats indicate that urothelial cells produce a layer of glycosaminoglycan (a polymer of carbohydrates and protein) that coats their surface.[11,69,82,122,152,174]

(1). Glycoaminoglycans are hydrophilic and attract an aqueous film of water or urine onto their surfaces.[125]

(2). In rabbits and guinea pigs, it covers that portion of the urinary tract from the distal renal tubules to the urethra.[198]

b. The surface coating of glycosaminoglycans and water nonspecifically inhibits bacterial adherence to urothelial cells and thus enhances the mechanical washout of bacteria during micturition.

c. Whether or not patients susceptible to UTIs have a deficiency in quantity or composition of urinary glycosaminoglycans is unknown.

d. Investigators have suggested that the protective glycosaminoglycan layer may be influenced by estrogens and progesterone in some species.

(1). In one study, an increase in the susceptibility of ovariectomized rabbits to bacterial UTIs was attributed to decreased effect of estrogen on this protective layer.[128]

(2). The same investigators also reported that bacterial UTI was more common in spayed than in intact female dogs.

e. Canine studies are needed to evaluate the value of synthetic glycosaminoglycans (pentosanpolysulfate) in the management of UTIs, especially those induced by catheterization.[125,159,172]

3. Intrinsic Mucosal Antimicrobial Properties.

a. The mucosa of the urinary bladder possesses intrinsic antibacterial properties in addition to locally secreted immunoglobulins (so-called mucosal factor). However, deeper layers of the bladder wall are more susceptible to experimental bacterial infection than are the mucosa and submucosa.[62]

b. Experimental studies in animals have demonstrated that the bladder mucosa kills or inhibits the growth of bacteria present in the minimal amount of residual urine remaining after normal voiding.[85,133,165]

(1). In one study of guinea pigs, the mechanism(s) whereby the urothelial surface killed the bacteria was not established, although it was apparently not related to the antibacterial activity of urine, the clumping of organisms on the bladder mucosa, phagocytosis by leukocytes, or bactericidal antibody in serum.[133]

(2). Authors have suggested that organic acids or other unidentified compounds produced by mucosal cells account for their antibacterial activity.[85]

(a). This activity has a finite capacity because it may be inhibited if the bacteria in the bladder are excessive, or if excessive residual urine in the bladder lumen following micturition dilutes its concentration.

(b). The residual volume of urine in the bladder of normal dogs following micturition has been estimated to be 0.2 to 0.4 mL of urine per kilogram body weight.[126]

c. At one time, investigators thought that once leukocytes entered urine their function was impaired to such a degree that they were no longer effective.

(1). However, recent studies of humans suggest that urine leukocytes maintain their phagocytic activity.[114]

(2). In combination with fixed macrophages in deeper layers of the bladder wall, leukocytes have an important role in the inflammatory process initiated by bacterial infection.[76,138]

(3). Leukocytes also assist in host defense following exposure of the kidneys to bacterial pathogens.[71]

4. Exfoliation of Cells.

a. The attrition and exfoliation of urothelial cells are normal phenomena that may be accelerated by abnormal conditions.

b. Results of experimental studies of infections with *Klebsiella pneumoniae* of rat bladders were interpreted to indicate that the exfoliation of epithelial cells that were altered or damaged by bacteria was an initial host response to pathogens.[38]

c. The desquamated cells and bacteria subsequently became trapped in amorphous and fibrin-like strands, and were removed from the urinary tract by voiding. Similar results have been reported by other investigators.[138]

5. Bacterial Interference.

a. Adherence of uropathogenic bacteria to uroepithelial cells is an essential prerequisite to UTIs.

b. The concept of bacterial interference is based on the assumption that bacterial commensals in the genital tract and distal urethra (see Table 40-1) prevent pathogenic bacteria from adhering to, and colonizing cells in these areas.[46,48,66]

(1). They may accomplish this by steric hindrance and competition for receptor sites on cell surfaces.[159]

(2). Investigators have proposed that commensal organisms may also interfere with the growth of alien bacteria by elaborating antimicrobial substances (bacteriocins) and utilizing essential nutrients.

(3). Studies in dogs and humans suggest that bacterial interference may have a role in the prevention of ascending colonization of the urinary tract with bacterial pathogens.[48,66]

F. Antimicrobial properties of urine.

1. Although urine may support bacterial growth under certain circumstances, urine from cats, dogs, and humans is frequently inhibitory and sometimes bactericidal for pathogens that cause UTIs.[39,75,85,89,97]

a. The antibacterial properties of urine are influenced by its composition.

b. Unfavorable physiologic conditions for growth of some types of aerobic bacteria include high osmolality, low or extremely high pH, high concentration of urea, and certain weak organic acids primarily derived from the diet. These factors have a variable effect on different types of bacteria.[22,89,145]

c. Urinary acidifiers have been commonly recommended as supportive therapeutic aids for bacterial UTI because most aerobic bacteria found in the urine of humans grow well at a neutral or mildly alkaline pH.[10]

d. As reviewed in Section IID, Renal Medullary and Cortical Defenses, the effects of high osmolality in the renal medulla may favor survival of some types of bacteria.

2. Tamm-Horsfall protein (also called uromucoid and urinary slime) is normally produced by tubular cells of the ascending limbs of the loops of Henle.

a. The fact that Tamm-Horsfall mucoprotein can bind to fimbriae on the surface of bacteria, and the fact that adhesive fimbriae are essential for many types of bacteria to adhere to uroepithelial cell receptors, has led to the hypothesis that Tamm-Horsfall mucoprotein is a urinary tract defense mechanism.[113,159]

b. Tamm-Horsfall protein may aggregate to produce a "fish-net"-like formation that traps microorganisms and facilitates their elimination from the urinary tract during the voiding phase of micturition.[20]

3. Small-molecular-weight carbohydrates (oligosaccharides) have been described in urine that have the potential to detach *Escherichia coli* bound to epithelial cells and to prevent attachment of *E. coli*

to cell surfaces.[159] Presumably these oligosaccharides in urine resemble sugar moieties on epithelial cell surface receptors and bind to bacteria.

G. Local and systemic immune responses.

1. Overview
   a. Because host-parasite relationships in UTIs are extraordinarily complex, the role(s) of immune components have been difficult to identify.[24]
   b. To date, the effects of local and systemic immunoglobulins in protection of the urinary tract against infections and in eradication of existing infections have been difficult to establish precisely.
2. Local Immunity
   a. Evidence suggests that locally produced antibodies may assist in the protection of the urinary tract from infection.[123,194]
   b. Genital mucosa, urethral mucosa, and, to a lesser extent, other mucosal surfaces of the urinary tract appear to produce a substantial quantity of secretory immunoglobulin A (IgA), an antibody known to be important in the protection of most mucous membranes of the body.[32,145]
      (1). Secretory IgA interferes with bacterial attachment to mucosal surfaces.[32]
      (2). The premise that much of the secretory IgA in urine originates from the urethral mucosa is a plausible explanation for why bacteria from the urethra normally have difficulty in ascending to the bladder.[196]
   c. Experimental studies in rats have revealed that prior infection with *E. coli* subsequently decreased the mucosal adherence of *Klebsiella pneumoniae,* a phenomenon attributed to local immune factors.[196]
      (1). Because of technical difficulties, correlation of the decreased bacterial adherence to urothelium with urinary immunoglobulin concentrations was not possible.
      (2). In another study in mice, local immunity appeared to minimize reinfection of the bladder.[134]
      (3). Likewise, vaccines against type 1 fimbriae of *Escherichia coli* prevented induction of pyelonephritis in rats.[176]
      (4). In yet another study, vaginal immunization of rats reduced the severity of bladder lesions following experimentally induced UTI.[195]
   d. Immunoglobulins (IgG, IgA, SIgA) in urine of human patients with pyelonephritis inhibit the in vitro adherence of *E. coli* to uroepithelial cells.[184]
      (1). Other studies have indicated that antibodies directed against bacterial O (somatic) antigens efficiently reduce adherence, whereas antibodies against capsular antigens are less efficient in this regard.[186]
      (2). Antibodies prepared in animals to purified P-fimbriae inhibit attachment of the strain of bacteria from which the fimbriae were isolated, as well as of bacterial strains with antigenically similar fimbriae.[135]
3. Systemic Immunity
   a. The role of systemic antibodies in the prevention and eradication of UTI also is unclear.
   b. Infection of the urinary tract in humans and animals is accompanied by an immune response characterized by an increase in the serum concentration of antibodies against antigens of the infecting organisms.[123]
   c. Renal infections typically provoke a much more significant rise in antibody titers against the infecting organisms than do infections confined to the urinary bladder.[59,76,145]
   d. The effectiveness of systemic humoral immune responses has been questioned because of the following observations.
      (1). The quantity of immunoglobulins in urine is comparatively small.
      (2). Urine lacks active complement components, and in addition, ammonium ions produced by the renal tubular cells may inactivate the fourth component of complement.[17]
      (3). Antibody-mediated opsonization, which facilitates phagocytosis, may be of little potential value because phagocytosis in urine may be impaired by the wide range of osmolality and toxic concentrations of metabolites.[31,138]
      (4). UTIs are not a major problem in patients with immunodeficiencies.
   e. The fact that production of host immunoglobulin is involved with the pathophysiology of UTIs, however, is suggested by experimental studies in dogs in which administration of immunosuppressive agents was associated with an increased susceptibility to UTI following (but not preceding) trauma to the mucosa of the urinary tract.[117] Also, long-term administration of glucocorticoids to dogs with dermatologic diseases resulted in an increased frequency of bacterial UTI.[70]
      (1). Partial immunosuppression of monkeys permitted the occurrence of *E. coli* pyelonephritis and allowed organisms to persist as L-forms for 18 days.[135]
      (2). In addition, experimental studies in rats revealed that active immunization with bacterial antigens resulted in production of immobilizing antibodies, detected in urine, that inhibited the spread of motile bacteria *(Proteus mirabilis)* to other portions of the urinary tract.[155]

(3). Results of other experimental studies in rats also suggest that systemic antibodies may have a role in protection of the kidneys from UTI.

(4). Experimental suppression of macrophages in monkeys enhanced the severity of *Escherichia coli*-induced pyelonephritis.[9]

(5). Following partial obstruction of their ureters, vaccination of rats with formalin-treated *E. coli* reduced the severity of unilateral retrograde *E. coli* pyelonephritis.[155]

(6). Studies in humans suggest that IgG and IgM may interact with IgA to reduce the susceptibility of women to recurrent UTI.[182]

f. Recently, the role of inflammation in resistance to UTI has been emphasized.

(1). Evidence suggests that inflammation helps to protect against UTI; genetic defects in the inflammatory response or administration of anti-inflammatory agents can render animals highly susceptible to UTI.

(2). The inflammatory response to UTI causes cytokines (e.g., interleukin-6 and interleukin-8) and inflammatory cells to appear in the urine, and susceptibility to UTI might be influenced by differences in the inflammatory response.

(3). Administration of corticosteroid drugs has been shown to promote development of UTI in dogs and cats; however, whether this outcome is the result of immunosuppressive, anti-inflammatory or other effects of these drugs is unknown.

III. BACTERIAL VIRULENCE FACTORS

A. Not all bacteria are pathogenic.

1. A group of investigators found that, of the more than 150 known serotypes of *E. coli*, only 5 accounted for the majority of UTI in humans.[60] Thus, strains of *E. coli* that infect the urinary tract are not necessarily the most prevalent organisms populating the intestinal or lower urogenital tracts.
2. Because *E. coli* are one of the most common bacterial uropathogens affecting humans and dogs, their virulence (pathogenicity) has been most extensively studied.[203]
3. Less is known about virulence factors of other uropathogens. However, uropathogens may have multiple virulence factors (Table 40–3). Therefore, absence of one factor does not necessarily result in loss of pathogenicity.
4. Bacteria that are nonpathogenic in normal individuals may become relatively virulent in patients with altered host defenses.

B. Some bacteria appear to have less ability to invade the urinary tract than do others.

1. Less-invasive bacteria include *Pseudomonas* spp, *Klebsiella* spp, and *Enterobacter* spp.

TABLE 40–3.
SOME FACTORS THAT MAY ENHANCE THE VIRULENCE OF UROPATHOGENIC BACTERIA

A. *Escherichia coli*
 1. Certain O (somatic) antigens
  a. Outer polysaccharide portion of bacterial envelope.
  b. Smooth colony morphology on culture plate.
  c. Indirect marker of virulence (human studies).
 2. Certain K (capsular) antigens
  a. The capsule surrounds the bacterium.
  b. May inhibit phagocytosis and complement-mediated bacteriocidal activity.
  c. Increased resistance to inflammation favors persistence of bacteria in tissue.
 3. Adhesive fimbriae (pili)
  a. Proteinaceous filamentous organelles that protrude from the surface of the bacterium.
  b. Specific types of fimbriae (P-fimbriae) enhance the ability of a bacterium to remain adherent to uroepithelium, despite cleansing action of the urinary system.
 4. Hemolysin
  a. Increases amount of free iron available for bacterial growth.
  b. May cause tissue damage.
 5. Aerobactin
  a. Iron binding protein.
  b. Facilitates bacterial growth.
 6. R-Plasmids promote resistance to antimicrobial agents.
 7. Resistance to serum bactericidal activity
 8. Short generation time in urine
B. *Proteus, Staphylococcus,* some *Klebsiella*
 1. Adherence factors
 2. Urease
  a. Bacterial enzyme that hydrolyzes urea to ammonia.
  b. Ammonia directly injures epithelium.
  c. Urease fosters production of magnesium ammonium phosphate uroliths.
 3. R-Plasmids
C. *Pseudomonas*
 1. Heavy mucoid polysaccharide capsule prevents antibody coating
 2. R-plasmids

2. When these bacteria are identified in urine by culture, one should have a high suspicion of complicated forms of UTI.

C. Bacterial virulence factors include their ability to survive and grow in urine.

1. Some bacteria are better able to survive in urine than are others. For example, cocci have greater capacity to survive in concentrated urine than do rod-shaped bacteria.[89,91,92]
2. Slowly growing bacteria are more likely to be voided before they adhere to and colonize cell surfaces than are bacteria that grow rapidly.

3. Some bacteria grow in the urine of patients treated with antimicrobial drugs because they have innate, or have gained acquired (often plasmid-mediated), resistance to the drugs.

D. Studies of humans and dogs suggest that uropathogenic bacteria may originate from the intestinal tract.[16,165] Once these or other bacteria ascend to various sites within the urinary tract, however, they apparently can induce infection of adjacent tissues only if they can adhere to cells.[185]

1. Adherence of bacteria to uroepithelial cells is the net result of multiple interactions between bacterial surface ligands (adhesins) and complementary epithelial cell structures (receptors).[159] This process has been likened to a lock-and-key process.
2. Bacterial adhesins are frequently, but not invariably, associated with proteinaceous hair-like projections from the surface of bacteria called pili, fimbriae (many gram-negative bacteria), or fibrillae (some gram-positive bacteria). Fimbriae and fibrillae recognize carbohydrate sequences (either glycolipids or glycoproteins) called cell receptors.
3. Nonpathogenic *Escherichia coli* may produce adhesins that bind to Tamm-Horsfall mucoprotein, secretory IgA, or phagocytic cells. However, uropathogenic bacteria produce adhesins that bind to epithelial cells, but not to phagocytic cells. Thus, uropathogens can resist elimination during the voiding phase of micturition while avoiding phagocytosis. Uropathogens apparently have the ability to produce or suppress fimbriae during various phases of growth (a phenomenon sometimes called phase variation). In addition to prevention of loss during voiding, close apposition to epithelial cells associated with adherence enhances the effect of bacterial toxins (e.g., urease, hemolysin).

E. Several different types of adhesins have been identified on uropathogenic *E. coli* obtained from infected dogs. They include type 1 fimbriae, P-fimbriae, and X-adhesins.[53,200]

1. In humans, type 1 fimbriae facilitate attachment of *E. coli* to vaginal and bladder epithelial cells.[159]
2. P-fimbriae facilitate adherence of *E. coli* to renal parenchymal cells, as do X-adhesins.

F. Variation is evident in both the ability of bacteria to adhere to cells and the receptivity (or stickiness) of mucosal cells to bacteria. The number and accessibility of cell receptors for bacterial adhesins apparently influence host susceptibility to some infectious agents.[167]

1. These observations may explain why some investigators have observed an increased receptivity to bacterial attachment by vaginal, periurethral, and uroepithelial cells obtained from human patients with recurrent UTI.[159]
2. Hormones may be one factor that influences cell receptivity to bacterial adherence.

G. Other virulence factors also exist.

1. Colicin is a bacterial product that increases vascular permeability and inflammation, and also inhibits host macrophage function.[132,151]
2. Hemolysin produced by *E. coli* may increase bacterial invasiveness by damaging tissue, and also increases the amount of iron available for bacterial growth.[30,53,132]

H. Another virulence factor produced by some bacteria is beta-lactamase, an enzyme that confers a high level of bacterial resistance to beta-lactam antibiotics (including penicillins and cephalosporins).

I. Several species of bacteria, including staphylococci, *Proteus* spp, and *Klebsiella* spp, produce the enzyme urease.

1. Urease hydrolyzes urea to ammonia, which in turn may damage the protective glycosaminoglycan covering of the bladder mucosa[154] and renal tubular epithelium.[23]
2. Administration of acetohydroxamic acid (a urease inhibitor) to dogs with staphylococcal UTI minimized the severity of inflammation of the urinary tract.[23,83,84]
3. Likewise, reduction of urinary excretion of urea by reducing dietary protein minimized the magnitude of urease-mediated inflammation in dogs with staphylococcal UTI.[1,148]

IV. ROUTES OF INFECTION

A. Ascending.

1. As a result of numerous experimental and clinical studies in animals and humans, the current general consensus is that UTIs are most commonly a consequence of the ascending migration of bacteria through the genital tract and urethra to the bladder, ureters, and one or both kidneys.[145]
2. In humans, the rectal, perineal, and genital bacterial flora are thought to serve as the principal reservoirs of infection.[35,155,165]
3. Results of studies in dogs have indicated that a similar situation occurs in this species.[111,170]
4. Although the intrinsic motility of some bacteria, including *Escherichia coli* and *Proteus* spp, may aid in their retrograde migration through the excretory pathway, bacteria ascend the urinary tract by brownian movement and may reach the kidneys in the absence of alterations of urine flow.[85]
5. However, in addition to gaining access to the urinary tract, bacteria must adhere to, and colonize the surface of, uroepithelial cells to induce infection. Thus, whether or not infection is established depends on the virulence and number of bacteria that reach the urinary tract, and on their interaction with uroepithelial cells.

B. Hematogenous.

1. Although hematogenous seeding of the kidneys as a result of systemic bacterial infection may cause UTI, this mechanism does not appear to be a major pathway of infection in dogs or cats.[79] The rela-

tionship between this observation and the observation that the renal cortex is more resistant to infection than is the medulla is logical inasmuch as the blood must first pass through the renal cortex before it enters the medulla.

2. Studies in rats have revealed that an average of only 1 of 10,000 organisms injected into the bloodstream lodge in the kidneys, unless the urinary tract is obstructed (intrarenal or extrarenal) or traumatized.[61] Obstruction may impair renal defense mechanisms against bacterial infection by interfering with renal microcirculation.[180]

C. Other. Exposure of the urinary tract via the lymphatics has been regarded as an unlikely route of infection. However, experimental studies in dogs and other animals suggest that this condition should be reevaluated.[40,68,170]

V. ABNORMAL HOST DEFENSE MECHANISMS

A. Uncomplicated versus complicated UTI.

1. Overview
   a. Although UTIs have been classified as acute or chronic, vague definitions of these terms add little to the understanding of their etiology and pathophysiology because their cause, lesions, and biologic behavior overlap considerably.
   b. Knowledge that UTI is acute or chronic may be helpful in formulating therapy and prognosis; however, in our opinion, classifying a UTI as uncomplicated or complicated is of much greater clinical benefit.
   c. Uncomplicated and complicated UTI may lead to substantial morbidity and mortality if untreated or improperly treated (Table 40–4).
2. Uncomplicated UTI
   a. An uncomplicated (or simple) UTI is defined as an infection in which no underlying structural, neurologic, or functional abnormality can be identified. Although useful, this classification may be somewhat misleading because it infers that bacterial infection is always the primary abnormality. This situation may occur if normal host defenses are overwhelmed by a large inoculum of pathogens.
   b. Most bacteria multiply and survive only when urinary tract host defenses are abnormal. A UTI usually represents a transient or persistent defect in the innate defense mechanisms of the patient, even though the underlying cause may escape detection.
   c. The clinical relevance of identification of an uncomplicated UTI is that it is more likely to be caused by a transient, self-limiting, and potentially reversible abnormality in host defenses than is UTI caused by identifiable abnormalities in local host defenses (complicated UTI).
3. Complicated UTI
   a. Complicated UTI occurs as a result of bacterial invasion of the urinary system secondary to identifiable diseases that interfere with normal defense mechanisms.
   b. Causes of complicated UTI include interference with normal micturition, anatomic defects, alterations of urothelium, altered volume, frequency, or composition of urine, and impaired immunocompetence (Table 40–5).
   c. The signs of UTI are often the first evidence of underlying congenital or acquired abnormalities.
   d. In general, the underlying cause must be removed or corrected if secondary bacterial infection is to be eradicated. Failure to do so is a common cause of recurrent (relapse, reinfection, or superinfection) UTI.[140]

TABLE 40–4.
POTENTIAL SEQUELAE TO BACTERIAL URINARY TRACT INFECTIONS

1. Lower urinary tract dysfunction (acute or chronic)
   a. Dysuria, pollakiuria
   b. "Urge" incontinence
   c. Damage to the detrusor muscle
   d. Damage to the urethra
2. Prostatitis (acute or chronic)
3. Struvite urolithiasis and its sequelae
4. Renal dysfunction (acute or chronic)
   a. Pyelonephritis
   b. Renal failure
   c. Septicemia (especially in patients with concomitant obstruction to urine outflow)

B. Some causes of complicated UTI.

1. Interference with Normal Micturition
   a. Interference with normal micturition often results in abnormal retention of urine (Table 40–5).
   b. The mechanisms whereby interference with urine flow increases the susceptibility of the urinary tract to infection have not been completely defined but appear to include several abnormalities.
      (1). Because of reduced movement of the urine and/or impaired contractility of the walls of the excretory pathway, the mechanical flushing action of normal voiding is impaired or lost.[108]
      (2). In addition, incomplete emptying and stasis of urine favor bacterial multiplication by lowering the ratio between the surface area of the bladder mucosa and the volume of urine exposed to it. A large residual volume of urine may keep bacteria in solution, thereby limiting access to intrinsic defense mechanisms of the urothelial surface.
   c. Overdistention of the urinary bladder as a

TABLE 40–5.
CLASSIFICATION OF SOME IDENTIFIABLE CAUSES OF COMPLICATED URINARY TRACT INFECTIONS

Causes	Potential For Surgical Correction
I. Interference with Normal Micturition	
A. Mechanical obstruction to outflow	
1. Uroliths and strictures (especially of urethra)	++++
2. Herniated urinary bladder	++++
3. Prostatic cysts, abscesses, or neoplasms	++
4. Obstructing urothelial neoplasms	+
B. Incomplete emptying of excretory pathway	
1. Damaged innervation	
a. Vertebral fractures, luxations, subluxations	++
b. Intervertebral disc disease	++
c. Vertebral osteomyelitis	–
d. Neoplasia	++
e. Vertebral or spinal cord anomalies	±
f. Reflex dyssynergia	–
2. Anatomic defects	
a. Diverticula of urethra, bladder, ureters, renal pelves (especially persistent urachal diverticula)	++++
b. Vesicoureteral reflux	±
II. Anatomic Defects	
A. Congenital or inherited	
1. Urethral anomalies	++
2. Ectopic ureters	++++
3. Persistent urachal diverticula	++++
4. Primary vesicoureteral reflux	+
B. Acquired	
1. Diseases of the urinary tract, especially lower portions	++++
2. Secondary vesicoureteral reflux	+
3. Urethrostomy, trigonal-colonic anastomosis, and other surgical diversion procedures	±
III. Alteration of Urothelium	
A. Trauma	
1. External force	++
2. Palpation	–
3. Catheterization and other instrumentation	±
4. Urolithiasis	++++
B. Metaplasia	
1. Administration of estrogens	–
2. Estrogen-producing sertoli cell neoplasms	++++
C. Neoplasia	++
D. Urinary excretion of cytotoxic drugs, such as cyclophosphamide	–
E. Others	?
IV. Alterations in the Volume, Frequency, or Composition of Urine	
A. Decreased urine volume	
1. Negative water balance	
a. Decreased water consumption	–
b. Vomiting and/or diarrhea	–
2. Primary oliguric renal failure	–
B. Voluntary or involuntary retention	+
C. Glucosuria	–
D. Formation of dilute urine*	–
V. Impaired Immunocompetence	
A. Diseases	
1. Congenital immunodeficiency?	–
2. Acquired	
a. Hyperadrenocorticism?	+
b. Uremia	–
B. Corticosteroids; immunosuppressant drugs	–

*Formation of dilute urine predisposes the patient to lower UTI, but may prevent or minimize bacterial infections of the renal medulla.
– = not applicable; ± = sometimes; + = low potential; ++++ = high potential.

result of obstruction to outflow may collapse the vessels in the bladder wall.

(1). Cells may be damaged by hypoxia, and the rate of delivery of WBCs, antibodies, complement, and other antimicrobial factors to the bladder may be impaired.[54,121,130]

(2). Studies of obstruction to urine outflow in rabbits revealed that overdistention of the bladder produced irreversible anatomic and functional changes that impaired micturition following relief of the obstruction.[108] In this study, the ability of the rabbits to eliminate bacteria following obstruction was decreased, a factor that predisposed them to recurrent UTI.

d. Once an infection becomes established, dysfunction in micturition may be further aggravated by bacteria, including *Escherichia coli* and *Pseudomonas* spp, that impair the contractility of smooth muscle.[55,190]

e. Vesicoureteral reflux (VUR) is associated with retrograde flow of urine from the urinary bladder into the ureters and renal pelves.

(1). The term primary VUR denotes an intrinsic maldevelopment of the ureterovesical junction. The term secondary VUR implies an acquired disorder of the ureterovesical junction.

(2). When the ureterovesical flap valve is damaged, VUR occurs as soon as intraluminal bladder pressure exceeds intraluminal ureteral pressure. Once infection becomes established in the urinary bladder, VUR allows ascending spread of bacteria to the kidneys.[158]

(a). In one study in dogs, natural and surgically induced VUR without concomitant persistent bladder infection was not associated with radiographic, gross, or microscopic changes in the kidneys or ureters.[131] When persistent infection of the urinary bladder was induced by implanting a foreign body in the bladder lumen, however, pyelonephritis and renal dysfunction developed.

(b). Similar results of experimental studies in dogs have been reported by other investigators, although they concluded that impaired ureteral peristalsis was also an important factor.[190]

(c). The requirement for refluxed urine to contain bacteria to establish an infection of the kidneys has also been observed in experimental studies in rats.[52]

(d). One need not postulate the existence of VUR to explain the ascent of bacteria from the urinary bladder to the kidneys in all circumstances, however, because ureteral peristalsis is not invariably unidirectional.[169]

(3). Studies of normal male and female dogs and cats in our laboratory have revealed that attempts to induce voiding by manual compression of the urinary bladder may induce VUR.

(a). Application of digital pressure to the urinary bladder for a prolonged period to initiate voiding was associated with greater occurrence of VUR than was application of pressure for a transient period.

(b). The greater the pressure, the more likely VUR was to occur.

(c). VUR associated with compression-induced voiding probably occurs as a result of lack of coordinated relaxation of the smooth muscle of the internal urethral sphincter mechanism and the striated muscle of the external urethral sphincter, which normally occurs during the voiding phase of spontaneous micturition.

(d). To prevent iatrogenic infection of the upper urinary tract, one should use appropriate caution when considering manual compression to obtain urine from a patient with lower bacterial UTI.

2. Anatomic Defects

a. Anatomic defects may predispose a patient to UTIs by interfering with normal micturition, altering the urethral high-pressure zone and surface characteristics of the urothelium, altering ureteral or urethral peristalsis, and interfering with the ureterovesical flap valve (Table 40–5).

b. Anatomic defects also may permit ascending migration of bacteria from lower to upper parts of the urinary tract.

(1). For example, turbulent urine flow induced by structural defects in the urethra may facilitate ascending migration of bacteria toward the urinary bladder.[134]

(2). Obstructive pyelonephritis was found 12 times more frequently than was nonobstructive pyelonephritis in an autopsy study of humans.[18]

c. Obstruction to urine outflow above the level of the urinary bladder may be less significant than urethral obstruction, because stasis of urine in the urinary bladder is more likely to be associated with ascending bacterial infection. However, obstruction of outflow to either kidney enhances the likelihood of upper UTI when bacteremia occurs secondary to infection elsewhere.

d. Vesicourachal diverticula are an anatomic abnormality deserving of further review.

(1). As described in detail elsewhere, macroscopic vesicourachal diverticula in dogs and cats appear to occur as a sequela to abnormal sustained increase in bladder intraluminal pressure associated with diverse diseases.[112,142,146]

(2). Persistence of asymptomatic microscopic urachal canals in the vertex of the bladders following birth of otherwise normal animals appears to be a prerequisite to their formation.

(3). Eradication or control of the underlying disease (including bacterial UTI) that predisposed to development of macroscopic vesicourachal diverticula often is followed by their spontaneous regression.

(a). Surgical extirpation may not be warranted to manage all vesicourachal diverticula in dogs or cats, even when associated with concomitant bacterial UTI.

(b). Diverticulectomy may only be indicated if macroscopic diverticula persist as a result of inability to eradicate or control the underlying cause (e.g., a persistent stricture of the urethra).

3. Alteration of Urothelium

a. Whether UTI develops subsequent to damage to the urothelium depends on several factors, including:

(1). The extent and depth of the lesion.

(2). The concomitant introduction of pathogens into the urinary tract by such procedures as catheterization and instrumentation.

(3). The size and virulence of the inoculum of bacteria that gains access to the urinary tract.

(4). The integrity of other host defense mechanisms (see Tables 40–2 and 40–5).[140]

b. UTI may be a cause or sequela of urolithiasis (see Table 40–4).

(1). Infections with urease-producing bacteria, especially staphylococci, predispose dogs and cats to magnesium ammonium phosphate urolithiasis.

(2). Urothelial trauma caused by so-called metabolic uroliths, such as urate, cystine, oxalate, and silica, also predisposes patients to UTI.

c. Urinary excretion of cytotoxic drugs, especially cyclophosphamide, has become a more prevalent cause of inflammation of the urinary tract because of the widespread use of these drugs in the treatment of malignant lesions in dogs and cats.[37]

d. Analgesics containing phenacetin have been reported to cause similar problems in humans.[64]

e. Generalized damage to the urothelium would be expected to be a predisposing cause of secondary bacterial infection.

f. Recent studies suggest that the mucoprotein coating of the urothelium is deficient in humans with recurrent bacterial UTI.[166] Disrupting the mucoprotein coating prior to bacterial challenge increased the incidence of bacterial UTI in rats.[34]

g. Alterations in urothelial cells induced by hormones have been incriminated as factors that predispose women to a higher incidence of UTIs as compared with men.[10,115,123,171]

(1). Hormonal changes also have been incriminated in the increased occurrence of UTIs in women taking oral contraceptive agents.[175,188]

(2). In one study, UTIs in women were linked to a reduced level of estrogens and to reduced estrogen/progesterone ratios.[115] Parodoxically estrogens have also been associated with increased adherence of bacteria to urogenital cells in humans and rats, a phenomenon linked to estrogen-induced increases in urothelial cell receptor sites.[159]

(3). Hormone-induced changes also have been found to be associated with a higher incidence of UTIs in female dogs.[80]

(4). Experience at the Veterinary Teaching Hospital at the University of Minnesota indicates that recurrent UTIs are common in male dogs with estrogen-secreting Sertoli's cell neoplasms.

(a). One can logically hypothesize that squamous metaplasia of the prostate gland is at least one underlying factor.

(b). Using a similar line of reasoning, administration of estrogens to male dogs in an attempt to control idiopathic incontinence might also be a risk factor for bacterial UTI.

4. Alterations in Volume, Frequency, or Composition of Urine.

a. As previously stated, the mechanical washout of bacteria from the excretory pathway depends on periodic, frequent, and complete voiding of an adequate volume of urine. Potential causes of decreased production of urine include pathologic oliguria (the urine is not concentrated) or anuria associated with some types of primary renal failure, especially nephrotoxic and ischemic renal failure.

b. Prolonged voluntary retention of urine by confined housebroken pets might also be considered as a cause of UTI. The low incidence of UTIs in the general dog and cat population, however, suggests that this phenomenon has an insignificant effect in most situations.

c. Physiologic, pharmacologic, and pathologic diuresis may enhance the susceptibility of patients to lower UTI.[63]

(1). Although the precise mechanisms explaining this association have not been established, diuresis may impair some host defenses.

(a). For example, rod-shaped bacteria generally attain higher survival rates in dilute compared to concentrated urine.[89,91,92]

(b). In one study of healthy cats, diuresis increased the frequency and severity of catheter-induced bacterial UTI.[103] The magnitude of bacteriuria in cats with dilute urine was 1000 times greater than that observed in cats with highly concentrated urine.

(c). Bacteria identified in cats with highly concentrated urine were primarily cocci.

(2). In contrast to the association of diuresis and lower UTI, diuresis may minimize or prevent infection of the renal medulla with certain types of bacteria by decreasing medullary hypertonicity and thereby improving migration and function of inflammatory cells.[2,6,74,77,78]

d. Results of studies in humans have been interpreted to indicate a significantly higher prevalence of bacteriuria in patients, especially women, with diabetes mellitus as compared with nondiabetic controls. A similar predisposition has been suggested in diabetic dogs.[101] Others have challenged the generality that UTIs are more common in diabetic patients, but agree that, once the UTIs occur, they are associated with increased morbidity.[26,165]

(1). Although the possibility that urine glucose would enhance the environment for bacterial growth seems plausible, the effect of glucosuria on development of UTI in diabetic humans and animals has not yet been defined. In vitro studies suggest that the addition of glucose to the urine enhances bacterial growth.[10]

(2). One author has suggested that the predisposition of diabetic patients to UTI is related to a generalized vulnerability to infection and to iatrogenic infection secondary to catheterization.[85]

(3). We have observed several cases of iatrogenic catheter-induced UTI in diabetic dogs.

(4). Studies suggest that age, degree of glucosuria, impaired perfusion caused by microvascular disease, and instrumentation of the urinary tract are major factors in the etiopathogenesis of UTI in human patients with diabetes mellitus.[158a]

(5). The point to be made is that care should be taken not to expose diabetic patients to unnecessary transurethral catheterization of the urinary bladder.

5. Impaired Immunocompetence

a. Although the significance of abnormalities in systemic and local, and humoral and cellular immunity of the urinary system has not been extensively investigated, the importance of such abnormalities in the homeostasis of other body systems is noteworthy.

(1). A relative state of immunodeficiency in infants as compared with that in adults was hypothesized to explain the observation that experimentally induced ascending *Escherichia coli* pyelonephritis persisted longer in infant than in adult monkeys.[162]

(2). In another study, partial immunosuppression of monkeys permitted the development of *E. coli* pyelonephritis and allowed organisms to persist as L-like forms for 18 days.[135]

(3). The reduction of host defense mechanisms by immunosuppression with cyclophosphamide was associated with an increased susceptibility to UTI following trauma to the mucosa of the urinary tract.[117]

b. UTIs are a common sequela of uremia, and may be associated, at least in part, with general debility, depressed cellular immunity, lymphopenia, structural and functional abnormalities of WBCs, dialyzable factors in uremic serum that inhibit migration of phagocytes, and depressed serum concentrations of immunoglobulins.[29,41,141,177] Dogs with hyperadrenocorticism appear to have an increased susceptibility to bacterial UTIs.[104,109] Likewise, prolonged administration of glucocorticoids to dogs also increases the risk of bacterial UTIs, including those caused by more than one type of bacteria (mixed infections).[70] Speculation that the enhanced susceptibility may be attributed to cortisol-induced immunosuppression, suppression of inflammation, and/or the formation of dilute urine is tempting. Reduction of the severity of associated clinical signs and pyuria in infected dogs exposed to excessive glucocorticoids may be related to their anti-inflammatory effects.

6. Catheter-Induced Infection

a. Catheterization, no matter how carefully performed, is always associated with an increased risk of bacterial infection of the urinary tract because catheters bypass all the local defenses in the urethra.

b. Catheterization may trigger development of recurrent UTI in some patients.

(1). Bacteria from the external environment, hair, skin, genital tract, and/or urethra that contaminate the catheter tip are carried into the urinary bladder lumen.

(2). If indwelling urethral catheters are used, bacteria may migrate to the bladder through the catheter lumen, or along the space between the outside of the catheter and the mucosal surface of the urethra.

c. The potential for catheter-induced UTI is illustrated by the following studies.

(1). Bacterial UTI developed in 20% (7 of 35) of healthy adult female dogs following intermittent catheterization, and in 33% (3 of 9) male dogs following repeated intermittent catheterization.[19]

(2). Bacterial UTI developed in 8 of 12 healthy male cats during 3 to 5 days of open indwelling urethral catheterization.[93]

(3). In a clinical study, indwelling closed catheterization developed in 52% (11 of 21) of dogs and cats.[13] The risk of infection increased with duration of catheterization.

d. Although catheter-induced bacterial UTI may undergo spontaneous remission following removal of catheters from patients with normal lower urinary tracts, 60% of cats with perineal urethrostomy in 1 study remained infected for months following catheter-induced bacterial UTI.[179]

e. Concomitant oral or parenteral administration of antimicrobial agents during indwelling urethral catheterization of dogs and cats may reduce the frequency of development of bacterial UTI, but alters the flora and promotes development of UTI caused by bacteria with resistance to multiple antimicrobial agents.[13,93]

f. The risk of catheter-induced bacterial UTI is influenced by several variables, including:

(1). The status of the urinary tract.

(2). Patient profile.

(3). The technique used.

g. The most important variables affecting the risk of catheter-induced UTIs are the anatomic and functional status of the urinary tract, especially the bladder and urethra.

(1). When diseases of the genital or urinary tract result in technically difficult catheterization, bacterial contamination of the catheter and/or catheter-induced trauma are likely.

(2). Patients with urinary tract diseases, especially of the lower urinary tract, are at increased risk for catheter-induced UTI because of compromised local host defenses.

h. The risk of catheter-induced complications is also associated with species, sex, size, temperament, and health status of the patient.

(1). Cats are generally more difficult to catheterize than are dogs.

(2). Dogs may be more susceptible to UTI than are cats.

(3). Regardless of species, males are easier to catheterize than are females. Perhaps this and other sex-related factors are associated with the greater risk of catheter-induced UTI in female as compared to male dogs.

(4). Concomitant diseases may also influence the risk of catheter-induced UTI. For example, dogs with hyperadrenocorticism, diabetes mellitus, and uremia are at risk for iatrogenic UTI.

i. Technique and catheter selection may influence the likelihood of catheter-induced UTI.

(1). Frequency and duration of catheterization also influence the risk of catheter-induced complications.

(2). Iatrogenic infection is least likely to occur as a consequence of a single brief catheterization.

(3). Studies of repeated intermittent brief catheterization have revealed that the risk of inducing infection is similar following each catheterization. Thus, the cumulative risk of catheter-induced UTI is proportional to the number of catheterizations.

j. Risk of iatrogenic infection is greatest during indwelling catheterization, especially when the portion of catheter protruding from the urethra is not connected to a receptacle (i.e., it is open).

(1). Closed sterile catheter drainage reduces the frequency of nosocomial UTI, but does not prevent it.[13,105]

(2). In general, the risk of infection during indwelling catheterization is proportional to the duration of catheterization.

(3). Concomitant administration of glucocorticoids during indwelling urethral catheterization is likely to increase the risk of bacterial UTI.

(4). When long-term catheterization is needed, intermittent catheterization is less likely to induce UTI than is indwelling catheterization. In some situations, however, risk of urethral trauma caused by repeated insertion of a catheter is sufficient to make indwelling catheterization the safer alternative.

(5). Indwelling catheters may cause continuous trauma to the urinary tract and may elicit a foreign body reaction in surrounding tissue.[94]

(6). The composition of the catheter may influence the ability of bacteria to adhere to its luminal and external surface.[161a]

C. Summary of relevance to clinical management of patients.

1. The interaction between host defense mechanisms and pathogenic microbes should be considered in the diagnosis, prognosis, and treatment of UTI.
2. Although pathogenic organisms must gain access to the urinary tract to promote UTIs, entrance into the urinary tract is not synonymous with infection.
3. Host defenses either must be overwhelmed as a result of inappropriate catheterization or must be transiently or persistently abnormal for bacterial colonization to occur.
4. Attempts should be made to detect abnormalities in host defense mechanisms of patients with UTIs, especially if infections are persistent or recurrent (relapse or reinfection).
5. Equally as important as antimicrobial therapy in the management of UTIs is the necessity to anticipate, prevent, and/or treat symptomatic and asymptomatic recurrences, because they may be associated with progressive and potentially irreversible disease.
6. The underlying causes of a complicated UTI must be eliminated or controlled by the host or the clinician if permanent eradication of bacterial pathogens is to be accomplished.
7. In some instances, urinary tract abnormalities predisposing to bacterial UTI may be surgically corrected.

VI. BIOLOGIC BEHAVIOR OF URINARY TRACT INFECTIONS

A. Course of disease.

1. Uncomplicated UTI usually resolves rapidly, provided proper therapy is formulated and administered. Although *unpredictable,* some patients with UTI associated with a transient defect in normal host defense mechanisms, and/or those in which normal host defenses have been temporarily overwhelmed by a large inoculum of bacteria (septic catheterization), may undergo spontaneous remission without therapy.
2. Long-term elimination of clinical and laboratory signs of disease in patients with UTI secondary to persistent abnormalities in host defense mechanisms by administration of antimicrobial agents is usually impossible. Either the signs persist despite therapy or they recur at a variable interval following withdrawal of therapy.

B. Recurrence resulting from relapse, reinfection, or superinfection.

1. Recurrence of clinical and/or laboratory signs of UTI following withdrawal of therapy may be classified as relapses, reinfections, or superinfections, as determined by follow-up urine cultures (Tables 40–6, 40–7, and 40–8).
2. Relapse
   a. Relapses (persistent infections) are defined as recurrences caused by the same species and serologic strain of microorganism within several weeks of the date of cessation of therapy.
   b. Relapses may be associated with one or more causes (Tables 40–6 and 40–7).
3. Reinfection
   a. Reinfections are defined as recurrent infections caused by a different pathogen(s). In contrast to relapses, most reinfections occur at a longer interval following cessation of therapy.
   b. Reinfection may be associated with several causes (Tables 40–6 and 40–8).
4. Superinfection
   a. Superinfections are defined as infections with

TABLE 40–6.
EXAMPLES OF PATTERNS OF BACTERIURIA DEMONSTRATED BY SEQUENTIAL URINE CULTURES PERFORMED TO MONITOR RESPONSE TO TREATMENT OF UTI

Timing of Urine Culture					
Before Rx	**3–5 Days After Initiating Rx**	**3–5 Days Before Finishing Rx**	**7–14 Days After Discontinuing Rx**	**≥3 Weeks After Discontinuing Rx**	**Interpretation**
Positive	Positive	NA	NA	NA	Persistent UTI Rx failure
Positive	Negative	Negative	Positive for same microbe	NA	Relapse
Positive	Negative	Negative	Negative	Negative	Cure
Positive	Negative	Negative	Negative	Positive for different microbe	Reinfection

Rx = treatment; NA = not applicable.

TABLE 40–7.
CHECKLIST OF POTENTIAL CAUSES OF PERSISTENT (RELAPSE) INFECTION WITH SAME TYPE OF BACTERIA

1. Use of improper antimicrobial susceptibility tests and/or misinterpretation of results.
2. Mixed infections in which all pathogens were not eradicated by antimicrobial therapy.
3. Failure to prescribe antimicrobial agents for a sufficient period to eradicate pathogens (a relapse occurs).
4. Failure to prescribe a proper dosage and/or maintenance interval for an antimicrobial agent that would otherwise be effective.
5. Failure or inability of owners to administer the prescribed dosage of antimicrobial agent(s) at the proper maintenance intervals and for sufficient duration.
6. Use of ineffective drugs.
   a. Ineffective against uropathogens.
   b. Fail to attain therapeutic concentration in urine.
   c. Fail to achieve therapeutic concentrations at infection sites (especially kidneys, prostate gland, and infection-induced uroliths).
7. Failure of the patient to absorb a portion or all of an orally administered drug because of ingesta or gastrointestinal dysfunction.
8. Premature assessment of therapeutic response.
9. Initiation of therapy at an advanced state in the evolution of the disease.
10. Formation of drug-resistant bacteria, including L-forms.

TABLE 40–8.
CHECKLIST OF POTENTIAL CAUSES OF REINFECTION WTH DIFFERENT BACTERIA

1. Invalid culture results caused by:
   a. Contamination of specimen during collection, transport, storage, or handling.
   b. Improper technique of bacterial culture of urine.
2. Continued dysfunction of host defense mechanisms (see Table 40–2).
3. Failure to recognize and eliminate a predisposing cause.
4. Iatrogenic infection, especially associated with catheterization.
5. Sequelae to surgical techniques that have modified host defenses, especially urethrostomies and urine diversion procedures.
6. Spontaneous reinfection.

an additional organism during the course of antimicrobial treatment.

b. They are most likely to occur in association with indwelling urethral catheters or as a sequela to urinary diversion techniques in which the urinary tract communicates with the intestinal tract and in which proximal portions of the urethra, the urinary bladder, or the kidneys communicate directly with the exterior (e.g., antepubic urethrostomy, tube cystostomy, percutaneous nephropyelostomy).

5. Summary
   a. Relapses of UTI in humans are usually associated with renal infections, whereas reinfections are most commonly associated with lower UTIs.[160,191] These observations may be related to persistence of foci of infection within the renal medulla and to impaired ability of natural host defense mechanisms to function in this environment.
   b. Empiric clinical observations suggest that bacterial infection of the prostate gland is a common source of recurrent UTI in dogs.

VII. CLINICAL MANIFESTATIONS

A. Overview.

1. UTI may be symptomatic or asymptomatic. Although asymptomatic UTI has been recognized in dogs and cats, the frequency of its occurrence has not been established. It has been recognized more frequently in dogs with hyperadrenocorticism and dogs given glucocorticoids for prolonged periods.[16,70,104]
2. Clinical signs associated with UTI are variable, depending on the interaction of:
   a. Virulence and numbers of causative organisms.
   b. The presence or absence of predisposing causes.
   c. The compensatory response of the body to infection.
   d. The duration of infection.
   e. The site(s) of infection (Table 40–9).
3. Information obtained from the history and physical examination may help to localize the source of clinical signs to the urinary system (Table 40–10), but additional evaluation is required to localize the specific site(s) responsible for clinical signs and to establish the underlying cause(s) (Table 40–9).
4. Clinical signs typical of UTIs are not pathognomonic for the disorder. Noninfectious diseases of the urinary system may cause similar signs.

B. Lower urinary tract infection.

1. Signs characteristic of lower UTI, including dysuria, frequent voiding of small quantities of urine, and impaired ability to void urine, may be combined with voiding of cloudy, foul-smelling or bloody urine. Gross hematuria that occurs predominantly at the end of micturition is indicative of urinary bladder involvement (Tables 40–9 and 40–11).
2. Abnormalities related to other body systems are usually absent in patients with uncomplicated infections. Temperature, pulse, and respirations are usually normal; affected animals are alert and active, and they usually have a normal appetite.

TABLE 40–9.
ABNORMALITIES THAT MAY AID IN LOCALIZATION OF BACTERIAL URINARY TRACT INFECTIONS

Sites of Infection	History	Physical Examination	Laboratory	Radiology and Ultrasound
Lower Urinary Tract	Dysuria; pollakiuria Urge incontinence Signs of abnormal detrussor reflex (overflow incontinence; residual urine) Gross hematuria at end of micturition No systemic signs of infection Recent catheterization; urethrostomy	Small, painful, thickened bladder (unless urethra obstructed) Palpable masses in urethra or bladder Flaccid bladder wall; residual urine in bladder lumen Abnormal micturition reflex ± Palpation of uroliths	Normal CBC Urinalysis reveals: pyuria hematuria proteinuria bacteruria Urine culture reveals significant bacteriuria	Kidneys usually not enlarged Structural abnormalities of lower urinary tract ± Urocystoliths and/or urethroliths ± Only thickening of bladder wall and irregularity of mucosa Rarely intramural gas formation (emphysematous cystitis)
Upper Urinary Tract	Polyuria and polydipsia ± Signs of systemic infection ± Signs of renal failure	± No detectable abnormalities ± Fever and other signs of systemic infection ± Abdominal (renal) pain Kidney size is normal, decreased, or increased	± Leukocytosis Urinalysis (variable) reveals: pyuria hematuria proteinuria bacteriuria WBC or granular cysts impaired concentration ± Azotemia and other abnormalities typical of renal failure	Increase or decrease in kidney size ± Abnormal kidney shape ± Nephrolithiasis ± Dilated renal pelves; dilated pelvic diverticula ± Evidence of outflow obstruction
Acute Prostatitis or Prostatic Abscess	Urethral discharge independent of micturition Signs of systemic infection ± Reluctance to defecate or micturate ± Hindlimb lameness or locomotor difficulty	± Fever and other signs of systemic infection ± Painful prostate and/or painful abdomen ± Enlarged or asymmetric prostate	± Leukocytosis Urinalysis reveals: pyuria hematuria proteinuria bacteriuria Cytology reveals infectious inflammation	± Indistinct cranial border; enlargement ± Cysts ± Reflux of contrast agent into prostate
Chronic Prostatitis	Recurrent urinary tract infections Urethral discharge independent of micturition ± Dysuria	Often no detectable abnormalities ± Enlarged or asymmetric prostate	Normal CBC Similar to acute prostatitis	± Similar to acute prostatitis ± Abnormal prostatic urethra ± Mineralization

Dogs with concomitant bacterial prostatitis and UTI may develop fever.

3. Palpable abnormalities associated with uncomplicated lower UTI include any combination of the following (degree of change usually occurs in proportion to the severity and duration of infection):
   a. No detectable abnormalities, pain.
   b. Spasm of the bladder musculature.
   c. An empty bladder or a bladder that contains only a small quantity of urine.
   d. Thickening of the bladder wall.
4. Palpable abnormalities associated with complicated lower UTI depend on the nature of the underlying cause(s) (see Tables 40–5, 40–9, and 40–10).

TABLE 40–10.
OUTLINE OF MINIMUM DATA BASE FOR DIAGNOSIS OF URINARY TRACT DISORDERS

I. History Checklist
- A. Diet: type? frequency of feeding? supplements?
- B. Water consumption: increased? decreased? no change? unknown?
- C. Duration of problem(s)?
- D. Recurrence of problems, and intervals involved?
- E. Observed by whom?
- F. Previous illness or injury?
- G. Other pets at home? Normal or abnormal?
- H. Exposure to other animals, potential toxins?
- I. Micturition:
  1. Character? frequency? quantity?
  2. Pollakiuria (dysuria, tenesmus)?
  3. Polyuria (polydipsia)?
  4. Oliguria?
  5. Anuria?
  6. Urinary incontinence?
  7. Micturition in unusual locations?
  8. Change in urine color:
     - a. Red (hematuria, hemoglobinuria, myoglobinuria)?
     - b. Other (brown, black, green)?
  9. Uroliths voided during micturition?
- J. Change in odor of urine?
- K. Licking vulva or prepuce?
- L. Association with other signs not directly related to urinary system:
  1. Vomiting?
  2. Diarrhea?
  3. Anorexia?
  4. Weight loss?
  5. Others?
- M. Are problem(s) increasing in severity, decreasing in severity, or remaining the same?
- N. Medication given? type? dose? response?

II. Physical Examination Checklist
- A. Temperature, pulse rate, and respiratory rate
- B. Body weight
- C. Skin pliability
- D. Mouth:
  1. Mucosal ulcers?
  2. Discoloration of tongue?
  3. Pallor mucous membranes?
  4. Evidence of vomitus?
  5. Loose or missing teeth?
  6. Enlargement of maxillary tissues?
  7. Xerostoma?
  8. Uremic breath?
- E. Rectal examination:
  1. Feces normal or abnormal?
  2. Palpation of urethra and periurethral tissues?
- F. Kidneys:
  1. Both palpable? bilaterally symmetric?
  2. Position in abdominal cavity?
  3. Shape, consistency, and surface contour?
  4. Size?
  5. Pain?
- G. Urinary bladder
  1. Position?
  2. Size, shape, and consistency?
  3. Grating or nongrating masses within or adjacent to bladder lumen?* If present, constant or variable in location?
  4. Pain?
  5. Thickness of bladder wall?
- H. Prostate gland
  1. Position?
  2. Size, shape, consistency?
  3. Pain?
- I. Urethra
  1. Examination of prepuce and penis in male dogs and cats; urethral or preputial discharge?
  2. Examination of perineal urethra in male dogs?
  3. Rectal examination of urethra for:
     - a. Position?
     - b. Size, shape, and consistency?
     - c. Periurethral abnormalities?
- J. Micturition
  1. Normal storage and voiding phases of micturition?
  2. Results of neurologic examination?
  3. Ease of inducing voiding by palpation?
  4. Residual urine following voiding?
  5. Evidence of incontinence?

III. Laboratory Data
- A. Complete blood count?
- B. Urinalysis?

*If overdistention with urine interferes with palpation of lumen, repalpate following removal of an appropriate quantity of urine.

C. Upper urinary tract infection.

1. Signs characteristic of upper UTI depend on the degree of renal parenchymal involvement and the duration of the disease (see Table 40–9).
2. Acute infections are uncommonly recognized in dogs and cats, but when present may be associated with fever, anorexia, depression, pain in the area of the kidneys, and leukocytosis. If both kidneys are involved, signs typical of renal failure may occur. Signs referable to a predisposing cause may also be detected.
3. Clinical signs associated with chronic generalized renal infection are often initially limited to polyuria and polydipsia, but may be indicative of more severe states of renal dysfunction.

VIII. URINALYSIS

A. Urine sediment should be evaluated for WBCs by utilizing standard techniques.[150] Dipstick leukocyte assays alone are unsatisfactory.[197]

1. Significant numbers of WBCs (which may be associated with RBCs and protein) in a properly collected urine sample suggest an active inflam-

matory lesion of the urinary tract. (See Section IC, Pyuria, in this chapter.) (Tables 40–12 and 40–13).

2. Detection of a significant number of bacteria in association with pyuria indicates that the inflammatory lesion is active and has been caused or complicated by bacterial infection. However, because bacteria are more difficult to detect than are WBCs, pyuria may appear to be unassociated with bacteria present in lower numbers.

3. On occasion, bacterial UTI occurs without detectable concomitant pyuria.

TABLE 40–11.
PROBABLE LOCALIZATION OF GROSS HEMATURIA

Hematuria Throughout Micturition
- R/O : Systemic clotting defect
- DX : Clotting profile; evaluation of other body systems for hemorrhage
- R/O : Hemoglobinuria
- DX : Examination of urine sediment for red blood cells; hemogram
- R/O : Renal disorder
- DX : Abdominal palpation; survey and contrast radiography; ultrasonography; biopsy; exploratory surgery
- R/O : Diffuse bladder lesions
- DX : Abdominal palpation; examination of urine sediment; survey and contrast radiography; catheter biopsy; exploratory surgery
- R/O : Focal ventral or ventrolateral bladder lesions in active patients
- DX : Abdominal palpation; examination of urine sediment; survey and contrast radiography; ultrasonography; catheter biopsy; exploratory surgery
- R/O : Severe prostatic or urethral lesions
- DX : Rectal and abdominal palpation; survey and contrast radiography; ultrasonography; catheter biopsy; aspiration biopsy; exploratory surgery

Hematuria Independent of or at the Beginning of Micturition
- R/O : Urethral lesions
- DX : Rectal and abdominal palpation; comparison of analysis of urine samples collected by voiding and cystocentesis; survey and contrast radiography; catheter biopsy; exploratory surgery
- R/O : Genital disease
- DX : Abdominal, rectal, and vaginal palpation; vaginal cytology; comparison of analysis of urine samples collected by voiding and cystocentesis; endoscopy; exploratory surgery

Hematuria at End of Micturition
- R/O : Focal ventral or ventrolateral bladder lesions in inactive patients
- DX : Abdominal palpation; examination of urine sediment; survey and contrast radiography; ultrasonography; catheter biopsy; exploratory surgery
- R/O : Renal disorder with intermittent hematuria in inactive patients
- DX : Abdominal palpation; survey and contrast radiography; ultrasonography; biopsy; exploratory surgery

R/O = rule out; Dx = diagnostic plan.
Modified from Osborne CA, and Klausner JS. A problem specific data base for urinary tract infections. Vet Clin North Am 1979;9:783.

TABLE 40–12.
FACTORS INFLUENCING NUMBERS OF WHITE BLOOD CELLS IN URINE SEDIMENT OF DOGS AND CATS WITH BACTERIAL URINARY TRACT INFECTIONS

1. Volume of urine produced*
2. Method of urine collection
3. Volume of urine centrifuged
4. Speed and time of centrifugation
5. Volume of urine in which sediment is resuspended
6. Magnitude of destruction of cells in alkaline urine
7. Ability to differentiate white blood cells from urothelial cells
8. Suppression of inflammation by endogenous (hyperadrenocorticism) or exogenous glucocorticoids
9. Ability of pathogen(s) to induce inflammation
10. Concomitant administration of antimicrobial drugs

*If the patient does not have pathologic oliguria, volume may be inferred by evaluation of urine specific gravity.

TABLE 40–13.
CHECKLIST OF POSSIBLE CAUSES OF INFLAMMATION DETECTED BY URINALYSIS BUT UNASSOCIATED WITH MICROSCOPIC BACTERIURIA

1. Noninfectious disease of the urinary tract.
2. Numbers of bacteria in urine too small for consistent detection (bacterial rods < 10,000/mL; bacterial cocci < 100,000/mL).
3. Male dogs with prostatitis.
4. Infections caused by mycoplasma, ureaplasma, or viruses.
5. Administration of antimicrobial agents prior to urinalysis.

B. Rod-shaped bacteria may be seen in unstained preparations of urine sediment if more than 10,000 bacteria per milliliter are present, but may not be consistently detected if they number less than 10,000/mL.[31a,96] Cocci are difficult to detect in urine sediment if they number less than 100,000/mL.

1. Although detection of bacteria in urine sediment suggests UTI, it should be verified by urine culture (Table 40–14).[4]
2. Gram's stain or new methylene blue stain may aid in detection of bacteriuria.
3. Failure to detect bacteria in urine sediment does not exclude their presence.
4. Detection of bacteria within the cytoplasm of phagocytes found in urine sediment suggests in

vivo phagocytosis rather than contamination of urine sample during collection or analysis.

C. Several factors, including diet and bacterial degradation of urea to ammonia, affect urine pH.

1. Although detection of persistently alkaline urine may be considered as an indication for further diagnostic study, it should not be considered as synonymous with UTI.
   a. Urine pH is persistently alkaline when UTI is caused or complicated by urease-producing bacteria (especially staphylococci, *Proteus* spp, and *Ureaplasma* spp).
   b. An alkaline urine pH in absence of pyuria, hematuria, and proteinuria is usually a normal finding.
2. Because many bacterial uropathogens are not urea splitters, urine pH may not be altered by ammonia production from urea. Acid or neutral urine pH values do not rule out the possibility of UTI.

D. Observation of WBC or bacterial casts indicates renal tubular involvement in the inflammatory and/or infectious process.

1. WBC casts may undergo degeneration to become granular casts.
2. In our experience, WBC casts are uncommonly associated with proven UTI.
3. Absence of WBC or granular casts does not exclude renal involvement in the inflammatory process.

E. Impaired capacity to concentrate urine, with or without azotemia, may be detected in dogs and cats with bilateral generalized infection of the kidneys. Variable degrees of proteinuria are typically associated with the inflammatory response.

IX. DIAGNOSTIC URINE CULTURE

Urine culture is the gold standard for diagnosis of UTIs. Diagnosis of bacterial UTI solely on the basis of clinical signs usually results in overdiagnosis. Failure to perform urine cultures or failure to interpret the results of urine cultures correctly may lead not only to diagnostic errors, but to therapeutic failures as well. Consult Chapter 8, Diagnostic Urine Culture, for further details.

TABLE 40–14.
CHECKLIST OF FACTORS THAT MAY EXPLAIN STERILE BACTERIAL URINE CULTURES WHEN BACTERIA WERE OBSERVED IN URINE SEDIMENT

1. Nonviable microbes in urine at time of collection (host defenses; antimicrobial drugs).
2. Urine sample utilized for urinalysis was contaminated following collection and then improperly preserved.
3. Fastidious uropathogens died between time of sample collection and urine culture.
4. Improper preservation of urine sample.
5. Improper culture technique.
6. Mistaken identity of nonbacterial structures in urine sediment.

X. RADIOGRAPHIC AND ULTRASONOGRAPHIC FINDINGS

A. Radiographic and ultrasonographic findings associated with UTI are not sufficiently distinctive to confirm a diagnosis. However, radiography and ultrasonography are of value in evaluation of the patient for predisposing factors that lead to persistent or recurrent infection, and in localizing the site(s) of anatomic abnormality in the urinary tract (see Table 40–9).

1. In general, ultrasonography provides a reliable means of assessing the urinary tract for changes in size and position of structures and for detection of cysts, abscesses, and uroliths. Affected kidneys may be characterized by areas of increased echogenicity, or they may be hypoechoic.
2. Contrast urography usually allows better examination of the integrity of the excretory pathway from the renal pelvis to the distal urethra.

B. Radiographic alterations that may be associated with lower UTI include:

1. None.
2. Diffuse thickening of the bladder caused by inflammation and/or underlying neoplasia.
3. Focal areas of bladder thickening.
4. Separation of bladder layers by gas (emphysematous cystitis).
5. Uroliths.
6. Alterations in the appearance of the prostate gland (see Table 40–9).

C. Acute pyelonephritis may be associated with:

1. No detectable radiographic changes.
2. Increased renal size.
3. Decreased opacity of the vascular phase of the nephrogram.
4. Decreased opacification of the renal pelvis and pelvic diverticula.
5. Dilation of the renal pelvis and ureters.
6. Findings associated with obstruction to urine outflow.[12]

D. Chronic pyelonephritis may be associated with:

1. Normal to decreased kidney size associated with destruction, scarring, and contraction of renal parenchyma.
2. Dilation of pelvic diverticula and retention of contrast medium within them.
3. Dilation of the proximal ureters.
4. Nephrolithiasis.

XI. URODYNAMIC STUDIES

A. Abnormalities of the storage and voiding phases of micturition may predispose to bacterial UTI. For example, abnormal quantities of

residual urine remaining in the bladder lumen (even when patients appear to void normally) facilitate bacterial adherence to the uroepithelium, and enhance the action of bacterial toxins on the urothelium. Normally only 0.2 to 0.4 mL of urine per kilogram of body weight remain in the bladder lumen following voiding.[126]

B. In addition to a neurologic examination, abnormalities in micturition may be evaluated with the aid of cystometrograms, urethral pressure profiles, uroflowmetry, and electromyography.[136,137]

XII. SPECIAL PROCEDURES FOR LOCALIZING UPPER AND LOWER UTI

A. The relevance of differentiating upper from lower UTIs is based on the presumption that lower UTI is a nuisance but not life threatening, whereas upper UTI may be life threatening if sufficient renal tissue is destroyed. In addition, prostatic and renal infections tend to be more difficult to eradicate than are bladder infections.

B. Several techniques have been used in humans to differentiate upper and lower UTI. These include:

1. Ureteral catheterization.[87]
2. A bladder washout technique in which microbes can be "washed out" if the infection is of bladder origin, but persist if the infection is of renal origin.[43] To date, bladder washout techniques have proved to be unreliable in localization of experimentally induced UTI in dogs.[44]
3. Antibody coating of bacteria in which bacteria of renal origin are coated with antibodies while bacteria of bladder origin are not.[79] To date, antibody coating of bacteria has proved to be unreliable in localization of experimentally induced UTI in dogs.[44,98]
4. Measurement of urine enzyme concentration.[157] Urinary enzymes have been utilized in dogs as an index of nephrotoxic renal damage, but apparently have not been evaluated in dogs or cats with bacterial UTI.[56]

C. Techniques of retrograde ureteral catheterization of female dogs[173] and direct aspiration of urine from the renal pelvis (percutaneous nephropyelocentesis) of dogs[97a] have been described. Bacterial culture of needle aspirates of renal parenchyma, culture and microscopic examination of needle punch biopsies of the kidney, and bladder biopsies obtained by cystoscopy may also be of value.

XIII. TREATMENT

A. Prevention.

1. Systemic and local host defenses are extremely effective barriers to naturally occurring UTIs. However, they are not impenetrable.
   a. Normal host defense mechanisms may be overwhelmed if large quantities of bacteria are introduced into the urinary tract during diagnostic and therapeutic maneuvers performed in patients with noninfectious urinary disorders or in patients with nonurinary disorders.
   b. Iatrogenic UTI is an especially common complication of use of open indwelling urinary catheters and urinary diversion techniques.
   c. Use of open indwelling urinary catheters during therapeutic diuresis is especially hazardous.[90,93] The problem may be further compounded if such patients are recovering from urinary tract surgery.
2. Efforts to prevent iatrogenic UTI in surgical patients should include:
   a. Avoiding indiscriminate use of urinary catheters.
   b. Use of closed systems if indwelling urinary catheters are deemed essential.
   c. Cautious use of indwelling urinary catheters in patients during therapeutic diuresis.
   d. Appropriate use and timing of antimicrobial agents to prevent or control iatrogenic UTI.
   e. Use of surgical techniques that minimize trauma and microbial contamination of the urinary tract.

B. Eradication of underlying cause(s).

1. Although antimicrobial agents are the cornerstone of therapy for UTIs, they should not be given haphazardly, or without follow-up evaluations. Likewise, caution must be used to prevent overtreatment; care must be used to avoid improper administration of antimicrobial agents for treatment of signs of urinary tract disease that are not caused by bacterial infection, because the underlying cause may persist.[14,21]
2. UTIs may be associated with transient reversible abnormalities in local host defenses. Such disorders are usually recognized as uncomplicated forms of UTI. In such patients, self repair of damaged host defenses may result in spontaneous resolution of UTI. However, remission of clinical signs is not necessarily synonymous with eradication of infection.
3. The status of host defense mechanisms is an extremely important determinant in the pathogenesis of UTIs (see Tables 40–2 and 40–5).
   a. Although UTI can be induced by overwhelming normal host defenses with a massive inoculum of pathogenic bacteria, such a phenomenon is uncommon in naturally occurring cases of UTI.
   b. Because bacteria can establish and propagate themselves when host defenses are inadequate, the underlying causes of complicated UTI must be eliminated or controlled if permanent eradication of pathogens is to be accomplished (Tables 40–5 and 40–15).
4. The success or failure of therapy should not be based solely on elimination or persistence of clinical signs, but rather should be monitored by serial

TABLE 40–15.
SUMMARY OF OBJECTIVES FOR TREATMENT OF PERSISTENT OR RECURRENT URINARY TRACT INFECTIONS

1. Predisposing or complicating causes of the UTI should be identified and eliminated or controlled.
2. Causative pathogens are identified by qualitative and quantitative culture, and antimicrobial drugs are selected on the basis of antimicrobial susceptibility tests. Ideally, the agent chosen should have the narrowest possible spectrum of antimicrobial activity.
3. Aggressive treatment with appropriate dosages of antimicrobials is indicated, especially when systemic sepsis is present.
4. Although usually unnecessary, urine pH can be altered to enhance antimicrobial activity (see Table 40–27).
5. Urine should be recultured 3 to 5 days following the initiation of therapy to check the efficacy of the antimicrobial agent in sterilizing urine.
6. Antimicrobial therapy is continued until there is clinical and laboratory evidence of response. The response of the patient is monitored by bacterial culture and urinalysis.
7. Because symptomatic or asymptomatic recurrences may be associated with irreversible and potentially progressive disease, they should be anticipated, prevented, and, if necessary, treated (see Table 40–4).

evaluation of urine cultures and urinalyses performed at appropriate intervals. Equally important is the necessity to anticipate, prevent, and/or treat symptomatic or asymptomatic recurrences because they may be associated with irreversible and potentially progressive disease.

C. Antimicrobial therapy.

1. Introduction. Selection of antimicrobial agents should encompass choice of drugs that are:
   a. Easy to administer.
   b. Associated with few, if any, adverse reactions.
   c. Inexpensive.
   d. Able to attain tissue or urine concentrations that exceed the minimum inhibitory concentration (MIC) for the pathogen involved by at least fourfold.
   e. Unlikely to adversely affect the fecal bacterial flora of the patient.
2. Antimicrobial Susceptibility Tests
   a. Evaluation of the susceptibility of infecting bacteria to antimicrobial drugs is advisable as a general guide for choice of therapeutic agents because bacteria isolated from dogs and cats with UTI may vary widely in their susceptibility to specific antimicrobial agents (Table 40–16). This generality is especially applicable when surgery of the urinary tract is being contemplated in patients with UTI.
      (1). *Escherichia coli, Proteus* spp, *Pseudomonas aeruginosa,* and *Enterobacter* spp are examples of urinary pathogens that may be associated with polyresistant strains.
      (2). When antimicrobial agents are selected on the basis of antibacterial susceptibility tests (preferably by determining MICs of the antimicrobial agent excreted in urine), good immediate response is most likely to occur.
      (3). Follow-up evaluation of the susceptibility of infecting bacteria to antimicrobial drugs may be indicated in patients with recurrent infections, especially if they have been treated with antimicrobial drugs, to determine whether changes in susceptibility have occurred (see Tables 40–7 and 40–8).
   b. Two main types of antimicrobial susceptibility tests are currently in common use.
      (1). The agar diffusion (Kirby-Bauer) method consists of Mueller-Hinton agar plates that have been inoculated with a standardized suspension of a single uropathogen (pure culture).
         (a). Paper discs impregnated with different antimicrobial drugs are then placed on the plate.
         (b). After incubation for 18 hours at 37°C, antimicrobial susceptibility is estimated by measurement of zones of inhibition of bacterial growth surrounding each disc.
         (c). Zones of inhibition are then interpreted in light of established standards and recorded as resistant, susceptible, or intermediate.

TABLE 40–16.
INDICATIONS FOR ANTIMICROBIAL SUSCEPTIBILITY TESTS

1. Patient has confirmed complicated UTI (see Table 40–5)
2. Patient has frequent recurrences of UTI (see Tables 40–6 to 40–8)
3. Clinical signs persist for more than 5 to 7 days after starting empiric therapy, or become substantially more severe at any time after initiation of therapy
4. Patient has been treated with antimicrobial drugs within past 4 to 6 weeks
5. Patient has been recently catheterized
6. Patient has high risk of morbidity
   a. Urinary outflow obstruction
   b. Uremia
   c. Diabetes mellitus
   d. Neurogenic bladder
   e. Hyperadrenocorticism
   f. Patient is receiving glucocorticoids

TABLE 40–17.
AVERAGE CANINE URINE CONCENTRATIONS OF SOME ANTIMICROBIAL AGENTS*

Drug	Daily Dosage (mg/kg)	Route of Administration	Mean Urine Concentration (± SD)
Amikacin	15	Subcutaneous	342 (± 143) μg/mL
Amoxicillin	33	Oral	202 (± 93) μg/mL
Ampicillin	77	Oral	309 (± 55) μg/mL
Cephalexin	55	Oral	500 μg/mL
Chloramphenicol	100	Oral	123.8 (± 39.7) μg/mL
Enrofloxacin	5	Oral	40 (± 10) μg/mL
Gentamicin	6.6	Subcutaneous	107.4 (± 33.0) μg/mL
Hetacillin	77	Oral	300.3 (± 156.1) μg/mL
Kanamycin	11	Subcutaneous	529.6) (± 150.5) μg/mL
Nitrofurantoin	15	Oral	100 μg/mL
Penicillin G	110,000†	Oral	294.9 (± 210.7) U/mL
Penicillin V	77	Oral	148.3 (± 98.5) μg/mL
Sufisoxazole	66	Oral	1466.3 (± 832.4) μg/mL
Tetracycline	5	Oral	137.9 (± 64.6) μg/mL
Tobramycin	3	Subcutaneous	66.0 (± 39.0) μg/mL
Trimethoprim-sulfadiazine	26	Oral	55.0 (± 19.2) μg/mL

*Data courtesy of Dr. Gerald V. Ling, University of California, Davis.
†Dosage of penicillin G expressed in units per kilogram.

(d). Because of differences in the ability of various antibiotics to diffuse through agar, the antibiotic disc surrounded by the largest zone of inhibition of bacterial growth is not necessarily the drug most likely to be effective.

(e). Because the concentration of antimicrobial drugs (except nitrofurantoin) in the paper discs is comparable to typical serum concentrations of drugs, drugs that are found to be resistant by the agar diffusion test may be effective in the urinary tract if they are excreted in high concentration in urine (e.g., ampicillin, cephalexin, chloramphenicol, enrofloxacin, oxytetracycline, penicillin G, and trimethoprim).

(f). Agar diffusion antimicrobial susceptibility tests may be useful for patients with renal infections and acute bacterial prostatitis because renal and prostate tissue concentrations of antibiotics are more likely to correspond to serum concentrations of antibiotics.

(2). Antibiotic dilution susceptibility tests are designed to determine the MIC of the antimicrobial drug.

(a). Following inoculation and incubation of uropathogens into wells containing serial twofold dilutions of antimicrobial drugs at concentrations achievable in tissues and urine of patients given usual drug dosages, the MIC is defined as the lowest antimicrobial concentration (or the highest dilution) without visible bacterial growth.

(b). The MIC is several dilutions lower than the minimum bactericidal concentration (MBC) of drugs.

(c). In general, the antimicrobial agent is likely to be effective if it can achieve a concentration of four times the MIC (Table 40–17). This observation is especially noteworthy because many antibiotics excreted by the kidneys attain a urine concentration that is 10 to 100 times greater than the serum concentration.

c. Although susceptibility tests are valuable, clinical and laboratory evidence of response to an antimicrobial drug is the ultimate parameter of success. Factors other than in vitro susceptibility may affect in vivo effectiveness of an antimicrobial agent; the role of natural host defense mechanisms should also be considered.

d. If UTI associated with more than one pathogen is identified and the organisms do not have similar antimicrobial sensitivities, initial treatment of the predominant pathogen with an effective drug is recommended. Urine should be recultured during therapy, and a therapeutic approach for the second pathogen should be devised if it is still present.

3. Empiric Choice of Antimicrobial Agents
   a. Bacterial culture and antimicrobial susceptibility tests are essential for patients:
      (1). Recently treated for UTI with antimicrobial drugs.
      (2). At high risk of morbidity as a result of UTI (e.g., diabetes mellitus, uremia).
      (3). Recently catheterized.
      (4). With frequently recurrent UTI.
   b. Treatment of an acute onset of uncomplicated bacterial UTI may be formulated without results of antimicrobial susceptibility tests provided patients have not been given antibacterial drugs in the past 4 to 6 weeks. In this situation, choice of drug should be based on known properties of antimicrobial agents in combating UTI caused by commonly isolated organisms (Tables 40–18 and 40–19), and their ability to attain a high concentration in urine (Table 40–17).
   c. Results of studies of the in vitro susceptibility of common urinary tract pathogens (obtained from previously untreated patients) to selected oral antimicrobial agents may be helpful.[96]
      (1). Almost 100% of the staphylococci and streptococci may be expected to respond to penicillin (daily dose = 50,000 IU/lb divided 3 times a day), or ampicillin (daily dose = 35 mg/lb divided 3 times a day).
      (2). Almost 80% of the *Escherichia coli* respond to trimethroprim-sulfa given at a daily dose of 12 mg/lb divided 2 times a day.
      (3). About 80% of the *Proteus mirabilis* respond to oral penicillin or ampicillin at the same dosages and maintenance intervals suggested for streptococci or staphylococci.
      (4). About 80% of the *Pseudomonas aeruginosa* respond to oral tetracycline given at a daily oral dose of 25 mg/lb divided 3 times a day.
      (5). More recent studies have revealed that more than 90% of the *Klebsiella pneumoniae* were susceptible to cephalexin given at a dose of 50 mg/lb divided 3 times a day.[103]
4. Serum Versus Urine Concentrations.
   a. Because of numerous variables, meaningful generalities about the relative importance of tissue, urine, and serum concentrations of antimicrobial agents in the treatment of UTIs are difficult to formulate.
   b. Serum or urine concentrations of antimicrobial agents do not necessarily reflect their tissue concentrations.
   c. With these limitations in mind, select agents that have high urine concentrations (at least four times the MIC) for treatment of lower UTIs.
   d. For treatment of acute bacterial infections of the prostate gland (Tables 40–20 and 40–21), or of bacterial infections of the kidneys, select antimicrobial agents that attain high concentrations in serum and (if possible) urine.
5. Bacteriostatic Versus Bacteriocidal Drugs.
   a. Urinary tract pathogens often respond satisfactorily to bacteriostatic (those that inhibit multiplication) and bactericidal (those that kill) antimicrobial agents (Table 40–22).
   b. Use of bactericidal agents appears superior if persistent impairment in the natural defense mechanism of the patient exists.
6. Dosage.
   a. In general, dosage and intervals between maintenance dosages should conform to the recommendations of the manufacturer (Table 40–

TABLE 40–18.
FREQUENCY OF ISOLATION OF DIFFERENT BACTERIA FROM DOGS WITH URINARY TRACT INFECTIONS*

Pathogen	Biberstein[18a] (n = 102) (%)	Finco, et al.[44] (n = 27) (%)	Ihrke, et al.[70] (n = 27) (%)	Kivisto, et al.[81] (n = 187) (%)	Ling, et al.[99] (n = 1400) (%)	Wooley and Blue[204] (n = 655) (%)
Bordetella bronchiseptica	0	0	3.7	0	0	0
Enterobacter spp	0	5.9	0	3	2.6	3.3
Escherichia coli	11.8	36	59	67	37.8	20.1
Klebsiella pneumoniae	2.9	5	7	0	8.1	3.4
Proteus mirabilis	10.8	32	11	3	12.4	15.4
Pseudomonas aeruginosa	2.9	2.7	0	0	3.4	6.9
Staphylococcus spp	56.9	19	11	21	14.5	9.6
Streptococcus spp	9.8	9	22	6	10.7	10.6

*Some columns add to greater than 100% because of multiple isolates per specimen.

TABLE 40–19.
GUESSTIMATE OF SUSCEPTIBILITY OF URINARY BACTERIAL PATHOGENS TO SOME COMMONLY USED ANTIMICROBIAL AGENTS*

Pathogen	Drug(s) of Choice	Alternatives
Enterobacter spp	Trimethoprim-sulfadiazine Enrofloxacin	Cephalosporins (1st and 2nd generation) Chloramphenicol Nitrofurantoin Gentamicin
Escherichia coli	Trimethoprim-sulfadiazine Nitrofurantoin Enrofloxacin	Cephalosporins (1st, 2nd, and 3rd generation) Chloramphenicol Gentamicin
Klebsiella spp	Cephalosporins (1st generation) Enrofloxacin	Trimethoprim-sulfadiazine Cephalosporins (2nd and 3rd generation) Amikacin Gentamicin
Mycoplasma, Ureaplasma	Enrofloxacin	Chloramphenicol Doxycycline Erythromycin Oleandomycin Tetracycline
Proteus spp	Ampicillin Amoxicillin Penicillin G Enrofloxacin	Cephalosporins (1st, 2nd, and 3rd generation) Chloramphenicol Nitrofurantoin Trimethoprim-sulfadiazine Gentamicin
Pseudomonas aeruginosa	Tetracycline Enrofloxacin	Carbenacillin Trimethoprim-sulfadiazine Cephalosporins (1st, 2nd, and 3rd generation) Gentamicin
Staphylococcus intermedius	Penicillin G Ampicillin Amoxicillin Enrofloxacin	Cephalosporins (1st generation) Chloramphenicol Nitrofurantoin Trimethoprim-sulfadiazine
Streptococcus	Penicillin G Ampicillin Amoxicillin	Cephalosporins (1st generation) Chloramphenicol Nitrofurantoin Trimethoprim-sulfadiazine

*Prior treatment with antimicrobial drugs may alter the susceptibility of bacterial pathogens to these drugs.

22).[57] Maintenance of high concentrations of antimicrobial agents in urine is emphasized. Although signs of UTI may subside following administration of suboptimum doses of an antimicrobial agent, bacteriuria may persist.

b. Because of the short therapeutic half-lives of many antimicrobial drugs used to treat bacterial UTI, and the relatively frequent voiding patterns of most dogs (3 to 5+ times/day), most drugs should be given in 2 to 3 equal subdoses per day.
    (1). However, this schedule of administration may be associated with poor owner compliance, resulting in administration of subtherapeutic dosages.
    (2). The ability of owners of companion animals to comply with recommendations must be considered when selecting dosage intervals.
    (3). To ensure adequate concentrations of the drug in the urinary tract during treatment intervals, daily doses should be administered shortly following micturition, and especially just prior to a period of confinement during which voiding is not permitted (such as overnight).

c. Available evidence suggests that azotemic patients with renal infection should be treated with drugs that obtain a high serum concentration, whereas patients with lower UTI should be treated with agents that attain a high concentration in urine. Special precautions must be taken for patients with renal failure to prevent adverse drug reactions.[143,161] These include adjustment of dosage and/or maintenance intervals.[156]

(1). Because the kidneys are the major route of excretion of active and metabolized drugs from the body, and because of the inherent nephrotoxicity of some drugs, there is an increase in the frequency and severity of drug intolerance in patients with renal insufficiency.

(2). Drugs should be selected for treatment of patients with UTI and renal failure only:

(a). After considering their nephrotoxic potential.

(b). On the basis of antimicrobial susceptibility tests.

(c). When the potential benefit to be gained from their use is known.

(d). With the advent of fluoroquinolone antimicrobials, the need for nephrotoxic aminoglycosides should be uncommon (Table 40–23).

d. Although single administration of large doses of antibiotics has been successfully used to treat certain types of superficial mucosal bladder infections of humans,[46,174] single-dose therapy has not proved to be effective in dogs with induced or spontaneously occurring UTI.[25,164,193]

(1). This implies that bacteria have invaded canine urinary tracts beyond the surface of the urothelium.

(2). Single-dose therapy is unlikely to be effective in eradicating infections of tissues adjacent to the urothelium. Because of difficulty in localizing the site(s) of UTI in

TABLE 40–20.
SOME ANTIMICROBIAL AGENTS THAT MAY REACH THERAPEUTIC CONCENTRATIONS IN PROSTATE GLANDS OF DOGS WITH CHRONIC BACTERIAL PROSTATITIS

Drug	Lipid Solubility	Chemical Nature	pKa	Plasma Protein Binding (%)	Dosage	Route
Carbenicillin Indanyl Sodium	Yes	?	?	50	15 mg/kg every 8 hours	IV
Chloramphenicol	Yes	NA	NA	53	45–60 mg/kg every 8 hours	PO, IM, IV
Ciprofloxacin	Yes	Base	?	Low	?	PO
Doxycycline	Yes	Ampholyte	3.4; 7.7; 9.7	88	3 mg/kg every 12 hours	PO
Enrofloxacin	Yes	Ampholyte	6.3; 7.7	?	2.5 mg/kg every 12 hours	PO
Erythromycin Base	Yes	Base	8.8	84	10–15 mg/kg every 8 hours	PO
Hetacillin Potassium	Yes	Base	?	18	10–20 mg/kg every 8 hours	PO
Minocycline	Yes	Ampholyte	7.8; 9.3	76	3–5 mg/kg every 8 hours	PO
Tetracycline	Yes	Ampholyte	3.3; 7.7; 9.7	65	25 mg/kg every 12 hours	PO
Trimethoprim	Yes	Base	7.3	35	3–5 mg/kg every 12 hours	PO
Trimethoprim-sulfadiazine	Yes	Acid	?	?	15 mg/kg every 12 hours	PO

NA = not applicable; IV = intravenous; PO = oral; IM = intramuscular.

TABLE 40–21.
SOME ANTIMICROBIAL AGENTS THAT MAY NOT REACH THERAPEUTIC CONCENTRATIONS IN PROSTATE GLANDS OF DOGS WITH CHRONIC BACTERIAL PROSTATITIS

Drug	Lipid Solubility	Chemical Nature	pKa	Plasma Protein Binding (%)	Dosage	Route
Ampicillin	No	Acid	2.5	20	20 mg/kg every 6–8 hours	PO, IV, IM
Cefadroxil	No	Acid	?	?	22 mg/kg every 12 hours	PO
Cephalexin	No	Acid	5.2, 7.3	14	20–30 mg/kg every 8–12 hours	PO
Cephalothin sodium	No	Acid	2.5	20	35 mg/kg every 8 hours	IV, IM
Cephapirin	No	Ampholyte	2.2	62	20 mg/kg every 6 hours	IV, IM
Sulfadiazine	No	Acid	?	?	110 mg/kg every 12 hours	PO

PO = oral; IV = intravenous; IM = intramuscular.

TABLE 40–22.
ANTIMICROBIAL AGENTS COMMONLY USED TO TREAT BACTERIAL URINARY TRACT INFECTIONS IN DOGS AND CATS

			Dosage*		
Agent	**Spectrum of Activity in Urine**	**Effect**	**Dog**	**Cat**	**Route of Administration**
Amoxicillin	Broad	Bactericidal	11 mg/kg every 8 hours	Same	Oral
Amoxicillin trihydrate/ clavulanate potassium	Broad	Bactericidal	10–20 mg/kg (combined) every 8 hours	Same	Oral
Ampicillin	Broad	Bactericidal	25 mg/kg every 8 hours	Same	Oral
		Bactericidal	8 mg/kg every 8 hours	Same	Subcutaneous, Intramuscular, Intravenous
Amikacin	Moderately Broad	Bactericidal	10 mg/kg every 12 hours	5–10 mg/kg every 8 hours	Subcutaneous
Cefadroxil	Broad	Bactericidal	10–20 mg/kg every 12 hours	Same	Oral
Cefotoxin†	Gram neg	Bactericidal	2.5–5.0 mg/kg every 8 hours	Same	Intramuscular, Intravenous
Cephalexin	Broad	Bactericidal	30–40 mg/kg every 8 to 12 hours	Same	Oral
Chloram-phenicol	Broad	Bacteriostatic	33 mg/kg every 8 hours	20 mg/kg every 8 hours for 1 week	Oral
Doxycycline	Broad	Bacteriostatic	5–11 mg/kg every 12 hours	Same	Oral
Gentamicin	Broad	Bactericidal	2–3 mg/kg every 8 hours for first day; then 1/2 mg/kg every 8 hours	Same	Subcutaneous, Intramuscular
Enrofloxacin	Broad	Bactericidal	2.5 to 5.0 mg/kg every 12 hours	Same	Oral
Hetacillin	Broad	Bactericidal	25 mg/kg every 8 hours	Same	Oral
Kanamycin	Moderately Broad	Bactericidal	6 mg/kg every 12 hours	Same	Intramuscular, Subcutaneous
Methenamine mandelate Methenamine hippurate	Moderately Broad	Bacteriostatic	10 mg/kg every 6 to 8 hours; urine pH must be below 6	Same?	Oral
Nitrofurantoin	Moderately Broad	Bacteriostatic	4 mg/kg every 6 to 8 hours	Same	Oral
Norfloxacin	Broad	Bactericidal	5–20 mg/kg every 12 hours	Same	Oral
Oxytetracycline	Broad	Bacteriostatic	20 mg/kg every 8 hours	Same	Oral
Penicillin G (Na or K)	Moderately Broad	Bactericidal	40,000 U/kg every 8 hours	Same	Oral
Sulfisoxazole	Broad	Bacteriostatic	20–30 mg/kg every 8 hours	Same	Oral
Tetracycline	Broad	Bacteriostatic	20 mg/kg every 8 hours	Same	Oral
Trimethoprim-Sulfadiazine	Broad	Bacteriostatic/ bactericidal	15 mg/kg (combined) every 12 hours	Unknown	Oral
Tobramycin	Moderately Broad	Bactericidal	1–2 mg/kg every 8 hours	Same	Subcutaneous

*Dosage for patients with normal hydration and normal renal function.
†Dosage recommended by Dr. David P. Aucoin, North Carolina State University.

companion animals with currently available diagnostic procedures, single high-dose administration of an antimicrobial drug is not recommended.

7. Duration of Therapy
   a. Data concerning the minimum and optimum duration of antimicrobial therapy for UTIs are not available. Therefore, no rigid generalities concerning the duration of treatment for acute, chronic, and recurrent UTI can be established. Duration of therapy must be individualized on the basis of serial clinical and laboratory findings, and therefore depends on patient response to therapy. The goals are to: 1) eliminate bacteria from urine and tissue and 2) allow the urinary tract and its defense mechanisms time to recover sufficient function to prevent recurrence of UTI.
   b. Selection of the proper antimicrobial drug, dosage, and frequency of administration usually eradicates bacteriuria within 2 to 5 days. However, if bacteria have gained access to tissues below the urothelium, the renal parenchyma, and/or the prostate gland, a longer course of therapy is usually required to eradicate them.
   c. Remission of clinical signs is not itself a reliable index of successful eradication of infection, nor is reduction in WBC, RBC, and protein detected by urinalysis. Duration of therapy should be based on the elimination of UTI as defined by urine cultures in addition to amelioration of pyuria and clinical signs.
   d. We recommend that the first episode of UTI should be treated for approximately 10 days to 2 weeks, whereas chronic or recurrent UTI should be treated for at least 4 to 6 weeks. Deep-seated and severe infections, and infections of the kidney or prostate gland, may require more prolonged therapy (Table 40–23).
      (1). We recognize that our recommendation regarding duration of therapy may be in excess of that required to eradicate bacterial pathogens in some patients, especially those with uncomplicated lower UTI.
      (2). Until convincing data become available to provide meaningful generalities about duration of therapy, we have chosen to err in the direction of giving antimicrobial agents for a period that is too long rather than too short.
8. Monitoring Response To Therapy (see Table 40–6). The following recommendations extrapolated from studies in humans are based on uncontrolled clinical observations.[178,180] They are guidelines only and should not be interpreted as rigid facts.
   a. Select the least expensive, least toxic, and most effective antimicrobial agent and begin therapy. Avoid indiscriminate administration of two or more antimicrobial drugs simultaneously (trimethoprim-sulfadiazine and amoxicillin with potassium clavulanate are exceptions).
   b. Culture a urine sample collected by cystocentesis 3 to 5 days following initiation of therapy.
      (1). Therapy is considered to be successful only if urine does not contain any pathogenic organisms.
      (2). Treatment is ineffective and relapse will occur if the colony count has only been reduced (e.g., from 10^8 to 10^2). Hematuria, pyuria, and proteinuria are likely to be present at this stage, although possibly of lesser magnitude.
   c. Consider evaluation of a urine culture and urinalysis 3 to 5 days (or sooner if necessary) prior to the scheduled discontinuation of therapy, especially if prophylactic antibiotics are to be used to prevent frequent reinfection. Therapy may be discontinued if the urine is sterile and the urine sediment is normal. If results indicate persistent infection, reevaluation of therapy is essential.
9. Management of Recurrent UTI
   a. If treatment appears to be effective, follow-up evaluation is required to detect recurrences.
      (1). Relapse caused by the same organism would be expected to occur shortly after cessation of antimicrobial therapy (see Table 40-7). Therefore, the results of a urinalysis and culture should be reevaluated 7 to 10 days following the discontinuation of therapy to detect recurrent relapses at a subclinical stage.
      (2). Recovery of the same organism from urine that is sterile during antimicrobial therapy is presumptive evidence that antimicrobial therapy failed to eradicate the infection and suggests lack of com-

TABLE 40–23.
CHARACTERISTICS OF FLUOROQUINOLONES THAT ARE DESIRABLE IN PATIENTS WITH COMPLICATED BACTERIAL UTI

1. Good tissue penetration
   a. Kidneys
   b. Prostate gland
2. High urine concentration
   a. Sustained for extended period
   b. Urine concentration may exceed MIC in patients with renal failure
3. Not nephrotoxic; wide safety margin
4. Extended spectrum of activity
5. Often effective against resistant bacteria
6. Plasmid mediated resistance extremely rare—not reported

TABLE 40–24.
ANTIMICROBIAL AGENTS THAT MAY BE EFFECTIVE IN PREVENTING RECURRENT BACTERIAL URINARY TRACT INFECTIONS FOLLOWING ERADICATION OF INFECTION BY CONVENTIONAL ANTIMICROBIAL THERAPY

Agent	Conventional Dose	Prophylactic Dose*	Route of Administration
Ampicillin	25 mg/kg every 8 hours	25 mg/kg every 24 hours	Oral
Cephalexin	10 mg/kg every 8 hours	10 mg/kg every 24 hours	Oral
Enrofloxacin	2.5 to 5.0 mg/kg every 12 hours	2.5 to 3.0 mg/kg every 24 hours	Oral
Nitrofurantoin	4 mg/kg every 8 hours	3–4 mg/kg every 24 hours	Oral
Trimethoprim-sulfadiazine	15 mg/kg (combined) every 12 hours	7–8 mg/kg every 24 hours	Oral

*Daily dosage to be administered shortly after micturition and prior to confinement to enhance duration of period during which the antimicrobial agent will be retained in the urinary tract. Urine of patient should be cultured for bacteria at appropriate intervals to ensure that infection has not recurred.

pliance or deep-seated infection (see Table 40–7).

(a). If the relapse occurred following a brief period of therapy, continue treatment for a longer period.

(b). If the relapse occurred 10 or more days following therapy, repeat therapy with a different antimicrobial agent selected on the basis of susceptibility tests and continue therapy for a longer period. The procedures to evaluate efficacy previously described should be repeated.

b. Reinfection caused by a different organism would be expected to occur later than a relapse (see Table 40–8). Therefore, the results of a urinalysis and culture should be re-evaluated approximately 4 weeks (and in some instances repeatedly) after cessation of antimicrobial therapy.

(1). Detection of frequent reinfections following antimicrobial therapy is an absolute indication to evaluate the patient for a predisposing cause (see Table 40–5).

(2). Reinfections should be managed by choosing antimicrobial agents on the basis of antimicrobial susceptibility tests. Each product should be used for a sufficient period of time (3 to 5 days) to evaluate its effectiveness in sterilizing urine.

(3). Elimination of bacterial pathogens associated with reinfections may require therapy of shorter duration than may recurrences associated with relapses.

(4). Infrequent recurrences (2 or 3 times per year) may be treated as single episodes (i.e., short course of a suitable antimicrobial agent).

c. Infections of the canine prostate gland are a common cause of recurrent UTI.

(1). Relapses appear to be related to poor penetration of antimicrobial drugs into prostatic secretions, but may also be related to drug resistance (see Table 40–7).

(2). Reinfections may be associated with persistent abnormalities in prostatic defenses against bacterial infections (see Table 40–8).

10. Prevention of Frequent Reinfections. In some patients with chronic UTI, elimination of predisposing causes may be impossible. The result is frequent reinfections. In such cases, low-dose (preventative) antibacterial therapy may be helpful for an indefinite period (6 months or more) with drugs primarily eliminated in urine (Table 40–24).

a. Reduced dosages (about one third of the therapeutic dosage) of drugs excreted in high concentration in urine may be utilized provided *bacterial pathogens have been completely eradicated by therapeutic dosages of appropriate drugs.*

b. Logically, preventative antimicrobial therapy would be inappropriate for management of patients with recurrent bacterial UTI caused by relapses.

c. Even though this preventative dosage regime does not result in MICs throughout the day, low concentrations of some drugs apparently interfere with production of fimbriae by some uropathogens.[159,183] This in turn interferes with the ability of potential pathogens to adhere to uroepithelial cells.

d. The administration of one daily preventative dose of the antibiotic is best at a time when the drug is likely to be retained in the urinary tract for several hours (i.e., prior to bedtime).

e. During preventative therapy, urine samples collected by cystocentesis (not by catheterization or voiding) should be recultured approximately once each month. If bacteria are identified, a "breakthrough" infection may have occurred. This infection may be associated with poor compliance. The patient should be treated again with therapeutic dosages of an antimicrobial drug selected on the basis of susceptibility tests. Once the infection has been eradicated and the associated inflammatory response subsides, preventative therapy may be resumed.

f. Following 6 to 9 months of consecutive negative urine cultures, therapy may be discontinued on a trial basis to determine if a relapse or reinfection will occur. If abnormalities in host defenses have healed, UTI may not recur. If UTI develops within a short period, the procedures previously outlined should be repeated.

g. Long-term use of antimicrobial agents is not without risk of adverse effects. For example, sulfadiazine-trimethoprim combinations have been associated with keratoconjunctivitis sicca,[37] folate deficiency anemia, and immune-complex reactions.[58,201]

11. Persistent Bacteriuria.

a. No evidence shows that long-term antimicrobial therapy in the presence of persistent bacteriuria (so-called suppressive therapy) is beneficial in preventing further episodes of progressive UTI. Long-term or continuous therapy in the presence of bacteria is of no value, but may cause other antibiotic-resistant strains to develop.

b. Continuous antimicrobial therapy of persistent UTI that is associated with sterilization of urine is of clinical value. Selection of drugs should be based on antimicrobial susceptibility tests and the likelihood that the drug will be well tolerated during long-term therapy.

XIV. ANCILLARY THERAPY

A. Many forms of ancillary therapy for UTIs have been developed and evaluated on an empiric basis. In terms of value to the patient, they usually rank behind antimicrobial therapy and correction of predisposing factors of UTIs.[154]

B. Ancillary forms of therapy include:

1. Urine acidifiers (Table 40–25).
2. Urinary antiseptics.
3. Local instillation of antimicrobial agents into the urinary bladder.
4. Altering urine volume.
5. Use of pharmacologic agents that affect the storage and voiding phases of micturition.

C. Catheterization performed solely for the purpose of local instillation of antimicrobial agents into the urinary bladder is not recommended because it is usually ineffective and may cause iatrogenic infection.

1. If antimicrobial agents are deemed to be indicated, oral or parenteral administration is usually best.
2. One experimental study in dogs implied that gentamicin could be infused into the bladder lumen without resulting in measurable blood levels of the drug.[120]

D. Water should not be withheld from the patient. Induction of diuresis may aggravate lower UTIs, especially when indwelling urethral catheters are present. The possible benefit of diuresis in management of upper UTI has not been evaluated in dogs or cats.

XV. SUMMARY OF THERAPEUTIC PROTOCOLS (TABLE 40–26)

A. Initial discovery of untreated UTI (without upper tract signs).

1. Try to determine the nature of uropathogen by examining Gram-stained urine sediment (see Table 40–18).
2. Select an effective antimicrobial drug (see Tables 40–17 and 40–19).
3. Administer the proper dosage of the drug at the proper maintenance intervals (see Table 40–22).
4. Continue treatment for 10 to 14 days.
5. Discontinue therapy if signs subside, but educate clients about recurrent UTI.
6. Consider follow-up urinalysis and/or urine culture 7 to 14 days after completing treatment to verify cure or to detect subclinical recurrent UTI.
7. Consider appropriate diagnostic studies and selection of a different antimicrobial drug on the basis of antimicrobial susceptibility tests if signs of lower UTI persist during therapy or recur following withdrawal of therapy.

B. Infrequent reinfections (see Table 40–8).

1. Identify bacterial pathogen, preferably by culture (see Table 40–18).
2. Consider diagnostic procedures to identify the underlying causes of infection (see Tables 40–5 and 40–9).
3. Select an effective antimicrobial drug (see Tables 40–17 and 40–19).
4. Administer the proper dosage of the drug at the proper maintenance intervals (see Table 40–22).
5. After 3 to 5 days of antimicrobial therapy:

TABLE 40–25.
URINE pH ASSOCIATED WITH OPTIMUM ANTIMICROBIAL ACTIVITY*

Acid	Alkaline	Either
Chlortetracycline	Erythromycin	Cephalosporins
Methenamine mandelate	Gentamicin	Chloramphenicol
Nitrofurantoin	Kanamycin	Nalidixic acid
Oxytetracycline	Neomycin	Sulfonamides
Penicillin G	Streptomycin	
Tetracycline	Fluoroquinolones	

*Reports concerning the optimum urine pH for activity of ampicillin are contradictory.

TABLE 40–26.
CHECKLIST FOR TREATMENT OF BACTERIAL UTI

I. Has bacterial UTI been confirmed?
  A. Simple or complicated?
  B. First episode or recurrent episode?
II. Select appropriate drug
  A. Antimicrobial susceptibility test?
  B. Upper or lower UTI? Prostatitis?
  C. Status of renal function?
III. Select appropriate dose and maintenance interval
  A. Client compliance?
  B. Status of renal function?
IV. Select appropriate duration of treatment
  A. Upper or lower UTI? Prostatitis?
  B. First episode or recurrent episode?
    1. Relapse?
    2. Reinfection?
  C. Simple or complicated UTI?
V. Consider need for ancillary treatment
VI. Monitor response
  A. Clinical signs
  B. Urinalysis
  C. Urine culture
VII. Consider prevention
  A. Status of host defenses?
  B. Preventative antibiotic treatment (reinfections)
  C. Suppressive antibiotic treatment (persistent infections)

a. Collect a urine sample by cystocentesis for bacterial culture.
b. If the sample is sterile, continue therapy for an additional 7 to 10 days. An inflammatory response may still be detected by urinalysis 3 to 5 days after initiating therapy, even if the sample is bacteriologically sterile.
c. If bacteria are cultured, even in low numbers, therapy should be considered ineffective. If the owners have been compliant in giving therapy, consider appropriate diagnostic studies and selection of a different antimicrobial drug on the basis of antimicrobial susceptibility tests.

6. Anticipate and evaluate for recurrence by periodically evaluating urinalyses and, when appropriate, urine cultures following discontinuation of therapy.

C. Relapses.

1. Attempt to identify abnormalities in host defenses by appropriate diagnostic procedures (see Tables 40–5, 40–7, and 40–9).
2. Because by definition the same type of bacteria is the cause of the relapse, determine its susceptibility to antimicrobial drugs.
3. Control or correct abnormalities predisposing to recurrence of UTI.
4. Select an effective agent, especially one that is able to attain MIC concentrations in the renal parenchyma, prostate gland, or tissue surrounding the urinary tract.
5. Administer the proper dosage at the proper maintenance intervals (see Table 40–22).
6. After 3 to 5 days of antimicrobial therapy, collect a urine sample by cystocentesis for bacterial culture.
   a. If the sample is sterile, continue therapy for a prolonged interval (6 to 8 weeks or more for renal infections and prostate infections).
   b. If bacteria are cultured, even in low numbers, therapy should be considered to be ineffective. If owners have been compliant, reevaluate susceptibility of the pathogen by dilution tests (MIC).
7. Following discontinuation of therapy, evaluate urinalyses and urine cultures at frequent intervals to detect relapses as early as possible.

D. Frequent reinfections.

1. Attempt to identify abnormalities in host defenses by appropriate diagnostic procedures (see Tables 40–5 and 40–8).
2. Identify the nature of uropathogens by *in vitro* culture, and determine their susceptibility to drugs by antimicrobial susceptibility tests.
3. Correct or control the abnormalities in host defenses, if possible.
4. Select an effective antimicrobial drug (see Tables 40–17 and 40–19).
5. Administer the proper dosage of the drug at the proper maintenance intervals (see Table 40–22).
6. After 3 to 5 days of antimicrobial therapy, collect a urine sample by cystocentesis for bacterial culture.
   a. If the sample is sterile, continue therapy for at least an additional 10 to 14 days. An inflammatory response may still be detected by urinalysis 3 to 5 days after initiating therapy, even if the sample is bacteriologically sterile.
   b. If bacteria are cultured, even in low numbers, therapy should be considered ineffective. If the owners have been compliant in providing therapy, consider additional diagnostic studies, re-evaluation of antimicrobial susceptibility tests, and/or alternate forms of therapy to correct predisposing causes.
7. If preventative antimicrobial therapy is to be subsequently used (see the following), collect a urine sample by cystocentesis for urinalysis and urine culture prior to discontinuation of therapeutic dosages of antimicrobial drugs. The urine should be sterile and have no evidence of inflammation. If infection persists, preventative therapy is inappropriate.
8. If preventative therapy is not to be given following withdrawal of antimicrobial drugs, anticipate recurrences by periodically evaluating urinalyses and urine cultures.

E. Prevention of frequent reinfections.

1. Evaluate a urinalysis and urine culture to ensure that bacterial UTI has been eliminated.

2. Select a drug that is excreted in high concentration in urine and is unlikely to cause adverse effects to the patient (see Table 40–24).
3. Give the drug at approximately one third of the normal daily therapeutic dosage.
4. Strive to give the drug immediately after the patient has voided, and at a time when the drug will be retained in the urinary tract for several hours (prior to bedtime).
5. Plan to give the drug for 6 to 8 months.
6. Collect urine samples, preferably by cystocentesis (never by catheterization), every 4 to 6 weeks for urinalysis and urine culture.
   a. If the urine is normal, continue preventative antimicrobial therapy.
   b. If bacterial UTI is identified (so-called breakthrough infection), repeat the therapeutic protocol outlined for frequently recurrent UTI. Check compliance of clients to determine if they are administering the proper dosage of the drug on a daily basis.
7. After 6 to 8 months, successful preventative therapy may be discontinued. At this time, the patient's own body may have repaired abnormalities in host defenses. In this situation, anticipate recurrences by periodically evaluating urinalyses and urine cultures.

F. Prevention and treatment of catheter-induced UTI (Table 40–27).

1. Consider administration of therapeutic dosages of antimicrobial drugs excreted in high concentration in urine at an interval of 8 to 12 hours prior to, and 2 to 3 days following, single brief catheterization of patients at high risk for UTI. Collect a urine sample by cystocentesis 2 to 3 days following catheterization to detect iatrogenic UTI at a subclinical stage of development. If UTI is present, select an antimicrobial drug on the basis of susceptibility tests and administer it for an appropriate period.
2. If indwelling urethral catheters must be used, avoid concomitant administration of antimicrobial drugs (and corticosteroids) unless UTI develops. Although antibiotics may decrease the frequency and delay the onset of UTI, the risk is high of promoting development of infections with one or more bacteria that are resistant to multiple drugs.
   a. Use a closed indwelling catheter system.
   b. Try to avoid inducing diuresis during indwelling catheterization, especially if an "open" system is used.
   c. Remove the catheter as soon as possible.
   d. Obtain a urinalysis, urine culture, and antimicrobial susceptibility test. Initiate therapy with an appropriate drug for 10 to 14 days if UTI is confirmed.
   e. If infection with more than one species of bacteria occurs, and if the microbes have different susceptibilities to drugs, treat the bacteria likely to be most virulent first. Then select the type of drug most likely to eliminate remaining pathogens.

TABLE 40–27.
GUIDELINES TO MINIMIZE IATROGENIC CATHETER-INDUCED URINARY TRACT INFECTIONS

1. Avoid unnecessary catheterization, especially in patients with increased risk for bacterial UTI and its sequelae. They include patients with:
   a. Urinary diseases, especially of the lower urinary tract
   b. Hyperadrenocorticism
   c. Diabetes mellitus
2. Urinary catheterization should be performed only by properly trained personnel.
3. If the need for catheterization spans more than a few hours, consider intermittent catheterization as an alternative to indwelling catheterization.
4. If single brief catheterization is required for high-risk patients, consider an antibiotic excreted in high concentration in urine, and administer it 8 to 12 hours before and 8 to 12 hours following catheterization.
5. Avoid overinsertion of catheters to minimize damage to the mucosa of the urinary bladder.
6. If indwelling urethral catheters are required, strive to maintain a closed system.
7. Select indwelling urethral catheters constructed of materials least likely to cause irritation and inflammation of the adjacent mucosa.
8. Consider administration of antibiotics during indwelling urethral catheterization only if evidence of infection is detected. Exercising such restraint minimizes the likelihood of infection with bacteria resistant to antimicrobial agents. If catheter-induced infection develops and remains asymptomatic, treat the infection following removal of the catheter.
9. Periodically perform urinalyses and bacterial cultures during the period of indwelling urethral catheterization and always at the time the catheter is removed.

REFERENCES

1. Abdullahi SU, et al. Evaluation of a calculolytic diet in female dogs with induced struvite urolithiasis. *Am J Vet Res.* 1984;45: 1508-1519.
2. Acquantella H, Little PJ, DeWardener HE, Coleman JC. The effect of urine osmolality and pH on the bactericidal activity of plasma. *Clin Sci.* 1967;33:471-480.
3. Alerman MH, Freeman LR. Experimental pyelonephritis. X. The direct injection of *E. coli* protoplasts into the medulla of the rabbit kidney. *Yale J Biol Med.* 1963;36:1.
4. Allen TA, Jones RL, Purvance J. Microbiologic evaluation of canine urine: Direct microscopic examination and preservation of specimen qualify for culture. *J Am Vet Med Assoc.* 1987;190: 1289-1291.

5. Andriole VT. Acceleration of inflammatory response of renal medulla by water diuresis. *J Clin Invest.* 1966;45:847-854.
6. Andriole VT. Effect of water diuresis on chronic pyelonephritis. *J Lab Clin Med.* 1968;72:1-16.
7. Andriole VT. Water, acidosis, and experimental pyelonephritis. *J Clin Invest.* 1970;49:21-30.
8. Andriole VT, Epstein FH. Prevention of pyelonephritis by water diuresis: Evidence for the role of medullary hypertonicity in promoting renal infection. *J Clin Invest.* 1965;44:73-79.
9. Angel JA, Roberts JA, Smith TW, DiLuzio N. Immunology of pyelonephritis. *J Urol.* 1982;128:624-628.
10. Asscher AW. Urine as a medium for bacterial growth. *Lancet.* 1966;2:1037-1041.
11. Balish MJ, Jensen J, Uehlina DT. Bladder mucin: A scanning electron microscopic study in experimental cystitis. *J Urol.* 1982;128:1060-1063.
12. Barber DL, Finco DR. Radiographic findings in induced bacterial pyelonephritis in dogs. *J Am Vet Med Assoc.* 1979;175: 1183-1190.
13. Barsanti JA, Blue J, Edmunds J. Urinary tract infection due to indwelling bladder catheters in dogs and cats. *J Am Vet Med Assoc.* 1985;187:384-388.
14. Barsanti JA, Finco DR, Shotts EB, Ross L. Feline urologic syndrome: Further investigation into therapy. *J Am Anim Hosp Assoc.* 1982;18:387-390.
15. Barsanti JA, et al. Feline urologic syndrome: Further investigation into etiology. *J Am Anim Hosp Assoc.* 1982;18:391-395.
16. Barsanti JA, Johnson CA. Genitourinary infections. In: Greene CE, ed. *Infectious Diseases of the Dog and Cat.* 2nd ed. Philadelphia, Pennsylvania: WB Saunders; 1990;157-183.
17. Beeson PB, Rowley D. The anticomplementary effect of kidney tissue: Its association with ammonia production. *J Exp Med.* 1959;110:685-697.
18. Bell ET. *Renal Diseases.* Philadelphia, Pennsylvania: Lea & Febiger; 1950.
18a. Biberstein EL. Urinary tract infections in dogs: Microbiological diagnosis. *Calif Vet.* 1977;31:10-17.
19. Biertuempfel PH, Ling GV, Ling GA. Urinary tract infection resulting from catheterization in healthy dogs. *J Am Vet Med Assoc.* 1981;178:989-991.
20. Bjugn R, Flood RR. Scanning electron microscopy of human urine and purified Tamm-Horsfall's glycoprotein. *Scand J Urol Nephrol.* 1988;22:313-315.
21. Booth DM. The practical aspects of treating bacterial infections in cats. *Vet Med.* 1989;84:884-904.
22. Bovee KC, Abt DA, Kronfeld DS. The effects of dietary protein intake on renal function in dogs with experimentally reduced renal function. *J Am Anim Hosp Assoc.* 1979;15:9-16.
23. Braude AI, Siemienski J. The role of bacterial urease in experimental pyelonephritis. *J Bacteriol.* 1960;80:171-179.
24. Brodeur GY. Diagnosis of ectopic ureter. *Canine Pract.* 1977;4: 25-28.
25. Brown SA, et al. Pharmacokinetics of norfloxacin in dogs after single intravenous and single and multiple oral administrations of the drug. *Am J Vet Res.* 1990;51:1065-1070.
26. Brown SA, Barsanti JA. Diseases of the bladder and urethra. In: Ettinger SJ, ed. *Textbook of Veterinary Internal Medicine.* 3rd ed. Vol 2. Philadelphia, Pennsylvania: WB Saunders; 1989:2108-2141.
27. Brown SG. Surgery of the canine urethra. *Vet Clin North Am.* 1975;5:457-470.
28. Brushim A, Lutsky I. Isolation of mycoplasmas from the canine genital tract: A survey of 108 clinical healthy dogs. *Res Vet Sci.* 1978;25:243-245.
29. Casciani CU, et al. Immunologic aspects of chronic uremia. *Kidney Int.* 1978;13:S49-S53.
30. Cavalier ST, Snyder IS. Cytotoxic activity of partially purified *Escherichia coli* alpha hemolysin. *J Med Microbiol.* 1982;15:11-21.
31. Chernew I, Braude AI. Depression of phagocytosis by solutes in concentrations found in the kidney and urine. *J Clin Invest.* 1962;41:1953-1954.
31a. Chew DJ, DiBartola SP. Diagnosis and pathophysiology of renal disease. In: Ettinger SJ, ed. *Textbook of Veterinary Internal Medicine.* 3rd ed. Vol 2. Philadelphia, Pennsylvania: WB Saunders; 1989;1893-1961.
32. Colleen SLY. The human urethral mucosa. An experimental study with emphasis on microbial attachment. *Scan J Urol Nephrol.* 1982;Suppl 68:10-55.
33. Collins BK, Moose CP, Hagee JH. Sulfonamide-associated keratoconjunctivitis sicca and corneal ulceration in a dog. *J Am Vet Med Assoc.* 1986;189:924-926.
34. Cornish J, et al. Host defense mechanism in the bladder. *Br J Exp Pathol.* 1988;69:759-770.
35. Corriere JN, McClure JM, Lipschultz LI. Contamination of bladder urine by urethral peristalsis during voiding: Urethrovesical reflux. *J Urol.* 1972;107:399-401.
36. Cox CE, Hinman F. Experiments with induced bacteriuria, vesical emptying and bacterial growth on the mechanism of bladder defense to infection. *J Urol.* 1961;86:739-748.
37. Crow SE, et al. Cyclophosphamide induced cystitis in the dog and cat. *J Am Vet Med Assoc.* 1977;171:259-262.
38. Davis CP, et al. Bladder response to *Klebsiella* infection: A scanning electron microscopic study. *Invest Urol.* 1977;15: 227-231.
39. Davis RF, Hain FR. Urinary antisepsis—the antiseptic properties of normal dog urine. *J Urol.* 1918;2:309.
40. Dieraut LA, Gowdey AC, Mulholland GS. Bacterial invasion of the urinary tract by way of the vaginal route in the rat. *Surg Gynecol Obstet.* 1974;138:62-64.
41. Eknoyan G, Weinman EJ. The kidney and infections. *Contrib Nephrol.* 1977;7:272.
42. Fair WR, Couch J, Wehner N. Prostatic antibacterial factor: Identity and significance. *Urology.* 1976;7:169-177.
43. Fairley KF, et al. Site of infection in acute urinary tract infection in general practice. *Lancet.* 1971;2:615-618.
44. Finco DR, Shotts EB, Crowell WA. Evaluation of methods for localization of urinary tract infection in the female dog. *Am J Vet Res.* 1979;40:707-712.
45. Forland M, Thomas V, Shelokov A. Urinary tract infections in patients with diabetes mellitus. *JAMA.* 1977;238:1924-1926.
46. Fowler JE. *Urinary Tract Infection and Inflammation.* Chicago, Illinois: Year Book Medical Publishers; 1989.
47. Fowler JE, Latta R, Stamey TA. Studies of introital colonization in women with recurrent urinary tract infections. VIII. The role of bacterial interference. *J Urol.* 1977;118:296-298.
48. Fowler JE, Stamey TA. Studies of introital colonization in women with recurrent urinary tract infections. VII. The role of bacterial adherence. *J Urol.* 1977;117:472-476.
49. Freedman LR. Experimental pyelonephritis. 13. On the ability of water diuresis to induce susceptibility to *E. coli* bacteriuria in the normal rat. *Yale J Biol Med.* 1967;39:255.
50. Freedman LR. Urinary tract infection, pyelonephritis, and other forms of chronic interstitial nephritis. In: Strauss NB, Welt LG, eds. *Diseases of the Kidney.* 2nd ed. Boston, Massachusetts: Little, Brown & Co; 1971.
51. Freedman LR, Beeson PB. Experimental pyelonephritis. IV. Observations on infections resulting from direct inoculation of

bacteria in different zones of the kidney. *Yale J Biol Med.* 1958;30:406.

52. Freeman RB, Murphy TE, Dickstein CD. Experimental renal infection. Acute and chronic studies of histology and function. *Kidney Int.* 1978;13:129-135.
53. Garcia E, et al. Isolation and characterization of dog uropathogenic *Escherichia coli* strains and their fimbriae. *Antonic van Leeuwenhoek.* 1988;54:149-163.
54. Gould F, Chang C, Lapides J. Rapid versus slow decompression of the distended urinary bladder. *Invest Urol.* 1976;14:156-158.
55. Grana L, Donnellan WL, Swenson O. Effects of gram negative bacteria on ureteral structure and function. *J Urol.* 1968;99: 539-550.
56. Greco DS, et al. Urinary gamma-glutamyl transpeptidase activity in dogs with gentamicin-induced nephrotoxicity. *Am J Vet Res.* 1985;46:2332-2335.
57. Greene CE. Dosages of antimicrobial drugs. In: Greene CE, ed. *Infectious Diseases of the Dog and Cat.* Philadelphia, Pennsylvania: WB Saunders; 1990:926-929.
58. Greene CE, Ferguson DC. Antibacterial chemotherapy. In: Greene CE, ed. *Infectious Diseases of the Dog and Cat.* Philadelphia, Pennsylvania: WB Saunders; 1990:461-493.
59. Gregory JG, Wein AJ, Sansone TC, Murphy JJ. Bladder resistance to infection. *J Urol.* 1971;105:220-222.
60. Gruneberg RH, Leigh DA, Brunfitt W. *Escherichia coli* serotypes in urinary tract infections. In: O'Grady F, Brumfitt W, eds. *Urinary Tract Infection.* London: Oxford University Press; 1968:68.
61. Guze LB, Beeson PB. Experimental pyelonephritis. I. Effect of ureteral ligation on the course of bacterial infection in the kidney of the rat. *J Exp Med.* 1956;104:803-815.
62. Harn SD, Keutel HJ, Weaver RG. Immunologic and histologic evaluation of the urinary bladder wall after group A streptococcal infection. *Invest Urol.* 1973;11:55-64.
63. Harrison G, Cornish J, Vanderwee MA, Miller TE. Host defense mechanisms in the bladder. I. Role of mechanical factors. *Br J Exp Pathol.* 1988;69:245-254.
64. Hesse VE, VanTonder H, Abrahams C. Analgesic cystitis: An unusual microangiopathy of the bladder. *J Urol.* 1976;116: 176-177.
65. Hinman F. Hydrodynamic aspects of urinary tract infection. In: Lutzeyer W, Melchior H, eds. *Urodynamics.* New York, New York: Springer Verlag; 1973.
66. Hinman F. Meatal colonization in bitches. *Trans Am Assoc Genitourinary Surg.* 1977;68:73.
67. Hirsch DC, Wiger N. The bacterial flora of the normal canine vagina compared with that of vaginal exudates. *J Small Anim Pract.* 1977;18:25-30.
68. Hjort EF. An experimental study on the pathogenesis of sporadic bacteriuria in the rat. *Scand J Urol Nephrol.* 1977; 11:271.
69. Hutch JA. The role of urethral mucus in the bladder defense mechanism. *J Urol.* 1970;103:165-167.
70. Ihrke PJ, Norton AL, Ling GV, Stannard AA. Urinary tract infection associated with long-term corticosteroid administration in dogs with chronic skin diseases. *J Am Vet Med Assoc.* 1985;186:43-46.
71. Johnston WH, Latta H. Acute hematogenous pyelonephritis in the rabbit. Electron microscopic study of *Escherichia coli* localization and early acute inflammation. *Lab Invest.* 1978;38: 439-446.
72. Jones SR, Smith JW, Sanford JP. Localization of urinary tract infections by detection of antibody-coated bacteria in urine sediment. *N Engl J Med.* 1974;290:591-593.
73. Kallenus G, Winberg J. Bacterial adherence to periurethral epithelial cells in girls prone to urinary-tract infections. *Lancet.* 1978;2:540-543.
74. Kaye D. The effect of water diuresis on spread of bacteria through the urinary tract. *J Infect Dis.* 1971;124:297-305.
75. Kaye D. Host defense mechanisms in the urine and urinary bladder. In: Griefer I, ed. *Bacteriuria and Urinary Tract Infections.* New York, New York: National Kidney Foundation; 1974.
76. Kaye D. Host defense mechanisms of the urinary tract. *Urol Clin North Am.* 1975;2:407-422.
77. Keane WF, Freedman LR. *Escherichia coli* pyelonephritis in mice during water diuresis. *Clin Res.* 1967;15:468.
78. Keane WF, Freedman LR. Experimental pyelonephritis. XIV. Pyelonephritis in normal mice produced by inoculation of *E. coli* into the bladder lumen during water diuresis. *Yale J Biol Med.* 1967;40:231.
79. Kelly DF. Pyelonephritis and renal response to infection. In: Bovee, KC, ed. *Canine Nephrology.* Media, Pennsylvania: Harwall; 1984:481-503.
80. Kivisto AK, Vasenius H, Sundholm M. Canine bacteriuria. *J Small Anim Pract.* 1977;18:707-712.
81. Kivisto AK, et al. Desorption assay. A function in vitro test for measuring the adhesion of *E. coli* on the urinary tract epithelium (of dogs). *Invest Urol.* 1978;15:412-415.
82. Koss LG. The asymmetric unit membranes of the epithelium of the urinary bladder of the rat. An electron microscopic study of a mechanism of epithelial maturation and function. *Lab Invest.* 1969;21:154-168.
83. Krawiec DR, Osborne CA, Leininger JR, Griffith DP. Effect of acetohydroxamic acid on dissolution of canine struvite uroliths. *Am J Vet Res.* 1984;45:1266-1275.
84. Krawiec DR, Osborne CA, Leininger JR, Griffith DP. Effect of acetohydroxamic acid on prevention of canine struvite uroliths. *Am J Vet Res.* 1984;45:1276-1282.
85. Kunin CM. *Detection, Prevention, and Management of Urinary Tract Infections.* 4th ed. Philadelphia, Pennsylvania: Lea & Febiger; 1987.
86. Lancaster MG, Allison F. Studies on the pathogenesis of acute inflammation. VII. The influence of osmolality upon the phagocytic and clumping activity of human leucocytes. *Am J Pathol.* 1966;49:1185-1200.
87. Leadbetter GW. Diagnostic urologic instrumentation. In: Walsh PC, Retik AB, Stamey TA, Vaughn ED, eds. *Campbell's Urology.* 4th ed. Vol 1. Philadelphia, Pennsylvania: WB Saunders; 1978.
88. Lees GE. Epidemiology of naturally occurring feline bacterial urinary tract infections. *Vet Clin North Am.* 1984;14:471-479.
89. Lees GE, Osborne CA. Antibacterial properties of urine: A comparative review. *J Am Anim Hosp Assoc.* 1979;15:125-132.
90. Lees GE, Osborne CA. Use and misuse of intermittent and indwelling urinary catheters. In: Kirk RW, ed. *Current Veterinary Therapy.* Vol 8. Philadelphia, Pennsylvania: WB Saunders; 1983.
91. Lees GE, Osborne CA, Stevens JB. Antibacterial properties of urine: Studies of feline urine specific gravity, osmolality and pH. *J Am Anim Hosp Assoc.* 1979;15:135-141.
92. Lees GE, Osborne CA, Stevens JB. Urine: A medium for bacterial growth. *Vet Clin North Am.* 1979;9:611-616.
93. Lees GE, Osborne CA, Stevens JB, Ward GE. Adverse effects of open indwelling urethral catheterization in clinically normal male cats. *Am J Vet Res.* 1981;42:825-833.
94. Lees GE, Osborne CA, Stevens JB, Ward GE. Adverse effects caused by polypropylene and polyvinyl feline urinary catheters. *Am J Vet Res.* 1980;41:1836-1840.
95. Lees GE, Rogers KS, Wolf AM. Diseases of the lower urinary

tract. In: Sherding RG, ed. *The Cat: Diseases and Clinical Management.* New York, New York: Churchill Livingstone; 1989:1397-1454.

96. Ling GV. Treatment of urinary tract infections with antimicrobial agents. In: Kirk RW, ed. *Current Veterinary Therapy.* Vol 8. Philadelphia, Pennsylvania: WB Saunders; 1983.

97. Ling GV. Therapeutic strategies involving antimicrobial treatment of the canine urinary tract. *J Am Vet Med Assoc.* 1984;185: 1162-1164.

97a. Ling GV, Ackerman N, Lowenstone LJ, Cowgill LD. Percutaneous nephropyelocentesis and nephropyelostomy in the dog. A description of the technique. *Am J Vet Res.* 1979;40:1605-1612.

98. Ling GV, Ackerman N, Ruby AL. Relation of antibody-coated urine bacteria to the site(s) of infection in experimental dogs. *Am J Vet Res.* 1980;40:686-690.

99. Ling GV, Biberstein EL, Hirsh DC. Bacterial pathogens associated with urinary tract infections. *Vet Clin North Am.* 1979;9: 617-630.

100. Ling GV, Kaneko JJ. Microscopic examination of canine urine sediment. *Calif. Vet.* 1976;30:14-18.

101. Ling GV, et al. Diabetes mellitus in dogs: A review of initial evaluation, immediate and long-term management, and outcome. *J Am Vet Med Assoc.* 1977;170:521-530.

102. Ling GV, Ruby AL. Aerobic bacterial flora of the prepuce, urethra and vagina of normal adult dogs. *Am J Vet Res.* 1978; 39:695-698.

103. Ling GV, Ruby AL. Cephalexin for oral treatment of canine urinary tract infection caused by *Klebsiella pneumoniae. J Am Vet Med Assoc.* 1983;182:1346-1347.

104. Ling GV, et al. Canine hyperadrenocorticism: Pretreatment clinical and laboratory evaluation of 117 cases. *J Am Vet Med Assoc.* 1979;174:1211-1215.

105. Lippert AC, Fulton RB, Parr AM. Nosocomial infection surveillance in a small animal intensive care unit. *J Am Anim Hosp Assoc.* 1988;24:627-636.

106. Lloyd-Davies WR, Hayes TL, Hinman F. Urothelial microcontour. I. Scanning electron microscopy of normal resting and stretched urethra and bladder. *J Urol.* 1971;105:236-241.

107. Lloyd-Davies WR, Hayes TL, Hinman F. Urothelial microcontour. III. Mucosal alteration by infection. *J Urol.* 1971;106: 81-83.

108. Lloyd-Davies WR, Hinman F. Structural and functional changes leading to impaired bacterial elimination after overdistention of the rabbit bladder. *Invest Urol.* 1971;9:136-142.

109. Lorenz MD. Diagnosis and medical management of canine Cushing's syndrome: A study of 57 consecutive cases. *J Am Anim Hosp Assoc.* 1982;18:707-716.

110. Louria DB. L forms, spheroplasts, and aberrant forms in chronic sepsis. *Adv Intern Med.* 1971;17:125.

111. Low DA, et al. Isolation and comparison of *Escherichia* strains from canine and human patients with urinary tract infections. *Infect Immun.* 1988;56:2601-2609.

112. Lulich JP, Osborne CA, Johnston GR. Nonsurgical correction of infection-induced struvite uroliths and a vesicourachal diverticulum in an immature dog. *J Small Anim Pract.* 1989;30: 613-617.

113. Lynn KL, et al. Antibodies to Tamm-Horsfall urinary glycoprotein in patients with urinary tract infection reflux nephropathy, urinary tract obstruction and paraplegia. *Kidney Int.* 1984; 26:242.

114. Maeda S, et al. Studies on the phagocytic function of urinary leukocytes. *J Urol.* 1983;129:427-429.

115. Marshall S, Linfoot J. Influence of hormones on urinary tract infections. *Urology.* 1977;9:675-679.

116. Masih BK, Drouin G, Hinman F. Voiding and intrinsic defenses of the lower urinary tract of the female dog. I. Effects of episiotomy, colostomy, dilatation, and urinary diversion. *J Urol.* 1970;104:130-136.

117. Masih BK, Hinman F. Voiding and intrinsic defenses on the lower urinary tract in the female dog. II. Effect of immunosuppressive drugs on canine urethral and vaginal flora. *Invest Urol.* 1971;8:494-498.

118. Mayo ME, Heine JP, Hinman F. Intrinsic urethral peristalsis. *Invest Urol.* 1974;12:1-4.

119. Mayo ME, Hinman F. Role of mid-urethral high pressure zone in spontaneous bacterial ascent. *J Urol.* 1973;109:268-272.

120. McGuire EJ, Savastano JA. Treatment of intractable bacterial cystitis with intermittent catheterization and antimicrobial installation. Case report. *J Urol.* 1987;137:495-496.

121. Mehrotra RML. Experimental study of the vesical circulation during distention and in cystitis. *Bacteriology.* 1953;66:79.

122. Monis B, Dorfman HD. Some histochemical observations on transitional epithelium of man. *J Histochem Cytochem.* 1967; 15:475.

123. Montgomerie JZ, Guze L. The renal response to infection. In: Brenner BM, Rector FC, eds. *The Kidney.* Vol 2. Philadelphia, Pennsylvania: WB Saunders; 1976.

124. Mooney JK, Mooney JS, Hinman F. The antibacterial effect of the bladder surface. An electron microscopic study. *J Urol.* 1976;115:381-386.

125. Mooreville M, Fritz RW, Mulholland SG. Enhancement of the bladder defense mechanism by an exogenous agent. *J Urol.* 1983;130:607-609.

126. Moreau PM. Neurogenic disorders of micturition in the dog and cat. *Comp Cont Educ.* 1982;4:2-21.

127. Mulholland SG, Perez JR, Gillenwater JY. The antibacterial properties of urine. *Invest Urol.* 1969;6:569-581.

128. Mulholland SG, Qureshi SM, Fritz RW, Silverman H. Effect of hormonal deprivation on the bladder defense mechanism. *J Urol.* 1982;127:1010-1013.

129. Nath KA, Hostetter MK, Hostetter TH. Pathophysiology of chronic tubulo-interstitial disease in rats. *J Clin Invest.* 1985;76: 667-675.

130. Nemeth CJ, Khan RM, Kirchner P, Adams R. Changes in canine bladder perfusion with distension. *Invest Urol.* 1977;15: 149-150.

131. Newman L, Bucy JG, McAlister WH. Experimental production of reflux in the presence and absence of infected urine. *Radiology.* 1974;111:591-595.

132. Nolan LK, et al. Comparison of virulence factors and antibiotic resistance profiles of *Escherichia coli* strains from humans and dogs with urinary tract infections. *J Vet Intern Med.* 1987; 1:152-157.

133. Norden CW, Green GH, Kass EH. Antibacterial mechanisms of the urinary bladder. *J Clin Invest.* 1968;47:2689-2700.

134. O'Grady F. Urinary tract infection: Initiation and ascent. In: Chisholm GD, Williams DI, eds. *Scientific Foundations of Urology.* 2nd ed. Chicago, Illinois: Year Book Medical; 1982:199-204.

135. O'Hanley P, Lark D, Falkow S, Schoolnik G. Molecular basis of *Escherichia coli* colonization of the upper urinary tract in Balb/c mice. *J Clin Invest.* 1985;75:347-360.

136. Oliver JE. Disorders of micturition. In: Oliver JE, Hoerlein BF, Mayhew IG, eds. *Veterinary Neurology.* Philadelphia, Pennsylvania: WB Saunders; 1987:342-352.

137. Oliver JE. Urodynamic assessment. In: Oliver JE, Hoerlein BF, Mayhew IG, eds. *Veterinary Neurology.* Philadelphia, Pennsylvania: WB Saunders; 1987:180-184.

138. Orikasa S, Hinman F. Reaction of the vesical wall to bacterial

penetration. Resistance to attachment, desquamation, and leukocytic activity. *Invest Urol.* 1977;15:185-193.

139. Osborne CA, et al. Comparison of perineal urethrostomy versus dietary management in prevention of recurrent lower urinary tract disease in male cats. *J Small Anim Pract.* 1991;32:296-305.

140. Osborne CA, Finco DR. Urinary tract infections: New solutions to old problems. In: *Scientific Proceedings of the 44th Annual Meeting of the American Animal Hospital Association.* South Bend, Indiana: American Animal Hospital Association; 1977.

141. Osborne CA, Finco DR, Low DG. Pathophysiology of renal disease, renal failure, and uremia. In: Ettinger SJ, ed. *Textbook of Veterinary Internal Medicine.* Philadelphia, Pennsylvania: WB Saunders; 1983.

142. Osborne CA, et al. Etiopathogenesis and biological behavior of feline vesicourachal diverticula. *Vet Clin North Am.* 1987;17: 633-697.

143. Osborne CA, Klausner JS. Adverse drug reactions in the uremic patient. In: Kirk RW, ed. *Current Veterinary Therapy.* Vol 6. Philadelphia, Pennsylvania: WB Saunders; 1977.

144. Osborne CA, Klausner JS, Hardy RM, Lees GE. Ancillary treatment of urinary tract infections. In: Kirk RW, ed. *Current Veterinary Therapy.* Vol 7. Philadelphia, Pennsylvania: WB Saunders; 1980.

145. Osborne CA, Klausner JS, Lees GE. Urinary tract infections: Normal and abnormal host defense mechanisms. *Vet Clin North Am.* 1979;9:587-609.

146. Osborne CA, et al. Medical management of vesicourachal diverticula in 15 cats with lower urinary tract disease. *J Small Anim Pract.* 1989;30:608-612.

147. Osborne CA, Kruger JM, Johnston GR, Polzin DJ. Feline lower urinary tract disorders. In: Ettinger SJ, ed. *Textbook of Veterinary Internal Medicine.* 3rd ed. Vol 2. Philadelphia, Pennsylvania: WB Saunders; 1989:2057-2082.

148. Osborne CA, et al. Struvite urolithiasis in animals and man. Formation, detection, and dissolution. *Adv Vet Sci Comp Med.* 1985;29:1-101.

149. Osborne CA, Polzin DJ, Feeney DA, Caywood DD. The urinary system: Pathophysiology, diagnosis, and treatment. In: Gourley IM, Vasseur PB, eds. *General Small Animal Surgery.* Philadelphia, Pennsylvania: JB Lippincott; 1985:479-658.

150. Osborne CA, Stevens JB. *Handbook of Canine and Feline Urinalysis.* St. Louis, Missouri: Ralston Purina Co.; 1981.

151. Ozanne G, Mathieu LG, Baril JP. Production of colicin V *in vitro* and *in vivo* and observations on its effects in experimental animals. *Infect Immun.* 1977;17:497-503.

152. Parsons CL, Greenspan C, Moore SW, Mulholland SG. Role of surface mucin in primary antibacterial defense of the bladder. *Urology.* 1977;9:48-52.

153. Parsons CL, Greenspan C, Mulholland SG. The primary antibacterial defense mechanism of the bladder. *Invest Urol.* 1975; 13:72-76.

154. Parsons CL, Stauffer C, Mulholland SG, Griffith DP. Effect of ammonium on bacterial adherence to bladder transitional epithelium. *J Urol.* 1984;132:365-366.

155. Pazin GJ, Braude AI. Immobilizing antibodies in urine. II. Prevention of ascending spread of *Proteus mirabilis. Invest Urol.* 1974;12:129-133.

156. Polzin DJ, Osborne CA, O'Brien TD. Diseases of the kidneys and ureters. In: Ettinger SJ, ed. *Textbook of Veterinary Internal Medicine.* 3rd ed. Vol 2. Philadelphia, Pennsylvania: WB Saunders; 1989:1962-2056.

157. Raeb WP. Diagnostic value of urinary enzyme determinations. *Clin Chem.* 1972;18:5-25.

158. Ransley PG. Vesicoureteral reflux: Continuing surgical dilemma. *Urology.* 1978;12:246-255.

158a. Rayfield EJ, et al. Infection and diabetes: The case for glucose control. *Am J Med.* 1982;72:439-450.

159. Reid G, Sobel JD. Bacterial adherence in the pathogenesis of urinary tract infection: A review. *Rev Infect Dis.* 1987;9:470-487.

160. Riley HD. Management of urinary tract infections in children. *Urol Clin North Am.* 1975;2:537-556.

161. Riviere JE. Checklist of hazardous drugs in patients with renal failure. In: Kirk RW, ed. *Current Veterinary Therapy.* Vol 8. Philadelphia, Pennsylvania: WB Saunders; 1983.

161a. Roberts JA, Fussell EN, Kaack MB. Bacterial adherence to urethral catheters. *J Urol.* 1990;144:264-269.

162. Roberts JA, Ricker P Experimental pyelonephritis in the monkey. VI. Infection of infants versus adults. *Invest Urol.* 1978;16:128-133.

163. Rocha H, et al. Experimental pyelonephritis. III. The influence of localized injury in different parts of the kidney to bacillary infection. *Yale J Biol Med.* 1958;30:341.

164. Rogers KS, Lees GE, Simpson RB. Effects of single-dose and three-day trimethoprim-sulfadiazine and amikacin treatment of induced *Escherichia coli* urinary tract infections in dogs. *Am J Vet Res.* 1988;49:345-349.

165. Rubin RH, Tolkoff-Rubin NE, Cotran RS. Urinary tract infection, pyelonephritis, and reflux nephropathy. In: Brenner BM, Rector CF, eds. *The Kidney.* 4th ed. Vol 2. Philadelphia, Pennsylvania: WB Saunders; 1991:1369-1429.

166. Ruggiers MR, et al. Defective antiadherence activity of bladder extracts from patients with recurrent urinary tract infections. *J Urol.* 1988;140:157-159.

167. Rutter JM, Burrows MR, Sellwood R, Gibbons RA. A genetic basis for resistance to enteric disease caused by *Escherichia coli. Nature (London).* 1975;257:135-136.

168. Schaeffer AJ, Stamey TA. The effect of hysterectomy on colonization of the vaginal vestibule with *Escherichia coli. Invest Urol.* 1976;14:10-12.

169. Schick E, Tanago EA. The effect of gravity on ureteral peristalsis. *J Urol.* 1973;109:187.

170. Schwartz H. Renal invasion by *E. coli* via a mucosal lesion of the sigmoid colon. A demonstration utilizing methods of autoradiography and group specific serologic typing. *Invest Urol.* 1968;6:98-113.

171. Seddon JM, Bruce AW. Cystourethritis. *Urology.* 1978;11:1-10.

172. Senior DF. Bacterial urinary tract infections: Invasion, host defenses, and new defenses, and new approaches to prevention. *Comp Cont Educ.* 1985;7:333-344.

173. Senior DF, Newman RC. Retrograde ureteral catheterization in female dogs. *J Am Anim Hosp Assoc.* 1986;22:831-834.

174. Shrom SH, Parsons CL, Mulholland SG. Role of urothelial surface mucoprotein in intrinsic bladder. *Urology.* 1977;9: 526-533.

175. Silk M, Perez-Varela MR. Effect of oral contraceptives on urinary bacterial growth rate. *Invest Urol.* 1970;8:239.

176. Silverblatt FJ, Cohen LS. Antipili antibody affords protection against experimental ascending pyelonephritis. *J Clin Invest.* 1979;64:333-336.

177. Siriwatratananonta P, Sinsakal V, Stern K, Slavin RG. Defective chemotaxis in uremia. *J Lab Clin Med.* 1978;92:402-407.

178. Smith TW, Roberts JA. Chronic pyelonephritis—electron microscopic study. II. Persistance of variant bacterial forms. *Invest Urol.* 1978;16:154-162.

179. Smith CW, et al. Effects of indwelling urinary catheters in male cats. *J Am Anim Hosp Assoc.* 1981;17:427-433.

180. Stamey TA. Pathogenesis and treatment of urinary tract infections. Baltimore, Maryland: Williams & Wilkins; 1980.

181. Stamey TA, Fair WR, Timothy MM. Antibacterial nature of prostatic fluid. *Nature.* 1968;218:444-447.

182. Stamey TA, Wehner N, Mihara G. The immunologic basis of recurrent bacteriuria. Role of cervicovaginal antibody in enterobacterial colonization of the introital mucosa. *Medicine.* 1978;57:47.

183. Stengvist K, et al. Effects of subinhibitory concentrations of antibiotics and antibodies on the adherence of *Escherichia coli* to human uroepithelial cells *in vitro. Scand J Infect Dis.* 1982; Suppl 33:104-107.

184. Svanborg Eden C, et al. Receptor analogues and anti-pili antibodies as inhibitors of bacterial attachment *in vivo* and *in vitro.* Ann NY Acad Sci. 1983;409:580-592.

185. Svanborg Eden C, et al. Host-parasite interaction in the urinary tract. *J Infect Dis.* 1988;157:421-425.

186. Svanborg-Eden C, Svennerholm AM. Secretory immunoglobulin A and G antibodies prevent adhesion of *Escherichia coli* to human urinary tract epithelial cells. *Infect Immun.* 1978;22: 790-797.

187. Svenson SB, et al. P-fimbriae of pyelonephritogenic *Escherichia coli. Eur J Clin Study Treat Infect.* 1983;11:61-67.

188. Takahashi M, Loveland DB. Bacteriuria and oral contraceptives. *JAMA.* 1974;227:762-765.

189. Tanagho EA, Meyers FH, Smith DR. Urethral resistance. Its components and implications. II. Striated muscle component. *Invest Urol.* 1969;7:195-205.

190. Tsuchida S, Sugawara H, Arai S. Ascending pyelonephritis in dogs induced by ureteral dysfunction. *Invest Urol.* 1973;10: 450-457.

191. Turck M. Localization of the site of recurrent urinary tract infections in women. *Urol Clin North Am.* 1975;2:433-441.

192. Turck M, Ronald AR, Petersdorf RG. Relapse and reinfection in chronic bacteriuria. II. Correlation between site of infection and pattern of recurrence in chronic bacteriuria. *N Engl J Med.* 1968;278:422-427.

193. Turnwald GH, et al. Comparison of single-dose and conventional trimethoprim-sulfadiazine therapy in experimental *Staphylococcus intermedius* cystitis in the female dog. *Am J Vet Res.* 1986;47:2621-2623.

194. Uehling DT. Urinary immunoglobulin excretion in induced urinary infection. *Invest Urol.* 1972;9:408-410.

195. Uehling DT, Jensen J, Balish E. Vaginal immunization against urinary tract infection. *J Urol.* 1982;128:1382-1384.

196. Uehling DT, Steihm ER. Elevated urinary secretory IgA in children with urinary tract infection. *Pediatrics.* 1971;47:40.

197. Vail DM, Allen TA, Weiser CA. Applicability of leucocyte esterase test strip in detection of canine pyuria. *J Am Vet Med Assoc.* 1986;189:1451-1453.

198. Walker SR, Callahan HJ, Fritz R, Mulholland SG. Distribution of rabbit mucosal glycoprotein throughout urinary tract. *Urology.* 1989;33:127-130.

199. Weiss RM. Ureteral function. *Urology.* 1978;12:114-133.

200. Westerlund R, et al. Characterization of *Escherichia coli* strains associated with canine urinary tract infections. *Res Vet Sci.* 1987;42:404-406.

201. Wilcke JR. Therapeutic application of sulfadiazine-trimethoprim in dogs and cats. A review. *Companion Anim Pract.* 1988;2:3-8.

202. Williams RC, Gibbons RJ. Inhibition of bacterial adherence by secretory immunoglobulin A: A mechanism of antigen disposal. *Science.* 1972;177:697-699.

203. Wilson RA, et al. Strains of *Escherichia coli* associated with urogenital disease in dogs and cats. *Am J Vet Res.* 1988;49: 743-746.

204. Wooley RE, Blue JL. Bacterial isolations from canine and feline urine. *Mod Vet Pract.* 1976;57:535-538.

205. Zimskind PD. The renal pelvis and calyces. In: Boyarsky S, et al., eds. *Urodynamics.* New York, New York: Academic Press; 1971.

CHAPTER 41

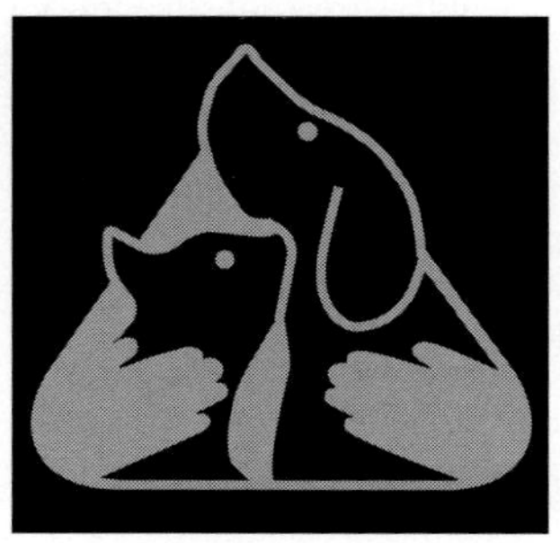

Canine and Feline Urolithiases: Relationship of Etiopathogenesis to Treatment and Prevention

CARL A. OSBORNE
JODY P. LULICH
JOSEPH W. BARTGES
LISA K. UNGER
ROSAMA THUMCHAI
LORI A. KOEHLER
KATHLEEN A. BIRD
LAWRENCE J. FELICE

I. INTRODUCTION

A. Urolithiasis may affect 1.5 to 3.0% of all dogs admitted for medical care and more than 25% of cats with lower urinary tract disorders. Recurrence of uroliths following their removal or dissolution is common. Uroliths are always the result of one or more underlying inherited, congenital, or acquired disorders; Therefore, the detection of uroliths should not be accepted as the end point of diagnostic investigation, but rather as the beginning.

B. During the past decade, medical protocols designed to promote dissolution of canine and feline struvite uroliths, canine ammonium urate uroliths, and canine cystine uroliths have been developed. Likewise, medical protocols designed to minimize urolith recurrence have been improved. Nonetheless, surgical removal remains the preferred method for removing all types of nephroliths and ureteroliths that obstruct urine flow and for active uroliths composed of calcium oxalate, calcium phosphate, or silica.

C. Our primary objective in this chapter is to review the etiology and pathophysiology of various types of urolithiasis, with the goal of applying these principles to diagnosis, treatment, and prevention of stones. Many clinical recommendations have been condensed into tabular form, to facilitate their clinical application.

II. CHEMICAL AND PHYSICAL CHARACTERISTICS OF UROLITHS

A. Terminology.

1. The urinary system is designed to dispose of body wastes in liquid form; however, some waste products are sparingly soluble and occasionally precipitate out of solution. In the past, confusion has resulted from the use of various terms to describe precipitates that form in urine. Depending on the size and consistency of the precipitates, they have been referred to as *crystals, sand, sabulous plugs, gravel, pebbles, stones, rocks, uroliths,* and *calculi.*
2. The word *crystal* is derived from the Greek word *krystallosus,* which means *ice* and is used to refer to the solid phase of substances having a specific

internal structure and enclosed by symmetrically arranged planar surfaces. The term *sabulous* is derived from the Latin word *sabulosus* meaning *sand.* The Latin word *calculus* means *pebble.* The Greek word *lithos* means *stone,* and *-uria* is a suffix derived from a Greek word *(ouron)* meaning *urine.* The preferred terminology for abnormal microscopic precipitates in urine is *crystalluria,* whereas macroscopic concretions are called *uroliths.*

3. Plugs are defined as objects of any composition that close or obstruct passageways or ducts. Pending further studies, urethral plugs should be described in terms that reflect their approximate proportions and type of minerals and matrix. Because there are physical and, probable etiopathogenic differences between feline uroliths and urethral plugs, these terms should not be used interchangeably. Uroliths are polycrystalline concretions composed primarily of minerals (organic and inorganic crystalloids) and smaller quantities of matrix. In contrast, feline urethral plugs commonly are composed of large quantities of matrix mixed with minerals.[8,155] Some urethral plugs are composed primarily of matrix, others primarily of aggregates of crystalline minerals, and some consist of sloughed tissue, blood, or inflammatory reactants (see Chapter 35, Disorders of the Feline Lower Urinary Tract).[147]
4. Uroliths may be named according to mineral composition (Tables 41–1 to 41–5), location—nephroliths (Figs. 41–1 to 41–4), renoliths, ureteroliths (Fig. 41–5), urocystoliths (Figs. 41–6, 41–7), vesical calculi, urethroliths (Fig. 41–7), or shape—smooth, faceted, pyramidal, laminated (Figs. 41–8 to 41–10), mulberry, jackstone, (Figs. 41–11 to 41–13), staghorn (Fig. 41–4) or branched (see Fig. 41–2).
5. Characteristic shapes of crystals and uroliths are influenced primarily by the internal structure of crystals and the environment in which they form.
   a. Crystals of calcium oxalate monohydrate tend to fuse, producing smoothly rounded or mamillated uroliths (Figs. 41–14, 41–15). Crystals of calcium oxalate dihydrate typically produce uroliths with sharp spiculated surfaces (Figs. 41–14, 41–15).
   b. Amorphous silica commonly produces stones that resemble small, pronged metal pieces used in the children's game of jacks, and thus the name *jackstone* (Figs. 41–11, 41–12, 41–13, 41–16).
   c. Ammonium urate usually forms tan to brown, smooth stones with concentric layers (Figs. 41–9, 41–14, 41–17).
6. Local factors influence the size and shape of uroliths.
   a. Number of uroliths.
   b. Degree and duration of contact of multiple uroliths with each other.
   c. Mobility or fixation of uroliths.
   d. Flow characteristics of urine.
   e. Anatomic configuration of the structure in which uroliths grow.
   f. Foreign bodies such as hair, suture material, and catheters around which lithogenic minerals precipitate (Figs. 41–18, 41–19).

B. Mineral composition.

1. Uroliths.
   a. The most common mineral found in uroliths of dogs and cats is magnesium ammonium phosphate (see Tables 41–1 to 41–5).[119]
   b. Calcium oxalate (monohydrate and dihydrate), ammonium acid urate, uric acid, xanthine, calcium phosphate, cystine, and silica occur much less frequently. In contrast, calcium-containing uroliths (calcium oxalate and calcium phosphate) are most prevalent in humans who live in developed countries of the world.
   c. Trace elements, including iron, copper, zinc, tin, lead, and aluminum, have been identified in human uroliths.[133] It is logical to suspect that they may also occur in animals' uroliths. These elements appear to be incorporated into uroliths by adsorption during growth. Some may play a role in initiation or growth of uroliths.[186]
   d. Even though a particular mineral usually predominates, the mineral composition of many uroliths may be mixed (see Tables 41–1 to 41–5). Different minerals may be intimately mixed with each other or separated into discrete bands or layers.
   e. On occasion, the center of a compound urolith may be composed of one type of crystalloid (e.g., silica), whereas outer layers are composed of a different crystalloid (especially struvite; Fig. 41–20).
   f. Detection, treatment, and prevention of the causes underlying urolithiasis depend on knowledge of the composition and structure of all portions of uroliths.
2. Nephroliths.
   a. Canine nephroliths (see Figs. 41–2, 41–3, and 41–21).
      (1). During a 12-year period, 17,610 canine uroliths were analyzed by quantitative methods at the Minnesota Urolith Center. Of these, 226 (1.3%) were nephroliths. Urolithiasis affected the kidneys alone in 154 of 226 cases, whereas in 72 of 226 cases, they affected the kidneys and other portions of the tract. Nephroliths composed of calcium salts comprised 43% of the total (see Table 41–3).
      (2). Calcium oxalate. Thirty-nine percent of the canine nephroliths were composed predominantly of calcium oxalate. They affected males (54%) more often than

TABLE 41–1.
MINERAL COMPOSITION OF 30,642 CANINE UROLITHS EVALUATED AT THE MINNESOTA UROLITH CENTER BY QUANTITATIVE METHODS, 1981 TO 1994

Predominant Mineral Type	Composition* (%)	Uroliths (No.)	Uroliths (%)
Magnesium ammonium phosphate $6H_2O$		16542	54.0
	100	(9654)	(31.5)
	70–99*	(6888)	(22.5)
Magnesium hydrogen phosphate $3H_2O$		2	<0.1
	100	(1)	(<0.1)
	70–99	(1)	(<0.1)
Calcium oxalate		8557	27.9
Calcium oxalate monohydrate			
	100	(2706)	(8.8)
	70–99	(2560)	(8.4)
Calcium oxalate dihydrate			
	100	(1009)	(3.3)
	70–99	(1194)	(3.9)
Calcium oxalate monohydrate and dihydrate			
	100	(767)	(2.5)
	70–99	(321)	(1.1)
Calcium phosphate		237	0.8
Calcium phosphate			
	100	(58)	(0.2)
	70–99	(85)	(0.3)
Calcium hydrogen phosphate $2H_2O$			
	100	(48)	(0.2)
	70–99	(45)	(0.2)
Tricalcium phosphate			
	70–99	(1)	(<0.1)
Purines		2130	7.0
Ammonium acid urate			
	100	(1546)	(5.1)
	70–99	(359)	(1.2)
Sodium acid urate			
	100	(112)	(0.4)
	70–99	(20)	(<0.1)
Sodium calcium urate			
	100	(33)	(0.1)
	70–99	(11)	(<0.1)
Ammonium calcium urate			
	70–99	(1)	(<0.1)
Uric acid			
	100	(11)	(<0.1)
	70–99	(7)	(<0.1)
Xanthine			
	100	(23)	(<0.1)
	70–99	(7)	(<0.1)
		405	1.3
Cystine	100	(389)	(1.3)
	70–99	(16)	(<0.1)
Silica		356	1.2
	100	(232)	(0.8)
	70–99	(124)	(0.4)
Dolomite	100%	1	<0.1
Mixed†		623	2.0
Compound‡		1755	5.7
Matrix		32	0.1
Drug metabolite		2	<0.1
Total		30,642	100

*The 70–99 indicates uroliths were composed of 70–99% of mineral type listed; no nucleus or shell detected.
†Uroliths did not contain at least 70% of mineral type listed; no nucleus or shell detected.
‡Uroliths contained an identifiable nucleus and one or more surrounding layers of a different mineral type.

TABLE 41–2.
MINERAL COMPOSITION OF 6335 FELINE UROLITHS EVALUATED BY QUANTITATIVE METHODS*

Predominant Mineral Type	Composition† (%)	Uroliths (No.)	Uroliths (%)
Magnesium ammonium phosphate $6H_2O$		3413	53.9
	100	(2904)	(45.8)
	70–99	(509)	(8.0)
Magnesium hydrogen phosphate $3H_2O$		16	0.3
	70–99	(16)	(0.3)
Calcium oxalate		2037	37.2
Calcium oxalate monohydrate			
	100	(738)	(11.6)
	70–99	(704)	(11.1)
Calcium oxalate dihydrate			
	100	(69)	(1.2)
	70–99	(234)	(3.7)
Calcium oxalate monohydrate and dihydrate			
	100	(269)	(4.2)
	70–99	(231)	(0.4)
Calcium phosphate		68	1.1
Calcium phosphate			
	100	(23)	(0.3)
	70–99	(29)	(0.5)
Calcium hydrogen phosphate $2H_2O$			
	100	(5)	(0.1)
	70–99	(9)	(0.2)
Tricalcium phosphate			
	100	(1)	(<0.1)
	70–99	(1)	(<0.1)
Uric acid and urates		432	6.8
Ammonium acid urate			
	100	(327)	(5.2)
	70–99	(97)	(1.5)
Sodium urate			
	70–99	(1)	(<0.1)
Uric acid			
	100	(4)	(0.1)
	70–99	(3)	(<0.1)
Cystine		22	0.3
Xanthine		9	0.1
Silica		0	0
Mixed‡		118	1.9
Compound§		115	1.8
Matrix		106	2.0
Total		6335	100

*Uroliths analyzed by polarized light microscopy and x-ray diffraction methods.
†The 70–99 indicates uroliths were composed of 70–99% of mineral type listed; no nucleus or shell detected.
‡Uroliths did not contain at least 70% of mineral type listed; no nucleus or shell detected.
§Uroliths contained an identifiable nucleus and one or more surrounding layers of a different mineral type.

females (44%). The gender of 2% of the patients with calcium oxalate nephroliths was not specified. The mean age of dogs with calcium oxalate nephroliths was 9.4 ± 2.4 years (range, 3.8 months to 14 years). Twenty-four different breeds had calcium oxalate nephroliths. The breeds most commonly affected were miniature schnauzers (18.2%), Lhasa Apsos (12.5%), Yorkshire terriers (11.4%), miniature poodles (11.4%), and Shih Tzus (10.2%). These breeds are apparently pre-

TABLE 41–3.
MINERAL COMPOSITION OF 226 CANINE NEPHROLITHS EVALUATED BY QUANTITATIVE METHODS

Predominant Mineral Type	Proportion of Predominant Mineral* (%)	Uroliths (No.)	Uroliths (%)
Calcium oxalate		88	39
Calcium oxalate 1H_2O	70–100	(70)	(31)
Calcium oxalate 2H_2O	70–100	(13)	(6)
Calcium oxalate 1H_2O and 2H_2O	70–100	(5)	(2)
Calcium phosphate		9	4
Calcium apatite	70–100	(8)	(4)
Calcium hydrogen phosphate 2H_2O	70–100	(1)	(<1)
Magnesium ammonium phosphate 6H_2O	70–100	79	35
Purines		18	8
Ammonium acid urate	70–100	(16)	(7)
Sodium acid urate	70–100	(1)	(<1)
Xanthine	70–100	(1)	(<1)
Silica	70–100	1	<1
Mixed†		17	8
Compound‡		9	4
Matrix		5	2
Total		226	100

*The 70–100 indicates uroliths were composed of at least 70% of mineral type listed; no nucleus or shell was detected.
†Uroliths contained less than 70% of predominant mineral; no nucleus or shell were detected.
‡Uroliths contained an identifiable nucleus and one or more surrounding layers of a different mineral.

TABLE 41–4.
MINERAL COMPOSITION OF 113 FELINE NEPHROLITHS EVALUATED BY QUANTITATIVE METHODS

Predominant Mineral Type	Proportion of Predominant Mineral* (%)	Uroliths (No.)	Uroliths (%)
Calcium oxalate		48	43
Calcium oxalate 1H_2O	70–100	(45)	(40)
Calcium oxalate 2H_2O	70–100	(1)	(1)
Calcium oxalate 1H_2O and 2H_2O	70–100	(2)	(2)
Calcium phosphate		17	15
Calcium apatite	70–100	(16)	(14)
Tricalcium phosphate	70–100	(1)	(1)
Magnesium ammonium phosphate	70–100	6	5
Mixed†		13	12
Compound‡		1	<1
Matrix		28	25
Total		113	100

*Uroliths were composed of at least 70% of mineral type listed; no nucleus or shell were detected.
†Uroliths contained less than 70% of predominant mineral; no nucleus or shell were detected.
‡Uroliths contained an identifiable nucleus and one or more surrounding layers of a different mineral.

TABLE 41–5.
MINERAL COMPOSITION OF 820 FELINE URETHRAL PLUGS ANALYZED BY QUANTITATIVE METHODS*

Predominant Mineral Type	Composition† (%)	Uroliths (No.)	Uroliths (%)
Magnesium ammonium phosphate $6H_2O$		636	77.6
	100	(540)	(65.9)
	70–99	(96)	(11.7)
Newberyite		3	0.4
	100	(1)	(0.1)
	77–99	(2)	(0.3)
Calcium oxalate		14	1.7
Calcium oxalate monohydrate			
	100	(4)	(0.5)
	70–99	(5)	(0.6)
Calcium oxalate dihydrate			
	100	(2)	(0.2)
	70–99	(2)	(0.2)
Calcium oxalate monohydrate and dihydrate			
		(1)	(0.1)
Calcium phosphate		21	2.6
Calcium phosphate			
	100	(11)	(1.3)
	70–99	(7)	(0.9)
Calcium hydrogen phosphate $2H_2O$			
	100	(2)	(0.3)
	70–99	(1)	(0.1)
Ammonium acid urate		6	0.7
	100	(6)	(0.7)
Xanthine		1	0.1
Sulfadiazine		1	0.1
Mixed‡		27	3.3
Matrix		113	13.4
Total		820	100

*Urethral plugs examined by polarizing light microscopy and x-ray diffraction methods.
†The 70–99 indicates uroliths were composed of 70–99% of mineral type listed; no nucleus or shell detected.
‡Uroliths did not contain at least 70% of mineral type listed; no nucleus or shell detected.

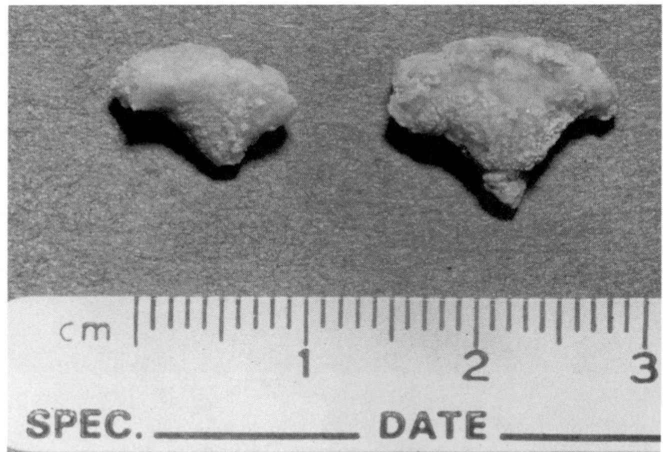

FIG. 41–1. Photograph of infected struvite uroliths removed from the renal pelves of a 5-year-old, female cat. (Courtesy of Dr. Lyle Hanson, Fond du Lac, Wisconsin.)

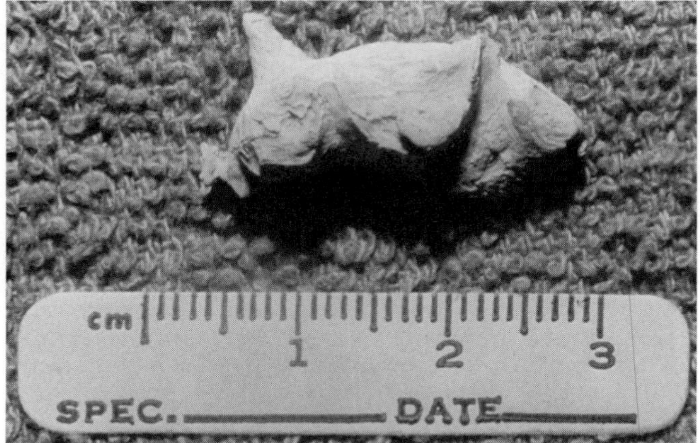

FIG. 41–2. Branched renolith composed of ammonium acid urate removed from the left kidney of a 2-year-old male Dalmatian. Note the branches shaped by diverticula of the renal pelvis. (*Vet Clin North Am.* 1986;16:1–207.)

disposed to calcium oxalate urolithiasis. Among 4,509 dogs with calcium oxalate uroliths, 91.5% of stones were located in the bladder and urethra, 3.1% affected the kidneys and ureters, and 1% were voided. The location of 4.4% of calcium oxalate uroliths removed from dogs was not specified.

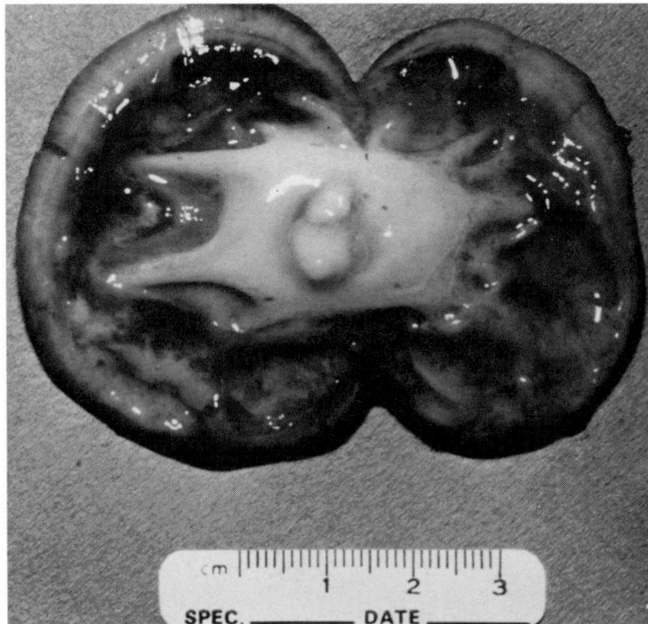

FIG. 41–3. Pyonephrosis associated with obstruction of the proximal ureter with *Staphylococcus*-induced struvite nephroliths in a 3-year-old female miniature schnauzer. Despite the relatively small size of the uroliths, obstruction to urine outflow combined with bacterial infection destroyed the kidney, necessitating nephrectomy.

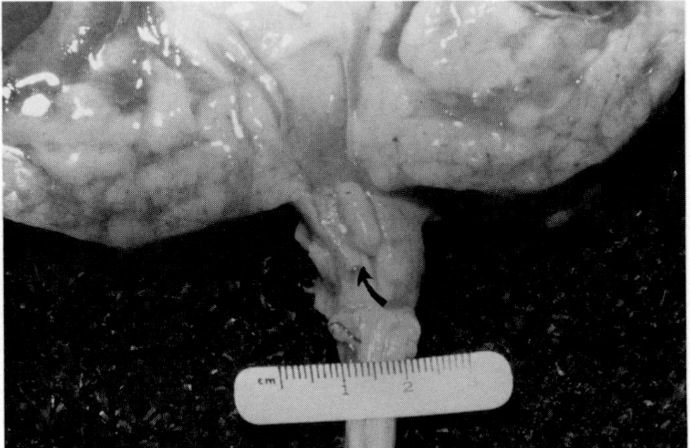

FIG. 41–5. Ureterolith *(arrow)* lodged in the proximal lumen of the left ureter of a 4-year-old female malamute. Most of the renal parenchyma has been destroyed by obstruction to urine outflow and secondary UTI with urease-producing *Proteus mirabilis.* (From Osborne CA, et al. Struvite urolithiasis in animals and man: Formation, detection, and dissolution. *Adv Vet Sci Comp Med.* 1985;29:1–101.)

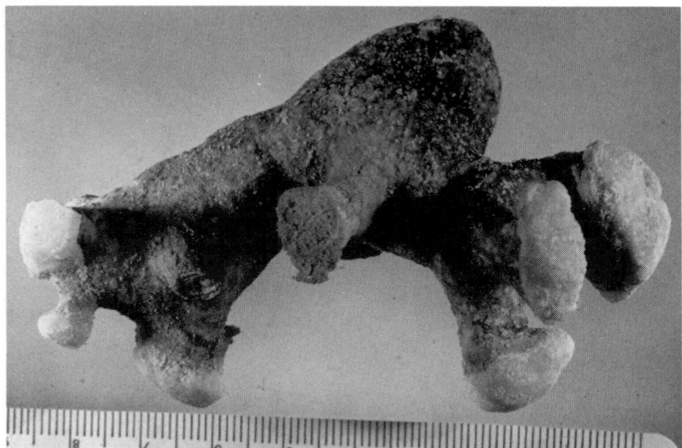

FIG. 41–4. Staghorn struvite urolith removed from the kidney of an adult human being. Animals with unipyramidal kidneys (such as dogs and cats) cannot form true staghorn uroliths. (Compare to Figs. 41–82 to 41–86; from Osborne CA (ed). Canine urolithiasis: etiopathogenesis, detection, treatment, and prevention. *Vet Clin North Am.* 1986;16:1–207.)

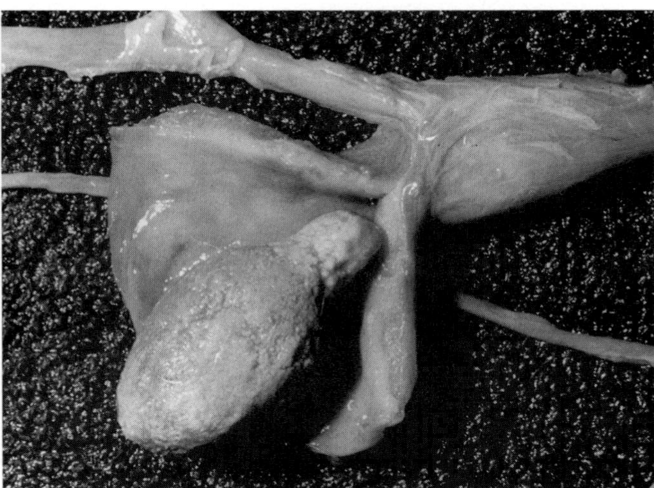

FIG. 41–6. Struvite urolith formed in the shape of the lumens of the urinary bladder and proximal urethra of a 9-year-old female Pekingese. (From Osborne CA (ed). Canine urolithiasis: etiopathogenesis, detection, treatment, and prevention. *Vet Clin North Am.* 1986;16:1–207.)

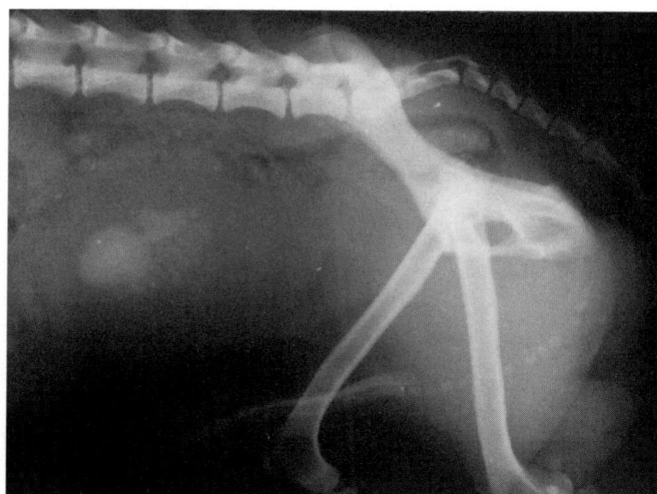

FIG. 41–7. Abdominal radiograph of a 7-year-old male Chihuahua with cystic and urethral calculi. The wall of the urinary bladder is markedly thickened. (From Piermattei DL, Osborne CA: Nonsurgical removal of calculi from the urethra of male dogs. *JAVMA*. 1971;159:1755–1757.)

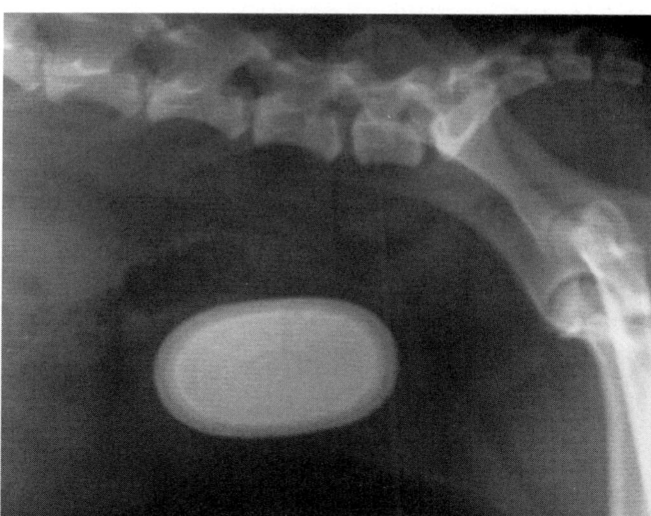

FIG. 41–8. Laminated urocystoliths in a 6-year-old spayed female pug. The urocystolith was caused by staphylococcal UTI. The laminated appearance is associated with varying quantities of matrix (which is not radiodense) mixed with struvite (which is radiodense).

(3). Struvite. Thirty-four percent of the canine nephroliths were composed of struvite. In contrast to calcium oxalate stones, those of struvite affected females (76%) more often than males (19%). The gender of 5% of the dogs with struvite nephroliths was not recorded. The higher prevalence of struvite urolithiasis in female dogs is likely associated with the higher prevalence of bacterial urinary tract infection (UTI) in females. The mean age of dogs with struvite nephrolithiasis was 7 ± 3 years (range, 17 months to 15 years). Twenty-

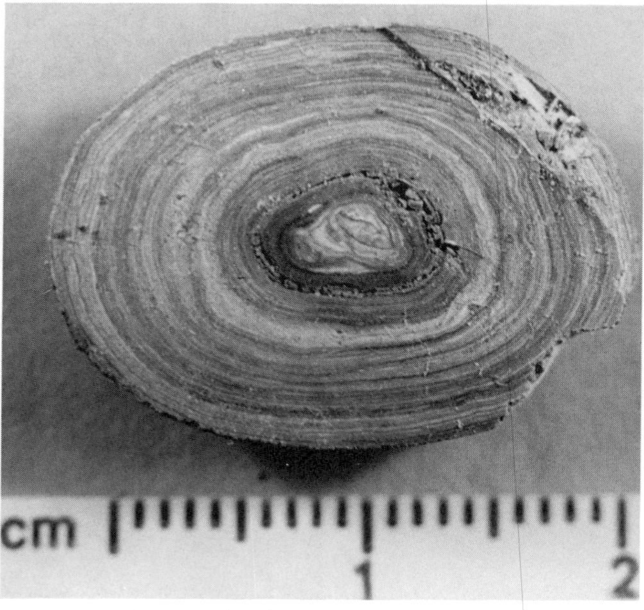

FIG. 41–9. Photograph of a cross section of a pure (100%) ammonium acid urate urocystolith removed from a 7-year-old spayed female Yorkshire terrier. Note the typical concentric laminations and central nucleus. (From Osborne CA (ed). Canine urolithiasis: etiopathogenesis, detection, treatment, and prevention. *Vet Clin North Am*. 1986;16:1–207.)

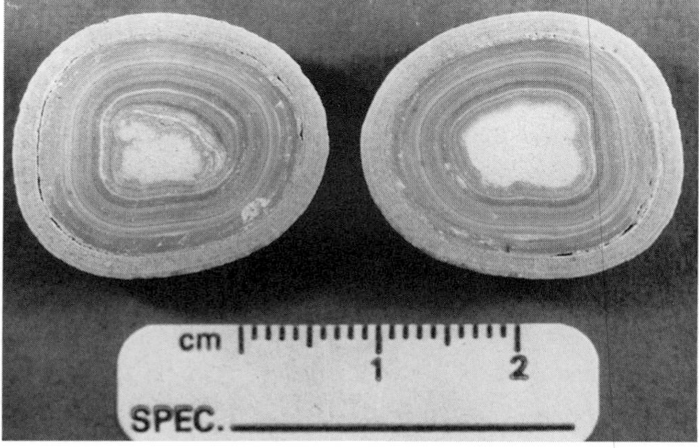

FIG. 41–10. Cross section of a urolith removed from the urinary bladder of a dog. The shell of the urolith is composed of 50% magnesium ammonium phosphate, 30% ammonium acid urate, and 20% calcium apatite. The nucleus was composed of an unidentified substance (perhaps a drug metabolite).

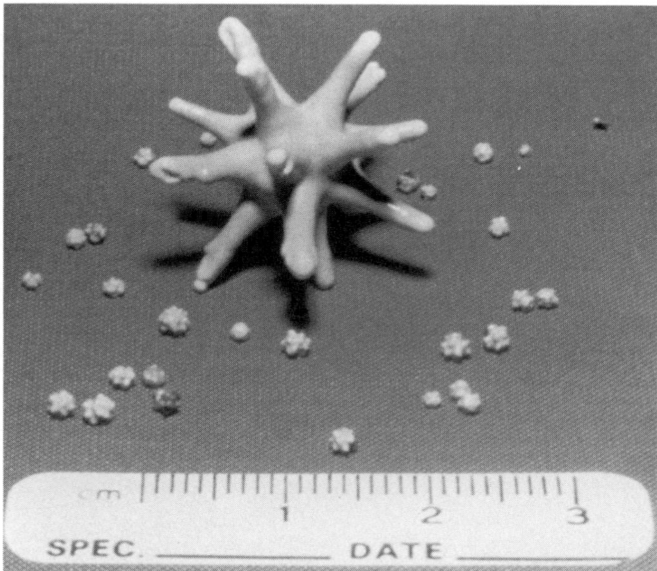

FIG. 41–11. Urocystolith with jackstone configuration removed from an 8-year-old miniature schnauzer. The urolith was composed of amorphous silica. (From Osborne CA (ed). Canine urolithiasis: etiopathogenesis, detection, treatment, and prevention. *Vet Clin North Am.* 1986;16:1–207.)

two different breeds had struvite nephroliths. The breeds commonly affected were miniature schnauzers (17.7%), bichon frise (10.1%), Shi Tzu (7.6%), Yorkshire terrier (6.3%), Lhasa Apso (6.3%), cocker spaniel (6.3%), and miniature poodle (6.3%). Among 9,927 dogs with struvite uroliths, 89.4% were located in the bladder and urethra, 4.6% were voided, and 1.2% were in the kidneys and ureters. The location of 4.9% of the struvite uroliths removed from dogs was not specified.

(4). Purines. Eight percent of the canine nephroliths were composed of ammonium urate, sodium urate, or xanthine. Purine nephroliths affected males (56%) more frequently than females (28%). The gender of 16% of the dogs with purine nephroliths was not specified. The mean age of dogs with purine nephroliths was 4.8 ± 3.5 years (range, 3 months to 12 years). Twelve different breeds had purine nephroliths. The breeds most commonly affected were dalmatian (18%), Yorkshire terrier (18%), and English bulldog (12%). Of 1,078 dogs' purine uroliths, 86% were located in the bladder and urethra, 7.1% were voided, and 2.1% affected the kidneys and ureters. The location of 4.8% of the purine uroliths removed from dogs was not specified.

b. Feline nephroliths (see Fig. 41–1).

(1). During a 12-year period, 3,989 feline uroliths were analyzed by quantitative methods at the Minnesota Urolith Center. Of these, 113 (2.8%) were nephroliths. Urolithiasis in 95 of 113 cases affected only the kidneys, whereas 18 of 113 affected the kidneys and other portions of the urinary tract. Nephroliths composed of calcium salts comprised 58% of the total (see Table 41–4).

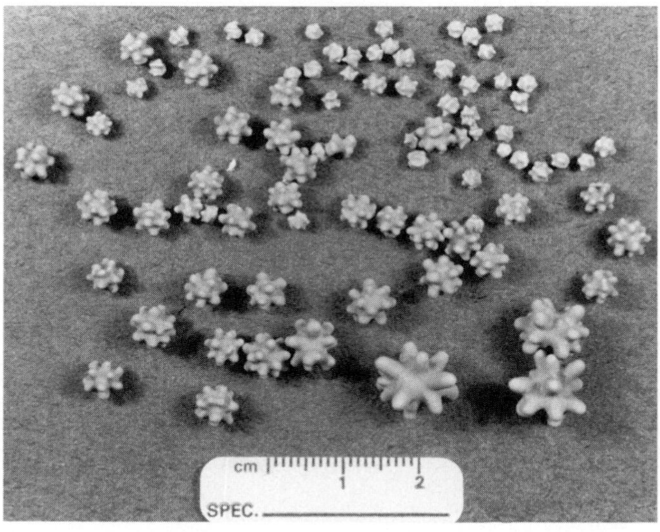

FIG. 41–12. Multiple silica urocystoliths with jackstone configuration removed from a 10-year-old border collie. (Courtesy of Dr. John McCarthy, New York, NY.)

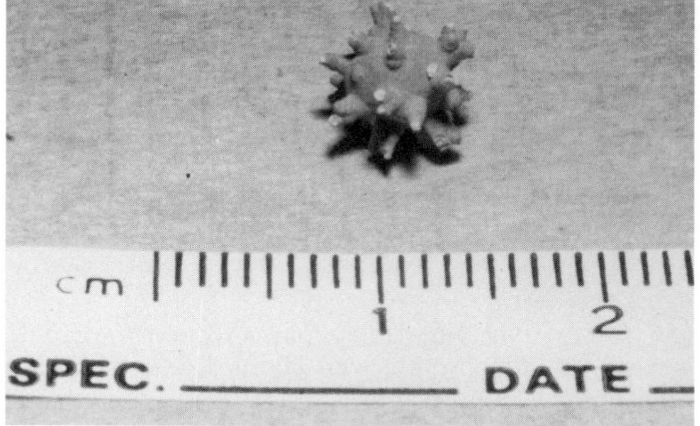

FIG. 41–13. Ammonium urate jackstone removed from the urinary bladder of a 9-year-old Persian cat. (Courtesy of Dr. C.P. Ryan.)

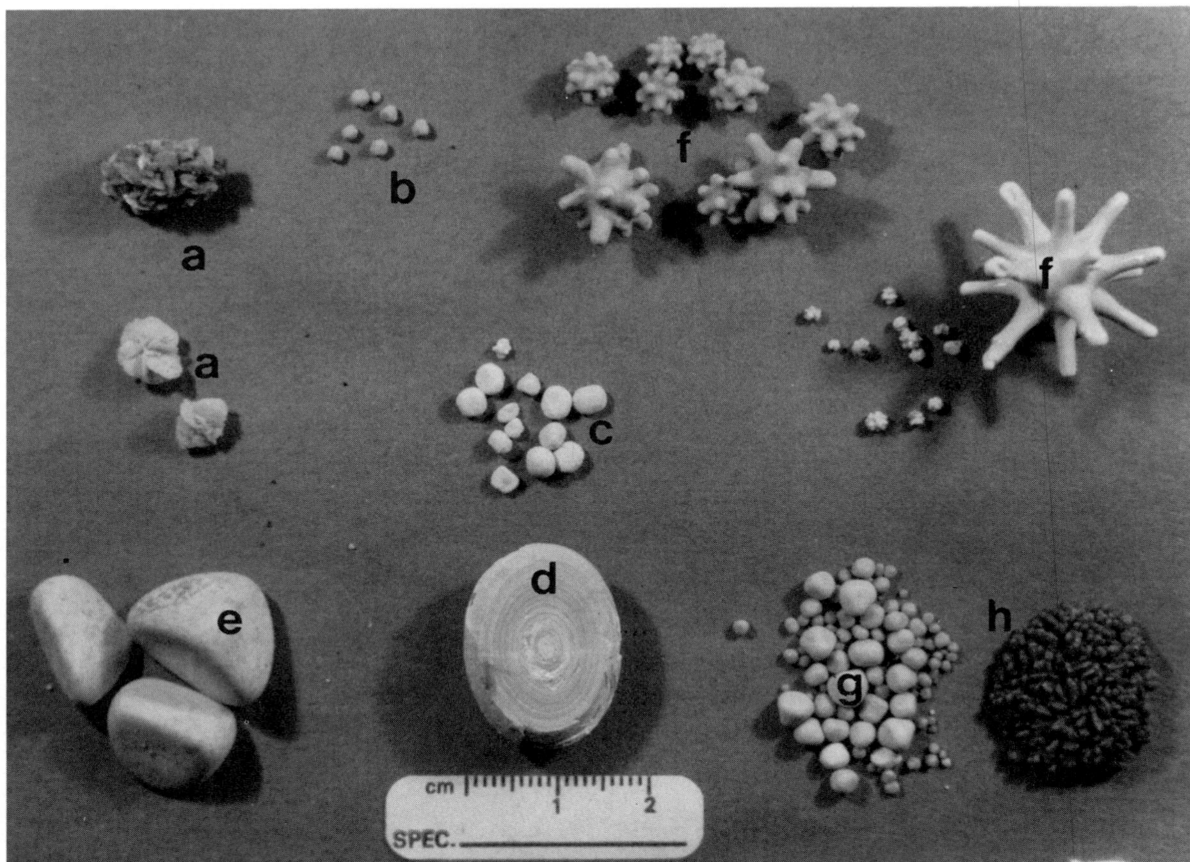

FIG. 41–14. Photograph of common shapes of some canine uroliths. Key: a, calcium oxalate dihydrate; b, calcium oxalate monohydrate; c, ammonium urate; d, cross section of ammonium urate; e, magnesium ammonium phosphate; f, silica; g, cystine; h, atypical cystine.

(2). Calcium oxalate. Forty three percent of the feline nephroliths were composed of calcium oxalate. Calcium oxalate stones affected males (54%) more often than females (42%). The gender of 4% of the patients with calcium oxalate nephroliths was not specified. The mean age of cats with calcium oxalate nephroliths was 7.9 years ± 3.9 (range, 2 to 18 years). Five different breeds had calcium oxalate nephroliths: domestic short-haired (52%), domestic long-haired, (15%), Siamese (6%), Persian (8%), and unknown (19%). Of 1,004 cats with calcium oxalate uroliths, 85.7% were located in the bladder and urethra, 6.6% in the kidneys and ureters, and 3.5% were voided. The location of 3.9% of the calcium oxalate uroliths removed from cats was not specified.

(3). Struvite. Surprisingly, only 5% of the feline nephroliths were composed of magnesium ammonium phosphate. Struvite nephroliths affected males (83%) more commonly than females (17%). The mean age of cats with struvite nephroliths was 6 ± 3.8 years (range, 2 months to 11 years). Four breeds had struvite nephroliths; those most affected were domestic short-haired (33%), domestic long-haired (17%), and unknown (33%). Of 2,467 cats' struvite uroliths, 90% were located in the bladder and urethra, 4% were voided, and 0.3% were located in the kidneys or ureters. The location of 5.4% of the struvite uroliths removed from dogs was not specified.

3. Urethral plugs.
   a. A variety of minerals have been identified in urethral plugs of cats (see Table 41–5).
   b. The mineral composition of urethral plugs should be used to describe them, since, often, therapeutic regimens are influenced by knowledge of their mineral composition (see Chapter 35, Disorders of the Feline Lower Urinary Tract).

C. Matrix composition.

1. The nondialysable portion of uroliths that remains after crystalline components have been dissolved with mild solvents is organic matrix.
   a. Uroliths consistently contain variable quantities of organic matrix substances in addition to crystalloids.[142]
   b. Organic matrix substances identified in human uroliths and produced experimentally in animals include matrix substances A, Tamm-Horsfall mucoprotein (uromucoid), serum albumin, and alpha- and gamma-globulins.[178] Of these, matrix substances A and Tamm-Horsfall mucoprotein appear to be quantitatively more significant than alpha- and gamma-globulins.
2. The macromolecular complex of diverse mucoprotein compounds comprising matrix substances has been hypothesized by some to represent the skeleton of uroliths.
   a. In vitro studies utilizing human urine revealed that polymerized Tamm-Horsfall protein is related to formation of calcium oxalate crystals.[32,181] Tamm-Horsfall mucoprotein may also play a role in the formation of feline urethral plugs.
   b. Although the physical characteristics of uroliths suggest an organized relationship between the matrix skeleton and crystalline building blocks, the role of each of these components in formation, retention, and growth of uroliths is still ill-understood.
3. In summary, different types of organic matrix may affect urolith formation by one or more of several mechanisms.
   a. Serving as a site for crystal formation (heterogenous nucleation).
   b. Acting as a template for organizing and modifying growth of crystals.
   c. Serving as a binding agent that cements calculus particles together and promotes retention of crystals.
   d. Protective colloids that prevent further growth of calculi.
   e. Remaining passive, having no effect on urolith formation or growth.

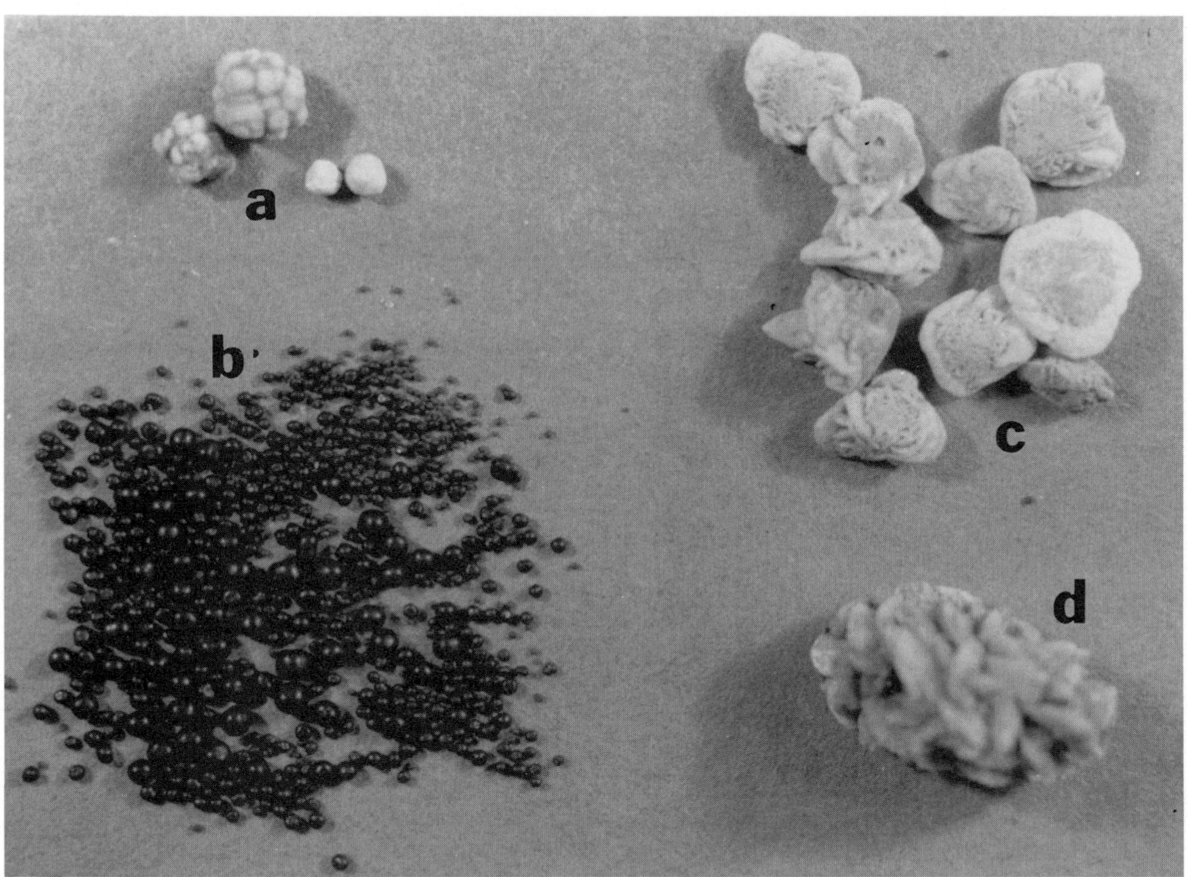

FIG. 41–15. Comparison of the smooth contour of uroliths composed of calcium oxalate monohydrate (a, b) to sharp-edged surface protrusions typical of uroliths composed of calcium oxalate dihydrate (c, d).

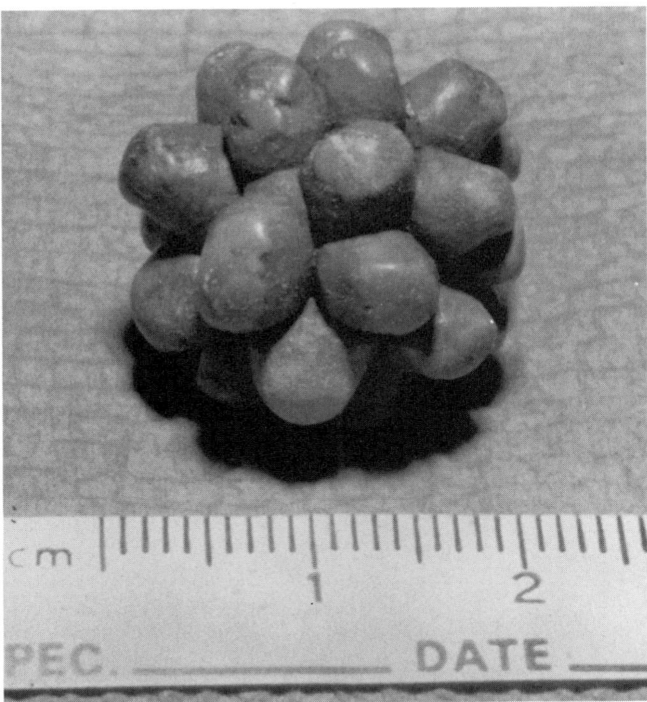

FIG. 41–16. Silica urocystolith with jackstone configuration removed from a 9-year-old male German shepherd. (From Osborne CA (ed). Canine urolithiasis: etiopathogenesis, detection, treatment, and prevention. *Vet Clin North Am.* 1986;16:1–207.)

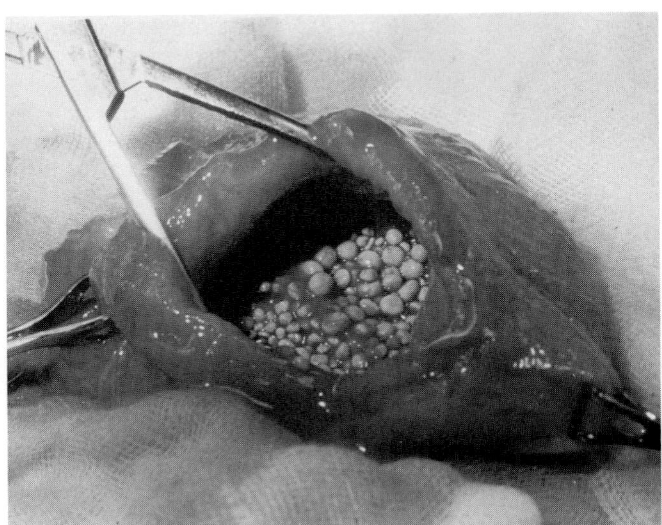

FIG. 41–17. Multiple ammonium acid urate uroliths in the urinary bladder of a 10-year-old male Dalmatian. (From Osborne CA (ed). Canine urolithiasis: etiopathogenesis, detection, treatment, and prevention. *Vet Clin North Am.* 1986;16:1–207.)

III. INITIATION AND GROWTH OF UROLITHS

A. Overview. Urolith formation is associated with two complementary but separate phases: initiation and growth.

1. It appears that initiating events are not the same for all types of uroliths.

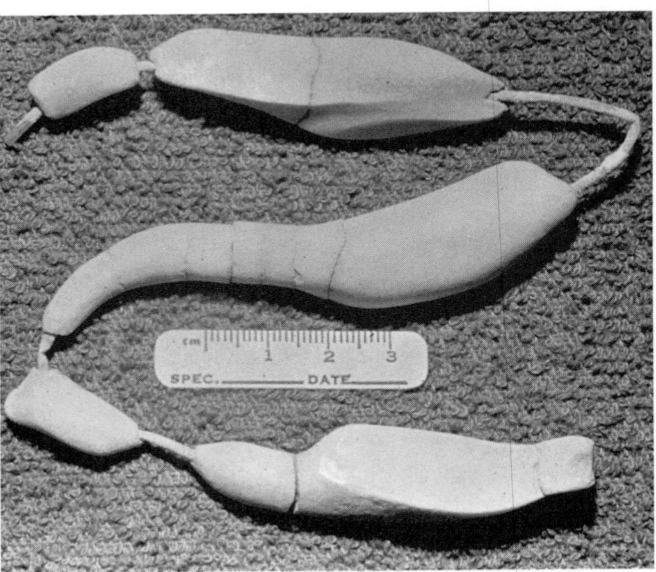

FIG. 41–18. Ammonium acid urate urolith formation around a portion of urinary catheter trapped in the urinary bladder of an adult male Dalmatian. (Courtesy of Christabel Frederick, Lake Bluff, Illinois.)

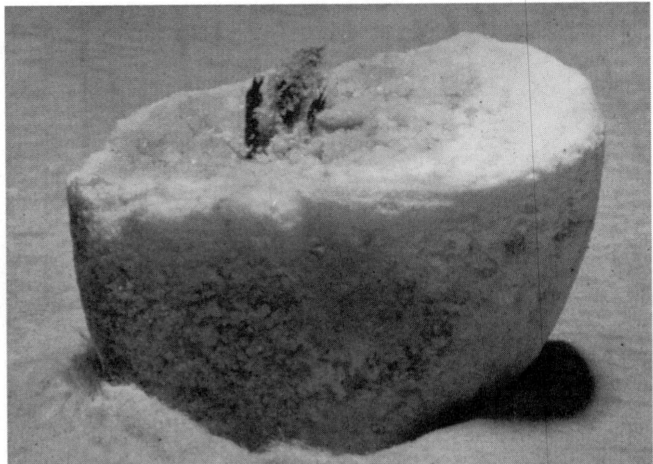

FIG. 41–19. Suture material in the center of a struvite urolith removed from the urinary bladder of an adult male mixed-breed dog. (From Osborne CA, Polzin DJ, Abdullahi SU, et al. Struvite urolithiasis in animals and man: Formation, detection and dissolution. *Adv Vet Sci Comp Med.* 1985;29:1.)

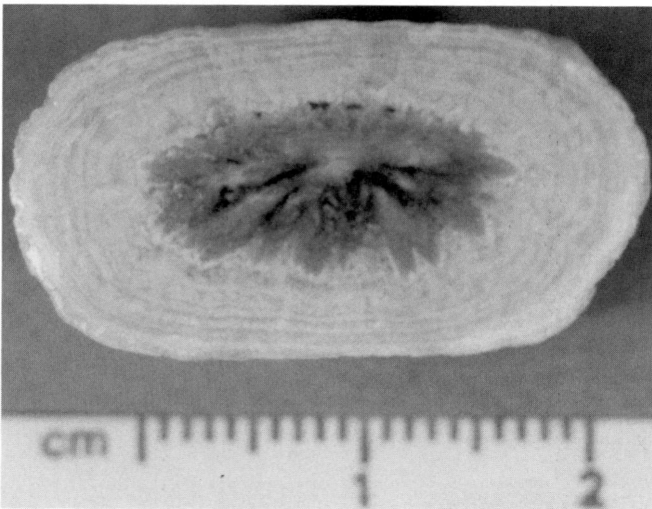

FIG. 41–20. Cross section of a compound urocystolith formed by a 12-year-old spayed female toy poodle with a staphylococcal UTI and struvite crystalluria. The nucleus of the urolith is composed of 100% calcium oxalate; the shell, of 70% struvite and 30% calcium apatite.

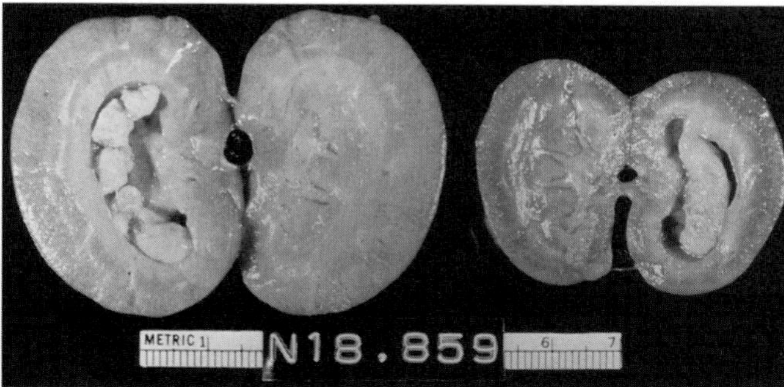

FIG. 41–21. Generalized pyelonephritis and hydronephrosis associated with struvite urolithiasis and UTI of a 15-year-old female toy Manchester terrier. (From Osborne CA (ed). Canine urolithiasis: etiopathogenesis, detection, treatment, and prevention. *Vet Clin North Am.* 1985;16:1–207.)

2. In addition, factors that initiate urolith formation may be different from those that allow them to grow.

B. Initiation.

1. The initial step in the development of a urolith is the formation of a crystal nidus (or crystal embryo). This phase of initiation of urolith formation (called *nucleation*) is dependent on supersaturation and oversaturation of urine with lithogenic crystalloids (Fig. 41–22). The degree of supersaturation may be influenced by the magnitude of renal excretion of the cystalloid, urine pH, and crystallization inhibitors in urine.
2. Determinants of further growth of the crystal nidus.
   a. Its ability to remain in the urinary tract.
   b. The degree and duration of supersaturation or oversaturation of urine with crystalloids identical to or different from that of the nidus.
   c. Physical characteristics of the crystal nidus.
3. Several theories have been proposed to explain the initiation of lithogenesis. Each theory emphasizes a single factor. On the basis of current knowledge, the most popular hypotheses are the precipitation-crystallization theory, the matrix-nucleation theory, and the crystallization-inhibition theory. These theories are not mutually exclusive.
   a. Precipitation-crystallization theory.
      (1). This hypothesis incriminates excessive supersaturation of urine with stone-forming crystalloids as the primary event in lithogenesis.
      (2). In this hypothesis, nucleation (initiation of urolith formation) is considered a physiochemical process of precipitation of crystalloids from a supersaturated solution.
      (3). Urolith formation is thought to be independent of preformed matrix or inhibitors of crystallization.
      (4). According to this hypothesis, production of urine excessively saturated with one or more urolith-forming crystalloids leads to spontaneous nucleation of the crystalloid.
      (5). If nucleated crystalloids become trapped in the urinary system during continued supersaturation, uroliths grow.
      (6). Mucoprotein matrix is thought to be nonspecifically incorporated into the urolith as urolith growth proceeds.
      (7). Oversaturation of urine with urolith-forming crystalloids may be associated with:
         (a). Increased renal excretion of crystalloids as a result of increased glomerular filtration, increased tubular secretion, or decreased tubular reabsorption (examples include hypercalciuria, hyperuricosuria, hyperoxaluria, cystinuria, and xanthinuria).
         (b). Negative body water balance associated with increased tubular reabsorption of water and subsequent urine concentration (examples include excessive water loss via other routes, lack of water consumption, and living in a hot, dry climate).
         (c). Urine pH favoring crystallization (examples include formation of alkaline urine by urease-producing bacteria, formation of alkaline urine as a result of renal tubular acidosis, formation of

UNIVERSITY OF MINNESOTA COLLEGE OF VETERINARY MEDICINE
UROLITH ANALYSIS REQUEST
*** USE THIS FORM FOR UROLITH SUBMISSIONS ***

PLEASE SUBMIT STONES **DRY** IN **UNBREAKABLE** CONTAINER (FOR FELINE URETHRAL PLUGS SEE BELOW)

SUBMITTED BY: Date ______
NAME:
CLINIC NAME:
ADDRESS:

PHONE NUMBER:
FAX NUMBER:

TEST REQUESTED: (check one)
1. Quantitative Analysis (__)
2. Other ______

Owner's Name ______
Owner's Address ______
______
Owner's Phone Number (____)______
Animal's Name/ID# ______
Species ______
Breed (specific) ______
Birth Date ______
Gender: M MC F FS Unk
Source: Renal Pelvis (__) (check all
Ureter (__) applicable)
Bladder (__)
Urethra (__)
Other ______

Date voided (__) or removed (__): ______
What diet was fed prior to urolith diagnosis?
______
Approximately how long was the animal fed this diet? ______
Was a prescription diet fed? Yes No
If yes, which one?
______
If yes, approximately how long was the prescription diet fed? ______

Was the urine cultured? Yes No
If yes, was it sterile? Yes No
Isolates: ______
______
______

Were antibiotics given? Yes No
If yes, type: ______
Dosage: ______
Were urinary acidifiers or alkalinizers given? Yes No
If yes, type: ______
Dosage: ______
Previous Uroliths? Yes No Unk
If yes, date of detection: ______
If yes, what was the composition?
______

Previous illness or injury:
Dx: ______; Date ______
Dx: ______; Date ______
Dx: ______; Date ______

FOR URETHRAL PLUGS ONLY
HOW WAS THE PLUG PRESERVED? (check)
1. No preservative (__)
2. 10% buffered formalin (__)
3. 3% gluteraldehyde (__)
4. Paraformaldehyde (__)
5. Other ______

MAIL TO:
MINNESOTA UROLITH CENTER
Dr. Carl Osborne
Dept. of Small Animal Clinical Sciences
College of Veterinary Medicine
University of Minnesota
St. Paul, MN 55108
612/625-4221

FIG. 41–29. Request form for quantitative analysis of uroliths.

nium urate and ammonium biurate) is the monobasic ammonium salt of uric acid.

c. Sodium acid urate (sodium urate) is the monobasic sodium salt of uric acid.

2. Dalmatians.
   a. Dalmatian dogs are predisposed to urate uroliths owing to their unique metabolism of purines. The ability of Dalmatians to oxidize uric acid to allantoin is intermediate between human beings and non-Dalmation dogs.[58,59,76]
      (1). Humans have a serum uric acid concentration of approximately 3 to 7 mg/dL and excrete approximately 500 to 700 mg of uric acid per day in their urine.

(2). Non-Dalmatian dogs have a serum uric acid concentration of less than 0.5 mg/dL and excrete approximately 10 to 60 mg of uric acid per day in their urine.

(3). Dalmatians have a serum uric acid concentration that is two to four times that of non-Dalmatians and excrete approximately 400 to 600 mg of uric acid per day.

b. Studies of the fate of uric acid in Dalmatians have revealed unique hepatic and renal pathways of metabolism.

(1). Of these two metabolic sites, reciprocal allogenic renal and hepatic transplantations between Dalmatians and non-Dalmatians indicate that the hepatic mechanism is quantitatively the most significant.[4,46,113] The liver of Dalmatians does not completely oxidize available uric acid, even though it contains a sufficient concentration of uricase. As compared with non-Dalmatians, Dalmatians convert uric acid to allantoin at a reduced rate. It has been hypothesized that hepatic cellular membranes are partially impermeable to uric acid.

(2). The proximal renal tubules of Dalmatians reabsorb less uric acid than other dogs; a small amount is secreted by the distal tubules. In non-Dalmatian dogs, 98 to 100% of the uric acid in glomerular filtrate is reabsorbed by the proximal tubules and returned to the liver for further metabolism. Uric acid in urine of non-Dalmatians is thought to be secreted by the distal tubules.[75]

c. The definitive cause of urate urolith formation in Dalmatian dogs remains unknown.

(1). Increased urate excretion is a risk factor rather than a primary cause. Whereas all Dalmatians excrete relatively large quantities of urate in their urine, only a small percentage (especially males) form urate stones.

(2). At one time, it was thought that stone-forming Dalmatians did not excrete greater quantities of urate in their urine than non–stone-forming Dalmatians; however, recent studies indicate that insensitive methods of measurement of urine uric acid concentration were responsible for this conclusion. When steps are taken to ensure that urine uric acid remains in solution, differences in urine uric acid concentrations between non–stone-forming Dalmatians and stone-forming Dalmatians may be expected.[67,185]

d. Even though ammonium urate uroliths commonly affect Dalmatian dogs, not all uroliths formed by Dalmatians are composed of ammonium urate. For example, of 387 uroliths formed by Dalmatian dogs, 82% were composed of purines (ammonium urate, sodium urate, uric acid, xanthine), 7% were of mixed composition, 3% were struvite, 3% calcium oxalate, 3% were compound uroliths, 0.5% cystine, and 0.3% calcium phosphate.[10,151]

3. Non-Dalmatian dogs (Figs. 41–30 to 41–34).

a. Many breeds of dogs have been affected with urate urolithiasis. Whereas urate uroliths are

TABLE 41–9.
CHECKLIST OF FACTORS THAT SUGGEST THE PROBABLE MINERAL COMPOSITION OF CANINE AND FELINE UROLITHS

1. Urine pH
   a. Struvite and calcium apatite uroliths, usually alkaline. Sterile struvite uroliths may be observed when urine pH is 6.5 or higher.
   b. Ammonium urate uroliths, acid to neutral.
   c. Cystine uroliths, acid*
   d. Calcium oxalate, often acid to neutral*
   e. Silica, acid to neutral* (only in canine)
2. Identification of crystals in uncontaminated fresh urine sediment, preferably at body temperature
3. Type of bacteria, if any, isolated from urine
   a. Urease-producing bacteria, especially staphylococci and less frequently *Proteus* spp., are typically associated with canine struvite uroliths. Ureaplasmas may cause struvite uroliths in dogs.
   b. Urinary tract infections often are absent in patients with calcium oxalate, cystine, ammonium urate, and silica uroliths.
   c. Calcium oxalate, cystine, ammonium urate, and silica uroliths may predispose patients to UTI; if infections are caused by urease-producing bacteria, struvite may precipitate around metabolic uroliths.
4. Radiographic density and physical characteristics of uroliths (see Table 41–7)
5. Serum chemistry evaluation
   a. Hypercalcemia may be associated with calcium uroliths.
   b. Hyperuricemia may be associated with uric acid or urate uroliths.
   c. Hyperchloremia, hypokalemia, and acidemia may be associated with distal RTA and calcium phosphate or struvite uroliths.
6. Urine chemistry evaluation
   a. Patient should be consuming a standardized diagnostic diet or the diet consumed when uroliths formed.
   b. Excessive quantities of one or more minerals contained in the urolith are expected. The concentration of crystallization inhibitors may be decreased.
7. Breed of dog or cat and history of uroliths in patient's ancestors or littermates.
8. Quantitative analysis of uroliths fortuitously passed during micturition, collected via catheter technique, or collected by voiding urohydropropulsion.

*Intercurrent infection with urease-producing microbes may result in formation of alkaline urine.

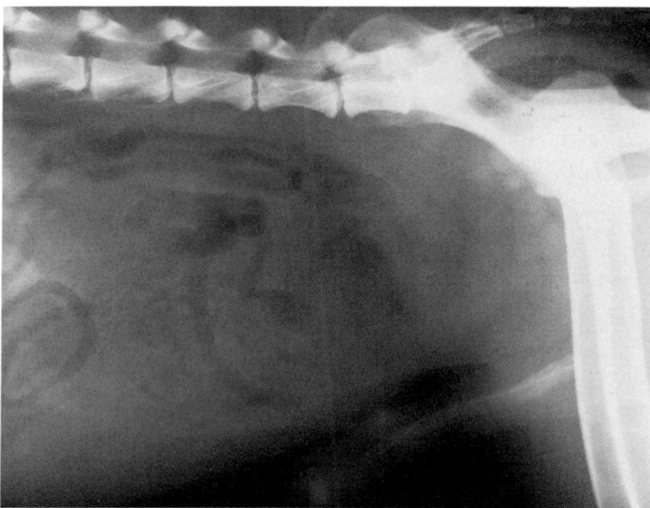

FIG. 41–30. Survey radiograph of the lateral abdomen of a 5-year-old male Alaskan malamute illustrates multiple radiopaque urate urocystoliths *(arrows).* Note the variable size and radio density of the uroliths (compare with Fig. 41–31). Quantitative analysis revealed the uroliths were composed of 100% ammonium acid urate. (From Osborne CA (ed). Canine urolithiasis: etiopathogenesis, detection, treatment, and prevention. *Vet Clin North Am.* 1985;16:1–207.)

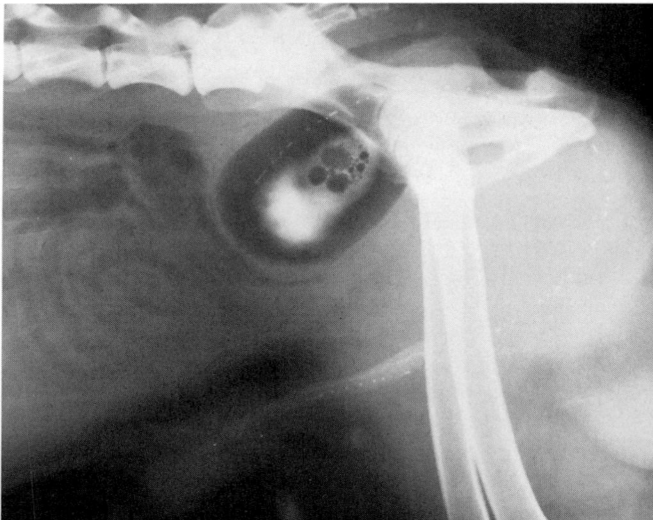

FIG. 41–31. Lateral abdominal view of a double-contrast cystogram of the dog described in Fig. 41–30. Note the additional radiolucent urinary bladder filling defects that, most likely, represent small urate uroliths not readily identified on survey abdominal radiographs. (From Osborne CA (ed). Canine urolithiasis: etiopathogenesis, detection, treatment, and prevention. *Vet Clin North Am.* 1985;16:1–207.)

commonly encountered in Dalmatian dogs, approximately 30 to 60% of all canine urate uroliths analyzed by quantitative methods are found in other breeds.[24,120,143]

b. Although other non-Dalmatian breeds have not been reported to have a significantly higher incidence of urate urolithiasis based on quantitative analyses, our observations indicate that bulldogs and Yorkshire terriers may have a high incidence of urate urolithiasis.[143] Of 94 uroliths formed by bulldogs, 47% were composed of purines.[10]

c. As in Dalmatians, urate uroliths in other breeds have been recognized most frequently in males. They have been detected throughout the life span of affected dogs but were most frequently detected in dogs 3 to 6 years of age.[112,143]

d. Comparatively little is known about urate lithogenesis in non-Dalmatian dogs that do not

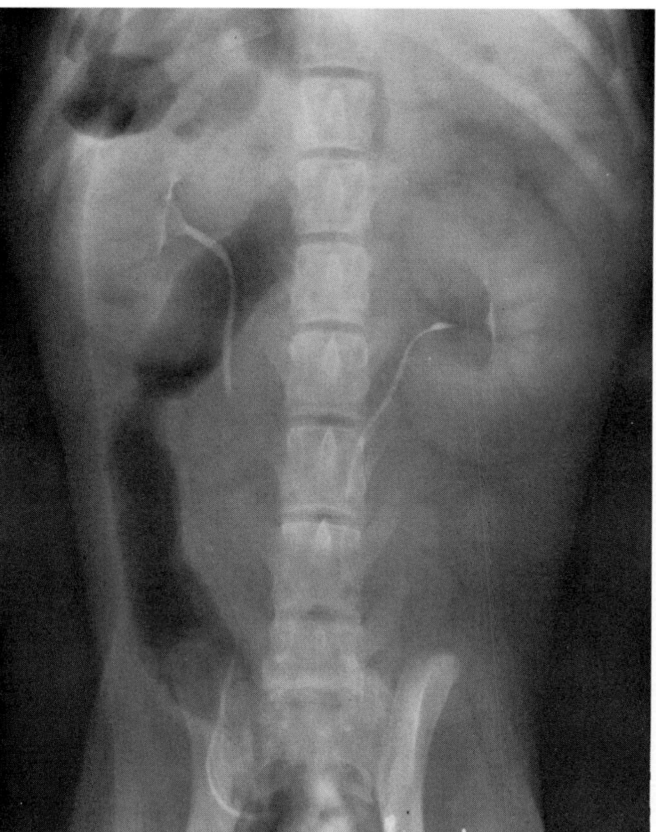

FIG. 41–32. Ventrodorsal view of an excretory urogram of a 7-year-old female Alaskan malamute illustrating a radiolucent nephrolith that is presumed to be composed of ammonium urate. Note the radiolucent filling defect in the right renal pelvis *(arrow).* The dog had a patient ductus venosus (portovascular anomaly). (From Osborne CA (ed). Canine urolithiasis: etiopathogenesis, detection, treatment, and prevention. *Vet Clin North Am.* 1985; 16:1–207.)

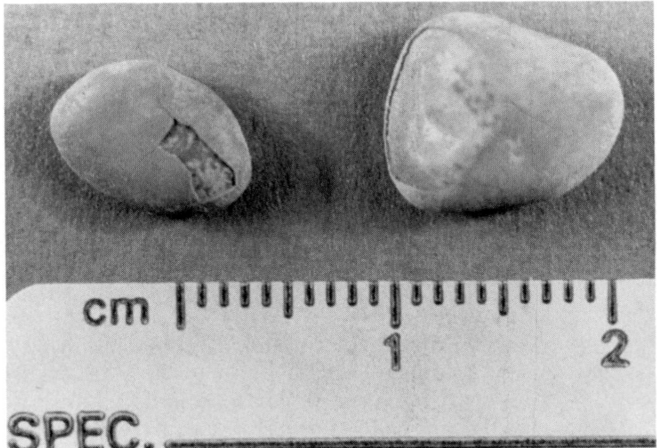

FIG. 41–33. Photograph of two ammonium urate urocystoliths removed from a 2-year-old female miniature schnauzer. Note the brittle laminated structure. Quantitative analysis revealed that the stone was composed of 70% ammonium acid urate and 30% magnesium ammonium phosphate, and the shell was composed of 100% ammonium acid urate. (From Osborne CA (ed). Canine urolithiasis: etiopathogenesis, detection, treatment, and prevention. *Vet Clin North Am.* 1985;16:1–207.)

have portovascular anomalies. Risk factors for urate lithogenesis in dogs include:

(1). Increased renal excretion and urine concentration of uric acid.
(2). Increased renal excretion, renal production, or microbial urease production of ammonium ion.
(3). Low urine pH.
(4). Presence of promoters or absence of inhibitors of urate urolith formation.[112]

e. Regardless of cause, severe hepatic dysfunction may predispose dogs to urate lithogenesis, especially ammonium urate uroliths.
   (1). Our observations, and evidence from other experimental models, suggest that prolonged consumption of severely protein-restricted diets may be associated with formation of urate uroliths in dogs.[112] Biochemical and histologic evaluations of these dogs suggest that longterm consumption of diets severely restricted in protein may induce hepatocellular dysfunction and concomitant hyperuricemia.
   (2). Hepatic cirrhosis has also been reported to be associated with urate uroliths in dogs and other species[183,211]; however, in our experience, cirrhosis, severely restricted protein diets, and other causes of hepatic dysfunction have been uncommon causes of ammonium urate urolithiasis. Nonetheless, their significance relative to ammonium urate lithogenesis deserves further study.

f. Clinical evaluation of eight male English bulldogs with confirmed ammonium urate urocystoliths revealed mild elevations in serum uric acid concentration. The size of their livers was normal, as was serum concentration of hepatic enzymes, blood concentration of ammonia, and bromosulphthalein retention.

4. Portal vascular anomalies.
   a. A high incidence of ammonium urate uroliths has been observed in dogs with portal vascular anomalies. They occur in both males and females, and usually are detected before age 3 years.[85,105,125]
   b. Direct communication between the portal and systemic vasculature bypasses blood around the liver, resulting in severe hepatic atrophy and diminished hepatic function. Hepatic dysfunction, in turn, is associated with reduced hepatic conversion of uric acid to allantoin and of ammonia to urea.
   c. The predisposition to urate urolithiasis of dogs with portal systemic shunts is probably associated with concomitant hyperuricemia, hyperammonemia, hyperuricuria, and hyperammonuria.[93,112]
      (1). Serum uric acid concentrations in 15 dogs with portal systemic shunts evaluated at the University of Minnesota, Veterinary Teaching Hospital were found to be increased (values ranged from 1.2 to 4.0 mg/dL).[93]
      (2). Concurrent hyperuricuria, hyperammonuria, hyperuricemia, and hyperammo-

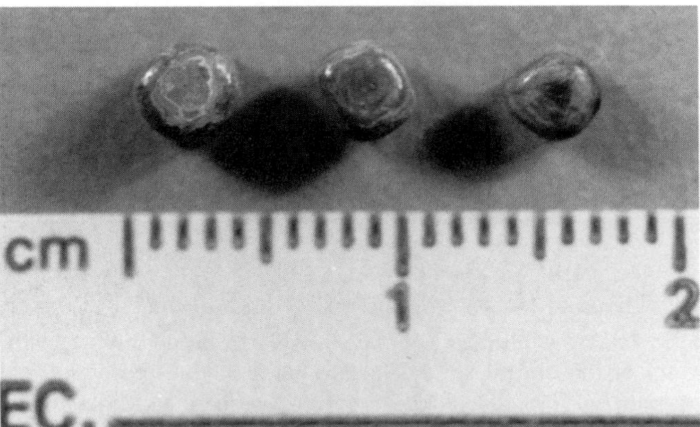

FIG. 41–34. Photograph of multiple ammonium urate urocystoliths removed from a 4-year-old male Pekingese. Quantitative analysis revealed the uroliths were composed of 100% ammonium acid urate. Note the typical smooth exterior and laminated structure. (From Osborne CA (ed). Canine urolithiasis: etiopathogenesis, detection, treatment, and prevention. *Vet Clin North Am.* 1985;16:1–207.)

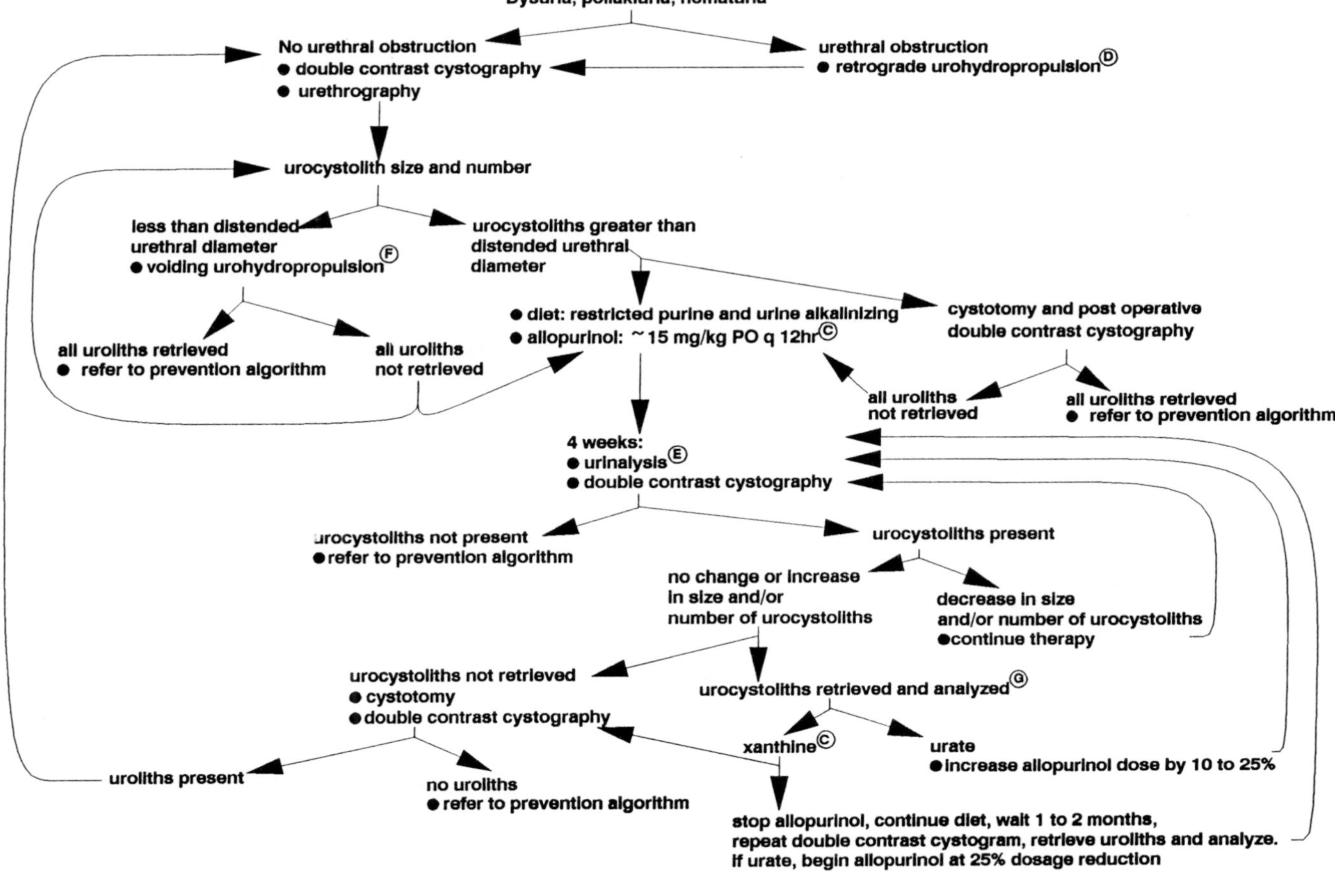

FIG. 41–35. Algorithm for medical management of canine ammonium urate urocystoliths.

nemia was observed in an 18-month-old Bernese mountain dog with recurrent ammonium urate uroliths associated with a portal vascular anomaly.[112] In this dog, urine uric acid concentrations were ± 42 mg/kg per 24 hours, and urine ammonia concentration was 3.2 mM/kg per 24 hr, during consumption of a protein-restricted diet.

d. Not all dogs with portal systemic shunts develop concurrent ammonium urate urolithiasis. Definition and characterization of other factors responsible for promoting or inhibiting urate lithogenesis in affected dogs requires further investigation.[79]

B. Treatment.

1. Dogs without portovascular anomalies (Figs. 41–35 to 41–39).
   a. Our current recommendations for medical dissolution of canine ammonium acid urate uroliths include a combination of these measures:
      (1). Calculolytic diet.
      (2). Administration of xanthine oxidase inhibitors (allopurinol).
      (3). Alkalinization of urine.
      (4). Eradication or control of UTI (Table 41–10).
      (5). Although formation of an increased quantity of dilute urine may also be useful, this may be accomplished by dietary modification.
   b. Calculolytic diets. The goal of dietary modification for patients with uric acid or ammonium acid urate uroliths is to reduce urine concentration of uric acid, ammonium ion, and hydrogen ion (Table 41–11). We utilize a purine-restricted nonacidifying diet that does not contain supplemental sodium (Prescription Diet Canine u/d, Hill's).[153]
   c. Xanthine oxidase inhibitors (Figs. 41–40, 41–42).
      (1). Allopurinol is a synthetic isomer of hypoxanthine.[91] It binds rapidly to and inhibits the action of xanthine oxidase, and

thereby decreases production of uric acid by inhibiting the conversion of hypoxanthine to xanthine and of xanthine to uric acid. The result is a reduction in serum and urine uric acid concentration within ap-

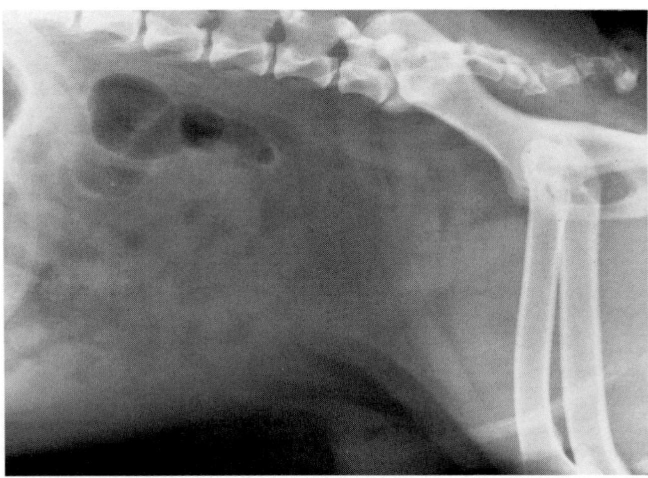

FIG. 41–36. Survey lateral radiograph of a 4-year-old male English bulldog with dysuria and hematuria. No radiodense uroliths can be detected in the urinary tract (see Figs. 41–37 to 41–39). (From Osborne CA, et al. Current status of medical dissolution of canine and feline uroliths. In: *Proceedings of the 7th Kal Kan Symposium.* Lawrenceville, NJ: Veterinary Learning Systems; 1984.)

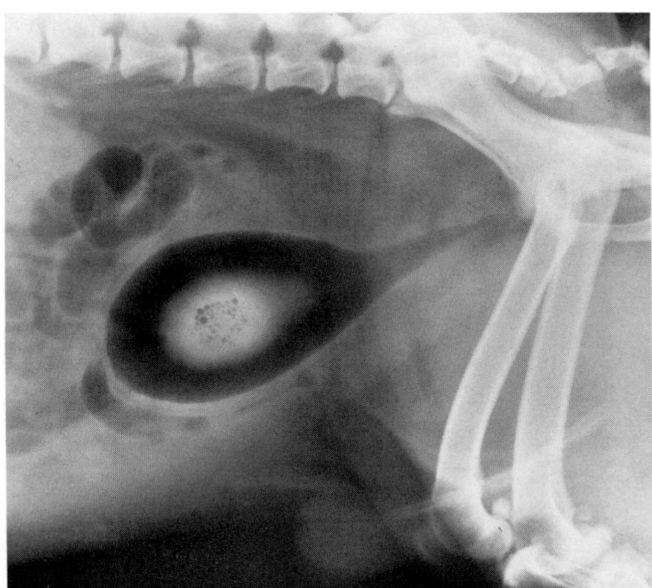

FIG. 41–37. Double-contrast cystogram of the dog described in Fig. 41–36. Multiple radiolucent uroliths are visible in the bladder lumen. Quantitative analysis of a urolith voided during micturition revealed that it was composed of 100% ammonium acid urate.

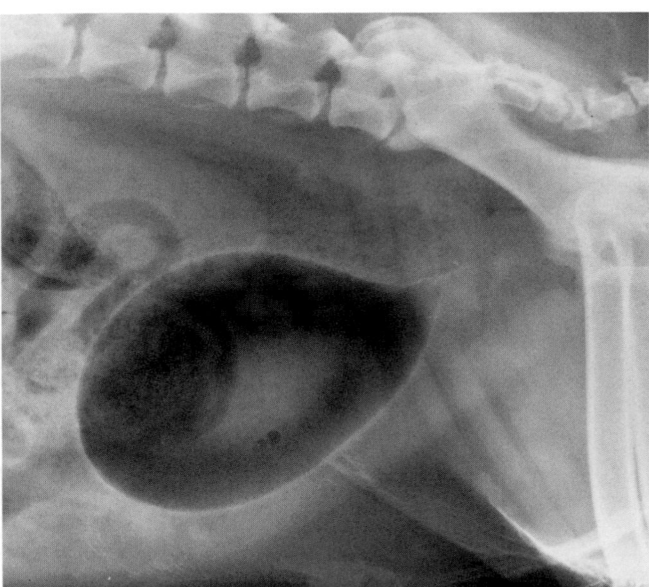

FIG. 41–38. Double-contrast cystogram of the dog described in Fig. 41–36. This cystogram was obtained approximately 7 weeks after initiation of calculolytic therapy. Only three uroliths can be identified.

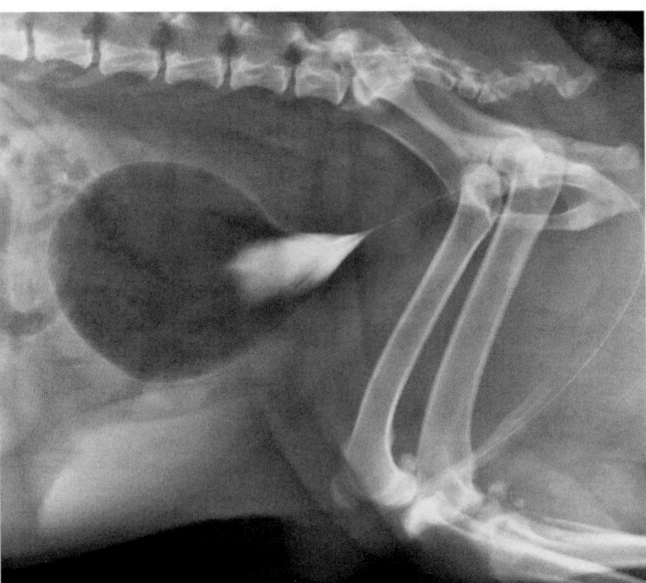

FIG. 41–39. Double-contrast cystogram of the dog described in Fig. 41–36. This cystogram was obtained approximately 11 weeks after initiation of calculolytic therapy. No uroliths can be identified in the lower urinary tract.

proximately 2 days and a concomitant but less pronounced increase in the serum concentrations of hypoxanthine and xanthine.[75,150] Although allopurinol has a short half-life in humans with normal renal function (approximately 90 minutes), its metabolic derivative oxypurinol is also a xanthine oxidase inhibitor and has a half-life of approximately 12 to 16 hours.[150] The elimination half-life of allopurinol in dogs is dose dependent (about 2½ hours following a 5-mg/kg dose, and 3 hours following a 10 mg/kg dose). The elimination half-life of oxypurinol in dogs was 3 to 5 hours.

(2). The dosage of allopurinol that we have used for dissolution of ammonium acid urate uroliths in dogs is 30 mg/kg/day divided into two or three doses.[150] According to the manufacturer, the drug has been given to normal dogs in this dosage for 1 year without causing significant abnormalities.[218] We have used this dosage for nonazotemic urate urolith–forming dogs for up to 6 months without detectable consequences, except formation of xanthine uroliths. Particularly when owners supplemented the diet with foods containing purine precursors, a layer of xanthine formed around ammonium urate uroliths (Figs. 41–40 to 41–43).[11]

(3). Although uncommon, allopurinol has caused adverse side effects in humans. They include gastrointestinal complaints, skin rashes, leukopenia, thrombocytopenia, vasculitis, and hepatitis.[2,132,163] Other than formation of xanthine uroliths, adverse reactions to allopurinol are apparently uncommon in dogs. We have not detected them and found no reports of their occurrence in dogs in the literature.

(4). Because allopurinol and its metabolites are dependent on the kidneys for elimination from humans, the dose is commonly reduced in patients with renal dysfunc-

TABLE 41–10.
SUMMARY OF RECOMMENDATIONS FOR MEDICAL DISSOLUTION OF CANINE AMMONIUM ACID URATE UROLITHS

1. Perform appropriate diagnostic studies, including complete urinalysis, quantitative urine culture, and diagnostic radiography. Determine precise location, size, and number of uroliths. The size and number of uroliths are not a reliable index of probable efficacy of therapy.
2. If available, determine mineral composition of uroliths. If unavailable, "guesstimate" their composition by evaluating appropriate clinical data.
3. Consider surgical correction if uroliths obstruct urine outflow.
4. Determine baseline pretreatment serum uric acid concentrations (and if possible 24-hour urine uric acid concentration).
5. Initiate therapy with a low-purine calculolytic diet (Prescription Diet Canine u/d). No other food supplements should be fed to the patient. Compliance with dietary recommendation is suggested by reduction in serum urea nitrogen concentration (usually <10 mg/dL).
6. Initiate therapy wth allopurinol at a dosage of 30 mg/kg per day in two equal doses (a smaller dose will be required for azotemic patients). Xanthine uroliths may form if a diet containing excessive purines is fed or if excessive allopurinol is given.
7. If necessary, administer sodium bicarbonate or potassium citrate orally, to eliminate aciduria. Strive for a urine pH of approximately 7.
8. If necessary, eradicate or control UTI with appropriate antimicrobial agents. Maintain antimicrobial therapy during, and for an appropriate period following, urate urolith dissolution.
9. Devise a protocol to monitor efficacy of therapy:
   a. Try to avoid diagnostic followup studies that require urinary catheterization. If they are required, give appropriate pericatheterization antimicrobial agents to prevent iatrogenic UTI.
   b. Evaluate serial urinalyses. Urine pH, specific gravity, and microscopic examination of sediment for urate crystals are especially important. Remember, crystals formed in urine stored at room or refrigeration temperatures may represent in vitro artifacts.
   c. Serially evaluate serum uric acid concentration and (if possible) fractional excretion of urine uric acid.
   d. Evaluate urolith(s) location(s), number, size, density, and shape at approximately monthly intervals. Intravenous urography may be utilized for radiolucent uroliths located in the kidneys, ureters, or urinary bladder. Retrograde contrast urethrocystography may be required for radiolucent uroliths located in the bladder and urethra.
   e. If necessary, perform quantitative urine cultures. They are especially important for patients that are infected before therapy and those catheterized during therapy.
10. Continue calculolytic diet, allopurinol, and alkalinizing therapy for approximately 1 month following disappearance of uroliths as detected by radiography.
11. Prevention: Urate uroliths are very often recurrent. Preventive therapy should be directed at keeping urine concentrations of ammonia and uric acid to a minimum. This may be achieved by feeding a diet low in protein that also promotes alkaline urine in dogs and a low-protein alkalinizing diet to cats. The effectiveness of dietary management for the prevention of ammonium urate uroliths in dogs with portosystemic shunts and in cats with and without portosystemic shunts is unknown. The longterm use of allopurinol is discouraged because of the potential for development of xanthine uroliths.

TABLE 41–11.
EXPECTED CHANGES ASSOCIATED WITH MEDICAL THERAPY OF AMMONIUM URATE UROLITHS

Finding	Before Therapy	During Therapy	Prevention Therapy
Polyuria	±	1+ to 3+	1+ to 3+
Pollakiuria	0 to 4+	↑ then ↓	0
Hematuria	0 to 4+	↓	0
Urine specific gravity	Variable	1.004–1.015	1.004–1.015
Urine pH	<7.0	>7.0	>7.0
Urine inflammation	0 to 4+	↓	0
Urate crystals	0 to 4+	0	Variable
Bacteriuria	0 to 4+	0	0
Bacterial culture of urine	0 to 4+	0	0
BUN (mg/dL)	Variable	≤15	≤15
Urolith size, number	Small to large	↓	0

Key: BUN, blood urea nitrogen; ± = sometimes; 1+ = small quantity; 4+ = large quantity.

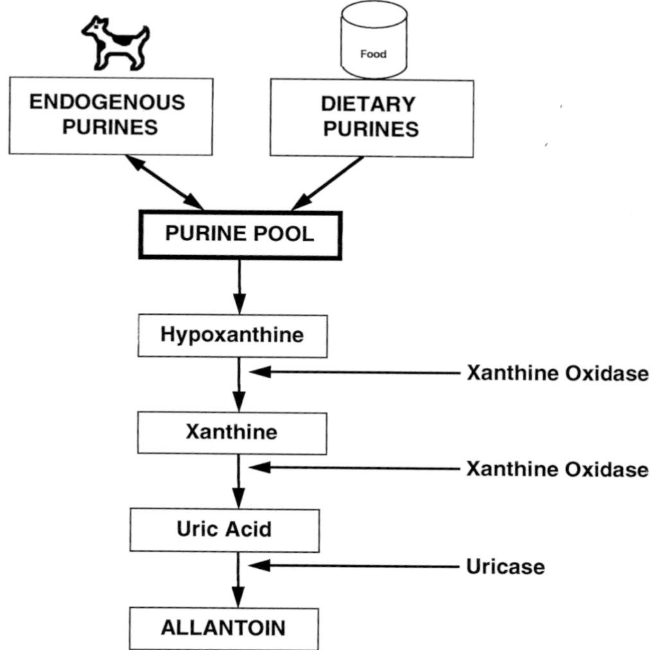

FIG. 41–40. Diagram of normal canine purine degradation.

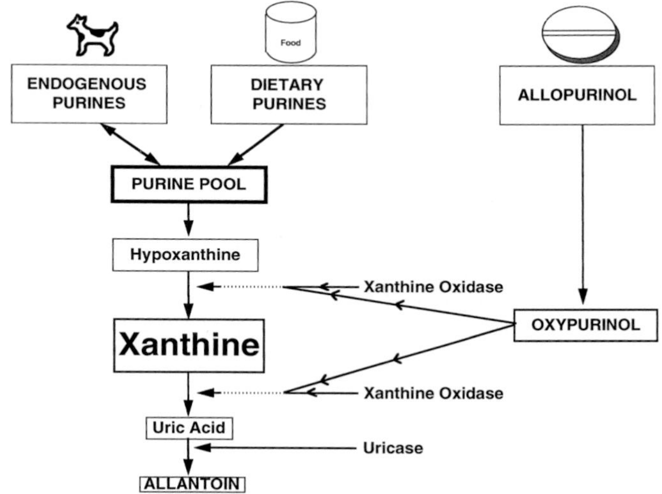

FIG. 41–41. Diagram of purine degradation in dogs fed a maintenance diet and given allopurinol.

tion. Allopurinol given to human patients with renal insufficiency has been reported to cause life-threatening erythematous desquamative skin rash, fever, hepatitis, eosinopenia, and further decline in renal function.[91] Pending further studies, appropriate precautions should be used when considering use of allopurinol in dogs with primary renal failure.

d. Alkalinization of urine.
 (1). Because ammonium ion and hydrogen ion appear to precipitate urates in dog urine, administration of alkalizing agents, such as oral sodium bicarbonate or potassium citrate, appear to be of value in preventing acid metabolites from increasing renal tubular production of ammonia. Under physiologic conditions associated with alkaluria, urine contains low concentrations of ammonia and ammonium ion.[206]
 (2). Dosage of urine alkalinizers should be individualized for each patient.
  (a). Preliminary dosages of sodium bicarbonate vary from approximately 10 to 90 grains per day, depending on

the size of the patient and pretreatment urine pH values.

(b). Alternatively, potassium citrate in wax matrix tablets may be given (Urocit-K, Mission Pharmacal).

(c). Administration of divided doses is suggested to maintain a consistently nonacidic environment in the urinary tract.

(3). The goal of treatment with urine alkalizers is to maintain a urine pH of approximately 7.0 (see Table 41–11).

(a). Values higher than 7.5 should be avoided until it is determined whether or not they provide a significant risk factor for formation of calcium phosphate uroliths.

(b). Deposition of a layer of calcium phosphate crystals around existing urate uroliths could impede stone dissolution. Owners may participate in monitoring urine pH with pH paper.

e. Eradication or control of urinary tract infection.

(1). Clinical studies indicate that UTI in dogs with ammonium acid urate uroliths usually occurs as a consequence of altered local host defenses. These alterations may be caused by urolith-induced trauma to the urothelium, or they may occur as a consequence of catheterization or other invasive diagnostic procedures. Every effort should be made to prevent, eradicate, or control them, since they may cause problems of equal or greater severity as the uroliths.

(2). Studies of ammonium acid urate uroliths in humans have been interpreted to suggest that UTI caused by urease-producing microbes may be a causative factor. In this circumstance, formation of ammonium ion as a consequence of urease-mediated hydrolysis of urea may result in formation of insoluble ammonium acid urate crystals. If a similar phenomenon occurs in dogs, eradication or control of potent urease-producing microbes (staphylococci, *Proteus* spp., and ureaplasmas) would be especially important.

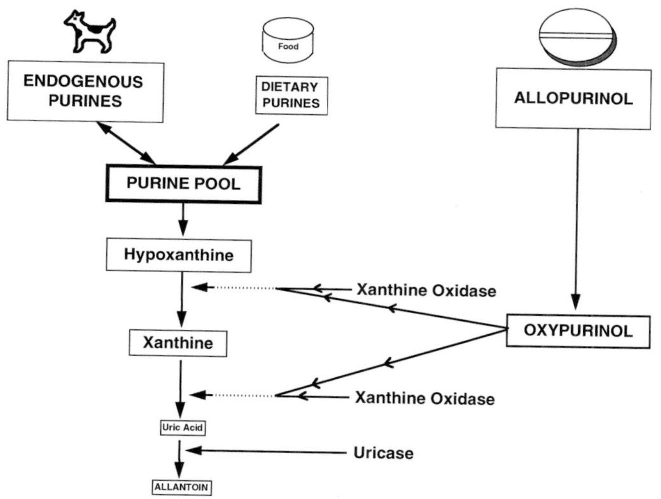

FIG. 41–42. Diagram of purine metabolism in dogs that consume a purine-restricted diet and are given allopurinol.

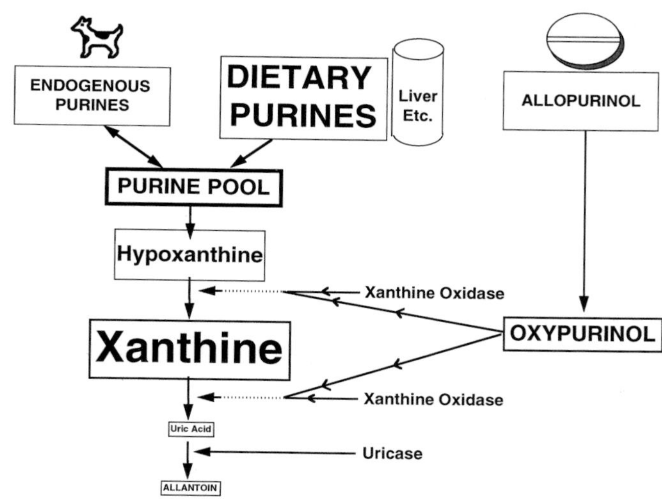

FIG. 41–43. Diagram of purine metabolism in dogs that consume a purine-rich diet and are given allopurinol.

(3). Appropriate antimicrobial agents selected on the basis of susceptibility or minimum inhibitory concentration tests should be used as therapeutic dosages. The fact that diuresis reduces the urine concentration of the antimicrobial agent should be considered when formulating antimicrobial dosages.

f. Augmenting urine volume.

(1). Augmenting urine volume with the goal of decreasing urine uric acid and ammonium concentration, and enhancing urine flow through the excretory pathway, appears to be a logical recommendation.

(2). Because the calculolytic diet designed for urate urolith dissolution impairs urine-concentrating capacity by decreasing renal medullary urea concentration, additional diuretic agents are not required.

(3). Excessive dietary sodium should be avoided, particularly if the urine pH is high, since excessive sodium excretion may cause hypercalciuria. This may in turn cause calcium phosphate crystals to form (see the section on calcium oxalate urolithiasis). It is of interest that oral sodium chloride given to normal human volunteers for 10 days did not alter urine uric acid concentration.[157]

(4). Longterm administration (up to 3 years) of hydrochlorothiazide to human patients with uroliths containing calcium salts resulted in a rise in serum and urine uric acid concentration.[170]

g. Canine clinical studies.

(1). In clinical studies performed at the University of Minnesota, the following results were obtained following use of dietary and allopurinol therapy of 32 dogs with urolithiasis.

(a). Of 25 dogs with ammonium urate uroliths, complete dissolution was obtained in nine (36%), partial dissolution in eight (32%), and no dissolution in eight (32%).

(b). Of seven dogs with sodium urate uroliths, complete dissolution was obtained in two (29%), partial dissolution in three (42%), and no dissolution in two (29%).

(2). Inability to dissolve urate uroliths was usually associated with formation of xanthine.

(3). The mean time of urate urolith dissolution in 11 dogs was 3.5 months (median, 1 month; range, 1 to 18 months).

(4). Following urolith dissolution, initiation of preventive therapy was associated with recurrence in six of 20 (30%) dogs with ammonium urate uroliths and recurrence in none of five dogs with sodium urate uroliths. Seven dogs were unavailable for followup studies.

2. Dogs with portovascular anomalies.

a. There apparently have been few studies of the biologic behavior of ammonium acid urate uroliths in dogs with portovascular anomalies. It is logical to hypothesize that elimination of hyperuricuria and reduction of urine ammonium concentration following surgical correction of anomalous shunts would result in spontaneous dissolution of uroliths composed primarily of ammonium acid urate. Appropriate clinical studies are needed to prove or disprove this hypothesis.[112]

b. We observed a substantial reduction of urine uric acid concentration in a 3-month-old female miniature schnauzer following surgical correction of an extrahepatic portacaval shunt.

c. Additional clinical studies are needed to evaluate the relative value of calculolytic diets, allopurinol, and alkalinization of urine in dissolving ammonium acid urate uroliths in dogs with portovascular anomalies. The efficacy of allopurinol may be altered in such dogs, since biotransformation of this drug, which has a very short half-life, to oxypurinol, which has a longer half-life, requires adequate hepatic function.[150]

3. Monitoring response to therapy (see Table 41–11).

a. In our experience, ammonium acid urate urocystoliths have a propensity to move into the urethra of dogs.

(1). This may be related to their small size, their round to ovoid shape, and their smooth surface.

(2). If small enough, they pass readily through the urethra.

(3). They often become lodged behind the os penis of males.

(a). Owners should be informed of this likelihood and given a written summary of associated clinical findings.

(b). When urethroliths cause clinical signs, they may be easily returned to the bladder lumen by urohydropropulsion.[154] The physical characteristics that promote their passage into the urethra also facilitate their removal from the urethra.

b. The size of the uroliths should be periodically monitored by survey and (if necessary) by double-contrast radiography.

(1). It is more difficult to monitor changes in the size and number of uroliths that are radiolucent.

(2). We have successfully used retrograde double-contrast urethrocystography to monitor dissolution of radiolucent urethrocystoliths without causing iatrogenic urinary tract infections. To utilize this technique a balloon catheter does not need to be inserted beyond the distal urethra.[99]

c. Urine pH should be monitored at appropriate intervals.

d. Periodic evaluation of urine sediment for crystalluria should also be considered. Ammonium acid urate crystals should not form in fresh urine if therapy has been effective in promoting formation of urine that is undersaturated with ammonia and uric acid.

e. Periodic evaluation of concentrations of serum urea nitrogen, serum uric acid, and (if possible) urine uric acid is recommended.

(1). Reduction of serum urea nitrogen concentration below pretreatment values (usually below 10 mg/dL in previously nonazotemic patients) indicates owner and patient compliance with recommendations to consume the calculolytic diet exclusively.

(2). Reductions in serum and urine uric acid concentrations also indicate compliance with recommendations for dietary and allopurinol therapy.

f. Since small uroliths may escape detection by survey radiography, we recommend that therapy be continued for approximately 1 month following documentation of urolith dissolution by survey radiography.

g. There is no rigid therapeutic interval after which response to dissolution therapy is unlikely.

(1). The fact that current medical protocols are not designed to induce dissolution of urolith matrix may be a factor that influences dissolution rate.

(2). The time required to induce dissolution of nine episodes of urate urolithiasis in our clinical study has ranged from 4 to 40 weeks (mean, 14.2 weeks).

(3). If uroliths increase in size during therapy or do not begin to decrease in size after approximately 8 weeks of appropriate medical therapy, re-evaluation of the diagnosis or alternative methods of management should be considered.

C. Prevention (see Table 41–10; Fig. 41–44).

1. Prophylactic therapy should be considered for dogs at high risk for recurrent urate uroliths.
2. As a first choice, diets that are restricted in purines and that promote formation of dilute alkaline urine should be considered. If urate crystalluria or hyperuricuria persists, serial evaluation of urine pH to ensure appropriate alkalinization is indicated.
3. If necessary, alkalinizing agents may be added to the protocol.
4. If difficulties persist, allopurinol (approximately 10 to 20 mg/kg body weight per day) may be given.

a. Recent studies performed at the University of California and the University of Minnesota indicate that prolonged administration of large doses (30 mg/kg body weight per day) of allopurinol may result in formation of xanthine uroliths.[9,117]

b. The risk of xanthine urolithiasis is enhanced if dietary purines are not restricted during allopurinol therapy. Therefore appropriate caution in longterm administration of this drug is indicated.

5. Since it is possible to induce dissolution of recurrent ammonium urate uroliths, it is unnecessary to risk prophylactic protocols that may themselves cause disorders.

Prevention algorithm for canine urate Ⓐ ***urocystoliths*** Ⓑ

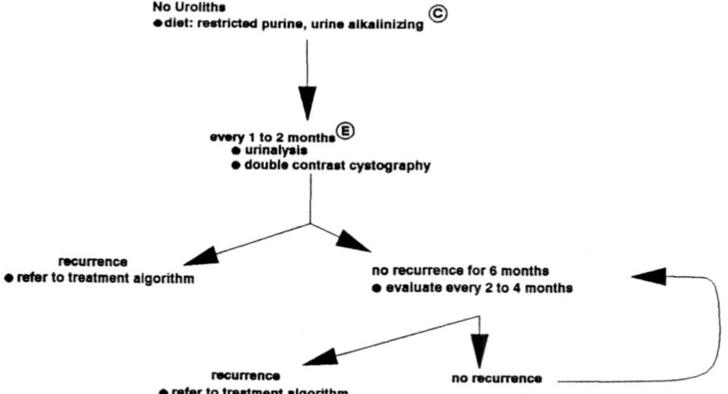

FIG. 41–44. Algorithm for prevention of canine ammonium urate uroliths.

VII. FELINE AMMONIUM URATE AND URIC ACID UROLITHIASIS

A. In our feline urolith series, ammonium urate and uric acid comprised approximately 7% of the total (see Table 41–2).

B. See Chapter 35, Disorders of the Feline Lower Urinary Tract.

VIII. CANINE CALCIUM OXALATE UROLITHIASIS

A. Etiopathogenesis (Tables 41–12, 41–13; Figs. 41–45 to 41–48).

1. Overview.

a. Calcium oxalate urolith formation is a sequela of a group of underlying disorders that result in precipitation of calcium oxalate in urine.

(1). Alterations in the balance between urine concentrations of calculogenic minerals (calcium and oxalate) and crystallization inhibitors (including citrate, phosphorus, magnesium, sodium, and potassium) have been associated with initiation and growth of calcium oxalate uroliths.[32,198]

(2). The fact that urolith formation is erratic and unpredictable emphasizes that several inter-related physiologic and pathologic factors are often involved.

(3). Identifying one or more factors that promote urolith formation may inform their management (see Table 41–12).

b. Calcium oxalate comprised approximately 28% of canine stones submitted to our laboratory, and approximately 39% of the canine nephroliths (see Tables 41–1 and 41–3).

(1). Although calcium oxalate uroliths have been recognized in many breeds of dogs, miniature schnauzers, Lhasa Apsos, Shih Tzus, Yorkshire terriers, and miniature poodles are most often affected. Infrequently affected breeds include boxers, English bulldogs, golden retrievers, and Labrador retrievers.

(2). Approximately 70% of calcium oxalate

TABLE 41–12.
RISK FACTORS FOR CALCIUM OXALATE UROLITHIASIS

		Therapeutic Management	
Risk Factor	**Etiopathologic Disorder**	**Goal**	**Method**
Hypercalciuria	Intestinal hyperabsorption		
	• Idiopathic	Reduce dietary calcium.	Provide diet with reduced calcium (Prescription Diet u/d).
	• Hvpophosphatemia	Normalize vitamin D production by sustaining a normal serum phosphorus concentration.	Provide phosphorus supplementation (Neutra-Phos-K; Willen).
	• Vitamin D excess	Limit excessive intestinal calcium absorption.	Avoid oral vitamin D supplementation.
	Renal leak		
	• Idiopathic	Promote renal calcium reabsorption.	Consider thiazide diuretic?
	• Renal tubular acidosis	Increase renal tubular reabsorption of bicarbonate to enhance calcium reabsorption	Provide oral alkali therapy (potassium citrate).
	• Dietary protein excess	Increase renal tubular reabsorption of bicarbonate to enhance calcium reabsorption and promote adequate citrate excretion.	Provide diet with reduced protein (Prescription Diet u/d).
	• Dietary sodium excess	Minimize renal sodium and calcium excretion.	Provide diets with reduced sodium (Prescription Diet u/d).
	• Glucocorticoid excess	Decrease glucocorticoid-enhanced bone resorption and urine calcium excretion.	Control hyperadrenocorticism, avoid glucocorticoid supplementation.
	Excessive Skeletal Resorption		
	• Primary hyperparathyroidism	Normalize skeletal calcium resorption, serum calcium concentration, and renal calcium filtration.	Parathyroidectomy.
	• Pseudohyperparathyroidism	Control paraneoplastic parathyroid hormone–like activity.	Eradicate neoplasm or induce remission.
	• Osteolytic lesions	Minimize release of excessive skeletal calcium.	Correct underlying bone disorder.
Hyperoxaluria	Dietary oxalate excess	Avoid foods of high oxalate content.	Provide diet low in oxalate (Prescription Diet u/d).
	Fat malabsorption	Decrease intestinal fat.	Provide diet with reduced fat.
	Vitamin C excess	Minimize precurser of oxalate.	Avoid vitamin C supplementation.
	Vitamin B_6 deficiency	Permit conversion of glyoxylate (an oxalate precurser) to glycine.	Provide adequate vitamin B_6
	Primary hyperoxaluria	Minimize oxalate synthesis.	Provide excess vitamin B_6?
Hypocitraturia	Idiopathic	Promote citrate excretion.	Provide oral potassium citrate (Urocit-K Mission Pharmacal).
	Acidosis	Minimize acidosis.	Provide oral alkali therapy (potassium citrate).
Defective macromolecular inhibitors	Inherited disorder?	Restore urinary concentration of effective inhibitors.	Not known.

TABLE 41–13.
SUMMARY OF DISTINGUISHING CLINICAL MANIFESTATIONS FOR DIFFERENT TYPES OF HYPERCALCIURIA

Feature*	AH	RH	PHPT
Serum calcium	N	N	↑
Serum PTH	↓/N	↑	↑
Serum phosphorus	N/↑	N	↓/↑**
Urine calcium			
Fasting	N	↑	↑a
Dx diet†	↑	↑	↑
Urine oxalate	N	N	N
Urine uric acid	N	N	N
Bone density	N	↓	↓
Calcium balance (total body)	Positive	Negative	Negative

*Key: AH, absorptive hypercalciuria; RH, renal-leak hypercalciuria; PHPT, primary hyperparathyroidism; PTH, parathyroid hormone.
†Dx Diet, Diagnostic diet used in the evaluation of normal and calcium oxalate urolith dogs.
‡As glomerular filtration rate declines, phosphorus is retained in serum.

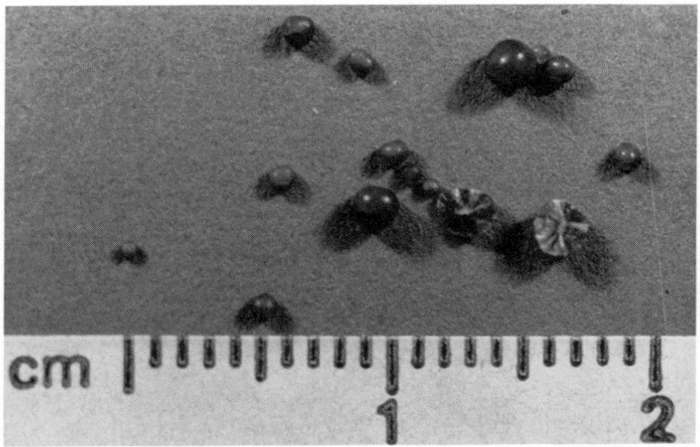

FIG. 41–45. Photograph of urocystoliths removed from a 14-year-old female miniature schnauzer. The uroliths, composed of 100% calcium oxalate monohydrate, are brown and have a smooth, polished surface. The cut surface of the urolith in the lower left-hand corner appears to have radial striations. (From Osborne CA (ed). Canine urolithiasis: etiopathogenesis, detection, treatment, and prevention. *Vet Clin North Am.* 1986;16: 1–207.)

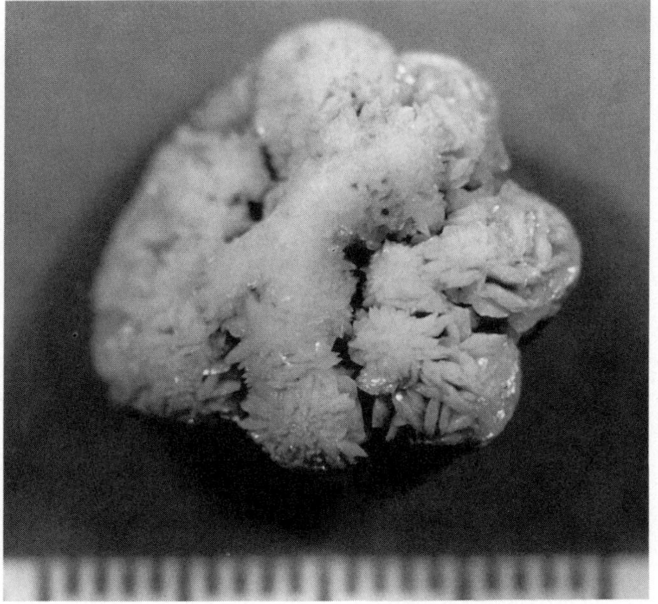

FIG. 41–46 Photograph of urocystolith removed from a 12-year-old male mixed-breed dog. The urolith, composed of 70% calcium oxalate dihydrate and 30% calcium oxalate monohydrate, is tan and has an irregular surface caused by protrusion of sharp-edged crystals. (Scale is in millimeters; from Osborne CA (ed). Canine urolithiasis: etiopathogenesis, detection, treatment, and prevention. *Vet Clin North Am.* 1986;16:1–207.)

uroliths have affected male dogs. Most were detected in adults (mean age, 8 to 9 years).

2. Hypercalciuria.
   a. For uroliths to form, urine must be supersaturated with calculogenic substances.
      (1). For example, increasing the urinary concentration of calcium promotes calcium oxalate crystal formation.
      (2). Hypercalciuria has been a significant finding in dogs with calcium oxalate uroliths.[124]
   b. Calcium homeostasis is achieved principally through the actions of parathyroid hormone (PTH) and 1,25 cholecalciferol (1,25-vitamin D) on bones, intestines, and kidneys.
      (1). For example, states of low serum ionized calcium concentration result in enhanced PTH– and 1,25-vitamin D–mediated mo-

bilization of calcium from the skeleton, absorption of calcium from the intestines, and conservation of calcium by the kidneys.

(2). High serum ionized calcium concentrations suppress release of PTH and production of 1,25-vitamin D. The result is decreased skeletal mobilization and intestinal absorption of calcium and enhanced renal calcium excretion.

(3). Hypercalciuria can result from increased renal clearance of calcium owing to several phenomena.

(a). Excessive intestinal absorption of calcium.

(b). Impaired renal conservation of calcium.

(c). Excessive skeletal mobilization of calcium (Table 41–13).

c. In dogs, normocalcemic hypercalciuria is thought to result from either intestinal hyperabsorption of calcium (so-called absorptive hypercalciuria) or decreased renal tubular reabsorption of calcium (so-called renal-leak hypercalciuria).[124,153] Hypercalcemic hypercalciuria results from increased glomerular filtration of mobilized calcium, which overwhelms normal renal tubular reabsorptive mechanisms (so-called resorptive hypercalciuria because excessive bone resorption is associated with increased serum calcium concentrations).

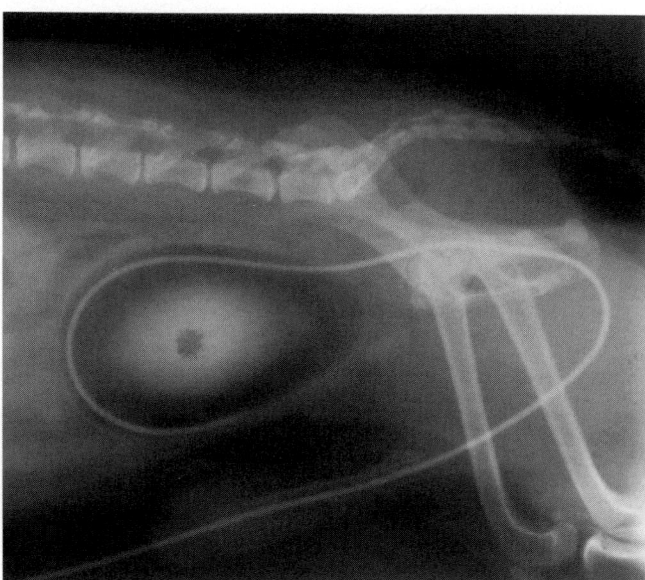

FIG. 41–47. Lateral abdominal view of a double-contrast cystogram of a 15-year-old male toy poodle, illustrates a urocystolith with a jackstone configuration. (Compare to Figs. 41–48, 41–90, 41–91).

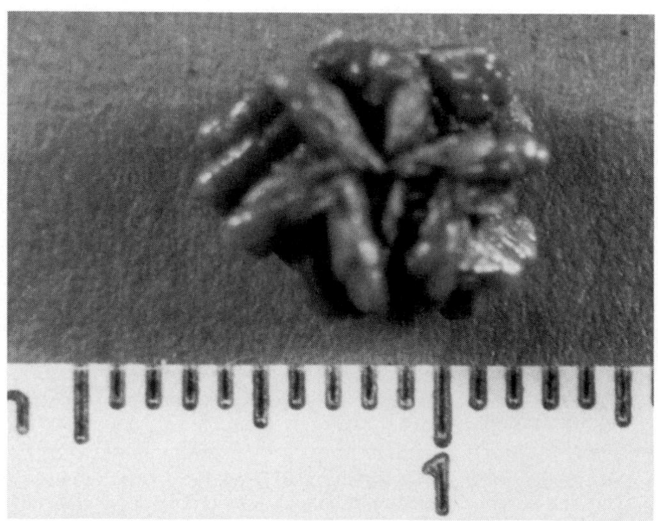

FIG. 41–48. Photograph of the urocystolith removed from the dog described in Fig. 41–47. The urolith was composed of 90% calcium oxalate monohydrate, 5% calcium oxalate dihydrate, and 5% calcium phosphate.

(1). Absorptive hypercalciuria is characterized by increased urine calcium excretion, normal serum calcium concentration, and normal or low serum PTH concentration.

(a). Because absorptive hypercalciuria depends on dietary calcium, urine calcium excretion during food fasting is normal or significantly reduced as compared with urine calcium excretion during nonfasting conditions.

(b). Mean 24-hour urine calcium excretion in 33 normal beagles was 0.32 ± 0.2 mg/kg per 24 hours during fasting and 0.52 ± 0.3 mg/kg per 24 hours when dogs consumed a standard diet (Prescription Diet Canine k/d; Hill's).[125]

(c). By comparison, mean urine calcium excretion in 5 miniature schnauzers with calcium oxalate urolithiasis and absorptive hypercalciuria was 1.0 ± 0.5 mg/kg per 24 hours during fasting and 2.84 ± 0.9 mg/kg per 24 hours during nonfasting urine collections.[121]

(d). A primary defect observed in human patients with absorptive hypercalciuria is intestinal hyperabsorption of calcium, which results in increased excretion of excess calcium in urine.[153] In addition to enhanced glomerular filtration of absorbed dietary calcium, decreased PTH secretion results in decreased renal tubular reabsorption of filtered calcium. The same phenomenon appears to occur in dogs with absorptive hypercalciuria.[124]

(e). Primary intestinal abnormalities in calcium absorption, disorders of 1,25-vitamin D production, and hypophosphatemia-induced hypervitaminosis D have been recognized as causes in humans.[153] A single pathogenic mechanism for absorptive hypercalciuria has not been identified in dogs we have evaluated; however, we did not observe hypophosphatemia or elevated levels of 1,25-vitamin D in five dogs with absorptive hypercalciuria.[124]

(2). In our studies of dogs, *renal-leak hypercalciuria* has been recognized, but less frequently than excessive intestinal absorption of calcium.[124]

(a). In our dogs, renal-leak hypercalciuria was characterized by normal serum calcium concentration, increased urine calcium excretion, and increased serum PTH concentration (Table 41–13). Unlike patients with absorptive hypercalciuria, urinary calcium loss did not decline during food fasting. As a result, urinary calcium excretion during fasting was similar to calcium excretion during nonfasting conditions. The underlying cause was not established.

(b). The defect in human patients with renal-leak hypercalciuria is associated with impaired tubular reabsorption of calcium. The resulting decline in serum calcium concentration causes enhanced secretion of PTH, which in turn increases synthesis of 1,25-vitamin D. The resulting increase in intestinal calcium absorption further contributes to hypercalciuria. In humans, disorders that alter the kidneys' ability to appropriately conserve calcium include distal renal tubular acidosis, acquired or congenital Fanconi's syndrome, chronic metabolic acidosis, glucocorticoid excess, and excessive dietary consumption of sodium or protein.[153]

(3). Resorptive hypercalciuria is characterized by excessive filtration and excretion of calcium in urine as a result of hypercalcemia.

(a). Increased serum calcium concentration, increased serum PTH concentration, and increased urinary calcium excretion are characteristic of dogs with resorptive hypercalciuria.

(b). In our experience, hypercalcemic disorders have been infrequently recognized causes of calcium oxalate uroliths in dogs.

3. Hyperoxaluria.

a. Oxalic acid is the end product of metabolism of ascorbic acid and amino acids (glycine and serine) derived from both endogenous and dietary sources. Oxalic acid forms soluble salts with sodium and potassium ions, but a relatively insoluble salt with calcium ions. Increases in urine oxalate concentration promote calcium oxalate urolith formation to a greater degree than comparable increases in urine calcium concentration.

b. Hyperoxaluria has not been documented in dogs with calcium oxalate uroliths; however, failure to recognize canine hyperoxaluria likely is related to the unavailability of a reproducible method of determining the concentration of oxalate in urine.

c. In humans, hyperoxaluria has been associated with inherited abnormalities of excessive oxalate synthesis (primary hyperoxaluria), increased consumption of foods containing large quantities of oxalate or oxalate precursors (leafy vegetables such as spinach, parsley, and rhubarb; soybean products; nuts; cocoa; some

TABLE 41–14.
EXPECTED CHANGES ASSOCIATED WITH MEDICAL THERAPY TO MINIMIZE RECURRENCE OF CALCIUM OXALATE UROLITHS

Finding	Before Therapy	Prevention Therapy
Polyuria	±	Variable
Pollakiuria	0 to 4+	0
Hematuria	0 to 4+	0
Urine specific gravity	Variable	1.004–1.015
Urine pH	<7.0	>7.0
Urine inflammation	0 to 4+	0
CaOx crystals	0 to 4+	0
Bacteriuria	0 to 4+	0
Bacterial culture of urine	0 to 4+	0
BUN (mg/dL)	>15	<15
Urolith size, number	Small to large	0

Key: CaOx, calcium oxalate; BUN, blood urea nitrogen; ± = sometimes; 1+ = small quantity; 4+ = large quantity.

diet colas), pyridoxine deficiency, and disorders associated with fat malabsorption.[216]

4. Hypocitriuria.
   a. Hypocitriuria is a common physiologic disturbance in humans with calcium oxalate urolithiasis.
   b. The role of low urine citrate concentration in the causation of calcium oxalate uroliths is not completely resolved.
      (1). Urine citrate has been recognized as one inhibitor of calcium oxalate urolith formation.
      (2). By complexing with calcium ions to form the relatively soluble salt of calcium citrate, citrate reduces the quantity of calcium available to bind with oxalate.
   c. Hypocitriuria has been observed in dogs with calcium oxalate uroliths.
      (1). Mechanisms responsible for decreased urinary citrate excretion are unknown.[124]
      (2). It is known that acid-base homeostasis influences the quantity of citrate excreted in urine.[190]
      (3). In normal dogs, acidosis is associated with decreased urinary citrate excretion, whereas alkalosis promotes urinary citrate excretion.
5. Defective macromolecular crystal growth inhibitors.
   a. In addition to urinary concentration of calculogenic minerals and other ions, large–molecular weight proteins in urine have a profound ability to enhance solubility of calcium oxalate.
   b. One such protein, called *nephrocalcin,* minimized calcium oxalate crystal growth in human urine.[137,137a]
      (1). Nephrocalcin is a macromolecular glycoprotein present in renal proximal tubule cells and the thick ascending limb of Henle's loop.[137,137a] Nephrocalcin can be adsorbed to calcium oxalate crystals, forming a macromolecular layer that inhibits crystal growth. Nephrocalcin also inhibits calcium oxalate crystal aggregation.
      (2). Nephrocalcin found in urine of human patients with calcium oxalate urolithiasis was structurally different from nephrocalcin found in healthy human urine. Nephrocalcin from urolith-forming patients lacked appropriate quantities of carboxyglutamic acid residues and was unable effectively to prevent crystal growth.
      (3). Preliminary studies of urine obtained from dogs with calcium oxalate uroliths have revealed that nephrocalcin also lacked appropriate numbers of carboxyglutamic acid residues as compared with nephrocalcin isolated from normal dog urine.

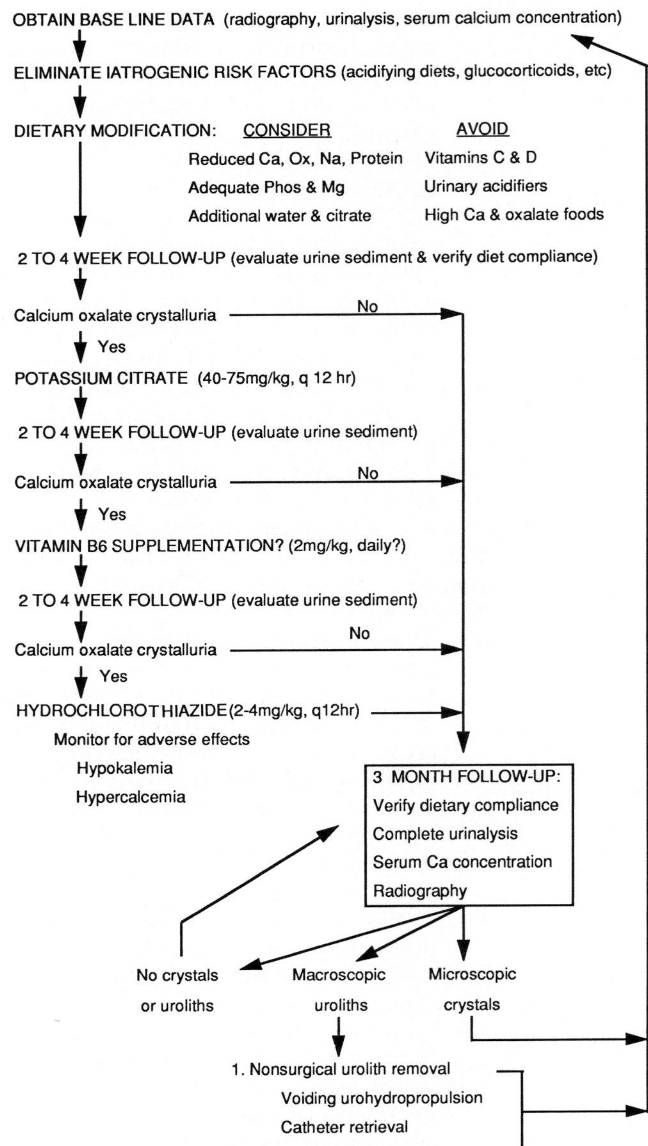

FIG. 41–49. Algorithm for medical management of calcium oxalate uroliths.

6. Nonpolymerized Tamm-Horsfall mucoprotein, which binds to crystal surfaces, is a stabilizing agent.[32,95] At low pH and in the presence of calcium and sodium chloride, Tamm-Horsfall mucoprotein in urine obtained from humans with urolithiasis has a tendency to polymerize, reducing its ability to interact with crystals.

B. Treatment and prevention (Table 41–12, 41–14; Fig. 41–49).

1. Overview.
   a. In contrast to struvite, urate, and cystine uroliths, which dissolve when oversaturation of urine with calculogenic substances is abol-

ished, we have been unable to consistently dissolve calcium oxalate uroliths in dogs.

b. Currently, surgery remains the most effective method for removing active canine calcium oxalate uroliths.

c. Medical protocols may be considered, to prevent further growth of uroliths that remain in the urinary tract or to minimize urolith recurrence following removal.

(1). In general, medical therapy should be formulated in an incremental fashion, with the initial goal of reducing the urine concentration of calculogenic substances. Medications that have the potential to induce a sustained alteration in body composition of metabolites, in addition to urine concentration of metabolites, should be reserved for patients with active or frequently recurrent calcium oxalate uroliths. Caution must be used so that side effects of treatment are not more detrimental than the effects of uroliths.

(2). In patients with hypercalcemia and resorptive hypercalciuria, the cause of hypercalcemia (for example, primary hyperparathyroidism) should be corrected (see Table 41–12).

(3). Whether calcium oxalate uroliths that remain in the patient following parathyroidectomy subsequently dissolve is not known; however, growth or recurrence of such stones is unlikely.

(4). In patients with normal serum calcium concentrations, an attempt should be made to identify risk factors for urolith formation. Amelioration or control of the consequences of risk factors (urine oversaturation with calculogenic minerals) should minimize urolith growth and recurrence (see Table 41–12).

2. Diet modification.

a. Although reduction of urine calcium and oxalate concentrations by reduction of dietary calcium and oxalate appears to be a logical therapeutic goal, it is not necessarily a harmless maneuver.

(1). Reducing consumption of only one of these constituents (e.g., calcium) may increase the availability of the other (e.g., oxalate) for intestinal absorption and subsequent urinary excretion.[81]

(2). In general, reduction in dietary oxalate should be accompanied by an appropriate reduction in dietary oxalate.

b. Humans with calcium oxalate uroliths are often cautioned to avoid milk and milk products because the carbohydrate component (lactose) of these products may augment intestinal absorption of calcium from any dietary source.[153] Likewise, they are often discouraged from consuming foods that contain relatively large quantities of oxalate (chocolate, nuts, beans, sweet potatoes, wheat germ, spinach, rhubarb). Although there is agreement that excessive consumption of calcium and oxalate should be avoided, the general consensus of urologists is that it is inadvisable to restrict dietary calcium unless absorptive hypercalciuria has been documented. Even then, only moderate restriction is advocated, to prevent negative balance of calcium in the body.

c. Consumption of large amounts of sodium may augment renal excretion of calcium.

(1). Twenty-four–hour urinary calcium excretion for normal dogs that consumed a diet with 0.8% sodium (dry weight analysis) was comparable to calcium excretion in dogs with calcium oxalate uroliths.

(2). Therefore, moderate dietary restriction of sodium (less than 0.3% sodium) is recommended for active calcium oxalate stone formers.

d. Studies of laboratory animals, dogs, and humans suggest that dietary phosphorus should not be restricted in patients with calcium oxalate urolithiasis because reduction in dietary phosphorus is often associated with augmentation of hypercalciuria.

(1). If calcium oxalate urolithiasis is associated with hypophosphatemia and normal serum calcium concentration, oral phosphorus supplementation should be considered.

(2). However, caution must be used, since excessive dietary phosphorus may predispose to formation of calcium phosphate uroliths.

e. Although supplemental dietary magnesium contributes to formation of magnesium ammonium phosphate uroliths in some species (cats and ruminants), urine magnesium apparently impairs formation of calcium oxalate crystals.

(1). For this reason, supplemental magnesium has been used in attempts to minimize recurrence of calcium oxalate uroliths in humans.

(2). However, we observed increased urinary excretion of calcium by normal dogs given supplemental magnesium.

(3). Pending further studies we do not recommend dietary magnesium restriction or supplementation for treatment of canine calcium oxalate uroliths.

f. Ingestion of foods that contain large quantities of animal protein may contribute to calcium oxalate urolithiasis by increasing urinary calcium excretion and decreasing urinary citrate excretion.

(1). Some of these consequences result from obligatory acid excretion associated with protein metabolism.
(2). We have observed hypercalciuria in normal dogs fed a high-protein diet (40% dry weight analysis).
(3). Therefore, excessive dietary protein consumption should be avoided in dogs with active calcium oxalate urolithiasis.

g. A diet moderately restricted in protein, calcium, oxalate, and sodium (such as Prescription Diet Canine u/d; Hill's) may be considered, to help prevent recurrence of active calcium oxalate uroliths in dogs. Ideally, diets should not be restricted or supplemented with phosphorus or magnesium.

h. Excessive levels of vitamin D (which promotes intestinal absorption of calcium), and ascorbic acid (a precursor of oxalate), should also be avoided.

i. A deficiency of pyridoxine should be avoided, since vitamin B_6 deficiency promotes endogenous production of oxalate.[153]

3. Thiazide diuretics.

a. Thiazide diuretics have been recommended to reduce recurrence of calcium-containing uroliths in humans, owing to their ability to reduce urine calcium excretion.[153] The exact mechanism(s) by which thiazide diuretics reduce urinary calcium excretion are not known; however, several factors appear to be involved.
(1). For instance, studies in rats revealed that thiazide diuretics directly stimulated distal renal tubular resorption of calcium.
(2). Although results of studies in humans suggest that thiazide diuretics potentiate the action of PTH, effects of thiazide diuretics on urinary calcium excretion were not altered in parathyroidectomized rats or dogs.
(3). Because the hypocalciuric response to thiazide diuretics was blocked when volume depletion was prevented by sodium chloride administration to humans, it was hypothesized that thiazide diuretics promote mild extracellular volume contraction and, thus promote proximal tubular reabsorption of several solutes, including sodium and calcium.

b. In dogs, urinary calcium excretion may increase, decrease, or remain unchanged following thiazide diuretic administration.
(1). In one canine study, fractional clearance of calcium increased following intravenous administration of chlorothiazide.
(2). In contrast, infusion of thiazide diuretics into the left renal artery of dogs resulted in a significant reduction in calcium clearance as compared with clearance by the right kidney.
(3). In another canine study, distal tubular concentrations of calcium did not change following intravenous administration of chlorothiazide.
(4). These results suggest that the effect of thiazide diuretics on urinary excretion of calcium in dogs is variable.
(5). When we evaluated the effect of chlorothiazide (21, 42, and 65 mg/kg every 12 hours) in six normal dogs, a hypocalciuric effect was not observed. In fact, the opposite occurred. As the dose of chlorothiazide was increased, daily urinary calcium excretion also increased.
(6). We have observed a beneficial reduction in urinary calcium excretion in dogs with calcium oxalate urolithiasis following administration of hydrochlorothiazide (2 to 4 mg/kg every 12 hours) for 2 weeks. Because thiazide diuretic administration can be associated with adverse effects (dehydration, hypokalemia, hypercalcemia), they should not be used without appropriate monitoring.

4. Citrate.

a. Citrate inhibits calcium oxalate crystal formation because of its ability to form soluble salts with calcium. This may explain why some humans with abnormally low quantities of urine citrate are at risk for development of calcium oxalate uroliths.

b. Oral administration of potassium citrate (approximately 90 mg/kg per day) to human patients has been associated with marked increases in urinary citrate excretion.

c. Administration of up to 150 mg/kg per day of potassium citrate to normal dogs was not associated with a consistent increase in urine citrate concentration. A dose-dependent rise in urine pH did occur.
(1). These results suggest that metabolism and excretion of potassium citrate in dogs may differ from those in humans. While 10 to 35% of filtered citrate is excreted in urine by humans, only 1 to 3% is excreted by dogs.[190]
(2). Even though oral administration of potassium citrate may not be associated with a sustained increase in urine citrate concentration, potassium citrate may be beneficial in management of calcium oxalate because of its alkalinizing effect.
(a). In dogs, chronic metabolic acidosis inhibits renal tubular reabsorption of calcium, whereas metabolic alkalosis enhances tubular reabsorption of calcium.

(b). Potassium citrate is preferred to sodium bicarbonate as an alkalinizing agent because oral administration of sodium enhances urine calcium excretion.

(c). A commercially available diet for the dissolution or prevention of urate, cystine, and calcium oxalate uroliths in dogs (Prescription Diet Canine u/d; Hill's) contains potassium citrate.

(d). If hypocitrituria is recognized in dogs (mean urinary citrate excretion of 33 normal beagles was 2.57 ± 2.31 mg/kg per 24 hours, median urinary citrate excretion of 33 normal beagles was 1.88 mg/kg per 24 hours), wax matrix tablets of potassium citrate may be considered.[125] We currently recommend a dosage of 100 to 150 mg/kg per day (in two doses); tablets should be crushed and then mixed with food.

5. Other agents have been suggested for management of calcium oxalate uroliths in humans, including:
   a. Allopurinol, to minimize heterogenous nucleation of calcium oxalate on uric acid crystals.

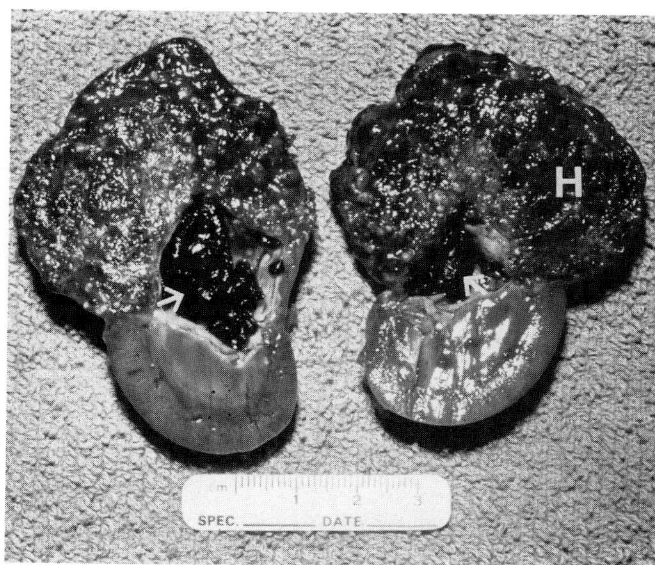

FIG. 41–51. Blood clots *(arrows)* mineralized with calcium phosphate in the renal pelvis of a kidney surgically removed from a 5-year-old spayed female poodle. A benign hemartoma (H) resulted in gross hematuria and formation of the blood clots. The mineralized blood clots were radiodense.

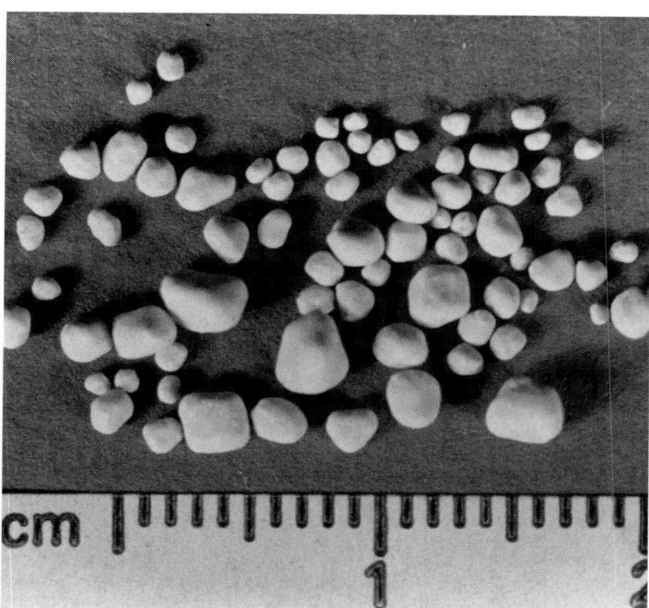

FIG. 41–50. Photograph of urocystoliths removed from a 5-year-old castrated male miniature schnauzer. Quantitative analysis revealed that the uroliths were 75% calcium apatite, 15% calcium oxalate monohydrate, and 10% calcium oxalate dihydrate. These uroliths are similar in radiodensity, size, and shape to calcium oxalate monohydrate. They are similar in size and shape to—but more radiodense than—cystine and some ammonium urate uroliths.

   b. Sodium cellulose phosphate, to bind intestinal calcium.
   c. Orthophosphates, to minimize calcium excretion. (Consult references for details and applications to veterinary medicine.[81,153,196])

IX. FELINE CALCIUM OXALATE UROLITHIASIS

A. In our most recent studies, calcium oxalate uroliths accounted for approximately 24% of the total (Table 41–2). They were detected in the kidneys, ureters, urinary bladder, and urethra. Calcium oxalate uroliths were also voided through the urethra.

B. Calcium oxalate was the most common mineral identified in feline nephroliths submitted to our laboratory (Table 41–4).

C. Medical protocols that promote dissolution of calcium oxalate uroliths in cats are as yet unavailable. Surgery remains the only alternative for removal of clinically active calcium oxalate uroliths. Some calcium oxalate uroliths, especially those in the kidneys, may remain clinically silent for months to years.

1. Because of the unavoidable destruction of nephrons during nephrotomy, this procedure is not recommended unless it can be established that the stones are a cause of clinically significant disease.
2. Serial urinalysis, renal function tests, serum electrolyte evaluations, and radiographic studies may be indicated to evaluate the clinical activity of calcium oxalate nephroliths.

TABLE 41–15.
GLOSSARY OF CALCIUM PHOSPHATE CRYSTALS THAT MAY OCCUR IN UROLITHS

Chemical Name	Crystal Name	Formula
Beta–tricalcium phosphate (calcium orthophosphate)	Whitlockite	Beta-$CA_2(PO_4)_2$
Carbonate apatite	Carbonate apatite	$Ca_{10}(PO_4CO_3OH)_6(OH)_2$
Calcium hydrogen phosphate dihydrate	Brushite	$CaHPO_42H_2O$
Calcium phosphate	Hydroxyapatite or calcium apatite	$Ca_{10}(PO_4)_6(OH)_2$

D. See Chapter 35, Disorders of the Feline Lower Urinary Tract, for additional details.

X. CANINE CALCIUM PHOSPHATE UROLITHIASIS

A. Etiopathogenesis (Figs. 41–50, 41–51).

1. Calcium phosphate uroliths are commonly called *apatite uroliths.*
   a. The most common forms of calcium phosphate observed in canine uroliths are hydroxyapatite, carbonate apatite, and brushite (Tables 41–1, 41–15). The name *carbonate apatite* is derived from the fact that carbonate ion may displace phosphate ion in some uroliths.
   b. Less common forms of calcium phosphate include whitlockite and octacalcium phosphate.
   c. Calcium carbonate apparently does not exist as a separate compound in canine and feline uroliths as it does in equine, rabbit, and guinea pig uroliths. In humans, dogs, and cats, the carbonate radical associates with the complex apatite structure to form a carbonate apatite lattice.
   d. More than one crystalline form of calcium phosphate may be present in a single urolith. In alkaline urine, brushite is readily transformed to apatite; it is possible that some apatite identified in uroliths originated from brushite.[168] In addition, mixtures of calcium phosphate and calcium oxalate often occur.
2. Calcium phosphate is commonly a minor component of struvite and calcium oxalate uroliths (see the appropriate sections of this chapter for additional information). Uroliths composed primarily of calcium phosphate are uncommon in dogs, accounting for about 1 to 2% of those submitted to stone centers (see Table 41–1).[106,120,143,149] Calcium phosphate accounted for approximately 4% of the canine nephroliths (see Table 41–3).
3. Epidemiology.
   a. Of 22,810 canine uroliths analyzed by polarizing light microscopy, infrared spectroscopy, and x-ray diffraction at the Minnesota Urolith Center, 195 were composed primarily (70 to 100%) of calcium phosphate. Of the 195 canine calcium phosphate uroliths, 99 were hydroxyapatite, 77 were brushite, 18 were carbonate apatite, and one was tricalcium phosphate.
   b. Hydroxyapatite. Of 99 canine hydroxyapatite uroliths, 46 were composed entirely (100%) of calcium phosphate and 53 were composed of at least 70% of this mineral. The mean age of dogs at the time of urolith retrieval was 7 ± 3.8 years (range, 1 month to 16 years). Males were affected (62%) more commonly than females (31%); the gender of 7% of the dogs was not recorded. Thirty-five different breeds were affected, including cocker spaniels (10%), mixed breeds (10%), miniature schnauzers (8%), German shepherds (6%), miniature poodles (5%), and springer spaniels (5%). Hydroxyapatite uroliths were more often removed from the lower urinary tract (77%) than the upper tract (7%); the location of 16% of the hydroxyapatite uroliths was not specified.
   c. Brushite. Of 77 calcium hydrogen phosphate dihydrate uroliths, 40 were composed entirely (100%) of this mineral and 37 were at least 70% of this mineral. The mean age of dogs at the time of urolith retrieval was 7.5 ± 2.8 years (range, 1 month to 16 years). Males were affected (77%) more commonly than females (16%); the gender of 7% of affected dogs was not recorded. Twenty-seven breeds were affected, including Yorkshire terriers (10%), bichon Frisé (7%), miniature poodles (7%), Shih Tzus (7%), and mixed breeds (5%). Brushite uroliths were more commonly retrieved from the lower urinary tract (94%) than the upper urinary tract (4%); the location of 3% of the brushite uroliths was not recorded.
   d. Carbonate apatite. Of 18 carbonate apatite uroliths, three were composed entirely (100%) of this mineral and 15 were composed of at least 70% of this mineral. The mean age of dogs at the time of urolith retrieval was 8 ± 4 years (range, 1 month to 12 years). Thirteen different breeds were affected. Females were affected (72%) more commonly than males (28%). Carbonate apatite uroliths were more commonly retrieved from the lower urinary tract (72%) than the upper urinary tract (28%).
4. Factors that decrease calcium phosphate solubility predispose to urolith formation (Table 41–16).

a. The solubility of calcium phosphates in urine is dependent on several variables:
   (1). Urine hydrogen ion concentration.
   (2). Urine calcium ion concentration.
   (3). Total urine inorganic phosphate concentration.
   (4). Urine concentration of inhibitors of calcium crystallization.
   (5). Urine concentration of potentiators of crystallization.

b. Urine pH. Urine pH has a profound effect on the solubility of some forms of calcium phosphate.[64] With the exception of brushite, calcium phosphate solubility markedly decreases in alkaline urine and increases in acid urine. Increased urine pH increases the availability of ionic PO_4^{3-} and HPO_4^{2-} for incorporation into calcium phosphates.[45] Apatite does not crystallize from human urine unless the pH is at least 6.6.[62] At a pH of 5.5, approximately 400 mg/L of calcium phosphate can be held in solution, whereas only 32 mg/L of calcium phosphate is held in solution at a pH of 7.8.[63] Therefore, human patients with disorders associated with persistent elevation of urine pH (such as distal renal tubular acidosis) are predisposed to calcium phosphate urolith formation. In contrast to carbonate apatite and hydroxyl apatite, brushite is less soluble in acid urine.

c. Hypercalciuria.
   (1). Hypercalciuria decreases calcium phosphate solubility and may result in oversaturation with calcium phosphate.[166] Hypercalciuria may result from excessive resorption of calcium from bone, enhanced intestinal absorption of calcium, impaired renal tubular reabsorption of calcium, or a combination of these factors. Urine specimens obtained from human patients with hypercalciuria and calcium uroliths are usually supersaturated with brushite.
   (2). Controversy exists over the relative importance of urine pH and hypercalciuria as determinants of calcium phosphate solubility in vivo. Some believe that calcium phosphate crystallization is governed primarily by changes in urine pH; these investigators minimize the importance of hypercalciuria.[62] However, it has been suggested that persistent hypercalciuria tends to raise the calcium phosphate saturation of urine so that small increases in urine pH result in calcium phosphate crystalluria. There have been no studies on the relative effect of hypercalciuria and urine pH on the solubility of different types of calcium phosphate in canine urine.

d. Crystallization inhibitors.
   (1). Normally, urine contains calcium phosphate crystal inhibitors. One mechanism by which inhibitors prevent urolith formation is by chelating with stone constituents, making them unavailable for nidus formation or crystal growth. In addition, crystallization inhibitors may alter crystalline structure in such a way that crystal growth and aggregation are prevented. Inhibitors of calcium phosphate crystallization include inorganic pyrophosphates, citrate, and magnesium ions.[16] These inhibitors provide 30 to 40% of the inhibitory capacity of normal human urine for calcium phosphate crystallization. The remaining 60 to 70% is provided by as yet unidentified low–molecular weight inhibitors.
   (2). Pyrophosphates increase the upper limit of urine calcium phosphate saturation at which spontaneous precipitation occurs, and they retard growth of hydroxyapatite crystals by adsorbing to their surfaces and blocking active growth sites. In addition, pyrophosphates inhibit transformation of amorphous calcium phosphate into crystalline form.[73] Citrate forms soluble complexes with calcium and thus decreases the availability of calcium for incorporation into crystals. Magnesium may replace calcium on the surface of growing crystals and thus block epitaxial growth.

e. Crystallization promoters. Formation of calcium phosphate uroliths may be promoted by epitaxy. Epitaxy is the process by which crystals of one salt induce the formation of crystals of another salt. Epitactic induction occurs between crystals of similar lattice dimensions. Calcium phosphate precipitation has been reported to be stimulated by calcium oxalate and monosodium urate crystals.[73]

5. Calcium phosphate uroliths may occur in patients with primary hyperparathyroidism, other hypercalcemic disorders, distal renal tubule acidosis, and idiopathic hypercalciuria (Table 41–16). Be-

TABLE 41–16.
DISORDERS THAT MAY PREDISPOSE TO THE FORMATION OF CALCIUM PHOSPHATE UROLITHS

Primary hyperparathyroidism	Distal renal tubular acidosis
Other hypercalcemia disorders	Normocalcemic hypercalciuria
Neoplasia	Intestinal hyperabsorption
Vitamin D intoxication	Renal leak
Excessive calcium intake	
Thyrotoxicosis	
Hyperadrenocorticism	
Immobilization	

cause the prevalence of calcium phosphate uroliths in dogs and cats is low, and because appropriate metabolic studies have rarely been performed in affected animals, the association of calcium phosphate uroliths with other canine and feline metabolic disorders is not as firmly established as it is in humans.

a. Primary hyperparathyroidism.

(1). Between 18 and 20% of patients with primary hyperparathyroidism have uroliths at the time of diagnosis.[138] In one study of 21 dogs with primary hyperparathyroidism, four (20%) had uroliths.[15] Uroliths from patients with primary hyperparathyroidism typically are composed of calcium phosphate, calcium oxalate, or mixtures of the two. Uroliths composed predominantly of calcium phosphate are more commonly identified in human patients and dogs with primary hyperparathyroidism; uroliths composed predominantly of calcium oxalate more often in humans and dogs with normocalcemic hypercalciuria. Bladder uroliths composed primarily of calcium phosphate have been induced experimentally in dogs following injections of parathyroid hormone.[106]

(2). Factors that predispose patients with primary hyperparathyroidism to calcium phosphate urolith formation include hypercalciuria, increased urine pH, and increased renal excretion of a substance that promotes spontaneous precipitation of calcium salts. Hypercalcemia results from parathyroid hormone–induced bone resorption and renal tubular reabsorption of calcium. In addition, increased intestinal absorption of calcium results from parathyroid hormone–stimulated conversion of 25-hydroxycholecalciferol to 1,25-dihydroxycholecalciferol.[166] Hypercalcemia results in increased glomerular filtration of calcium and hypercalciuria, which in turn enhances the likelihood of urolith formation by increasing urine saturation with brushite and calcium oxalate.[16] The urine of most hypercalciuric humans with primary hyperparathyroidism is supersaturated with brushite and calcium oxalate. Hypercalciuria has been documented in dogs with primary hyperparathyroidism and calcium uroliths.[11,12]

(3). Persistent elevation in urine pH may predispose some patients with primary hyperparathyroidism to calcium phosphate urolithiasis. Urine pH is elevated in these patients because of impaired renal tubule reabsorption of bicarbonate. This abnormality may explain, at least in part, the increased incidence of calcium phosphate uroliths in patients with primary hyperparathyroidism as compared with patients with other hypercalciuric disorders. It has been suggested that some patients with primary hyperparathyroidism excrete a substance in their urine that facilitates calcium phosphate and calcium oxalate precipitation.[166] The specific nature of this urolithiasis-promoting factor has not been determined.

b. Other hypercalcemic disorders. In addition to primary hyperparathyroidism, other hypercalcemic disorders are occasionally associated with formation of calcium phosphate uroliths. Uroliths have been identified in human patients with hypervitaminosis D, neoplastic disorders, Cushing's syndrome, and in patients who are immobilized for long periods.[195] Although calcium phosphate is the most frequently identified mineral in uroliths obtained from these patients, calcium oxalate may also be present. Because the prevalence of uroliths in patients with these hypercalcemic disorders is low, it is likely that factors other than hypercalcemia are involved.

c. Distal renal tubule acidosis.

(1). Nephrolithiasis is a common manifestation of hereditary distal renal tubular acidosis (Type I) in humans.[109] Uroliths typically are composed entirely of calcium phosphate, though calcium oxalate and struvite stones have also been identified.[109] Urolith formation has not been observed in patients with acquired distal renal tubular acidosis or proximal renal tubular acidosis (Type II).

(2). Hypercalciuria, alkaline urine, low urine citrate concentration, and excessive urinary phosphate excretion contribute to formation of calcium phosphate uroliths observed in patients with distal renal tubular acidosis. Hypercalciuria and hyperphosphaturia tend to raise urine saturation with calcium phosphate. Acidosis increases calcium mobilization from bone, causing an increase in the quantity of calcium excreted in urine. In addition, acidosis decreases renal tubular fractional reabsorption of calcium and further increases calcium excretion.[106] Acidosis may alter renal tubular calcium transport, the response of the tubules to parathyroid hormone, or both.

(3). Distal renal tubular acidosis results from functional inability of the distal nephron to establish a hydrogen ion gradient between blood and tubule fluid, regardless of the severity of acidemia. In humans, the disorder is characterized by inability to lower urine pH below 5.4, hypokalemia, hyperchloremia, hypophosphatemia, hypocalcemia, metabolic acidosis, osteomalacia, nephrocalcinosis, and urolithiasis.[52]

(4). Elevated urine pH increases the availability of PO_4^{3-} and HPO_4^{2-}, which may be incorporated into ionic octacalcium phosphate and brushite, respectively.[45] Increased urine pH is considered more important than hypercalciuria in predisposing to calcium phosphate urolith formation in patients with distal renal tubular acidosis.[45]

(5). Patients with distal renal tubular acidosis excrete decreased amounts of citrate in their urine. Citrate is reabsorbed more avidly in proximal convoluted tubules as a consequence of intracellular acidosis.[52] Because citrate is a major chelator of calcium, decreased citrate concentration decreases calcium solubility.

(6). In humans, distal renal tubular acidosis sometimes occurs as an incomplete form in which uroliths form in the absence of systemic acidosis.[13] Urolithiasis may be the only clinical manifestation of this disorder. The tubular defect can be recognized only by abnormal response to the ammonium chloride–loading test.

d. Normocalcemic hypercalciuria. Normocalcemic hypercalciuria is a syndrome characterized by normal serum calcium concentration, increased urinary excretion of calcium, absence of systemic disease, and increased tendency for formation of calcium phosphate or calcium oxalate uroliths. Approximately 33% of human calcium stone formers have normocalcemic hypercalciuria.[45] Normocalcemic hypercalciuria has been recognized in dogs (see the section on calcium oxalate urolithiasis for details).

e. Mineralization of blood clots (see Fig. 41–51).

(1). We have on numerous occasions observed nephroliths, urocystoliths, and urethroliths composed of blood clots mineralized with calcium phosphate.

(2). They occur primarily in cats, and most often are found in the renal pelvis and the renal pelvic diverticula. Formation of very concentrated urine may favor formation of blood clots in patients with gross hematuria. Contrary to one theory, these black-colored uroliths are not composed of bile metabolites.

B. Treatment and prevention.

1. Surgery remains the most reliable way to remove calcium phosphate uroliths from the urinary tract; however, we emphasize that surgery may be unnecessary for clinically inactive calcium phosphate uroliths. Small urocystoliths may be removed by voiding urohydropropulsion.[123]
2. Because the likelihood of recurrence after removal of calcium phosphate uroliths is not well-established, patients should be periodically monitored by urinalysis, appropriate radiographic procedures, and, if indicated, laboratory tests of blood and urine (Table 41–17). If recurrent urocystoliths are detected when small, they may be nonsurgically removed by voiding urohydropropulsion or by aspiration through a urinary catheter.[122,152]
3. Medical therapy of patients with recurrent calcium phosphate uroliths should then be directed at removing or minimizing risk factors that contribute to supersaturation of urine with calcium phosphate (Table 41–18). Although calcium-chelating agents have been reported to be useful in dissolving calcium phosphate uroliths in humans, the feasibility of this type of therapy has not been reported in dogs or cats.
4. Primary hyperparathyroidism.
   a. Patients with primary hyperparathyroidism usually require surgery.[15] Parathyroidectomy may result in dissolution of uroliths and generally prevents recurrence.
   b. In a dog with primary hyperparathyroidism and recurrent calcium phosphate uroliths, parathyroidectomy resulted in decreased urinary calcium excretion and prevention of new urolith formation.[104a]
5. Distal renal tubule acidosis.
   a. To our knowledge, medical dissolution of calcium phosphate uroliths has not been attempted in dogs with distal renal tubule acido-

TABLE 41–17.
PROBLEM-SPECIFIC DATA BASE FOR DOGS AND CATS WITH CALCIUM PHOSPHATE UROLITHS

Blood tests	Complete urinalysis, including careful evaluation of pH and crystals
SUN and/or serum creatinine	Bacterial culture of urine
Calcium	Consider 24-hr urine collection*
Phosphorus	Volume
Sodium	Creatinine
Chloride	Calcium
Potassium	Phosphorus
Blood gas or total CO_2	Magnesium
Intact PTH (if serum Ca is elevated)	Citrate (if possible)
25-hydroxyvitamin D	Oxalate (if possible)
Magnesium (if possible)	
Uric acid (if possible)	

Key: PTH, parathyroid hormone.
*A standardized diet should be fed as described in text.

TABLE 41–18.
SUMMARY OF RECOMMENDATIONS FOR MANAGEMENT OF CALCIUM PHOSPHATE UROLITHS

1. Whereas surgery remains the most reliable way to remove active calcium phosphate uroliths from the urinary tract, we emphasize that surgery may be unnecessary for clinically inactive calcium phosphate uroliths. Small urocystoliths may be removed nonsurgically by voiding urohydropropulsion or by aspiration through a urinary catheter (Table 41–24). Medial therapy of patients with recurrent calcium phosphate uroliths should then be directed at removing or minimizing risk factors that contribute to supersaturation of urine with calcium phosphate.
2. Patients with hypercalcemia and primary hyperparathyroidism usually require surgery. Parathyroidectomy may result in dissolution of uroliths, and it generally prevents recurrence.
3. Several different medical protocols have been reported to be of value in humans with normocalcemic hypercalciuria. Ideally, choice of therapy should be based on the cause of idiopathic hypercalciuria (see Tables 41–12, 41–13).
   a. There is little clinical experience in the use of drugs in dogs and cats with calcium phosphate uroliths; however, medications that can enhance calcium excretion, such as glucocorticoids, furosemide and those containing large quantities of sodium, should be avoided, if possible.
   b. Diets designed to avoid excessive protein, sodium, calcium, and vitamin D may be of benefit. Excessive restriction or supplementation of dietary phosphorus probably should be avoided. Enhancement of urine volume by feeding a canned diet (and/or a protein-restricted diet to dogs to reduce renal medullary urea) and encouraging water consumption may also be of benefit. Although understandably difficult in some patients, fluid intake should be encouraged throughout the day, to promote constantly large urine volume. In humans, high-fiber diets have been shown to reduce intestinal absorption and urinary excretion of calcium.
   c. With the exception of brushite, calcium phosphates tend to be less soluble in alkaline urine. Whether or not patients so affected would benefit by use of appropriate doses of acidifiers is not known. Acidification tends to enhance urine calcium excretion and is a risk factor for calcium oxalate urolith formation. Pending further studies, we are not now able to recommend routine use of urine acidifiers for patients with calcium phosphate urolithiasis.
4. To our knowledge, medical dissolution of calcium phosphate uroliths has not been attempted in dogs with distal RTA. Diets designed to dissolve struvite uroliths generally would not be expected to promote dissolution of calcium phosphate uroliths, in part because they may tend to promote acidemia and aciduria, thus potentially enhancing hypercalciuria and hypocitraturia. Correction of hypercalciuria, hyperphosphaturia, and hypocitraturia by alkalinization therapy with potassium citrate might promote dissolution of these uroliths in patients with complete or incomplete distal RTA. Longterm alkalinization therapy appears to be beneficial in preventing calcium phosphate urolith formation in humans with distal RTA. Such therapy has been advocated for patients with complete or incomplete forms of distal RTA because it decreases urolith formation and nephrocalcinosis and increases urine citrate concentration. Oral administration of sodium chloride, long recommended for all forms of urolithiasis, may promote hypercalciuria and calcium phosphate urolith formation. Thus, oral salt therapy is not recommended to promote diuresis in dogs whose uroliths contain calcium salts.

sis (RTA). Diets designed to dissolve struvite uroliths would generally not be expected to promote dissolution of calcium phosphate uroliths, in part because they tend to promote acidemia and aciduria, thus potentially enhancing hypercalciuria and hypocitraturia. Correction of hypercalciuria, hyperphosphaturia, and hypocitraturia by alkalinization therapy with potassium citrate might, however, promote dissolution of these uroliths in patients with complete or incomplete distal RTA.

b. Longterm alkalinization therapy appears to be beneficial in preventing calcium phosphate urolith formation in humans with distal RTA. Such therapy has been advocated for patients with complete or incomplete forms of distal RTA because it decreases urolith formation and nephrocalcinosis and increases the urine citrate concentration. Oral administration of sodium chloride, long recommended for all forms of urolithiasis, may promote hypercalciuria and calcium phosphate urolith formation; therefore, oral salt therapy is not recommended to promote diuresis in dogs with uroliths containing calcium salts.

6. Normocalcemic hypercalciuria.
   a. Several different medical protocols have been reported to be of value in humans with normocalcemic hypercalciuria.[45] Ideally, the choice of therapy should be based on the cause of idiopathic hypercalciuria. There has been little clinical experience with the use of drugs in dogs and cats with calcium phosphate uroliths; however, medications that can enhance calcium excretion, such as glucocorticoids, furosemide, and those containing large quantities of sodium should be avoided, if possible.
   b. Dietary modification.
      (1). Diets designed to avoid excessive protein, sodium, calcium, and vitamin D may be of benefit.
      (2). Excessive restriction or supplementation of dietary phosphorus should probably be avoided.
      (3). Enhancement of urine volume by feeding

a canned diet (and/or a protein-restricted diet to dogs to reduce renal medullary urea) and encouraging water consumption may also be of benefit. Though this is understandably difficult in some patients, fluid intake should be encouraged throughout the day to promote constantly high urine volume.

(4). In humans, high-fiber diets have been shown to reduce intestinal absorption and urinary excretion of calcium.

c. Urine acidifiers.

(1). With the exception of brushite, calcium phosphates tend to be less soluble in alkaline urine. Whether or not such patients would benefit from appropriate doses of acidifiers is not known. Acidification tends to enhance urine calcium excretion and is a risk factor for calcium oxalate urolith formation. Pending further studies, we are unable to recommend routine use of urine acidifiers for patients with calcium phosphate urolithiasis.

(2). Because calcium hydrogen phosphate dihydrate (brushite) is less soluble in acid urine, it might seem logical to promote formation of alkaline urine by patients with brushite uroliths. However, in alkaline urine brushite may be converted to other insoluble forms of calcium phosphate. Use of potassium citrate, an alkalinizing agent, might be rationalized on the basis of minimizing acidosis-induced hypercalciuria and formation of the soluble calcium citrate rather than insoluble calcium phosphate in urine. We emphasize that the beneficial or detrimental effects of orally administered potassium citrate to dogs and cats with calcium phosphate urolithiasis have not been carefully evaluated. Consult the section on canine calcium oxalate urolithiasis for additional therapeutic information about potassium citrate.

d. Thiazide diuretics.

(1). Because thiazide diuretics decrease renal calcium excretion, they may be considered to minimize renal leak hypercalciuria.

(2). Hydrochlorothiazide may be given on a trial basis to dogs with recurrent calcium phosphate urolithiasis in doses of 2 to 4 mg/kg every 12 hours. Because administration of thiazide diuretics may be associated with unwanted side effects (dehydration, hypercalcemia, hypokalemia, and magnesium depletion) patients should be appropriately monitored during therapy.

(3). Thiazide therapy is not recommended to treat absorptive hypercalciuria because it does not correct the hyperabsorptive state and may promote positive systemic calcium balance with possible soft-tissue calcification.

e. Other agents.

(1). Other drugs have been utilized in attempts to minimize hypercalciuria in humans.

(2). Sodium cellulose phosphate, the sodium salt of the phosphoric ester of cellulose, is an ion-exchange cellulose with special affinity for divalent ions. In the gastrointestinal tract, it exchanges sodium for dietary calcium, which is then eliminated in the feces. It also binds calcium secreted into the gastrointestinal tract, minimizing its resorption.

(3). Oral administration of orthophosphates to humans with normocalcemic hypercalciuria reduces urinary excretion of calcium and increases urine crystal inhibitory activity by increasing the urine concentration of pyrophosphates.

XI. FELINE CALCIUM PHOSPHATE UROLITHIASIS

A. In our current series, calcium phosphate accounted for 1.3% of naturally occurring feline uroliths (see Table 41–2).

B. As was the situation with nephroliths composed of calcium oxalate, calcium phosphate nephroliths were more common than struvite nephroliths (see Table 41–4).

C. We have documented nephroliths composed of blood clots mineralized with calcium phosphate.

1. Such mineralized blood clots may be found in renal pelvic diverticula and in the renal pelvis.
2. Formation of highly concentrated urine by patients with gross hematuria may favor formation of blood clots.
3. In one persistently hematuric patient, such nephroliths remained inactive (i.e., did not increase in number or size, or cause outflow obstruction, or predispose to bacteria urinary tract infection) over a 3-year period of evaluation.

D. See Chapter 35, Disorders of the Feline Lower Urinary Tract, for additional information.

XII. CANINE CYSTINE UROLITHIASIS

A. Etiopathogenesis (Fig. 41–52).

1. Cystinuria is an inborn error of metabolism characterized by abnormal transport of cystine (a nonessential sulfur-containing amino acid composed of two molecules of cysteine) and other amino acids by the renal tubules. The name cystine was coined because this substance was first identified from urine removed from the urinary bladder (or urocyst) and thus was thought to have originated from the bladder.[187]

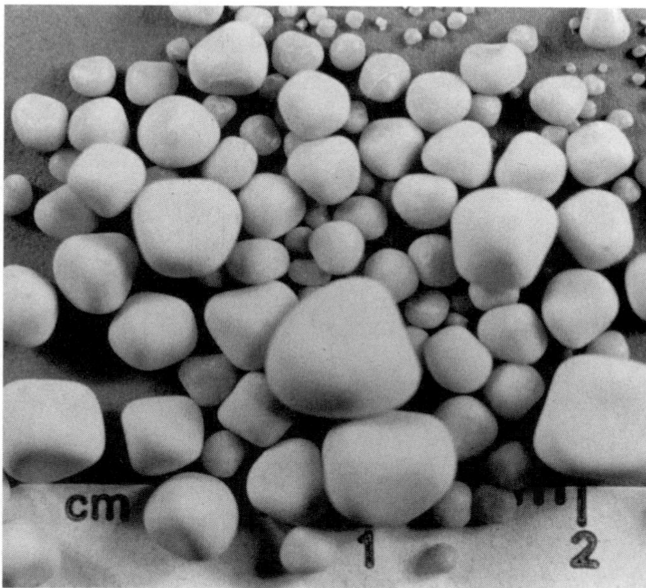

FIG. 41–52. Multiple smooth cystine urocystoliths removed from a 6-year-old male bull mastiff. (From Osborne CA (ed). Canine urolithiasis: etiopathogenesis, detection, treatment, and prevention. *Vet Clin North Am.*1986;16:1–207.)

2. Cystine is normally present in low concentrations in plasma. Normally, circulating cystine is freely filtered at the glomerulus and most is actively reabsorbed in the proximal tubules. The solubility of cystine in urine is pH dependent. It is relatively insoluble in acid urine but becomes more soluble in alkaline urine.
3. Unlike normal dogs, cystinuric dogs reabsorb a much smaller proportion of the amino acid from glomerular filtrate.[21,22] Some may even have net cystine secretion.
   a. The exact mechanism of abnormal renal tubular transport of cystine in dogs is not known.
   b. Plasma concentration of cystine in affected dogs is normal, indicating faulty tubule function rather than hyperexcretion.[22,23] Concentrations of plasma methionine, a precursor of cystine, have been found to be elevated in cystinuric dogs.
   c. Some studies in humans suggest that tubular reabsorption of cysteine, the immediate precursor of cystine, may be abnormal.[12] In this situation, the increase in urine cystine concentration may result from dimerization of two cysteine molecules in tubule urine.
   d. In dogs with cystinuria, the exact pattern of amino aciduria reported by various investigators has been variable.[23,40,48,49] Two populations of cystinuric dogs have been reported.[22]
      (1). One group had cystinuria without the loss of other amino acids.
      (2). Another group had cystinuria and a lesser degree of lysinuria.
   e. Unless protein intake is severely restricted, cystinuric dogs have no detectable abnormalities associated with amino acid loss except for formation of cystine uroliths.
      (1). This occurs because cystine is sparingly soluble at the usual urine pH range of 5.5 to 7.0.
      (2). Cystinuria would be a medical curiosity if cystine were not the least soluble naturally occurring amino acid. The major causes of morbidity and mortality associated with this disorder are the sequelae of urolith formation.
   f. The exact mechanism of cystine urolith formation is not known.
      (1). Because not all cystinuric dogs form uroliths, cystinuria is a predisposing, rather than a primary, cause of cystine urolith formation.
      (2). In one study, 4 of 14 dogs with a history of cystine urolith formation had urine cystine concentrations that fell within the range of those found in control dogs.[23]
      (3). Many breeds of dogs have been reported to develop cystine uroliths, especially dachshunds. English bulldogs also have an unexpectedly high prevalence of cystine uroliths.
   g. With two exceptions, cystine uroliths have been reported only in male dogs.[29,120]
      (1). We have observed cystine urocystoliths in a 9-month-old female Scottish terrier.
      (2). Cystinuria has also been observed in female dogs.[22]

B. Treatment (Figs. 41–53 to 41–55).

1. Objectives. Current recommendations for dissolution of cystine uroliths encompass reduction in the urine concentration of cystine and increasing the solubility of cystine in urine. Utilizing the following protocol, we have induced dissolution of 11 episodes of canine cystine urocystoliths in a mean interval of 81 (range, 29 to 217) days: (1) dietary modification, (2) alkalinization of urine, administration of drugs containing thiol (Table 41–19).[44]
2. Dietary modification.
   a. Reduction of dietary protein has the potential of minimizing formation of cystine uroliths. By decreasing intake of methionine, some decrease in urine cystine excretion might occur. An even more important indirect effect would be a reduction in renal medullary urea concentration and associated reduction in urine concentration.
   b. A protein-restricted alkalinizing diet (Prescription Diet Canine u/d, Hill's) was observed to have a beneficial effect in promoting reduction

in cystine urocystolith size in a 3-year-old male dachshund (see discussion of thiol drugs).

3. Alkalinization of urine.
   a. The solubility of cystine is pH dependent.
      (1). In dogs, the solubility of cystine at urine pH of 7.8 has been reported to be approximately twice that at urine pH of 5.0.[209]
      (2). Changes in urine pH that remain in the acidic range have minimal effect on cystine solubility.
   b. A quantity of potassium citrate or sodium bicarbonate should be given orally in divided doses sufficient to sustain a urine pH of approximately 7.5.
   c. Data derived from studies in cystinuric humans suggest that dietary sodium may enhance cystinuria.[98] Therefore, potassium citrate may be preferable to sodium bicarbonate as a urine alkalinizer. Further studies are required to evaluate the effect of dietary sodium on urinary excretion of cystine in dogs.
   d. It is of interest that UTI caused by urease-producing bacteria in an adult man with cystine nephroliths resulted in extreme urine alkalinity and subsequent urolith dissolution.[89]
4. Thiol-containing drugs.
   a. D-Penicillamine (dimethylcysteine) is a nonmetabolizable degradation product of penicillin that may combine with cysteine to form cysteine-D-penicillamine disulfide. This disulfide exchange reaction is facilitated by alkaline pH. The resulting compound has been reported to be 50 times more soluble than free cystine. The cysteine-D-penicillamine complex does not react with nitroprusside as cystine does, providing a mechanism to titrate dosage of the drug.[164]

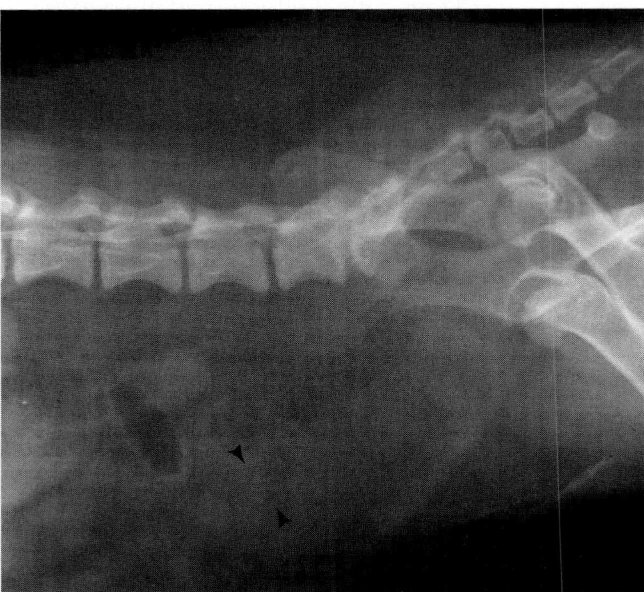

FIG. 41–53. Survey abdominal radiograph of a 3-year-old male dachshund obtained 1 month after a cystotomy. At least six slightly radiodense uroliths *(arrows)* can be identified in the craniad portion of the urinary bladder.

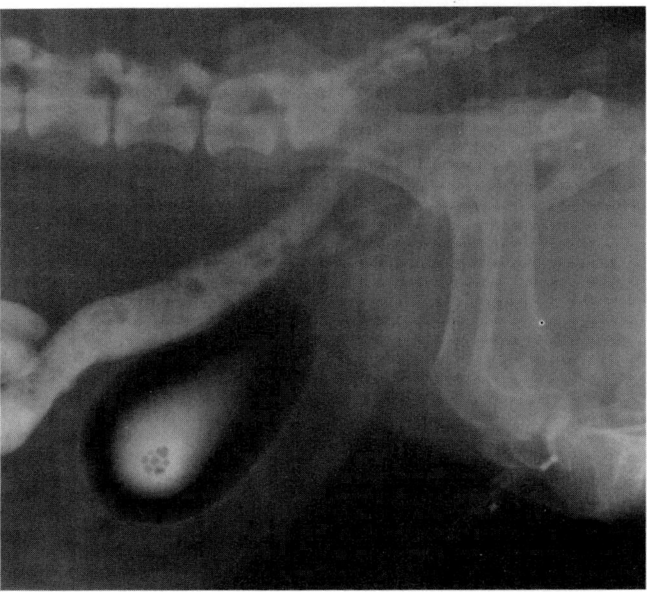

FIG. 41–54. Double-contrast urocystogram of the dog described in Fig. 41–53. Seven uroliths can be seen surrounded by contrast medium.

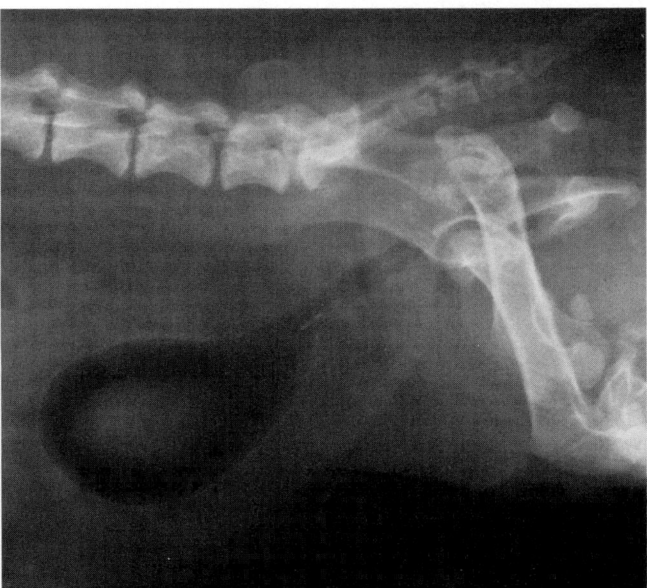

FIG. 41–55. Double-contrast cystogram of the dog described in Fig. 41–53 obtained following management with Hill's Prescription Diet Canine u/d and 2 MPG. There are no uroliths in the bladder lumen, and contrast urethrography revealed no uroliths in the urethral lumen.

TABLE 41–19.
SUMMARY OF RECOMMENDATIONS FOR MEDICAL DISSOLUTION AND PREVENTION OF CANINE CYSTINE UROLITHS

1. Perform appropriate diagnostic studies, including complete urinalysis, quantitative urine culture, and diagnostic radiography. Determine precise location, size, and number of uroliths. The size and number of stones are not reliable indexes of probable efficacy of therapy.
2. Determine mineral composition of uroliths; determine their composition by evaluating appropriate clinical data (see Table 41–9).
3. Consider surgical correction if uroliths are obstructing urine outflow or if correctable abnormalities that predispose to recurrent UTI are identified by radiography or other means. Small urocystoliths may be removed by voiding urohydropropulsion (see Table 41–24).
4. Initiate therapy with a calculolytic diet (Prescription Diet Canine u/d). No other food or mineral supplements should be fed to the patient. Compliance with dietary recommendations is suggested by reduction in serum blood urea nitrogen concentration (usually <10 mg/dL).
5. Initiate therapy with *N*-(2-mercaptopropionyl)-glycine (MPG) at a daily dosage of approximatey 30 mg/kg body weight (divided into 2 equal subdoses).
6. If necessary, administer potassium citrate orally, to eliminate aciduria. Strive for pH of approximately 7.5.
7. If necessary, eradicate or control UTI with appropriate antimicrobial agents.
8. Devise protocol for followup therapy.
   a. Try to avoid diagnostic followup studies that require urinary catheterization. If they are required, give appropriate pericatheterization antimicrobial agents to prevent iatrogenic UTI.
   b. Evaluate serial urinalyses. Urine pH, specific gravity, and microscopic examination of sediment for crystals are especially important. Remember, crystals formed in urine stored at room or refrigeration temperatures may represent in vitro artifacts.
   c. Perform serial radiography at monthly intervals to evaluate stone location(s), number, size, density, and shape. Intravenous urography may be utilized for radiolucent uroliths in the kidneys, ureters, or urinary bladder. Antegrade contrast cystourethrography may be required for radiolucent uroliths located in the bladder and urethra.
9. Continue calculolytic diet, 2 MPG, and alkalinizing therapy for approximately 1 month following disappearance of uroliths as detected by radiography.
10. Prevention: A low-protein diet that promotes alkaline urine has been effective in preventing cystine urolith recurrence. If necessary, small doses of 2 MPG may also be utilized.

(1). The most commonly utilized dosage of D-penicillamine for dogs has been 30 mg/kg per day in two doses.[77] Larger doses frequently cause vomiting and may cause other undesirable reactions. If nausea and vomiting occur with the aforementioned dosage, the drug may be mixed with food or given at mealtimes. In some instances, it may be necessary to prevent gastrointestinal disturbances by initiating therapy with small doses and gradually increasing them until the full dose is reached.

(2). D-Penicillamine has been associated with a variety of adverse reactions in humans, including immune-complex glomerulonephropathy, fever, lymphadenopathy, and skin hypersensitivity.[164] Fever and lymphadenopathy have been found in a dachshund given D-penicillamine at a dosage of 30 mg/kg per day. The signs subsided following withdrawal of the drug and administration of glucocorticoids.

b. *N*-(2-mercaptopropionyl)-glycine (MPG) decreases the concentration of cystine by a thiol disulfide exchange reaction similar to that of D-penicillamine.[96,164,169]

(1). Studies in humans indicate that the drug is highly effective in reducing urinary cystine concentration and is less toxic than D-penicillamine.[169]

(2). Oral administration of MPG in daily doses of approximately 30 mg/kg body weight (in two equal doses) was effective in inducing dissolution of multiple cystine urocystoliths in three of four dogs evaluated.[46] Dissolution required 2 to 4 months' therapy. One dog developed nonpruritic vesicular skin lesions following 3 months' therapy. One month after reduction of the daily dose of MPG from 30 to 25 mg/kg body weight, the skin lesions healed.

c. Dissolution of multiple cystine urocystoliths was induced in a 3-year-old male dachshund by a combination of diet (Prescription Diet Canine u/d, Hill's), urine alkalinization (with sodium bicarbonate), and MPG therapy (30 mg/kg per day in two equal doses).

(1). MPG was utilized because the dog had a history of hypersensitivity to D-penicillamine.

(2). Initial therapy with the diet and sodium bicarbonate resulted in reduction of urolith size by 50% over a 10-week period; however, further reduction in urolith size did not occur during the following month. Therefore, MPG was added to the regimen. When the dog was evaluated by contrast urethrocystography 1 month later, there was no evidence of uroliths.

(3). Cystine urocystoliths recurred approximately 1 year after dissolution. Treatment of the dog with the identical regimen (Prescription Diet Canine u/d, sodium bicarbonate, and MPG) resulted in uro-

TABLE 41–20.
EXPECTED CHANGES ASSOCIATED WITH MEDICAL THERAPY OF CYSTINE UROLITHS

Finding	Before Therapy	During Therapy	Prevention Therapy
Polyuria	±	1+ to 3+	1+ to 3+
Pollakiuria	0 to 4+	↑ then ↓	0
Hematuria	0 to 4+	↓	0
Urine specific gravity	Variable	1.004–1.014	1.004–1.014
Urine pH	<7.0	>7.0	>7.0
Urine inflammation	0 to 4+	↓	0
Urate crystals	0 to 4+	0	Variable
Bacteruria	0 to 4+	0	0
Bacterial culture of urine	0 to 4+	0	0
BUN (mg/dL)	Variable	<15	≤15
Urolith size and number	Small to large	↓	0

Key: BUN, blood urea nitrogen; ± = sometimes; 1+ = small quantity; 4+ = large quantity.

cystolith dissolution in approximately 1 month; though at that time the dog developed Coombs'-positive regenerative spherocytic anemia. Withdrawal of the MPG and oral administration of prednisone was associated with rapid remission of the anemia.

(4). These results suggest that dogs with a history of hypersensitivity to D-penicillamine may also have hypersensitivity to MPG. Appropriate evaluations for adverse reactions should be performed during use of MPG in dogs with a history of D-penicillamine hypersensitivity.

d. We have had excellent results in dissolving 18 episodes of cystine urocystoliths affecting 14 dogs with a combination of dietary and 2-MPG therapy. The mean time required to dissolve the cystine uroliths was 78 days (range 11 to 211 days).

C. Prevention (Tables 41–19, 41–20).

1. Because cystinuria is an inherited metabolic defect, and because cystine uroliths recur in a large percentage of stone-forming dogs within 1 year after surgical removal,[21] prophylactic therapy should be considered.
2. Dietary therapy combined with urine alkalinization may be initiated with the objective of minimizing cystine crystalluria and promoting a negative cyanide-nitroprusside test result.
3. If necessary, MPG or D-penicillamine may be added to the regimen in sufficient quantity to keep the urine concentration of cystine below approximately 200 mg/L. If dosage cannot be titrated by measurement of urine cystine concentration, dosages of 30 mg/kg per day of MPG, or 20 to 30 mg/kg per day of D-penicillamine may be considered. Continuous therapy of stone-free cystinuric dogs with MPG has been effective in preventing formation of cystine uroliths in studies in Sweden.

$$NH_2\text{-}\overset{\displaystyle O}{\overset{\|}{C}}\text{-}NH_2 + H_2O \xrightarrow{\text{urease}} 2NH_3 + CO_2$$

$$CO_2 + H_2O \longleftrightarrow H_2CO_3 \longleftrightarrow H^+ + HCO_3^- \longleftrightarrow CO_3^=$$

$$NH_3 + H_2O \longleftrightarrow NH_4^+ + OH^-$$

FIG. 41–56. Schematic illustration of factors leading to the formation of struvite, calcium apatite, and carbonate apatite as a consequence of degradation of urea by microbial urease.

XIII. FELINE CYSTINE UROLITHIASIS

A. We have encountered 22 urocystoliths composed of cystine (see Table 41–2).

B. See Chapter 35, Disorders of the Feline Lower Urinary Tract, for additional information.

XIV. CANINE STRUVITE UROLITHIASIS

A. Etiopathogenesis.

1. Overview.
   a. Struvite is the most common type of mineral detected in canine uroliths (see Table 41–1).
   b. Urine must be supersaturated with magnesium ammonium phosphate (MAP) for struvite uroliths to form. Supersaturation of urine with MAP may be associated with several factors, including UTI with urease-producing microbes, alkaline urine, genetic predisposition, and diet.[155]
2. Infection-induced struvite.
   a. When UTIs with urease-producing microbes (especially staphylococci, *Proteus* spp., and ureaplasmas) occurs in dogs that form urine with a sufficient quantity of urea, the unique combination of concomitant elevation in

the concentrations of ammonium and carbonate (CO_3^{2-}) in an alkaline environment may develop. These conditions favor formation of uroliths containing struvite ($MgNH_4PO_4 \cdot 6H_2O$), calcium apatite [$Ca_{10}(PO_4)6(OH)_2$], and carbonate apatite [$Ca_{10}(PO_4)_6CO_3$]. The following mechanisms are involved (Figs. 41–56 to 41–59):

(1). Urease, a metalloenzyme containing nickel and produced by bacteria or ureaplasmas, hydrolyzes urea to form two molecules of ammonia and a molecule of carbon dioxide. Since urease is not consumed during this reaction, a single urease molecule may catalyze the hydrolysis of multiple urea molecules.

(2). The ammonia molecules react spontaneously with water to form ammonium and hydroxyl ions (pK NH_3, 9.03), which alkalinize urine by reducing its hydrogen ion concentration. Ammonia also damages the glycosaminoglycan lining of the urothelium, increasing the ability of bacteria and crystals to adhere to mucosa. The

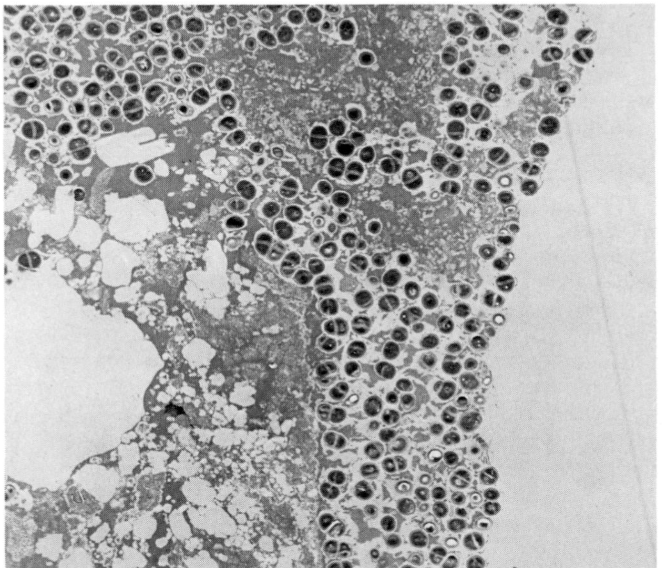

FIG. 41–58. Transmission electron micrograph of a struvite urocystolith removed from an adult female beagle. The clear spaces were occupied by struvite crystals. Note the numerous staphylococci in the matrix of the urolith. (26,000 × original magnification.)

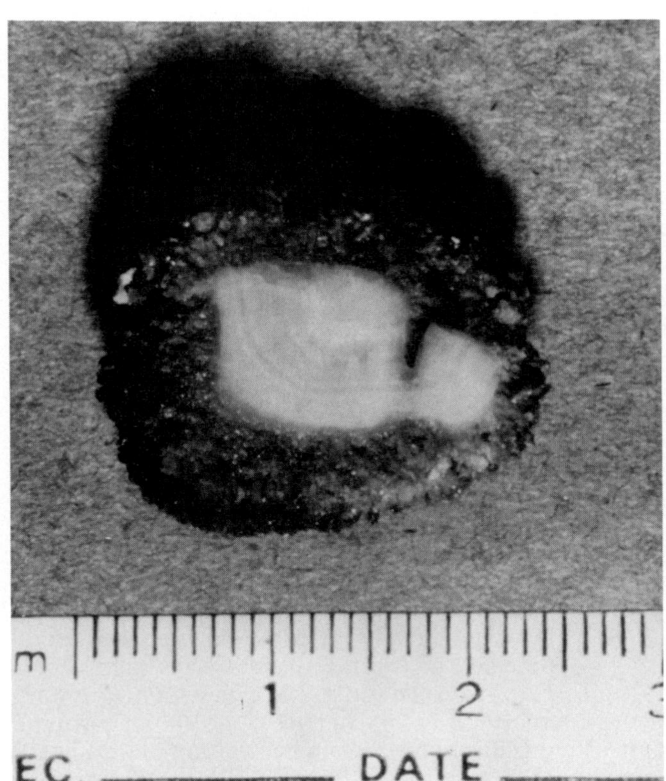

FIG. 41–57. Cross section of a urolith formed in the urinary bladder of an adult female beagle dog as a result of experimental infection with urease-producing *Proteus* spp. The nucleus of the urolith consists of struvite and was transplanted into the bladder before induction of infection. The shell also consists of struvite formed after induction of infection. The darker color of the shell was caused by hematuria. (From Osborne CA, Polzin DJ, Abdullahi SU, et al. Struvite urolithiasis in animals and man: Formation, detection and dissolution. *Adv Vet Sci Comp Med.* 1985;29:1.)

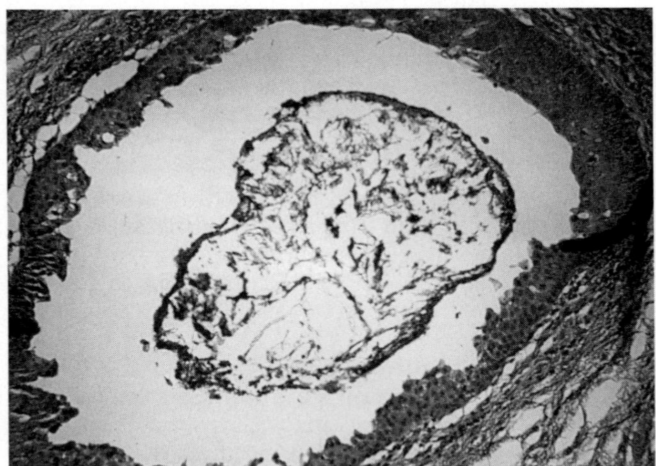

FIG. 41–59. Photomicrograph of a "subvisual" struvite urolith located in the lumen of a urachal diverticulum of a 2-year-old female Sealyham terrier. The matrix of the urolith contained countless gram-positive urease-producing staphylococci. The open spaces in the urolith represent the sites of dissolved struvite crystals.

solubility of struvite (and calcium apatite) decreases in alkaline urine. In addition to alkalinization of urine, the newly generated ammonium ion is available for formation of MAP crystals.

(3). The newly generated molecule of carbon dioxide combines with water to form carbonic acid, which in turn dissociates to form bicarbonate (pK, 10.1). Anions of carbonate may displace anions of phosphate in calcium apatite crystals, to form carbonate apatite crystals.

(4). In the progressively alkaline environment induced by microbial hydrolysis of urea, dissociation of monobasic hydrogen phosphate ($H_2PO_4^-$) results in an increased concentration of dibasic hydrogen phosphate (HPO_4^{2-}) and anionic phosphate (PO_4^{3-}). Given a constant concentration of total phosphate, a change in pH from 6.80 to 7.40 increases the PO_4^{3-} concentration by a factor of approximately six. Anionic phosphate is then available in increased quantities to combine with magnesium and ammonium to form struvite or with calcium to form calcium apatite.

(5). Ammonium ions may combine with urates to form ammonium acid urate.

b. The quantity of dietary protein catabolized for energy influences formation and dissolution of infection-induced struvite uroliths. Consumption of dietary protein in quantities that exceed daily protein requirements for anabolism results in the formation of urea from catabolism of amino acids. Hyperammonuria, hypercarbonaturia, and alkaluria mediated by microbial urease is dependent on the quantity of urea (the substrate of urease) in urine.

c. Abnormal urinary excretion of minerals as a result of enhanced glomerular filtration rate, reduced tubular reabsorption, and/or enhanced tubular secretion is not required for initiation and growth of infection-induced struvite uroliths; however, metabolic and anatomic abnormalities may induce struvite uroliths indirectly by predisposing to UTIs.

3. Sterile struvite (Fig. 41–60).

a. Clinical studies indicate that microbial urease is not involved in formation of struvite uroliths in some dogs.[11,155] Several observations suggest that dietary or metabolic factors may be involved in the genesis of sterile struvite uroliths in these species.

(1). Pilot studies of clinical cases of sterile struvite in dogs revealed a population of patients (nine of 20) whose urine was frequently alkaline but that contained no identifiable bacteria or detectable quantities of urease.[11,155]

(2). Microscopic examination of demineralized Gram-stained sections of some struvite uroliths removed from dogs with bacteriologically sterile urine revealed no gram-positive bacteria.

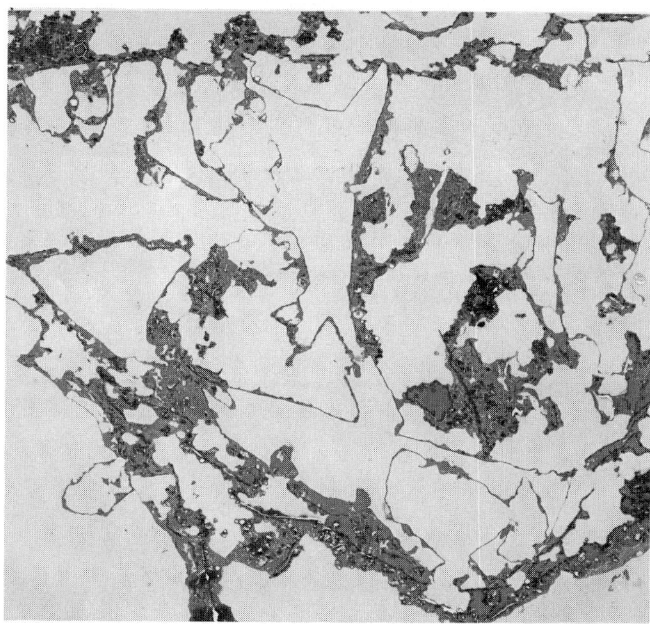

FIG. 41–60. Transmission electron micrograph of struvite urocystolith removed from an 8-year-old male miniature schnauzer. Bacteria were not cultured from the urine, bladder wall, or inside of the urolith. Bacteria were not detected within the stone matrix by electron microscopy. Note the paucity of matrix as compared with the infection-induced struvite urolith described in Fig. 41–59). Clear spaces represent areas occupied by struvite crystals. (2640 × original magnification)

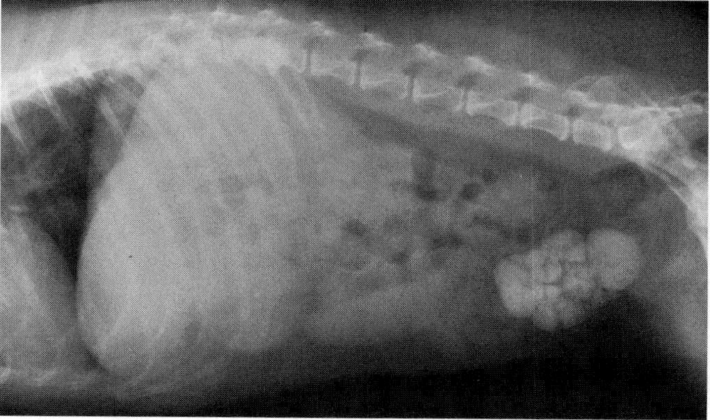

FIG. 41–61. Lateral view of a survey abdominal radiograph of a 12-year-old spayed female miniature schnauzer with numerous urinary bladder uroliths likely to be composed of struvite, and staphylococcal UTI.

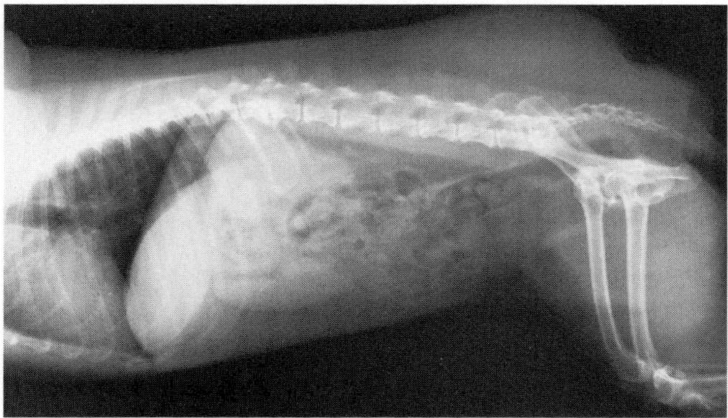

FIG. 41–62. Lateral view of a survey abdominal radiograph of the dog in Fig. 41–61 obtained approximately 15 weeks after initiation of therapy with ampicillin and a calculolytic diet. There are no radiodense uroliths in the urinary tract. (Many staphylococci are resistant to ampicillin.)

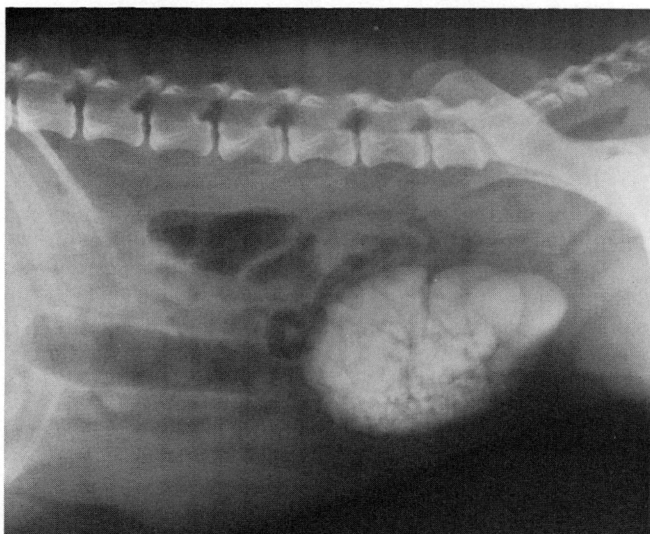

FIG. 41–63. Survey abdominal radiograph of a 2-year-old female miniature schnauzer with urease-positive staphylococcal UTI and urolithiasis (see Figs. 41–64 to 41–69; (From Osborne CA (ed). Canine urolithiasis: etiopathogenesis, detection, treatment, and prevention. *Vet Clin North Am.* 1986;16:211–407.)

(3). Whereas infection-induced human struvite uroliths frequently contain calcium apatite or carbonate apatite, a large number of the canine sterile uroliths were 100% struvite.

(4). Recurrent struvite urocystolithiasis has been evaluated in three related English cocker spaniels, a sire, and two male offspring from different litters and dams.[11] Episodes of struvite urocystolithiasis were associated with alkaluria but not with bacterial UTI, urease activity in urine, or distal RTA.

b. Although struvite is less soluble in alkaline than in acidic urine, the mechanism(s) of sterile struvite urolith formation in dogs is not clear.

(1). Under physiologic conditions associated with alkaluria, urine contains low concentrations of ammonia (and thus of ammonium ion). Thus, alkaline urine formed in the absence of ureolysis would not be expected to favor formation of crystals that contain ammonia ion (such as

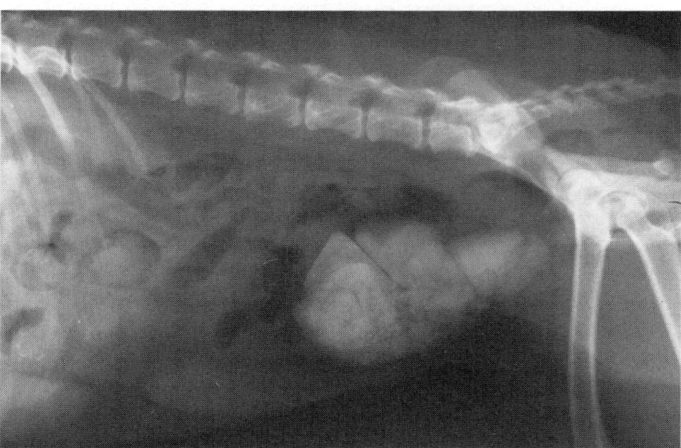

FIG. 41–64. Survey abdominal radiograph of the dog described in Fig. 41–63 that was obtained 5 weeks after initiation of therapy with a calculolytic diet and orally administered ampicillin.

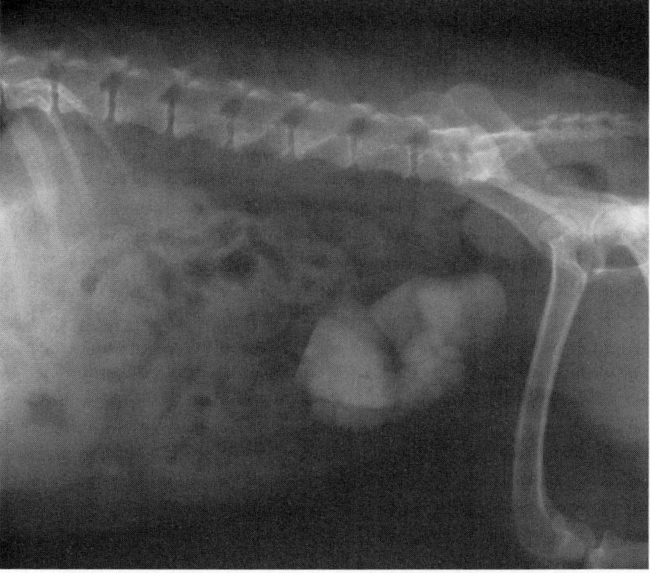

FIG. 41–65. Survey abdominal radiograph of the dog described in Fig. 41–63 obtained 9 weeks after initiation of therapy with a calculolytic diet and orally administered ampicillin.

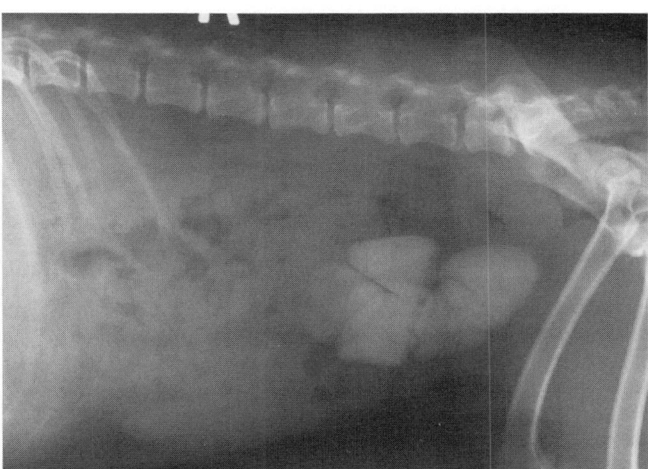

FIG. 41–66. Survey abdominal radiograph of the dog described in Fig. 41–63 obtained 13 weeks after initiation of therapy with a calculolytic diet and orally administered ampicillin.

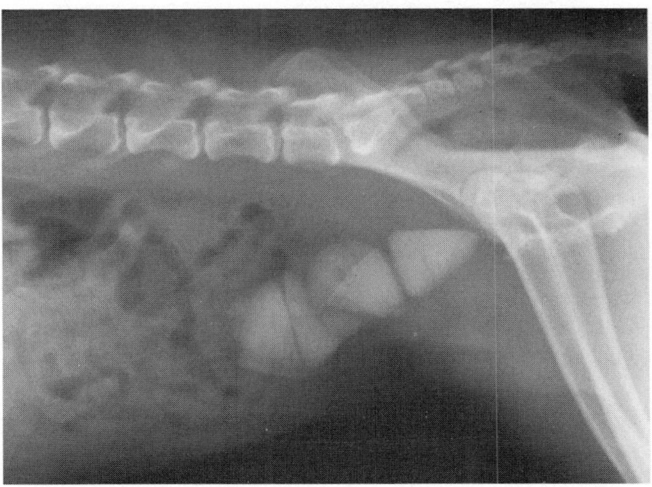

FIG. 41–67. Survey abdominal radiograph of the dog described in Fig. 41–63 that was obtained 16 weeks after initiation of therapy with calculolytic diet and orally administered ampicillin.

magnesium ammonium phosphate hexahydrate). Clinical studies of naturally occurring urolithiasis in human patients support this generalization.

(2). Formation of persistently alkaline urine in the absence of urease-mediated ureolysis may predispose to formation of uroliths containing hydroxylapatite $[Ca_{10}\ (OP_4)_6\ (OH)_2]$, but not carbonate apatite.

c. In vitro studies consisting of addition of magnesium ($Mg\ SO_4$), ammonium (NH_4Cl), or phosphate ($NH_4\ H_2\ PO_4$ or $NaH_2\ PO_4$) to sterile human urine ranging in pH from 5.0 to 9.6 revealed that struvite crystals could be induced in an acid or an alkaline environment.[19] High ammonia concentrations were not necessary for formation of struvite crystals, provided the concentration of $Mg \times [NH_4] \times [PO_4]$ was of sufficient magnitude at a given pH. Corresponding studies in vivo in dogs have not yet been performed.

B. Treatment (Figs. 41–61 to 41–80).

1. Overview of therapy of struvite urolithiasis.
   a. Elimination of existing uroliths.
   b. Eradication or control of UTI.
   c. Prevention of recurrence of uroliths.[156,202]
2. Infection-induced struvite uroliths (Figs. 41–61 to 41–80).
   a. Current recommendations include eradication or control of UTI with appropriate antimicro-

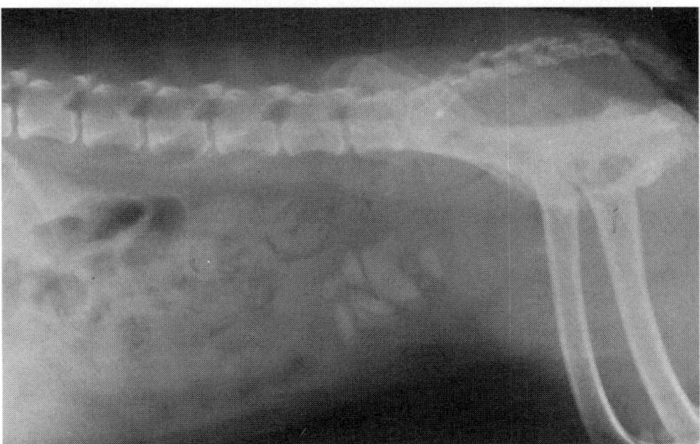

FIG. 41–68. Survey abdominal radiograph of the dog described in Fig. 41–63 that was obtained 21 weeks after initiation of therapy with a calculolytic diet and orally administered ampicillin.

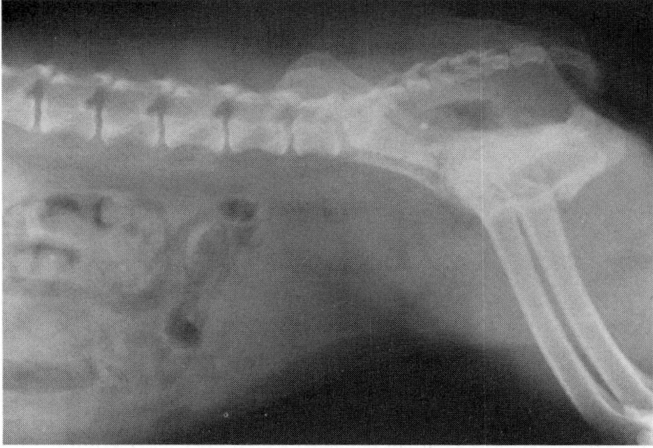

FIG. 41–69. Lateral survey abdominal radiograph of the dog described in Fig. 41–63 that was obtained approximately 7 months after initiation of therapy. There are no radiodense uroliths in the urinary tract.

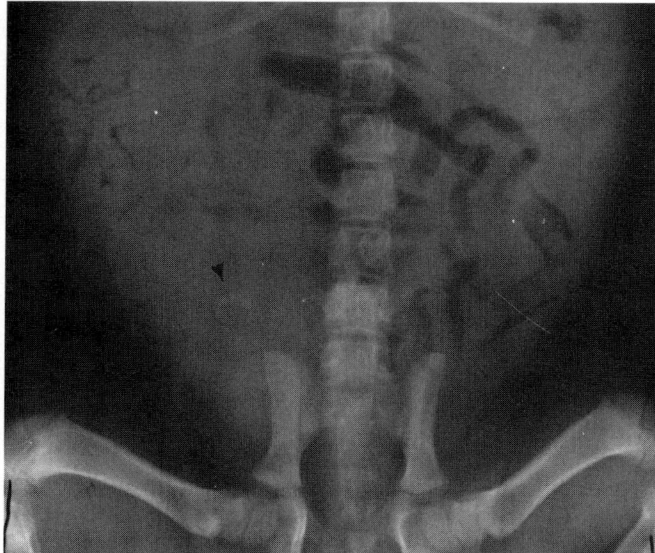

FIG. 41–70. Ventrodorsal abdominal radiograph of a 9-week-old male dog illustrating multiple radiodense urocystoliths *(arrows)*. The dog had a staphylococcal UTI (from Lulich JP, Osborne CA, Johnston GR. Nonsurgical correction of infection-induced struvite uroliths and a vesicourachal diverticulum in an immature dog. *J Sm Anim Pract.* 1989;30:613–617.)

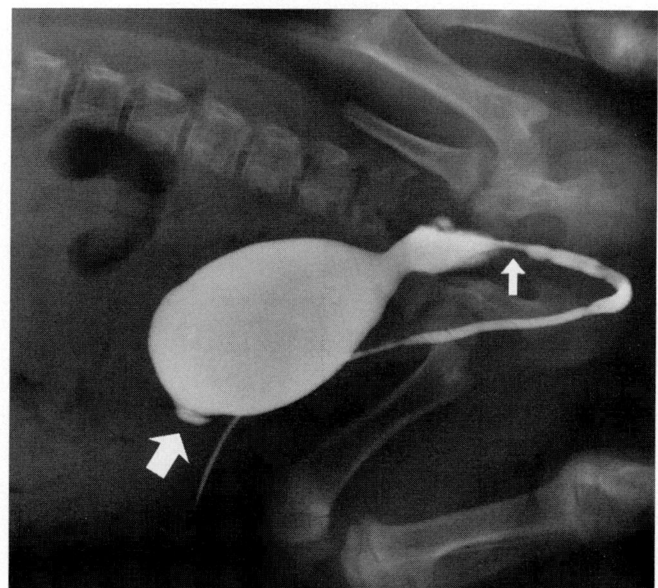

FIG. 41–71. Positive-contrast retrograde urethrocystogram of the dog described in Fig. 41–70. Note the vesicourachal diverticulum *(large arrow)* and narrowing of the proximal portion of the urethra *(small arrow)*.

bial agents, calculolytic diets, and urease inhibitors (acetohydroxamic acid) to patients with *persistent* UTI caused by urease-producing microbes (Table 41–21).[155]

(1). The importance of UTI with urease-producing bacteria in the formation of most struvite uroliths in dogs emphasizes the importance of therapy to eradicate or control them. Because of the quantity of urease produced by bacterial pathogens, it may be impossible to acidify urine with urine acidifiers administered in doses that prevent systemic acidosis. Therefore, sterilization of urine appears to be an important objective in creating a state of struvite undersaturation that may prevent further growth of uroliths or that promotes their dissolution.

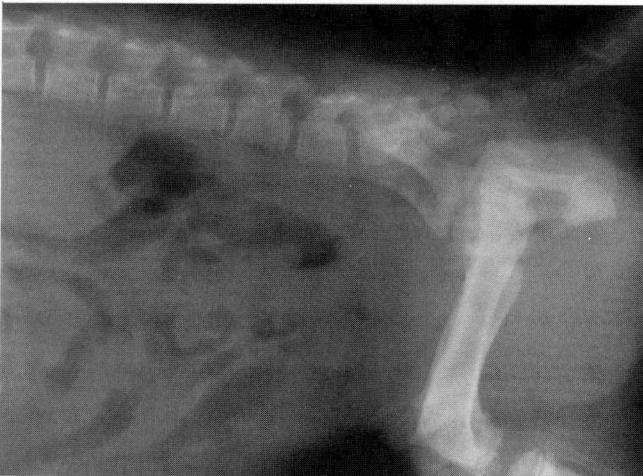

FIG. 41–72. Lateral abdominal radiograph of the dog described in Fig. 41–70, obtained 10 days after initiation of therapy with an antibiotic and Hill's Prescription Diet Canine s/d. Radiodense uroliths cannot be detected in the urinary tract.

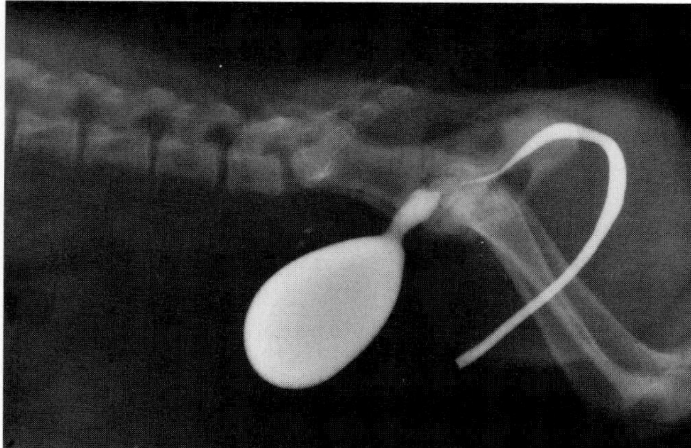

FIG. 41–73. Positive-contrast retrograde urethrocystogram of the dog described in Fig. 41–70 obtained 39 days following diagnosis of uroliths and a vesicourachal diverticulum. There is no evidence of a vesicourachal diverticulum, but narrowing of the lumen of the proximal urethra is still present.

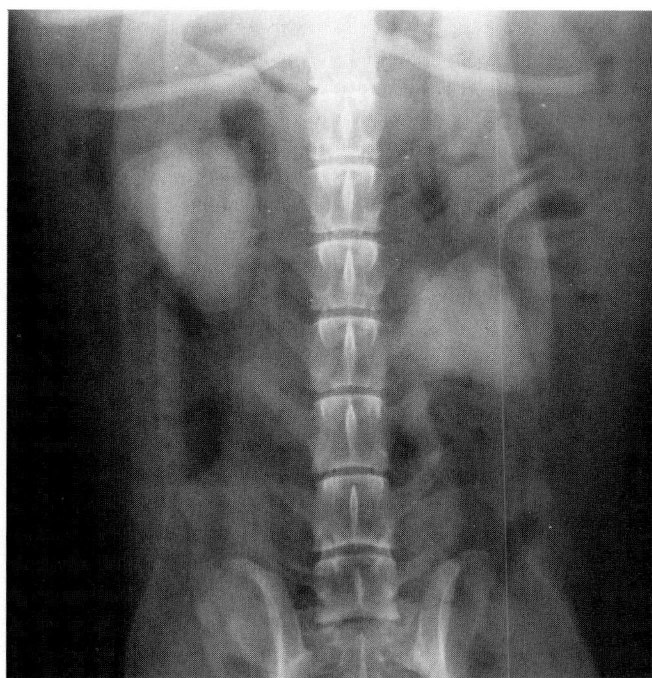

FIG. 41–74. Ventrodorsal survey abdominal radiograph of a 6-year-old female basset hound. Two large, radiodense uroliths, presumed to be composed of struvite, are present in the renal pelves. Significant numbers of non–urease-producing *Escherichia coli* and *Enterococcus* spp. were cultured from urine collected by cystocentesis. Subsequently, significant numbers of urease-producing ureaplasmas were isolated from urine (From Osborne CA (ed). Canine urolithiasis etiopathogenesis, detection, treatment, and prevention. *Vet Clin North Am.* 1986;16: 211–407.)

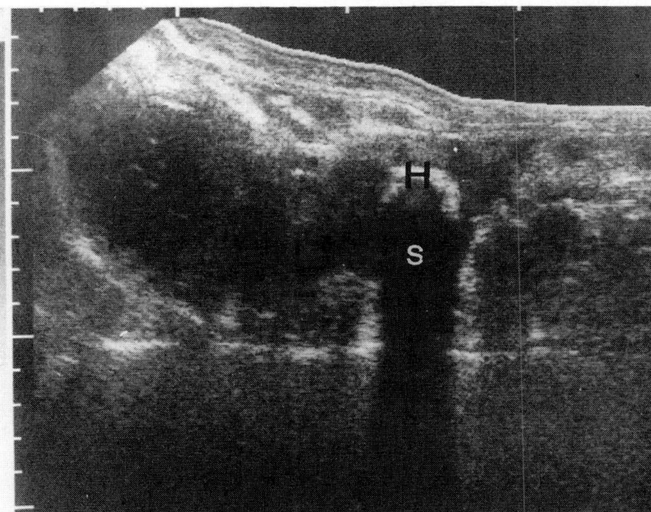

FIG. 41–75. Sagittal ultrasonogram of the right kidney of the dog described in Fig. 41–74. Note the hyperechoic nephrolith (H) and its acoustic shadow(s).

(a). Appropriate antimicrobial agents selected on the basis of susceptibility or minimum inhibitory concentration tests should be used in therapeutic doses.

(1′). The fact that diuresis reduces the urine concentration of the antimicrobial agent should be considered when formulating antimicrobial dosages.

(2′). Antimicrobial agents should be administered as long as the uroliths can be identified by survey radiography. This recommendation is based on the fact that bacterial pathogens harbored inside uroliths may be protected from antimicrobial agents (see Fig. 41–58). Whereas the urine and surface of uroliths may be sterilized by appropriate antimicro-

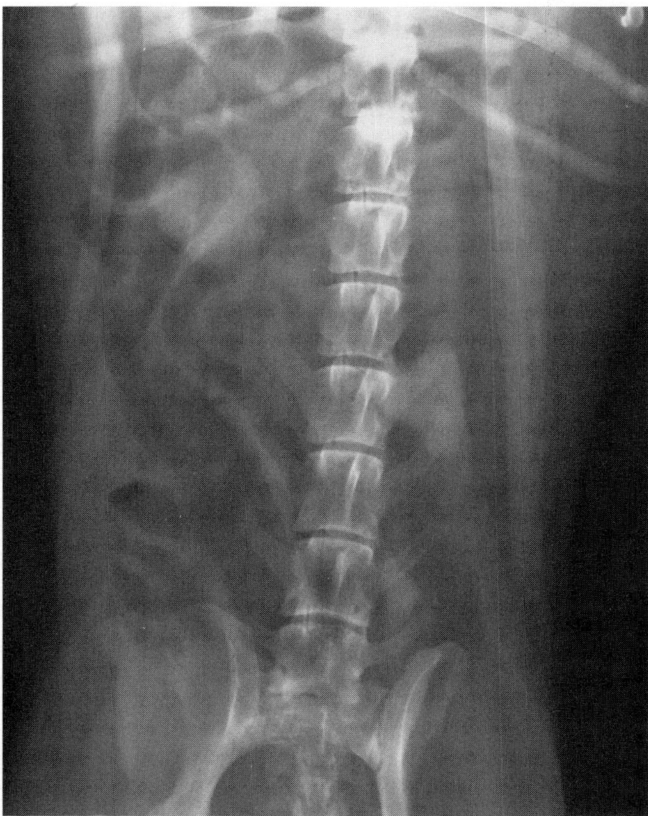

FIG. 41–76. Ventrodorsal survey abdominal radiograph of the dog described in Fig. 41–74 that was obtained approximately 5 weeks after initiation of therapy with a calculolytic diet and oral ampicillin. Using the length of the second lumbar vertebra as a comparative landmark, it can be seen that the nephroliths are smaller.

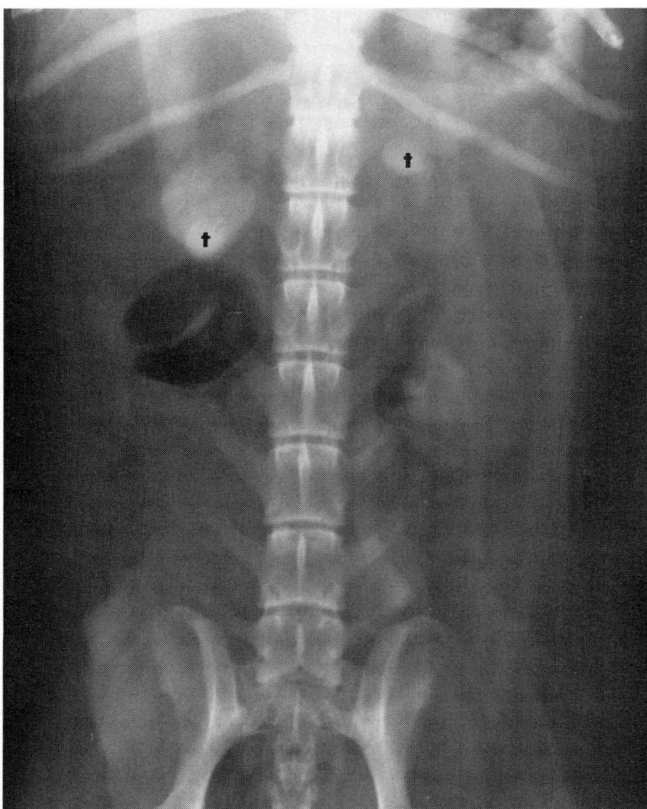

FIG. 41–77. Ventrodorsal survey abdominal radiograph of the dog described in Fig. 41–74 that was obtained approximately 21 weeks after initiation of therapy with a calculolytic diet and ampicillin. The nephroliths are smaller (note that a larger thela [*t*] is superimposed over the urolith in the right kidney).

bial therapy, the original pathogen can remain viable below the surface of the urolith. Discontinuing antimicrobial therapy may result in relapse of bacteriuria and UTI.

(b). Although antimicrobial therapy alone may dissolve struvite uroliths in some patients, experimental studies in rats and dogs and clinical studies in humans indicate that this phenomenon represents the exception, rather than the rule.[155] In addition to the unpredictable response to this form of therapy, the time required to induced urolith dissolution with antimicrobial agents is usually measured in multiples of months, rather than of weeks.

b. The goal of calculolytic diets is to reduce urine concentration of urea (the substrate of urease), phosphorus, and magnesium. A calculolytic diet (Prescription Diet Canine s/d, Hill's) was formulated that contains a reduced quantity of high-quality protein and reduced quantities of phosphorus and magnesium. The diet was supplemented with sodium chloride, to stimulate thirst and induce compensatory polyuria. Reducing hepatic production of urea from dietary protein reduces renal medullary urea concentration and contributes to further diuresis.

(1). The efficacy of the aforementioned diet in inducing dissolution of infected struvite uroliths has been confirmed by controlled experimental and clinical studies in dogs.[1,155,162] When a combination of calculolytic diet and antimicrobial agents was given to 11 dogs with naturally occurring urease-positive UTI and urocystoliths presumed to be composed of struvite, uroliths dissolved. The mean interval required to induce urocystolith dissolution was approximately 3 months (range, 2 weeks to 7 months).[155]

(2). Consumption of a calculolytic diet by dogs with infection-induced struvite uroliths

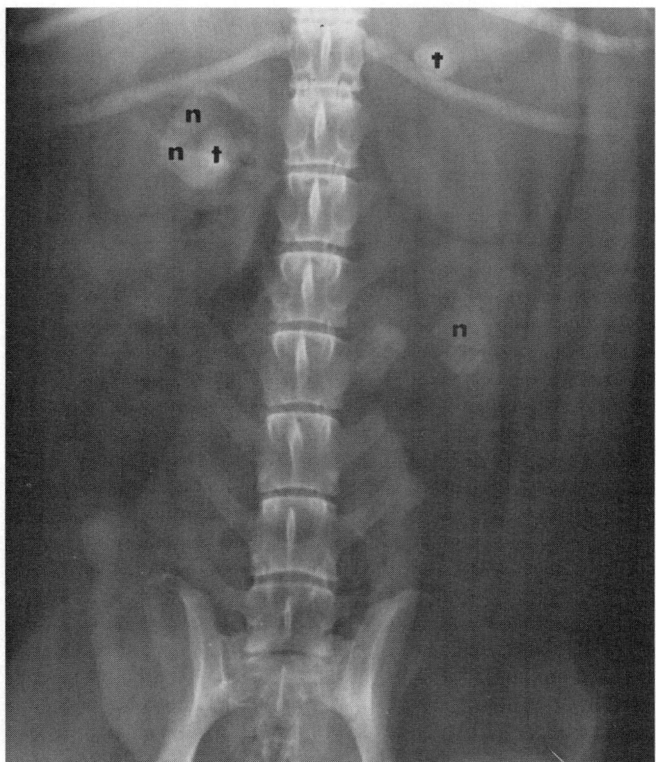

FIG. 41–78. Ventrodorsal survey abdominal radiograph of the dog described in Fig. 41–74 that was obtained approximately 29 weeks after initiation of therapy with a calculolytic diet and ampicillin. The nephroliths are smaller and less dense. Key: *t,* thela; *n,* nephrolith. (Compare Figs. 41–74 to 41–77.)

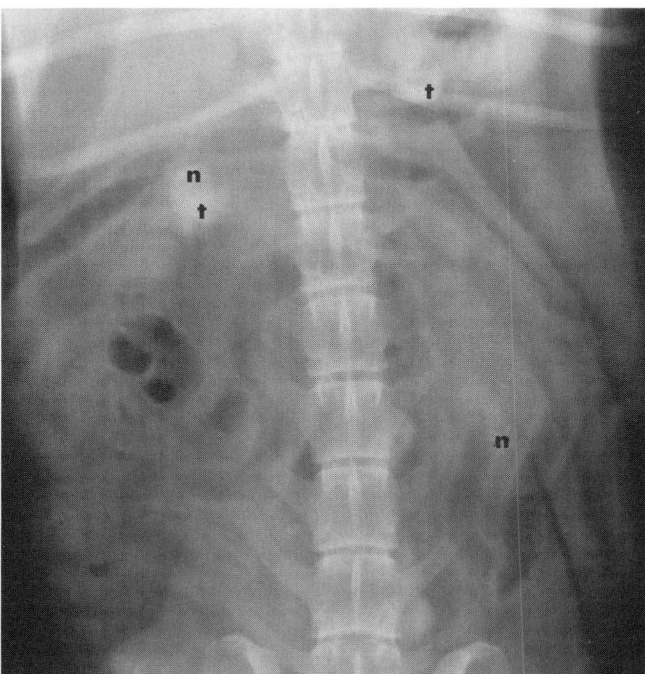

FIG. 41–79. Ventrodorsal abdominal radiograph of the dog described in Fig. 41–74 that was obtained approximately 45 weeks after initiation of therapy with a calculolytic diet and orally administered ampicillin. The nephroliths are barely discernible. Key: *t,* thela; *n,* nephrolith.

typically is associated with a marked reduction in the concentration of serum urea nitrogen and with mild reductions in the serum concentrations of magnesium, phosphorus, and albumin (Table 41–22).[1,155,162] A mild increase in the serum activity of hepatic alkaline phosphatase isoenzyme may also be observed. These alterations in serum chemistry values were of no detectable clinical consequence during 6-month experimental studies or during clinical studies. They underscore the fact that the diet is designed for short-term (weeks to months) dissolution therapy rather than longterm (months to years) prophylactic therapy. Changes in serum urea nitrogen concentrations are one index of client and patient compliance with dietary recommendations.

c. Experimental and clinical studies in dogs have revealed that administration of microbial urease inhibitors in pharmacologic doses are capable of inhibiting struvite urolith growth and/or promoting struvite urolith dissolution. Acetohydroxamic acid (AHA) given orally to dogs at a dosage of 25 mg/kg (divided into two daily subdoses) will reduce urease activity, struvite crystalluria, and urolith growth (Fig. 41–81).[103] By reducing the pathogenicity of staphylococci, it may also mitigate the severity of dysuria, bacteriuria, pyuria, hematuria, and proteinuria.
   (1). Although larger doses of AHA may result in urolith dissolution, they are not recommended, since they may cause reversible hemolytic anemia and abnormalities in bilirubin metabolism.[110] Because it is teratogenic, AHA should not be administered to pregnant bitches.[6]
   (2). We have not utilized AHA routinely to promote dissolution of infection-induced struvite uroliths in dogs, because of the efficacy of calculolytic diet and antimicrobial therapy. We have used AHA in combination with calculolytic diets and antimicrobial agents with refractory urease-producing UTIs. If after an appropriate trial of therapy with diet modification and antimicrobial agents, infection-induced struvite uroliths do not dissolve, AHA may be added to the therapeutic regimen.

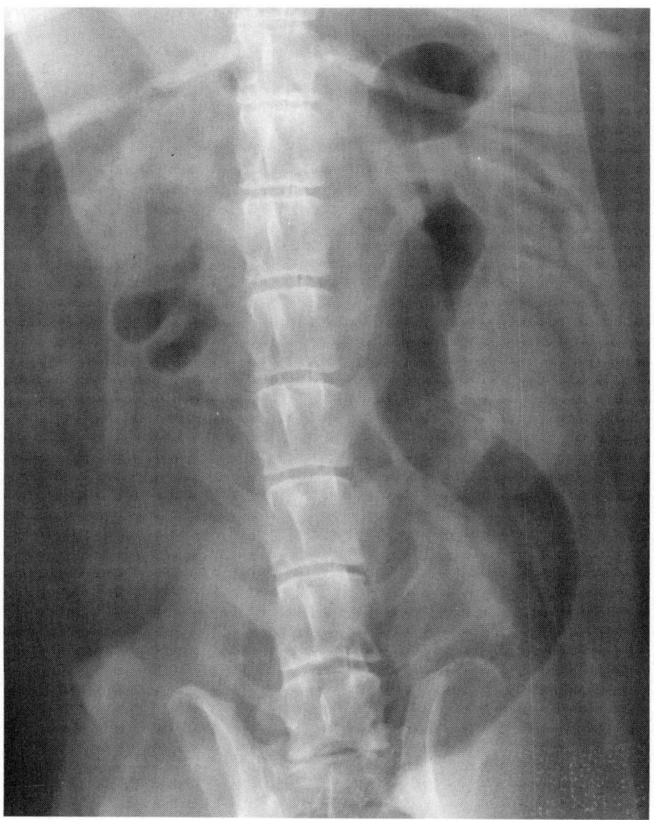

FIG. 41–80. Ventrodorsal abdominal radiograph of the dog described in Fig. 41–74 that was obtained approximately 1 year after initiation of therapy with a calculolytic diet and ampicillin. There is no evidence of radiodense uroliths in the urinary tract.

TABLE 41–21.
SUMMARY OF RECOMMENDATIONS FOR MEDICAL DISSOLUTION OF CANINE STRUVITE UROLITHS

A. Adult dogs with UTI
1. Perform appropriate diagnostic studies, including complete urinalysis, quantitative urine culture, and diagnostic radiography. Determine precise location, size, and number of uroliths. (Size and number of stones are not reliable indexes of probable efficacy of therapy.)
2. If available, determine mineral composition of uroliths; If unavailable, "guesstimate" their composition by evaluation of appropriate clinical data (see Table 41–9).
3. Consider surgical correction if uroliths are obstructing urine outflow or if correctable abnormalities that predispose to recurrent UTI are identified by radiography or other means. Small urocystoliths may be removed by voiding urohydropropulsion (see Table 41–24).
4. Eradicate or control UTI with appropriate antimicrobial agents. Maintain antimicrobial therapy during, and for 3 to 4 weeks after, urolith dissolution.
5. Initiate therapy with a calculolytic diet. No other food or mineral supplements should be fed to the patient. Compliance with dietary recommendations is suggested by reduction in serum urea nitrogen concentration (usually <10 mg/dL).
6. Devise a protocol to monitor efficacy of therapy.
   a. Try to avoid diagnostic follow-up studies that require urinary catheterization. If they are required, give appropriate pericatheterization antimicrobial agents, to prevent iatrogenic UTI.
   b. Evaluate serial urinalysis. Urine pH, specific gravity, and microscopic examination of sediment for crystals are especially important. Remember, crystals formed in urine stored at room or refrigeration temperature may represent in vitro artifacts.
   c. Perform serial radiography monthly to evaluate stone location(s), number, size, density, and shape.
   d. If necessary, perform quantitative urine cultures. They are especially important in patients that are infected before therapy and in those that are catheterized during therapy.
   e. Feed patients a calculolytic diet for 1 month following disappearance of uroliths as detected by survey radiography.
   f. If, during dietary management, uroliths grow or do not begin to decrease in size after approximately 4 to 8 weeks of appropriate medical management, alternative methods should be considered. Difficulty in inducing complete dissolution of uroliths by creating urine that is undersaturated with the suspected calculogenic crystalloid should prompt consideration that: (1) the wrong mineral component was identified, (2) the nucleus of the uroliths is a different mineral than other portions of it, and (3) the owner of the patient is not complying with medical recommendations.
7. Consider administration of acetohydroxamic acid (25 mg/kg/day divided into two equal doses) to patients with persistent uroliths and persistent urease-producing microburia, despite the use of antimicrobial agents and calculolytic diets.

B. Adult dogs with persistently sterile urine
1. Follow the protocol described above, but do not administer antimicrobial agents or acetohydroxamic acid.
2. Periodically, culture urine specimens obtained by cystocentesis to detect secondary UTI. If UTI develops, initiate antimicrobial therapy.

C. Immature dogs
1. Use caution in consideration of use of protein-restricted diets in growing pups.
2. Short-term therapy with calculolytic diets has been effective in dissolving struvite urocystoliths, but if such management is instituted, the patient must be monitored for evidence of nutritional deficiencies, especially protein malnutrition.
3. Acetohydroxamic acid has not been evaluated in growing pups.
4. Small urocystoliths may be removed by voiding urohydropropulsion (see Table 41–24). Pending further studies, surgery remains the safest means of removing large uroliths from immature dogs.

3. Infection-induced struvite nephroliths (see Figs. 41–74 to 41–80).
   a. Nephroliths or ureteroliths that cause outflow obstruction and substantial impairment of the function of the associated kidney should be managed by surgical intervention or (if possible) percutaneous nephropyelonephrostomy, especially if they are associated with concomitant bacterial infection. Medical therapy designed to induce urolith dissolution over a period of several weeks is unlikely to be effective in patients with poorly functioning kidneys, since the urolith(s) are not continually bathed with newly formed urine modified to induce litholysis.
   b. We have successfully induced dissolution of nephroliths presumed to be composed of infection-induced struvite in six dogs.
      (1). The mean time required for dissolution was 184 ± 99 (range, 67 to 300) days.
      (2). Though the dogs had varying degrees of impaired capacity to concentrate urine as a result of pyelonephritis, none had primary renal azotemia when therapy with calculolytic diet and antimicrobial agents was instituted. This point is emphasized

TABLE 41–22.
EXPECTED CHANGES ASSOCIATED WITH MEDICAL THERAPY OF STRUVITE UROLITHS

Finding	Before Therapy	During Therapy	Prevention Therapy
Polyuria	±	1+ to 3+	0
Pollakiuria	1+ to 4+	↑ then ↓	0
Hematuria	1+ to 4+	↓	0
Urine specific gravity	Variable	1.004–1.014	Normal
Urine pH	>7.0	≤6.5	Variable
Urine inflammation	1+ to 4+	↓	0
Struvite crystals	0 to 4+	0	Variable
Bacteruria	0 to 4+	↓ to 0	0
Bacterial culture of urine	0 to 4+	↓ to 0	0
BUN (mg/dL)	>15	≤10	Variable
Urolith size and number	Small to large	↓	0

Key: BUN, blood urea nitrogen; ± = sometimes; 1+ = small quantity; 4+ = large quantity.

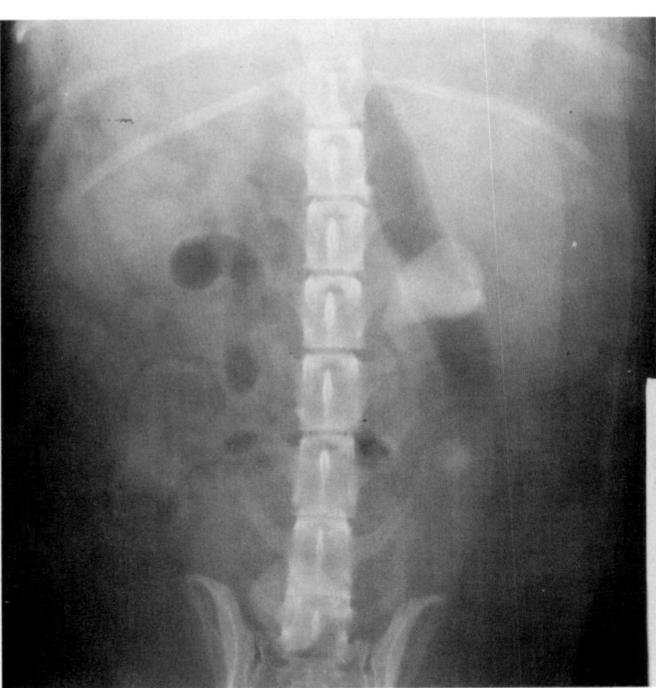

FIG. 41–82. Survey ventrodorsal abdominal radiograph of a 9-year-old female cocker spaniel illustrates radiodense uroliths in the pelvis of the left kidney and the urinary bladder. Though the dog had adequate renal function, she had signs of UTI and septicemia: temperature 105.6°F, depression, immature leukocytosis. A significant number of *Enterobacter* spp. were cultured from a urine sample collected by cystocentesis.

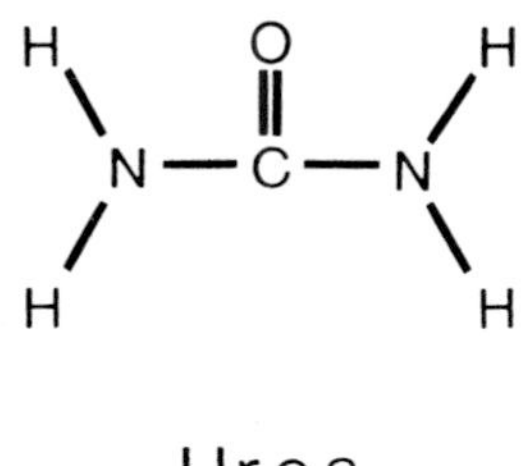

H O OH
H—C—C—N
H H

Acetohydroxamic Acid

FIG. 41–81. Schematic illustration of similarity in structural configuration of urea and acetohydroxamic acid (Lithostat).

because, for anabolism, dogs with moderate to severe primary renal failure require more protein than normal. The calculolytic diet used in our studies (Prescription Diet Canine s/d, Hill's) could induce or aggravate protein malnutrition if given for prolonged periods to dogs with moderate azotemic primary renal failure, or other concomitant disorders associated with protein malnutrition.[174]

(3). In general, we would not expect dietary and antimicrobial therapy to be effective in dissolving struvite ureteroliths causing partial outflow obstruction (Fig. 41–82 to 41–86). To be dissolved, uroliths must be completely surrounded by urine that is undersaturated with struvite for long periods. Intermittent passage of urine through a partially obstructed ureter logically would preclude dissolution of struvite ureteroliths.

4. Sterile struvite uroliths (Figs. 41–87 to 41–89).
   a. Current recommendations include use of calculolytic diets and utilization of urine acidifiers (see Table 41–21).

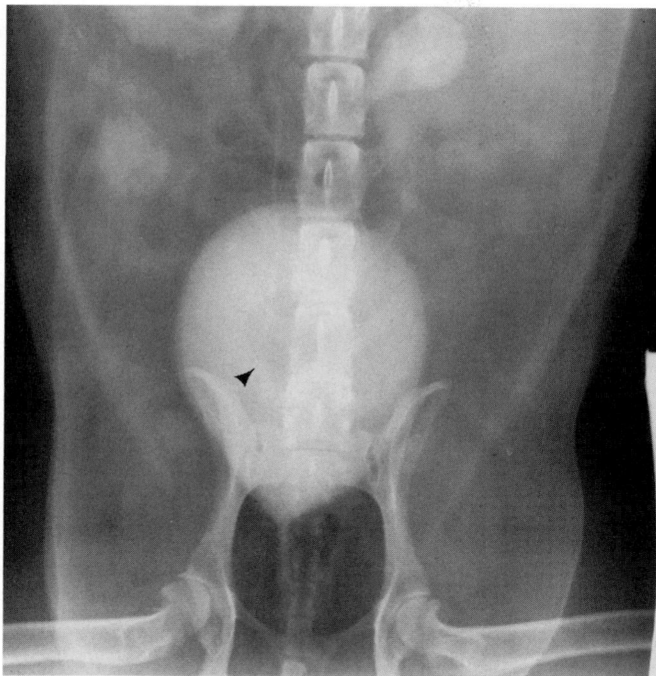

FIG. 41–83. Ventrodorsal view of 20-minute intravenous urogram of the dog described in Fig. 41–82. The left kidney has not excreted significant quantities of contrast medium. The right kidney is normal in appearance. The urocystolith appears radiolucent in the urinary bladder filled with contrast medium *(arrow)*.

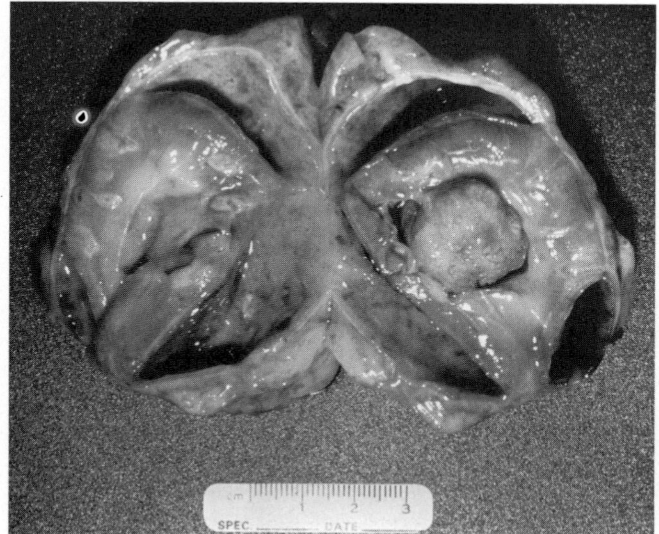

FIG. 41–84. Cross section of the left kidney removed from the dog described in Fig. 41–82. Obstruction of urine outflow caused by the nephrolith, combined with UTI, resulted in almost complete destruction of the renal parenchyma and formation of a perinephric abscess.

(1). Controlled experimental and clinical studies have confirmed the efficacy of calculolytic diets (Prescription Diet Canine s/d, Hill's) in inducing sterile struvite urolith dissolution.[155,160,162]

(a). Unless secondary UTI develops, anti-

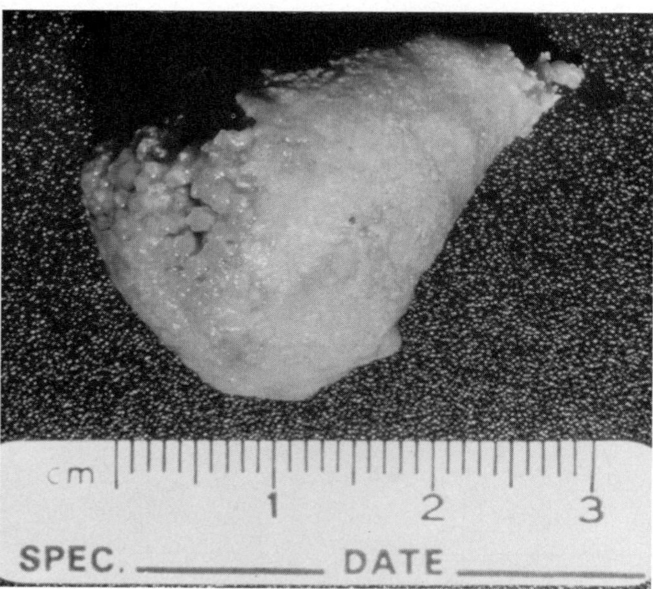

FIG. 41–85. Photograph of the renolith found in the right kidney of the dog described in Figs. 41–82 to 41–84. Because the kidneys of dogs are unipyramidal, they do not form "staghorn" renoliths. (Compare Figs. 41–1 to 41–4).

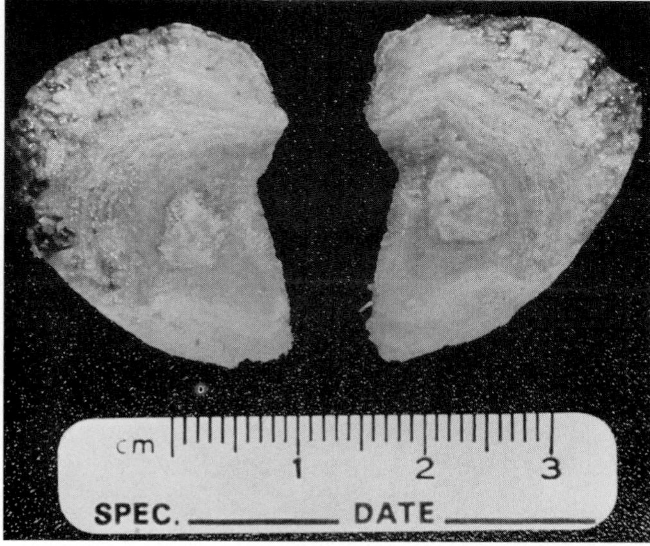

FIG. 41–86. Cross section of the struvite renolith described in Figs. 41–82 to 41–85 illustrating laminated structure. Despite differences in appearance of the nucleus and outer laminations, the mineral composition of both was struvite.

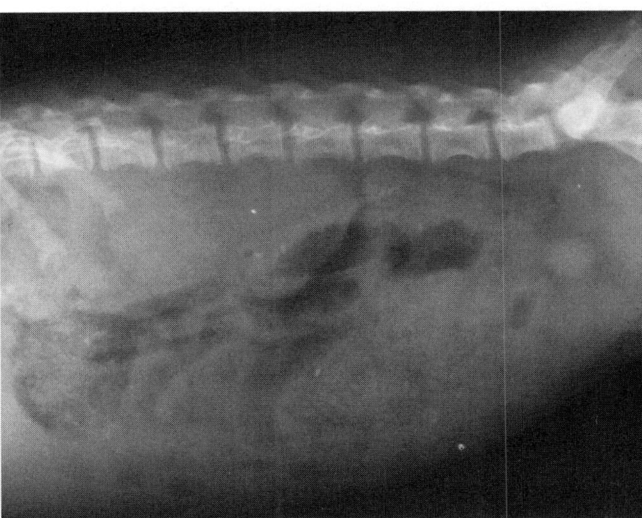

FIG. 41–87. Survey abdominal radiograph of a 12-week-old female miniature dachshund with a urocystolith presumed to be composed of struvite. Aerobic bacteria were not cultured from serial urine samples. (From Osborne CA (ed). Canine urolithiasis: etiopathogenesis, detection, treatment, and prevention. *Vet Clin North Am.* 1986;16:211–407.)

biotics and urease inhibitors are not needed.

(b). Sterile struvite stones usually dissolve more rapidly than infection-induced struvite stones.

(c). When the calculolytic diet was given to nine dogs, naturally occurring sterile uroliths presumed to be composed of struvite dissolved in a mean time of 6 weeks (range, 1 month to 3 months).[139,155]

(d). Management of six episodes of naturally occurring sterile struvite urocystoliths with calculolytic diet in two related male English cocker spaniels resulted in urolith dissolution in a mean interval of 38.5 ± 12.8 days.[11]

(e). Preliminary studies indicate that protein restriction is not essential for dissolution of canine sterile struvite uroliths.

(2). Acidification of urine to approximately pH 6.0 has been effective in promoting sterile struvite urolith dissolution.[158] In this respect, they are similar to feline sterile struvite uroliths.

b. Studies are in progress to evaluate the efficacy of magnesium- and phosphorus-restricted acidifying diets in dissolving canine sterile struvite stones.

5. Monitoring response to therapy (see Table 41–22).

a. The size of uroliths should be monitored periodically by survey radiography (Figs. 41–61 to 41–80 and 41–87 to 41–89).

(1). We recommend radiography at monthly intervals.

(2). Survey radiography is usually preferable to retrograde contrast radiography, since use of catheters during retrograde

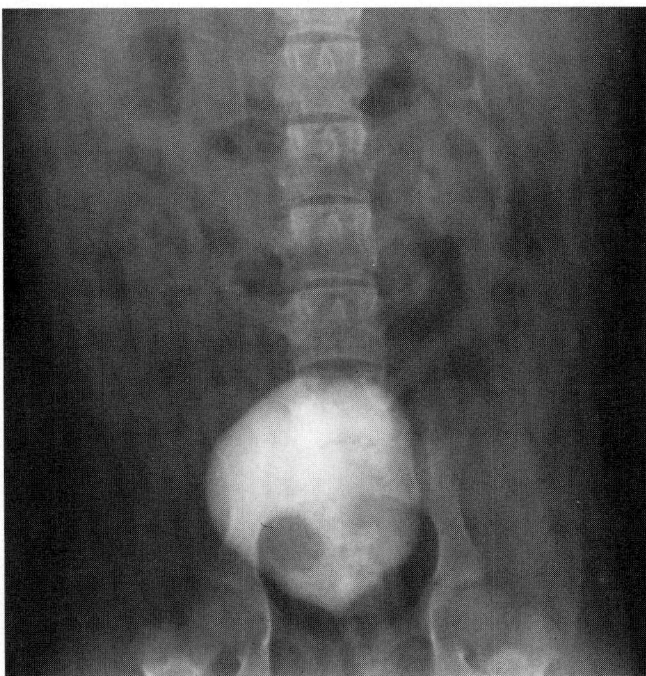

FIG. 41–88. Ventrodorsal view of the abdomen of the dog described in Fig. 41–87. Following intravenous urography, the solitary urocystolith appears to be radiolucent.

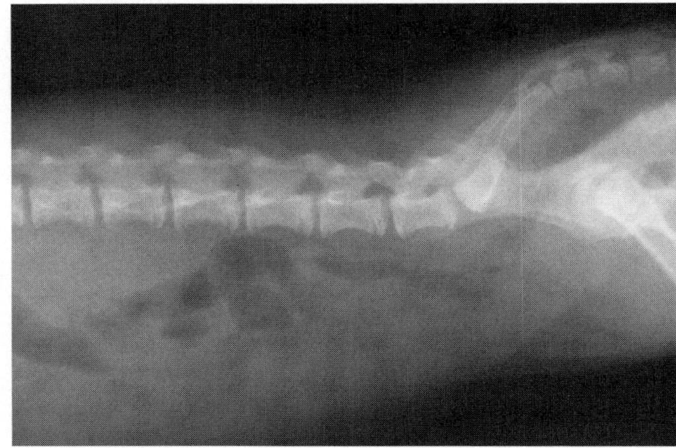

FIG. 41–89. Survey abdominal radiograph of the dog described in Fig. 41–20 that was obtained 2 weeks after initiation of therapy with a calculolytic diet. There are no radiodense structures in the urinary tract.

radiographic studies may result in iatrogenic UTI.

(3). Alternatively, intravenous urography may be considered.

b. Periodic evaluation of urine sediment for crystalluria also may be considered (see the section on Crystalluria in this chapter). If therapy effectively promotes formation of urine that is undersaturated with magnesium ammonium phosphate, struvite crystals should not form.

c. UTI may persist, despite antimicrobial therapy in patients with infection-induced struvite uroliths consuming the calculolytic diet.

(1). In most patients, the magnitude of bacteriuria is usually reduced substantially (i.e., from more than 10^5 bacteria per milliliter of urine to 10^2 or 10^3 bacteria per mL of urine), and the associated inflammatory response progressively subsides.

(2). Difficulty in eradicating infection while uroliths persist may be related to persistence of viable microbes harbored within the stones.

(3). Diet-induced diuresis should be considered when formulating dosages of antimicrobial agents intended to achieve minimum inhibitory concentrations in urine.

(4). Despite persistent bacteriuria during antimicrobial and dietary treatment of patients infected with struvite stones, we have had excellent success in inducing urolith dissolution. Concomitant use of calculolytic diet, antimicrobial agents, and acetohydroxamic acid in this situation was the most effective method of inducing urolith dissolution.

d. Since small uroliths may escape detection by survey radiography, we recommend that the calculolytic diet—and, if necessary, antimicrobial therapy—be continued for at least 1 month following radiographic documentation of urolith dissolution. This maneuver is likely to prevent rapid recurrence of radiographically detectable uroliths and bacterial UTI after cessation of therapy.

e. If, during therapy, uroliths increase in size or do not begin to dissolve after approximately 8 weeks of appropriate medical therapy, alternative methods of management should be considered.

(1). Small uroliths that become lodged in the urethra of male or female dogs during therapy may readily be returned to the urinary bladder lumen by urohydropropulsion.

(2). Complete obstruction of a ureter or renal pelvis, especially with concomitant UTI, is an absolute indication for surgical intervention.

f. Difficulty in inducing complete dissolution of uroliths by creating urine that is undersaturated with the suspected calculogenic crystalloid should prompt certain considerations:

(1). The wrong mineral component was identified.

(2). The nucleus of the uroliths might have a different mineral composition than outer portions of the urolith.

(3). The owner or the patient might not have complied with therapeutic recommendations.

6. Precautions.

a. The diet designed to dissolve canine struvite uroliths (Prescription Diet Canine s/d, Hill's) is restricted in protein and supplemented with sodium chloride. Therefore, it should not be given to patients with concomitant diseases associated with positive fluid balance (e.g., heart failure, nephrotic syndrome) or hypertension.

b. Nonobstructing struvite nephroliths have been dissolved in patients with nonazotemic renal failure caused by ascending pyelonephritis.[155,159] Protein-restricted calculolytic diets should be used with caution in patients with azotemic primary renal failure. The diet could induce protein malnutrition if given for prolonged periods to dogs with moderate azotemic primary renal failure.[171]

c. Inducing diuresis by augmenting water consumption appears to be a logical method of decreasing the urine concentration of struvite and other calculogenic substances; however, additional salt is not recommended for dogs fed the calculolytic diet previously described, because it has been formulated to contain supplemental sodium chloride. In addition, depletion of renal medullary urea as a consequence of dietary protein restriction is associated with obligatory diuresis.[1]

d. The protein-, phosphorus-, and magnesium-restricted diet designed to promote dissolution of struvite uroliths does not dissolve uroliths of calcium oxalate, calcium phosphate, silica, or cystine. See appropriate sections of this chapter for current recommendations about medical management of these forms of uroliths.

C. Prevention.

1. Infection-induced struvite uroliths.

a. Eradication or control of UTIs caused by urease-producing bacteria is the most important factor in preventing recurrence of most infection-induced struvite uroliths. If recurrent UTI persists, indefinite therapy with prophylactic doses of antimicrobial agents eliminated in high concentration in urine is indicated.[205] These include nitrofurantoin and trimethoprim-sulfadiazine.

b. In light of the effectiveness of diet in inducing dissolution of struvite uroliths, using dietary modification to prevent recurrence of uroliths is logical and feasible. Nevertheless, before reliable recommendations can be established, further studies must be performed to evaluate the longterm effects of low-protein calculolytic diets in dogs. Because they induce polyuria, some degree of hypoalbuminemia, and mild alteration in hepatic enzymes and morphology, we recommend longterm use of severely protein-restricted calculolytic diets *only* if patients develop recurrent urolithiasis despite augmented fluid intake, urine acidification, and attempts to control infection.

c. Studies to evaluate the effectiveness of acetohydroxamic acid in the prevention of struvite urolithiasis in dogs with persistent UTI with urease-producing bacteria have been encouraging. Administration of 25 mg of AHA per kilogram per day to dogs with urinary bladder foreign bodies (zinc discs) and experimentally induced urease-positive staphylococcal UTI have been effective in preventing formation of uroliths and in minimizing the growth rate of uroliths (see Fig. 41–81).[111] Acetohydroxamic acid has also been reported to be effective in preventing struvite uroliths induced in rats by urease-producing mycoplasmas.[114]

d. Studies are in progress to evaluate the preventative efficacy of mild to moderate restriction of protein, magnesium, and phosphorus of acidifying diets. Caution must be used in deciding whether or not to induce prophylactic diuresis in patients with a history of struvite uroliths induced by recurrent UTI. Although formation of dilute urine tends to minimize supersaturation of urine with calculogenic crystalloids, it tends to counteract innate antimicrobial properties of urine. Experimental studies performed in rats and cats indicate that diuresis tends to minimize pyelonephritis but enhance lower UTIs.

2. Sterile struvite uroliths.
   a. As compared to infection-induced struvite uroliths in patients whose UTI has been eradicated or controlled, sterile struvite uroliths have a greater tendency to recur.
   b. If the urine pH of patients with sterile struvite urolithiasis remains alkaline, administration of urine acidifiers should be considered.
   c. The prophylactic value of concomitant restriction of dietary phosphorus and magnesium has not yet been determined.

XV. FELINE STRUVITE UROLITHIASIS

A. Struvite is the most common mineral identified in feline uroliths (Table 41–2).

B. Surprisingly, feline struvite nephroliths are uncommonly encountered (Table 41–4).

C. See Chapter 35, Disorders of the Feline Lower Urinary Tract, for specific details.[66,177]

XVI. CANINE SILICA UROLITHIASIS

A. Etiopathogenesis (Figs. 41–11, 41–12, 41–14, 41–16, 41–90 to 41–92).

1. When naturally occurring silica jackstones were first encountered in dogs in the mid-1970s, they

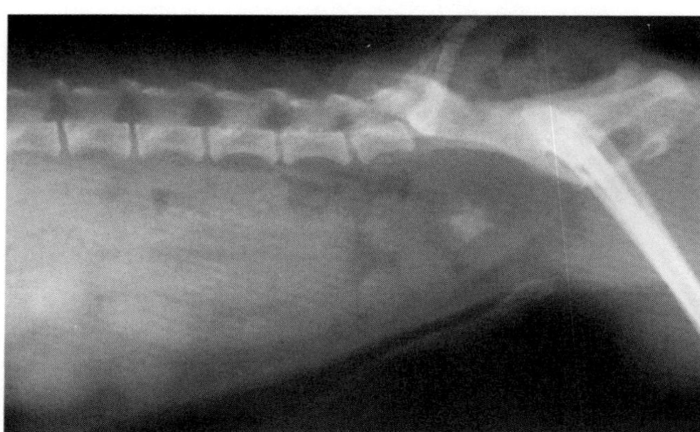

FIG. 41–90. Survey lateral abdominal radiography of a 7-year-old male Yorkshire terrier. A radiodense jackstone in the bladder lumen. (Compare Figs. 41–47 and 41–48).

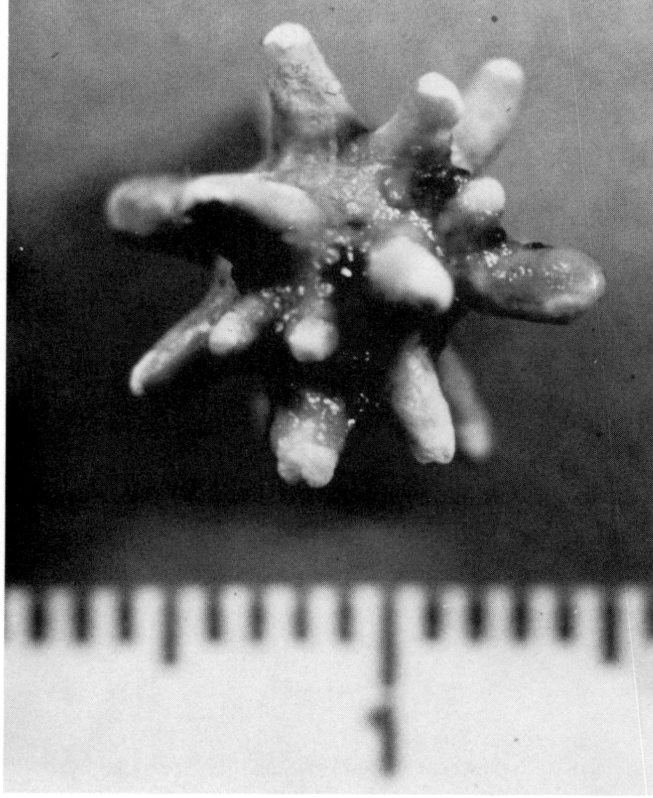

FIG. 41–91. Amorphous silica jackstone surgically removed from the urinary bladder of the dog described in Fig. 41–90.

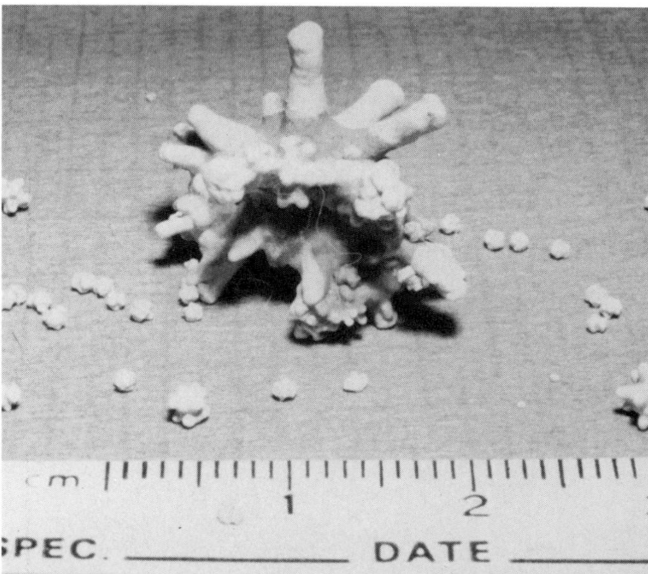

FIG. 41–92. Multiple jackstone urocystoliths removed from a 5-year-old miniature schnauzer. The irregular shape of the large silica jackstone in the center was caused by deposition of outer layers of *Staphylococcus*-induced struvite. (From Osborne CA, et al. Canine silica urolithiasis. *JAVMA*. 1981;178:809–813.)

TABLE 41–23.
SUMMARY OF RECOMMENDATIONS FOR PREVENTING CANINE SILICA UROLITHS

Perform appropriate diagnostic studies, including complete urinalysis, quantitative urine culture, and diagnostic radiography. Determine precise location, size, and number of uroliths.
If possible, determine mineral composition of uroliths. If unavailable, determine their composition by evaluation of appropriate clinical data (see Table 41–9).
Small urocystoliths may be removed by voiding urohydropropulsion (see Table 41–24). Consider surgical removal of larger uroliths that cause clinical disease.
Prevent further growth of existing silica uroliths or prevent recurrence of surgical removed silica uroliths:
- Avoid diets containing substantial plant proteins; especially, avoid those containing soybean hulls or corn gluten feed.
- Enhance diuresis by adding moisture to the diet or stimulating thirst with supplemental sodium chloride.
- Do not deliberately attempt to acidify urine.

If necessary, attempt to eradicate or control UTIs with appropriate antimicrobial agents.

were confined to the United States and Canada.[144] In 1985, canine silica jackstones were recognized in Japan, and shortly thereafter they were recognized in Europe. Calcium magnesium aluminum silicate uroliths without a jackstone configuration were identified in dogs native to Kenya in 1977.[27]

2. Available clinical information provides a strong link between canine silica uroliths and dietary ingredients. Diets that contain substantial quantities of corn gluten feed and/or soybean hulls are especially suspect.[144,158]
3. For reasons as yet unexplained, more than 95% of the canine silica uroliths have affected male dogs.[144] We hypothesize that the low rate of detection of silica uroliths in female dogs is related to their voiding small uroliths during micturition, before they induce clinical signs.
4. Twenty-nine of the 107 (27%) dogs affected by silica uroliths in one series were German shepherds; the remainder were of 32 other breeds.[144] The explanation for this apparently high prevalence of silica uroliths in German shepherd dogs is unknown, but it may be related to their popularity as a large breed. Larger-breed dogs are often fed

TABLE 41–24.
VOIDING UROHYDROPROPULSION: A NONSURGICAL TECHNIQUE FOR REMOVING SMALL UROCYSTOLITHS

1. Perform appropriate diagnostic studies, including complete urinalysis, quantitative urine culture, and diagnostic radiography. Determine location, size, surface contour, and number of urocystoliths.
2. Anesthetize the patient, if necessary.
3. If the urinary bladder is not distended with urine, moderately distend it with a physiologic solution (e.g., saline, lactated Ringer's) injected through a transurethral catheter. To prevent overdistention, palpate the bladder per abdomen during infusion. Remove the catheter.
4. Position the patient so that the vertebral spine is approximately vertical.
5. Gently agitate the urinary bladder wtih the objective of promoting gravitational movement of urocystoliths into the bladder neck.
6. Induce voiding by manually expressing the bladder. Use steady digital pressure rather than intermittent squeezing motion.
7. Collect urine and uroliths in a cup. Compare the number and size uroliths to those detected by radiography and submit them for quantitative analysis.
8. If necessary, repeat Steps 3 through 7 until the number of uroliths detected by radiography are removed or until uroliths are no longer voided.
9. Perform double-contrast cystography, to ensure that no uroliths remain in the urinary bladder. Repeat voiding urohydropropulsion if small urocystoliths remain.
10. Administer prophylactic antimicrobials for 3 to 5 days or, if necessary, for a longer period.
11. Monitor for adverse complications (hematuria, dysuria, bacterial UTI, and urethral obstruction with uroliths).
12. Formulate appropriate recommendations to minimize urolith recurrence or to manage those that remain in the urinary tract on the basis of quantitative mineral analysis of voided urocystoliths.

dry foods that contain relatively large quantities of plant ingredients (e.g., corn gluten feed). Soybean hulls are sometimes added to reducing diets as a non-nutritive ingredient.

B. Treatment and prevention (Table 41–23).

1. Effective medical protocols to induce dissolution of canine silica jackstones have not yet been developed. Calculolytic diets that do not contain vegetable proteins, and that induce diuresis, may prevent further growth of silica uroliths. Voiding urohydropropulsion may be utilized to remove small urocystoliths (Table 41–24). Surgery remains the only viable alternative for removing large silica uroliths.
2. Because initiating and perpetuating causes of silica urolithiasis are not known, only nonspecific measures to reduce the degree of supersaturation of urine with calculogenic substances can be recommended for prevention. At this time, our recommendations include these: change of diet, augmentation of urine volume, and consideration of altering urine pH (see Table 41–23).[144]
   a. Though the role of diet in the genesis of canine silica uroliths is speculative, it seems reasonable to recommend that the diet of affected patients be changed, especially if the problem is recurrent.
      (1). Even though empirical, this maneuver is unlikely to be harmful—and may be helpful.
      (2). Based on the assumption that the primary source of excessive silica in diets is vegetable matter (especially soybean hulls and corn gluten feed), selection of a diet with reduced quantities of vegetable protein and non-nutritive plant ingredients is recommended.
   b. For dogs with recurrent silica uroliths, increasing the volume of urine produced by increasing water consumption increases the volume of urine in which calculogenic substances are dissolved or suspended. Oral administration of sodium chloride has been a favored empirical method to induce diuresis in dogs with uroliths.
      (1). Depending on the size of the dog, the quantity of urine produced before therapy, and the functional status of the cardiovascular system, we recommend oral administration of 0.5 to 10 g of sodium chloride per day.
      (2). A satisfactory response is suggested by reduction of previously elevated specific gravity value to a range below 1.020 to 1.030. Provided that consumption of sodium chloride is effective in inducing formation of less concentrated urine and is tolerated by the patient, it may be continued.
   c. Silica is less soluble in acid than in alkaline water, and currently available information suggests that silica is less soluble in acid than in alkaline biologic environments.[144]
      (1). It is noteworthy that the urine pH of eight infection-free dogs with silica uroliths was acidic or neutral at the time of diagnosis (mean, 6.0; range, 5.0 to 7.0).[144]
      (2). Whether or not alkalinization of urine is of benefit in increasing the solubility of silica or silicates in urine is unknown. Likewise, the effects of orally administered alkalinizing agents (e.g., sodium bicarbonate) on the absorbability of silica from the gastrointestinal tract have not been evaluated.
         (a). Nonetheless, it seems prudent to recommend that deliberate efforts to acidify the urine of dogs with recurrent silica uroliths be avoided.
         (b). Mild alkalinization of the urine (but not of the digestive system) might be considered for dogs affected by silica uroliths that recur frequently.
         (c). We emphasize, however, that we have had no experience with this form of therapy.

XVII. COMPOUND UROLITHS

A. Compound uroliths (i.e., nucleus of one mineral type and shells of different mineral types) occurred in approximately 7% of canine and 1% of feline uroliths analyzed in our series (see Tables 41–1 to 41–4). Examples follow.

1. A nucleus of 100% calcium oxalate monohydrate surrounded by a shell of 80% magnesium ammonium phosphate and 20% calcium phosphate.
2. A nucleus composed of 95% magnesium ammonium phosphate and 5% calcium phosphate surrounded by a shell of 95% ammonium acid urate and 5% magnesium ammonium phosphate.
3. Sulfadiazine comprised 30% of the shell of one compound urocystolith removed from a 7-year-old female domestic shorthair cat.

B. Because risk factors that predispose to precipitation (nucleation) of different minerals vary, the occurrence of compound uroliths poses a unique challenge in terms of prevention of recurrence. In the absence of clinical evidence to the contrary, it seems logical to recommend management protocols designed principally to minimize recurrence of nucleation of minerals comprising the nucleus (rather than the shells) of compound uroliths. Followup studies designed to evaluate efficacy of preventive protocols should include complete urinalysis, radiography, and, if available, evaluation of the urine concentrations of calculogenic metabolites.

XVIII. NONSURGICAL AND PERCUTANEOUS TECHNIQUES FOR MANAGEMENT OF NEPHROLITHS AND URETEROLITHS

A. Obstruction of the upper urinary tract.

1. Obstruction to urine outflow may cause varying degrees of damage to the upper urinary tract (see Figs. 41–3, 41–5, 41–21, 41–23, 41–82 to 41–86). For example, persistent obstruction of the urethra or of both ureters of a patient with previously normal renal function leads to death within a few days. Therefore, reestablishment of urine outflow should receive emergency priority. Likewise, unilateral ureteral or renal pelvic obstruction caused by uroliths associated with bacterial UTI may rapidly (within a few days) lead to acute generalized pyelonephritis, septicemia, and, possibly, death. Prolonged persistent obstruction of one ureter in the absence of infection usually is not an immediate threat to life, but it causes progressive and irreversible destruction of the associated kidney.
2. Results of experimental and clinical studies underscore the fact that some degree of renal function may be recovered following elimination of the cause of obstruction. For example, in one study of dogs with unilateral renal obstruction of 2, 4, or 6 weeks' duration, there was 38.7% recovery of renal function after 2 weeks' obstruction, 9.8% recovery after 4 weeks', and 2% after 6 weeks' obstruction.[80] In another study of dogs, glomerular filtration rate (GFR) returned to 68% of normal values after 7 days of complete unilateral ureteral obstruction.[102]
3. Sequential studies in dogs with unilateral ureteral obstruction revealed that recovery of renal function is inversely proportional to the duration of obstruction.[103] After 28 days of complete unilateral obstruction, GFR was only 22% of the preobstruction value; however, after contralateral nephrectomy, GFR in the previously obstructed kidneys increased 95 to 114% of control values. It is obvious that, in absence of infection, kidneys have remarkable ability to recover function after relatively long periods of obstruction. Increased renal function after contralateral nephrectomy is also noteworthy.
4. Results of these studies have great clinical significance: They prevent adoption of an overly pessimistic view about recovery of renal function following correction of obstruction. In the absence of conclusive evidence of irreversibility, efforts to decompress the urinary tract and to eliminate the cause(s) of obstruction should be considered, because at least partial restoration of renal function is likely.

B. Percutaneous nephropyelostomy.

1. Use of percutaneous nephropyelostomy techniques to decompress the upper urinary tract and to detect, localize, extract, and/or dissolve nephroliths and ureteroliths has gained widespread attention in humans.[191] With the aid of fluoroscopy, contrast radiography, real-time ultrasound, or computer axial tomography, needles, catheters, cannulas, nephroscopes (endourology), and stone baskets are inserted percutaneously through the renal parenchyma into the renal pelves and ureters.[115,135,136,199]
2. The key to successful percutaneous extraction or dissolution of nephroliths and ureteroliths is the capacity to introduce relatively large tubes into the renal pelvis. Once access to the upper urinary tract has been attained, uroliths may be removed by several means, including:
   a. Mechanical extraction with stone baskets.[36]
   b. Mechanical extraction following fragmentation by hydraulic shock waves initiated by an electrical discharge (electrohydraulic lithotripsy),[31,41,42,174,207]
   c. Mechanical extraction following fragmentation with ultrasound (ultrasonic lithotripsy).[3,128]
   d. Flushing with stone solvents (chemolysis).[57,189,192]
3. Techniques of percutaneous nephropyelostomy applicable to dogs have been reported,[7,56,118] but the technique is more difficult to perform in dogs than in human beings owing to greater mobility of the kidneys and smaller size of the renal pelves. Although it may be used to decompress the upper urinary tract, further studies are needed to develop a procedure that permits passage of catheters large enough to remove or dissolve renoliths and ureteroliths in dogs and cats. Electrohydraulic ureterolithotripsy has been used under experimental conditions to disintegrate ureteral stones in dogs.[172]

C. Extracorporeal shock-wave lithotripsy.

1. Extracorporeal shock-wave lithotripsy (ESWL) has been developed as a noninvasive technique of disintegrating human uroliths.[33–35,70]
2. Basically, the technique involves disintegration of uroliths by subjecting them to repeated (1,000 to 2,000) focused shock waves generated outside the body. The focused shock waves are generated in a tub of water (containing the patient) by an electrical discharge across a spark gap positioned at the first focal point of a hemiellipsoidal reflector. Pressure (or shock-) waves originating from the first focal point are reflected so that they (and their energy) are focused at the second focal point of the ellipse. With the aid of fluoroscopy, the urolith to be disintegrated is placed precisely at the second focal point of the ellipsoid.
3. ESWL has been used successfully to treat unilateral and bilateral calcium oxalate nephroliths in dogs.[18] At this time, use of special equipment requires collaboration between veterinarians and physicians.

XIX. RETROGRADE AND ANTEGRADE PROPULSION

A. Overview.

1. Within 2 or 3 days, persistent complete obstruction of the urethra by uroliths is fatal. Thus, reestablishing urine outflow should receive emergency priority.
2. Palpation of the entire urethra (including evalua-

tion per rectum) and appropriate radiography and/or ultrasonography should always be performed to establish the site(s) and cause of outflow obstruction.

3. If the patient has signs of systemic illness, or if the history suggests prolonged outflow obstruction, pretreatment urine and blood samples should be obtained to assess renal function, electrolyte, and acid-base status.
4. Regardless of the techniques employed, appropriate care must be utilized to minimize pain, trauma to various components of the urinary tract, and iatrogenic UTI.

B. Summary of procedure:

1. Obtain appropriate diagnostic information to localize the sites, number, size, and surface characteristics of urethroliths.

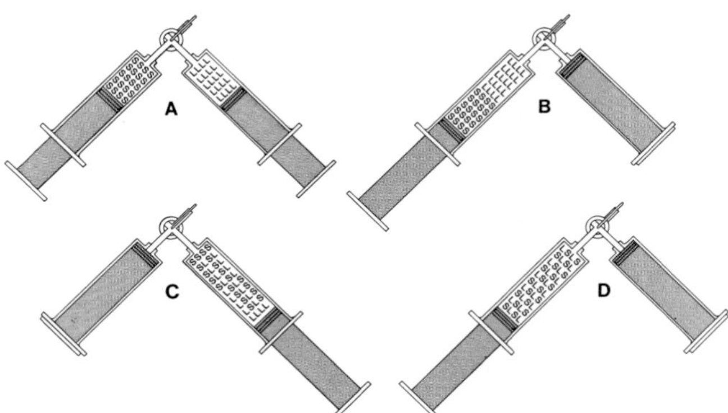

FIG. 41–93. Schematic diagram illustrates technique for mixing sterilized aqueous lubricant (L) with physiologic saline solution (S) in two syringes connected by a three-way valve. (From Osborne CA, et al. Nonsurgical removal of uroliths from the urethra of female dogs. *JAVMA.* 1983;182:47–50.)

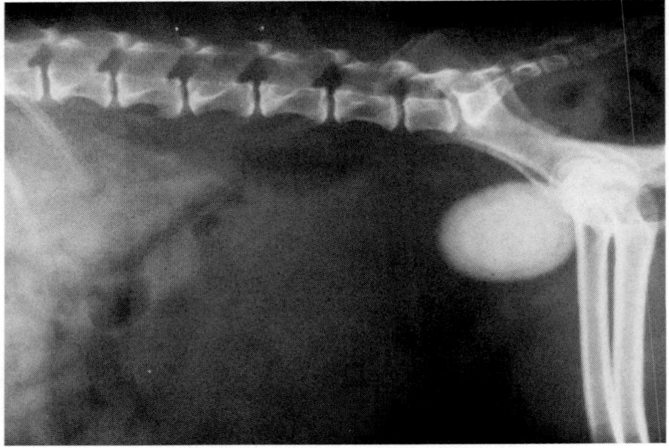

FIG. 41–94. Survey lateral abdominal radiograph of a 5-year-old spayed female miniature schnauzer with obstruction of the proximal urethra and distal ureters caused by a large struvite–calcium apatite urocystolith. The urocystolith was dislodged following lubrication and digital palpation through the abdomen.

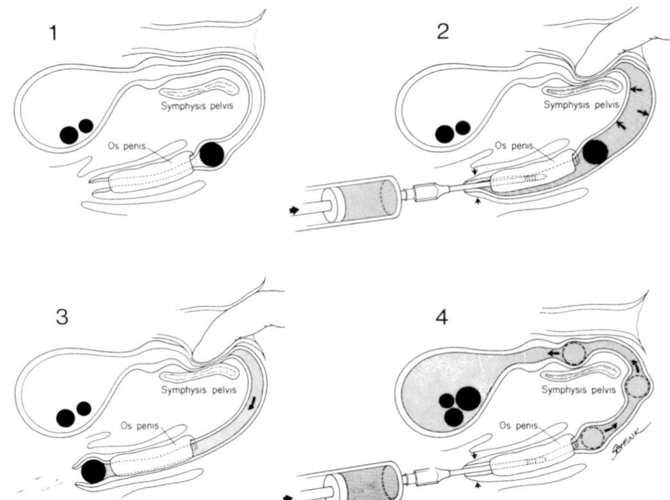

FIG. 41–95. Removal of urethrolith in a male dog by urohydropropulsion: (1) Urethrolith originating from the urinary bladder has lodged behind the os penis. (2) Dilation of the urethral lumen is achieved by injecting fluid with pressure. Digital pressure applied to the external urethral orifice and the pelvic urethra has created a closed system. (3) Sudden release of digital pressure at the external urethral orifice and subsequent movement of fluid and urethroliths toward the external urethral orifice. (4) Sudden release of digital pressure at the pelvic urethra and subsequent movement of fluid and urethrolith toward the urinary bladder. (From Piermattei DL, Osborne CA. Urohydropropulsion: Nonsurgical removal of urethral calculi in male dogs. In: Kirk RW, ed. *Current Veterinary Therapy.* Vol. 6. Philadelphia: WB Saunders; 1977:1195–1196.)

2. Decompress the urinary bladder by cystocentesis. Save aliquots of pretreatment urine for urinalysis and urine culture.
3. If indicated, collect pretreatment blood samples for hematologic and biochemical evaluation.
4. Lubricate the urethral lumen to facilitate movement of uroliths.
5. Attempt to move the uroliths by palpation.
6. Perform urohydropropulsion.

C. Cystocentesis.

1. If obstruction to urine outflow causes overdistension of the urinary bladder, it may be decompressed by cystocentesis.
2. Decompressive cystocentesis should generally be performed before urohydropropulsion.
3. See Chapter 35 for specific details.
4. The need for prophylactic antibacterial therapy following cystocentesis must be determined on the basis of the status of the patient and retrospective evaluation of technique. If it is likely that the dog has a UTI infection, or if subsequent restoration of urethral patency requires intermittent or indwelling catheterization, antimicrobial therapy should be considered. Pretreatment urine samples must be collected for urinalysis and bacterial urine culture.

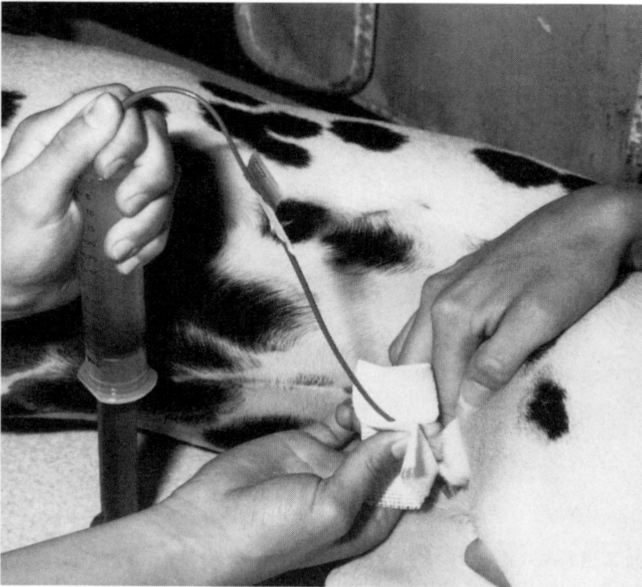

FIG. 41–96. Photograph illustrates use of a flexible urinary catheter and position of a saline-filled syringe to facilitate distension of the urethral lumen. It is important to ensure attachment of the urinary catheter to the syringe tip by using digital pressure.

D. Lubrication (Fig. 41–93).

1. A liberal quantity of 1:1 mixture of sterilized physiologic saline solution (or a comparable non-irritating physiologic saline solution) and aqueous lubricant should be injected through a catheter into the urethral lumen adjacent to the uroliths. This maneuver helps to lubricate the urolith(s) and the urethral mucosa, which is often inflamed and swollen.
2. We recommend that this mixture be prepared by connecting the tips of two large-capacity syringes, one partially filled with an aqueous lubricant and the other partially filled with saline solution, using a three-way valve. Injecting these materials back and forth between the syringes allows rapid mixing without compromising sterility (see Fig. 41–93).
3. Aqueous lubricants should not be injected into the urinary tract of patients known to have tears in the wall of the urethra or urinary bladder, because lubricants have been implicated in the formation of periurethral granulomas in humans[152] and rabbits.[17]

E. Palpation (Fig. 41–94).

1. Unidirectional massage of a urethral urolith with a finger inserted into the vagina or rectum of female dogs is frequently effective in dislodging urethral uroliths. Likewise, manipulation of a urolith lodged in the neck of the bladder and proximal urethra by palpation per abdomen usually restores urine outflow (see Fig. 41–94).
2. Gentle palpation of urethroliths in male dogs may help to dislodge them from adjacent swollen and inflamed mucosa.
3. Caution must be used to avoid inducing iatrogenic swelling and trauma of such magnitude that it further reduces the size of the urethral lumen.

F. Urohydropropulsion (Figs. 41–95 to 41–100).

1. Uroliths lodged in the urethra of male and female dogs may be moved back into the lumen of the urinary bladder by urohydropropulsion,[141,152] a

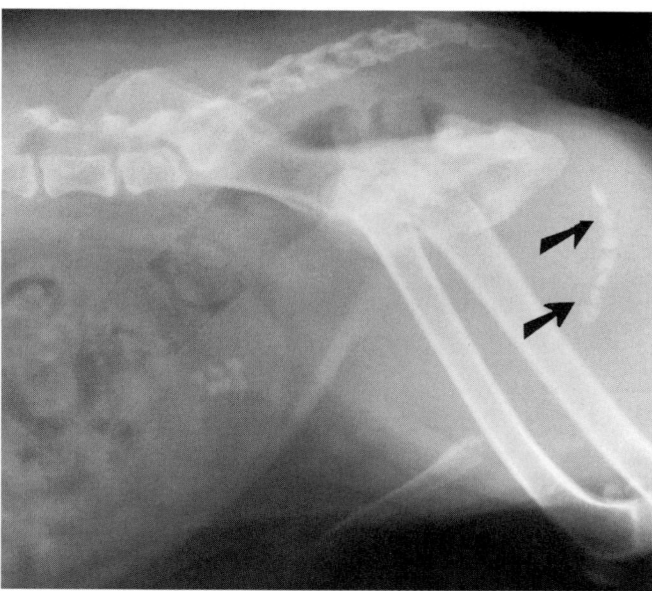

FIG. 41–97. Lateral survey abdominal radiograph of a 9-year-old male miniature schnauzer illustrates irregularly shaped calcium oxalate uroliths in the urethra *(arrows)* and urinary bladder.

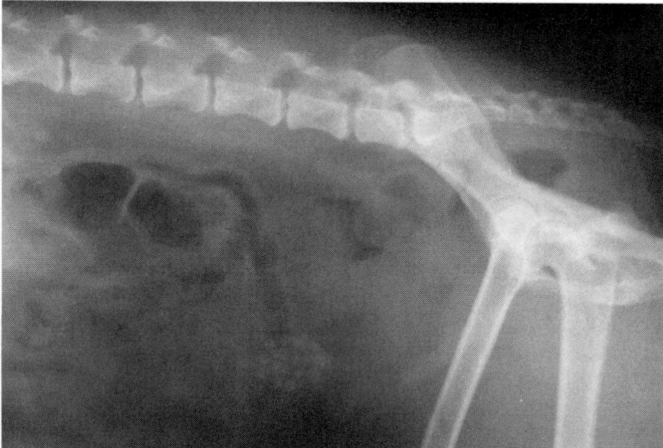

FIG. 41–98. Lateral survey abdominal radiograph of the dog described in Fig. 41–97 following retrograde voiding urohydropropulsion. Quantitative analysis of surgically removed urocystoliths revealed that they were composed of 90% calcium oxalate monohydrate and 10% calcium oxalate dihydrate.

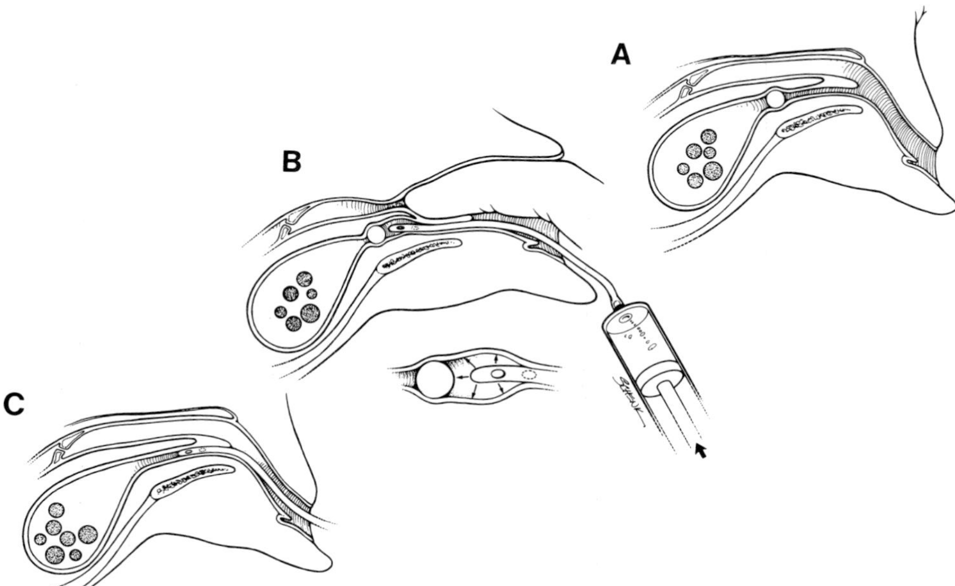

FIG. 41–99. Schematic illustration of urohydropropulsion in a female dog with a solitary urethrolith using a conventional urinary catheter. **A,** Urolith originating from the urinary bladder has become lodged in the urethra. **B,** Small portion of the urethral lumen distal to the urethrolith and proximal to a site occluded by digital pressure applied through the vaginal wall has been expanded by injecting saline solution through a catheter. **C,** The urolith has been forced back into the bladder lumen, eliminating obstruction to urine outflow. (From Osborne CA, et al. Nonsurgical removal of uroliths from the urethra of female dogs. *JAVMA.* 1983;182:47–50.)

technique based on dilatation of a portion of the urethra with fluid under pressure.

2. Restraint and anesthesia.
   a. The disposition of the patient may warrant sedation or general anesthesia. Pharmacologic agents dependent on renal metabolism or excretion for inactivation and elimination from the body should be avoided. If an uncooperative patient is an anesthesia risk because of a uremic crisis, topical application of lidocaine gel to the urethral mucosa in combination with parenteral administration of a small dose of analgesic may afford adequate patient restraint.
   b. General anesthesia should be used if uroliths cannot be removed from the urethra of nonanesthetized patients by urohydropropulsion. Appropriate caution should be used, since patients in renal failure are more sensitive than normal patients to general anesthesia. Short-acting barbiturates (e.g., thiamylal) may be used, as they are inactivated primarily by the liver. Propofol, an ultra–short-acting anesthetic, is often an excellent choice.[97] Inhalant anesthetics such as halothane may also be considered because they are not dependent on the kidneys for inactivation and excretion from the body.

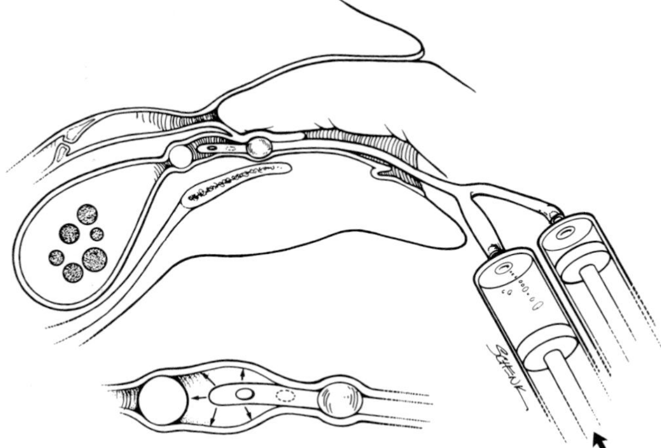

FIG. 41–100. Schematic illustration of urohydropropulsion utilizing a Swann-Ganz balloon catheter. Inflation of the balloon with air helps to prevent reflux of saline solution out of the external urethral orifice. (From Osborne CA, et al. Nonsurgical removal of uroliths from the urethra of female dogs. *JAVMA.* 1983;182:47–50.)

3. Male dogs: To remove uroliths by urohydropropulsion, follow this procedure:
   a. Inject a liberal quantity of a 1:1 mixture of sterilized saline solution and aqueous lubricant

through a flexible catheter into the urethral lumen adjacent to the uroliths.

b. Next, have an assistant insert an index finger into the rectum and firmly occlude the lumen of the pelvic urethra by applying digital pressure against the ischium, through the ventral wall of the rectum (see Fig. 41–95).

c. A flexible catheter or a bovine-teat cannula with an attached 35- to 60-ml syringe filled with sterilized saline should then be inserted into the lumen of the penile urethra via the external urethral orifice. The penile urethra should be compressed by digital pressure around the shaft of the catheter or cannula. As a result of these maneuvers, a portion of the urethra from the external urethral orifice to the bony pelvis becomes a closed system.

d. Saline should be injected into the urethra until a marked increase in the diameter of the pelvic urethra is perceived by the assistant (see Fig. 41–95). If a flexible urethral catheter is used, we recommend that the plunger be placed on the table while the barrel of the syringe is pushed down on the plunger (see Fig. 41–95). This maneuver generates greater pressure in the urethral lumen. Confirmation that the urethra has been markedly distended is very important because the urethra must be distended to its maximum capacity before enough pressure can be created in the urethral lumen to advance the uroliths. The chance of rupture of the urethral lumen is minimal, since the path of least resistance for fluid is into the urinary bladder or out the external urethral orifice. Caution must be used to avoid overdistending the urinary bladder.

e. At this point, the lumen of all portions of the isolated urethra, except in the ventral groove of the os penis, is markedly dilated (see Fig. 41–95). Dilation of the lumen of the segment of the urethra in the ventral groove of the os penis is limited to stretching of the ventral portion of the urethral wall (see Fig. 41–95).

f. If the uroliths are very small, at this point in the maneuver the catheter or cannula may be removed rapidly from the distal urethra. Simultaneously, digital pressure applied to the distal penile urethra should be released rapidly, to permit forceful expulsion of saline from the urethra (see Fig. 41–95). Digital pressure applied to the pelvic urethra must be sustained. If the uroliths are small enough to pass through the distended portion of the urethra in the ventral groove of the os penis, they will be carried with the fluid toward the external urethral orifice. It is usually necessary to repeat the procedure several times to move the urolith(s) from the caudal end of the os penis to the external urethral orifice. Movement of uroliths within the urethral lumen may be monitored with the aid of a urethral catheter, or, if necessary, radiographically.

g. If the urethroliths are too large to pass through the ventral groove of the os penis, the procedure should be modified: Instead of releasing digital pressure on the distal portion of the urethra, digital pressure to the pelvic urethra should be rapidly released (see Fig. 41–95). Pressure should be maintained in the urethral lumen by forcing the syringe plunger forward, even after the assistant has released digital pressure applied through the rectal wall. This variation in technique forcibly advances fluid, and usually urethroliths, into the urinary bladder (see Figs. 41–95, 41–97, 41–98). Sometimes, the urolith is suddenly freed from adjacent tissues and rapidly returns to the bladder lumen; however, as with antegrade flush, it may be necessary to repeat the procedure several times before the uroliths reach the urinary bladder. If the technique is repeated, it is often necessary to repeat decompressive cystocentesis, to prevent overdistension of the bladder lumen with fluid. The position of the urolith(s) may be monitored by palpating the perineal and pelvic urethra, with the aid of a urethral catheter, or by means of radiography.

h. A combined procedure utilizing cystotomy and retrograde flushing of the urethra to remove silica uroliths in the bladder and urethra has been described.[61] The objective is to obviate urethrotomy in addition to cystotomy for patients whose uroliths are lodged in the urethra. Following cystotomy and removal of urocystoliths, a relatively small catheter is advanced to the site of obstructing uroliths. The catheter should be narrow enough to allow passage of urethral uroliths while the catheter is positioned in the urethra. Large quantities of a nonirritating isotonic solution are then injected into the urethra in an attempt to flush the uroliths back into the bladder lumen. To facilitate retrograde flushing of the urethra, it may be necessary to have an assistant occlude the distal end of the urethra with digital pressure to the tip of the penis.

4. Female dogs: Urohydropropulsion may be used to remove uroliths lodged in the urethra.[141]

   a. Inject into the urethral lumen adjacent to the uroliths a liberal quantity of 1:1 mixture of a sterilized solution and aqueous lubricant through a flexible catheter (see Fig. 41–93). With an index finger in the rectum (or preferably the vagina), firmly occlude the lumen of the distal end of the urethra around a catheter (see Fig. 41–99). This creates a closed system between the occluding urolith and the site of digital compression of the urethra.

b. Next, inject saline solution through the catheter to distend the urethra to its maximal diameter. Dilation of the urethra, combined with pressure generated by the intraluminal saline solution, usually causes the urolith to move back into the bladder lumen. Gentle digital manipulation of the urolith may aid in moving it toward the bladder lumen.

c. Movement of a large urolith lodged in the neck of the bladder and proximal portion of the urethra may require digital manipulation of the urolith per abdomen by an assistant while saline solution is injected through the catheter.

d. If, owing to reflux of saline solution through the external urethral orifice intraurethral pressure is lost, it may be necessary to repeat the procedure several times before the uroliths reach the urinary bladder. The position of the urolith(s) may be monitored by digital palpation, attempts to advance the catheter, or radiography.

e. If difficulty is encountered in occluding the external urethral orifice around the catheter, a No. 4 to No. 7 French Swan-Ganz balloon catheter or pediatric Foley catheter may be used (see Fig. 41–100). Inflation of the balloon after it has been inserted into the urethra, combined with firm digital pressure, may be effective in minimizing reflux of saline solution through the external urethral orifice.

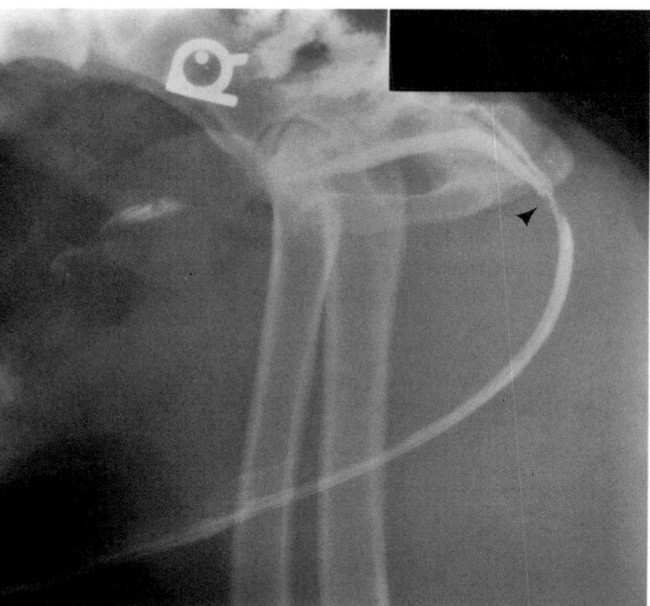

FIG. 41–101. Lateral view of a retrograde positive-contrast urethrogram of an 8-year-old male Labrador retriever. The tip of the urinary catheter has penetrated the caudodorsal aspect of the urethral wall at a site just distal to a urethrolith *(arrow)*. (From Osborne CA, et al. Nonsurgical removal of uroliths from the urethra of female dogs. *JAVMA*. 1983;182:47–50.)

G. Urethral catheterization.

1. Attempts to dislodge urethroliths.

a. Though urethral uroliths may be pushed back into the bladder with the aid of a catheter, this technique is often unsuccessful and is associated with risk of urethral trauma and secondary infection (Fig. 41–101). If the urolith can be moved easily by inserting a catheter into the urethral lumen, our experience has been that it also can be moved readily by digital pressure applied through the vaginal or rectal wall.

b. As a last resort, judicious use of a catheter to attempt to dislodge urethral uroliths may be justified. The diameter of the catheter should be as large as is consistent with atraumatic technique. A rigid catheter is more likely to be associated with success than a flexible one; it is also more likely to cause urethral injury. The catheter should be liberally coated with sterilized, water-soluble lubricant. Unless there is a tear in the urethral wall, a liberal quantity of a 1 : 1 saline solution plus water-soluble lubricant should be injected through the catheter as the urolith is advanced toward the urinary bladder (see Fig. 41–93). If there is a tear in the urethra, only nonirritating isotonic solution, such as physiologic saline solution or lactated Ringer's solution, should be used. Caution must be used to avoid trauma to the urethra; excessive force should never be used.

c. Stone baskets have been designed to retrieve small uroliths from the ureters of human beings. The Mitchell stone basket (C.R. Bard Co., Murray Hill, New Jersey) has been used to remove uroliths from the urethra of male dogs. Ability to entrap the urolith in a stone basket may be enhanced by dilating the urethral lumen with fluid in a fashion similar to that used for antegrade and retrograde urohydropropulsion. Stone baskets may be useful in small female dogs with urethral uroliths; however, we have had no clinical experience with this technique. Flexible foreign body forceps (R. Wolf Medical Instruments Corp., Rosemount, Illinois) may also be useful in some patients.

2. Temporary bypass of urethroliths.

a. At one time, a commonly used nonsurgical method for attempting to reestablish patency of a urethra occluded with one or more uroliths was attempts to pass a catheter around them. This technique is associated with a high risk of urethral trauma (abrasion, contusion, laceration, or puncture) or secondary UTI, inflammatory constriction of the urethral lumen at the site where the catheter was forced past the urolith, and a high rate of failure. Nonetheless, it may be considered if attempts to remove urethroliths by other nonsurgical methods have failed and there is an immediate need to re-establish urethral patency. If a catheter cannot be advanced beyond a urethrolith without excessive trauma, attempts should be abandoned in favor of other nonsurgical or surgical methods (e.g., cystocentesis, tube cystotomy).

b. Successful insertion of a catheter beyond the site of an obstructing urethrolith may be enhanced as follows:
   (1). Selecting human ureteral catheters with tips (spiral filiform tips) designed to bypass narrowed lumens.
   (2). Proper restraint and/or sedation of the patient.
   (3). Injecting a liberal quantity of a 1 : 1 mixture of saline solution and water-soluble lubricant around the urolith(s).
   (4). Manipulation of the catheter tip and urolith through overlying tissues by palpation.
   (5). If necessary, dilation of the urethral lumen by the same techniques used for urohydropropulsion.
   (6). Gradual dilation of the urethral lumen adjacent to the urolith by application of firm and steady pressure on the catheter (in contrast to intermittent and forceful pressure).

c. Catheters, lubricants, irrigating solutions, specula, and other instruments should be sterile; however, because the distal portion of the urethra normally contains a commensal population of bacteria, it is impossible to catheterize the patient aseptically.[116,140] Ascending migration of bacteria through the lumen of the catheter may be minimized by use of closed drainage systems that prevent reflux of urine from the collection receptacle back into the urinary tract.[116] If an open system of indwelling catheterization is used, the question is not *whether* UTI will occur, but rather *when* it does.

d. If the purpose of the indwelling catheter is to bypass the site of urethral obstruction, if the detrusor muscle is functional, and if the micturition reflex is intact, there is usually no need to extend the tip of the catheter into the bladder lumen. Inserting a catheter too far should be avoided, to minimize trauma to the bladder and/or prevent the catheter from becoming knotted or entangled in the bladder or urethral lumens.

XX. VOIDING UROHYDROPROPULSION (FIGS. 41–102 TO 41–106)

A. Overview.

Historically, cystotomy has been considered an effective method of removing all types of uroliths from the urinary bladder; however, a non-

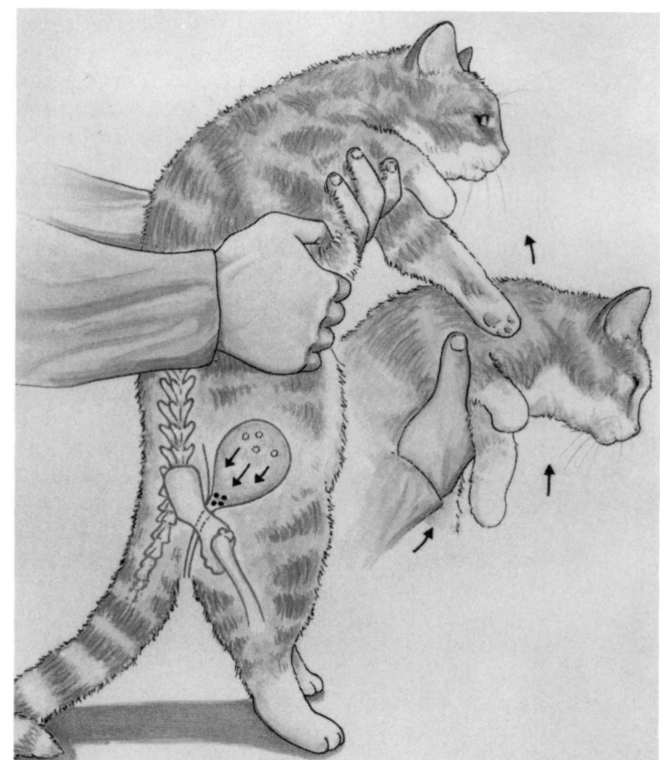

FIG. 41–102. To remove urocystoliths by voiding urohydropropulsion, the patient is positioned so that the vertebral column is approximately vertical. The urinary bladder is then gently agitated, in an effort to promote gravitational movement of urocystoliths into the bladder neck. (Adapted by Ralston Purina from Lulich JP, Osborne CA, Carlson M, et al. Nonsurgical removal of uroliths in dogs and cats by voiding urohydropropulsion. *JAVMA.* 1993;203:660–663.)

surgical alternative has been developed called urohydropropulsion.[123] The effectiveness of voiding urohydropropulsion depends on altering the patient's body position before micturition, to take advantage of the gravitational force necessary for urolith repositioning and expulsion. Voiding urohydropropulsion permits safe and rapid removal of small to medium-sized urocystoliths of any mineral composition from dogs and cats. The procedure does not require special equipment; uroliths can be removed from some patients without anesthesia.

B. Indications (Figs. 41–104 to 41–106).

1. Proper selection of patients for voiding urohydropropulsion enhances removal of urocystoliths.
2. The relationship of the size, shape, and surface contour of urocystoliths to the luminal diameter of the urethra are important factors.
   a. Uroliths that are larger than the smallest diam-

eter of any portion of the distended urethral lumen are unlikely to be voided.

b. In our clinical case series, the diameter of the largest urolith expelled from the urinary bladder was 7 mm from a 7.4-kg female dog, 5 mm from a 9-kg male dog; 5 mm from a 4.6-kg female cat, and 1 mm from a 6.6-kg male cat.[123]

c. It is logical to hypothesize that uroliths greater than 1 mm in diameter could be voided from a male cat with a perineal urethrostomy.

3. Compared to uroliths with an irregular contour, smooth uroliths pass more readily through the urethra.
   a. This may be related, at least in part, to the fact that uroliths with sharp surface projections are more likely to adhere to the urethral mucosa.
   b. In addition, contact of the surface of smooth uroliths with the urethral mucosa may form a continuous seal, which would prevent voiding of saline solution without concomitant advancement of the urolith. Fluids can bypass a urolith of irregular contour and projections without forcing it through the urethral lumen.
4. Because uroliths can be removed from conscious animals, voiding urohydropropulsion may be considered for patients at high risk for anesthesia-related morbidity and mortality. Even if anesthesia is needed for patient restraint, it is often of shorter duration than that required for cystotomy.
   a. The mean time required to complete voiding urohydropropulsion and postvoiding double-contrast cystography in 15 patients from whose uroliths were all completely removed was 22 minutes.
   b. In one female dog, it took 7 minutes to remove a solitary urolith and to complete followup cystography.
5. Uroliths larger than the smallest diameter of any portion of the distended urethral lumen are unlikely to be voided. Thus, voiding urohydropropulsion may be ineffective in patients whose uroliths are lodged in the urethra at the time of diagnosis. However, *canine* uroliths composed of magnesium ammonium phosphate, ammonium urate, or cystine, and *feline* uroliths composed of magnesium ammonium phosphate that initially are too large to be voided may be easily removed once their size has been reduced by medical therapy.
6. If the size of urocystoliths can be reduced by electrohydraulic shock wave lithotripsy, voiding urohydropropulsion can be used to facilitate their removal from the urinary bladder.
7. As compared with cystotomy, voiding urohydropropulsion offers several advantages.
   a. Because a surgical incision is unnecessary, healing time is reduced and post-technique dysuria and hematuria may be less severe.
   b. Voiding urohydropropulsion also may be more effective than surgery in removing small uro-

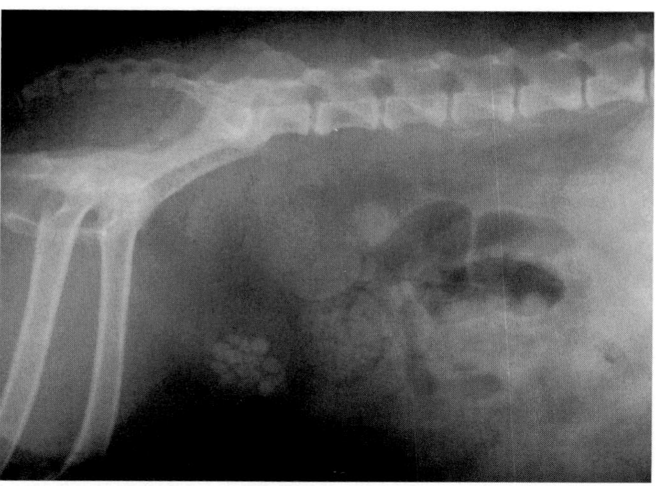

FIG. 41–104. Lateral survey abdominal radiograph of a 13-year-old female miniature schnauzer with multiple urocystoliths before voiding urohydropropulsion.

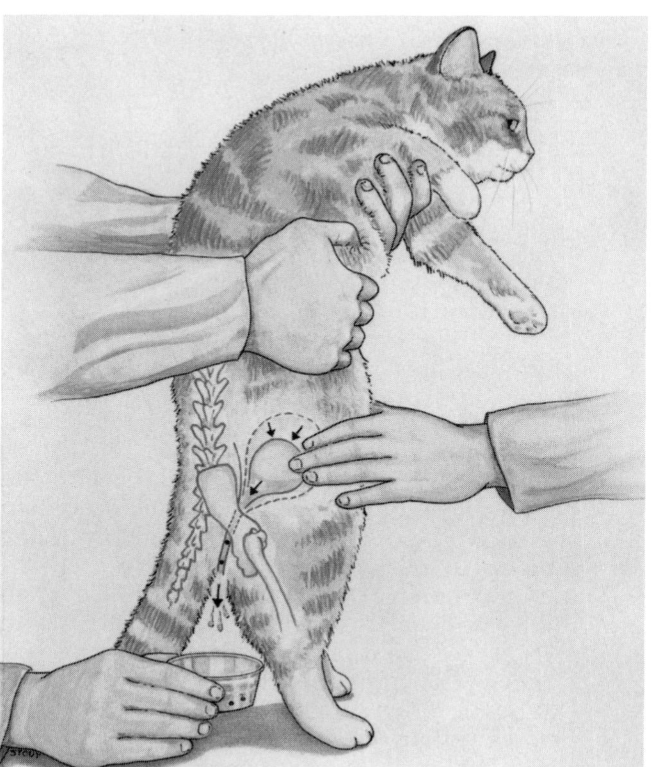

FIG. 41–103. To expel urocystoliths, voiding is induced by applying steady pressure to the urinary bladder. (Adapted by Ralston Purina from Lulich JP, Osborne CA, Carlson M, et al. Nonsurgical removal of uroliths in dogs and cats by voiding urohydropropulsion. *JAVMA*. 1993;203:660–663.)

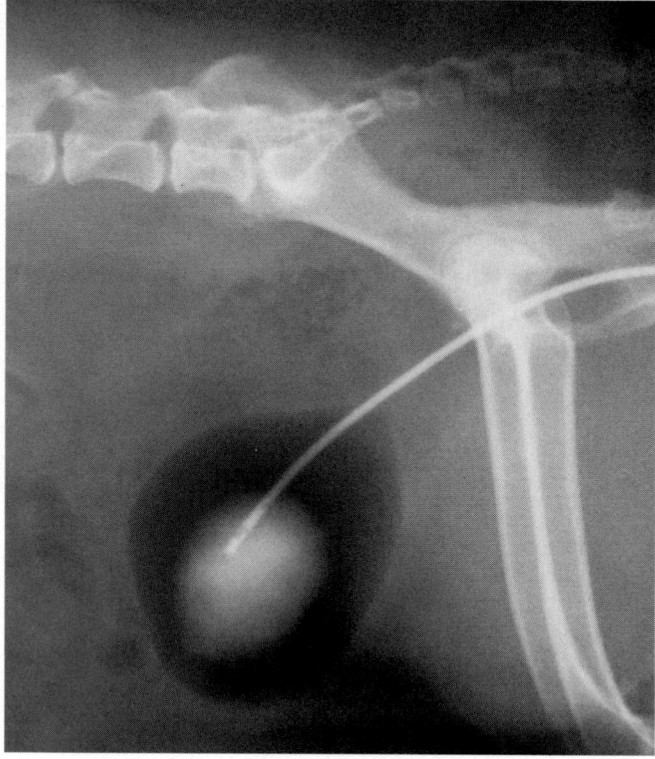

FIG. 41–105. Double-contrast cystogram of the female miniature schnauzer described in Fig. 41–104. All urocystoliths were voided through the urethra.

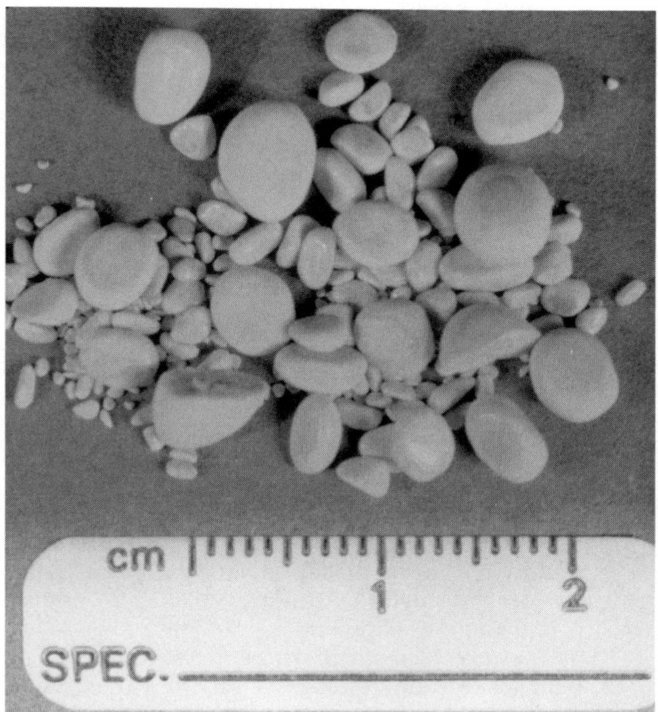

FIG. 41–106. By voiding urohydropropulsion, 417 calcium oxalate monohydrate urocystoliths removed from the dog described in Fig. 41–104.

liths, which often remain in the lower urinary tract following cystotomy.[126]

c. In some cases, voiding urohydropropulsion can be performed without anesthesia. Even if it's needed, the anesthetic period typically is much briefer than that required for cystotomy.

C. Contraindications.

1. Uroliths that obviously are too large to pass through a dilated urethra cannot be removed by voiding urohydropropulsion.
2. Voiding urohydropropulsion should not be used if manual compression of the urinary bladder is likely to cause extravasation of urine into the peritoneal cavity. Consequently, this procedure should not be used during the period of healing after urinary bladder surgery.
3. Manual compression of the urinary bladder to induce voiding is not without risk in patients with UTIs. If excessive pressure is applied to the urinary bladder, vesicoureteral reflux of urine and bacteria can occur.[65] Therefore, UTI should be controlled before voiding urohydropropulsion is applied. (See Chapter 33, Vesicoureteral Reflux, for additional details.)

D. Equipment.

1. No special equipment is needed to perform voiding urohydropropulsion. In fact, no equipment is needed if the urinary bladder already is distended with urine.

2. For patients whose urinary bladders are not sufficiently filled at the time of voiding, a urinary catheter, syringe, and physiologic saline are the only materials needed.
3. The assistance of one or two additional people should be considered, to properly position the patient and monitor anesthesia.

E. Patient restraint.

1. Anesthesia is not necessary in all patients to perform voiding urohydropropulsion. The advantage of performing voiding urohydropropulsion without anesthesia is that the micturition response is not affected by pharmacologic agents. As a result, voiding is facilitated by contraction of bladder smooth muscle and relaxation of urethral smooth muscle.
2. Sedation facilitates positioning of the patient and palpation of the urinary bladder. In addition, greater force is often required to initiate voiding in conscious animals as compared with anesthetized ones. We have not been able to determine if increased digital pressure applied to the urinary bladder of conscious animals is associated with a greater degree of hematuria and dysuria immediately following the procedure.
3. When anesthetics are used, we recommend agents that provide analgesia and muscle relaxation.
   a. In dogs, a combination of IM oxymorphone (0.1 to 0.2 mg/kg) followed by IV propofol, titrated to effect, has provided the proper the degree and duration of anesthesia.
   b. In cats, oxymorphone (0.05 to 0.1 mg/kg) and a tranquilizer (midazolam, 0.05 to 0.1 mg/kg) are administered intramuscularly before propofol titration.
   c. Because these drugs depress respiration, patients should be appropriately monitored.
   d. Once uroliths have been removed, the effects of oxymorphone can be antagonized with nalbuphine HCl (0.03 to 0.1 mg/kg, IV), if continued analgesia is desired, or if naloxone (0.002 to 0.02 mg/kg, IV) if respiratory depression is of greater concern.
   e. For small urocystoliths unlikely to induce urethral discomfort, we typically use propofol as the sole anesthetic. Propofol induced anesthesia is easily titrated, and recovery is rapid and smooth.[97] Inhalant anesthetics (isofluorane or halothane) also provide good analgesia and muscle relaxation.

F. Technique (Table 41–24; Figs. 41–102 to 41–107).

1. To enhance movement of urocystoliths by gravity, the urinary bladder should be moderately distended. If the urinary bladder is not distended with urine, it can be moderately distended with a physiologic saline solution (0.9% NaCl) injected through a transurethral catheter.
   a. As a general guideline, the normal empty canine or feline urinary bladder can be distended moderately by injecting 4 to 6 mL of fluid for every kilogram of body weight.
   b. To minimize overdistension of the bladder, its size should be assessed by abdominal palpation during infusion.
   c. After the bladder is distended, the catheter is removed.
2. Next, the dog or cat should be positioned so that the vertebral column is approximately vertical (see Fig. 41–102).
3. The urinary bladder is then gently agitated by palpation, to promote gravitational movement into the bladder neck of all urocystoliths.
4. By applying steady digital pressure to the urinary bladder to induce micturition, urine and uroliths are voided through the urethra and into a cup (see Fig. 41–103).
5. If the number of uroliths voided is fewer than that previously detected by radiography, the procedure can be repeated.
6. If uroliths detected by radiography were too numerous to count, voiding urohydropropulsion should be repeated until uroliths are no longer voided by induced micturition.
7. Before discontinuing voiding urohydropropulsion, double-contract cystography should be performed to ensure that all urocystoliths have been removed.

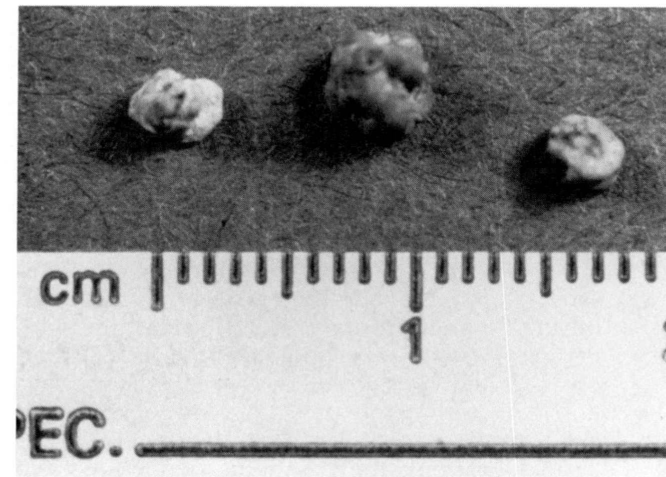

FIG. 41–107. Photograph of urocystoliths removed from the urinary bladder of a 5-year-old male Chihuahua. The uroliths contained primarily calcium oxalate dihydrate and sulfadiazine. (From Osborne CA (ed). Canine urolithiasis: etiopathogenesis, detection, treatment, and prevention. *Vet Clin North Am.* 1986; 16:207–411.)

G. Recommended followup care.

1. Following voiding urohydropropulsion, we routinely perform double-contrast cystography, to determine if any uroliths remain in the bladder. Survey radiography or ultrasonography can also

be used to determine the success of voiding urohydropropulsion. If the presence or absence of urocystoliths is not verified immediately after completion of the procedure, later it is impossible to distinguish between urolith recurrence or incomplete removal.

2. For patients with urocystoliths unassociated with bacterial UTI, antimicrobials are not needed, provided that normal host defenses have not been disrupted by transurethral catheterization. In most of our cases, catheters were used either during the procedure or for postprocedural radiography. To minimize catheter-induced UTI, clinicians should consider administering therapeutic doses of antimicrobial drugs excreted in high concentrations in urine 4 to 8 hours before, and for 2 to 5 days after, catheterization.[146] Urine collected by cystocentesis 3 to 7 days later can be cultured to verify that the urinary tract has not become infected.
3. If urocystoliths persist despite voiding urohydropropulsion, urethral obstruction may occur, especially if the patient is dysuric. If urethral obstruction occurs, uroliths can easily be moved back into the urinary bladder by retrograde urohydropropulsion. They can then be dissolved with medical management or surgically removed.

H. Complications.

1. Visible hematuria is a common complication of voiding urohydropropulsion and probably is induced by manual compression of an inflamed urinary bladder.
   a. In our experience, visible hematuria resolved within 4 hours in dogs; dysuria has not been observed in dogs.
   b. In cats, hematuria and dysuria can persist as long as 2 days.[123]
2. Urethral obstruction with uroliths is a potential complication, especially when dysuria persists in animals that still harbor uroliths in the urinary bladder.
3. Use of urinary catheters has been associated with UTI. Catheter-induced infection can be minimized by providing antimicrobials some 4 to 8 hours before catheter use and for 2 to 5 days thereafter.

XXI. SURGICAL MANAGEMENT OF UROLITHS

A. Indications.

1. Detection of uroliths is not, in itself, an indication for surgery; however, along with medical management, surgical intervention has a vital role in therapy of urolithiasis. Surgical candidates include these:
   a. Patients with urolith-induced obstruction to urine outflow that cannot be corrected by nonsurgical techniques, especially in patients with concomitant UTI (Figs. 41–3, 41–5, 41–21, 41–23, 41–82 to 41–86).
   b. Patients with uroliths that are refractory to current methods of medical dissolution (e.g., silica, calcium oxalate, and calcium phosphate uroliths).
   c. Patients with uroliths that are growing or multiplying, despite medical therapy designed to inhibit their growth or dissolve them (especially if they are causing obstruction to urine outflow and/or progressive deterioration in renal function).
   d. Patients with nephroliths and renal dysfunction such that the time it takes to induce medical dissolution is likely to be associated with more renal dysfunction than that associated with surgical procedures.
   e. Patients with anatomic defects of the urogenital tract that predispose to recurrent UTI and urolithiasis and that are amenable to surgical correction when uroliths are removed.
   f. Patients unable to respond to medical management because of poor client- or patient compliance with therapeutic recommendations.
2. Complete obstruction to urine outflow caused by uroliths in patients with concomitant UTI should be regarded as a surgical emergency. In this situation, rapid spread of infection and associated damage to the urinary tract (especially the kidneys) is likely to induce septicemia and peracute renal failure caused by a combination of obstruction and pyelonephritis (see Figs. 41–82 to 41–86).
3. Unilateral renoliths and/or ureteroliths that have caused outflow obstruction and substantial impairment of function of the associated kidney should be managed by surgical intervention or, if possible, by percutaneous nephropyelonephrostomy. Medical therapy designed to induce urolith dissolution during a several week period in patients with poorly draining kidneys is unlikely to be effective since the urolith(s) are not continually bathed with sufficient newly formed urine modified to induce litholysis. The same concept applies to urethroliths that cannot be removed by nonsurgical methods.
4. Combined use of surgical removal of uroliths, followed by medical protocols, may help some patients. Examples include patients whose uroliths or fragments of uroliths persist after surgery and patients with crystalluria of a character and magnitude that indicate rapid recurrence is likely.

B. Limitations.

1. Surgery has been a time-honored approach for management of all types of urolithiasis in dogs and cats. Though surgery has been an effective method that provides immediate elimination of uroliths, it is associated with several limitations, including:
   a. Persistence of underlying causes and high rate of recurrence of uroliths, despite surgery.

b. Patient factors that enhance adverse consequences of general anesthesia or surgery.
c. Inability to remove all uroliths or fragments of uroliths during surgery.
d. Situations in which owners of companion animals do not consent to surgical therapy but will consider medical therapy.
e. Asymptomatic uroliths.

2. Despite the feasibility of dissolution of uroliths, we emphasize that this form of therapy is associated with potential hazards. Uroliths are always a predisposing cause of UTI, and always predispose the patient to obstructive uropathy. Both risks and benefits of medical—versus surgical and medical—therapy must be considered for each patient.

C. Goals.

1. Goals of surgery.
   a. Removal of all uroliths.
   b. Preservation of organ function.
   c. Elimination of partial or complete obstruction to urine outflow.
   d. Correction of structural deformities that have predisposed to infection and/or urolithiasis (Tables 41–25, 41–26).
2. Every effort should be made to minimize damage to the renal parenchyma and pelvis and to their blood supply.
3. When all uroliths cannot be removed surgically, a combination of surgical and medical therapy should be considered.

D. Surgical removal of nephroliths.

1. Overview.
   a. Surgical procedures that may be considered for removal of renoliths in dogs and cats include nephrolithotomy, pyelolithotomy, and nephrectomy.[156,203] Techniques utilized in humans that may have application for selected cases of nephrolithiasis in dogs and cats include percutaneous nephropyelostomy and autotransplantation. The procedure of choice is determined primarily by the likelihood of complete removal of the urolith(s) and depends on the location(s), size, and shape of the urolith(s). Other important factors include the structural and functional integrity of affected

TABLE 41–25.
GENERAL PRINCIPLES AND CONSIDERATIONS FOR SURGICAL MANAGEMENT OF UROLITHS

Preoperative considerations
- Obtain all blood and urine samples before administration of diagnostic (radiopaque contrast media) or therapeutic (e.g., antibiotics, fluids) agents. Quantitatively evaluate renal function.
- Always image the entire urinary tract to determine the location and number of uroliths. Contrast radiography and/or ultrasonography should be considered, to evaluate the patency of the excretory pathway. Thoroughly evaluate the entire urinary tract for correctable anatomic abnormalities that may have initiated UTIs and subsequent struvite urolithiasis.

Operative considerations
- Preserve renal function. Avoid using mattress sutures to repair nephrotomy incisions, because they cause additional irreversible loss of renal function due to infarction.
- In patients with multiple uroliths, remove renoliths before removing cystoliths. If ureteroliths are present, or if small or fractured renoliths subsequently pass into the ureters, they may be flushed into the bladder from the renal pelvis. Obtain urine samples for routine analysis and microbial culture if they could not be obtained before surgery. Collect biopsy samples of the urinary tract at the time of nephrotomy, pyelotomy, cystotomy, or urethrotomy. Evaluation of biopsy samples may have diagnostic and prognostic significance.
- Make a special effort to remove all uroliths. Thoroughly flush the affected lumen of the urinary tract with a sterile isotonic solution to remove small uroliths. Bacteria harbored inside struvite uroliths allow UTIs to persist and predispose to recurrence of struvite uroliths.
- When possible, do not allow suture material to penetrate the lumen of the urinary tract. Suture material may serve as a nidus for urolith formation by lowering the formation product. Nonabsorbable and multifilament sutures are more calculogenic than absorbable or monofilament sutures.
- Save all uroliths for mineral analysis, possible culture, and possible microscopic examination. Culturing uroliths may help detect a bacterial organism in patients receiving antimicrobial therapy before diagnostic urine culture and antimicrobial susceptibility tests are performed.

Postoperative considerations
- Avoid using indwelling catheters, because they are a common cause of iatrogenic UTIs. If one must use an indwelling catheter, a closed system should be used when possible, as it minimizes retrograde migration of pathogens through the catheter lumen.
- If multiple uroliths are present, evaluate the urinary tract radiographically after surgery. Immediate detection of uroliths that were inadvertently allowed to remain in the urinary tract is prognostically significant. It may be assumed (erroneously) that the patient is highly predisposed to recurrent urolithiasis if residual uroliths are first detected on radiographs taken several weeks after surgery. Appropriate medical and/or surgical therapy should be formulated to manage residual uroliths.
- Therapy should be designed to promote postoperative diuresis in patients undergoing nephrolithotomy. Increased urine flow minimizes formation in the renal pelves of blood clots that have the potential to obstruct urine outflow or mineralize.

TABLE 41–26.
DIFFICULTIES, *DO'S* AND *DON'TS* IN UROLITH MANAGEMENT

Difficulties in diagnosis of uroliths
- Wrong "guesstimate" of mineral type (see Table 41–9)
- Improper analysis (retrieval, submission, qualitative rather than quantitative technique)
- Uroliths composed of multiple minerals
- Uroliths not composed of minerals (matrix, drugs, foreign material)

Difficulties in treating uroliths
- Owner or patient noncompliance
- Inability to correct or control underlying disease process
- Improper therapy
- Composition of uroliths changed during therapy
- Undesired influence of drug therapy
- Inadequate surgical retrieval

Difficulties in preventing uroliths
- Owner or patient noncompliant
- Inability to correct or control underlying disease process
- No short-term or longterm plan to prevent urolith recurrence
- Improper therapy

Urolith management *Do's* and *Don'ts*
- *Do*
  - Analyze uroliths by quantitative methods.
  - Obtain baseline data before therapy.
  - Serially monitor patient's response to therapy.
  - Monitor compliance of owners and patients.
  - Retrieve and analyze recurrent uroliths.
  - Radiograph the urinary tract following surgery to remove uroliths.
- *Don't*
  - Rely on incomplete data.
  - Treat without obtaining baseline data.
  - Treat without serially monitoring the patient.
  - Assume owner or patient compliance.

and unaffected kidneys, the presence of concomitant but unrelated disorders that affect anesthesia and surgical risks, and the skill of the surgeon.

b. Nephroliths may be bilateral, forcing the surgeon to choose between a simultaneous procedure or staged unilateral procedures. This decision should be based on the following factors:
   (1). The renal function of the patient.
   (2). Whether the renoliths are causing partial or complete obstruction to urine flow.
   (3). Whether or not one kidney has severe infection resulting in systemic signs.
   (4). The overall condition of the patient.

c. If staged unilateral procedures are necessary, in the absence of obstruction to urine flow, the choice of which kidney to repair *first* is a matter of personal judgment. The surgeon should choose the kidney that is most likely to sustain the patient and least likely to be compromised by surgical intervention.
   (1). If, after the first operation, the second kidney is considered unsalvageable, it may be removed with the knowledge that the first kidney is more likely to provide adequate function.
   (2). Staged unilateral procedures should be separated by several weeks in patients with renal dysfunction. Nephrotomy further compromises the patient because of the irreversible loss of nephrons caused directly by the incision and indirectly by damage to transected vessels. The patient's renal function is assessed after the first surgery; plans for the second procedure are based on results of this reevaluation.

d. It is of interest that there have been two reports of spontaneous dissolution of struvite nephroliths in dogs with bilateral nephrolithiasis and renal dysfunction a few weeks after nephrotomy to remove stones from one kidney.[104,105]

e. Recent observations in our veterinary teaching hospital indicate that the longterm consequences of nephrotomy on renal function should be evaluated in normal dogs and cats. We observed progressive reduction in the size of the right kidney of an 8-year-old female domestic shorthair cat during a 3-year period following nephrotomy to remove multiple calcium phosphate nephroliths. Although a similar number of calcium phosphate nephroliths in the left kidney were not removed, the kidney did not change in size or morphology during the 3-year period of study. There has apparently been only one short-term (6 weeks) study of the effect of nephrotomy in normal dogs.[78] Results of that study revealed a 20 to 40% decline in glomerular filtration rate as compared with presurgical values. Would further decline in renal function have been observed if the dogs had been evaluated for a longer period?

2. Nephrolithotomy.[5,37,78,82–85,156,173,200,201,203,215]
   a. Nephrolithotomy should be considered when one or more active uroliths are present in functional kidneys (see the discussion on Biologic Behavior of Uroliths). Access to the kidney may be obtained by ventral midline or paralumbar celiotomy. In most instances, ventral midline celiotomy is chosen because it permits evaluation of both kidneys, the remaining portion of the urinary tract, and adjacent structures. It also facilitates dissection of the renal vascular pedicle and ureter and provides better access to major vessels in the event

of vascular accidents. A ventral midline celiotomy must be used if simultaneous operative management is to be performed on patients with bilateral nephrolithiasis or nephrolithiasis associated with ureteroliths, cystoliths, or urethroliths.

b. Appropriate caution should be used to prevent fragmentation of the urolith(s) during removal, especially those that are friable or that have branches protruding into pelvic diverticula. Residual stone fragments (especially those composed of infected struvite) often (but not invariably) lead to rapid recurrence of clinical signs.

c. The renal pelvis and ureter should be thoroughly flushed with a warm isotonic solution, to attempt to remove tiny stone fragments and "subvisual" uroliths. Addition of 1000 units of heparin per liter of irrigating solution helps to minimize formation of blood clots in the excretory pathway.[82] If appropriate, a small-gauge flexible catheter may be inserted into the proximal ureter to permit flushing of its lumen and assessment of its patency. Flexible nephroscopes have been designed to permit evaluation of the renal pelves of human beings and may have applications for canine or feline patients with large renal pelves.[42] Intraoperative radiography also is utilized extensively for human patients.

3. Anatrophic nephrolithotomy.
   a. Anatrophic (prevention of atrophy) nephrolithotomy is a refined technique of nephrolithotomy in which the site of incision into the renal parenchymal is chosen on the basis of its arterial blood supply.[182,197]
   b. Because renal arteries are end arteries without significant collateral blood supply, and because their anatomic site is predictable, anatrophic incisions can be made between vascular segments without damaging major intrarenal arterial branches. The precise segmental nature of the arterial blood supply in each patient is determined by preoperative and intraoperative identification of segmental vessels with the aid of indicator dyes.
   c. Since intrarenal veins have widespread anastomoses, they can be transected without causing damage to the parenchyma they supply. After identification of the segmental arterial supply to the affected kidney, the remaining portion of the procedure is similar to that employed for conventional nephrolithotomy.
4. Pyelolithotomy.
   a. Pyelolithotomy may be considered for removal of uroliths located within renal pelves that have been dilated to such a degree that they protrude beyond the normal confines of the renal hilus.[85] This technique has the advantage of minimizing further operative destruction of nephrons. It is the technique of choice to remove nephroliths from humans. Unfortunately, the technique is not applicable to dogs or cats unless the proximal urinary tract is markedly enlarged.
   b. A "coagulum" consisting of cryoprecipitate has been designed to form an extractable cast of the renal pelvis of dogs.[71,72] The cryoprecipitate was injected into and removed from the renal pelvis through an incision in its wall. The goal of the technique is to minimize the possibility of fragmentation of uroliths during their removal and to enhance removal of small uroliths. This technique, called "coagulum pyeleolithotomy," has been used successfully in humans.[55]
   c. Operative nephroscopy utilizing fiberoptic endoscopes inserted into the renal pelvis via a pyelotomy has been used to remove renoliths from humans.[42,131,134] Small uroliths and fragments of large ones have been successfully extracted from the renal pelvis with the aid of direct visualization through the nephroscope.
5. Nephrectomy.
   a. Nephrectomy should be considered for severe unilateral hydronephrosis, pyonephrosis, or multiple renal abscesses, provided the opposite kidney is capable of sustaining sufficient function to maintain homeostasis. It may also be considered when recurrent unilateral obstructive nephrolithiasis is unresponsive to various combinations of medical and surgical intervention.
   b. Compensatory hypertrophy of the contralateral kidney following unilateral nephrectomy is a well-documented event; however, substantial additional compensatory hypertrophy should not be anticipated in patients with a kidney that has been functionally destroyed by chronic nephrolithiasis, since it can reasonably be expected that viable nephrons have already been maximally stimulated to compensate.
6. Autotransplantation.
   a. Removal of a kidney affected with extensive nephrolith formation for "bench" surgery during in vitro perfusion with a protective cold perfusate has been reported in humans.[20,210]
   b. The technique is designed to provide excellent exposure and facilitates intraoperative radiography; however, if the patients have a UTI, postoperative complications can occur.
   c. Successful use of this procedure requires experience with the vascular surgery required to transplant the kidney to the region of the iliac fossa.[47,208]
7. Management of residual postsurgical uroliths.
   a. If fragments of uroliths remain within the renal

pelvis or if uroliths are inadvertently missed, medical therapy designed to dissolve them should be instituted following surgery.

b. If the stones are refractory to medical dissolution, the decision to perform another surgical procedure should not be made until it is recognized that the uroliths are clinically significant (i.e., clinically active). Although residual stones and stone fragments predispose to UTI and recurrence of clinical signs, this is not an invariable consequence.

E. Surgical management of ureteroliths.

1. Overview.

a. Ureteroliths originate from the renal pelves and are commonly associated with nephroliths. Because small ureteroliths may pass through the ureteral lumen and be flushed from the bladder and urethra during micturition, detection of ureteroliths is not an absolute indication for surgical intervention. Certain factors determine whether a ureterolith will pass spontaneously, including:

(1). The size and shape of the urolith.
(2). The diameter of the ureteral lumen.
(3). The state of ureteral peristalsis.
(4). The magnitude of intraluminal hydrostatic pressure proximal to the ureterolith.
(5). The magnitude of inflammation and/or muscle spasm of the ureteral wall adjacent to the urolith.

b. Immobility of a ureterolith may be inferred from detection of significant hydroureter and hydronephrosis. If proximal portions of the urinary system are not substantially dilated, immobility of the ureterolith should be confirmed by serial radiography or ultrasonography before surgery.

c. Surgery should be considered for uroliths trapped in the ureteral lumen, especially if they are associated with UTI. Surgical procedures that are commonly used for ureteroliths in dogs include ureterolithotomy, ureterectomy, and nephrectomy. Surgical procedures that may have application in selected situations include ureteroureterostomy, transureteroureterostomy, ureteroneocystotomy, vesicoureteroplasty creating a bladder flap extension, and renal autotransplantation.

2. Ureterolithotomy.[38,60,82,200,202,203]

a. Ureterolithotomy should be considered for patients that do not have irreversible functional damage to the ureter or associated kidney.

b. In patients with hydroureter, it may be possible to massage the urolith into the dilated portion of the ureter. Either a transverse or a longitudinal incision may be made into the ureteral wall, to facilitate urolith removal. The longitudinal incision may be closed with a transverse suture pattern, to minimize the danger of problems caused by postoperative stricture.

3. Ureterectomy. Ureterectomy and nephrectomy should be considered for obstructing ureteroliths that are associated with irreversible damage to the ureter and/or associated kidney, provided the contralateral kidney and ureter are capable of sustaining homeostasis.

4. Reconstructive procedures.

a. Reconstructive procedures provide an alternative for management of ureteroliths associated with irreversible damage to a portion of the adjacent ureter. For best results, most of these techniques require familiarity and experience with microsurgery.

b. Surgical techniques that may have application for repair of proximal ureteral injuries:

(1). Ureteroureterostomy (end-to-end ureteral anastomosis incorporating spatulation or Z-plasty of the transected portions of the ureter).[13,101,175]
(2). Autotransplantation into the iliac fossa.[47,208,210]
(3). Substitution of a portion of the ureter with a section of ileum (ureteroenterostomy) or prosthetic material.[87,212]

c. In addition to ureteroureterostomy, lesions of the midportion of the ureter may be managed by transureteroureterostomy (oblique end-to-side anastomosis of the proximal portion of one ureter to the contralateral one).[13,50]

d. Lesions affecting distal portions of ureters may be repaired by ureteroneocystotomy (transplantation of the shortened ureter into a new site in the bladder wall),[180] or bladder flap ureteroplasty (excision of the distal portion of the ureter and reimplantation into a bladder flap).[175]

F. Surgical removal of urocystoliths.

1. Although cystotomy to remove uroliths is not technically difficult, appropriate caution should be taken to remove all uroliths from the bladder, bladder neck, and urethra. Anatomic defects that have predisposed to urolithiasis (e.g., urachal diverticulum, patent urachus) should be corrected if possible.

2. Following cystotomy, uroliths may be removed with the aid of spoons, forceps, gauze sponges, or suction.

a. The lumen of the bladder and bladder neck should be explored with a finger to detect remaining large uroliths.

b. The lower portion of the excretory pathway should be flushed with an isotonic solution to dislodge urethroliths and to remove "subvisual" ones. Patency of the urethra may be evaluated by inserting a flexible catheter through its lumen via the urinary bladder.

Injection of an isotonic solution through the catheter may force uroliths out the distal urethral orifice.

c. If the urethral lumen has been occluded with uroliths, they may be flushed back into the bladder lumen by injecting large quantities of fluid through a catheter placed in the urethra. The external urethral orifice should be occluded around the catheter, to facilitate flushing of urethroliths back into the bladder lumen. If the distal urethral is not occluded, fluid may flow around small urethroliths without moving them into the bladder lumen. This will result in incomplete removal of uroliths.

d. If retrograde flushing techniques are used to flush urethroliths into the bladder with the aid of a catheter inserted into the distal urethral orifice, appropriate caution must be used, to minimize retrograde flushing of bacteria that normally colonize the mucosa of the distal urethra and genital tract.

3. As an alternative to cystotomy, small uroliths may be aspirated from the bladder lumen of dogs and cats by voiding urohydropropulsion, or with the aid of a urinary catheter.[122,152] In addition, urocystoliths may be retrieved from female dogs via cystoscopy.[188]

G. Surgical management of urethroliths.

1. Overview.
   a. Urethroliths originate from the urinary bladder and, thus, are commonly associated with bladder stones. They are common in male and female dogs, and also occur in male and female cats. Although uroliths commonly pass through the urethral lumen of female dogs and cats, they rarely become lodged there.
   b. Nonsurgical procedures are frequently successful in removing uroliths from the urethra and in most patients should be attempted before resorting to surgery.
   c. Although properly performed surgical techniques are very effective in removing uroliths, they may be associated with complications:[14]
      (1). Postoperative hemorrhage.
      (2). UTI.
      (3). Strictures.
      (4). Urine scald dermatitis.
      (5). Periurethral extravasation of urine. If periurethral extravasation of urine occurs because of devitalized tissue or faulty technique, it is likely to induce substantial inflammation.
   d. Inability to remove urethroliths by urohydropropulsion or other nonsurgical techniques is not a mandate for surgery. Small stones lodged in the urethra may remain asymptomatic if they do not substantially interfere with micturition; however, they always represent a potential cause of urinary outflow obstruction and UTI. Because urethroliths are not continuously exposed to urine, medical therapy is not effective in inducing dissolution.
   e. Surgery should be considered for uroliths trapped in the urethral lumen if they cause dysuria, UTI, or outflow obstruction. Complete obstruction to urine outflow combined with urosepsis should be regarded as a surgical emergency. Immediate relief of outflow obstruction in severely depressed patients may be accomplished by urine diversion utilizing cystocentesis or antepubic indwelling catheterization of the bladder lumen (tube cystostomy). Uroliths in the penile or membranous urethra may be removed by urethrotomy. Removal of stones lodged in the pelvic urethra may require a combination of cystotomy and urethrotomy. Permanent urethrostomy may be considered for patients that have uncontrollable recurrence of symptomatic urethroliths or patients with irreversible damage to the urethra (especially strictures) that interferes with micturition.
2. Prescrotal (prepubic) urethrotomy.[28,51,200,201,203]
   a. Prescrotal urethrotomy may be performed to remove canine uroliths lodged at or near the caudal end of the os penis, if necessary, with local anesthesia. However, general anesthesia facilitates relaxation of the skeletal component of the urethral musculature and minimizes the patient's discomfort.
   b. The prescrotal urethrotomy site does not need to be repaired with sutures; it will heal by granulation. By allowing the urethrotomy incision to remain open for several days following surgery, additional small uroliths that remain in the bladder are less likely to reobstruct the urethra at this site; however, suture closure of the urethral mucosa and surrounding tunica albuginea may reduce postoperative hemorrhage.[213] The urethrotomy site may be closed with 4–0 to 5–0 suture material. A urethral catheter often facilitates repair of the incision. Following closure, urine should be diverted away from the incision via tube cystostomy or an indwelling urethral catheter.
   c. A prescrotal urethrotomy may be converted to a prescrotal urethrostomy by suturing the urethral mucosa to the overlying skin. The permanent opening in the urethra should be approximately 2 cm long; however, if a permanent urethrostomy is desired, scrotal urethrostomy should be considered.
3. Perineal urethrotomy.[5,51]
   a. Perineal urethrotomy may be considered for removal of uroliths lodged between the region of the scrotum and the ischial arch. The tech-

nique is similar to that described for prescrotal urethrotomy. In this area, the urethra lies a considerable distance from the skin and is surrounded by the bulbocavernosus muscle. Identification of the urethra may be facilitated by use of a urethral catheter. The urethrotomy incision may be repaired with suture material or allowed to heal by granulation.

   b. Perineal urethrostomies are not routinely recommended in dogs because of problems associated with hygiene during micturition and urine scald dermatitis.

4. Tube cystostomy (prepubic catheterization).[53,54,176,200,203]
   a. In dogs and cats that cannot tolerate anesthesia or the surgery required to remove urethral uroliths, newly formed urine may be diverted temporarily from the urinary bladder via a Foley catheter placed into its lumen through a small celiotomy incision.
   b. Alternatively, intermittent decompressive cystocentesis may be performed. Extravasation of urine through needle tracts into the peritoneal cavity can be avoided by performing cystocentesis often enough to prevent distension of the bladder lumen with urine. Definitive surgery should be performed as soon as risks associated with anesthesia and surgery are acceptable.
5. Cystotomy and urethrostomy.
   a. A combination of cystotomy and prescrotal or perineal urethrotomy may be required to remove uroliths lodged in proximal portions of the male canine urethra.
   b. The uroliths may be dislodged by alternate catheterization and flushing through the bladder and urethrotomy site with a large volume of isotonic fluid.
6. Scrotal urethrostomy.[28,51,176,193,200,203]
   a. If a new permanent urethral opening is desired caudal to the os penis of male dogs, scrotal urethrostomy usually is the procedure of choice.
   b. Advantages of a scrotal urethrostomy over a prescrotal or perineal urethrostomy include:
      (1). The diameter of the scrotal urethra may be larger than more distal portions of the urethra.
      (2). The scrotal segment of the urethra is surrounded by less erectile tissue than more distal portions.
      (3). The scrotal urethra is more superficial than the perineal urethra.

REFERENCES

1. Abdullahi SU, Osborne CA, Leininger JR, et al. Evaluation of a calculolytic diet in female dogs with induced struvite urolithiasis. *Am J Vet Res.* 1984;45:1508.
2. Al-Kawas FH, Seelf LB, Berendson RA, et al. Allopurinol hepatotoxicity. *Ann Int Med.* 1981;95:588.
3. Alken P. Percutaneous ultrasonic destruction of renal calculi. *Urol Clin North Am.* 1982;9:145.
4. Appleman RM, Hallenbeck GA, Shorter RG. Effect of reciprocal allogenic renal transplantation between Dalmatian and non-Dalmation dogs on urinary excretion of uric acid. *Proc Soc Exp Biol Med.* 1966;121:1094.
5. Archibald J, Owen RR. Urinary system. In: Archibald J, ed. *Canine Surgery.* 2nd ed. Santa Barbara, Calif: American Vet. Publ. 1974.
6. Baillie NC, Osborne CA, Leininger JR, et al. Teratogenic effect of acetohydroxamic acid in clinically normal beagles. *Am J Vet Res.* 1986;47:2604.
7. Barbaric ZL, Gothlin JH, Davies RS. Transluminal dilatation and stent placement in obstructed ureters in dogs through use of percutaneous nephropyelostomy. *Invest Radiol.* 1977;12:534.
8. Barsanti JA, Finco DR. Feline urologic syndrome. In: Breitschwerdt EB, ed. *Contemporary Issues in Small Animal Practice—Nephrology and Urology.* Vol. 4. New York: Churchill Livingstone; 1986.
9. Bartges JW, Osborne CA, Felice LJ. Acquired canine xanthine uroliths. In: Bonagura JD, Kirk RW, eds. *Current Veterinary Therapy XI.* Philadelphia: WB Saunders; 1992;900–905.
10. Bartges JW, Osborne CA, Lulich JP, et al. Prevalence of cystine and urate uroliths in bulldogs and urate uroliths in Dalmations. *JAVMA.* 1994; 204:1914–1918.
11. Bartges JW, Osborne CA, Polzin DJ. Recurrent sterile struvite urocystolithiasis in three related cocker spaniels. *J Am Anim Hosp Assoc.* 1992;28:459–469.
12. Bartter FC, Lotz M, Thier S, et al. Cystinuria. *Ann Intern Med.* 1965;62:796.
13. Baumgartner GT, Rich RR, Albers DD. Vascular obstruction of ureter after transureteroureterostomy. *Urology.* 1977;9:266.
14. Bellah JR. Problems of the urethra. Surgical approaches. *Probl Vet Med.* 1989;1:17.
15. Berger B, Feldman EC. Primary hyperparathyroidism in dogs: 21 cases (1976–1986). *JAVMA.* 1987;191:350–356.
16. Bisaz S, Felix R, Newman WF, et al. Quantitative determination of inhibitors of calcium phosphate precipitation in whole urine. *Mineral Electrolyte Metab.* 1978;1:74.
17. Blaine G. Experimental observations on absorbable alginale products in surgery. *Ann Surg.* 1947;125:102–114.
18. Block G, Adams LG, Widmer WR, Lingeman JE. Use of extracorporeal shock-wave lithotripsy for treatment of spontaneous nephrolithiasis in dogs. *J Vet Intern Med.* 1994;8:166.
19. Boistelle R, Abbona F, Berland Y, et al. Growth and stability of magnesium ammonium phosphate in acidic sterile urine. *Urol Res.* 1984;12:79.
20. Bondevik H, Albrechtsen D, Sodal G, et al. Extracorporeal surgery and autotransplantation for complicated renal calculus disease in 108 kidneys. *Scand J Urol Nephrol.* 1990;24:301.
21. Bovee KC. Canine cystine urolithiasis. *Vet Clin North Am.* 1986;16:211.
22. Bovee KC. Urolithiasis. In: Bovee KC, ed. *Canine Nephrology.* Media, PA: Harwal; 1984:335.
23. Bovee KC. Genetic and metabolic diseases of the kidney. In: Bovee KC, ed. *Canine Nephrology.* Media, PA: Harwal; 1984:339.
24. Bovee KC, McGuire T. Qualitative and quantitative analysis of uroliths in dogs. Definitive determination of chemical type. *JAVMA.* 1984;185:983.
25. Bovee KC, Segal S. Canine cystinuria and cystine calculi. In: Proceedings of the 21st Gaines Veterinary Symposium. White Plains, NY: Gaines Dog Research Center; 1971:3–7.
26. Brodey RS. Canine urolithiasis. A survey and discussion of fifty-two clinical cases. *JAVMA.* 1955;126:1.

27. Brodey RS, Thomson R, Sayer P, Eugster B. Silicate renal calculi in Kenyan dogs. *J Small Anim. Pract.* 1977;18:523.
28. Brown SG, Greiner TP. Surgery of the urethra of the dog. In: Bojrab MJ, ed. *Current Techniques in Small Animal Surgery.* Philadelphia: Lea & Febiger; 1975.
29. Brown NO, Parks JL, Greene RW. Canine urolithiasis: Retrospective analysis of 438 cases. *JAVMA.* 1977;170:415.
30. Brown NO, Parks JL, Greene RW. Recurrence of canine urolithiasis. *JAVMA.* 1977;170:419.
31. Bulow H, Frohmuller GW. Electrohydraulic lithotripsy with aspiration of the fragments under vision. *J Urol.* 1981;126:454.
32. Cao LC, Boeve ER, de Bruijn WC, et al. A review of new concepts in renal stone research. *Scanning Microscopy.* 1993;7: 1049–1065.
33. Chaussy C, Brendel W, Schmiedt E. Extracorporeally induced destruction of kidney stones by shock waves. *Lancet.* 1980;2: 1265–1268.
34. Chaussy C, Schmiedt E. Shock wave treatment for stones in the upper urinary tract. *Urol Clin North Am.* 1983;10:743–750.
35. Chaussy C, Schmiedt E, Jocham D. Extracorporeal shock-wave lithotripsy for treatment of urolithiasis. *Urology.* 1984;23:59–66.
36. Casteneda-Zuniga WR, Miller RP, Amplatz K. Percutaneous removal of kidney stones. *Urol Clin North Am.* 1982;9:113.
37. Christie BA. Kidneys. In: Slatter DH, ed. *Textbook of Small Animal Surgery.* Vol. 2. Philadelphia: WB Saunders; 1985:1764.
38. Christie BA. Ureters. In: Slatter DH, ed. *Textbook of Small Animal Surgery.* Vol. 2. Philadelphia: WB Saunders; 1985:1777.
39. Clark WT. The distribution of urinary calculi and their recurrence following treatment. *J Small Anim Pract.* 1974;15:437.
40. Clark WT, Cuddeford D. A study of amino acids in urine from dogs with cystine urolithiasis. *Vet Rec.* 1971;88:414.
41. Clayman RV. Techniques in percutaneous removal of renal calculi: Mechanical extraction and electrohydraulic lithotripsy. *Urology.* 1984;23:11–19.
42. Clayman RV, Miller RP, Reinke DB, Lange PH. Nephroscopy: Advances and adjuncts. *Urol Clin North Am.* 1982;9:51.
43. Coe FL. Treated and untreated recurrent calcium nephrolithiasis in patients with idiopathic hypercalciuria, hyperuricosuria, or no metabolic disorders. *Ann Intern Med.* 1977;87:404.
44. Coe FL. *Nephrolithiasis, Pathogenesis and Treatment.* Chicago: Year Book; 1978.
45. Coe FL, Flavus MJ. Nephrolithiasis. In: Brenner BM, Rector FC, eds. *The Kidney.* 4th ed. Vol 12. Philadelphia: WB Saunders, 1991:1728–1767.
46. Cohn R, Dibbel DG, Laub DR, et al. Renal allotransplantation and allantoin excretion of Dalmatians. *Arch Surg.* 1965;91:911.
47. Collins DL, Christensen RM. Kidney transplantation in the dog: Surgical technique. *Can J Surg.* 1966;9:308.
48. Cornelius CE, Bishop JA, Schaffer MH. A quantitative study of amino aciduria in dachshunds with a history of cystine urolithiasis. *Cornell Vet.* 1967;57:177.
49. Crane CW, Turner AW. Amino acid patterns of urine and blood plasma in a cystinuric Labrador dog. *Nature.* 1956;177:237.
50. Crane SW, Waldron DR. Ureteral function and healing following microsurgical transureteroureterostomy in the dog. *Vet Surg.* 1980;9:108.
51. Dean PW, Hedlund CS, Lewis DD, Bojrab MJ. Canine urethrotomy and urethrostomy. *Compend Contin Ed.* 1990;12:1541.
52. Defronzo RA, Their SO. Inherited disorders of renal function. In: Brenner BM, Rector FC Jr, eds. *The Kidney.* Philadelphia: WB Saunders, 1981:1816–1871.
53. Dhein CR, Person MW. Prepubic (suprapubic) catheterization of eight dogs with lower urinary tract disorders. *J Am Anim Hosp Assoc.* 1989;25:272.
54. Dhein CR, Person MW, Leathers CW, Gavin PR. Prepubic (suprapubic) catheterization of the dog. *J Am Anim Hosp. Assoc.* 1989;25:261.
55. Demler JW, Dennis MA, Finlayson B. Bilateral nephrolithiasis: Simultaneous operative management. *J Urol.* 1983;129:263.
56. Donner GS, Ellison GW, Ackerman N, Senior DF, Campbell G. Percutaneous nephrolithotomy in the dog. An experimental study. *Vet Surg.* 1987;16:411.
57. Dretler SP, Pfister RC. Percutaneous dissolution of renal calculi. *Annu Rev Med.* 1983;34:359–366.
58. Duncan H, Wakin KG, Ward LE. The effects of intravenous administration of uric acid in its concentration in plasma and urine of Dalmation and non-Dalmatian dogs. *J Lab Clin Med.* 1961;58:876.
59. Duncan H, Curtiss AS. Observations on uric acid transport in man, the Dalmatian, and the non-Dalmation dog. *Henry Ford Hosp Med J.* 1971;19:105.
60. Dupre GP, Dee LG, Dee JF. Ureterotomies for treatment of ureterolithiasis in two dogs. *J Am Anim Hosp Assoc.* 1990; 26:500.
61. Egger EL, Rigg DL. Treatment of silica urethral obstruction in a dog by retrograde urohydropropulsion. *Compend Contin Ed Pract Vet.* 1983;5:147–150.
62. Elliot JS. Solubility and crystallization in urinary stone disease. In : Hodgkinson A, Nordin BEC, eds. *Proceedings of the Renal Stone Research Symposium.* London: J & A Churchill, 1968:199–207.
63. Elliot JS. Urinary calculus disease. *Surg Clin North Am.* 1965;45: 1393–1404.
64. Elliott JS. Calcium phosphate solubility in urine. *J Urol.* 1957; 77:269.
65. Feeney DA, Osborne CA, Johnston GR. Vesicoureteral reflux induced by manual compression of the urinary bladder. *J Am Vet Med Assoc.* 1983;182:795.
66. Feldman BM, Kennedy BM, Schlstraeta M. Dietary minerals and feline urologic syndrome. *Feline Pract.* 1977;7:39.
67. Felice LJ, Dombrovskis D, Lafond E, et al. Determination of uric acid in canine serum and urine by high performance liquid chromatography. *Vet Clin Pathol.* 1990;19:86.
68. Finlayson B. Renal lithiasis in review. *Urol Clin North Am.* 1974;1:1818.
69. Finlayson B. Calcium stones: Some physical and chemical aspects. In: David DS, ed. *Calcium Metabolism in Renal Failure and Nephrolithiasis.* New York: John Wiley & Sons; 1977.
70. Finlayson R, Thomas WC. Extracorporeal shock-wave lithotripsy. *Ann Intern Med.* 1984;101:387–389.
71. Fischer CP, Sonda LP. Cryoprecipitate: Its use and effects in canine coagulum pyelolithotomy. *Invest Urol.* 1979;16:266.
72. Fischer CP, Sonda LP, Diokno AC. Further experience with cryoprecipitate coagulum in renal calculus surgery: A review of 60 cases. *J Urol.* 1981;126:432.
73. Fleisch H. Inhibitors and promoters of stone formation. *Kidney Int.* 1978;13:361–371.
74. Fleisch H, Russel RGG. Experimental and clinical studies with pyrophosphate and diphosphonates. In: David DS, ed. *Calcium Metabolism in Renal Failure and Nephrolithiasis.* New York: John Wiley & Sons; 1977.
75. Foreman JW. Renal handling of urate and other organic acids. In: Bovee KC, ed. *Canine Nephrology.* Media, PA: Harwal; 1984;144.
76. Friedman M, Byers SO. Observations concerning the causes of excess excretion of uric acid in the Dalmatian dog. *J Biol Chem.* 1948;175:727.
77. Frimpter GW, Thouin P, Ewalds BH. Penicillamine in canine cystinuria. *J Am Vet Med Assoc.* 1967;151:1084.

78. Gahring DR, Crowe DT, Powers TE, et al. Comparative renal function studies of nephrotomy closure with and without sutures in dogs. *JAVMA.* 1977;171:537.
79. Garcia del Pena E, Cifuentes Dellatte L. Forms of ammonium urate presentation in urinary calculi of non-infectious and infectious origin. In: Smith LH, ed. *Urolithiasis: Clinical and Basic Research.* New York: Plenum Press; 1981:935.
80. Gillenwater JY. Clinical aspects of urinary tract obstruction. *Semin Nephrol.* 1982;2:46–54.
81. Goldfarb S. Dietary factors in the pathogenesis and prophylaxis of calcium nephrolithiasis. *Kidney Int.* 1988;34:544.
82. Gourley IMG. Nephrectomy and nephrolithotomy. *Vet Clin N Amer.* 1975;5:401.
83. Gourley IMG, Leighton RL, Swanwick PM. Surgical procedures for nephrotomy and ureterotomy in the dog. *Pract Vet.* 1971; 43:11.
84. Grainger R, Webb DR, Alken P, et al. The sapphire crystal infrared photocoagulator and polyglactin (vicryl) mesh: Two alternatives to the suturing of radial nephrotomies. *Br J Urol.* 1986;58:484.
85. Greenwood KM, Rawlings CA. Removal of canine renal calculi by pyelolithotomy. *Vet Surg.* 1981;10:12.
86. Gregory JG, Park KY, Burns TC. Effect of alkalinizing agents on calcium oxalate stone formation in a rat model. *Urol Res.* 1984;12:48.
87. Griffith DP, Moseleu WG, Beach PD. Experimental studies in ureteral substitution. *Invest Urol.* 1973;11:239.
88. Groen J. An experimental syndrome of fatty liver, uric acid kidney stones, and acute pancreatic necrosis produced in dogs by exclusive feeding of bacon. *Science.* 1948;107:425.
89. Gutierrez Millet V, Praga M, Miranda B, et al. Ureolytic *Citrobacter freundii* infection of the urine as a cause of dissolution of cystine renal calculi. *J Urol.* 1985;133:443.
90. Hallson PC, Rose GA. Uromucoids and urinary stone formation. *Lancet.* 1979;1:1000.
91. Hande K, Reed E, Chabner B. Allopurinol kinetics. *Clin Pharmacol Ther.* 1978;23:598.
92. Hansen NM, Felix R, Bisaz S, et al. Aggregation of hydroapatite crystals. *Biochem Biophys Acta.* 1976;451:549.
93. Hardy RM, Klausner JS. Urate calculi associated with portal vascular anomalies. In: Kirk RW, ed. *Current Veterinary Therapy.* 8th ed. Philadelphia: WB Saunders; 1983;1073.
94. Hardy RM, Osborne CA, Cassidy FC, et al. Urolithiasis in immature dogs. *Vet Med Small Anim Clin.* 1972;67:1205.
95. Hess B, Nakagawa Y, Parks JH, et al. Molecular abnormality of Tamm-Horsfall glycoprotein in calcium oxalate nephrolithiasis. *Am J Physiol.* 1991;260:F569–F578.
96. Hoppe A, Denneberg T, Kagedal B. Treatment of normal and cystinuric dogs with 2-mercaptopropionylglycine. *Am J Vet Res.* 1988;49:923.
97. Ilkiw JE. Other potentially useful new injectable agents. *Vet Clin North Am Small Anim Pract.* 1992;22:281.
98. Jaeger P, Portman L, Saunders A, et al. Anticystinuric effects of glutamine and of dietary sodium restriction. *N Engl J Med.* 1986;315:1120.
99. Johnston GR, Jessen CR, Osborne CA. Retrograde contrast urethrography. In: Kirk RW, ed. Current Veterinary Therapy. 6th ed. Philadelphia: WB Saunders; 1977:1189.
100. Johnston GR, Walter PA, Feeney DA. Radiographic and ultrasonographic features of uroliths and urinary tract filling defects. *Vet Clin North Am.* 1986;16:261.
101. Jonas D, Kramer W, Weber W. Splintless microsurgical anastomosis of the ureter in the dog. *Urol Res.* 1981;9:271.
102. Kerr WS, Jr. Effect of complete ureteral obstruction for one week on kidney function. *J Appl Physiol.* 1954;6:762–772.
103. Kerr WS Jr. Effects of complete ureteral obstruction in dogs on kidney function. *Am J Physiol.* 1956;184:521–526.
104. Kirby R, Crane S, Schaer M. Dissolution of a nephrolith in a dog. *JAVMA.* 1983;178:827.
104a. Klausner JS, O'Leary TP, Osborne CA. Calcium urolithiasis in two dogs with parathyroid adenomas. *JAVMA.* 1987;191:1423.
105. Klausner JS, Osborne CA. Dissolution of a struvite nephrolith in a dog. *JAVMA.* 1979;174:1100.
106. Klausner JS, Osborne CA. Canine calcium phosphate uroliths. *Vet Clin North Amer.* 1986;16:171.
107. Klausner JS, Osborne CA, O'Leary TP, et al. Experimental induction of struvite uroliths in miniature schnauzer and beagle dogs. *Invest Urol.* 1980;18:127.
108. Klausner JS, Osborne CA, O'Leary TP, et al. Struvite urolithiasis in a litter of miniature schnauzer dogs. *Am J Vet Res.* 1980;40: 712.
109. Konnak JW, et al. Renal calculi associated with incomplete renal tubular acidosis. *J Urol.* 1982;128:900–902.
110. Krawiec DR, Osborne CA, Leininger JR, Griffith DP. Effect of acetohydroxamic acid on dissolution of canine uroliths. *Am J Vet Res.* 1984;45:1266.
111. Krawiec DR, Osborne CA, Leininger JR, Griffith DP. Effect of acetohydroxamic acid on prevention of canine struvite uroliths. *Am J Vet Res.* 1984;45:1276.
112. Kruger JM, Osborne CA. Etiopathogenesis of uric acid and ammonium urate uroliths in nonDalmatian dogs. *Vet Clin North Am.* 1986;16:87.
113. Kuster G, et al. Uric acid metabolism in Dalmatians and other dogs. *Arch Intern Med.* 1972;129:492.
114. Lamm DL, et al. Medical therapy of experimental infection stones. *Urology.* 1977;10:418.
115. Leadbetter GW. Diagnostic urologic instrumentation. In: *Campbell's Urology.* 4th ed. Vol. 1. Philadelphia: WB Saunders; 1978.
116. Lees GE, Osborne CA. Use and misuse of intermittent and indwelling urinary catheters. In: Kirk RW, ed. *Current Veterinary Therapy.* Vol. 8. Philadelphia: WB Saunders; 1983:1097–1100.
117. Ling GV. Unpublished data. Department of Medicine, School of Veterinary Medicine, University of California, 1987.
118. Ling GV, Ackerman N, Lowenstone LJ, Cowgill LD. Percutaneous nephropyelocentesis and nephropyelostomy in the dog. A description of the technique. *Am J Vet Res.* 1979;40:1605.
119. Ling GV, Franti CE, Ruby AL, Johnson DL. Epizootiologic evaluation and quantitative analysis of urinary calculi from 150 cats. *JAVMA.* 1990;196:1459.
120. Ling GV, Ruby AL. Canine uroliths: Analysis of data derived from 813 specimens. *Vet Clin North Am.* 1986;16:303.
121. Lotz M, Potts JT Jr, Bartter FC, et al. D-Penicillamine therapy in cystinuria. *J Urol.* 1966;95:257.
122. Lulich JP, Osborne CA. Catheter assisted retrieval of canine and feline urocystoliths. *JAVMA.* 1992;201:111–113.
123. Lulich JP, Osborne CA, Carlson M, et al. Nosurgical removal of uroliths in dogs and cats by voiding urohydropropulsion. *JAVMA.* 1993;203:660–663.
124. Lulich JP, Osborne CA, Nagode LA, et al. Evaluation of urine and serum analytes in miniature schnauzers with calcium oxalate urolithiasis. *Am J Vet Res.* (accepted for publication).
125. Lulich JP, Osborne CA, Parker ML, et al. Urine chemistry values in nonfasted and fasted normal beagle dogs. *Am J Vet Res.* (accepted for publication).
126. Lulich JP, Osborne CA, Polzin DJ, et al. Incomplete removal of canine and feline urocystoliths by cystotomy. (Abstract) *J Vet Intl Med.* 1993;7:124.
127. Malek RS, Boyce WH. Observation on the ultrastructure and genesis of urinary calculi. *J Urol.* 1977;117:336.

128. Marberger M. Disintegration of renal and ureteral calculi with ultrasound. *Urol Clin North Am.* 1983;10:729–742.

129. Marretta SM, Park AJ, Greene RW, et al. Urinary calculi associated with portosystemic shunts in six dogs. *JAVMA.* 1981;178:133.

130. McCullagh KG, Ehrhart LA. Silica urolithiasis in laboratory dogs fed semisynthetic diets. *JAVMA.* 1974;164:712.

131. McAninch JW, Fay R. Flexible nephroscope in calculous surgery. *J Urol.* 1977;128:5.

132. Medline A, Cohen LB, Tobe BA, et al. Liver granulomas and allopurinol. *Br Med J.* 1978;1:1320.

133. Meyer JL, Angino EE. The role of trace elements in calcium lithiasis. *Invest Urol.* 1977;14:347.

134. Miki M, Inaba Y, Machida T. Operative nephroscopy with fiberoptic scope: Preliminary report. *J Urol.* 1978;119:166.

135. Miller RP, Reinke DB, Clayman RV, Lange PH. Percutaneous approach to the ureter. *Urol Clin North Am.* 1982;9:31.

136. Mitty HA, Gribetz ME. The status of interventional uroradiography. *J Urol.* 1982;127:2.

137. Nakagawa Y, Abram V, Hall SL, et al. Isolation from human calcium oxalate renal stones of nephrocalcin, a glycoprotein inhibitor of calcium oxalate growth. *J Clin Invest.* 1987;79:1782–1787.

137a. Nakagawa Y, Abram V, Kezdy FJ, et al. Purification and characterization of the principal inhibitor of calcium oxalate monohydrate crystal growth in human urine. *J Bio Chem.* 1983;258.

138. Nikkila MT, et al. Clinical and biochemical features of primary hyperparathyroidism *Surgery.* 1989;105:148–153.

139. Osborne CA. Unpublished data. College of Veterinary Medicine. University of Minnesota, St. Paul, 1987.

140. Osborne CA. Bacterial infections of the canine and feline urinary tract: cause, cure and control. In: Bojrab MJ, ed. *Disease Mechanisms in Small Animal Surgery.* 2nd ed. Philadelphia: Lea & Febiger; 1993:458.

141. Osborne CA, Abdullahi S, Klausner JS, et al. Nonsurgical removal of uroliths from the urethra of female dogs. *JAVMA.* 1983;182:47–50.

142. Osborne CA, Clinton CW. Urolithiasis: Terms and concepts. *Vet Clin North Am.* 1986;16:3.

143. Osborne CA, Clinton CW, Bamman LK, et al. Prevalence of canine uroliths: Minnesota Urolith Center. *Vet Clin North Am.* 1986;16:27.

144. Osborne CA, Clinton CW, Kim KM, et al. Etiopathogenesis, clinical manifestations and management of canine silica urolithiasis. *Vet Clin North Am.* 1986;16:185.

145. Osborne CA, Davis LS, Sanna J, et al. Identification and interpretation of crystalluria in domestic animals. A light- and scanning electron microscopic study. *Vet Med.* 1990;85:18.

146. Osborne CA, Hoppe A, O'Brien TD. Medical dissolution and prevention of cystine urolithiasis. In: Kirk RW, Bonagura JD, eds. *Current Veterinary Therapy.* Vol. 10. Philadelphia: WB Saunders, 1989:1189.

147. Osborne CA, Johnston GR, Polzin DJ, et al. Redefinition of the feline urologic syndrome: Feline lower urinary tract disease with heterogeneous causes. *Vet Clin North Am.* 1984;14:409.

148. Osborne CA, Klausner JS, Clinton CW. Analysis of canine and feline uroliths. In: Kirk RW, ed. Current Veterinary Therapy. 8th ed. Philadelphia: WB Saunders; 1983:1061.

149. Osborne CA, Klausner JS, Lulich JP. Canine and feline calcium phosphate urolithiasis. In: Bonagura JD, ed. *Current Veterinary Therapy.* Vol. 12. Philadelphia: WB Saunders; (in press).

150. Osborne CA, Kruger JM, Johnston GR, Polzin DJ. Dissolution of canine ammonium urate uroliths. *Vet Clin North Am.* 1986;16:375.

151. Osborne CA, Lulich JP, Bartges JW, Felice LJ. Medical dissolution and prevention of canine and feline uroliths: Diagnostic and therapeutic caveats. *Vet Record.* 1990;127:369.

152. Osborne CA, Lulich JP, Unger LK. Nonsurgical retrieval of uroliths for mineral analysis. In: Bonagura JD, Kirk RW, eds. *Current Veterinary Therapy.* Vol. 11. Philadelphia: WB Saunders; 1992:886.

153. Osborne CA, Poffenbarger EM, Klausner JS, et al. Etiopathogenesis, clinical management of canine calcium oxalate urolithiasis. *Vet Clin North Am.* 1986;16:133.

154. Osborne CA, Polzin DJ. Nonsurgical management of canine obstructive urolithopathy. *Vet Clin North Am.* 1986;16:333.

155. Osborne CA, Polzin DJ, Abdullahi SU, et al. Struvite urolithiasis in animals and man: Formation, detection and dissolution. *Adv Vet Sci Comp Med.* 1985;29:1.

156. Osborne CA, Polzin DJ, Feeney DA, Caywood, DD. The urinary system: Pathophysiology, diagnosis, and treatment. In: Gourley IM, Vasseur PB, eds. *General Small Animal Surgery.* Philadelphia: JB Lippincott; 1985:479.

157. Osborne CA, Polzin DJ, Johnston GR, O'Brien TD. Canine urolithiasis. In: Ettinger SJ, ed. *Textbook of Veterinary Internal Medicine.* 3rd ed. Vol. 2. Philadelphia: WB Saunders; 1989:2083.

158. Osborne CA, Polzin DJ, Johnston GR, et al. Medical management of canine uroliths with special emphasis on dietary modification. *Companion Anim Pract.* 1987;1:72.

159. Osborne CA, Polzin DJ, Kruger JM, et al. Medical dissolution of canine struvite uroliths. *Vet Clin North Am.* 1986;16:349.

160. Osborne CA, Polzin DJ, Lulich JP, et al. Relationship of nutritional factors to the cause, dissolution, and prevention of canine uroliths. *Vet Clin North Am Small Anim. Pract.* 1989;19:583.

161. Osborne CA, O'Brien TD, Ghobrial HK, et al. Crystalluria. Observations, interpretations and misinterpretations. *Vet Clin North Am.* 1986;16:45.

162. Osborne CA, Polzin DJ, Kruger JM, Abdullahi S. Medical dissolution and prevention of canine struvite uroliths. In: Kirk RW, ed. *Current Veterinary Therapy.* 9th ed. Philadelphia: WB Saunders; 1986:1177.

163. O'Sullivan WJ. Metabolic side-effects of allopurinol. *Progr Biochem Pharmacol.* 1974;9:174.

164. Pahira JJ. Management of the patient with cystinuria. *Urol Clin North Am.* 1987;14:339.

165. Pak CYC. *Calcium Urolithiasis. Pathogenesis, Diagnosis and Management.* New York: Plenum; 1978:25.

166. Pak CYC. Primary hyperparathyroidism and other causes of hypercalciuria. In: Pak CYC, ed. *Calcium Urolithiasis: Pathogenesis, Diagnosis and Management.* New York: Plenum; 1978:81–117.

167. Pak CYC. *Calcium Urolithiasis: Pathogenesis, Diagnosis and Management.* New York: Plenum; 1978.

168. Pak CYC, et al. Spontaneous precipitation of brushite in urine: Evidence that brushite is the nidus of renal stones originating as calcium phosphate. *Proc Natl Acad Sci USA.* 1971;68:1456–1460.

169. Pak CYC, Fuller C, Sakhaee K, et al. Management of cystine nephrolithiasis with alpha mercaptopropionyl glycine. *J Urol.* 1986;136:1003.

170. Pak CYC, Tolentino R, Stewart A, et al. Enhancement of renal excretion of uric acid during long-term thiazide therapy. *Invest Urol.* 1978;16:191.

171. Polzin DJ, Osborne CA, Hayden DW, Stevens JB. Effects of modified protein diets in dogs with chronic renal failure. *JAVMA.* 1983;183:980.

172. Purohit GS, Pham D, Raney AM, Bogaev JH. Electrohydraulic ureterolithotripsy: An experimental study. *Invest Urol.* 1980;17:462.

173. Pyrah LN. *Renal Calculus.* New York: Springer-Verlag; 1979.
174. Raney AM, Handler JH. Electrohydraulic nephrolithotripsy. *Urology.* 1975;6:439.
175. Rawlings CA. Repair of the traumatized ureter. In: Bojrab MJ, ed. *Current Techniques in Small Animal Surgery.* 2nd ed. Philadelphia: Lea & Febiger; 1983.
176. Rawlings CA, Wingfield WE. Urethral reconstruction in dogs and cats. *J Am Anim Hosp Assoc.* 1976;12:850.
177. Rich LJ, Dysart I, Chow FC, Hamar DW. Urethral obstruction in cats: Experimental production by addition of a magnesium and phosphate to diet. *Feline Pract.* 1974;4:44.
178. Roberts SR, Resnick MI. Urinary stone matrix. In: Wickham JEA, Buck AC, eds. *Renal Tract Stone: Metabolic Basis and Clinical Practice.* New York: Churchill Livingstone; 1990:59.
179. Robertson WG, Parcock M, Nordin BEC. Calcium oxalate crystalluria and urine saturation in recurrent renal stone formers. *Clin Sci.* 1971;40:365.
180. Robins GM, Presnell KR. Ureteroneocystotomy in the dog. *J Small Anim Pract.* 1974;15:185.
181. Rose AG, et al. Tamm-Horsfall mucoproteins promote calcium oxalate crystal formation in urine. *J Urol.* 1982;127:177.
182. Roth RA. Current surgical management of branched renal calculi. *Surg Clin North Am.* 1976;56:753.
183. Rothuizen J, Van Den Ingh TSGAM, Voorhoot G, et al. Congenital porto-systemic shunts in sixteen dogs and three cats. *J Small Anim Pract.* 1982;23:67.
184. Ruby AL, Ling GV. Bacterial culture of uroliths: Techniques and interpretation of results. *Vet Clin North Am.* 1986;16:325.
185. Schaible RH. Genetic predisposition to purine uroliths in Dalmatian dogs. *Vet Clin North Am.* 1986;16:127.
186. Scott R. The role of trace elements in renal stone disease. In: Wickham JEA, Buck AC, eds. *Renal Tract Stone: Metabolic Basis and Clinical Practice.* New York: Churchill Livingstone; 1990:103.
187. Segal S, Thier SO. Cystinuria. In: Stanbury JB, Wyngaarden JB, eds. *The Metabolic Basis of Inherited Disease.* 5th ed. New York: McGraw-Hill; 1983:1774.
188. Senior DF. Electrohydraulic shock-wave lithotripsy in experimental struvite bladder stone disease. *Vet Surg.* 1984;13:143.
189. Sheldon CA, Smith AD. Chemolysis of calculi. *Urol Clin North Am.* 1982;9:121.
190. Simpson DP. Citrate excretion: A window on renal metabolism. *Am J Physiol.* 1983;244:F223.
191. Smith AD. Symposium on endourology. *Urol Clin North Am.* 1982;9:15.
192. Smith AD, Lee WJ. Percutaneous stone removal procedures including irrigation. *Urol Clin North Am.* 1983;10:719–727.
193. Smith CW. Surgical diseases of the urethra. In: Slatter DH, ed. *Textbook of Small Animal Surgery.* Vol. 2. Philadelphia: WB Saunders; 1985:1799.
194. Smith LH. Medical evaluation of urolithiasis. Etiologic aspects and diagnostic evaluation. *Urol Clin North Am.* 1974;1:241.
195. Smith LH. Urolithiasis. In: Earley LE, Gottschalk CW, eds. *Strauss and Welt's Diseases of the Kidney.* 3rd ed. Boston: Little, Brown; 1979:893–903.
196. Smith LH. The pathophysiology and medical treatment of urolithiasis. *Semin Nephrol.* 1990;10:31.
197. Smith MJ, Boyce WH. Anatrophic nephrotomy and plastic calyrhaphy. *J Urol.* 1968;99:521.
198. Spector AR, Gray A, Prien EL. Kidney stone matrix. Differences in acidic protein consumption. *Invest Urol.* 1976;13:387.
199. Stables DP. Percutaneous nephrostomy: Techniques, indications, and results. *Urol Clin North Am.* 1982;9:15.
200. Stone EA. Surgical management of urolithiasis. *Comp Contin Ed.* 1981;3:627.
201. Stone EA. Nephrolithotomy. In: Bojrab MJ, ed. *Current Techniques in Small Animal Surgery.* 2nd ed. Philadelphia: Lea & Febiger; 1983.
202. Stone EA. Surgical therapy for urolithiasis. *Vet Clin North Am.* 1984;14:77.
203. Stone EA, Barsanti SA. *Urologic Surgery of the Dog and Cat.* Philadelphia: Lea & Febiger; 1992.
204. Sutor DJ, Percival JM, Doonan S. Isolation and identification of some urinary inhibitors of calcium phosphate formation. *Clin Chem Acta.* 1978;89:273.
205. Svenson SB, Hultberg H, Kallenius G, et al. P-fimbriae of pyelonephritogenic *Escherichia coli. Eur J Clin Study Treat Infect.* 1983;11:61.
206. Tannen RL. Ammonia and acid-base homeostasis. *Med Clin North Am.* 1983;67:781.
207. Tessler AN, Kossow J. Electrohydraulic stone disintegration. *Urology.* 1975;5:470.
208. Thompson AE. Comparative aspects of renal transplantation in man and dog. *J Small Anim Pract.* 1971;12:575.
209. Treacher RJ. Urolithiasis in the dog. II. Biochemical aspects. *J Small Anim Pract.* 1966;7:537.
210. Turini D, Nicita G, Fiorelli C, et al. Staghorn renal stones: Value of bench surgery and autotransplantation. *J Urol.* 1977;118:905.
211. Ungar H, Ungar R. Further studies on the pathogenesis of urate calculi in the urinary tract of white rats. *Am J Pathol.* 1952;28:291.
212. Varady S, Friedman E, Yap WT, et al. Ureteral replacement with a new synthetic material: Gore-Tex. *J Urol.* 1982;128:171.
213. Waldron DR, Hedlund CS, Tangner CH, et al. The canine urethra: A comparison of first and second intention healing. *Vet Surg.* 1985;14:213.
214. Wickham JEA. The matrix of renal calculi. In: Williams DI, et al. *Scientific Foundations of Urology.* Vol. 1. Chicago: Year Book; 1976:323.
215. Williams HE. Nephrolithiasis. *N Engl J Med.* 1975;290:33.
216. Williams HE, Smith LH. Primary hyperoxaluria. In: Stanbury JB, Wyngaarden JB, Fredickson DS, et al., eds. *The Metabolic Basis of Inherited Disease.* 5th ed. New York: McGraw-Hill; 1983:204.
217. Zinn KR, Glascock MD, Schmidt DA. Instrumental neutron-activation analysis of canine urinary calculi. *Am J Vet Res.* 1986;47:2536.
218. Zyloprim Product Insert. Burroughs Wellcome Co., North Carolina, November 1981.

CHAPTER 42

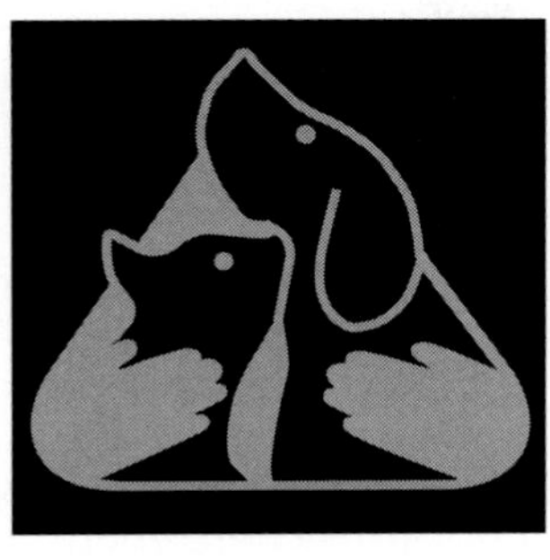

Obstructive Uropathy and Hydronephrosis

DELMAR R. FINCO

I. INTRODUCTION

A. Definitions[6].

1. Obstructive uropathy refers to abnormalities in structure or function of the urinary tract caused by impairment of normal flow of urine.
   a. Structural changes may impede urine outflow by blocking the lumen of the urinary outflow tract.
   b. Functional obstruction may occur without blockage. Urine is moved from the pelves to the bladder via rhythmic ureteral contractions initiated by a pacemaker in the pelves. A flaw in this system or in detrusor action can render propulsion of urine through the outflow tract ineffective. Ureteral dilation by this mechanism probably occurs with bacterial pyelitis or ectopic ureters.
2. Obstructive nephropathy refers to the renal damage caused by obstruction.
3. Hydronephrosis refers to dilatation of the pelvis of the kidney from obstructed urine outflow.

B. Significance.

1. Specific data on incidence of obstructive uropathy are not available for dogs and cats, but cases are relatively commonly observed.
2. Clinical consequences of obstruction may be broadly categorized as obstruction leading to acute uremia or obstruction without uremia.
   a. Complete obstruction caused by bladder or urethral outflow obstruction affects both kidneys and causes acute uremia within a few days after obstruction. Early detection and removal of the obstruction results in prompt disappearance of signs of uremia, although renal abnormalities may persist much longer. (See section II of this Chapter.) Urethral obstruction also may lead to bladder detrusor muscle dysfunction. (See Chapter 11, Diagnostic Imaging of the Urinary Tract, and Chapter 38, Urethral Diseases of Dogs and Cats.)
   b. Gradual or partial unilateral ureteral obstruction may result in insidious dilatation of the renal pelvis and destruction of renal parenchyma, while the patient remains nonazotemic so long as the contralateral kidney functions normally.
   c. Either unilateral or bilateral obstruction may be partial, and the degree of obstruction may change with time (e.g., growth of bladder trigone squamous cell carcinoma).

C. Causes of obstructive nephropathy and hydronephrosis in dogs and cats.

1. Most causes are lower tract disease.
2. A compilation by cause is given in Table 42–1.

II. PATHOPHYSIOLOGY OF OBSTRUCTIVE UROPATHY.

A. Introduction.

1. Several factors can influence the effects of obstructive uropathy.
   a. Species affected.

TABLE 42–1.
CAUSES OF OBSTRUCTIVE UROPATHY IN DOGS AND CATS

Urethra and bladder diseases
- Urethral uroliths (dogs and cats)
- Urethral mucus and/or crystals (cats, rarely dogs)
- Detrusor malfunction
  - Sequela to urethral obstruction
  - Traumatic or atraumatic neurologic disease
- Neoplasia
  - Bladder trigone transitional cell carcinoma
  - Prostatic neoplasms
  - Urethral neoplasms
- Blood clots
  - Trauma
  - Infection
  - Clotting defects
- Trauma
  - Blood clots
  - Soft tissue swelling
  - Fracture of the pelvis or os penis
- Dislocation of bladder (perineal, inguinal hernia)
- Urethral foreign body
- Urethral valves(?)

Ureteral and kidney diseases
- Ureteral or pelvic uroliths
- Trauma, inflammation
  - Soft tissue swelling
  - Outflow tract rupture
  - Blood clots
- Blood clots
  - Trauma
  - Clotting defects
- Ectopic ureters
- Surgical sequela
  - Ureteral neocystostomy
  - Urinary diversion
- Dioctophyma renale
- Invasive neoplasia
- Profuse polyuria (i.e., diabetes insipidus)*
- Papillary necrosis
- Congenital(?)
- Ureteral valve, polyp, stricture(?)

*Mild, reversible hydroureter

(1). Dogs, rats, rabbits, and cats have been used for most studies on pathophysiology of urinary tract obstruction.[6–8]

(2). Some differences in response between species have been noted.

b. Degree of obstruction. Most studies on pathophysiology have been done with total obstruction. Pathophysiology of partial obstruction is not as well understood.

c. Site of obstruction. Most studies on pathophysiology have been done with ureteral obstruction. Lower tract obstruction should have the same renal effects once bladder filling is maximal.

d. Duration of obstruction. Progressive damage to the upper and lower urinary tract occurs with time.

e. Urine flow rate. With polyuria, more urine traverses the tubular and outflow system per unit of time. Rapid flow rate accentuates the outflow problem at all levels between the glomerular filter and the site of the obstruction.

B. Effects of obstruction on renal blood flow (RBF) and glomerular filtration rate (GFR) of dogs.

1. Factors determining GFR (see Chapter 2, Applied Physiology of the Kidney) indicate that an increase in pressure in Bowman's space opposes glomerular filtration. With obstruction, there is potential for pressure buildup proximal to the site of obstruction, which opposes the hydraulic pressure causing filtration.
2. While these intratubular pressure effects exist, studies have demonstrated that renal changes occurring with obstruction are far more complex, involving vasoactive substances that affect glomerular afferent and efferent arteriolar resistance. Adding to the complexity is the finding that differences in pathophysiology exist between unilateral and bilateral obstruction.
3. Total, abrupt ureteral obstruction in dogs.
   a. In a normal dog, intraluminal ureteral pressure is about 7 mm Hg at rest and about 17 mm Hg during peristalsis.[12,14]
   b. Within 1 hour of obstruction, intraureteral pressure increases to about 50 mm Hg and peristalsis ceases, resulting in all pressure being transmitted to Bowman's space.
   c. With bilateral obstruction, the increase in pressure persists beyond 24 hours, but with unilateral obstruction, intraureteral pressure is normal at 24 hours.[13]
   d. Immediately after ureteral obstruction, there is a period of a few hours during which RBF increases owing to decreased afferent arteriolar resistance that is mediated by release of vasodilatory prostaglandins.[1]
   e. During this hyperemic phase, GFR is decreased, but only to 80% of normal because afferent arteriolar dilatation increases intraglomerular pressure to counter the increased Bowman's space pressure.[6]
   f. After 24 hours, GFR decreases further, despite a decrease in Bowman's space pressure. The decrease is caused by two major vasoconstrictors, thromboxane and angiotensin II, and possibly by a decrease in endothelium-derived relaxing factor (EDRF).[6–8]
      (1). Thromboxane is produced by infiltrating cells (blood monocytes and T-lymphocytes) and possibly by mesangial cells.[8] Thromboxane causes constriction of afferent arterioles.

(2). Although angiotensin II causes efferent arteriole constriction, which should increase GFR, blockade of angiotensin II increases GFR. The mechanism whereby these angiotensin II effects occur during obstruction may be a decrease in GFR via mesangial cell contraction and a decrease in the ultrafiltration coefficient.

g. In limited studies, total obstruction of 1 ureter resulted in GFR values of 43% of normal at 24 hours,[18] 17% of normal at 1 week, 14% of normal at 2 weeks, and 3% of normal at 4 weeks.[17]

h. Some glomerular filtration persists during total obstruction because filtrate that is formed is totally reabsorbed by renal tubules.

C. Recovery of GFR in dogs following relief of unilateral ureteral obstruction.

1. As anticipated, longer periods of obstruction are more harmful to the kidneys, so recovery of GFR following relief of obstruction decreases as duration of obstruction increases.
2. With complete ureteral obstruction and a normal contralateral kidney, recovery of GFR was 100% with obstruction of 1 week, 70% with 2 weeks, 30% with 4 weeks, and 0% when obstruction lasted 6 or 7 weeks. Time for recovery of maximum function was 26 weeks.[5]
3. Relief of complete ureteral obstruction followed later by contralateral nephrectomy reduced the interval to restoration of maximum GFR.[5]
4. In dogs, partial ureteral occlusion for 14 to 60 days resulted in 100% recovery of GFR with 14 days occlusion, 31% with 28 days, and 8% with 60 days. This recovery may not have been maximal, because it was measured 28 days after relief of obstruction.[10]
5. Studies in dogs indicated that hippuran-131 scans performed before release of obstruction reliably predicted recovery potential for GFR.[4]
6. Studies in rats suggest that outer cortical nephrons may recover better from obstruction than do juxtamedullary nephrons.[6] No studies have been done in dogs or cats to compare their response to that of rats.

D. Effects of obstruction on tubular functions.

1. Complete urinary obstruction precludes study of tubular functions during obstruction.
2. Clinically, partial ureteral obstruction is known to be associated with several tubular abnormalities, which are reviewed in subsequent sections.
3. The degree and nature of tubular effects, and their recovery, depend on whether obstruction is unilateral or bilateral.
   a. With unilateral obstruction, body water and electrolyte homeostasis are not compromised so long as contralateral renal function is normal.
   b. With bilateral complete obstruction, anuria creates the potential for marked abnormalities in water, electrolyte, and acid-base balance. Once obstruction is relieved, renal functions may reflect either programmed homeostatic responses or aberrant consequences of renal injury.
4. The following information pertains to tubular functions following relief of bilateral obstruction that may reflect the responsiveness of the kidneys to homeostatic needs.
   a. Sodium, potassium, phosphate, magnesium, and proton retention may have occurred during obstruction; the normal renal response is to enhance urinary excretion by increasing fractional excretion of retained materials.
   b. Water balance may be positive; polyuria ensues as the body tries to excrete the excess fluid.
5. Tubular damage during obstruction may compromise renal tubular functions once obstruction is released. Damage is reflected as defects in urine concentration, electrolyte homeostasis, and acid-base homeostasis.

E. Urine concentration defect.

1. The term postobstruction diuresis has been used to describe profuse polyuria that sometimes follows release of obstruction.
2. Initial diuresis with relief of obstruction may be attributed partly to homeostatic efforts for resolution of positive water and electrolyte balance and diuresis associated with renal excretion of urea and other nitrogenous wastes.
3. However, water homeostasis may be defective, because dehydrated patients cannot conserve water once obstruction is removed.[3]
4. The ability of the kidney to concentrate urine is markedly impaired, whereas the ability to dilute urine is less affected.
5. It is hypothesized that impaired concentrating ability is caused by increased medullary blood flow and washout of the medullary hypertonic gradient, and also by impaired response of the medullary collecting ducts to antidiuretic hormone (ADH).
6. Some data suggest that accumulation of atrial natriuretic factor (ANF) during bilateral obstruction may play a role.

F. Urine-acidifying defect.

1. Immediately after removal of obstruction of 24 hours' duration, dogs have impaired distal tubule proton secretion.[16]
2. Dogs studied after recovery from long-term obstruction were able to both acidify and alkalinize urine following ammonium chloride and bicarbonate loading,[5] thus suggesting at least partial recovery of proton secretory function.

G. Urinary potassium excretion.

1. The fractional excretion of potassium increases following relief of obstruction.
2. Although initially this may be interpreted as a

homeostatic response to hyperkalemia, some animals develop hypokalemia during the post obstruction period. This observation indicates that there is an impairment of normal homeostatic mechanisms.
3. Increased urinary potassium excretion may be caused by increased delivery of sodium to the distal tubule, where sodium-potassium exchange occurs during sodium reabsorption.
4. The medullary collecting duct may be the major site of the defect in potassium homeostasis.

III. CLINICAL SIGNS

A. Signs of obstructive uropathy vary considerably, depending on several factors—anatomic site of the primary lesion, degree of urine outflow impairment, duration of disease, and presence of secondary infection.

B. Anatomic site.
1. Azotemia and uremia may be the prominent findings if urine outflow from both kidneys is obstructed.
2. Unilateral ureteral obstruction may remain asymptomatic and may be detected only when hydronephrosis results in a marked increase in kidney size. However, acute ureteral obstruction may lead to intense pain.

C. Degree of urine outflow impairment.
1. Complete outflow obstruction (both ureters, bladder trigone, or urethral obstruction) usually causes uremia within 3 to 4 days.
2. Partial obstruction of the lower tract may not interfere with outflow enough to cause uremia but may cause lower tract signs, such as dysuria.
3. Partial ureteral obstruction may initially be asymptomatic.

D. Duration of disease.
1. Partial outflow obstruction may not impair renal functions sufficiently to ever cause uremia.
2. Bilateral partial ureteral obstruction may slowly cause progressive destruction of nephrons.
   a. As functional renal mass decreases, urine-concentrating ability is lost and polyuria may be noted.
   b. The polyuria may accelerate renal damage because increased urine volume increases ureteral pressure proximal to the obstruction.
   c. With progressive loss of renal mass, polyuria may soon be accompanied by azotemia and uremia.

E. Presence of secondary bacterial infection.
1. Outflow obstruction predisposes the urinary tract to ascending bacterial infection. (See Chapter 40, Bacterial Infections of the Canine and Feline Urinary Tract.)
2. Bacterial pyelonephritis may impair the urine-concentrating mechanism, leading to polyuria.
3. Signs of lower urinary tract infection (pyuria, hematuria, dysuria) also may be present.
4. Renal damage and its consequences are accelerated when bacterial infection accompanies obstructive uropathy. Septicemia also is a risk with obstructive uropathy.

F. Complications of obstructive uropathy.
1. Bacterial infection is a common complication of obstructive uropathy.
   a. Infection is difficult to eradicate in the presence of urinary stasis.
   b. Infection may persist after relief of obstruction or may be introduced as a consequence of procedures used to remove obstruction.
2. Associated with infection, urea-splitting organisms may render the urine alkaline, thereby predisposing the patient to struvite urolithiasis.
3. Hypertension and polycythemia have been observed as complications of obstructive uropathy in humans; their prevalence in dogs and cats is unknown.

IV. DIAGNOSIS OF OBSTRUCTIVE UROPATHY

A. Physical examination.
1. Diagnostic information can be obtained by physical examination, which allows localization of lesions or an etiologic diagnosis.
2. Urethral obstruction results in bladder distention; palpation of a markedly distended urinary bladder and inability to pass a urinary catheter of appropriate size confirm the presence of urethral obstruction.
3. Trigone lesions of the urinary bladder may cause unilateral or bilateral ureteral obstruction. Palpation of a soft tissue bladder mass should raise the index of suspicion for hydroureter and hydronephrosis.
4. Although benign prostatic hyperplasia is not associated with impingement on the urethra, either prostatic neoplasia or a large prostatic mass (cyst or abscess) may cause obstructive uropathy.
   a. Prostatic neoplasms may impinge on the lumen of the urethra.
   b. Massive cysts or abscesses may compromise urethral patency by mechanically interfering with urine outflow through the urethra.
5. Severe, acute paralumbar pain has been associated with acute unilateral urethral obstruction associated with renal calculi moving into the ureter (Fig. 42-1).
6. Chronic hydronephrosis should be considered whenever increased size of one or both kidneys is detected by physical examination.

B. Interpretation of azotemia.
1. Azotemia is categorized as prerenal, renal, or postrenal. Postrenal azotemia may be caused by either outflow obstruction or lower urinary tract rupture.
2. Postrenal azotemia occurs only with outflow obstruction of both kidneys or with unilateral disease associated with other causes of contralateral renal disease.
3. Because azotemia is a relatively insensitive index

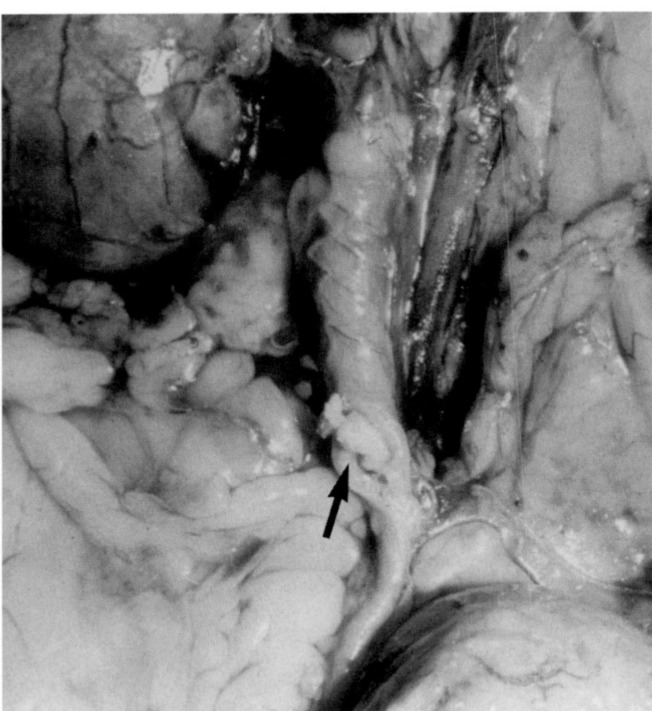

FIG. 42-1. Unilateral hydroureter and mild hydronephrosis secondary to obstruction by a urinary calculus (arrow). Engorgement of subcapsular renal vessels (upper left) is typical of hydronephrosis. Severe pain may accompany acute ureteral obstruction.

lower urinary tract obstruction. (See Chapter 11, Diagnostic Imaging of the Urinary Tract.)

V. PATHOLOGY

A. Urethra and bladder.

1. Complete urethral obstruction may lead to death from acute uremia and its complications.
   a. Urethral swelling, hemorrhage, and epithelial denudation may be present at the site of, and proximal to, the obstruction.
   b. The urinary bladder may be distended and hemorrhagic and its epithelium denuded.
2. Similar but milder lesions are likely in nonfatal cases.

B. Kidneys and ureters.

1. Mild hydroureter and hydronephrosis may or may not be noted with acute lower tract obstruction.
2. Unilateral partial or complete obstruction may lead to progressive loss of renal parenchyma while life is sustained by the opposite kidney.
   a. A thin "shell" of renal parenchyma may be all that persists (see Fig. 45-3).
   b. Histologically, glomeruli are preserved more readily than are tubular elements, leading to a preponderance of glomeruli in residual cortical tissue. Fibrosis and cellular infiltration occur.
3. Unilateral ureteral obstruction may lead to irreversible loss of renal function, partial occlusion of ureteral outflow may cause a mild to moderate degree of hydronephrosis without causing azotemia.

C. Imaging studies (see Chapter 11, Diagnostic Imaging of the Urinary Tract).

1. Survey and contrast radiography are valuable tools for diagnosis of hydronephrosis and hydroureter.
   a. With upper tract obstruction, dilation of the urinary outflow system leads to accumulation of contrast medium, making the contrast between the outflow tract and surrounding soft tissue more distinctive (Figure 42–2).
   b. Mild obstructive nephropathy that is otherwise indetectable is best diagnosed by contrast intravenous urography.
   c. When renal damage is extensive because of chronic obstruction, functional residual tissue does not facilitate filtration of large amounts of contrast medium into the outflow tract, making visualization of the dilated outflow tract more difficult.
2. Sonography also may be used for diagnosis of hydronephrosis, but it is less discriminating than is contrast intravenous urography.[2]
3. Retrograde urethrography may help to detect

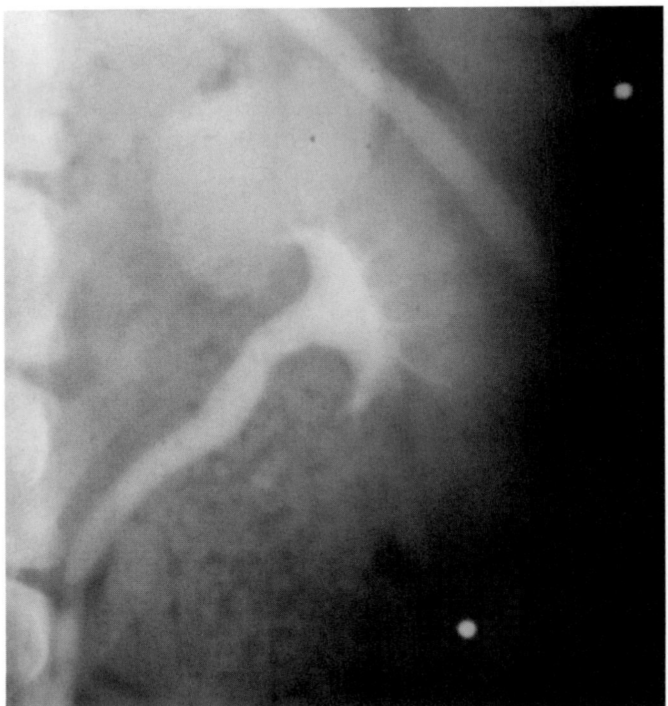

FIG. 42-2. Mild hydroureter secondary to induced bacterial pyelonephritis. Ureteral dilation exists in the absence of ureteral obstruction.

versible ureteral dilatation proximal to the obstruction.

VI. TREATMENT

A. Introduction.

1. Owing to wide range of causes and manifestations of obstructive uropathy, a standard protocol of treatment is not applicable to all cases.
2. Treatment should be based on findings of each individual case.

B. Life-threatening consequences of obstruction should be reversed. (See Chapter 22, Acute Renal Failure: Ischemic and Chemical Nephrosis; Chapter 28, Conservative Medical Management of Chronic Renal Failure; and Chapter 31, Application of Peritoneal Dialysis and Hemodialysis in the Management of Renal Failure.) These maneuvers entail treatment of (1) hyperkalemia, (2) acidemia, and/or (3) uremia.

C. Palliative procedures for preservation of renal parenchyma and bladder function should be employed (i.e., indwelling catheters to maintain urine flow and decompression).

D. Procedures for removal of the primary problem should be employed. (See Table 42–1 and the chapters that correspond to the disease diagnosed.)

REFERENCES

1. Allen JT, Vaughan ED, Gillenwater JY. The effect of indomethacin on renal blood flow and ureteral pressure in unilateral ureteral obstruction in awake dogs. *Invest Urol.* 1978;15: 324–327.
2. Dodd GD, Kaufman PN, Bracken RB. Renal arterial duplex Doppler ultrasound in dogs with urinary obstruction. *J Urol.* 1991;145:644–646.
3. Finco DR, Cornelius LM. Characterization and treatment of water, electrolyte, and acid-base imbalances of induced urethral obstruction in the cat. *Am J Vet Res.* 1977;38:823–830.
4. Gillenwater JY. Clinical aspects of urinary tract obstruction. *Semin Nephrol.* 1982;2:46–54.
5. Kerr WS. Effects of complete ureteral obstruction in dogs on kidney function. *Am J Physiol.* 1956;184:521–526.
6. Klahr S, Harris KP. Obstructive uropathy. *In:* Seldin DW, Giebisch GG, ed. *The Kidney.* New York, New York: Raven Press, 1992.
7. Klahr S. Pathophysiology of obstructive nephropathy: A 1991 update. *Semin Nephrol.* 1991;2:156–168.
8. Klahr S. New insights into the consequences and mechanisms of renal impairment in obstructive nephropathy. *Am J Kidney Dis.* 1991;18:689–699.
9. Kochin EJ, et al. Evaluation of a method of ureteroneocystistomy in cats. *J Am Vet Med.* 1993;202:257–260.
10. Leahy AL, et al. Renal injury and recovery in partial ureteric obstruction. *J Urol.* 1989;142:199–203.
11. McCarthy RJ, Lipowitz AJ, O'Brien TD. Continent jejunal reservoir (Koch pouch) for urinary diversion in dogs. *Vet Surg.* 1992;21:208–216.
12. Moody TE, Vaughan ED, Gillenwater JY. Relationship between renal blood flow and ureteral pressure during 18 hours of total unilateral ureteral occlusion. *Invest Urol.* 1975;13:246–251.
13. Moody TE, Vaughan Ed, Gillenwater JY. Comparison of the renal hemodynamic response to unilateral and bilateral ureteral occlusion. *Invest Urol.* 1977;14:455–459.
14. Rose JG, Gillenwater JY. Pathophysiology of ureteral obstruction. *Am J Physiol.* 1973;225:830–837.
15. Ross LA, Lamb CR. Reduction of hydroureter associated with ectopic ureters in two dogs after ureterovesical anastomosis. *J Am Vet Med Assoc.* 1990;196:1497–1499.
16. Thirakomen K, Koslov N, Arruda JA, Kurtzman NA. Renal hydrogen ion secretion after release of unilateral ureteral obstruction. *Am J Physiol.* 1976;231:1233–1239.
17. Vaughan ED, Gillenwater JY. Recovery following complete chronic unilateral ureteral occlusion: Functional, radiographic and pathologic alterations. *J Urol.* 1971;106:27–35.
18. Yarger WE, Griffith LD. Intrarenal hemodynamics following chronic unilateral ureteral obstruction in the dog. *Am J Physiol.* 1974;227:816–826.

CHAPTER 43

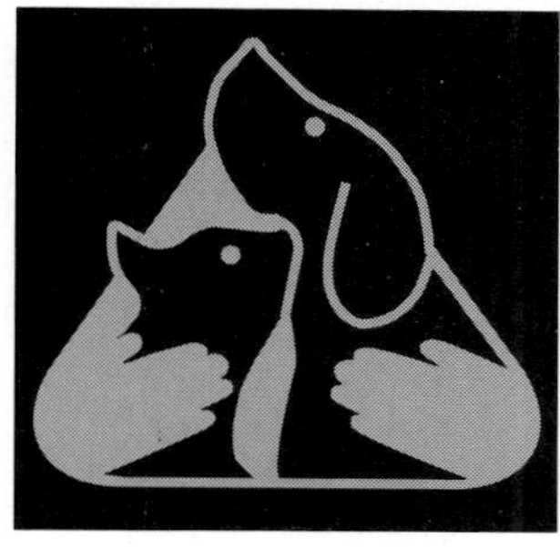

Physical Injuries to the Urinary Tract

WAYNE E. WINGFIELD
DEBORAH R. VAN PELT
SUZANNE BARKER

I. TRAUMA

A. Treatment priorities.

1. Emergency management of urologic injuries is influenced by many factors, including type of trauma, anatomic site, associated injuries, clinical status, and patient stability.
   a. Standard treatment priorities prevail; associated injuries of the respiratory, cardiovascular, and nervous system command priority attention.
2. Treatment priorities in trauma.
   a. Arterial bleeding is the highest priority in trauma. Realistically, this principle is more didactic than practical.
      (1). If arterial hemorrhage is profuse, it is unlikely that the animal will survive to be admitted to the hospital.
      (2). If arterial bleeding is identified, a compression bandage is applied for temporary control.
   b. The respiratory system is the most important organ system in trauma. A dyspneic traumatized animal should be investigated for pneumothorax, hemothorax, pulmonary contusions, and diaphragmatic hernia.
      (1). Initial therapy for treatment of shock must consider respiratory emergencies.
      (2). Fluid therapy must often be adjusted to avoid overhydration, hemodilution, and exacerbation of pulmonary hemorrhage or edema.
   c. The cardiovascular system is investigated for cardiac pump function and volume depletion.
      (1). Cardiac trauma may result in dysrhythmias affecting pump function. Unfortunately, owing to release of catecholamines secondary to pain, shock, and excitement, the dysrhythmias are rarely diagnosed until 12 to 48 hours after the traumatic event. These catecholamines drive the cardiac pacemaker at a rate higher than the depolarization rate of the ectopic injury focus.
      (2). Shock is defined as abnormal tissue perfusion leading to abnormal cellular metabolism. In trauma, the abnormal tissue perfusion begins with hypovolemia and redistribution of available fluid volumes. Treatment is directed to rapid volume replacement with crystalloid solutions, or occasionally colloids. Shock volumes of crystalloids are 90 mL/kg/h in dogs and 44 ml/kg/h in cats.
   d. Control of hemorrhage and consideration of transfusion are next in priority with trauma. If hemodilution is excessive (packed cell volume [PCV] $< 20\%$; total solids $< 50\%$ of initial

value), then whole blood or plasma/colloids should be substituted for the crystalloids.

e. Brain, spinal cord, and peripheral nerve injuries should be identified and emergency treatment instituted. At this point of triage, the goal is to control hemorrhage that might exacerbate neurologic injuries. Additionally, treatment is implemented for edema of the neurologic system.

f. Fractures and luxations are rarely a life-threatening emergency. Although the injury is often quite apparent, one should concentrate on blood loss and tissue injuries associated with the fracture or luxation.

g. Other injuries, a catch-all category, includes investigation for possible abdominal hemorrhage and for urologic trauma.

(1). Abdominal hemorrhage is usually a result of laceration of the liver or spleen. The diagnosis is generally made from abdominocentesis. The PCV of abdominal hemorrhage material is greater than the PCV in the peripheral circulation. Management of abdominal hemorrhage is controversial. At this time, a conservative approach, with attention to fluids, electrolytes, transfusions, and the application of an abdominal compression bandage, is successful.

(2). Management of urinary tract trauma is often temporizing, but it must anticipate subsequent surgery.

B. Physical injuries to the urinary tract.

1. Automobile trauma is the cause of most urinary tract trauma in dogs and cats.

a. The prevalence of urinary injury is largely unknown. In a study of 600 dogs victims of automobile trauma, 2.5% had urinary tract injuries.[14]

b. Approximately 40% of dogs with pelvic fractures showed evidence of urinary tract injury.[24]

c. In decreasing order of prevalence, ruptured urinary bladder, kidney, urethra, ureter, and perirenal hematoma are the most frequent traumatic urinary tract injuries.[13,17]

2. Other physical injuries to the urinary tract include those resulting from urinary catheterization, gunshot and other penetrating wounds, and physical abuse.

II. RENAL TRAUMA

A. Classification.

1. Renal injuries may be classified by causative factor as penetrating or nonpenetrating injuries.

2. Another classification scheme is based on clinical severity; Class V is the most severe.[12,29]

a. Class I: Renal contusion (Fig. 43–1A).

(1). Studies are not available in small animals, but contusions are most likely the most common renal injury.

(2). Renal contusions account for 60 to 80% of all renal injuries in humans.[9,29]

(3). Contusions to the kidney are caused by the compression of the kidney between the ribs and vertebral column and are most often the result of automobile trauma.

b. Class II: Cortical laceration (Fig. 43–1B).

(1). A cortical laceration is a tear of the renal parenchyma with extravasation of both urine and blood into the retroperitoneal space.

c. Class III: Renal pelvis laceration (Fig. 43–1C).

(1). A laceration through the renal cortex and medulla, extending to the renal pelvis is a more serious injury. Commonly, the fibrous capsule is torn and a hematoma forms in the perirenal area.

d. Class IV: Complete renal tear or fracture (Fig. 43–1D).

(1). This very serious injury involves rupture of both poles and the midportion of the kidney. There is generally extravasation of both urine and blood into the retroperitoneal space. Occasionally, the trauma is severe enough also to rupture the peritoneum; then, blood and urine empty into the abdominal cavity.

e. Class V: Vascular pedicle injury (Fig. 43–1E).

(1). These, most serious types of renal trauma involve a tear or laceration to the renal vasculature.

(2). No data are available to document the prevalence in small animals.

(3). In humans, this injury accounts for only 6 to 20% of all renal trauma cases.[29]

(4). Because the kidney receives 10 to 25% of the cardiac output, massive hemorrhage in the retroperitoneal space results. In humans, the survival rate with this type of injury is extremely low.

B. Recognition.

1. Physical examination.

a. Trauma to the thorax, abdomen, or flank should arouse suspicion of possible renal trauma. In humans, 50 to 60% of blunt renal injuries and 80 to 90% of penetrating renal injuries are associated with injuries to other organ systems.[9]

b. No clinical evidence of trauma was present in 13 of 39 dogs that exhibited radiographic evidence of damage to the urinary tract.[24]

c. Abdominal rigidity is usually present, but it may also reflect other abdominal injuries.

d. Because of the blood loss, shock is usually evident when lacerations of the renal pedicle are severe.

e. Blood around the urinary meatus warrants investigation of the urinary tract.

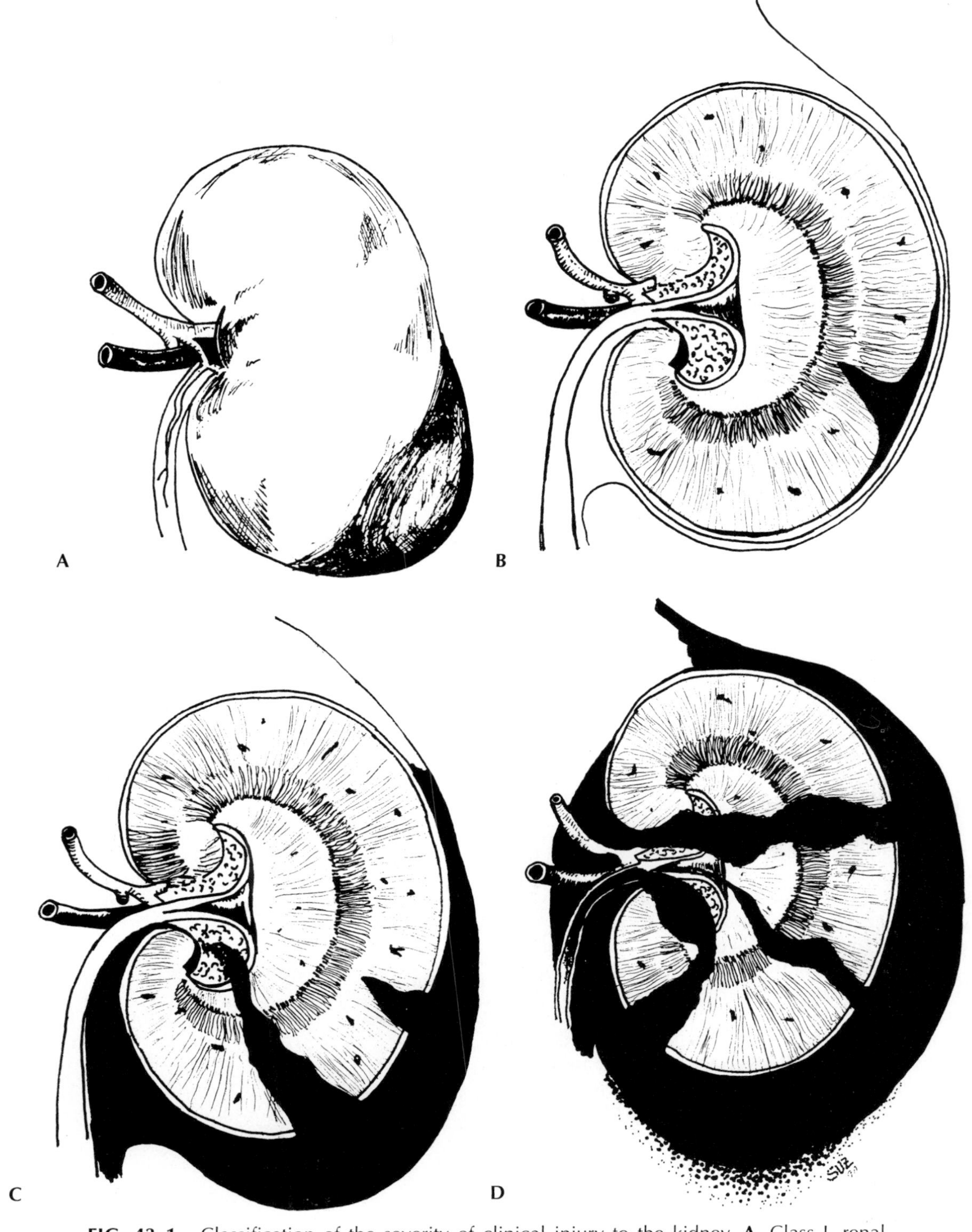

FIG. 43–1. Classification of the severity of clinical injury to the kidney. **A,** Class I, renal contusion; **B,** Class II, cortical lacerations; **C,** Class III, renal pelvis laceration; **D,** Class IV, complete renal tear or fracture; *continued on next page*

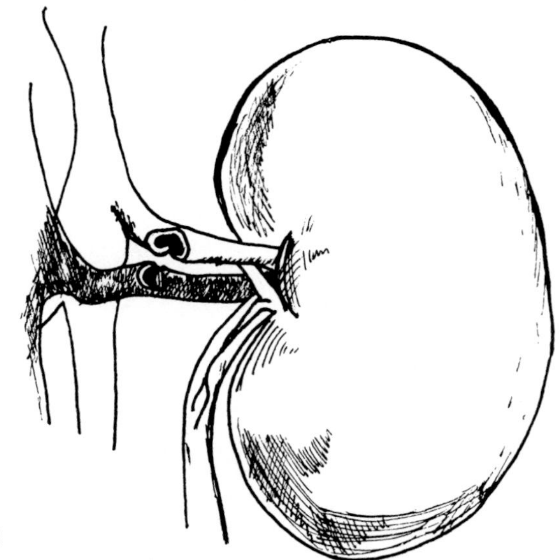

FIG. 43–1. cont'd. **E,** Class V, vascular pedicle injury.

f. Hematuria, either gross or microscopic, is the most frequent finding with urinary tract injury.
   (1). Absence of hematuria does not exclude even major renal injury, because with some injuries, occlusion or severance of the vascular pedicle or complete disruption of the ureter may prevent the passage of urine and blood into the lower urinary tract.[5]
   (2). Hematuria may be transient and cease after a few hours, or it may continue for days. Gross hematuria often clears within hours.
   (3). Cessation of hematuria is not evidence of healing of the injury. Blood clots may obstruct the source of bleeding, or the injured kidney may actually decrease its output and finally cease to function.

g. Auscultation of the abdomen should be performed. Absence of bowel sounds may indicate reflex paralytic ileus caused by extravasation of blood, bacteria, or chemicals that irritate the peritoneum.

h. Tympany should predominate in percussion of the abdomen. Dullness on percussion indicates accumulation of fluid in the abdominal cavity. Percussion may induce muscle guarding, localized pain, or rebound tenderness. If the volume of fluid is adequate, succussion may be detected by ballottement.

2. Diagnostic procedures.
   a. Laboratory studies that aid in the diagnosis of renal trauma include hematologic and coagulation studies, serum electrolytes, blood urea nitrogen (BUN), creatinine, and arterial blood gases.
      (1). Results supportive of renal trauma include mildly elevated white blood cell count with increased neutrophils, low hematocrit, and elevated BUN and creatinine levels.[29]
      (2). The most relevant laboratory study with renal trauma is urinalysis. Gross or microscopic hematuria occurs in 80 to 90% of all blunt renal trauma cases in humans.[9]
   b. If hematuria is present, its origin is determined radiographically.
      (1). Survey radiographs are useful in suggesting the diagnosis of urologic trauma.[13,29]
         (a). The presence of intra-abdominal effusion, retroperitoneal density changes, intestinal ileus, displacement or asymmetry of the kidneys, and loss of renal shadow all suggest trauma to the kidney.
         (b). The most useful survey radiographic finding is a retroperitoneal space effusion.[24]
         (c). The reported prevalence of false-negative findings of urologic trauma is 36%.[24]
      (2). The most common special radiographic procedure is the intravenous pyelogram (IVP), also known as an excretory urogram.
         (a). The IVP evaluates parenchymal integrity and excretory capacity of the kidneys.
         (b). The outline of the kidneys is visualized, followed by those of the renal pelves, ureters, and bladder.
         (c). An abnormal IVP shows extravasation of radiopaque contrast dye outside the normal excretory pathways, nonfunction or distortion of the renal pelves, incomplete filling, or delayed excretion or visualization (Fig. 43–2).

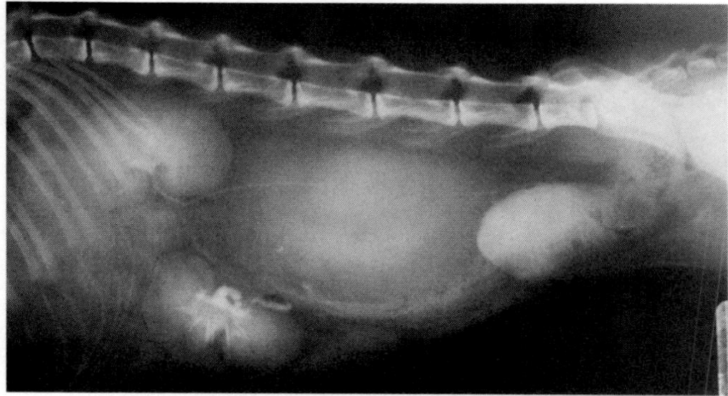

FIG. 43–2. Extravasation of positive-contrast material for a traumatized kidney in a cat. Note the accumulation of contrast material in the sublumbar musculature.

(d). Indications for an IVP include strong evidence of renal injury and gross hematuria.[10,18,19,26]

(3). Renal arteriography can be used to evaluate the integrity of the renal vasculature.

c. Abdominal ultrasonography has been shown to be extremely reliable in the diagnosis of renal trauma in humans.[8] This will likely become a valuable aid as ultrasound becomes more widely available to veterinary emergency clinics and hospitals.

d. Abdominocentesis may occasionally be helpful. (See Section IV in this chapter.)

C. Treatment.

1. Some 80 to 90% of all human renal trauma patients do not require surgery.[9,11,29]
2. Animals with Class I or Class II injuries to the kidney are usually managed conservatively, with cage rest and intravenous fluids.
3. Major injuries (Class III, IV, and V) may require surgery.
   a. Criteria for surgery include deterioration of physical status, inability to control shock from continued blood loss, and detection of free urine in the abdominal cavity.[27]
   b. If the renal trauma is extraperitoneal, criteria for surgery include deterioration of condition, radiographic evidence of extravasation of dye into the perirenal space, disruption of the renal pelvis, shock, and an expanding sublumbar soft tissue swelling.
   c. Surgery for renal trauma includes either total or partial nephrectomy.

D. Sequelae.

1. In humans, the most common sequela to renal trauma is systemic hypertension. This has not been investigated in animals.
   a. Renal injury causes scarring and devitalization of renal parenchyma. This can cause a narrowing of the renal vasculature, resulting in decreased renal blood flow.
   b. Reduced blood flow secondary to a chronic narrowing of vasculature leads to sustained stimulation of the renin-angiotensin mechanism and increased blood pressure.[9,29]
2. Additional possible complications include infection, secondary hemorrhage, and tissue necrosis. Acute renal failure following crush injuries results from release of globulins, which may have an obstructive effect on the kidney. Hemorrhage, hypotension, and decreased glomerular filtration rate (GFR) may also increase the risk of ischemic acute renal failure.

III. URETERAL TRAUMA.

A. Recognition.

1. Blunt trauma that causes injury to the ureters is rare in dogs and cats. Most commonly the injury results in damage to the ureter, close either to the kidney or to the urinary bladder.
2. Penetrating trauma is more likely to result in ureteral injury.
   a. In humans, some 3 to 17% of abdominal gunshot wounds result in ureteral injury, and some 90% of ureteral injuries are a consequence of gunshot wounds.[21]
   b. Up to 90% gunshot wounds that injure the ureter in humans produce major injury to nonrenal intra-abdominal organs (with stabbings, 60%), including bowel, colon, liver, spleen, blood vessels, and pancreas.[16]
3. Physical examination.
   a. Definitive findings of a ruptured ureter are lacking.
   b. Clinical symptoms of peritonitis result if urine is leaking into the abdominal cavity.
   c. In humans, gross or microscopic hematuria is absent in 50% of cases of confirmed ruptured ureter.[21]
4. Excretory urography is diagnostically accurate in 56 to 90% of human cases.[16]
   a. Urography characteristically demonstrates ureteral extravasation and the approximate site of the injury.
5. With unilateral ureteral rupture, only mild azotemia may be seen, because the opposite kidney is still quite functional and able to control this azotemia.

B. Treatment.

1. Treatment for ureteral injury is surgery. The procedure is complicated, and repair should probably be conducted by a surgical specialist.
   a. In the past, nephrectomy and ligation of the ureter at the urinary bladder were the treatment for ureteral lacerations or avulsion. Before such surgery, excretory urography should be performed to ensure that the opposite kidney is functional.
   b. Ureteral surgery requires careful suturing and use of stents for adequate repair.

C. Sequelae.

1. In humans, failure to use ureteral stenting during surgery was associated with a 91% complication rate.[7]
2. With ureteral stents, the surgical complication rate was 15%.[7]

IV. URINARY BLADDER TRAUMA.

A. Types of injury.

1. The most common severe traumatic urinary tract injury is rupture of the urinary bladder.[13]
   a. Pelvic bone fracture is the injury most commonly associated with rupture of the urinary bladder.
   b. Male and female dogs that sustain pelvic fractures have nearly equal rates of bladder rupture.[24]
2. Classification of urinary bladder rupture.
   a. Intraperitoneal ruptures in the fundus of the bladder are most common.

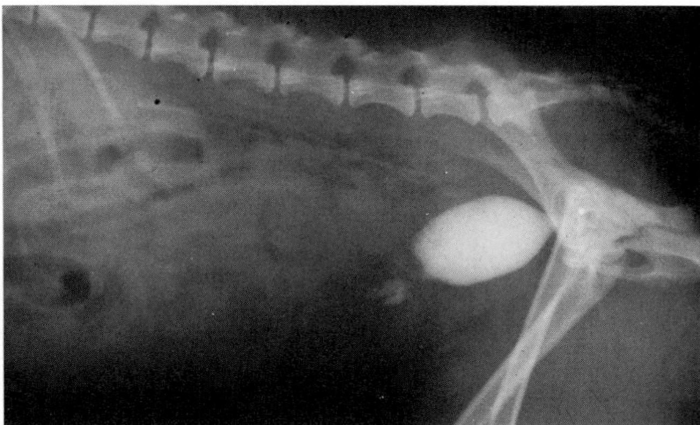

FIG. 43–3. Positive-contrast excretory urogram of bladder rupture in a dog. Note the leakage of contrast medium from the cranial portion of the urinary bladder.

b. Extraperitoneal bladder rupture involves the area of the bladder trigone. Urinary extravasation follows fascial planes and may lead to cellulitis.

B. Recognition.

1. Leakage of urine from the intraperitoneal urinary bladder rupture results in signs of chemical peritonitis, with abdominal pain and vomiting.
   a. Abdominal distention and uremia appear 1 to 3 days after initial presentation.[2,4]
   b. Although in experimental canine bladder rupture the mean time to death is 2½ days, with an intermittent or small leak, appearance of signs may be longer delayed.[4]
   c. Hematuria is the most common clinical sign of urinary tract trauma.[24] (See Section II of this chapter.)
   d. Rapid development of abdominal distention following parenteral fluid therapy may be seen with intraperitoneal urinary bladder rupture.
2. Examination of the abdominocentesis fluid aids in the diagnosis of urinary bladder rupture.
   a. Urea and creatinine are more concentrated in the urine than in serum or in transudates.[23] Thus, intraperitoneal extravasation of urine should result in high urea and creatinine levels in fluid obtained by abdominocentesis.
   b. Urea nitrogen and creatinine concentrations are significantly higher in fluid obtained by abdominocentesis than in serum in association with acute rupture of the bladder in dogs.[23]
   c. After 45 hours, the creatinine levels in abdominocentesis fluid are higher than serum levels, whereas the urea nitrogen is nearly the same as the serum value.[4]
      (1). With bladder rupture of 48 hours' duration or longer, creatinine may be a more sensitive marker than urea nitrogen, as urea nitrogen is a smaller molecule (molecular weight, 60 Kd) than creatinine (molecular weight, 113 Kd). Urea is cleared back into the bloodstream more rapidly than is creatinine, owing to its ability to cross the peritoneal membrane.[23,25]
   d. Diagnostic peritoneal lavage is reported to be unreliable for intraperitoneal bladder rupture in humans, the false-negative rate can be as great as 33%.[6]
3. Radiographic findings indicated that the majority of dogs with a ruptured bladder had evidence of ascites, ileus, and peritonitis.[4]
   a. Excretory urography is not reliable for diagnosing a ruptured bladder. In humans, findings of the cystographic phase of excretory urography have an inaccuracy rate as great as 85%, owing to dilution and depressed renal function.[3]
   b. Reliable diagnosis of intraperitoneal bladder rupture is provided by retrograde positive cystography. It is important to fully distend the bladder, to avoid missing small tears.
      (1). Extraperitoneal extravasation is represented as contrast medium escaping from the bladder base adjacent to the pubis but remaining relatively confined.
      (2). Visible contrast material outside the bladder, outlining loops of bowel and pooling under the liver or spleen, reflects intraperitoneal rupture (Fig. 43–3).

C. Treatment.

1. Emergency treatment for ruptured bladder first involves the stabilization of the metabolic and electrolyte status of the patient, plus treatment for shock.
   a. Because fluid therapy is part of the initial management, intraperitoneal bladder rupture often results in abdominal distention as the urine leaks into the abdominal cavity.
   b. In the early stages of trauma, use of anesthetic agents is risky. Thus, an abdominal drain is quite useful for stabilizing a patient prior to anesthesia. Usually No. 8 F balloon-tipped catheter (Foley catheter) is inserted into the abdomen, and urine is collected into a continuous, closed urinary collection system. These drains usually work well for 12 to 24 hours before becoming occluded by omentum. During this time, the metabolic abnormalities of the patient are resolving and the animal becomes a more satisfactory risk for anesthesia.
   c. Careful placement of a urinary catheter to the area of the bladder trigone has been tried as a means for draining the urine from a ruptured

bladder. Results of this technique have not been rewarding.

2. A ruptured bladder usually requires surgical repair. In the case of an extraperitoneal bladder rupture, use of a urinary catheter as a temporary stent is useful.
   a. Following repair, the abdominal fluid should be collected for culture and sensitivity testing, the abdomen generously lavaged with warm saline, and the abdominal wall closed for first-intention wound healing.
   b. Abdominal drains usually are not required.

D. Sequelae.

1. Peritonitis and cellulitis are the most common postoperative complications of intra- and extraperitoneal bladder rupture, respectively.
2. The animal should be encouraged to micturate frequently, to avoid overdistention and stress on the suture lines.
3. Appropriate antibiotic therapy is based on results of the culture and sensitivity tests.

V. RUPTURED URETHRA.

A. Recognition.

1. Traumatic rupture of the urethra is most common in male dogs and cats with pelvic fractures.[20,24] Other causes of ruptured urethra include bite wounds, poor catheterization technique, urolithiasis, and os penis fractures.
2. Rupture of the urethra most frequently occurs near the junction with the bladder, and it results in accumulation of urine in the retroperitoneal, perineal, or subcutaneous tissues of the associated fascial planes.[13]
3. Dysuria, stranguria, and local swelling after trauma suggest the need to investigate the lower urinary tract for evidence of injury.
4. Positive-contrast urethrography is the examination of choice to evaluate urethral injury (Fig. 43–4).
   a. Aqueous organic iodides are diluted to a 10 to 15% solution and often are mixed with a sterile lubricant (K-Y jelly).
   b. Leakage of this contrast material from the urethra locates the site of the urethral tear. Air should not be used as a negative contrast agent, as it carries the risk of urethrocavernous reflux and the potential for fatal embolization of instilled air.[1]

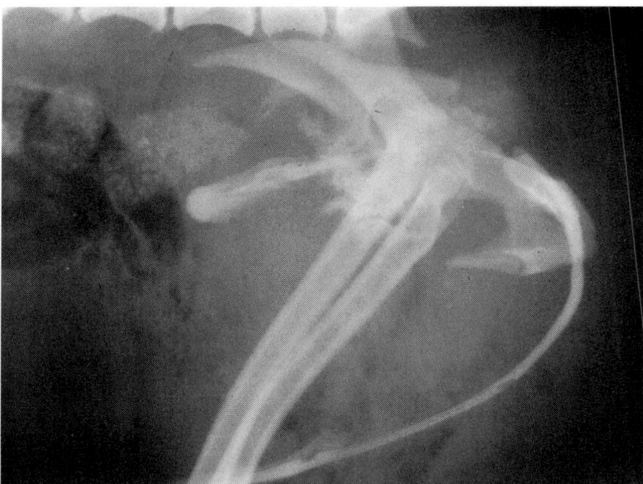

FIG. 43–4. Positive-contrast urethrogram with extravasation of contrast from a ruptured pelvic urethra.

B. Treatment.

1. Small urethral lacerations may heal if an appropriate sized catheter is left in place for 7 to 21 days.[17]
2. Primary urethral repair, extrapelvic anastomosis of the bladder to the urethra (for male dogs), antepubic urethrostomy, or urinary diversion procedures are alternatives for management of severe urethral rupture.[2,15,22,28]
3. Pelvic urethral tears usually require surgery.

C. Sequelae.

1. Urethral stricture is the most common complication.
   a. Stricture is most common with inaccurate suturing or when the urethra is distended with a catheter.
   b. Urinary incontinence is common when surgery involves the proximal pelvic urethra or prostatectomy following severe urethral damage.
   c. Fracture of the os penis may lead to stricture secondary to callus formation. Surgical repair generally involves fragment removal, prescrotal urethrostomy, or scrotal urethrostomy.

REFERENCES

1. Ackerman N, Wingfield WE, Corely EA. Fatal air embolism associated with pneumourethrography and pneumocystography in a dog. *J Am Vet Med Assoc.* 1972;160:1616.
2. Bjorling DE. Traumatic injuries of the urogenital system. *Vet Clin North Am.* 1984;14:61.
3. Bretan PN Jr, et al. Computerized tomography staging of renal trauma. *J Urol.* 1986;136:561.
4. Burrows CA, Bovee KC. Metabolic changes due to experimentally induced rupture of the canine urinary bladder. *Am J Vet Res.* 1974;35:1083.
5. Engel RME. Trauma of the genitourinary system. *In:* Zuidema GD, Rutherford RB, Ballinger WF II, eds. *The Management of Trauma.* 3rd ed. Philadelphia, Pennsylvania: WB Saunders, 1979.
6. Fischer RP, Beverlin BC, Engrav LH. Peritoneal lavage: Fourteen years and 2586 patients later. *Am J Surg.* 1978;136:701.
7. Franco I, et al. Value of proximal diversion and ureteral stenting in management of penetrating ureteral trauma. *Urology.* 1988; 32:99.
8. Furtschegger A, Egender G, Jakse G. The value of sonography in the diagnosis and follow-up of patients with blunt renal trauma. *Br J Urol.* 1988;62:110.
9. Guerriero WG. Management of urologic injuries. *Trauma Q.* 1984;1:52.

10. Guice K, et al. Hematuria after blunt trauma. *J Trauma.* 1983;23:305.
11. Kenner CV, White KM. The critically ill adult following trauma. *In:* Kenner CV, Guzzelta CE, Dorsey BM, eds. *Critical Care Nursing: Body Mind Spirit.* 2nd ed. Boston, Massachusetts: Little, Brown; 1985:1054–1056.
12. Kidd P. Genitourinary trauma patients. *Topics Emerg Med.* 1987; 9:71.
13. Kleine LJ, Thornton GW. Radiographic diagnosis of urinary tract trauma. *J Am Anim Hosp Assoc.* 1971;7:318.
14. Kolata RJ, Johnson DE. Motor vehicle accidents in urban dogs: A study of 600 cases. *J Am Vet Med Assoc.* 1975;12:850.
15. Knecht CD, Slusher R. Extrapelvic anastomosis of the bladder and penile urethra in a dog. *J Am Anim Hosp Assoc.* 1970;6:247.
16. Mendez R. Renal trauma. *J Urol.* 1977;118:698.
17. Morgan RV. Urogenital emergencies. *Comp Contin Educ Pract Vet.* 1982;11:908.
18. Nicolaisen GS, et al. Renal trauma. *J Urol.* 1985;133:183.
19. Oakland CD, Britton JM, Charlton CA. Renal trauma and the intravenous urogram. *J Soc Med.* 1987;80:21.
20. Peckman RD. Urinary trauma in dogs and cats: A review. *J Am Anim Hosp Assoc.* 1982;18:33.
21. Peterson NE. Emergency management of urologic trauma. *Emery Clin North Am.* 1988;6:579.
22. Rawlings CA, Wingfield WE. Urethral reconstruction in dogs and cats. *J Am Anim Hosp Assoc.* 1976;12:850.
23. Rubin MJ, et al. Diagnosis of intraperitoneal extravasation of urine by peritoneal lavage. *Ann Emerg Med.* 1985;14:433.
24. Selcer BA. Urinary tract trauma associated with pelvic trauma. *J Am Anim Hosp Assoc.* 1982;19:785.
25. Sulivan MJ, Lackner LH, Banowsky LHW. Intraperitoneal extravasation of urine. *JAMA.* 1972;221:491.
26. Thomason RB, et al. Microscopic hematuria after blunt trauma. Is pyelography necessary? *Ann Surg.* 1989;55:145.
27. Van Allen H, Bruhl P, Porst H. Pediatric blunt trauma—surgical or conservative treatment? *Eur Urol.* 1988;14:407.
28. Yoshioka MM, Carb A. Antepubic urethrostomy in the dog. *J Am Anim Hosp Assoc.* 1982;18:290.
29. Zoller GW. Genitourinary trauma. *In:* Rosen P, ed. *Emergency Medicine: Concepts and Clinical Practice.* St. Louis, Missouri: CV Mosby; 1988:551–561.

CHAPTER 44

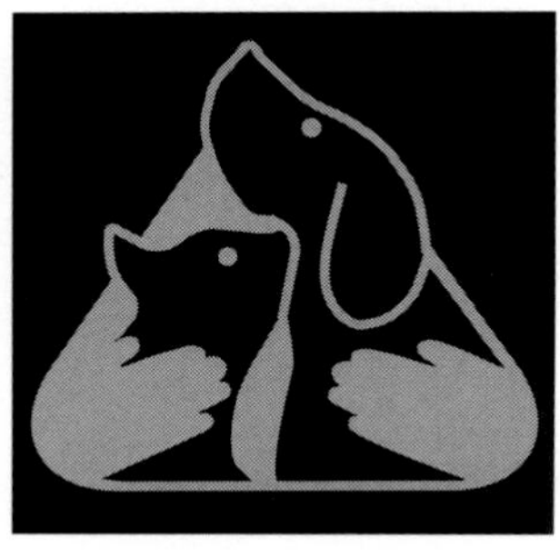

Neoplasms of the Urinary Tract

JEFFREY S. KLAUSNER
DENNIS D. CAYWOOD

I. KIDNEY

A. Epidemiology and etiology.

1. Benign renal neoplasms are less common than malignant ones in dogs and cats. Benign neoplasms are observed principally in older animals. No breed or sex predilections have been identified.[1–6]
2. Renal adenomas are one of the more common benign neoplasms of the kidney (Table 44–1). Other benign neoplasms that have been reported include hemangiomas, papillomas, lipomas, fibromas, and renal interstitial cell tumors.
3. Renal tubular cell carcinoma is the most common primary malignant neoplasm of the kidney.[1–7] As in humans, the renal tubular cell carcinoma more often affects males (Tables 44–1, 44–2). The tumor may be hormonally induced.
4. Bilateral and multiple renal cystadenocarcinomas have been associated with a syndrome of generalized nodular dermatofibrosis described primarily in German shepherd dogs.[8–10] The disease appears to be heritable probably in an autosomal dominant pattern.
5. Nephroblastomas occur more often in young dogs and cats, though many cases have been observed in dogs and cats aged 4 years or older (see Tables 44–1, 44–2). No breed or sex predilection is apparent.
6. Transitional cell and squamous cell carcinomas are much less common in the renal pelvis than in the urinary bladder and are rare in cats. No breed or sex predilection has been observed (see Tables 44–1, 44–2).
7. Renal fibrosarcomas, hemangiosarcomas, and undifferentiated sarcomas are frequently encountered in the kidneys of dogs (see Table 44–1). Other sarcomas are less common than nephroblastomas and transitional cell or squamous cell carcinomas (see Tables 44–1, 44–2).
8. Metastatic neoplasms are commonly found in the kidneys.[5,11–13] Renal lymphomas are generally considered metastatic neoplasms and are the most common renal neoplasm of cats.[2,13,14]

B. Pathology and biologic behavior.

1. Renal interstitial cell tumor, a benign neoplasm, arises from the fibroblast-like cells of the renal stroma. The tumors are common in humans and have been reported in dogs.[15] Renal interstitial cell tumors are multiple, and generally bilateral, located near the corticomedullary junction.
2. It has not been determined whether renal tubular cell carcinomas arise directly from renal tubular cells, by evolution through adenomatous hyperplasia, or from renal cortical adenomas.[12]
3. Renal tubular cell carcinomas spread by direct extension through the renal capsule or renal pelvis and by invasion of intrarenal veins and lymphatics.[2,5,6,12] Invasion and growth into renal

TABLE 44–1.
TYPE, AGE, AND SEX OF 523 DOGS WITH A PRIMARY RENAL NEOPLASM*

		Sex			Age (yr)		
Tumor Type	**Cases (No.)**	**Male**	**Female**	**Not Determined**	**Mean**	**Range**	**Not Determined**
Epithelial tissue							
Adenoma	16	9	6	1	10.2	3–15	1
Renal carcinoma	280	148	103	29	7.7	1–15	37
Transitional cell carcinoma	18	7	11	0	8.2	5–13	0
Squamous cell carcinoma	11	8	3	0	8.6	4–14	0
Connective tissue							
Fibroma	4	3	1	0	9.5	5–13	0
Fibrosarcoma	40	25	15	0	9.35	1–15	0
Lipoma	7	0	7	0	7.7	1–13	0
Liposarcoma	1	0	1	0	—	5	0
Chondroma	1	1	0	0	13	13	0
Osteoma	2	2	0	0	4	3–5	0
Myxoma	1	1	0	0	—	8	0
Reticulum cell sarcoma	1	1	0	0	—	3	0
Unclassified sarcoma	17	8	9	0	9.1	½–15	0
Muscle tissue							
Rhabdomyosarcoma	1	1	1	0	—	12	0
Leiomyoma	1	1	0	0	—	—	1
Leiomyosarcoma	3	2	0	1	9	5–13	1
Vascular tissue							
Hemangioma	7	4	3	0	11.3	8–5	0
Hemangiosarcoma	67	35	32	0	10.8	5–15	3
Mixed tissue							
Nephroblastoma	40	19	16	5	5.6	½–13	0
Teratoma	4	2	2	0	2.8	1–5	0
Hamartoma	1	1	0	0	—	5	0

*Data from the Veterinary Medical Data Program and the literature.[28]

veins can occur and may account for the high incidence of lung metastases. The most common sites of metastases in dogs and cats are the lungs, lymph nodes, liver, brain, and bone.[2,5,6,12]

4. Polysystemic signs occasionally observed with renal adenomas and renal tubular cell carcinomas may be related to production of excessive quantities of erythrocyte-stimulating factor, renin, parathormone, prostaglandins, and other hormones.[16–18]
5. Nephroblastoma is a congenital neoplasm derived from the pluripotential metanephrogenic blastema, which allows production of epithelial and connective tissue elements.[5,19,20] It is regarded as part of the developing kidney and is associated with continued growth but abnormal differentiation.[5,19,20]
6. Nephroblastomas are usually unilateral; however, bilateral involvement is reported.[2] If the tumor penetrates the renal capsule, local invasion of perinephric fat, posterior abdominal muscles, the diaphragm, and neighboring organs may occur.[4,19,21] Distant metastasis occurs via the lymphatics into pararenal and para-aortic lymph nodes or, more commonly, by venous metastasis from the renal vein into the vena cava. The most common site of metastasis is the lung, followed by liver, mesentery, and lymph nodes.[2,4,20–25]
7. Several urothelial carcinomas, adenocarcinomas, transitional cell carcinomas, and squamous cell neoplasms are observed because the urothelium maintains the embryonic potential to produce mucus-secreting glandular, transitional, and squamous epithelium.[12] Studies of humans, dogs, and laboratory animals have revealed that urothelial cell hyperplasia antedates formation of many malignant transitional cell neoplasms.[2,12,26]
8. Metastatic kidney neoplasms are common, possibly because of the large blood volume that perfuses the kidneys. Rarely are they clinically significant and usually they are incidental necropsy findings.

9. In cats, the alimentary form of lymphoma may be associated with extensive renal involvement. Both kidneys are usually affected.[2,13,14]

C. **Clinical findings.**

1. Historical findings.
   a. Benign renal neoplasms are rarely of clinical significance and usually are incidental necropsy findings. An exception is the renal hemangioma, which is frequently associated with constant or intermittent gross hematuria.[2,6]
   b. Neoplasms of the renal pelvis (i.e., transitional cell and squamous cell carcinomas) are usually associated with local signs such as hematuria and hydronephrosis, which precede polysystemic signs.[1,2,4,6] In contrast, hematuria is not usually a preclinical finding in patients with renal parenchymal neoplasms.[1,2,4,6]
   c. Polysystemic signs unrelated to the urinary tract are common and may be the first clinical signs of renal carcinomas.[2,27] In a study of 54 dogs with primary renal neoplasms, the most common historical findings were anorexia, depression, and weight loss.[4]
   d. Cats with alimentary tract lymphomas may have extensive renal involvement. Nonspecific clinical signs include progressive weight loss, depression, anorexia, vomiting, and diarrhea. Cachexia, fever, anemia, and secondary infections occur in the terminal phases.[2,13,14,28,29]
2. Physical examination findings.
   a. Early and small benign neoplasms are not often detected by physical examination; however, an abdominal mass is palpated in 43% of dogs with renal neoplasms, and pyrexia is commonly reported.[4]
   b. Bilateral renal involvement is common with feline renal lymphoma. Kidneys are palpable as enlarged asymmetric structures in the abdominal cavity.[2,13,14,28,29]
   c. Hypertrophic osteopathy has been reported in dogs with renal tumors. Characteristic bone lesions are observed as painful swellings of the distal limbs.[22,30,31]
   d. Clinical signs may be caused by metastatic lesions, and on occasion they are the first evidence of a neoplasm.
3. Laboratory findings.
   a. Anemia is commonly reported, and hematuria and proteinuria are the most consistent urinalysis findings.[2,4,6,32–35]
   b. Polycythemia has been observed in dogs and cats with renal adenomas and renal tubular carcinomas that elaborated excessive quantities of erythrocyte-stimulating factor.[16–18]
   c. Microscopic hematuria and neoplastic cells may be detected on cytologic examination of urine sediment.[2,6]
   d. Complete blood counts and chemistry profiles are usually within normal limits.[4]
   e. Even though both kidneys may be involved, a sufficient quantity of functional renal paren-

TABLE 44–2.
TYPE, AGE, AND SEX OF 71 CATS WITH A PRIMARY RENAL NEOPLASM*

		Sex			Age (yr)		
Tumor Type	**Cases (No.)**	**Male**	**Female**	**Not Determined**	**Mean**	**Range**	**Not Determined**
Epithelial tissue							
Adenoma	3	1	2	0	—	13	2
Renal carcinoma	31	15	6	10	9.2	1–13	6
Transitional cell carcinoma	6	5	1	0	10.8	6–15	1
Squamous cell carcinoma	3	2	1	0	—	13	2
Connective tssue							
Lipoma	2	1	1	0	4	3–5	0
Fibrosarcoma	2	2	2	0	9	5–13	0
Unclassified sarcoma	10	1	2	7	6.8	½–13	8
Muscle tissue							
Leiomyosarcoma	2	0	1	1	—	22	1
Vascular tissue							
Hemangiosarcoma	1	1	1	0	—	3	0
Mixed tissue							
Nephroblastoma	11	3	1	7	4.3	1–8	5

*Data from the Veterinary Medical Program and the literature.[28]

chyma may persist to prevent signs of renal failure. Extensive bilateral involvement of the kidneys that destroys 70 to 75% or more of the nephrons is associated with signs of progressive renal insufficiency.[2,6]

f. Renal failure caused by bilateral renal lymphoma is more common in cats than in dogs.[14,22]

4. Radiographic and ultrasonographic findings.
   a. Survey abdominal radiographs often allow visualization of an abdominal mass. In one study evaluating abdominal radiographs of 43 dogs with renal neoplasms, abdominal masses were detected in 81.4% and correctly identified as kidney in 53.5%.[4]
   b. In the same study, an abdominal mass was identified by ultrasound in 100% of the dogs evaluated with renal neoplasms and correctly identified as kidney in 84.6%.[4]
   c. Intravenous urography allowed visualization of renal mass in 96.2% of the dogs evaluated in the study.[4]
   d. Intravenous urography not only allows localization of the neoplasm but may permit estimation of the extent of renal parenchymal involvement. Distortion in the shape of the renal pelvis and diverticula and retention of contrast medium are generally seen in the neoplastic kidney. Lack of excretion of detectable quantities of radiopaque contrast material suggests severe hydronephrosis.[2,6]
   e. Selective angiography may be performed to delineate the precise site and extent of renal destruction.[2,6]

D. Diagnosis and clinical staging.

1. History, physical examination, blood studies, urinalysis, cytologic examination of urine sediment, and imaging procedures provide a presumptive diagnosis of renal neoplasia. Histologic evaluation of the affected tissue is required for a definitive diagnosis and to determine tumor cell type.[2,6,28]
2. Thoracic radiographs should be taken when a renal neoplasm is suspected, to aid in clinical staging for therapy.[2,6,28]
3. Needle biopsy of a unilateral renal neoplasm may be inadvisable if treatment by surgical extirpation is contemplated, since the potential for iatrogenic metastasis exists.
4. In case of unilateral renal involvement, exploratory celiotomy is performed and biopsy tissue is obtained by nephrectomy. The abdomen is explored for metastases.[2,6,28]

E. Treatment.

1. Therapy should be based on clinical staging of the neoplasm (Table 44–3).[36] If the tumor has not metastasized, and if the opposite kidney is not neoplastic and has adequate function, nephrectomy and partial ureterectomy are indicated.

TABLE 44–3.
WHO CLINICAL STAGES OF CANINE TUMORS OF THE KIDNEY*

T: Primary tumor
- T0 No evidence of tumor
- T1 Small tumor without deformation of the kidney
- T2 Solitary tumor with deformation and/or enlargement of the kidney
- T3 Tumor invading perinephric structures (peritoneum) and/or pelvis, ureter, and/or renal blood vessels (renal vein)
- T4 Tumor invading neighboring structures

N: Regional lymph nodes (RLN) (lumbar LN)
- N0 No RLN involved
- N1 Ipsilateral RLN involved
- N2 Bilateral RLN involved
- N3 Other LN involved (abdominal and pelvic LN)

M: Distant metastasis
- M0 No evidence of metastasis
- M1 Distant metastasis—specify sites
- M1a Single metastasis
- M1b Multiple metastasis in one organ
- M1c Multiple metastasis in various organs

*Data from the World Health Organization. Report of the Second Consultation of the Biological Behavior and Therapy of Tumors of Domestic Animals. Geneva: WHO, 1979.

2. Nephroureterectomy.
   a. Preoperative abdominal palpation should be restricted to prevent rupture of the tumor and abdominal seeding of the abdomen.[2,12,20,21,28]
   b. Adequate surgical exposure, careful manipulation of the affected kidney, and ligation of the renal vein are advised before mobilizing the tumor, to prevent release of neoplastic cells into the bloodstream.[2,12,20,21,28]
   c. The kidney and the entire ureter should be removed, since metastasis may occur anywhere along its length.[2,12,20,21,28]
   d. If the lymph nodes are enlarged and appear abnormal, systematic dissection and excision of regional lymph nodes is advised, to prevent incomplete removal of tumor cells within the lymphatics.[2,12,20,21,28]
3. Radiation therapy.
   a. There is little information in the veterinary literature about the use of radiation therapy for renal tubular cell carcinoma. Clinical and experimental studies in humans suggest limited success.[11]
   b. Use of radiotherapy for nephroblastomas in veterinary medicine has been limited, but it has significantly improved survival in humans.[12,20,23] Cancer cells dislodged during surgery or left behind because of incomplete excision may be destroyed by radiation therapy.

4. Chemotherapy.
   a. In humans, aggressive or invasive renal tubular cell carcinomas are treated with adjuvant cytotoxic chemotherapy. Combinations of 5-fluorouracil, doxorubicin, and cyclophosphamide have been used in dogs, but evidence of an objective response is lacking.[11]
   b. Medroxyprogesterone has been used in humans with some degree of success in causing partial regression or arresting the growth of renal tubular cell carcinomas.[11]
   c. Chemotherapy has been very effective in the management of nephroblastomas in humans. Actinomycin D has prevented metastasis.[24,37–40] In addition to laboratory evidence for a direct tumoricidal effect, this drug is also a radiosensitizer that potentiates the effect of radiation.[20,25,39] Vincristine has also been used. It is less toxic than actinomycin D and has a synergistic effect when combined with it.[12,20,25,38]
   d. A unilateral nephroblastoma with metastases was successfully controlled in a 1-year-old female mixed-breed dog by surgical extirpation of the tumorous kidney, local irradiation of tissue adjacent to the kidney, and periodic administration of actinomycin.[22] Combination therapy—surgical management, radiotherapy, and chemotherapy—has resulted in reported cure rates of 70 to 80% in human patients with metastatic nephroblastomas.[12,20,25,38]
   e. In one study, feline renal lymphoma has been treated with combination chemotherapy, consisting of vincristine, L-asparaginase, cyclophosphamide, methotrexate, cytosine arabinoside, and prednisone. Degree of response was related to clinical stage and the presence or absence of a positive feline leukemia virus (FeLV) test (Tables 44–4, and 44–5).[29]

TABLE 44–4.
CLINICAL STAGING SYSTEM FOR FELINE LYMPHOMA AT THE DONALDSON-ATWOOD CANCER CLINIC*

Stage	Description
Stage 1	Single tumor (extranodal) or single anatomic area (nodal) Includes primary intrathoracic tumors
Stage 2	Single tumor (extranodal) with regional lymph node involvement Two or more nodal areas on the same side of the diaphragm Two (extranodal) tumors with or without regional lymph node involvement on the same side of the diaphragm A primary, resectable, gastrointestinal tract tumor, usually in the ileocecal area, with or without involvement of associated mesenteric lymph nodes only
Stage 3	Two tumors (extranodal) on opposite sides of the diaphragm Two or more nodal areas cranial and caudal to the diaphragm All extensive primary unresectable intra-abdominal disease All paraspinal or epidural tumors, regardless of other tumor site(s)
Stage 4	Stages 1 to 3 with liver and/or spleen involvement
Stage 5	Stages 1 to 4 with initial involvement of CNS and/or bone marrow

*Data adapted from Mooney SC, Hayes AA, Matus RE, MacEwen EG. Renal lymphoma in cats: 28 cases (1977–1984). *JAVMA.* 1987;191:1473.

TABLE 44–5.
SURVIVAL TIME OF 28 CATS WITH RENAL LYMPHOMA, ACCORDING TO STAGE OF DISEASE*

Stage	Cats (No.)	Mean Survival Time (days)	Mean Survival Time for FeLV-Positive Cats (days)	Mean Survival Time for FeLV-Negative Cats (days)
2	11	396+	4/168	7/526+
3	5	30	4/27	3/31
4	6	213+	2/105	4/267+
5	6	321+	6/321+	267+

*Data adapted from Mooney SC, Hayes AA, Matus RE, MacEwen EG. Renal lymphoma in cats: 28 cases (1977–1984). *JAVMA.* 1987;191:1473.

F. Prognosis.
1. Prognosis depends on the type, location, and extent of neoplastic involvement, the presence or absence of metastasis, and the biologic behavior of the neoplasm.
2. Longterm survival has been reported for cases following surgical extirpation of a unilateral malignant neoplasm. Unfortunately, early diagnosis is not the rule and metastasis is often established, particularly with parenchymal tumors.
3. In cases with bilateral renal involvement or metastases, or in untreated cases, a guarded to poor prognosis should be offered.
4. Survival data.
   a. In a study of dogs with primary renal neoplasms undergoing nephrectomy that were alive 21 days following surgery, a mean survival time with renal tubular cell carcinomas was 6.8 months, with renal transitional cell carcinomas 11.0 months, and 2 dogs with nephroblastomas survived 4 and 21 months, respectively.[4]
   b. In a study of 28 cats whose renal lymphoma was diagnosed, staged, and treated, cats with

TABLE 44–6.
TYPE, AGE, AND SEX OF 21 DOGS WITH A PRIMARY NEOPLASM OF THE URETER*

Tumor Type	Cases (No.)	Sex			Age (yr)		
		Male	Female	Not Determined	Mean	Range	Not Determined
Epithelial tissue							
Papilloma	1	1	0	0	—	2	0
Transitional cell carcinoma	18	6	12	0	9	5–15	0
Muscle tissue							
Leiomyoma	2	0	2	0	13	11–15	0

*Data from the Veterinary Medical Data Program and the literature.[28]

Stage 2 lymphoma that were FeLV-test negative had the best prognosis as compared to other stages: mean survival times were longer than 526 days (see Tables 44–4, 44–5).[29]

II. URETER

A. Primary neoplasms of the ureter are rare in dogs and have not been reported in cats.[2,6,41–43]

B. They are more common in females, and transitional cell carcinoma is the most common type (Table 44–6).

C. Clinical signs are generally associated with hydronephrosis.[2,6,41–43]

D. A good prognosis is associated with nephroureterectomy of benign and malignant neoplasms confined to the ureter.

NEOPLASMS OF THE BLADDER AND URETHRA

III. URINARY BLADDER

A. Epidemiology and etiology.

1. Though neoplasms of the urinary bladder are the most frequently identified urinary tract tumor in dogs and cats, they account for fewer than 1% of all canine and feline neoplasms.[44–47]
2. The prevalence of bladder neoplasms is greater in dogs than in cats. The reason for the increased risk in dogs is unknown, but a difference in the metabolism of carcinogenic substances such as tryptophan has been suggested.[48]
3. Bladder tumors are identified more frequently in female dogs than in males.[27,46,47,49] In contrast, in humans, bladder tumors are more frequent in men than in women.[50]
4. Bladder tumors are more common in older animals, except for rhabdomyosarcomas, which typically are identified in young dogs.[27,47,49,51] The average age of dogs with bladder cancer is 8.3 years and of cats, 9.1 years.
5. Breeds with a high risk of bladder cancer include Scottish terriers, Shetland sheepdogs, beagles, and collies.[46] Rhabdomyosarcomas are prevalent in large-breed dogs, especially St. Bernards.[52]
6. Prolonged contact of carcinogenic substances in urine with the bladder mucosa is suspected to be a significant factor in the development of bladder cancer. Benzidine, 1-naphthylamine and 2-naphthylamine have been identified as primary agents.[53] Bladder tumors have been produced in dogs by administration of numerous carcinogens, including nitrosamines,[54–56] aminobiphenyl,[57] and orthoaminodiphenyl.[58]
7. The use of tobacco and occupational exposures (e.g., to dye, rubber, leather, paint, and organic chemical industries) increase the risk of bladder cancer in humans. The role of industrial carcinogens in causing bladder cancer is also supported by studies in humans and dogs that demonstrate an increased risk in those who reside in areas of intensive industrial activity.[53,59] In a recent report, topical insecticide exposure and obesity, but not sidestream cigarette smoke, increased bladder cancer risk in dogs.[60] Obesity was hypothesized to increase the risk of cancer, because insecticides stored in body fat would be gradually excreted in the urine, resulting in prolonged contact with the bladder mucosa.
8. In dogs and humans, an association has been noted between the administration of cyclophosphamide and the subsequent development of transitional cell carcinomas of the urinary bladder.[61–63]

B. Pathology and biologic behavior.

1. Malignant epithelial tumors are identified more frequently than benign tumors or sarcomas (Tables 44–7, 44–8). Metastatic tumors are rare.
2. Papillomas, which may be single or multiple, typically are identified in older animals.[27] Persistent hematuria results from ulceration of the tumor and/or urinary tract infection. Clinically, papillomas may be difficult to distinguish from inflammatory polyps.[64]
3. Fibromas are frequently associated with urinary

tract infection and urocystoliths.[65,66] Surgical removal usually is curative.

4. Transitional cell carcinomas, the most frequently identified bladder tumor, typically arise as broad-based, solitary projections from the trigone.[27,51,67] Tumor invasion of the bladder wall and extensive replacement of the mucosa and muscle layers by tumor cells are often noted. Extension of the tumor may result in ureteral and/or urethral obstruction. Transitional cell carcinomas typically grow slowly and metastasize late in their course.[11] Metastasis has been recognized in 50% of canine and 40% of feline cases.[27,67] Metastasis may be widespread: lungs, regional lymph nodes, kidney, liver, and prostate are frequent sites of metastasis.[27] Spread to long bones, skull, and eyes have also been noted.[68–70]
5. Leiomyosarcoma is the most frequently identified urinary bladder sarcoma. Diffuse invasive growth and a high rate of metastasis characterize bladder sarcomas.[27]
6. Rhabdomyosarcomas originate from a pluriopotential mesodermal stem cell arising from the urogenital ridge. Young, large-breed dogs are predisposed.[52,71–74] Typically, rhabdomyosarcomas are located at the neck of the bladder, are locally invasive, often do not metastasize, and frequently result in hypertrophic osteopathy.
7. Secondary bladder tumors are uncommon, comprising only 5% of urinary tract neoplasms.[27] Most secondary bladder tumors arise from the urethra or the prostate.[51]

C. Clinical findings.

1. Historical findings.
   a. Hematuria, increased frequency of urination, dysuria, and urinary incontinence are frequently associated with bladder tumors.[27,49] Signs may be present from a few days to months before a diagnosis is established. None of the signs is pathognomonic for neoplasia; animals with bacterial urinary tract infection, urolithiasis, and other disorders of the lower urinary tract may have similar signs.
   b. Dogs with tumors that cause partial or complete urethral obstruction make frequent attempts to urinate but pass little or no urine.

TABLE 44–7.
TYPE, AGE, AND SEX OF 1164 DOGS WITH A PRIMARY NEOPLASM OF THE URINARY BLADDER*

		Sex			Age (yr)		
Tumor Type	**Cases (No.)**	**Male**	**Female**	**Not Determined**	**Mean**	**Range**	**Not Determined**
Epithelial tissue							
Papilloma	36	9	23	4	10.6	3–15	3
Adenoma	3	1	1	1	10.3	8–13	1
Adenocarcinoma	78	43	35	0	8.9	2–15	0
Squamous cell carcinoma	50	11	38	1	9.9	5–15	1
Transitional cell carcinoma	797	287	507	3	10.9	½–15	7
Unclassified carcinoma	42	8	13	21	8.9	4–13	15
Muscle tissue							
Leiomyoma	12	1	2	9	12.7	12–13	7
Leiomyosarcoma	50	26	24	0	9.4	1–15	0
Botryoid rhabdomyosarcoma	20	7	10	3	1.3	½–5	4
Connective tissue							
Myxoma	1	1	0	0	13	—	0
Fibroma	12	1	2	10	7	4–11	7
Neurofibroma	6	0	6	0	10.5	3–13	0
Fibrosarcoma	21	7	13	1	8.6	1-15	1
Unclassified sarcoma	16	7	7	2	3.5	1–8	1
Vascular tissue							
Hemangioma	2	1	0	1	10	—	1
Hemangiosarcoma	18	11	7	0	9.7	2–15	0

*Data from the Veterinary Medical Data Program and the literature.[28]

TABLE 44–8.
TYPE, AGE, AND SEX OF 69 CATS WITH A PRIMARY NEOPLASM OF THE URINARY BLADDER*

		Sex			Age (yr)		
Tumor Type	**Cases (No.)**	**Male**	**Female**	**Not Determined**	**Mean**	**Range**	**Not Determined**
Epithelial tissue							
Papilloma	5	3	1	1	6.7	1/3–15	0
Cystadenoma	1	0	1	0	—	12	0
Adenocarcinoma	6	1	4	1	9.2	5–15	1
Squamous cell carcinoma	2	1	0	1	—	8	1
Transitional cell carcinoma	41	17	21	3	10.4	3–15	1
Unclassified carcinoma	5	3	0	2	13.3	13–14	2
Connective tissue							
Myxosarcoma	1	1	0	0	—	6	0
Fibrosarcoma	2	0	2	0	6.5	5–8	0
Muscle tissue							
Leiomyoma	4	1	3	0	6	1–12	0
Leiomyosarcoma	2	0	2	0	9.8	8.5–11	0

*Data from the Veterinary Medical Data Program and the literature.[28]

Residual urine and decreased bladder tone may predispose to urinary tract infection. If obstruction results in postrenal uremia, vomiting, depression, and decreased appetite may be noted.

c. Unilateral ureteral obstruction may result in hydronephrosis, which will probably be asymptomatic unless pyelonephritis is present. Obstruction of the ureter in the presence of infection can result in rapid destruction of the kidney. Bilateral ureteral obstruction may cause postrenal azotemia or uremia.

d. Polydypsia, which has been noted in up to 33% of dogs with bladder tumors, is thought to be psychogenic, because concentrated urine is usually produced following a water deprivation test.[11,51]

2. Physical examination findings.
   a. Early—and potentially curable—neoplasms typically do not produce abnormalities that can be detected by physical examination alone.
   b. Later, thickening of the bladder wall or a firm mass within the bladder can be detected by abdominal palpation. In addition, abdominal palpation may reveal cystic calculi, and, occasionally, enlargement of sublumbar lymph nodes.
   c. Distension of the urinary bladder associated with the passage of only small quantities of urine suggests urethral obstruction.
   d. Swollen, painful extremities resulting from hypertrophic osteopathy (HOA) has been noted in dogs with transitional cell carcinomas, rhabdomyosarcomas, and neurofibrosarcomas. HOA is most often seen in dogs with rhabdomyosarcomas and typically is not associated with pulmonary lesions.[31,72,73,75]
3. Laboratory findings.
   a. Complete blood counts and chemistry profiles are usually within normal limits, unless obstructive uropathy and postrenal azotemia are present.
   b. Microscopic examination of urine sediment typically reveals hematuria. Pyuria may be observed, especially if urinary tract infection is present.
   c. Cats are typically negative for the FeLV.[67]
   d. Cytologic examination of the urine sediment is very useful in establishing a diagnosis, especially in patients with transitional cell carcinomas.[49,51,76] Typically, one observes clusters of large anaplastic epithelial cells with prominent nuclear membranes and nucleoli, high nuclear-cytoplasmic ratio and variability in nuclear size. Because similar cells occasionally are observed in urine samples from animals with severe inflammatory cystitis, results should always be interpreted with other clinical and laboratory findings.[2] In dogs with rhabdomyosarcoma, evaluation of urine sediment

typically reveals large numbers of inflammatory cells and small numbers of small tumor cells with an eccentric nucleus and one or two prominent nucleoli.[73]

e. Material for cytologic examination can also be obtained by catheter biopsy[77] or percutaneous aspiration of bladder masses.
f. Evaluation of cytologic specimens should be performed before contrast radiology, because hypertonic contrast solutions can distort normal epithelial cells.
g. In humans, use of monoclonal antibodies directed against antigens expressed on the surface of tumor cells obtained from bladder washings has proven useful in the diagnosis of bladder cancer.[78]

4. Radiographic and ultrasonographic findings.
   a. Radiographic evaluations can provide presumptive evidence of bladder cancer, are helpful in accessing the clinical stage of disease, can aid in therapeutic planning, and can demonstrate urethral or ureteral obstruction and hypertrophic osteopathy.
   b. Survey radiographs of the abdomen may be normal or may reveal calcification of the bladder wall, urolithiasis, bladder distension, bladder displacement, or enlarged sublumbar lymph nodes.[49,51]
   c. Contrast cystography (pneumocystography, positive contrast cystography, or double-contrast cystography) usually demonstrates bladder tumors. Carcinomas typically arise from the trigone and protrude into the bladder lumen. In some instances, a diffuse increase in bladder wall thickness is noted. Severe inflammatory cystitis may be associated with lesions that mimic those produced by neoplasia. This is especially true in patients with polypoid cystitis.[64] Polypoid lesions that do not involve the trigone are likely to be benign.[79]
   d. Ureteral obstruction can be demonstrated by intravenous urography and urethral obstruction by voiding cystography.
   e. Thoracic radiographs aid in determining the presence of metastatic disease. In a study of 11 dogs with pulmonary metastases from transitional cell carcinomas of the bladder or urethra, four radiographic patterns were noted: (1) diffuse unstructured increase in interstitial density; (2) localized interstitial or alveolar infiltrates; (3) multiple interstitial nodules; and (4) normal pulmonary opacity.[80] The most common abnormality was the diffuse unstructured pattern, which can be confused with normal pulmonary changes of aging. Hilar lymphadenopathy was noted in one dog.
   f. Ultrasonographic evaluation of the bladder can be used to demonstrate tumors, determine the extent of bladder wall involvement, and document ureteral obstruction.[81] Compared to cystography, ultrasonography does not require injection of contrast media and usually does not require sedation.

D. Diagnosis and clinical staging.

1. Information obtained from the history, physical examination, urinalysis, cytologic examinations, and imaging procedures often provides a presumptive diagnosis of bladder cancer. Histopathologic evaluation of bladder tissue is required for a definitive diagnosis and to determine tumor cell type.
2. Samples for histopathologic examination can be obtained by catheter biopsy of the tumor,[77] cystoscopy,[82] or exploratory celiotomy.
3. To adequately determine the clinical stage in animals with bladder cancer (Table 44–9), one must ascertain the amount of bladder wall invasion, invasion into local organs such as the uterus or prostate, and spread to regional lymph nodes and lung. Survey and contrast radiography, ultrasonography, and computed tomography are helpful in determining stage, but at present celiotomy is required for a definitive determination.

E. Treatment.

1. The choice of therapy for bladder cancer depends on tumor type, extent and location of the tumor within the bladder, invasion into adjacent structures, and metastasis to regional lymph nodes or distant organs. In addition, concurrent problems such as renal failure, urinary tract infection, ure-

TABLE 44–9.
WHO CLINICAL STAGES OF CANINE TUMORS OF THE URINARY BLADDER*

T: Primary tumor†
- T1s Carcinoma in situ
- T0 No evidence of primary tumor
- T1 Superficial papillary tumor
- T2 Tumor invading the bladder wall, with induration
- T3 Tumor invading neighboring organs (prostate, uterus, vagina, anal canal)

N: Regional lymph nodes (RNL; internal and external iliac LN)
- N0 No RLN involved
- N1 RLN involved
- N2 RLN and juxtaregional nodes involved

M: Distant metastasis
- M0 No evidence of metastasis
- M1 Distant metastasis present (specify sites)

*Data from the World Health Organization. Report of the Second Consultation of the Biological Behavior and Therapy of Tumors of Domestic Animals. Geneva: WHO, 1979.

†The symbol "m" added to the appropriate T category indicates multiple tumors

thral or ureteral obstruction, and urolithiasis must be considered.

2. Benign tumors can be successfully treated by surgical removal, especially if the tumor does not involve the trigone. Following partial cystectomy, seven dogs with papillomas, two with hemangiomas and two with leiomyomas were alive 6 months to 5 years after surgery.[51] Ninety-five percent of dogs with fibromas were symptom free at least 3 months following tumor excision, and longterm survival has been reported for cats with leiomyomas and fibromas.[49,66]
3. The optimal therapy for animals with malignant bladder tumors has not been determined. Many treatment regimens have been attempted, including surgery (partial cystectomy or total cystectomy with urinary diversion), radiation therapy, chemotherapy, immunotherapy, and various combinations. Extensive disease at the time of diagnosis and a high rate of metastatic disease have limited survival times.
4. Partial cystectomy.
   a. Partial cystectomy can be employed to remove tumors that do not involve the trigone. Full-thickness cystectomy should be performed and an attempt made to remove a wide margin of normal tissue. Tumor handling should be minimized, to prevent seeding of tumor cells into the abdominal cavity or incision line.[83] More than 80% of the bladder can be removed without significant loss of capacity.[79] If the trigone is involved, one or both ureters can be transplanted into the bladder apex, but it may be difficult to obtain tumor-free margins.
   b. Benign tumors can be cured by partial cystectomy. Survival time for animals with malignant tumors tend to be short because of tumor recurrence or metastatic disease.[49]
5. Total cystectomy and urinary diversion.
   a. Complications from the diversion procedure or metastatic disease have limited the usefulness of total cystectomy.[84–87]
   b. Five months was the longest survival time for 10 dogs with transitional cell carcinomas of the bladder or urethra following complete removal of the bladder and proximal urethra and ureterocolonic anastomosis.[87] Six dogs had metastatic disease at the time of death. Complications of the diversion procedure included vomiting, anorexia, neurologic abnormalities, hyperchloremic metabolic acidosis, and pyelonephritis.
6. Radiation therapy.
   a. Both external-beam and intraoperative radiation therapy have been attempted in small numbers of animals. Overall, tumor control has been relatively short lived and complication rates high.
   b. Thirteen dogs received intraoperative radiation therapy following partial tumor excision.[88] Sixty-one percent were alive at 1 year, 46% at 18 months, and 23% at 2 years. One dog survived longer than 70 months. Persistence or recurrence of tumor was noted in 46% and metastasis in 39%. Significant complications from radiation therapy included increased frequency of urination (46%), urinary incontinence (46%), cystitis (38%), and stranguria (15%). Bladder wall fibrosis and resultant decreased bladder capacity were thought to be responsible for many of the adverse reactions.
   c. Fractionated external-beam radiation was used in seven dogs following partial tumor excision.[89] Mean survival time in dogs that completed therapy was 5 months; no dog lived longer than 13 months. Viable tumor was identified in five of the six dogs that were "necropsied." Hydroureter and urinary incontinence were frequent complications.
   d. Fractionated external beam radiation therapy combined with cisplatin was used in two dogs.[90] Tumor shrinkage and clinical improvement were noted in both dogs, but survival time was less than 7 months.
7. Chemotherapy.
   a. Intravesical chemotherapy (with agents including doxorubicin, triethylene thiophosphoramide, and mitomycin C) has been used in human patients with superficial bladder tumors.[53] Therapy has been useful in reducing recurrence rates in some patients.
   b. Systemic chemotherapy has resulted in complete or partial remission rates of 45 to 70% in humans with invasive disease. Chemotherapeutic protocols consisting of combinations of cisplatin, methotrexate, cyclophosphamide, and 5-fluorouracil have been found to be most effective.
   c. Few reports are available on use of systemic or local chemotherapy in animals, and only palliative benefits have been documented.
   d. In eight dogs with bladder or urethral transitional cell carcinomas, systemic cisplatin therapy resulted in one partial response and stabilization of disease in four dogs for 7½ to 8½ months.[91]
   e. In seven dogs, partial relief of symptoms was noted following therapy with combinations of intravesicular instillations of triethylene thiophosphoramide and/or 5-fluorouracil and systemic administration of 5-fluorouracil, doxorubicin, or cyclophosphamide.[92]
8. Immunotherapy.
   a. In mice, immunotherapy with bacillus Calmette-Guérin (BCG) significantly inhibited the growth of chemically induced bladder tumors.[93] In humans with superficial bladder tumors, intravesical and percutaneous BCG

immunotherapy decreased the rate of tumor recurrence.[94]

b. Injection of BCG into bladders of previously sensitized dogs resulted in inflammatory cystitis.[95] Clinical benefit was demonstrated in two of seven dogs treated with BCG at the time of partial tumor excision.[79]

9. Laser photodynamic therapy.
   a. Administration of photodynamic therapy involves a photosensitizer, usually a porphyrin compound, that is taken up by the tumor. A laser, then aimed at the photosensitizer, kills the tumor cells.
   b. Photodynamic therapy has been used successfully to treat superficial bladder cancer in humans.[96]
   c. In 10 dogs with transitional cell carcinomas, photodynamic therapy resulted in complete remission of stranguria and restored normal frequency of urination. Clinical remissions varied from 5 weeks to 4 months, but malignant cells and hematuria persisted in urine samples.[97]
10. Vitamin A derivatives and piroxicam.
   a. Vitamin A and synthetic retinoids block phenotypic expression, inhibit growth, and induce differentiation in many malignant cell types. The anticancer effect of retinoids may result from a modulating effect on protein kinase C.[98] Some of the retinoids that have been evaluated for clinical efficacy include tretinoin, etretinate, isotretinoin, and arotinoid.
   b. Retinoids have been demonstrated to have a chemoprotective effect against experimental urinary bladder tumors in mice and rats.[99]
   c. Etretinate and isotretinoin have induced complete and partial remission in 30 to 100% of human bladder cancer patients.[98]
   d. Piroxicam, a nonsteroidal anti-inflammatory drug that inhibits arachidonic acid metabolism, has been demonstrated to have a chemopreventive effect in experimental colon cancer in rats.[100]
   e. Piroxicam was used to treat 24 dogs with transitional cell carcinomas of the bladder. Four dogs had partial remissions, eleven had stable disease, and eight had progressive disease.[101] Mild gastrointestinal toxicity occurred in four dogs. Median survival time was 150 days, which was similar to that achieved with cisplatin chemotherapy.
11. Palliative therapy.
   a. Palliation of clinical signs is possible with currently available treatment methods and supportive care.
   b. Urothelial damage and urinary retention predispose animals with bladder cancer to bacterial urinary tract infection. Invasive procedures, such as catheterization, should be kept to a minimum. Urine should be cultured frequently and urinary tract infection treated vigorously with antibiotics chosen on the basis of sensitivity tests.

F. Prognosis.

1. The prognosis is good for benign tumors that can be completely excised.
2. The longterm prognosis for most animals with bladder tumors is poor, owing to extensive bladder wall invasion at the time of diagnosis and a high prevalence of metastatic disease. Surgery, chemotherapy, or radiation therapy may reduce the tumor burden enough to induce short-term improvement in clinical signs.
3. Treatment of complicating factors such as urolithiasis and urinary tract infection also alleviates clinical signs and improves short-term prognosis.

IV. URETHRA

A. Epidemiology and etiology.

1. Primary urethral tumors are rare in dogs and cats.
2. More females are affected than males; tumors are usually identified in older animals (mean age in dogs, 10.4 years).[102–104] The cause of the female predominance has not been determined.
3. Beagles may be at increased risk.[104]
4. The cause of urethral neoplasia in animals has not been established. In humans, chronic urethral irritation has been suggested as a possible risk factor.[105]

B. Pathology and biologic behavior.

1. Urethral tumors occur most frequently in the prostatic urethra in males and in the distal urethra, or throughout the urethra, in females.
2. Transitional cell carcinomas and squamous cell carcinomas are the most common urethral tumors identified (Table 43–10).
3. Urethral tumors tend to grow slowly, invade surrounding organs, and metastasize late in their course. Local invasion into the bladder occurs in about one third of cases.[104] Metastasis to local lymph nodes and/or the lung has been identified in approximately 30% of canine cases.[103]

C. Clinical findings.

1. Chronic dysuria is the clinical sign most frequently identified. Hematuria, urinary incontinence, and urethral discharge may also be noted. Signs of uremia may indicate obstructive uropathy.
2. A posterior abdominal mass and bladder distension may be noted on physical examination. In many cases, the urethral tumor can be palpated per rectum. The entire urethra may feel turgid, or a discrete mass may be palpated.
3. Vaginoscopy may reveal a mass protruding from the urethral orifice. Urethral catheterization may be difficult or impossible.

D. Diagnosis.

1. Neoplastic cells may be identified in the urine sediment.
2. Survey abdominal radiographs may reveal a pos-

TABLE 44–10.
TYPE, AGE, AND SEX OF 340 DOGS WITH A PRIMARY NEOPLASM OF THE URETHRA*

Tumor Type	Cases (No.)	Sex			Age (yr)		
		Male	Female	Not Determined	Mean	Range	Not Determined
Epithelial tissue							
Adenoma	5	1	0	4	—	5	4
Adenocarcinoma	17	5	11	1	11.3	5–15	1
Squamous cell carcinoma	35	5	30	0	10.5	5–13	0
Transitional cell carcinoma	275	36	239	0	7	6mo–15yr	5
Unclassifed carcinoma	1	0	1	0	—	15	0
Connective tissue							
Fibroma	1	1	0	0	—	5	0
Myxoma	1	1	0	0	—	13	0
Myxosarcoma	1	0	1	1	—	9	0
Muscle tissue							
Leiomyoma	1	0	1	0	—	8	0
Rhabdomyosarcoma	1	1	0	0	—	3	0
Vascular tissue							
Hemangiosarcoma	2	0	2	0	9.5	9–10	0

*Data from the Veterinary Medical Data Program and the literature.[28]

terior abdominal mass, sublumbar lymphadenopathy, or vertebral lysis.

3. Urethral tumors usually can be demonstrated by contrast radiography. If the urethra can be catheterized, a positive-contrast urethrogram is the technique of choice. If catheterization is not possible, a positive-contrast vaginogram or intravenous urogram may allow visualization of the urethra. Typical lesions include multiple, poorly marginated intraluminal masses that result in a generalized moth-eaten appearance of the urethra.[106] Contrast media may extend into the periurethral tissues.
4. Chest radiographs should be taken to rule out pulmonary involvement.
5. History, physical findings, and radiographic studies usually localize the disease to the urethra. Urethral tumors can be definitively diagnosed by biopsy. Material for histopathologic examination can be obtained by catheter biopsy of urethra[77] or by surgical exploration of the pelvic urethra. A pelvic osteotomy may be required to adequately visualize the tumor and to evaluate its extent.

E. Treatment.

1. By the time of diagnosis, urethral involvement is usually extensive, and an optimal method of therapy has not been determined.
2. Therapeutic options include surgical excision, radiation therapy, and chemotherapy.
3. Survival times up to 22 months following partial urethrectomy have been reported in dogs with involvement limited to the cranial third of the urethra.[102]
4. Complete urethrectomy, cystectomy, and urinary diversion is associated with the same problems described in the treatment of bladder neoplasia.
5. Radiation therapy may result in short-term improvement of clinical signs and may delay tumor progression. Survival times of 4 months were reported in two dogs treated with intraoperative radiation therapy.[89]
6. Chemotherapy has been evaluated in small numbers of animals. Cisplatin produced stabilization of disease in two dogs, for 4 and 8 months, respectively (authors' data).[91]

F. Prognosis.

1. Longterm prognosis for dogs with urethral tumors is poor because of extensive local disease at the time of diagnosis and a high rate of metastatic disease.
2. Radiation therapy and/or chemotherapy may result in reduction of clinical signs and increase survival time by several months.

REFERENCES

1. Baskin GB, DePaoli A. Primary renal neoplasms of the dog. *Vet Pathol.* 1977;14:591.
2. Caywood DD, Osborne CA, Johnston GR. Neoplasms of the

canine and feline urinary tract. In: Kirk RW, ed. *Current Veterinary Therapy* VII. Philadelphia: WB Saunders, 1980.

3. Hayes HM, Fraumeni JF. Canine renal neoplasm: Epidemiologic features. *Cancer Res.* 1977;37:2553.
4. Klein MK, et al. Canine primary renal neoplasms: A retrospective review of 54 cases. *J Am Anim Hosp Assoc.* 1988;24:443.
5. Moulton JR. *Tumors of the Urinary System.* Berkley: University of California Press, 1978.
6. Osborne CA, Low DG, Finco DR, eds. *Canine and Feline Urology.* Philadelphia, WB Saunders, 1972.
7. Peterson ME. Inappropriate erythropoietin production from a renal carcinoma in a dog with polycythemia. *JAVMA.* 1981; 179:995.
8. Cosenza SF, Seely JC. Generalized nodular dermatofibrosis and real cystadenocarcinomas in a German shepherd dog. *JAVMA.* 1986;189:1587.
9. Luim B, Moe L. Hereditary multifocal renal cystadenocarcinomas and nodular dermatofibrosis in the German shepherd dog: Macroscopic and histopathologic changes. *Vet Pathol.* 1985;22:447.
10. Suter M, Lott-Stolz G, Wild P. Generalized nodular dermatofibrosis in six Alsatians. *Vet Pathol.* 1983;20:632.
11. Crow SE. Urinary tract neoplasms in dogs and cats. *Comp Contin Ed.* 1985;7:607.
12. Rickham PP. Malignant tumors involving the genitourinary system. In: Johnston JH, Scholtmyer RJ, eds. *Problems in Pediatric Urology.* Amsterdam: Excerpta Medica, 1972.
13. Willson JE, Gillmore CE. Malignant lymphoma in a cat with involvement of the kidneys demonstrated radiographically. *JAVMA.* 1962;140:1068.
14. Osborne CA, Johnson KH, Hurtz HJ, Hanlon GF. Renal lymphoma in the dog and cat. *JAVMA.* 1971;158:2058.
15. Diters RW, Wells M. Renal interstitial cell tumors in the dog. *Vet Pathol.* 1986;23:74.
16. Brown NO. Paraneoplastic syndromes of humans, dogs and cats. *J Am Anim Hosp Assoc.* 1981;17:911.
17. Gorse MJ. Polycythemia associated with renal fibrosarcoma in a dog. *JAVMA.* 1988;192:793.
18. Waters D, Prueter JC. Secondary polycythemia associated with renal disease in the dog: two case reports and review of the literature. *J Am Anim Hosp Assoc.* 1988;24:109.
19. Balsaver AM, Gibley CW, Tessurer CF. Ultrastructural studies in Wilms' tumors. *Cancer.* 1968;22:417.
20. Rickham PP. Wilms' tumor. In: Rob C, Smith R, eds. *Operative Surgery.* London: Butterworth, 1972.
21. Ladd WE. Embryoma of the kidney (Wilms' tumor). *Ann Surg.* 1938;108:885.
22. Caywood DD, et al. Hypertrophic osteoarthropathy associated with an atypical nephroblastoma in a dog. *J Am Anim Hosp Assoc.* 1980;16:855.
23. D'Angio GJ. Radiation therapy in Wilms' tumor. *JAMA.* 1968; 204:124.
24. Garrett RA, Donohue JI, Arnold TL. Metastatic renal nephroma: Survival following therapy. *J Urol.* 1967;98:444.
25. James DH, Austu O, Wren EL, Johnston WW. Childhood malignant tumors—concurrent chemotherapy with dactinomycin and vincristine sulfate. *JAMA.* 1966;197:1043.
26. Mulligan RM. Comparative pathology in human and canine cancer. *Ann NY Acad Sci.* 1963;108:642.
27. Osborne CA, et al. Neoplasms of the canine and feline urinary bladder: Incidence, etiologic factors, occurrence and pathologic features. *Am J Vet Res.* 1968;29:2041.
28. Caywood D, Klausner J, Walter P. Tumors of the urinary system. In: Slatter D, ed. *Textbook of Small Animal Surgery.* 2nd ed. Vol 2, Philadelphia: WB Saunders; pp 2200–2212, 1993.
29. Mooney SC, Hayes AA, Matus RE, MacEwen EG. Renal lymphoma in cats: 28 cases (1977–1984). *JAVMA.* 1987;191: 1473.
30. Brody R, Craig PH. Hypertrophic osteoarthropathy in a dog with pulmonary metastasis arising from a renal adenocarcinoma. *JAVMA.* 1958;132:231.
31. Brody RS, Riser WH, Allen H. Hypertrophic pulmonary osteoarthropathy in a dog with carcinoma of the urinary bladder. *JAVMA.* 1973;162:474–478.
32. Burger GT, et al. Renal carcinoma in a dog. *JAVMA.* 1977; 171:282.
33. Habermann RT, Williams FP. Papillary cystic adenocarcinoma of a kidney in a dog. *JAVMA.* 1963;142:1011.
34. Nielson S, Archiblad J. Canine renal disorders. III. Renal carcinoma in 3 dogs. *North Am Vet.* 1955;36:36.
35. Zontinue WJ. Renal neoplasia and hematuria. *Pulse.* 1966;8:8.
36. World Health Organization. *Report of the Second Consultation of the Biological Behavior and Therapy of Tumors of Domestic Animals.* Geneva: WHO, 1979.
37. Farber S, D'Angio G, Evans A, Metus A. Clinical studies of actinomycin D with special reference to Wilms' tumor in children. *Ann NY Acad Sci.* 1960;89:421.
38. Greene FL, Donaldson MH. Chemotherapy of Wilms' tumor. *New Physician.* 1970;19:598.
39. Howard R. Actinomycin D in Wilms' tumor: Treatment of lungs metastasis. *Arch Dis Child.* 1965;40:200.
40. Schweisquth O, Schleiger MJ. Actinomycin D associated with irradiation in the treatment of Wilms' tumor. *Ann Radiol.* 1967;10:657.
41. Berzon JL. Primary leiomyosarcoma of the ureter of a dog. *JAVMA.* 1979;175:374.
42. Hanika C, Rebar AH. Ureteral transitional cell carcinoma in the dog. *Vet Pathol.* 1980;17:643.
43. Liska WD, Rebar AH. Leiomyoma of the ureter of a dog. *J Am Anim Hosp Assoc.* 1977;13:83.
44. Jabara AG. Three cases of primary malignant neoplasms arising in the canine urinary system. *J Comp Pathol.* 1968;78:335.
45. Cotchin E. Spontaneous carcinoma of the urinary bladder of the dog. *Br Vet J.* 1959;115:431–435.
46. Hayes HM. Canine bladder cancer: epidemiologic features. *Am J Epidemiol.* 1976;104:673.
47. Wimberly HC, Lewis RM. Transitional cell carcinoma in the domestic cat. *Vet Pathol.* 1979;16:223.
48. Brown RR, Price JM. Quantitative studies on metabolites of tryptophan in the urine of the dog, cat, rat, and man. *J Biol Chem.* 1956;219:985.
49. Schwarz PD, Green RW, Patnaik AK. Urinary bladder tumors in the cat: A review of 27 cases. *J Am Anim Hosp Assoc.* 1985;21:237.
50. Raghavan D, et al. Biology and management of bladder cancer. *N Engl J Med.* 1990;322:1129.
51. Burnie AG, Weaver AD. Urinary bladder neoplasia in the dog: A review of seventy cases. *J Small Anim Pract.* 1983;24:129.
52. Kelly DF. Rhabdomyosarcoma in the urinary bladder of a dog. *Vet Pathol.* 1973;18:375.
53. Richie JP, Shipley WU, Yagoda A. Cancer of the urinary bladder. In: DeVita S, Hellman M, Rosenberg SA, eds.*Cancer: Principles and Practice of Oncology.* 2nd ed. Philadelphia: JB Lippincott, 1989.
54. Bryan G. The pathogenesis of experimental bladder cancer. *Cancer Res.* 1977;37:2813.
55. Okajima E, et al. Urinary bladder tumors induced by *N*-butyl-*N*-(4-hydroxybutyl)nitrosamine in dogs. *Cancer Res.* 1981;41: 1958.
56. Suzuki E, et al. Species variations in the metabolism of

N-butyl-*N*-(4-hydroxybutyl) nitrosamine and related compounds in relation to urinary bladder carcinogenesis. *Gann.* 1983;74:60.

57. Rippe D, et al. Urinary bladder carcinogenesis in the dog: Preliminary studies on cellular immunity. *Transplant Proc.* 1975;7:495.
58. Harzmann R, et al. Induction of a transplantable urinary bladder carcinoma in dogs. *Invest Urol.* 1980;18:24.
59. Hayes H, Hoover R, Tarone R. Bladder cancer in pet dogs: A sentinel for environmental cancer? *Am J Epidemiol.* 1981; 114:229.
60. Glickman L, Schofer F, McKee L. Epidemiologic study of insecticide exposures, obesity, and risk of bladder cancer in household dogs. *J Toxicol Environ Health.* 1989;28:407.
61. Macy DW, Withrow SJ, Hoopes J. Transitional cell carcinoma of the bladder associated with cyclophosphamide administration. *J Am Animal Hosp Assoc.* 1983;19:965.
62. Weller RE, Wolf AM, Oyejide A. Transitional cell carcinoma of the bladder associated with cyclophosphamide therapy in a dog. *J Am Anim Hosp Assoc.* 1979;15:733.
63. Stillwell T, Benson R. Cyclophosphamide-induced hemorrhagic cystitis. A review of 100 patients. *Cancer.* 1988;61:451.
64. Johnston SJ, Osborne CA, Stevens JB. Canine polypoid cystitis. In: Kirk RW, ed. *Current Veterinary Therapy VII.* Philadelphia: WB Saunders, 1980.
65. Birchard SJ, et al. Fibroma of the urinary bladder of a dog. *J Am Anim Hosp Assoc.* 1982;18:63.
66. Esplin DG. Urinary bladder fibromas in dogs: 51 cases (1981–1985). *JAVMA.* 1987;190:440.
67. Patnaik AK, Schwartz PD, Green RW. A histopathologic study of twenty urinary bladder neoplasms in the cat. *J Small Anim Pract.* 1986;27:433.
68. Stone EA. Urogenital tumors. *Vet Clin North Am.* 1988;15:597.
69. McCaw DL, Hogan PM, Shaw DP. Canine urinary bladder transitional cell carcinoma with skull metastasis and unusual pulmonary metastases. *Can Vet J.* 1988;29:386.
70. Perry R, et al. Transitional cell carcinoma of the bladder with skeletal metastases in a dog. *J Am Anim Hosp Assoc.* 1989;25:547.
71. Halliwell WH, Ackerman N. Botryoid rhabdomyosarcoma of the urinary bladder and hypertrophic osteoarthropathy in a young dog. *JAVMA.* 1974;165:911.
72. Pletcher JM, Dalton L. Botryoid rhabdomyosarcoma in the urinary bladder of a dog. *Vet Pathol.* 1981;18:695.
73. Rozel JF. Cytology of urine from dogs with botryoid sarcoma of the bladder. *Acta Cytol.* 1972;16:443.
74. Stamps P, Harris DL. Botryoid rhabdomyosarcoma of the urinary bladder of a dog. *JAVMA.* 1968;153:1064.
75. Mandel M. Hypertrophic osteoarthropathy secondary to neurofibrosarcoma of the urinary bladder in a cocker spaniel. *VM/SAC.* 1975;70:1307.
76. Rozengurt N, et al. Urinary cytology of a canine bladder carcinoma. *J Comp Pathol.* 1986;96:581.
77. Melhoff T, Osborne CA. Catheter biopsy of the urethra, urinary bladder and prostate gland. In: Kirk RW, ed. Current Veterinary Therapy VI. Philadelphia: WB Saunders, 1977.
78. McCabe R, et al. Monoclonal antibodies in the detection of bladder cancer. In: Kupchik H, *Cancer Diagnosis in vitro Using Monoclonal Antibodies.* New York: Marcel Dekker; 1988.
79. Withrow SJ. Tumors of the urinary system. In: Withrow SJ, MacEwen EG, eds. *Clinical Veterinary Oncology.* Philadelphia, JB Lippincott, 1989.
80. Walter PA, et al. Radiographic appearance of pulmonary metastases from transitional cell carcinoma of the bladder and urethra of the dog. *JAVMA.* 1984;185:411.
81. Abu-Yousef MM. Ultrasound of bladder tumors. *Semin Ultrasound CT MR.* 1986;7:275.
82. Cooper JE, et al. Cystoscopic examination of male and female dogs. *Vet Rec.* 1984;115:571.
83. Anderson WI, et al. Presumptive subcutaneous surgical transplantation of urinary bladder transitional cell carcinoma in a dog. *Cornell Vet.* 1989;79:263.
84. Bjorling DE, Mahaffey MB, Crowell WA. Bilateral ureteroileostomy and perineal urinary diversion in dogs. *Vet Surg.* 1985;14:204.
85. Bovee KC, et al. Trigonal-colonic anastomosis: A urinary diversion procedure in dogs. *JAVMA.* 1979;174:184.
86. Montgomery RD, Hankes GH. Ureterocolonic anastomosis in a dog with transitional cell carcinoma of the urinary bladder. *JAVMA.* 1987;190:1427.
87. Stone EA, et al. Ureterocolonic anastomosis in ten dogs with transitional cell carcinoma. *Vet Surg.* 1988;17:147.
88. Walker M, Breider M. Intraoperative radiotherapy of canine bladder cancer. *Vet Radiol.* 1987;28:200–204.
89. Withrow SJ, et al. Intraoperative irradiation of 16 spontaneously occurring canine neoplasms. *Vet Surg.* 1989;18:7.
90. McCaw DL, Lattimer JC. Radiation and cisplatin for treatment of canine urinary bladder carcinoma—a report of two case histories. *Vet Radiol.* 1988;29:264.
91. Shapiro W, et al. Cisplatin for treatment of transitional cell and squamous cell carcinomas in the dog. *JAVMA.* 1988;193: 1530.
92. Crow SE, Klausner JS. Management of transitional cell carcinomas of the urinary bladder. In: Kirk RW, ed. *Current Veterinary Therapy VIII.* Philadelphia: WB Saunders, 1983.
93. Lamm D, Harris S, Gittes, R. Bacillus Calmette-Guerin and dinitrochlorobenzene immunotherapy of chemically induced bladder tumors. *Invest Urol.* 1977;14:369.
94. Lamm D, et al. Bacillus Calmette-Guerin immunotherapy of superficial bladder cancer. *J Urol.* 1980;124:38.
95. Bloomberg SD, et al. The effects of BCG on the dog bladder. *Invest Urol.* 1975;12:423.
96. Benson R. Laser photodynamic therapy for bladder cancer. *Mayo Clin Proc.* 1986;61:859.
97. Beck E, et al. Response of canine transitional cell carcinomas to photodynamic therapy. *J Vet Intern Med.* 1990;4:119.
98. Lippman S, Meyskens FJ. Vitamin A derivatives in prevention and treatment of human cancer. *J Am Col Nutr.* 1988;7:269.
99. Moon R, Metha R. Chemoprevention of experimental carcinogenesis in animals. *Prev Med.* 1989;18:576.
100. Boone C, Kelloff G, Malone W. Identification of candidate cancer chemopreventive agents and their evaluation in animal models and human clinical trials. *Cancer Res.* 1990;50:2.
101. Knapp D, et al. Piroxicam therapy in twenty-four dogs with transitional cell carcinoma of the bladder. *J Vet Intern Med.* 1991;5:140.
102. Davies JV, Read HM. Urethral tumors in dogs. *J Sm Anim Pract.* 1990;31:131.
103. Tarvin G, Patnaik A, Green R. Primary urethral tumors in dogs. *JAVMA.* 1978;172:931.
104. Wilson GP, Hayes HM, Casey HW. Canine urethral cancer. *J Am Anim Hosp Assoc.* 1979;15:741.
105. Grabstald H. Tumors of the urethra in men and women. *Cancer.* 1973;32:1236.
106. Ticer G, Spencer CP, Ackerman N. Transitional cell carcinoma of the urethra in four female dogs: Its urethrographic appearance. *Vet Radiol.* 1980;21:12.

CHAPTER 45

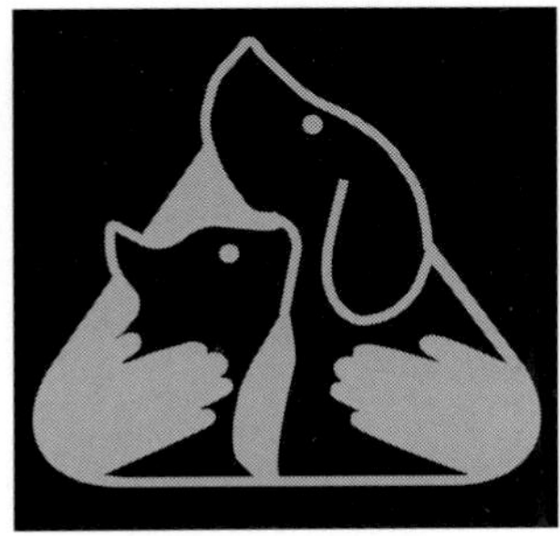

Parasites of the Upper and Lower Urinary Tract of Dogs and Cats

DONALD G. LOW

I. DIOCTOPHYMA RENALE

A. Introduction.

1. *Dioctophyma renale,* the largest known nematode, occurs throughout the world and has been reported in many species of animals, including dogs, mink, coyotes, jackals, raccoons, foxes, wolves, beech marten, pine marten, polecat, otters, weasels, seals, other wild carnivores, pigs, horses, cattle, and humans. Minks, the most commonly infected mustelids, are the principal definitive host. Up to 50% of minks may be infected in some areas.[4,10,15]

B. Morphology.

1. In dogs, the male worm can be as long as 45 cm and 4 to 6 mm in diameter, whereas the female may be up to 103 cm long and 5 to 12 mm in diameter (Figs. 45–1 and 45–2). In smaller hosts, such as the mink, the parasite is smaller. In minks, the length of the female may be about 30 cm.[4] Both males and females are blood red.

C. Life cycle.

1. If they are to complete the life cycle, both male and female parasites must be located in the same kidney of the host, and that kidney must be patent to the exterior.
2. The brownish-yellow eggs are barrel shaped. They are pitted, except at the poles.
3. The eggs measure 71 to 84 μm by 45 to 52 μm.[10,15]
4. Eggs are passed in the urine of the host.
5. The eggs embryonate slowly in water and require 1 to 7 months, depending on the temperature of the water, to produce first-stage larvae. The eggs may remain viable as long as 5 years.[9,15]
6. They hatch only after being swallowed by the intermediate host, an annelid worm.
7. The free-living oligochaete annelid, *Lumbriculus variegatus,* is the only intermediate host required to complete the life cycle. A developmental period of more than 100 days in the annelid is needed. Second-stage larvae develop and encyst in the annelid worm.
8. The definitive hosts may become infected by ingesting the infective larvae in annelids.[9,15]
9. Paratenic hosts may occur in the life cycle. In the United States, the northern black bullhead, *Ictalurus nebulosus,* is an important paratenic host, whereas in other countries, frogs and pike are frequent paratenic hosts. Pumpkin seed fish, *Lepomis gibbosus,* have recently been found to carry infective larvae.[11]
10. The larvae encyst in the liver, mesentery, stomach wall, or abdominal muscles of the paratenic host.
11. The definitive host becomes infected by ingesting raw fish or frogs, by eating viscera from a paratenic host, or by ingesting the free-living annelid worms.[10,13,15]
12. In the final host, the infective larvae penetrate the bowel wall and develop in the body cavity.
    a. After being swallowed by the definitive host, the infective larvae penetrate the stomach or

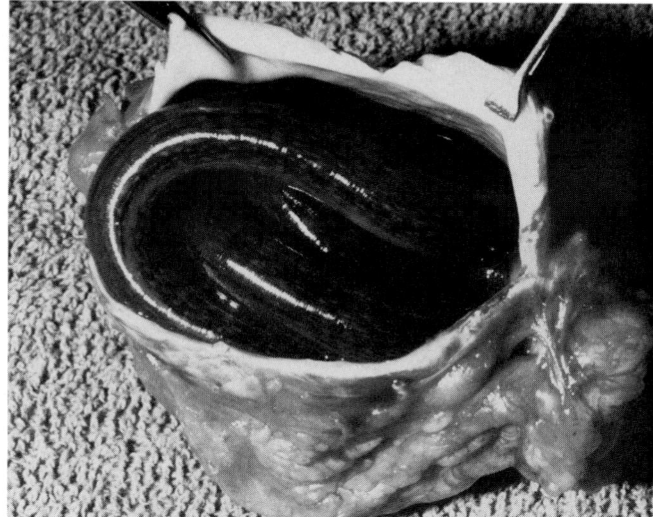

FIG. 45–1. Adult male and female *Dioctophyma renale* in the right kidney of a 15-month-old golden retriever dog (see Fig. 45–2). (Osborne CA, et al. *Dioctophyma renale* in the dog. *J Am Vet Med Assoc.* 1969;155:605–620.)

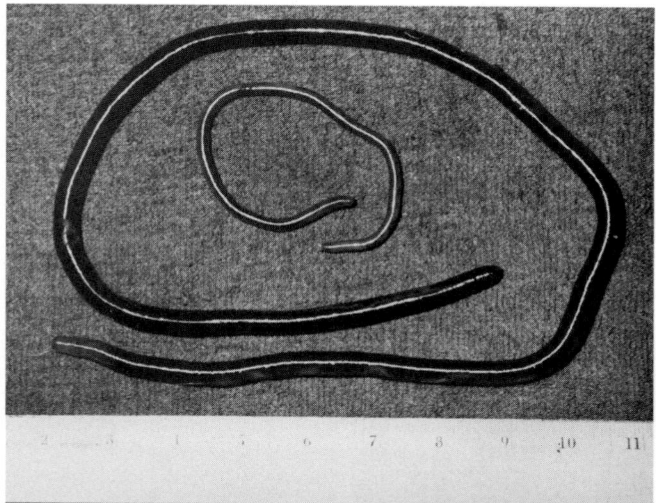

FIG. 45–2. Male and female *Dioctophyma renale* obtained from the right kidney of the dog described in Figure 45-1. (Osborne CA, et al. *Dioctophyma renale* in the dog. *J Am Vet Med Assoc.* 1969;155:605–620.)

bowel wall to the submucosa. After approximately 5 days, they migrate to the liver and remain there for about 50 days. Migration to the kidney (usually the right kidney) follows.[13]

b. In dogs, the parasite often fails to reach the kidney and instead is found free in the abdominal cavity or between lobes of the liver.[6,8]

c. The time required for infective larvae to become mature gravid females in the definitive host is 3½ to 6 months.[4]

d. The parasites survive in dogs for 1 to 3 years.[4]

D. Lesions.

1. The worms destroy the parenchyma of the kidney after entering at the pelvis. The exact mechanism of destruction is not known, but obstruction and secondary hydronephrosis are important factors, as is pressure necrosis (Figs. 45–3 and 45–4).
2. Most often, only one kidney is invaded and the host is able to survive nicely on the opposite kidney while the parenchyma of the affected kidney is destroyed.[12]
3. The affected kidney is reduced to a sac containing the worm or worms, plus a sanguinopurulent fluid containing red blood cells, parasite eggs, white blood cells, and epithelial cells (see Fig. 45–3).
4. Worms may be found free in the peritoneal cavity, where they commonly cause adhesions and chronic peritonitis. They may also destroy liver parenchyma.[3]
5. If both kidneys are parasitized, or if one kidney is parasitized and the opposite kidney is failing, lesions associated with renal failure may be present.[12]
6. If some renal parenchyma remains in a parasitized kidney, it may become partially calcified.[15]
7. In minks, 84 adult worms were distributed as follows[9]:

Right kidney	86%
Left kidney	5%
Abdominal cavity	5%
Omentum	1%
Partially emerged from duodenum	1%
Among fold of liver	2%

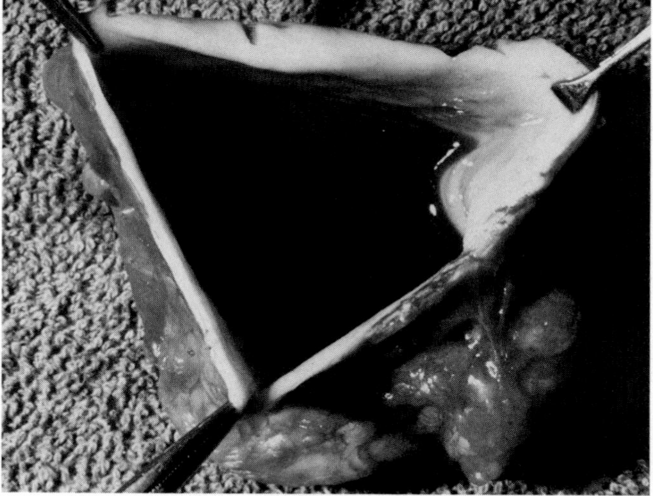

FIG. 45–3. Right kidney of the dog described in Figure 45-1 following removal of the male and female *Dioctophyma renale* organisms described in Figure 45-2.

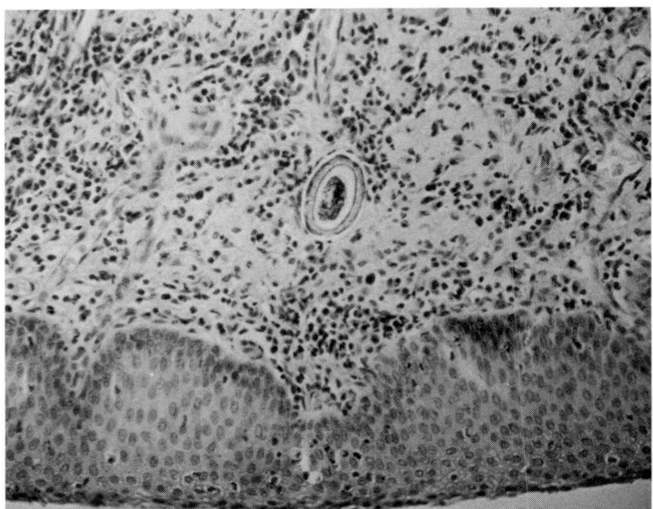

FIG. 45–4. Photomicrograph of a section of the hydronephrotic kidney described in Figures 45-1 and 45-3. An egg of *Dioctophyma renale* can be seen in the wall of the kidney beneath hyperplastic transitional epithelium of the renal pelvis. (Hematoxylin and eosin stain, 400× original magnification.)

8. In dogs, the following distribution was reported from 204 cases[12]:

Abdominal cavity only	58
Right kidney*	43
Left kidney*	15
Undesignated	108

* Sum greater than 204 because some dogs with adult worms in one kidney had other adult worms at other locations.

E. Clinical signs.

1. When only one kidney has been invaded with *D. renale* and the opposite kidney is normal, dogs often show few signs of infection.
2. Careful palpation of the abdomen may detect the enlarged hydronephrotic kidney.
3. Hematuria and dysuria have been observed by some owners and are especially noticeable at the end of micturition.
4. If both kidneys are parasitized, or if one is parasitized and the other is diseased, signs of chronic renal failure may be evident.
5. Rectal temperatures as high as 104° F have been reported in association with the presence of *D. renale* free in the abdominal cavity. Severe abdominal pain has also been reported in that circumstance.[3]

F. Laboratory findings.

1. When a gravid female worm is present in a kidney that has a patent track to the exterior, a microscopic examination of urine sediment from that host usually reveals the ova of *D. renale.* (See Chapter 7, A Clinician's Analysis of Urinalysis.) Other signs of inflammation are usually also found. This includes red blood cells, white blood cells, and protein.
2. Renal function tests may reveal results that are typical of chronic renal failure when both kidneys are parasitized or when one kidney contains parasites and the contralateral kidney is seriously diseased.

G. Other tests.

1. Radiography may reveal the enlarged hydronephrotic kidney. If intravenous urography is performed, it may demonstrate inability of the parasitized kidney to excrete the contrast agent.
2. Ultrasonography may show that the affected kidney is enlarged and contains excessive fluid.

H. Diagnosis.

1. If the gravid female parasite is located in a kidney that has a patent ureter, the diagnosis is based on the characteristic ova found by microscopic examination of the urine sediment.
2. When the worms are free in the peritoneal cavity, the diagnosis is usually made through exploratory laparotomy. The adult worms are often found between lobes of the liver.[3]

I. Treatment.

1. Nephrectomy is usually the treatment of choice when only one kidney is affected and the opposite kidney is capable of good function.
2. In patients with parasites in both kidneys nephrotomy with removal of the parasites may be indicated if sufficient functional tissue remains to sustain life. No report of such a procedure being performed in this situation was found.
3. If parasites are found free in the peritoneal cavity, they are removed at exploratory surgery.

J. Prevention.

1. Dogs and cats should not be permitted to eat raw fish or fish viscera, especially in areas where *D. renale* is known to exist.

II. CAPILLARIA PLICA, CAPILLARIA FELISCATI

A. Introduction.

1. *Capillaria plica* is widely distributed throughout the world. It is found in the urinary bladder, and less frequently in the ureters and renal pelves, of dogs, cats, foxes, raccoons, martens, badgers, otters, bobcats, and wolves. *Capillaria feliscati* is found less commonly in the urinary bladder of cats. The two species have similar biologic properties.[2,4] Several species of wild animals appear to be the primary host; for example, 48% of 320 British wild red foxes were infected with *C. plica.*[1] It was found in 64% of 70 raccoons in western Kentucky.[2]

B. Morphology.

1. The adult worm is a small, fragile, thread-like yellowish parasite. Males are generally 13 to 30 mm long, whereas females are 30 to 60 mm long.[4,5]

2. The eggs have bipolar plugs, are colorless, and have a slightly pitted shell. (See Chapter 7, A Clinician's Analysis of Urinalysis.) They measure 63 to 68 by 24 to 27 μm [4,5,7]

C. Life Cycle.

1. The eggs, which contain a single cell, are passed in the urine.
2. The first-stage larvae develop in approximately 1 month but do not hatch unless they are ingested by an earthworm.
3. The definitive host becomes infected by eating earthworms that have first-stage larvae in their tissues.
4. Eggs first appear in the urine of the definitive host about 2 months after ingestion of infective larvae.
5. Direct transmission by feeding embryonated eggs to foxes failed to accomplish infection, but ingestion of earthworms completed the life cycle.
6. Ingestion of embryonated eggs by beagle puppies failed to cause infection, whereas ingestion of earthworms collected from yards of a kennel caused patent infection 61 to 68 days later. The dogs did not find earthworms palatable and may ingest them inadvertently during grooming.[14] Foxes and racoons may find earthworms more acceptable as food than do dogs and cats.
7. Eggs were not found in the urine voided by pups younger than 8 months of age.

D. Lesions.

1. Adult worms weave the anterior portion of their bodies into the mucous membrane of the urinary bladder, and at times into the mucous membrane of the ureters and renal pelvis.
2. Submucosal edema of the urinary bladder has been reported in the vicinity of adult worms.[4,14]

E. Clinical signs.

1. Most often, dogs and cats with urinary capillariasis are asymptomatic.[4]
2. Some animals may exhibit signs of pollakiuria, polydipsia, urinary incontinence, and inappropriate micturition.[14]

F. Laboratory findings.

1. Urinalysis.
   a. Signs of inflammation may be present.
      (1). Microscopic hematuria has been reported.
      (2). Many transitional epithelial cells may be observed in the urine sediment.[14]
   b. *C. plica* eggs are easily seen, though at times are few in number. The mean width of *C. plica* eggs is about 28.5 ± 1.4 μm, whereas the length is 63 ± 3.1 μm.[14]
   c. Twenty-four-hour egg counts from 8 infected dogs yielded mean counts ranging from 666 to 25,333.[14]
   d. Twenty-four-hour egg counts from 3 infected dogs isolated in cages for 84 days diminished until, eventually, eggs were undetectable. This was interpreted as suggesting that a *Capillaria* infection, in the absence of reinfection, may be self-limiting.[14]

G. Diagnosis.

1. The diagnosis is made by finding typical eggs via microscopic examination of urine sediment.

H. Treatment.

1. Urinary capillariasis is most often asymptomatic and, in the absence of reinfection, may be self-limiting.
2. Suggested treatments.
   a. Levamisole, 2.5 mg/kg daily for 5 days.
   b. In a cat treated for *C. feliscati* infection, success was reported following administration of 2 doses of levamisole, 145 mg, at an interval of 1 week.[7]
   c. An oral dose of fenbendazole, 50 mg/kg/d for 3 days, has been reported to be effective.[5] However, several recent reports indicate that fenbendazole is not efficacious against urinary capillariasis.[8]
   d. Several dogs appear to have been cured by single doses of ivermectin, 0.2 mg/kg, administered by subcutaneous injection.[8]
   e. Prolonged treatment with albendazole was effective in 85% of dogs infected with *C. plica*. The urine was negative for eggs 30 days after treatment began. Oral doses of 50 mg/kg of albendazole were given twice daily for 10 to 14 days.[14]
   f. Because some evidence shows that, in the absence of reinfection, urinary capillariasis may be self-limiting, isolation of an animal from earthworms would seem to be sufficient to eliminate a *Capillaria* bladder infection in fewer than 90 days.[14]

I. Prevention.

1. Dogs and cats must be prevented from ingesting earthworms.

REFERENCES

1. Beresford-Jones WP. Observations on the helminths of British wild red foxes. *Vet Rec.* 1961;73:882–883.
2. Cole RA, Shoop WL. Helminths of the raccoon *(Procyon lotor)* in western Kentucky. *J Parasitol.* 1987;73:762-768.
3. Ehrenford FA, Snodgrass TB. Incidence of canine dioctophymiasis (giant kidney worm infection) with a summary of cases in North America. *J Am Vet Med Assoc.* 1955;126:415–417.
4. Georgi JR, Georgi ME. *Parasitology for Veterinarians* 5th ed. Philadelphia, Pennsylvania: WB Saunders, 1990:206.
5. Gillespie D. Successful treatment of canine *Capillaria plica* cystitis. *Vet Med/Small Anim Clin.* 1983;78:681.
6. Harkema R, Miller GC. Helminth parasites of the raccoon, *Procyon lotor* in the southwestern United States. *J Parasitol.* 1964;50:60–66.
7. Harris Lloyd F. Feline bladderworm. *Vet Med/Small Anim Clin.* 1981;76:844.
8. Kirkpatrick CE, Nelson GR. Ivermectin treatment of urinary capillariasis in a dog. *J Am Vet Med Assoc.* 1987;191:701–702.
9. Levine ND. Nematode parasites of domestic animals and of man. Minneapolis, Minnesota: Burgess Publishing; 1980:461-464.
10. Mace TF, Anderson RC. Development of the giant kidney worm,

Dioctophyma renale (Goeze, 1782) (Nematoda: Dioctophymatoidea). *Can J Zool.* 1975;53:1552–1568.

11. Measures LN, Anderson RC. Centrarchid fish as paratenic hosts of the giant kidney worm, *Dioctophyma renale* in Ontario, Canada. *J Wildlife Dis.* 1985;21:11–19.
12. Osborne CA, et al. *Dioctophyma renale* in the dog. *J Am Vet Med Assoc.* 1969;155:605–620.
13. Schmidt GD, Roberts LS. *Foundations in Parasitology.* 4th ed. St. Louis, Missouri: Times Mirror/Mosby College Publishing; 1989: 424–427.
14. Senior DF, et al. *Capillaria plica* infections in dogs. *J Am Vet Med Assoc.* 1980;176:901–905.
15. Soulsby EJL. *Helminths, Arthropods, and Protozoa of Domesticated Animals.* Philadelphia, Pennsylvania: Lea & Febiger; 1982.

Index

Note: Page numbers in italics indicate figures; page numbers followed by t indicate tables. Material specific to dogs and cats can be found under specific disorders, techniques, and breeds.